*Recent Progress in
Anaesthesiology and Resuscitation*

Recent Progress in Anaesthesiology and Resuscitation

Proceedings of the IV European Congress of Anaesthesiology, Madrid, Spain, 5–11 September, 1974

Editors:

A. ARIAS
R. LLAURADO
M. A. NALDA
J. N. LUNN

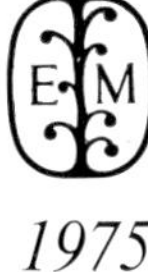

1975

Excerpta Medica, Amsterdam–Oxford
American Elsevier Publishing Co., Inc., New York

International Congress Series No. 347

ISBN Excerpta Medica 90 219 0269 9

ISBN American Elsevier 0 444 15134 6

Publisher:

Excerpta Medica

305 Keizersgracht

Amsterdam

P.O. Box 1126

Sole Distributors for the USA and Canada:

American Elsevier Publishing Company, Inc.

52 Vanderbilt Avenue

New York, N.Y. 10017

Printed in The Netherlands by Casparie Alkmaar bv

Letter of introduction by the President, IV European Congress of Anaesthesiology

My dear Colleagues,

On behalf of the Organizing Committee of the IV European Congress of Anaesthesiology, especially of its Scientific Commission and Commission of Scientific Publications, and on my own behalf, I am very pleased to introduce this Proceedings Volume with a few words of thanks to all the people connected with its appearance. First, to the many colleagues who came from all over the world, helping with their presence and that of their families to turn our meeting into an unprecedented success. Secondly, to those doctors connected with the field of anaesthesiology and resuscitation, who have contributed with their experience and research, and made this book possible. And finally, to our editors and their staff, whose wide experience and diligence has once more been proven by the high quality of this publication.

No meeting of this kind can be the success it proved to be without the cooperation, enthusiasm and good will of all its participants. My final thanks go to you, for the great 'simpatía' shown during your stay with us in Madrid.

Dr Alfredo Arias, President

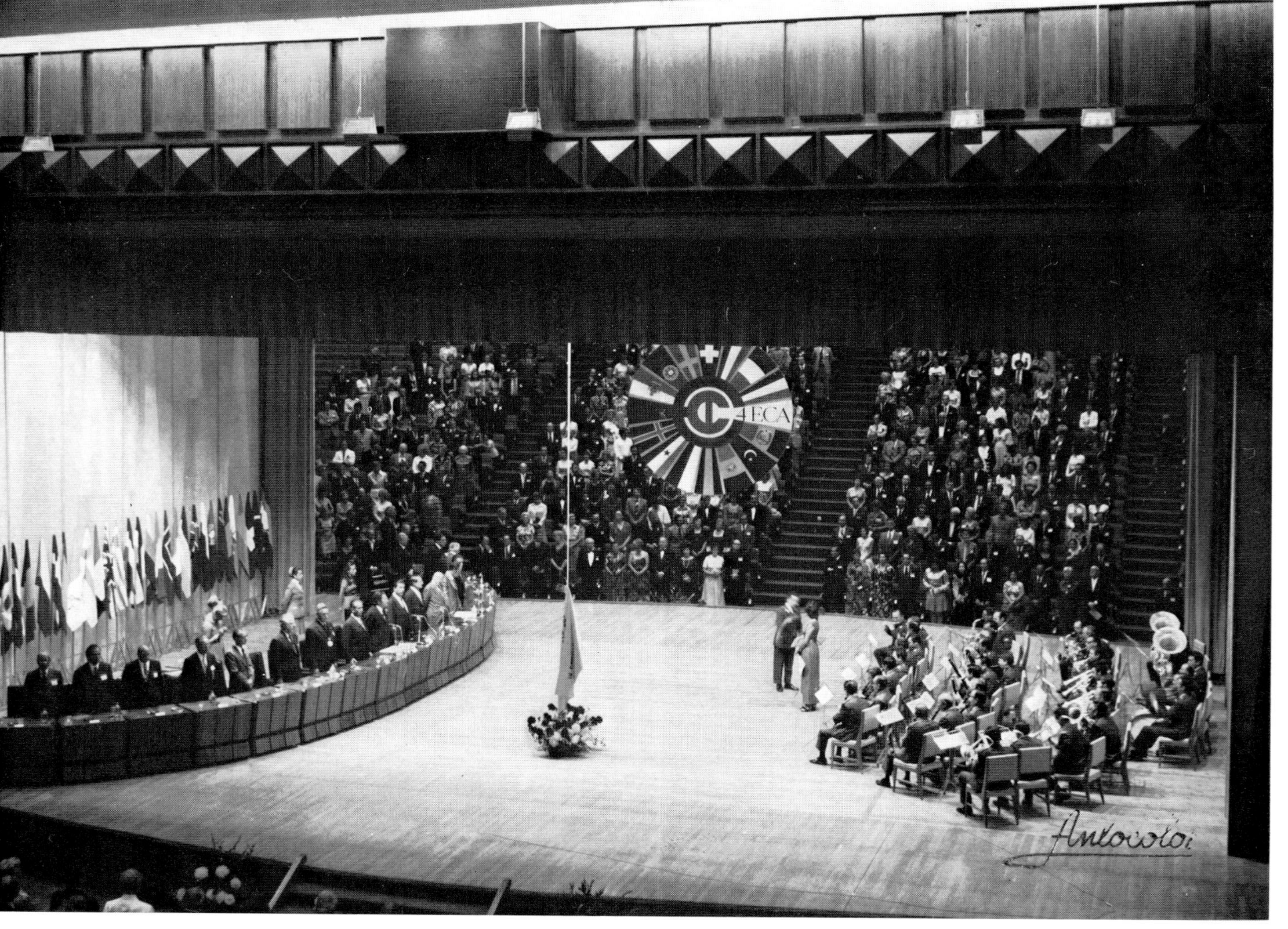

Opening ceremony

Official opening of the
IV European Congress of Anaesthesiology

During the evening of 5th September, 1974, the Under-Secretary for Education and Science, Prof. Don Federico Mayor Zaragoza, representing the head of the department, Sr. Martínez Esteruelas, performed the Opening Ceremony of the IV European Congress of Anaesthesiology in the Congress and Exhibition Hall of Madrid.

Those presiding over the occasion were the Director General of Health, Don Federico Bravo Morate; the President of the Congress, Dr Alfredo Arias; the President of the Spanish Society of Anaesthesiologists, Prof. Miguel Angel Nalda Felipe; the President of the European Section of the World Federation of Anaesthesiologists, Dr Douglas D. C. Howat; and the President of the World Federation of Anaesthesiologists, Dr Otto Mayrhofer.

After the Air Force Band had played the National Anthems of the 31 European countries represented, the President of the Congress, Dr Arias, delivered an address, followed by Drs Nalda Felipe, Howat and Mayrhofer. Prof. Mayor Zaragoza also said a few words of welcome.

Thereafter Congress medals were conferred upon a number of participants for their distinguished work in the field of Anaesthesiology. Following this, while the Air Force Band played the anthem specially composed for the Congress, Dr Arias hoisted a flag also designed for the occasion.

The Under-Secretary for Education and Science declared open the Congress whose working sessions in a tightly packed programme, continued until the 11th of September.

Speech by the President of the IV European Congress of Anaesthesiology at the Opening Ceremony

Welcome to you all. Nothing gives greater pleasure than seeing so many well-known faces gathered together from all corners of the world. Thank you for such a turn-out for the opening ceremony.

For four years, since the last European Congress in Prague, we have been looking forward to having you amongst us. Today, at last, the long-awaited moment of our being surrounded by colleagues has arrived. Many of you have come from a great distance, without considering the loss of valuable time and the expense it represents.

You have come not only to contribute to the scientific success of this Congress with the latest results of your researches or to take an interest in the development and content of certain symposia and free communications, but also to meet your colleagues and friends, to exchange ideas and to cement or create bonds of friendship and fellowship.

We make up a large family which grows from day to day, and its unity depends on us all. We must not slacken our efforts to consolidate this bond; not only to justify it, but also to succeed in the development of better anaesthesia for the world's sufferers. For years now anaesthesiology has been well established in many countries, but the tiller must be held with a steady hand so that its prestige may not decline. Other countries still need moral, scientific and material support from all sides to make its development possible. In our work, with the three-fold obligation to attend, to teach and to carry out research we should all strive for the achievement of the aims outlined by the World Federation of Societies of Anaesthesiologists (WFSA), collaborating with its members and placing our full trust in the governing body which tries with all its might, hopes and means to enhance the reputation, regard, and scientific level of all anaesthesiologists in the world. I trust that this Fourth European Congress of Anaesthesiology will contribute to the strengthening of this union and to the improvement of our scientific standards.

A great number of studies are to be presented in the course of the coming days. Apart from the symposia which form the core of the scientific structure of this congress, there are a large number of free communications of great interest, some related to the main themes, others grouped in special sections according to content. Finally, there are miscellaneous sessions comprising heterogeneous subject matter. As papers are presented simultaneously in different rooms, we hope that the individual congress member will choose what interests him most for these five days of intense work, and that he will have time as well to exchange ideas with his colleagues. It is precisely this sharing of ideas and comment that is the essence of every gathering or congress. Apart from the basic benefit obtained by attending the sessions, the booklet of summaries which you have for your convenience in your folders, as well as the Proceedings volume shortly to be published, will make it possible to read the papers presented at the congress.

In the progress of our own specialized subject the contribution made by the advance of pharmacology is quite extraordinary. New anaesthetics and drugs keep enriching our arsenal, and will contribute to clearer anaesthetic indications for each patient and situation. The amount of clinical evaluation and research accompanying these new preparations is extensive, and will, I hope, direct us as to their use. No one will better appreciate the pharmacological effect of new drugs and weigh the advantages and disadvantages of each one than the anaesthetist, constant observer of physiological reactions. Clinical experience has taught him to be cautious over the introduction and use of new anaesthetics and new techniques. Perhaps most surprising has been in recent years the contribution made by technical development towards perfecting the method of administration of anaesthetics, and the constant monitoring of patients. Every day improvements are seen for equipment and accessories in daily use, which not only improve the technique and skill of the anaesthetist, but which also guarantee the patient safe application. A thorough inspection of the different stands at the Technical, Scientific and Pharmacological Exhibition will satisfy the most exacting minds, given the number of innovations exhibited. We all need to bring ourselves regularly up to date with the most recent apparatus, so continuous is the perfection and appearance of new models. During this visit you will also be able to acquaint yourselves with projects outlined for the future. Our thanks go to the laboratories and firms responsible for the displays at this magnificent exhibition, and for their collaboration in this congress.

We hope that the social side of the congress will give pleasure to everyone, and will help you to enjoy your stay among us. Our wives and families who so unselfishly live with our problems and worries the whole year round deserve a few days of real enjoyment. Excursions in Madrid and its surroundings have been organized for them, so that they may get to know the outstanding features of this capital and of the old Castilian towns.

In Prague you entrusted us with the organization of this congress, and now is the moment to give an account of the work carried out to this end. We have attempted to solve most of the problems. We know there will be errors and inadvertent mistakes and that you will forgive us for them. We are here to solve any problems that may arise and are brought to our notice. Our firm intent is to make your stay among us as pleasant as possible.

Before finishing I want to express our gratitude to the Organizing Committees for the work they have done over these years, as well as to the secretaries for their immense task of putting into motion and bringing to fruition all the details which every large congress carries with it. Also, to the Sociedad Organizadora de Congresos for the most valuable contribution of its experience in setting up and coordinating the scheme and development of the organization; to the Companía Aérea Transportista for its invaluable collaboration in distributing promotion material, as well as facilitating the travel of the congress members; to the Agencia Oficial de Viajes for their incalculable help in giving publicity to the congress through their world chain of agencies, for the reservation of hotels, and for the efficient transport system which operates nowadays for everyone's convenience. Lastly, our everlasting and sincere gratitude to all those who, regardless of expense to themselves, or simply by moral support have collaborated in one way or another in the organization of the Fourth European Congress of Anaesthesiology.

One request: from this moment we can all contribute to the success of this congress, turning ourselves into a nucleus of action, widening our sympathies and enlarging the circle of our friendships. In this way, we will all feel the warmth of fellowship. To all of you, BIENVENIDOS, WELCOME, BIENVENUE, WILLKOMMEN!

Dr. Alfredo Arias Alvarez

Speech by the President of the Spanish Society of Anaesthesiology and Reanimation at the Opening Ceremony

The honour of presiding over the Spanish Society of Anaesthesiology and Reanimation has fallen to me at the time when the responsibility of the organization and realization of the Fourth European Congress of Anaesthesiology was entrusted to it.

First of all we would like to express our gratitude to the European Section of the World Federation of Societies of Anaesthesiologists and through it to the WFSA itself, for the honour that was bestowed on us when, during the for us memorable Assembly held during the European Congress in Prague, we were entrusted with the vessel of the Fourth European Congress of Anaesthesiology so that we might bring it to the haven of our hospitality, our sunshine and our peace, handling the tiller with a firm hand, according to our scientific and human capacities.

In the four years which have gone by since then, we have navigated through calm periods and through storms shaking the world, without losing our faith in ultimate success. For our only beacon was that of science and dedication, its light being the desire to improve the care of the sick, to give them ever more certainties, and to relieve their pain.

This congress has had an outstanding captain, Alfredo Arias, a man whose integrity and physical and spiritual strength have been able to keep course during the difficulties we have come through, who from the first moment understood what was wanted and fought for it boldly, until able to shape it into the marvellous reality which unites us here today, although at the cost of many anxieties and the sacrifice of many hours of private life.

It is a matter of satisfaction to me to see that all of you have responded to our invitation in the certainty that this congress will be a success, not only because of our work, but also because of the dignity, the scientific value and the human warmth that you will communicate.

We hope that your stay among us will leave you with an indelible memory so that when the moment of separation comes you will leave your new friends with something of regret and that scientific conclusions will be reached during this congress furthering the advancement of Anaesthesiology-Reanimation, covered with the fruits from that branch of the tree of Science which is our Speciality.

Welcome, and may your dreams and hopes see themselves fulfilled during your stay in this land of hidalgos and quijotes who fed the five continents with their blood and their culture, which today opens wide to you the doors of its heart full of affection and good will.

Prof. M. A. Nalda Felipe

X

Speech by the President of the World Federation of Societies of Anaesthesiologists at the Opening Ceremony

Although I know that I could speak today in my mother tongue, German, I would like to address you in Castellano, hoping that my Spanish friends and the translators will understand me. I am very proud to be an Honorary Member of the Spanish Society of Anaesthesiology and Reanimation, and I beg you to consider this attempt of mine as a gesture of gratitude and courtesy.

It is a great honour and a great pleasure for me to take part in this Fourth European Congress of Anaesthesiology, and to bring you, on behalf of the World Federation of Societies of Anaesthesiologists, the greetings and best wishes of our colleagues the world over.

The medal of the President of the Federation displays an image symbolizing our function as watchers over our patients, holding up the torch of life in the darkness of the unconscious state during operation. I believe that it really is a very important function and one which gives much satisfaction. The fact that death in the operating theatre is very rare nowadays, is without doubt primarily the accomplishment of the specialists in modern anaesthesiology.

We have a particular obligation, in my view, to continue this development, important as it is for the future benefit of the sick. International Congresses such as this provide important opportunities to exchange experience and professional knowledge.

Four years ago in Prague I helped to influence the decision in favour of Madrid because I was sure that our Spanish colleagues were very competent in organizing international congresses. The proof of it is this Opening Ceremony. Allow me, dear friends and colleagues, to wish you good and successful participation at this Fourth European Congress of Anaesthesiology.

Thank you!

Prof. Otto Mayrhofer

Speech by the President of the European section of the World Federation of Societies of Anaesthesiologists at the Opening Ceremony

It gives me great pleasure to be able, as Chairman of the European Section, to say how happy we are to be here in Madrid and to express our appreciation of all the efforts of Dr. Alfredo Arias and his organising committee to make us welcome at this, the Fourth European Congress of Anaesthesiology. It is already obvious that they have planned a meeting in the same fine tradition as those we enjoyed so much in Vienna, Copenhagen and Prague. How fortunate we are that Madrid has this fine new Congress Hall in which to hold it.

I know very well how long it takes and how hard one has to work in order to receive some 3,000 visitors, even under the best conditions, and I feel the greatest sympathy with those who have had so much to do in the last few years and particularly in the last twelve months. I know, too, the satisfaction they must be feeling at this moment, as they begin to see the fruits of all their labours.

The scientific programme shows every promise and I suspect that our only complaint will be that it is physically impossible to attend every session. The exhibitions, technical and scientific, are an important part of every meeting of anaesthetics and I trust you will not fail to visit them. I am sure you need no inducement from me to attend the social programme. I should like to congratulate the organisers on the high quality of the publications we have received and also, if I may, on the excellence of the English translation.

Sometimes it seems that modern methods of communication only exaggerate the troubles of the world, but I think we should remember that they also help to bring people together. I hope the day is not far distant when we shall all be able to travel freely and when common high standards of training will permit European anaesthetists to work anywhere in the continent. The Spanish Society of Anaesthesiology and Reanimation can be proud of the part it is playing towards this goal.

Dr. D. D. C. Howat

Speech by His Excellency the Under-Secretary for Education and Science at the Opening Ceremony

My first words at this magnificent opening ceremony of the European Congress of Anaesthesiology, are to pass on to you warm greetings on behalf of H. R. H. the Prince of Spain and the Minister for Education and Science. They would have liked to be here with you to convey personally their satisfaction at the organization of this congress in Madrid and to welcome you to our country, but last-minute obligations have prevented this, and thus it is all the greater an honour for me to represent them and to address you at the official opening of such an important gathering.

Allow me first of all to congratulate those who have borne the burden of making it possible to hold this international congress in Madrid. When a congress of this magnitude is initiated, it culminates in exhaustive work for the organizing committee who attend to all the details, who study in anticipation all aspects which contribute to ensure that, collectively and individually, the congress will be scientifically fruitful, will contribute to the consolidation of friendships and scientific contacts, and will also provide a pleasant memory of the hospitality received in a country. To the organizing committee therefore, I extend my warmest congratulations, in the certainty that the results of this congress will compensate for the immense hard work which has gone into making it possible.

A cordial welcome to all of you who have accepted the invitation to make public your contributions to the field of anaesthesiology, one of the most attractive, exciting, and unexplored facets of modern science. It would be useless for me to attempt to discuss the importance of anaesthesiology in the progress of medicine, to the extent of influencing to a large degree the development of surgery. Progressive improvement in techniques and systems of anaesthesia have constituted and will continue to constitute an indispensable condition for the development of new surgical possibilities, a condition of ever increasing knowledge, which is characteristic for the progress of science in general and medicine in particular, in our continual, never ending struggle to relieve the suffering of man.

As Under-Secretary for Education and Science it is my duty to urge you wholeheartedly to continue your researches with enthusiasm and to improve the teaching of this important subject, because, in the last resort, improved medical care will depend on new knowledge and adequate diffusion of new knowledge.

As a specialist in biochemistry, I am aware of the multiple intriguing lacunae still existing in the understanding of the pharmacological action of anaesthetics and the mechanism of action of each product capable of effecting the transitory loss of consciousness characteristic of the anaesthetic.

Many disciplines combine in successful anaesthesia: science and technique, the widest knowledge and the perfected apparatus are the two means upon which depends the success of the important mission entrusted to you.

XIII

Your specialized knowledge presents very varied facets in undefined areas being in danger of interfering in man's privacy, lines are crossed beyond which not only sensibility is affected, but also other faculties proper to human nature. The moral aspects and, therefore, ethical implications are worthy of serious study, as is reflected in the programme of this congress.

Welcome all of you to Madrid. Welcome to Spain, all of you who come from other countries. I want this congress to make an important contribution towards health care, one of the most definite signs of true progress, for it promotes common well-being by reducing the suffering and helping to make life more bearable.

In these early autumn days Madrid and its surroundings offer you the attractions of the fascinating beauty of Castile, the incomparable historical inheritance of its ancient people, witnesses to a past of great renown with an important artistic production, being at the same time a platform, we hope, for a powerful future in which we can continue to contribute worthily to the development of science and civilization.

It is now 21 years since the Spanish Association of Anaesthesiology and Reanimation was formed in Granada. The level of development reached by the Spanish Society, to the point of constituting today the seat for this important international reunion, is obvious, and I consider it a duty of objectivity and justice alike to congratulate the Spanish anaesthesiologists whose competence is so adequately reflected in this fact. You will have occasion to observe, especially those of you who are visiting our country for the first time, the high standards which we have reached in many fields, on a foundation, as in the case of anaesthesiology, of hard work, dedication and sacrifice.

When one looks at a gathering like this and studies a programme such as you are going to work through in the next few days, it is unavoidable to bring to mind, with the solemnity proper at these moments, the hard and often anonymous work of all the scientists of all the countries in the world who have made it possible, through their contributions in the course of time, to reach the present stage and degree of progress in this particular aspect of science.

Allow me finally to address special words of welcome to the wives accompanying the participants at this congress. Doing so is not only an act of courtesy which in any event is becoming from the country welcoming you here today, but also provides an opportunity to express our appreciation of the qualities of those who share your life, without the compensation of distinction and professional success.

Mr. D. F. Mayor Zaragoza

Contents

I. New methods in regional anaesthesia

II. Pain treatment

III. New agents in intravenous anaesthesia

"

IV. New agents in inhalation anaesthesia

V. Advances in neuromuscular transmission and new blocking drugs

VI. Pharmacological incompatibilities and medicinal interferences in anaesthesia and resuscitation

VII. Anaesthesia and the endocrine glands

VIII. Anaesthesia and postoperative care for organ transplantation

IX. Anaesthesia and postoperative care in coronary surgery

X. The role of the anaesthesiologist in the treatment of multiple injuries

XI. Problems in long-term respiratory treatment

XV. Documentation in anaesthesiology

XVI. Acupuncture

XVII. Ethical aspects of resuscitation

XVIII. Neuroanaesthesia

XIX. Miscellaneous

Chapter I

New methods in regional anaesthesia

Cervical peridural anaesthesia

L. LECRON, J. DE CASTRO and D. LEVY

Hôpital de Stage Universitaire de Bruxelles, Montignies le Tilleul, and
Institut des Mutuelles Socialistes, La Hestre, Belgium

A French physician, J. Forestier, used this technique around 1921, when treating obstinate cervicobrachial neuralgia and others followed suit. The technique was abandoned because the apparatus was makeshift, the drugs imperfect and the physiological consequences unknown. There were no means of avoiding possible accidents, such as hypotension or cardio-respiratory failure through spinal anaesthesia.

New techniques have been developed which are both safer and more precise, using the Tuohy needle, and drugs which are more powerful and which enable better control of physiological disturbances (blood volume, hypotension, respiratory depression).

Spinal anaesthesia is often contraindicated in neck and chest wall surgery because of the risk of anaesthesia of the cardio-respiratory centres in spite of perfect technique. Profound anaesthesia is necessary and so general anaesthesia must be used.

Peridural anaesthesia has several advantages: The anaesthetic effects can be gradually changed from analgesia to anaesthesia and vice versa by using different concentrations of drug. The extent of analgesia is volume determined. The duration of anaesthesia can be extended by the use of a catheter. There is no risk to the vital centres because the technique is accurate. Bromage has shown convincingly that the drug penetrates the dura mater, but no effect on the vital centres occurs because the concentration is too low. Phrenic nerve involvement is rare and unlikely because of its diameter.

INDICATIONS

The method may be used for surgical or medical cases.

Surgery

Surgery of the neck (thyroidectomy, limited surgery of the carotid artery), to minimize the effect of operating on a very reflexogenic area.

Shoulder and upper limb surgery. Anaesthesia is complete and easier to perform than brachial or cervical plexus techniques. It may be applied in chest wall surgery (Alstedt technique) to prevent a ventilatory insufficiency.

Bleeding is decreased.

Medicine

Raynaud's disease.
Post-amputation pain.

Cervical or brachial neuralgia which is resistant to the traditional treatments (massage, physiotherapy).

The onset of pain relief is rapid and profound; later on, the classical treatment may follow.

Corticoids may be added to the anaesthetic solution and the results can be dramatic.

Surgical decompression is not free of risk and cervical peridural analgesia should first be tried.

TECHNIQUE

It may appear to be spectacular and delicate or dangerous. However, when practised by an experienced anaesthetist, there is no risk. In our opinion, it is easier than lumbar peridural anaesthesia; indeed, in most cases deformities in the cervical column are less than those in the lumbar region.

The location of the peridural space must be very precise and demands several tests, but it is not a major difficulty.

When the injection is made, the patient should be sitting or lying in the ventral or lateral decubitus.

The cervical vertebrae must be stretched by bending the vertebral column so as to maximize the interspinous space and to ensure puncture almost perpendicular to the skin. The area chosen is usually C6–C7 or C7–D1, according to the area to be anaesthetized. Sitting is the most convenient posture and the patient rests his forehead on folded arms.

The technique is classical; after the skin has been infiltrated, a Tuohy needle is slowly pushed, almost perpendicular to the skin but with a 75° slant.

The needle (17 gauge) is mounted on a syringe filled with physiologic serum. *Air must be kept out to avoid embolism.*

The classical jerk shows that the peridural space has been reached:

Negative pressure is very obvious in cervical peridural anaesthesia. Some physiological serum is dropped occasionally on the hub of the needle and this is obviously sucked in.

Either the injection is performed or the catheter is introduced in the general direction of the patient's head.

In the lateral position, the vertebral column is kept straight with pillows. In this position, the anaesthetic solution spreads unevenly and may be lateralized to one side. For the treatment of pain this disadvantage can be utilized to direct the solution to the painful area.

The ventral position can also be used and the patient rests with a pillow under his chest so that C7 area juts out maximally. The technique of injection is similar. Afterwards, the patient resumes the dorsal decubitus. A horizontal position favours anaesthesia of the cervical roots. An inclined position results in the solution travelling downwards, according to the slope of the table and the volume injected.

DRUGS

It is important to avoid motor anaesthesia of the upper intercostal nerves and the choice of drug must be careful. Etidocaine is unsuitable because it readily passes through the dura mater.

For anaesthesia, bupivacaine 0.5% is used and for medical use, bupivacaine 0.25% is indicated. Epinephrine may be added (1/200,000). Two millilitres per vertebral segment is required.

The anti-inflammatory effects result from simultaneous injection of corticoids (methyl-prednisolone 124 mg).

ACCIDENTS

Spinal anaesthesia may occur. The injection must be interrupted immediately and artificial ventilation applied if necessary. This incident is not dangerous and it should be remembered that a few years ago Greene performed high spinal anaesthesia combined with general anaesthesia.

Horner's syndrome appears fairly often.

If anaesthesia reaches the T_1-T_6 area, the cardiac accelerating fibres are affected, but so is the vagus nerve and there is an equilibrium of effects.

CONCLUSION

This anaesthetic technique has a lot of advantages:

It is more reliable than cervical plexus block. It is less difficult than the supraclavicular route to the brachial plexus, more easily carried out and the danger of puncturing the pleural dome is avoided.

Since the anaesthesia is bilateral, it is an advantage for midline surgery of the neck and the upper part of the chest. It is also useful in bilateral arm injuries.

In vascular surgery, this limited anaesthesia is justified because it protects the patient undergoing operation in a reflexogenic area.

For the surgeon also, in some cases, it is useful for a patient to keep awake in order to test the results of the tying of the internal carotid artery.

Evaluation of myocardial function by measuring systolic time intervals before and during anesthesia (general, spinal and peridural) for cesarean section and gynecological procedures

FERNANDO RODRIGUEZ [1], SERGIO MORA [1],
JOSE AREVALO [1] and P. J. GARCIA [2]

[1] Department of Anesthesia, Hospital de Gineco-Obstetricia No. 2, and
[2] Section of Biostatistics and Experimental Signs, Centro Medico Nacional, IMSS, Mexico, DF

Myocardial contractility is perhaps the most important characteristic of cardiac function. It is related to the cardiac output and is an important physiological parameter which should be evaluated more frequently under stress such as in the obstetric patient. Changes in myocardial function can occur in pregnant women submitted to cesarean section with or without associated disease. Changes in cardiac performance could appear as a result of a move from the supine to the lateral position or during anesthesia and surgery, before or simultaneously with, the other common parameters such as blood pressure, heart rate, and central venous pressure.

A useful noninvasive technique consists of simultaneous recording of the electrocardiogram, phonocardiogram and the carotid pulse. It has been demonstrated that the systolic-time intervals obtained from these recordings are related to the stroke volume, cardiac output and the clinical state of the patient with cardiac disease (Bieniarz et al., 1968; Garrad et al., 1970; Heikkila et al., 1971; Jezek, 1963; Kitchner et al., 1973; Rodriguez et al., 1973; Talley et al., 1971; Weissler et al., 1961, 1968, 1969; Weissler and Schoenfeld, 1970).

The pre-ejection period (PEP), left ventricular ejection time (LVET) and the ratio PEP/LVET were found to be correlated with the ejection fraction (EF), and the end-diastolic volume (EDV) as determined angiographically in patients with cardiac disease (Bonica, 1967). Kumar and Spodick (1970) and Martin et al. (1971) demonstrated a linear relationship between the systolic-time intervals and the internal indices of left ventricular function in man. Jezek (1963) and Fishleder (1966) report that the common sign of left ventricular failure consisted of a prolongation of the pre-ejection phase and abbreviation of the ejection period while total electromechanical systole remained unaltered (62). Subsequently, similar changes were reported in several other studies (Heikkila et al., 1971; Talley et al., 1971; Weissler et al., 1961, 1969) and it is probable that these changes reflect a diminution in the rate of rise in left ventricular pressure during systole (dP/dt). Garrad et al. (1970) suggested that impaired left ventricular contractile performance is the most plausible explanation for changes in PEP/LVET ratio and the EF. Henderson et al. (1972) studied the effect of anesthesia on the heart using the method of systolic-time intervals. However, no other reports of the use of these techniques in obstetric patients have been found. This is a very important field which deserves more investigation.

MATERIAL

One hundred and twenty-nine patients were selected; the ages ranged between 17 and 74 years, and the patients were divided into 9 groups:
   (1) 29 patients without associated disease having cesarean section under lumbar peridural block; (2) 3 patients having cesarean section under spinal anesthesia; (3) 18 patients having cesarean section under peridural block with supplementation; (4) 38 patients with toxemia having cesarean section under lumbar peridural block; (5) 5 patients having cesarean section under general anesthesia; (6) 7 patients without associated disease having cesarean section under general anesthesia because of insufficient blockade; (7) 7 patients with associated cardiac disease having cesarean section under lumbar peridural block; (8) 9 patients having cesarean section under general anesthesia because of insufficient blockade associated with toxemia; (9) 14 patients having gynecological procedures under spinal or peridural anesthesia.

METHOD

Blood pressure was monitored by a cuff sphygmomanometer. The systolic-time intervals were obtained from simultaneous recordings of the electrocardiogram, phonocardiogram and carotid pulse tracing at a paper speed of 100 mm/sec using a 3-channel direct writing system. The phases of the cardiac cycle were measured according to previous workers (Jezek, 1963; Kumar and Spodick, 1970; Weissler et al., 1961, 1968) and are illustrated in Figure 1. Measurements were made with the patient in the supine and lateral position before, during, and after anesthesia; at rest and after exertion in patients undergoing gynecological procedures. The intervals measured were: the electromechanical systole QS_2, left-ventricular ejection time, the pre-ejection period, the PEP/LVET ratio and the ejection fraction. PEP and LVET were corrected according to the heart rate and sex.
   Lumbar peridural block was performed according to established techniques (Bonica, 1967; Bromage, 1961; Moore, 1964). A small pillow was used under the right hip to avoid compression of the inferior vena cava by the uterus (Marx, 1974; Moore, 1964). Spinal

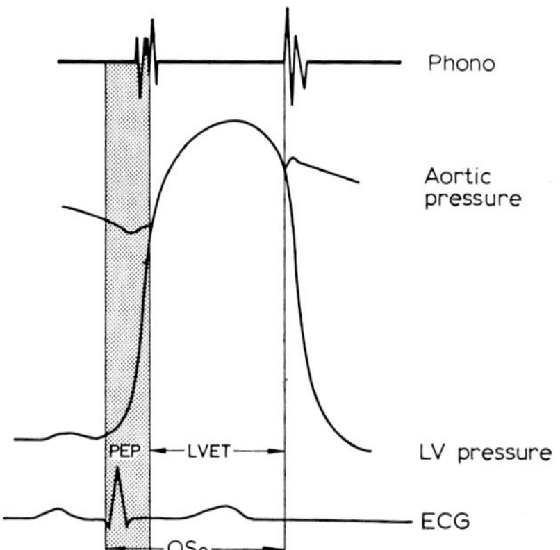

Fig. 1.   *Relation of the measured systolic-time intervals to the cardiac cycle. Simultaneous registration of phonocardiogram (phono), aortic pressure tracing, left ventricular (LV) pressure tracing and electrocardiogram. (PEP=pre-ejection phase; LVET=left ventricular ejection time; QS_2=total electromechanical systole.)*

anesthesia was administered following previously described methods (Bonica, 1969; Moore, 1964; Shnider, 1970). General anesthesia was administered by recommended techniques (Bonica, 1967, Marx, 1974; Shnider, 1970), and the anesthetic agents used were cyclopropane, halothane and methoxyflurane. Supplementation of the blockade was with ketamine as required. A vein was cannulated with a 14 gauge Bardic Intracath for fluid administration.

RESULTS

Group 1

The mean B.P. fell by 10% on moving from the supine to the lateral position but the heart rate was unchanged. Ejection fraction (EF) was below normal in the supine position (60%), but it increased 10% (normal) in the lateral position. During anesthesia a 10% fall in B.P. and a consistent increase of EF (74%) occurred.

Group 2

A similar fall in mean B.P. on changing from the supine to the lateral position. A more marked fall followed the spinal (20%) but this increased by the end of the procedure. EF was below normal in the supine position (65%) but increased to above normal (75%) in the lateral position. The heart rate was unchanged. EF remained normal during the procedure but increased by the end to 76%.

Group 3

The B.P. fell 5% on changing from the supine to the lateral position without any change in heart rate, while the EF increased from 63% to normal in the lateral position. During the procedure there were no changes in B.P., slight changes in the heart rate and a consistent increase in EF – to 75% – throughout the operation.

Group 4

There was a marked fall in B.P. on changing from the supine to the lateral posture and an increase of the EF from 55% to 67% but this is below normal. During the procedure the B.P. was in the normal range, the heart rate steady, and there was an increase in EF to 71% at the end of the procedure.

Group 5

There was no change in B.P. on changing position from supine to lateral, and a slight increase of EF although still below normal. No further changes occurred during the procedure and the EF remained below normal (62).

Group 6

There was a fall in B.P. on changing from the supine to the lateral position with no changes in the heart rate but an increase in EF from 58% to 70%. During the procedure there was only a slight fall in B.P., and a consistent increase in ejection fraction – to 71%.

Group 7

There was a fall in B.P. on changing from the supine to the lateral position and an increase in EF from 55% to 66%. During the procedure the B.P. remained steady and EF was slightly below normal 67%.

Group 8

A 10% fall in B.P. on change of posture and an increase of EF from 50% to 71%. During the procedure the B.P. remained steady but the EF was below normal.

Group 9

There was a slight increase of B.P., heart rate and EF after exertion. During the procedure all parameters were within the normal range.

DISCUSSION

Since measurement of cardiac output and cardiac catheterization are very expensive and complicated procedures which may limit their routine use in evaluating myocardial contractility, we believe that the measurement of systolic-time intervals represents a convenient, sensible noninvasive method of rapid assessment of myocardial function as expressed by the PEP/LVET ratio which is an excellent index of cardiac function by virtue of its very good correlation with the EF (Garrad et al., 1970; Talley et al., 1971; Weissler et al., 1969).

Some important features deserve our attention: (1) Almost all obstetric patients have a fall in B.P. and a remarkable increase in EF on changing from the supine to the lateral position. (2) Group 1 had stable myocardial function throughout the procedure perhaps due to the decrease in peripheral resistance and the beta effect of the epinephrine added to the local anesthetic agents. Spinal anesthesia produced more marked hypotension than the epidural, but the EF remained higher than normal. The addition of ketamine caused the mean B.P. to remain higher than in the patients without ketamine and the EF was above normal at 75%. In Group 4, the toxemic patients had a lower EF than the normal patients despite the elevated arterial pressure. This improved in the lateral position but remained higher despite the supine position for the procedure perhaps due to the reduced peripheral resistance, but the EF remained below normal probably due to the reduced circulating blood volume. The Group 5 patients, under general anesthesia, with placenta previa and fetal death, were hypovolemic and the EF remained lower than normal (62%) due possibly to the negative inotropic action of the anesthetic agent which was more marked with halothane and methoxyflurane than with cyclopropane. In Group 6 general anesthesia was given and there were no changes and the EF remained as high as in the patients who had blockade only. The patients (Group 7) with cardiac disease in whom the EF remained nearly normal indicate that lumbar peridural blockade can improve myocardial function. The toxemic patients (Group 8) under general anesthesia showed greater depression of the myocardium due to the adverse effects of general anesthetics. Cardiac reserve was measured in the patients (Group 9) for gynecological procedures. All the patients had cardiac function below normal but the use of peridural or spinal blocks allowed myocardial function to be maintained above normal during the procedure. The supine hypotension syndrome was present in 20% of the patients and was treated with rapid administration of fluids and uterine displacement. All the patients received fluids necessary to maintain an adequate circulating blood volume. Other data for future publication on Apgar scores, peridural drug dosage, PEP, LVET, their ratio, and urinary output during the procedure are available.

CONCLUSION

A noninvasive technique is helpful in anesthetic management of the obstetric patient and conduction anesthesia is a good procedure if it is handled with care.

REFERENCES

Bieniarz et al. (1968): *Amer. J. Obstet. Gynec.*, *100/2*, 203.

Bonica, J. J. (Ed.) (1967): In: *Principles and Practice of Obstetric Analgesia and Anesthesia, Vol. 1*, p. 689. F. A. Davis Co., Philadelphia, Pa.

Bonica, J. J. (Ed.) (1969): In: *Principles and Practice of Obstetric Analgesia and Anesthesia, Vol. 2*, pp. 1127, 1338. F. A. Davis Co., Philadelphia, Pa.

Braunwald, E. (1971): *Circulation*, *53*, 171.

Bromage, P. R. (1961): *Canad. med. Ass. J.*, *85*, 1138.

Garrad et al. (1970): *Circulation*, *42*, 455.

Fishleder, B. L. (Ed.) (1966): In: *Exploracion Cardiovascular y Fonomecanocardiografia Clinica*, Chapter 5, p. 92.

Heikkila et al. (1971): *Circulation*, *54*, 343.

Henderson et al. (1972): In: *Scientific Progress Abstracts, 46th International Congress of the Anesthesia Research Society*, p. 27.

Jezek, V. (1963): *Cardiologia*, *43*, 298.

Kitchner et al. (1973): *Chest*, *54/6*, 711.

Kumar, S. and Spodick, D. H. (1970): *Amer. Heart J.*, *80*, 401.

Martin et al. (1971): *Circulation*, *44*, 419.

Marx, G. F. (1968): In: *Obstetric Complications, Vol. 6*, p. 829. Editor: H. Ebner. Little, Brown and Co., New York – Boston – Toronto.

Marx, G. F. (1974): In: *The Anesthesiologist, Mother and Newborn*, p. 86. Editors: S. M. Shnider and F. Moya. Williams and Wilkins Co., Baltimore, Md.

Moore, D. C. (1964): In: *Anesthesia Techniques for Obstetric Anesthesia and Analgesia, 1st ed.*, Part 3, pp. 293, 322. Charles C. Thomas, Springfield, Ill.

Rodriguez et al. (1973): *Crit. Care Med.*, *1/3*, 141.

Shnider, S. M. (Ed.) (1970): In: *Obstetrical Anesthesia. Current Concepts and Practice*, p. 94. Williams and Wilkins Co., Baltimore, Md.

Smith, B. (1974): In: *The Anesthesiologist, Mother and Newborn*, p. 100. Editors: S. M. Shnider and F. Moya. William and Wilkins Co., Baltimore, Md.

Talley et al. (1971): *Amer. J. Cardiol.*, *27*, 384.

Weissler, A. M. and Schoenfeld, C. D. (1970): *Amer. J. med. Sci.*, *259*, 4.

Weissler et al. (1961): *Amer. Heart J.*, *62*, 367.

Weissler et al. (1968): *Circulation*, *37*, 149.

Weissler et al. (1969): *Amer. J. Cardiol.*, *27*, 384.

An evaluation of etidocaine for epidural analgesia in surgery and obstetrics

PHILIP R. BROMAGE, PETER O'BEIRN and SANJAY DATTA

Department of Anaesthesia, McGill University, and Royal Victoria Hospital, Montreal, Canada

The 2 long-acting local anaesthetic agents bupivacaine (a homologue of mepivacaine) and etidocaine (a homologue of lidocaine) have been compared in 362 cases of epidural analgesia for surgery or obstetrics.

The results of this investigation show that the 2 agents differ markedly in their clinical characteristics, and that there are quite clear cut limitations to each agent, with different indications and contraindications to their use.

METHODS

Bupivacaine HCl 0.5% and 0.25% was compared with etidocaine HCl 1.0% and 0.5% in epidural blockade, for general surgery. The range of solutions was extended to include 0.25% etidocaine in obstetrical epidural analgesia. Epinephrine 1/200,000 was added to all solutions, with the exception of 42 obstetrical epidurals.

Epidural analgesia was induced at the 6th thoracic interspace in 52 cases, but in the remainder it was induced at the 2nd lumbar interspace. A catheter was inserted in every case. All times for onset and duration were taken from the moment of completing the induction injection.

In each case a segment-time diagram was constructed for the onset and regression of analgesia and the following results were subjected to statistical analysis: (a) onset profile; (b) dose requirements, in terms of milligrams of drug per spinal segment; (c) duration of action, from the time of complete spread of analgesia, until analgesia regressed by 2 spinal segments; (d) intensity of motor block in terms of voluntary power in the lower limbs – 100%=unable to move knees or feet, 66%=unable to move knees, but able to move feet, 33%=partial flexion of knees, and full movement of feet, 0%=full flexion of knees and movement of feet.

In obstetrics, the quality of sensory analgesia was scored simply as 100% success if labour and delivery were pain-free with the epidural alone. If any supplementary general or local analgesia was required the epidural was scored as zero.

RESULTS

Surgical epidural analgesia

Analysis of the mean profiles for onset of lumbar epidural analgesia showed that the onset and spread of 1.0% etidocaine were nearly twice as fast as 0.5% bupivacaine and that with etidocaine, a salient of delay at L_5 and S_1 was almost eliminated.

Average dose requirements, in terms of the induction dose in milligrams, divided by the number of analgesic segments, were plotted against age, and it was seen that both these agents obey the general rule that dose requirements lessen with increasing age. It was also noted that the thoracic cases required about 30–40% less drug per segment than the lumbar cases.

Etidocaine produced a very profound degree of motor paralysis – about twice as intense as with bupivacaine; on the other hand, the latter proved to be slightly longer acting than the former.

Obstetrical anaesthesia

In obstetrics, bupivacaine provided a longer period of pain relief than etidocaine. Omission of epinephrine shortens the action of etidocaine appreciably.

A comparison of the duration of obstetrical analgesia provided by 100 mg of bupivacaine and 200 mg of etidocaine in various concentrations showed that bupivacaine is somewhat more efficient in equivalent doses.

The most striking differences between bupivacaine and etidocaine were found in the dissociation of motor paralysis and sensory blockade. Etidocaine caused a disproportionately intense paralysis in comparison to the quality of sensory blockade. The 0.5% solution with epinephrine led to 74% motor block and caused flaccid paresis of the legs and lower abdomen, and the patients were unable to move about freely, or to make effective bearing-down efforts. The presence of epinephrine added significantly to the quality of sensory analgesia and to the intensity of motor block. The plain solutions of etidocaine gave unacceptably low sensory scores, and for this reason they are judged to be unsuitable for obstetrical epidural analgesia.

In contrast, bupivacaine in 0.5% and 0.25% concentration gave very satisfactory sensory scores in the range of 96–100%, with motor block of less than 15%. These patients had comfortable deliveries, and were able to move about freely, and co-operate actively in the management of their labour.

DISCUSSION

Bupivacaine is characterised by a very slow onset of blockade, and by causing relatively little motor blockade in relation to the degree of sensory analgesia. These qualities make it well suited for segmental blockade in postoperative pain relief and in obstetrics, since the aim of treatment in both of these situations is to provide an active pain-free patient. On the other hand, the slow onset of bupivacaine makes it poorly suited for operative analgesia, either in the epidural space or in a plexus blockade.

Etidocaine has a very rapid onset with profound paralysis, and this makes it a very suitable choice for operative surgery. However, the intense motor blockade renders it useless in any situation where voluntary activity and co-operation are required, and so etidocaine is quite unsuited to postoperative pain relief, or to the management of labour and vaginal delivery. However, performance in caesarean section using 1% solution has been satisfactory in our hands.

The obstetrical series shows that the clinical performance of etidocaine is markedly affected by the addition of epinephrine. Plain etidocaine is relatively evanescent, with a very poor analgesic performance. On the other hand earlier studies have shown that bupivacaine is much less affected by the presence or absence of epinephrine.

*Lower limb reflex changes in segmental epidural analgesia**

PHILIP R. BROMAGE

Department of Anaesthesia, McGill University, and Royal Victoria Hospital, Montreal, Canada

Corning's original attempts at spinal analgesia in 1885 were based on the conceptual premise that medications injected close to the cord would be taken up by the substance of the spinal cord. Subsequent clinical and laboratory data discredited Corning's hypothesis, and led to the idea that subarachnoid and epidural analgesia acted primarily upon elements of the peripheral nervous system, such as spinal roots, ganglia and nerve trunks, and not upon elements of the neuraxis itself. However, animal experiments with radioactive tracers have shown that injected local anaesthetic agents can be demonstrated in the peripheral parts of the spinal cord after both epidural and subarachnoid injection. While similar direct experiments are not feasible in humans, indirect evidence of blockade of major descending pathways within the cord should be demonstrable by suitable neurological tests.

Segmental epidural analgesia confined to the cervical or thoracic regions presents the interesting possibility that the effects of any spinal cord involvement might be observed in unanaesthetized segments remote from the area of blockade. Thoracic blockade of descending pathways would then produce characteristic reflex changes in the legs, below the lowest limits of sensory anaesthesia. This paper is concerned with changes of lower limb reflexes that have been observed after segmental thoracic epidural block, and that strongly suggest partial interruption of long descending pathways. These observations were part of a larger enquiry into the clinical qualities of a new local anaesthetic agent, etidocaine [2-(N-ethylpropylamino)-2',6'-butyroxylidide hydrochloride] a drug with unusually high lipid solubility.

METHODS

Lower limb reflexes were observed in 35 patients between the ages of 23 years and 87 years (average age: 49 years) undergoing abdominal surgery after segmental epidural analgesia induced at the 6th or 7th thoracic interspace. All the patients in this series were free from neurological disease. Epidural puncture was performed using an 18-gauge thin-walled Bromage needle, with the patient in the sitting position. The epidural space was identified by the hanging-drop sign, and the calculated dose of local anaesthetic was injected through the needle in a single bolus. The following solutions were used: (*a*) 1% etidocaine (30 cases), (*b*) 2% lidocaine hydrochloride (3 cases), (*c*) 2% CO_2-lidocaine (2 cases). All solutions contained 1/200,000 adrenaline. Dosage was calculated in relation to age, and was approximately 40% less than the calculated dose for administration at the 2nd lumbar

* This study was partially supported by Grant No. MA. 1008 from the Medical Research Council of Canada.

13

interspace. The doses chosen were inversely proportional to age, and varied between 40 mg and 160 mg for etidocaine, and 120 mg and 220 mg for lidocaine. A vinyl plastic catheter (external diameter 1 mm) was passed until a length of 4 cm lay within the epidural space, and the needle was withdrawn, and the catheter taped in place. The patient was then placed in the supine position.

The onset of cutaneous anaglesia, and its subsequent regression were followed by pin-prick, and the area of analgesia plotted against time in a segment-time diagram. Subsequently, blockade was allowed to regress for a few segments before being reinstated by a reinforcing dose of local anaesthetic solution injected up the epidural catheter. The quantity of reinforcing dose was half the initial induction dose.

The following reflexes were tested in each limb: (*a*) Knee jerk. (*b*) Ankle jerk. Tendon reflexes were scored on a 4-point scale of absent (0), normal (1), brisk (2), and very brisk (3). (*c*) Ankle clonus. Ankle clonus was scored as the number of tonic beats following sharp passive dorsiflexion of the ankle. More than 20 beats were scored as 'sustained clonus'. (*d*) Plantar reflex, elicited as Babinski or Oppenheim reflex. Observations were made in the conscious patient before induction of epidural analgesia, and at frequent intervals for 20–45 min after induction of blockade, and then for a period of 2–6 hr in the postoperative period. All patients received light thiopentone and nitrous oxide anaesthesia during operation, in addition to the epidural block, and so observations of reflex changes were discounted during the 1st postoperative hr, in view of the emergence pattern of reflex change that lasts for 20–40 min after general anaesthesia. The lower limb reflexes were tested again on the following day, 24 hr after regression of anaesthesia.

RESULTS

Motor power and sensation to touch and pin-prick were normal in all segments below the lower limit of segmental analgesia. The knee jerks tended to be inhibited in all instances where the lower level of blockade extended caudally beyond the 1st lumbar dermatome; in these cases the tendon reflexes were scored after the sensory block had receded to the groin.

The lower limb reflexes began to show signs of upper motor neurone suppression within 10–15 min of epidural injection. The intensity of this change was usually symmetrical, but occasionally one leg would show more profound changes than the other. In some instances sustained clonus and an upgoing toe were present in one leg while reflexes remained normal in the other.

Increased briskness of the knee and ankle jerks were usually the first signs to appear, except in those patients where the lower level of blockade spread rapidly downwards to involve the 2nd and 3rd lumbar segments, when the knee jerks became obtunded at an early stage. This was occasionally followed by the onset of ankle clonus a few minutes later. The incidence and intensity of clonus were noted and it was seen that this sign was often absent. Even when present it was only mildly developed, except in 3 ankles where sustained clonus was obtained.

The plantar reflexes were the last to change, and the toes became upgoing about 20 min or longer after the induction of epidural block. In 6 patients the plantar reflexes did not change after the induction dose, but they did become upgoing after the 2nd or reinforcing epidural dose given 2–3 hr later. In all 35 patients the reflexes had returned to normal on the following day.

DISCUSSION

The results of this study demonstrate that certain descending pathways in the spinal cord are reversibly affected by segmental epidural analgesia. The sequence of reflex changes described in this series is a mirror-image of the pattern seen on emergence from general anaesthesia uncomplicated by the addition of muscle relaxants. The first sign on emergence from general anaesthesia and areflexia is a positive Babinski sign, followed shortly after by clonus and exaggerated tendon reflexes. The positive Babinski then progresses to a normal downgoing toe in 5–10 min but a condition of hyperreflexia persists for 15–25 min and then gradually subsides.

The pattern of reflex emergence after general anaesthesia is thought to be related to events occurring at intracranial levels, and acting upon inhibitory pathways restraining corticospinal impulses. In segmental epidural blockade the reflex changes could conceivably be due to local anaesthetic absorbed by the blood stream in sufficient amounts to cause a comparable degree of cerebral depression to that seen on emergence from general anaesthesia. However, this explanation seems extremely improbable, since the dosage of local anaesthetic was very small, and insufficient to cause any signs of central depression or impairment of alertness and intellectual activity. Although blood concentrations of local anaesthetic were not estimated in this investigation, published figures from other series strongly suggest that the doses used could not have given rise to significant concentrations in the blood.

Thus, it seems reasonable to assume that the reflex changes observed were due to events taking place at a spinal site, and probably within the segmental area of blockade. The question arises, what sites in the cord are involved, and why does the progression of reflex changes so closely resemble the reverse of the pattern seen after general anaesthesia?

Radioassay studies of cord, spinal roots and meninges in dogs have indicated that epidural analgesia produces the highest concentrations of local anaesthetic in spinal roots and pia-arachnoid, but in addition significant amounts of local anaesthetic enter the substance of the cord itself. Autoradiographs show that distribution of local anaesthetic is in the peripheral parts of the cord, and penetration does not extend very far into the deeper layers. Nevertheless, penetration is probably deep enough to affect a significant proportion of ascending and descending tracts. Therefore, the pathways involved in the observed lower limb reflex changes probably run relatively close to the surface of the cord, where they are likely to be included in the peripheral field of local anaesthetic diffusing inwards from the perimeter.

Identification of the long pathways implicated in the observed reflex changes can only be speculative at the present time. Lower limb reflexes might be affected by conduction changes in either ascending or descending pathways, or both. Interruption of ascending pathways may modulate distant segmental reflexes indirectly by long rostral circuits affecting corticospinal or propriospinal pathways. On the motor side, 2 major and separate descending pathways terminate in the grey matter of the cord. First, a medial system originating in the brain stem (the ventromedial subcortical spinal pathway), and running downwards close to the surface of the anterior median fissure to terminate in the dorsomedial and adjacent parts of the intermediate zone of the spinal grey matter, i.e. Rexed's laminae VIII and IX. This comprises the pontine reticulospinal fibres, and the vestibulospinal tract and the anterior funicular pyramidal fibres. Second, a lateral system consisting of the corticospinal and medullary reticulospinal fibres running relatively deeply in the lateral white matter to terminate on cells in the lateral and dorsal parts of the intermediate zone of the spinal grey matter, i.e. Rexed's laminae V, VI, and VII. In addition, some rubrospinal fibres lie relatively superficially in the lateral white matter of the lower thoracic cord.

The most superficial, and the most vulnerable would seem to be the reticulospinal fibres, the vestibulospinal tract, and the anterior direct pyramidal tract lying close to the anterior median fissure, in the sulcomarginal zone, together with the superficial fibres of the lateral corticospinal and rubrospinal tracts in the lateral columns. Wall has shown that the crossed pyramidal tract in the dorsolateral funiculus of the cat is markedly affected by reversible cold block applied to the surface of the cord. It is possible that some of the more superficial of these fibres in man are also affected by local anaesthetics diffusing inwards from a segmental epidural block.

It is tempting to suggest that the observed sequence of reflex change, hyperreflexia → clonus → positive Babinski, is the consequence of blockade of progressively deeper layers of descending fibres. If this is so then it is suggestive that superficial fibres in the sulco-marginal fasciculus may be largely concerned with the earlier hyperreflexia and clonus, while the lateral and deeper pyramidal fibres are concerned with the positive Babinski that appears later in the sequence of reflex changes.

This simple concept of inward diffusion affecting fibre tracts sequentially at increasing depth is supported by the author's original tracer studies and autoradiographs that suggested a relatively symmetrical pattern of peripheral uptake from the surface of the cord. However, this view may be unduly naive in the light of Cohen's subsequent work on the quantitative regional distribution of local anaesthetics in the cord after subarachnoid injection. Cohen found substantial differences in the concentration of local anaesthetic in different parts of the spinal white matter, with about twice as much drug present in the dorsal and lateral columns as in the anterior columns. Cohen has suggested that this uneven distribution may be due to different lipid characteristics and local anaesthetic affinities in the various regions of the cord.

There is a need to extend clinical observations and Cohen's quantitative analyses to enquire whether a similar pattern of selective uptake of local anaesthetic occurs within the cord after epidural injection. The emergence of a coherent chart of selective affinities within the spinal cord would be of importance in designing appropriate anaesthetic molecules for selective inhibition of spinal pathways, and for specific clinical tasks. Such a chart of neuraxial local anaesthetic affinities might throw light on some presently unexplained paradoxes of performance in epidural blockade. For example, certain local anaesthetics show an unexplained lack of correlation between the intensity of motor block and the quality of sensory anaesthesia that they provide. Thus, tetracaine produces a more profound degree of motor blockade than bupivacaine, and yet the quality of sensory analgesia produced by bupivacaine is superior. Recent studies with etidocaine show that etidocaine is somewhat similar to tetracaine in this respect. This dichotomy between quality of motor and sensory performance is not explicable in terms of neurophysiological considerations of fibre size within the nerves and nerve roots. However, these differences of motor and sensory performance might be explained by specific patterns of regional affinities and local anaesthetic distribution within the architecture of the cord. After the passage of nearly a century, the process of investigation would then come a little closer to Corning's original concept of intraspinal medication and spinal anaesthesia proposed in his paper entitled '*Spinal Anesthesia and Local Medication of the Cord.*'

ACKNOWLEDGEMENTS

The author wishes to thank Miss Lorna Dunford, R.N., for technical assistance. Supplies of etidocaine were provided by Astra Chemicals Ltd., Canada.

Duranest® and Marcaine®: A comparison of the long-acting local anesthetic agents

P. C. LUND, J. C. CWIK and R. T. GANNON

Department of Anesthesiology, Conemaugh Valley Memorial Hospital, Johnstown, Pa., U.S.A.

The structural formulae of Duranest and Marcaine which differ only slightly from that of lidocaine are quite similar. The physical and chemical properties of these agents are also similar but the plasma protein binding capacity and the partition coefficient of Duranest are both higher than those of Marcaine. The difference in these 2 very significant factors probably accounts for the major difference in their pharmacologic action. Our series, which exceeds 3000 cases of all forms of conduction anesthesia, suggests that regardless of the results found by animal studies, clinically, the therapeutic ratios of the new long-acting local anesthetic agents are lower than those of the short-acting local anesthetic agents.

CLINICAL PHARMACOLOGY

A comparison of various clinically significant factors following peridural administration of equipotent concentration and volumes of Duranest and Marcaine indicates the following: (1) Duranest has a slightly more rapid onset time averaging 5 min or less while that of Marcaine approaches 7 min. (2) The development of maximal or complete analgesia occurs more rapidly with Duranest than Marcaine, the average time being 17 and 21 min respectively. (3) Marcaine appears to have a slightly longer two segment regression time than Duranest combined with a slightly shorter duration of analgesia. (4) Duranest definitely produces a more intense degree and duration of motor blockade than Marcaine but Marcaine produces a greater intensity of sensory blockade. This factor has little clinical significance because of the lower systemic toxicity of Duranest. (5) The 1% solution of Duranest or the 0.75% solution of Marcaine produces adequate relaxation for abdominal and pelvic procedures, if sufficient volumes are administered. (6) The peak venous blood plasma concentration curves of Duranest are lower than those of Marcaine when equal volumes and concentrations are compared. This is probably due to the higher lipid solubility of etidocaine which results in its sequestration in various fat depots throughout the body.

SYSTEMIC TOXIC REACTIONS

The incidence of systemic toxic reactions has been very low with both agents. Those which have occurred have been secondary to partial intravascular injection during caudal or peridural anesthesia or the administration of excessively large doses in the presence of arteriosclerosis and senility. The more favorable margin of safety or the lower potential systemic toxicity of Duranest than Marcaine has also been demonstrated clinically by the intravenous administration of up to 125 mg of these agents in human volunteers. Four of five subjects showed signs of central nervous toxicity after Marcaine followed Duranest.

CONCLUSIONS

1.   Both are excellent, new very long-acting local anesthetic agents which fulfil a definite need today.

2.   Duranest has a more rapid onset of action but Marcaine is more potent.

3.   Duranest produces a greater intensity of motor blockade and Marcaine more intense sensory analgesia.

4.   Duranest has a lower systemic toxicity combined with a higher margin of safety or therapeutic index than Marcaine.

Duranest® - etidocaine

P. C. LUND, J. C. CWIK and R. T. GANNON

Department of Anesthesiology, Conemaugh Valley Memorial Hospital, Johnstown, Pa., U.S.A.

Duranest is a new stable local anesthetic agent synthesized by Astra (U.S.A.) in 1971 which is closely related chemically to lidocaine but differs considerably in anesthetic activity. It is available in 0.25, 0.5, 1 and 1.5% solutions. The pharmacologic actions of this agent are primarily related to a marked lipid solubility combined with a very high protein binding capacity. It has a rapid onset time combined with a slow regression period and a remarkably prolonged duration of action exceeding that of tetracaine. We have evaluated the clinical effectiveness and safety of Duranest for peridural (single dose and continuous technics), caudal, brachial plexus and miscellaneous nerve blocks in a total series exceeding 2500 cases. A dose response study conducted with peridural anesthesia indicated that the frequency of adequate surgical anesthesia was very high and directly proportional, within specific limits, to the dose administered; for example, 30 ml of 1% Duranest or 20 ml of 1.5% Duranest (300 mg) is required to produce adequate relaxation for major abdominal surgery. Thirty ml of the 0.5% solution is adequate for brachial plexus or caudal blocks. Sensory analgesia which was particularly prolonged following brachial plexus blocks frequently exceeds 12–18 hr.

The low peak venous blood plasma concentration levels of Duranest following various routes of administration which are unaffected by epinephrine indicate a wide margin of safety or therapeutic index. This is probably primarily due to the high partition coefficient (141) or lipid solubility which results in preferential accumulation in various fat depots including the peridural space. A nonlinearity of venous blood plasma concentration curves following peridural administration of various doses of Duranest indicates that the percentage of absorption increases as the total dose increases. The high plasma protein binding capacity also leaves less free drug available for access to the brain or cardiac tissue and in addition there is evidence of an unusual, rapid redistribution of this agent.

There is an absence of neurological sequelae or tissue irritation and an exceedingly low incidence of systemic toxicity was encountered. It also became apparent that the therapeutic ratio of this agent is lower than that of the other commonly used local anesthetic agents despite evidence to the contrary in small-animal studies. Dissipation of peridural analgesia unlike the onset of analgesia, does not follow a segmental pattern but tends to follow a horizontal pattern which surrounds the body like a belt. It was concluded that Duranest is an excellent new local anesthetic agent which in addition to having a prolonged duration of action, produces a particularly intense degree of motor blockade combined with adequate sensory analgesia. It has high potency, low toxicity, superior penetration or diffusion characteristics and a very rapid onset of action and therefore fulfils a definite need today.

NOTE ADDED IN PROOF:

Our total series now exceeds 3,500 cases.

Dorsal epidural analgesia: A double blind study between bupivacaine and etidocaine

H. RENCK and H. EDSTRÖM

Departments of Anesthesiology and Intensive Care, Centrallasarettet, Halmstad, and
Medical Department, Astra Läkemedel, Södertälje, Sweden

Dorsal epidural analgesia is not very frequently employed in clinical anesthesia. During recent years, however, an increasing interest in this type of blockade in connection with postoperative pain relief has become evident. The present study was undertaken to evaluate the sensory and motor blockade obtained with long-acting local anesthetic agents in dorsal epidural analgesia.

MATERIAL AND METHODS

40 patients scheduled for elective upper abdominal surgery were investigated in a double blind study. An epidural catheter was introduced through one of the T5 to T8 vertebral interspaces and 4–10 ml of a codified test solution (0.5% bupivacaine or 1.0% etidocaine, both with adrenaline 1 : 200,000) were injected. The patients were tested for analgesia to pin prick every 2nd min after injection and the upper and lower limits of segmental analgesia were charted on graph paper. Surgery was then performed under combined regional and general anesthesia. Postoperatively the patients were tested in the same way every 15th min until only 2 segments remained blocked. The patients' expiratory efforts (peak expiratory flow = PEF) were investigated pre- as well as postoperatively.

Table 1. *Onset characteristics of dorsal epidural analgesia*

Group		Initial onset (min)	Complete spread (min)	Maximum segmental spread		Dose		No segments blocked	Segmental dose (mg)
				upper	lower	ml	mg		
Bupivacaine (19 pats)	M	< 2	14.3	C 7.1	L 2.0	5.7	28.6	15.0	2.03
	SD	–	5.1	3.1	1.2	1.5	7.5	4.0	0.8
Etidocaine (21 pats)	M	< 2	11.2	C 8.1	L 1.7	5.6	55.7	13.7	4.35
	SD	–	5.8	2.0	1.2	1.6	16.4	3.0	1.9

Table 2. *Duration of action (in min) of dorsal epidural analgesia*

Group	Recession of 2 segments	Total duration	Complete analgesia	Supplementary analgetics
Bupivacaine				
M ± SD	225 ± 69	583 ± 255	233 ± 121	229 ± 44
n	18	18	15	13
Etidocaine				
M ± SD	249 ± 119	600 ± 310	195 ± 64	280 ± 159
n	21	21	13	17

Total duration = latency to recession to 3 or less segments. Complete analgesia = latency to experience slight wound pain at PEF. Supplementary analgetics = latency to supplementary administration of pentazocine.

Table 3. *Expiratory efforts after institution of dorsal epidural analgesia (PEF, in % of control)*

At min	0	5	10	15	20	25	30
Bupivacaine M	100.0	100.1	103.0	102.2	102.9	106.7	106.6
SD	–	11.2	15.0	15.8	13.9	11.4	15.4
Etidocaine M	100.0	98.4	97.0	97.3	96.2	98.4	96.5
SD	–	8.8	8.2	9.8	12.4	6.1	9.5

Table 4. *PEF in liters per minute*

		Ex I	Ex II	Ex III	Ex IV
Bupivacaine	M ± SD	364 ± 112	154 ± 93	108 ± 60	183 ± 101
	n	19	18	8	17
Etidocaine	M ± SD	371 ± 98	148 ± 65	130 ± 51	158 ± 64
	n	20	17	11	17

Ex I = control. Ex II = 30 min after arrival to recovery room. Ex III = 30 min prior to first pentazocine administration. Ex IV = 90 min after arrival to recovery room.

Table 5. *Control, maximum and minimum values (M ± SD) for arterial systolic blood pressure (B.P.) and heart rate (HR) after institution of dorsal epidural analgesia*

	Bupivacaine			Etidocaine		
	Control	Maximum	Minimum	Control	Maximum	Minimum
B.P. mm Hg	139 ± 25	139 ± 30	111 ± 24	140 ± 23	139 ± 24	111 ± 24
%	(100)	(0 ± 14)	(−18 ± 17)	(100)	(0 ± 10)	(−18 ± 14
HR b.p.m.	78 ± 13	86 ± 11	70 ± 11	80 ± 15	80 ± 14	68 ± 13
%	(100)	(+11 ± 13)	(−10 ± 10)	(100)	(0 ± 15)	(−17 ± 11)

RESULTS

Latency of initial onset, latency of complete spread – as defined by Bromage (1965) – *maximal segmental spread* and *segmental dose requirements* are given in Table 1. Various data expressing the *duration of action* are given in Table 2. *PEF* values during the first 30 min after institution of the block are stated in Table 3 and in the early postoperative period in Table 4. Changes of arterial *blood pressure* and *heart rate* are reported in Table 5.

DISCUSSION

The sensory blockade was measured according to Bromage (1965). With the exception of latency to complete spread, no significant differences between the 2 agents studied could be established. On the other hand dorsal epidural analgesia differs from lumbar epidural analgesia in onset time, segmental spread and duration. For comparison the results of Engberg et al. (1974) are given in Table 6.

Table 6. *Measures for sensory blockade in lumbar epidural analgesia**

Agent	Initial onset (min)	Complete spread (min)	Segmental dose (mg)	Recession of 2 segments (min)	Total duration (min)
Bupivacaine					
M ± SD	9.2 ± 4.0	22.9 ± 4.7	4.4	157 ± 69	284 ± 111
Etidocaine					
M ± SD	7.6 ± 2.2	16.4 ± 5.7	11.4	134 ± 68	225 ± 71

*   According to Engberg et al. (1974).

In this study PEF was investigated in attempts to evaluate the relaxation of the abdominal wall. No significant changes were noticed in the 2 groups studied, but PEF in relation to control values was significantly lower in the etidocaine than in the bupivacaine group at 25 and 30 min after institution of the blocks. This might in part be due to the more pronounced muscle relaxing properties of this agent as compared to bupivacaine (cf. Engberg et al., 1974). The changes of arterial blood pressure and heart rate were essentially in agreement with those published by Sjögren and Wright (1972).

Thus dorsal epidural analgesia obtained with long-acting local anesthetic agents of the amide type provides a widespread analgesia to pin prick of long duration with essentially no effects upon the patients' expiratory efforts and only minor effects upon systolic arterial blood pressure and heart rate. In addition puncture of the dorsal epidural space is considered to be safe in experienced hands providing a 5 % failure rate is accepted as necessary. Consequently dorsal epidural analgesia might seem to be a panacea for postoperative pain relief. However, in the present study the segmental spread was unnecessarily wide and the number of segments blocked was unaffected by dose reductions. The duration of complete analgesia was on the average about 40 % of the total duration. The reductions of the patients' expiratory efforts in the early postoperative period were essentially the same as we have seen in non-blocked patients after similar surgical procedures performed under general anesthesia alone. From a clinical point of view the efficacy of the sensory block when it was waning was not convincing. The duration varies widely between patients (total duration 180–4740 min). Only complete analgesia can be used as an indicator of the patients' need for further pain relief.

Our experience of dorsal epidural analgesia with long-acting local anesthetic agents of the amide type can be characterized by 3 dimensions – vertical, transversal and longitudinal – which differ from the corresponding dimensions of lumbar epidural analgesia. The vertical dimension is distinguished by the wide segmental spread which is not to any predictable extent influenced by the volume of local anesthetic injected, age, sex, or the weight of the patient. With these agents a limited segmental spread around an abdominal incision cannot be obtained. The transverse dimension – the intensity of the blockade – in dorsal epidural analgesia is not so intense that any significant muscle relaxation occurs. During regression of the blockade the intensity is reduced much more rapidly than the spread in contrast to lumbar epidural analgesia. The longitudinal dimension is characterized by, in several cases, an extremely long total duration of action.

REFERENCES

Bromage, P. R. (1965): *Acta anaesth. scand., Suppl. 16,* 55.
Engberg, G., Holmdahl, M. H:son and Edström, H. (1974): *Acta anaesth. scand., 18,* 277.
Sjögren, S. and Wright, B. (1972): *Acta anaesth. scand., Suppl. 46,* 5.

Chapter II

Pain treatment

*Acupuncture and pain mechanisms**

RONALD MELZACK

Department of Psychology, McGill University, Montreal, Quebec, Canada

The technique of acupuncture, which originated in ancient China, is being used increasingly in the Orient to induce profound analgesia so that even major surgical procedures can be performed without chemical anesthetics. Over the centuries, acupuncture has been used as a form of therapy for virtually every ailment (Mann, 1967). It is the more recent technique of producing surgical analgesia (Dimond, 1971; Brown, 1972) that has intrigued Western scientists and laymen alike. The possibility of a nonchemical form of analgesia, particularly in the case of elderly patients, may be a valuable contribution of acupuncture. Equally important is its potential for controlling a variety of pathological pain syndromes such as the neuralgias, causalgia or phantom-limb pain.

MAJOR CHARACTERISTICS OF ACUPUNCTURE ANALGESIA

There are three major characteristics of acupuncture analgesia, which at first glance seem to defy Western scientific theory. These are: (*a*) moderately intense somatic stimulation by acupuncture needles, which cannot possibly block neural transmission by any known pharmacological action, nevertheless produces analgesia; (*b*) insertion of needles at given skin sites produces an effect at distant body parts that are not segmentally interconnected; and (*c*) pain is relieved for hours after stimulation has stopped. Although these properties appear to be inexplicable in terms of traditional medical practice, they are in fact well documented in Western medical literature.

Control of pain by intense stimulation

One of the oldest methods of pain control is generally known as 'counter-irritation'. This method is characterized by intense stimulation on the body surface and it sometimes produces pain relief for variable periods of time. It includes such folk treatments as application of mustard plasters, ice packs, or blistering fluids.

Although these methods are still frequently used, it is only recently that any theoretical or physiological explanation for their effectiveness has been proposed. Usually, such placebo mechanisms as suggestion or distraction of attention are invoked, but neither seems adequate to account for both the power of the methods nor the long duration of pain relief which is achieved.

However, there is considerable evidence to show that brief, somewhat painful stimulation

* Supported by Grant No. A7891 from the National Research Council of Canada, and by the Advanced Research Projects Agency of the Department of Defense and monitored by the Office of Naval Research under contract N00014-70-C-0350 to the San Diego State College Foundation.

produces marked relief of more severe pathological pain for periods of time that extend far beyond the duration of stimulation (see Melzack, 1973). For example, tic douloureux, which is characterized by painful, convulsive spasms of the face and mouth, may be permanently abolished by vigorous massage of the sensory nerve which innervates the lower head and jaw. Similarly, an injection of hypertonic saline into the interspinous tissues of the back produces a sharp brief pain which may be followed by long-term relief of phantom limb pain. This may also be achieved by saline injections into the stump itself. Experimental evidence also suggests that one pain may produce a marked rise in threshold (the lowest stimulus intensity at which pain is reported) to other types of pain. The threshold to pain produced by electrical stimulation of the teeth is raised by about 30% by the application of painful cold to the shin of either leg. Furthermore, this effect may last as long as two hours. Likewise, paraplegics who suffer pain have a higher threshold to experimentally induced pain than pain-free paraplegics.

Distant body sites

The phenomena of referred pain and trigger zones provide a model for examining the effects of acupuncture at distant body sites. Patients with cardiac disease often develop referred pain in the shoulder, chest, and arm. Pressure on trigger spots in these areas frequently produces intense pain which may last for several hours. It is interesting to note that examination of subjects who do not suffer heart disease also reveals a similar pattern of trigger areas (Kennard and Haugen, 1955). When moderate pressure is applied, pain may be evoked which lasts for several minutes. The pain may actually increase in intensity for a few seconds following removal of the pressure. Similar patterns of referred pain are observed in other areas of the body (Travell and Rinzler, 1952).

Referred pain patterns and trigger zones are frequently used in Western medical practice for both diagnosis and treatment. The patterns of referred pain are highly consistent from one person to another, as are the small trigger spots within these areas. The application of pressure to these trigger spots evokes pain in the referred area and often in the related diseased visceral structure. Injections of anesthetic drugs such as novocaine may relieve both the referred pain and the pain in the viscera. A single such injection may not only reduce the frequency of painful attacks but may relieve it permanently.

We have found a high degree of correspondence between the various trigger areas and acupuncture spots for pain. What is particularly fascinating is that in most cases these spots are specified in relation to the same pathological pain patterns. Surprisingly, physicians have also found that intense stimulation of trigger areas may abolish referred pain. This usually involves dry needling of the trigger spot but may include such stimulation as the application of intense cold (Travell and Rinzler, 1952).

Central nervous system lesions also reveal something of the interactions between distant body areas (Nathan, 1956). Patients who have undergone anterolateral spinal cordotomy, usually for relief of pain due to malignancy, report pain at some distant area (such as the chest or abdomen) when pricked by a pin on an analgesic area (such as the leg). These pains can be evoked on the same or the opposite side of the body. In some cases the pain is evoked at the site of an earlier injury.

Pain relief outlasts stimulation

Pain is relieved for varying periods of time after acupuncture needles have been withdrawn. Actually, many pathological pain patterns involve unusual temporal characteristics, in which brief intense stimulation may evoke prolonged pain (see Melzack, 1973). On the other hand, a single temporary anesthetic block or a brief increase in stimulation may abolish pains that have persisted for months or years. These phenomena suggest a much more complex temporal relationship between stimulus and pain than that indicated by specificity theory.

That temporal patterns of pain do not bear a simple one-to-one relationship to the duration of stimulation is further substantiated by medical records. Referred pain may be evoked, by stimulating the tissues in the nasal sinuses, in teeth which have been drilled and filled without local anesthetic as long as 70 days prior to the stimulation. A single injection of novocaine into the appropriate nerve of the jaw abolishes this effect permanently. It is difficult to attribute this phenomenon to chronic local irritation due to trauma since the anesthetic block could not have affected the teeth themselves. These observations suggest prolonged changes in central neural activity which can be triggered by a brief, painful input and stopped permanently by a single anesthetic block.

All of these characteristics of acupuncture analgesia, which at first glance seem magical and puzzling, are consistent with the 'gate-control' theory of pain.

A PSYCHOPHYSIOLOGICAL EXPLANATION

The 'gate-control' theory of pain, which is based on current knowledge of central neural function, suggests that the transmission of pain signals from the body to the spinal cord and brain is not a fixed, immutable process but a dynamic one capable of plasticity and modulation (Melzack and Wall, 1965). According to the theory, a gate-like mechanism exists in the pain signalling system. This gate may be opened or closed in varying degrees so that, under certain circumstances, signals from injured tissues may be blocked and fail to reach the brain. The gate control theory describes three ways by which pain can be modulated (see Melzack, 1973).

Within somatic sensory nerves there are large and small fibers which have different effects on the transmission of pain signals. Physiological studies (Wall, 1964) suggest that stimulation of large fibers tend to 'close the gate' and block pain signals, whereas small-fiber activity tends to 'open the gate'. Acupuncture stimulation, at low-intensity levels, would generally activate a greater proportion of large fibers than small fibers, thereby blocking the transmission of pain signals. This hypothesis gains support from the fact that acupuncture stimulation loses its analgesic effect if the skin sites are first injected with local anesthetic. This explanation of how acupuncture blocks pain, however, is only plausible if the needles are inserted near the painful area. It does not clarify how acupuncture needles affect distant body areas.

A second modulating mechanism of the 'gate-control' theory involves the powerful inhibitory influence of portions of the brainstem over the pain-transmission system (Reynolds, 1969; Mayer et al., 1971). This inhibitory effect may operate via descending fibers which act on the spinal gating system or on fibers which project to other transmission areas in the brain. The brainstem reticular formation receives inputs from widely distributed parts of the body. Furthermore, when certain areas of the reticular formation are electrically stimulated, a profound analgesia is produced in a large part of the body. These data provide an explanation for the observation that stimulation at sites in one part of the body may produce analgesia of a distant part. In studies with rats, profound analgesia can be produced in a quarter or half of the body by electrical stimulation of certain regions of the reticular formation. These rats can be shocked, pinched or pin-pricked without responding in any way that indicates pain. Moreover, the duration of the analgesic effect in these studies often outlasts the period of stimulation by as long as 20 min. These findings suggest that the neural activities triggered by stimulation may 'close the gate' for prolonged periods of time.

The third way the nervous system modulates pain perception involves descending fibers from the cortex. Psychological processes, such as expectation, anxiety, suggestion, and memory of past experiences, all have a profound effect on pain. It is well known that increased anxiety enhances pain perception while decreases in anxiety diminish the intensity of perceived pain. The important role of anxiety and fear is evident in the observation that morphine has a greater analgesic effect when pain is accompanied by anxiety, but has little analgesic effect in the non-anxious patient. The placebo effect also demonstrates the importance of these psychological processes in pain perception. Pharmacologically inert substances, such as sugar or salt, may produce postoperative pain relief in one-third of patients who believe they are receiving an analgesic. The stronger the suggestion that a given procedure will reduce pain, the more likely it will have an effect. Strong suggestion, faith in the doctor and his techniques, relaxation and distraction all contribute to the diminution of pain and anxiety. The fact that suggestion and belief in the analgesic properties of acupuncture is highly explicit in the Chinese hospital environment undoubtedly contributes to its effectiveness.

Taken together, these three modulating mechanisms of the gate-control theory provide a plausible explanation of how acupuncture analgesia works. In particular, the inhibitory effects of the brainstem reticular formation on the transmission of pain signals in the spinal cord or at higher transmission levels seems to provide a powerful explanatory concept. Intense stimulation through acupuncture needles could activate this inhibitory brainstem system, thereby closing the gate to pain signals.

In conclusion, it is evident that we have only partial information about acupuncture. Apparently, the technique is not used routinely on all patients. Which patients, then, are good candidates and which are not? Conventional preoperative analgesic and relaxant medications are usually administered to patients undergoing acupuncture analgesia (Brown, 1972). The interaction between these drugs and the actual acupuncture procedure has not been determined. However, their effect, together with the faith in the procedure and the belief that no pain will be felt, which is engendered by long cultural tradition, would greatly diminish anxiety. This predisposition, then, would make it possible for the patient to feel little or no pain when the acupuncture needles are inserted and the tissues are stimulated electrically or manually. The stimulation of the needles either by twirling or mild electricity would produce nerve impulses which, in turn, would activate parts of the brainstem reticular formation. This activation would block the transmission of pain signals from the site of the surgery.

This explanation of acupuncture analgesia is based on the meager amount of knowledge we currently have available. With the increased dialogue that is developing between China and other countries we should, in the near future, have more scientific information and a greater understanding of acupuncture analgesia. Research which is being stimulated in this field will undoubtedly provide valuable knowledge of pain mechanisms in general and new approaches to pain relief in particular.

REFERENCES

Brown, P. R. (1972): *Lancet, 1,* 1328.
Dimond, E. G. (1971): *J. Amer. med. Ass., 218,* 1558.
Kennard, M. A. and Haugen, F. P. (1955): *Anesthesiology, 16,* 297.
Mann, F. L. (1967): *The Treatment of Disease by Acupuncture.* William Heinemann Medical Books, Ltd., London.
Mayer, D. J., Wolfle, T. L., Akil, H., Carder, B. and Liebeskind, J. C. (1971): *Science, 174,* 1351.
Melzack, R. (1973): *The Puzzle of Pain.* Basic Books, Inc., New York–London.
Melzack, R. and Wall, P. D. (1965): *Science, 150,* 971.
Nathan, P. (1956): *J. Neurol. Neurosurg. Psychiat., 19,* 88.
Reynolds, D. B. (1969): *Science, 164,* 144.
Travell, J. and Rinzler, S. (1952): *Postgrad. Med., 11,* 425.
Wall, P. D. (1964): *Progr. Brain Res., 12,* 92.

Subarachnoid alcohol injections for the management of chronic pain

JORDAN KATZ

Department of Anesthesiology,
University of Wisconsin Medical Center, Madison, Wisc., U.S.A.

The procedure of subarachnoid alcohol injection for the management of chronic pain was introduced almost a half century ago by Dogliotti (1931). In the original description of the technique a volume of alcohol was introduced into the lumbar subarachnoid space in an attempt to destroy pain fibers coming from affected areas of the body. Many authors used the procedure to treat chronic pain of various etiologies in the succeeding 10–20 years. Although the procedure was effective in producing pain relief, the medical community found the inherent dangers of the originally described procedure to be too great and hence the procedure was practically abandoned. Since alcohol was injected in the lumbar space, where the fused motor and sensory components of a nerve run, it was obvious that a percentage of patients would develop complications secondary to destruction of the motor fibers. Indeed this was found with a high percentage, approaching 40% in some series, having leg paralysis or paresis of the bladder and/or bowel.

A refinement of this technique has been used successfully by myself and others over the past several years. In this paper, I will describe the technique which I currently use, present results, and discuss the indications for this type of therapy.

TECHNIQUE

The technique used is based on several anatomic considerations. Both dorsal and ventral roots are separated by definitive space as they emerge from the spinal column. Therefore if the patient is positioned correctly, it would be possible to inject a lytic solution so that only one of these pairs of rootlets would be primarily affected. A second factor is that all spinal rootlets originate at the level of L1 (the end of the spinal cord) or higher. Therefore when a particular segment or segments require blocking their appropriate location on the cord must first be determined. For example, the T10 nerve has its origins approximately opposite the T7 thoracic interspace. This then is the area where the block should be attempted.

Technical considerations for the performing of the block are as follows. (1) *Position* The patient should be positioned so that the dorsal rootlets of the affected dermatome lie at the highest portion of the spinal canal. To achieve this the patient is put on an operating table over the break in the table. The table is then flexed putting those aspects of the spinal cord at the apex of the neuraxis. This then would place the affected dorsal and ventral roots over the flexion of the table. Since it is only the dorsal (sensory) roots that we are interested in blocking the patient is rotated 45° prone which rotates the dorsal rootlets superiorly. (2) *Agents* Although alcohol and phenol are both being used intrathecally I would like to report on the experiences that we have with alcohol. Alcohol, being extremely hypobaric (a specific gravity less than 0.8), if injected slowly into the subarachnoid space would tend to rise in the cerebral spinal fluid. If the patient is positioned as described above it will collect in the area immediately over and next to the affected dermatome. (3) *Methods of doing the block* A 20 or 22 gauge spinal needle is introduced into the subarachnoid space with extreme care noting the fact that the substance of the spinal cord is immediately beneath the arachnoid. Only after a clear drip of cerebral spinal fluid occurs or, in those cases where cerebral spinal pressure is low, aspiration of the fluid is easily obtained, a test dose of 0.1–0.2 ml of absolute alcohol is injected very slowly using a tuberculin syringe. The patient receives no anesthesia and only minimal sedation prior to the procedure. The patient is told that he will probably experience a severe burning sensation over some part of his body and is cautioned not to move but rather to relate where this paresthesia occurs. Usually, if the position of the patient is correct, the burning will be in the same location as the pain. If it is either below or above this, the horizontal position of the table is corrected. After it has been established that the position of the needle is proper a volume of absolute alcohol, usually not exceeding 1 ml for each segment, is injected very slowly, no more than a quarter of a ml per minute again using a tuberculin syringe. Once the correct volume of alcohol is injected the patient remains in position for a minimum of 20 min, in order to have the alcohol fixed and not diffuse throughout the entire spinal canal. He is then returned to his room where an additional 6 hr of bed rest is required. Ambulation with assistance is then accomplished and the patient is returned to normal ward activities by the next morning.

RESULTS

Using this technique several large series have been reported with incidences of up to 80% good to excellent relief being reported. My own personal experience in about 150 cases supports this high success rate. This is particularly true when the source of pain can be easily delineated, that is where lesions, such as metastases, can be localized to a specific area. Another factor which would aid in the percent of success would be the location of the pain. Pain in the thorax with its rather simple innervation is usually more easily treated than pelvic pain, in which the nerve supply might be quite diffuse and variable.

Complications of 5% have been reported in the literature. In my series I have had only one patient have anything more than just a temporary post-block headache and perhaps a slight degree of meningismus. This particular patient had paresis in his leg which lasted until his death as well as a temporary weakness of his bladder.

INDICATIONS FOR THE BLOCK

The use of subarachnoid alcohol is indicated in patients with chronic pain secondary to known severe organic pathology. I believe the quoted 5% risk makes this procedure too dangerous to those patients in whom organic pathology is not easily demonstrated. Although the duration of the block may be limited from 2–6 months in the average patient it should not be withheld until the patient is moribund. If pain recurs the block can be repeated.

In addition the block should be only considered if a single site of pain is noted. Where multiple sites of pain are noted one observes that relief of this primary area of pain is insufficient therapy since the other areas of pain soon become dominant and the overall improvement that the patient receives is negligible. In those cases in which pain is bilateral and at the same level the block can be done with the patient in the prone position, a bilateral chemical dorsal root rhizotomy thus being performed.

In the patient who has multiple sites of pain it is best to combine subarachnoid alcohol if indicated at all with some other type of procedure. For example, if the patient has diffuse metastases and pain at several sites on the right side of the body and only a single area on the left a percutaneous cervical chordotomy could be performed to relieve the right sided discomfort and a subarachnoid alcohol injection for the left. This may provide the patient with adequate pain relief. In addition it removes the possible complications inherent in bilateral chordotomies.

SUMMARY

The procedure of subarachnoid alcohol is an effective method of producing pain relief in patients with chronic pain secondary to cancer, if used in the manner described above. The complication rate is small, less than 5% in most series, and below the ranges described for most neurosurgical procedures. It is the opinion of the author that, when the indications are present, subarachnoid alcohol is the first choice in trying to relieve chronic discomfort.

REFERENCE

Dogliotti, A. M. (1931): *Presse méd., 39*, 1249.

An assessment of intrathecal chlorocresol

MARK SWERDLOW

Department of Anaesthesia, Hope Hospital, Salford, United Kingdom

The intrathecal injection of neurolytic agents is now a universally accepted method for the relief of intractable pain. Alcohol was the first agent to be used for this purpose (Dogliotti, 1931) and it is still much used in many clinics. In 1955 Maher introduced the use of phenol for subarachnoid injection, and many workers have found this a more satisfactory agent. The fundamental difference between these two agents is that phenol is hyperbaric while alcohol is lighter than the CSF. The consensus of opinion is that control and localization are easier with phenol and that this agent impairs sphincter activity less than alcohol (Jacobs and Howland, 1966; Tank et al., 1963; Maher, 1955). More recently Maher (1963) has advocated another hyperbaric agent, chlorocresol (parachlormetacresol). He claims that this agent gives superior results to phenol – in particular that it produces better nerve penetrability and fewer complications.

I have been using both phenol and chlorocresol for several years and the present paper analyses the results obtained in the most recent 140 completed cases. The two agents have been used in a non-selective manner although not on a strictly alternate patient basis.

Of the 140 patients treated, 124 were suffering from malignant disease while 16 had intractable pain due to non-malignant conditions – 71 were male and 69 female. Table 1

Table 1. *Age of patients*

Age (yr)	No. of patients
21–30	3
31–40	13
41–50	20
51–60	36
61–70	47
71–80	19
81–90	2

Table 2. *Number of injections required for pain relief*

No. of injections	No. of patients receiving
1	79
2	44
3	11
4	4
5	0
6	2

shows the ages of the patients, while Table 2 analyses the number of injections which were required to produce adequate relief of pain. Sixty-two patients received phenol, 62 were given chlorocresol, while 16 cases had one or more injections of each of the agents. In the early cases 5% phenol in glycerine and 1 in 50 chlorocresol in glycerine were used. In all the more recent cases, the concentrations employed in glycerine were 7% phenol and 1 in 40 chlorocresol. Table 3 details the site(s) of pain for which the treatment was being administered.

Table 3. *Sites of pain*

Site (nerve dermatomes)	No. of patients
Thoracic only	35
Lumbar only	76
Sacral only	17
Thoracic+lumbar	5
Lumbar+sacral	7

METHOD

Patients for intrathecal injections are admitted to hospital usually on the day before commencement of treatment. Before starting treatment a note is made of any existing neurological deficiencies such as paraesthesiae, paresis and bladder and rectal function abnormalities (Swerdlow, 1967). No premedication is given unless the patient is abnormally fearful, (*a*) because we want the pain to be present for 'identification' purposes, (*b*) because the patient's full co-operation and alertness are necessary to achieve accurate placement of the neurolytic solution. When the pain is bilateral the side with most pain is tackled first. With extensive pain or pains in numerous separate sites, the area of most severe pain is treated first. For all except perineal pain the patient lies in the lateral lumbar puncture position with the painful side underneath. Lumbar puncture is performed at the interspinous space corresponding to the level of the middle of the pain bearing dermatomes. When treating perineal pain the patient is placed in the sitting position with the spine flexed and lumbar puncture is carried out in the 4–5 lumbar space. In all cases, when the needle has just punctured the dura and CSF exudes the patient is leaned backwards so that his back makes an angle of 45° with the plane of the table. A 1 ml tuberculin syringe containing the neurolytic agent is now attached to the needle and 0.2 ml of solution is injected. The patient is asked to report the onset of symptoms – which are variously described as paraesthesiae, burning, prickling, etc. The appearance of diminished pinprick sensation over the buttock, or muscular weakness, or of appreciable symptoms on the contralateral side are indications for discontinuing the injection prematurely. It is frequently necessary to tilt the table to approximate the reported symptoms to the desired spinal level. When this has been achieved the remainder of the dose is injected. The total dose employed with both chlorocresol and phenol was 0.5–0.7 ml for sacral roots, 0.5–0.8 ml for lumbar roots, 0.6–1 ml for thoracic nerve roots. It should be noted that when chlorocresol is being employed the patient commonly does not feel any sensations with the first dose and it is necessary to await the onset of analgesia and numbness to ascertain the level of block.

After completion of the injection the patient is maintained in the injection position for 35 min after phenol and for 45 min after chlorocresol. The patient is then returned to bed and lies flat for 24 hr. He is seen 24–48 hr after treatment and if inadequate relief has been obtained a further injection is given. If the other side or another area of pain requires treatment the injection is now carried out.

RESULTS

The results reported here were assessed 3 months after completion of treatment or at death if this occurred at an earlier date. In fact 40 patients had died within 3 months of treatment. Table 4 analyses the results obtained.

Table 4.   *Results of treatment*

Agents	No. of cases	Degree of relief (%)		
		Good	Moderate	Little or none
Phenol	62	50	23	27
Chlorocresol	62	53	30	17
Phenol and chlorocresol	16	56	25	19
Total	140			

The present results tend to confirm the trend found in an earlier report (Swerdlow, 1973). It will be seen that the results obtained with chlorocresol are rather better than those after phenol. Table 5 shows the complications encountered in the 140 patients. Most of these are of short duration and of a relatively minor nature. Some of the patients had more than one complication while about half had no complications at all. The more serious complications are urinary and rectal dysfunction and paresis and in the few cases where these effects have persisted for longer than a week or so, they have presented serious problems in management. Expert nursing and intensive physiotherapy are invaluable therapeutic measures.

Table 5.   *Complications*

Agent	Retention of urine	Paral. rectal sphincter	Numbness	Paresis	Headache	Paraesthesiae	Others *
Phenol	13	4	5	1	5	3	1
Chlorocresol	11	2	14	8	4	3	5
Phenol and chlorocresol	5	1	5	5	4	0	0
Total	29	7	24	14	13	6	6

* 'Others' included backache, involuntary limb movement, and hyperaesthesia.

DISCUSSION

The assessment of the results of intrathecal injections is by no means a simple matter. Patients with intractable pain, especially those suffering from malignant disease, are often beset with a multitude of physical and psychological problems. When only a part of the pain is relieved they often complain bitterly of the remnant of pain, even though this is much less than the amount of pain which was present before the injection. In some cases the intrathecal injection produces only partial relief because visceral pain remains and requires a coeliac plexus block for its relief. Finally it may be difficult to decide whether pain in the post-injection period is due to the occurrence of further secondary deposits

Table 6. *Results of subarachnoid phenol blocks*

Author	No. of cases	Degree of relief (%)		
		Good	Fair	Little or none
Maher (1972)*	433	62	6	32
Stovner and Endresen (1972)	151		77	23
Brown (1972)*	114	68	5	27
Swerdlow (1974)	62	50	23	27
Wilkinson et al. (1964)	30		70	30
Tank et al. (1963)	23	48	18	34

* Personal communication.

or to inadequate persistence of the effects of the block. In an appreciable number of patients the initial injection is ineffective. Alexander and Lewis (1963) found that about two thirds of intrathecal alcohol blocks must be repeated at least once before good pain relief is obtained in any segment. In the present series 61 patients required more than one injection to produce adequate pain relief, although in many there was bilateral pain and/or pain in more than one region. Nathan et al. (1965) believe that the clinical success of chemical rhizotomy is due not to selective destruction of afferent fibres but depends rather on destruction of an adequate number of them. This must explain at least in part the relatively good results in the patients of the present series who received both chlorocresol and phenol and who thus had at least two treatments. The present results obtained with phenol are similar to those obtained in other reported studies, as can be seen from Table 6. As to chlorocresol there are as yet no other similar data available except for the initial report of Maher (1963). However Mehta (1973), in a preliminary communication, has recently reported promising results using a mixture of equal volumes of 5% phenol and 2% chlorocresol in glycerine. The evidence obtained to date with chlorocresol suggests that it merits further trial as an intrathecal neurolytic agent.

REFERENCES

Alexander, F. A. D. and Lewis, L. W. (1963): In: *Anesthesiology*, p. 801. Editor: D. E. Hale. Blackwell, Oxford.
Dogliotti, A. M. (1931): *Presse méd.*, *67*, 11.
Jacobs, R. G. and Howland, W. S. (1966): *J. Ky med. Ass.*, *64*, 408.
Maher, R. M. (1955): *Lancet*, *1*, 18.
Maher, R. M. (1963): *Lancet*, *1*, 965.
Mehta, M. (1973): *Intractable Pain*, p. 271. Saunders, London.
Nathan, P. W., Sears, T. A. and Smith, M. C. (1965): *J. neurol. Sci.*, *2*, 7.
Stovner, J. and Endresen, R. (1972): *Acta anaesth. scand.*, *16*, 17.
Swerdlow, M. (1967): *Anaesthesia*, *22*, 568.
Swerdlow, M. (1973): *Anaesthesia*, *28*, 297.
Swerdlow, M. (Editor) (1974): In: *Relief of Intractable Pain*, p. 148. Excerpta Medica, Amsterdam.
Tank, T. M., Dohn, D. F. and Gardner, W. J. (1963): *Cleveland Clin. Quart.*, *30*, 111.
Wilkinson, H. A., Mark, V. H. and White, J. C. (1964): *J. chron. Dis.*, *17*, 1055.

Percutaneous cervical cordotomy

SAMPSON LIPTON

Centre for Pain Relief, Department of Medical and Surgical Neurology,
Walton Hospital, Liverpool, United Kingdom

Spiller and Martin (1912) realised the possibility of treating persistent pain by surgical section of the anterolateral tract of the spinal cord. The technique has persisted in essentially unaltered form to the present date. It depends on the anatomical and physiological facts that pain fibres enter the posterior root of the spinal cord, ascend (or sometimes descend) a variable number of segments and then cross to the contralateral side where they ascend to form the anterolateral (spinothalamic) tract.

Section of this tract on one side produces loss of the sensation of pain (i.e. analgesia) on the opposite side of the body, combined with loss of the sensations of heat and cold. There is no loss of the sensation of touch. After a variable period, but of the order of two years, the degree and level of analgesia may decrease and even disappear entirely. If, after this time the process producing the original pain is still present, pain recurs. A further section of the anterolateral tract will again produce analgesia.

Thus it is fairly obvious that this technique of relieving pain is eminently suitable in those patients with a shortened expectation of life, which is usually due to cancer. In this class of patient fading of analgesia is not usually a feature as the patients tend to die before enough time has elapsed for this to happen.

There is another factor to this technique being used in cancer pain. The patients have usually undergone one or more serious operations and may not be in good physical condition. In fact the hazard of the major operation of surgical cordotomy may in itself drastically shorten the patients' already shortened life. For this reason many patients who could benefit from such an operation are not offered it, and in addition many patients are reluctant to submit to additional major surgery.

In 1963 Mullan et al. placed a radioactive strontium-90 tipped needle across the dura at the cervical vertebrae 1–2 level and irradiated the anterolateral tract. This produced radionecrosis of part of the anterolateral tract and thus relief of pain in the lower limb.

Later (Mullan et al., 1965a, b) the direction of the introducing needle was altered to aim directly at the anterolateral tract and an electrode was inserted down this and pushed on until it entered the spinal cord. A direct electrical current was used to produce an electrolytic destruction of cells in this region. The anterolateral tract was disrupted and analgesia was produced in the contralateral body and limbs. The electrolytic lesion produced in this fashion took about 20 min to appear in a fully developed form.

Rosomoff et al. (1965) described a method of producing the same results using a radio-frequency current (i.e. a diathermy current). In this way destruction of the anterolateral tract was produced, by means of a heat lesion, in a much quicker time. Certain safeguards were introduced to avoid the dangers inherent in this more rapid production of the cord lesion.

These dangers are twofold. Firstly if the lesion is produced too quickly, the heat evolved may not dissipate quickly enough and the tissues can boil. This produces an explosion which may disrupt the spinal cord. Secondly, although the pain fibres are usually quite separate from the corticospinal motor fibres, the distances involved are quite small. They are of the order of a few millimetres. Thus there can be some overlapping effect on the motor fibres from an adequate and safe lesion in the anterolateral tract. This will produce a, more or less marked, degree of weakness in the ipsilateral body or limbs, as at this level the motor tract has already crossed.

Fortunately the demarcation of the anteriorly placed anterolateral pain tract from the posteriorly placed corticospinal motor tract is approximately on the line of the dentate ligament. Thus if the position of this ligament can be found, the positions of the pain and motor tracts are known.

The modern percutaneous cervical cordotomy is a refined and safe technique (Lipton, 1974). The patient lies in the dorsal recumbent position. Local anaesthesia is used to insert an 18 gauge thin walled spinal needle between the C1 and C2 vertebrae from the lateral aspect. The tip of this needle is placed anterior to the dentate ligament as shown by an emulsion of radio-opaque material (iophendylate B.P., saline and air) injected down the needle. If necessary the needle is reinserted until it is anterior to the dentate ligament.

By means of a suitable elevator the hub of the needle is raised. This depresses the tip until it is 1 or 2 mm anterior to the dentate ligament. An electrode is then inserted down the needle and its 2 mm exposed pointed tip is pushed into the spinal cord. The accuracy of this position is easily determined by using an impedance measurement of the electrical resistance through the electrode. When the electrode tip is wholly or partially in the cerebrospinal fluid the impedance is low. When the electrode tip is wholly in the spinal cord tissue the impedance is high. This difference is easily seen on an impedance meter.

Once the electrode is in proper position tests are performed to check that the electrode tip is not in the motor tract. This is done by stimulation tests through the electrode at a frequency of 2 Hz. A satisfactory position occurs when pulsing of the ipsilateral neck muscles is produced. Pulsing of any other muscles in the body or limbs means that the electrode is in, or is near to, the corticospinal tract, and the position must be altered.

After this a similar stimulation test is performed at 100 Hz. If the electrode is placed correctly the patient will feel 'sensations' on the contralateral body or limbs.

When the correct position of the electrode has been obtained a radiofrequency current lesion is produced. This is done in a progressive and cumulative fashion by either using a constant time and varying the current, or using a constant current and varying the time. Whichever method is used the patient is tested for the development of analgesia on the contralateral body and for motor weakness on the ipsilateral body.

The procedure is terminated when an adequate level of analgesia for the pain suffered is produced. If motor weakness develops the position of the electrode is either altered or the procedure is terminated.

The method is an excellent one for cancer pain. Pain is relieved in 80–85% of patients treated, until they die. The overall mortality depends on the condition of the patients treated but is of the order of 6% when all except terminal cases are accepted.

Motor weakness is absent or minimal in 50% of cases. In a further 20% the lower limb is noticeably weak but does not stop the patient walking fairly normally on the first post-operative day. Another 20% have weakness of the lower limb more marked than this and need to take care when walking in the first two postoperative weeks. 8% need a knee brace or walking aid for up to one month and 2% have motor weakness until they die.

The great hazard of the percutaneous cervical cordotomy is in bilateral procedures, or when a unilateral one is carried out in the presence of respiratory disease. The reason is that the ascending and descending respiratory reticular fibres are situated near the anterior horn of the spinal cord. Bilateral destruction of this region produces a form of apnoea which may not respond to treatment (Rosomoff, 1969; Tenicella et al., 1968). A new approach was devised by Lin et al. (1966) to overcome this hazard. The spinal needle is inserted below the outflow of the phrenic nerve through the C5-6 or C6-7 disc space, and enters the spinal canal at that level from an anterior approach. Through this needle an electrode is inserted into the anterolateral tract and coagulated after stimulation tests, in exactly the same way as described for the C1–C2 cordotomy. The problem with this method is that once the needle enters the disc space its position cannot be altered without withdrawing and reinserting. Thus the line of insertion of the spinal needle must allow the electrode to reach the target point. This is a difficult procedure but can be performed manually as in the Lin technique, or a stereotactic method can be used (Lipton et al., 1973).

Pain tracts can also be interrupted at the cervico-medullary junction by using a stereotactic frame attached to the skull (Hitchcock, 1969). This method involves the insertion of an electrode across the cervico-medullary junction from a posterior approach between the base of skull and the first cervical vertebra. This method is not in common use.

REFERENCES

Hitchcock, E. (1969): *Lancet, 1*, 705.
Lin, P. M. et al. (1966): *J. Neurosurg., 25*, 553.
Lipton, S. et al. (1973): Paper read at the Symposium on Pain, Seattle, U.S.A. In press.
Lipton, S. (1974): In: *Relief of Intractable Pain*, Chapter 9, p. 195. Editor: M. Swerdlow. Excerpta Medica, Amsterdam.
Mullan, S. et al. (1963): *J. Neurosurg., 20*, 931.
Mullan, S. et al. (1965a): *J. Neurosurg., 22*, 531.
Mullan, S. et al. (1965b): *J. Neurosurg., 22*, 548.
Rosomoff, H. L. et al. (1965): *J. Neurosurg., 23*, 639.
Rosomoff, H. L. (1969): *J. Neurosurg., 31*, 41.
Spiller, W. G. and Martin, E. (1912): *J. Amer. med. Ass., 58*, 1489.
Tenicella, F. et al. (1968): *Anaesthesiology, 29*, 7.

Pain relief by transcutaneous nerve stimulation

J. SPIERDIJK [1], R. VAN SEVENTER [1], W. LUIJENDIJK [2], B. ZAPLETAL [2],
J. R. GRAVELOTTE-MULDER [3] and L. MENGES [3]

[1] Department of Anaesthesiology, [2] Department of Neurosurgery, and
[3] Department of Psychology, Academisch Ziekenhuis, Leiden, The Netherlands

In his book '*The Puzzle of Pain*', Melzack (1973) lists a number of pain syndromes which cannot be explained satisfactorily and which are therefore also difficult to treat. They are: phantom limb pain, causalgia, neuralgia, and posttraumatic pain.

The features of these pain syndromes are: (1) Summation. Non-noxious somatic stimuli can trigger excruciating pain. (2) Multiple causes. The pain in these syndromes cannot be attributed to any simple single cause. (3) Delay. Pain in hyperalgesic skin areas often occurs after a long delay and continues long after removal of the stimulus. (4) Persistence. The duration of these painful states often exceeds the time required for tissues to heal or for injured nerve fibres to regenerate. (5) Spread. The pain and trigger zones may spread unpredictably to unrelated parts of the body where there is no pathology. (6) Resistance to surgical control. Surgical lesions in the peripheral and control nervous systems have been singularly unsuccessful in permanently abolishing these pains. (7) Relief by modulation of the sensory input. The most promising method of treatment of these pains appears to be the modulation of the sensory input by either increasing or decreasing it.

The peripheral input can be modulated in various ways: (1) local anaesthetic block; (2) counter-irritation; this could be an injection of a hypertonic solution or vigorous vibration; (3) electrical stimulation.

Today we wish to discuss one form of electrical stimulation.

Neuromodulation can be produced in various ways:

1. *Transcutaneous nerve stimulation.* Electrodes of conductile rubber are taped to the painful part of the body or along the course of the nerve fiber which innervates the painful region. The skin is then stimulated electrically.

2. *Percutaneous nerve stimulation.* A flexible wire electrode is inserted with a needle percutaneously in the desired position. An indifferent electrode is taped to the skin. With this method, stimulation of a peripheral nerve or the dorsal column is possible.

3. *Stimulation of the dorsal column.* By means of laminectomy at the desired level, a small monopolar electrode is implanted subdurally or intradurally, the electrode is connected to a radio receiver which is generally placed subcutaneously, usually under the clavicle. The radio transmitter with antenna is normally carried externally. The patient can regulate voltage and frequency himself.

HISTORY

Wall and Sweet (1967) electrically stimulated peripheral nerves of patients with various localized pain syndromes. Temporary pain relief, which continued after stimulation, was obtained.

In accordance with the theory that the 'gate' is best influenced via the dorsal column where the thick myelinated nerve fibres are separated anatomically from the thin fibres, Shealy et al. (1970, 1974) developed a neurosurgical procedure for stimulation of the dorsal column to alleviate pain. As a selection method for dorsal column stimulation he used transcutaneous nerve stimulation. Shealy concluded, on the basis of his experiences with more than 750 patients, that transcutaneous nerve stimulation is a very valuable method for the alleviation of pain.

Hosobuchi et al. (1972) introduced percutaneous dorsal column stimulation as a selection method for implantation of a permanent dorsal column stimulator. Long (1974) stimulated 400 patients with chronic complaints of pain transcutaneously and was successful in 30% of the cases; Meyer and Fields (1972) reported that out of 8 patients with causalgia selected from a number of U.S. Vietnam patients with peripheral nerve injury, 6 experienced dramatic pain relief by means of transcutaneous nerve stimulation. Burton and Maurer (1974) described good results in more than half of a series of 50 patients with chronic pain. A dorsal column stimulator was later implanted in 25 of these patients.

TRANSCUTANEOUS NERVE STIMULATION

The following indications for transcutaneous nerve stimulation are given in the literature:

Chronic pain

Causalgia, neuralgia, posttraumatic pain, phantom limb or stump pain, arthritis-arthrosis, chronic low back pain, thalamic pains, pain due to cancer, various types of headache and facial neuralgia (Meyer and Fields, 1972; Burton and Maurer, 1974; Long, 1974; Shealy et al., 1974; Shealy and Maurer, 1974).

Acute pain

(*a*) Pain as a result of injury or wounds less than one week old (Shealy et al., 1974).
(*b*) Postoperative pain. After thoracotomy and abdominal surgery. Atelectasis and ileus occurred much less frequently than in the control group (Hymes et al., 1974).

TECHNIQUE

Patients indicated for electrical transcutaneous nerve stimulation first undergo a complete physical examination to confirm or establish the diagnosis of the cause of the pain. In addition the possibility of other, more definitive, therapy is also studied carefully. Standard treatment of pain relief had, more or less, failed in these patients or was accompanied by many difficulties. Our psychologists carry out a psychological examination to determine whether there are psycho-social factors which could affect the results of the treatment in a specific manner.

In addition to taking the history, the psychologist also uses the following tests: (1) Hooper Visual Organization Test. (2) Groninger Intelligence Test. (3) Thematic Perception Test. (4) Amsterdam Biographical Questionnaire. (5) The MMP Pain List.

Since we have recently commenced this management schedule the number of patients is limited and evaluation is impossible. The final decision regarding the treatment with the neurostimulator rests with our multidisciplinary pain group.

The transcutaneous nerve stimulator developed by Medtronic is used. The transcutaneous nerve stimulator consists of a battery-operated pulse generator connected to 2 soft conductile rubber electrodes. The apparatus (Fig. 1) is simple to handle. The pulse frequency (12–100/min) and voltage (0–99 V) are regulated by means of 2 external knobs. The current reaches a maximum of 76 mA at 500 Ω.

The Neuromod gives a biphasic asymmetrical spike pulse wave (Fig. 2). The patients are told that the apparatus stimulates the skin electrically for the purpose of pain relief. The electrodes were generally attached at the location of the pain (Fig. 3). Frequency, voltage and localization were varied until a maximum alleviation of the pain was achieved without unusual or unpleasant sensations. This was sometimes a time-consuming procedure. Initially we ask about the strength of the stimulation or 'vibration' during stimulation; later, questions about pain perception are also casually introduced.

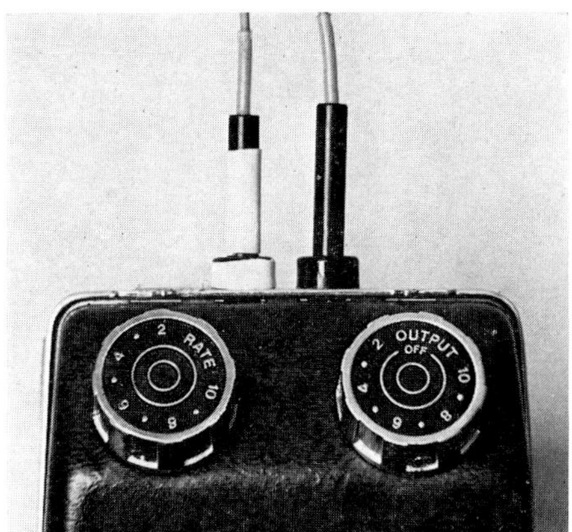

Fig. 1.   *The apparatus.*

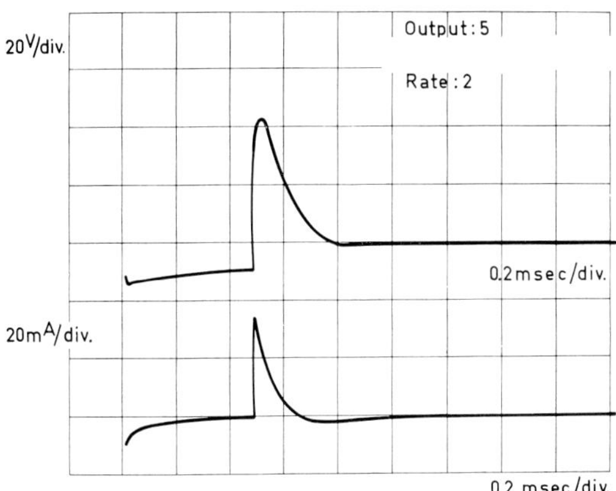

Fig. 2.   *Biphasic asymmetrical spike pulse waves.*

During subsequent stimulations the patient was usually permitted after initiation of the stimulation to regulate the frequency and voltage himself since these parameters are very specific. Most patients were treated in the out-patient clinic – stimulation usually lasted one hr and took place once a week. Stimulation was stopped or continued in the hospital if the results were insufficient after 3 sessions in the out-patient clinic. The treatment was continued in the out-patient department if moderate to good pain relief was obtained. The treatment was continued by the patient himself at home if the results were excellent.

Seventeen out of 26 patients were admitted to the hospital for several days of further evaluation. Three patients took the device home. All patients, except one, tolerated the apparatus well. Side-effects such as skin irritation did not occur. Muscle fasciculations were noted occasionally but these did not bother the patients at all. No difficulties occurred with the device, apart from a torn electrode.

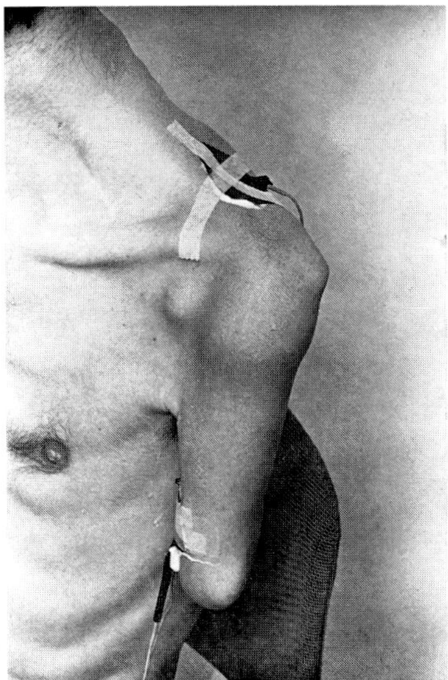

Fig. 3.   *Electrodes attached at the location of the pain.*

Table 1.   *Results of treatment*

	Number	Excellent	Good	Not sure	No
Phantom limb pain	4	1	2	1	–
Posttraumatic pain	3	–	–	1	2
Causalgia	1	1	–	–	–
Neuralgia	5	–	2	1	2
Arthralgia	2	1	1	–	–
Low back pain	9	–	1	1	7
Miscellaneous	2	–	1	1	–
Total	26	3	7	5	11

The results of treatment are given in Table 1. The results are excellent when the patients who have the device at home are free from pain for 24 hr. Good results are when the patients are free of pain during stimulation and for a period after stimulation. The term 'not sure' is used when the reactions of the patients differ from day to day, in which case the patients should be re-evaluated regularly.

The results of our study are such that, in our opinion, a further scientific investigation is justified.

REFERENCES

Burton, C. and Maurer, D. D. (1974): *J.E.E.E. Trans. biomed. Engng, 21/2*, 81.

Hosobuchi, Y., Adams, J. E. and Weinstein, P. R. (1972): *J. Neurosurg., 37*, 242.

Hymes, A. C., Raab, D. E., Yonchiro, E. G., Nelson, G. D. and Prunty, R. N. (1974): In: *Advances in Neurology, Vol. 4*, p. 671. Editor: J. J. Bonica. Raven Press, New York, N.Y.

Long, D. M. (1974): *Minn. Med., 3*, 195.

Melzack, R. (1973): *The puzzle of pain*. Penguin Science of Behaviour.

Meyer, G. A. and Fields, H. L. (1972): *Brain, 95*, 163.

Shealy, C. N., Beckner, T. F. and Prieto, A. (1974): In: *Advances in Neurology, Vol. 4*, p. 775. Editor: J. J. Bonica. Raven Press, New York, N.Y.

Shealy, C. N. and Maurer, D. D. (1974): *Surg. Neurol., 2/1*, 45.

Shealy, C. N., Mortimer, J. T. and Hagfors, N. (1970): *J. Neurosurg., 32/5*, 560.

Wall, P. D. and Sweet, W. H. (1967): *Science, 155*, 108.

Organization and function of a pain clinic

JOHN J. BONICA

Department of Anesthesiology and Anesthesia Research Center and Pain Clinic,
University of Washington School of Medicine, Seattle, Wash., U.S.A.

In dealing with complex pain problems, it is often necessary for the patient's physician to enlist the aid of one or more medical specialists and health professionals. One of the most efficient methods of managing such problems is through team approach, or a pain clinic group composed of health professionals of different disciplines working and collaborating in a well-coordinated manner. Although I proposed this concept over a quarter of a century ago and subsequently described it in many publications (Bonica, 1952, 1953, 1954, 1955a, b, 1974; Bonica and Black, 1974), until recently it was virtually ignored by the medical profession. During the past 2 years there has been a remarkable surge of interest in this team approach and multidisciplinary pain clinics have been organized in several medical centers throughout the world. I will briefly describe the organization and function of the Pain Clinic at the University of Washington as an example of this concept.

Currently the Pain Clinic Group is composed of 20 individuals representing 13 disciplines: anesthesiology, general practice, neurology, neurosurgery, nursing, oral surgery, orthopedics pharmacology, psychiatry, psychology, radiology, sociology, and surgery. The goals and missions of this group are: (*a*) to work as a well-coordinated team to provide optimal care to patients with chronic pain problems; (*b*) to carry on an effective teaching program for undergraduate, graduate, and postgraduate health professionals; and (*c*) to encourage independent and collaborative basic and clinical investigation. Although these objectives can be achieved through individual efforts, our experience suggests that the team approach is more efficient and productive.

ORGANIZATION

A key to the success of such complex multidisciplinary efforts is in effective organization of the personnel and ample physical facilities, equipment, and financial resources. The organization of our own group is shown in Figure 1. Our experience prompts me to make the following suggestions about personnel and facilities in order to have a highly effective operation.

Personnel

Director
The Director should have the capability of providing vigorous medical, scientific, and administrative leadership to the group. Since the team is composed of individuals who have appointments (and consequently allegiance) to their parent departments, it is essential that the Director possess those qualities necessary to bring a heterogeneous group together and have it function as a single, efficient unit. He must possess a superior knowledge

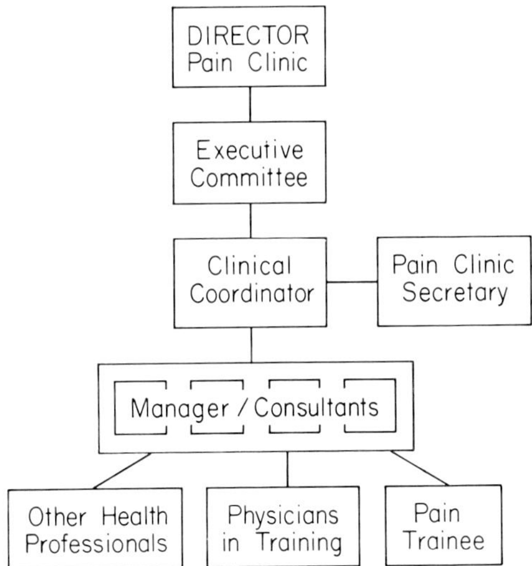

Fig. 1.   *Organizational chart of the Pain Clinic at the University of Washington. (From: Bonica and Black, 1974.)*

and skills in a special area of pain, and his performance in patient care, teaching, and research must be such as to accrue him the respect of all his colleagues.

Clinic Coordinator

The Clinic Coordinator is a professional who devotes most of his time to coordinating the functions and activities of the pain clinic. In addition to the day-to-day activities, this person must coordinate and execute plans for teaching activities by the clinic group and scheduling of case presentations. It is essential that all inpatient and outpatient admissions to the clinic, as well as patient consultations, be processed through the Clinic Coordinator so that he can organize these activities most efficiently. In our own Pain Clinic Group, the Clinic Coordinator is an anesthesiologist who spends most of his clinical time in the Pain Clinic.

Patient's manager

Each patient admitted to the Pain Clinic should be assigned a physician who has the responsibility for the initial examination of the patient, for making decisions as to which consultants the patient should be referred to, coordinating these consultations, and acting as a liaison between the patient, his own personal physician, and the rest of the Pain Clinic Group. The Manager is the first physician to see the patient, to obtain a thorough history, and to carry out a comprehensive physical examination. Based upon the information obtained, he decides which other members of the Pain Clinic should be consulted and in which order the consultants should see the patient. If the patient is presented in conference, the Manager presents a summary of the patient's work-up to the group and after the conference he relays the recommendations of the group to the patient and to the referring physician. He also has the responsibility of writing progress reports and follow-up of the case.

Consultants

Consultants are individual medical specialists, usually members of the Pain Clinic Group, who devote a significant portion of their clinical time to the care of patients with chronic pain. As previously mentioned, in order to be members of the Pain Clinic Group they must have special interest in, and ample knowledge of, pain syndromes, and must possess specialized diagnostic and therapeutic skills in a particular field. If the Pain Clinic Group does not have a representative from the various specialties, it may be necessary to refer the patient to a consultant outside the group.

Other personnel

Health professionals other than physicians whom we consider essential to the success of this type of effort include clinical psychologists, pharmacologists, neurophysiologists, sociologists, and nurse specialists with a particular interest in pain. These individuals serve in the same capacity as consultants and often provide valuable information which is not obtained by other consultants.

Resident physicians and surgeons who rotate through the Pain Clinic, Special Fellows in pain, and other health professionals assigned to the Clinic as part of their training constitute an important cadre of personnel which helps with the work-up and day-to-day care of these patients. The teaching program for these individuals is briefly described at the end of this paper.

Secretaries are extremely important members of the Pain Clinic Group because of their interface with the public and in managing details of clinic visits and admissions.

Space and equipment

To function optimally, the Pain Clinic Group requires space and equipment of three varieties: (*a*) space in the outpatient clinic; (*b*) inpatient hospital beds; and (*c*) specialized space and equipment to meet the peculiar needs of a team actively engaged in patient care and teaching.

FUNCTION

Patient care

The Pain Clinic accepts only patients referred by a physician. The sources of referral are: (*a*) inpatients of the University Hospital being cared for by another faculty; (*b*) patients referred by physicians outside the hospital. Usually the patient is referred to a specific member of the Pain Clinic Group, but a significant number are referred nonspecifically to the program.

Procedure for admission

Upon receipt of a request to admit a patient, the referring physician is asked to send a summary of all the diagnostic and therapeutic procedures done to date, including X-rays and operative reports. He is informed that the patient will be placed on a waiting list pending receipt of the information and evaluation of the data by the Clinic Coordinator, who then decides whether or not the patient is a suitable candidate for care by the group. The information not only helps in screening the patients, but also avoids excessive delay for the out-of-town patients who otherwise will need to wait while their records are being collected. Once the screening is completed and a decision is made to accept the patient, the referring physician and the patient are notified of the appointment date. In many cases the patient is asked to keep a two-week diary on a special form supplied by the Pain Clinic, pertaining to drug medication and daily activities including 'up time' (the amount of time the patient is up and active) and 'down time' (the amount of time the patient is in bed or inactive).

The initial visit

A patient referred to a specific member of the Clinic is seen by him, and he becomes his 'manager'. A patient who is not referred to a specific physician is assigned a manager by the Clinic Coordinator. At the time of admission the patient is asked to prepare a two-page description of the pain and his family history on a special form and also to complete the Minnesota Multiphasic Personality Inventory (MMPI) form. The information is then reviewed by the Patient's Manager and subsequently the patient is seen and informed in detail about the procedure of the Clinic work-up and how the Clinic functions. A very detailed history of the pain and of the patient's past medical history, family history, home and work environment, and other pertinent information is obtained. This is followed by an examination of the painful region and a general physical examination, and usually a neurologic and orthopedic examination.

The information is evaluated by the managing physician, who then determines what other consultations are necessary. Usually patients referred to the Clinic are seen by a psychologist and a psychiatrist and one or more other consultants. Coordination of the patient's visits with the consultants is a function of the Pain Clinic secretary.

After all of the consultants have seen the patient the information is studied by the Manager in an attempt to make a diagnosis. If the diagnosis and therapy are clear-cut, the patient is either referred back to the physician or is cared for by members of the Pain Clinic Group at the University of Washington Hospital.

The conference

Patients in whom the diagnosis or therapy or both are uncertain are presented at the weekly conference of the Pain Clinic Group. Prior to the conference a synopsis of each case is distributed to members of the group. Usually two patients are considered during each conference, which lasts 1.5 hours.

The conference is chaired by the Director or Clinic Coordinator of the Pain Clinic. The Patient's Manager or his House Officer presents a summary of the history and physical findings and then calls upon the consultants who have seen the patient to provide additional information. Members of the Clinic who have not seen the patient are given an opportunity to ask questions and make comments.

The patient and spouse are then brought into the room for further questions by members of the Clinic. This gives an opportunity to those members of the Clinic who have not seen the patient to ask specific questions or carry out brief examinations. Similarly, the patient and spouse are given an opportunity to ask questions of members of the Clinic. After this is completed, the patient and spouse leave the conference room and there is further discussion among members of the Clinic. Often the discussion is vigorous and continues until there is a consensus about diagnosis and therapeutic strategy. After the conference, the Patient's Manager sees the patient and informs him or her of the decision made by the group. He advises the referring physician as soon as possible about the medical details of the decision.

Experience has confirmed our deep conviction that this face-to-face group discussion is much more effective and productive in making a correct diagnosis and formulating the appropriate therapeutic strategy than communication by letter or telephone or through fragmented independent efforts inherent in traditional medical practice. In addition to providing highly specialized consultant service to the referring physician and the patient, these conferences serve as an excellent forum for exchange of ideas and information, and thus constitute a highly effective teaching mechanism.

TEACHING AND RESEARCH

Members of the Pain Clinic carry out active teaching programs for residents (registrars) from various disciplines who wish special rotation on pain and for special fellows of the pain service. The period of training varies from one month to one year depending on the objectives of the trainee.

Members of the Pain Clinic are active in basic laboratory research and/or clinical investigation. A number of members of the Pain Clinic participate in collaborative research.

REFERENCES

Bonica, J. J. (1952): *J. Amer. med. Ass., 150*, 1581.
Bonica, J. J. (1953): *The Management of Pain.* Lea and Febiger, Philadelphia, Pa.
Bonica, J. J. (1954): *Proc. roy. Soc. Med., 47*, 1029.
Bonica, J. J. (1955a): *Anaesthesist, 4*, 88.
Bonica, J. J. (1955b): *Minerva anest., 21/3*, 24.
Bonica, J. J. (1974): In: *Proceedings, International Symposium on Pain, Advances in Neurology, Vol. 4*, p. 433. Editor: J. J. Bonica. Raven Press, New York, N.Y.
Bonica, J. J. and Black, R. G. (1974): In: *Relief of Intractable Pain*, Chapter 5, p. 116. Editor: M. Swerdlow. Excerpta Medica, Amsterdam.

Postoperative pain relief: A reappraisal

THOMAS B. BOULTON

Department of Anaesthesia, Royal Berkshire Hospital, Reading, United Kingdom

Keats (1956) described postoperative pain as 'the most frequent and most neglected painful state in the hospital situation'. Many others, including intelligent and informed patients, have echoed this sentiment (Simpson and Parkhouse, 1961; Parkhouse et al., 1961; Editorial, *Lancet*, 1964; Smith, 1964; Cottingham, 1964; Smith, 1969; Foster, 1969) but postoperative pain relief is still all too often left to the junior physician's 'cautiously administered opiate and the balm that comes from time alone' (Editorial, *Brit. med. J.*, 1953).

THE NEED FOR POSTOPERATIVE MEDICATION

Most civilised men today would surely concede that there is a need for the relief of postoperative pain on humanitarian grounds alone. There are, however, other obvious reasons for mitigating the discomfort of the patient; these include the need to promote deep breathing and co-operation with the physiotherapist and the desirability of early mobilisation to avoid deep venous thrombosis (Editorial, *Brit. med. J.*, 1953; Editorial, *Lancet*, 1964).

REACTION TO POSTOPERATIVE PAIN

It must be remembered that the experience of pain is a central nervous system (CNS) reaction to a *peripheral* nervous stimulus and, further, that the intensity and quality of the reaction to stimuli of identical intensity will vary greatly from patient to patient. Some patients do not require postoperative pain relief, even after major operations (Jaggard et al., 1950; Papper et al., 1952; Keats, 1956; Parkhouse et al., 1961), but frightened patients may need a great deal of pharmacologically induced analgesia (Roe, 1963; Editorial, *Lancet*, 1964).

The vicious circle of pain-fear-muscle spasm-pain can be broken centrally, peripherally or in the nervous conductive pathways between the brain and the periphery.

The importance of the psychological attitude to pain

Roe (1963) showed how preoperative education and psychological preparation alone can greatly reduce the postoperative narcotic requirement and Beecher (1962) has demonstrated marked placebo reactions in his classical studies.

Children require proportionately less postoperative analgesia than adults. This is probably because they often do not have the same anticipatory fear of pain as adults (Editorial, *Lancet*, 1964).

CENTRAL PHARMACOLOGICAL RELIEF OF POSTOPERATIVE PAIN

Most pharmacological methods of postoperative pain relief are general analgesics directed towards central depression of the reception of pain impulses by the CNS but sedatives and tranquillizers which modify the attitude of the patient to the receipt of pain impulses can also be effective (Keats and Beecher, 1950; Keats, 1956).

General analgesics may be given orally, by intramuscular or intravenous injection or by inhalation.

The oral route

Oral administration may be ineffective or inappropriate in the early postoperative period (Comroe and Dripps, 1948).

Intramuscular and intravenous administration

The effectiveness of parenteral agents like morphia and pethidine has been greatly assisted in recent years by the introduction of recovery and intensive care areas; it is now feasible for the anaesthetist to routinely administer narcotics intravenously to achieve an immediate optimum effect rather than having to wait for an intramuscular injection to act. Lowenstein et al. (1969) demonstrated that surprisingly large amounts of narcotic can be given intravenously to pain-free individuals without dangerous cardiopulmonary depression but, in practice, adequate analgesia from parenteral agents often leads to impaired respiratory function and pulmonary sequelae (Muneyuki et al., 1968; Spence and Smith, 1971).

Continuous intravenous infusion of general analgesics or local analgesics acting generally is satisfactory but careful supervision is required to avoid overdosage (McLachlin, 1945; Pooler, 1949; De Clive-Lowe et al., 1954; Krogh, 1970; Ito and Ichiyanagi, 1974).

Inhalation methods

Methods involving the inhalation of limited concentrations of nitrous oxide and oxygen, trichloroethylene and methoxyflurane can be effective but only with considerable patient education and co-operation. They are most appropriate for intermittent use to provide pain relief for physiotherapy (Parbrook et al., 1964; Ellis and Bryce-Smith, 1965; Hovell et al., 1965; Yakaitis et al., 1972).

REGIONAL ANALGESIA FOR THE RELIEF OF POSTOPERATIVE PAIN

Regional analgesia offers a method of keeping a patient alert and co-operative but free from pain. Workers in this field prior to the introduction of bupivacaine (Marcain) in 1963 (Telivuo, 1963) were handicapped because they did not have the use of a truly long-acting local analgesic which would span the first 8–12 postoperative hours during which analgesia is most required (Parkhouse et al., 1961).

Neurolytic agents and depot solutions

Neurolytic agents and depot solutions were employed by earlier workers. Crile is reported to have used a mixture of urea and quinine infiltrated locally into the operative wound, but this was abandoned because of tissue necrosis (Allen, 1918; Bickham, 1924; Bonica, 1953), and Labat (1930) employed alcohol to block the intercostal nerves.

Various oily and non-oily depot solutions were compounded with the intention of promoting the gradual release of short-acting agents (Yeomans et al., 1928; Morgan, 1935; Roualle, 1952; Rutter, 1952; Editorial, *Brit. med. J.*, 1953) but most of these subsequently proved to be neurolytic rather than true depot solutions; there were disastrous consequences when they were administered in the vicinity of the spinal cord because of the benzyl alcohol and other solvents which they contained (Bonica, 1953; Roualle, 1953; Bryce-Smith, 1960). The mixture of lignocaine (Lidocaine) and dextron (Loder, 1962) was possibly not neurolytic although it was not used for paravertebral or extradural injection.

Repeated injection with shorter-acting local analgesics

Repetitive intercostal or paravertebral blocks with short-acting analgesics were advocated by some workers (Bonica, 1953; Gius, 1940) but repetitive multiple injections are tedious for the patient and time consuming for the medical practitioner.

Intermittent injections with shorter-acting local analgesics

Intermittent injection techniques are a better proposition. Various workers placed needles or plastic catheters or cannulae in the rectus sheath (Capelle, 1935; Blades and Ford, 1950; Gerwig et al., 1951; Lewis and Thompson, 1953; Samaraji and Clarke, 1973), in the intercostal spaces (Ablondi et al., 1966), or in the caudal (Hingson and Edwards, 1943), lumbar and thoracic sections of the extradural (epidural) space (Simpson et al., 1961; Green and Dawkins, 1966; Dawkins and Steel, 1971). Many ingenious devices have been invented to maintain sterility in these techniques (Capelle, 1935; Simpson and Salt, 1961; Atherley, 1961; Cole, 1964).

Intermittent extradural (epidural) injection

Intermittent extradural injection is still an important technique for postoperative pain relief, particularly after complex major abdominal surgery and in patients who have preoperative respiratory complications or insufficiency. The number of injections required is, of course, greatly reduced now that long-acting bupivacaine is available (Spence and Smith, 1971).

Single injection techniques with bupivacaine

It has been emphasised earlier in this paper that the greatest requirement for pain relief is in the first 6–12 hr (Parkhouse et al., 1961). Local analgesia with bupivacaine will usually last to some degree over such a period (Telivuo, 1963). Single injection techniques with bupivacaine are therefore valuable for the relief of postoperative pain in uncomplicated cases. No supervision or repetitive action is required by physician or nurse.

Many of the procedures which can be used are simple and can be undertaken with the minimum of apparatus and preparation. The undoubted benefits of local analgesia in the postoperative period can therefore be extended to a great many more patients than is possible with intermittent catheter techniques.

Thorax

The intercostal nerves can easily be injected under direct vision at thoracotomy. The spaces through which drains are inserted should not be forgotten. Delikan et al. (1973) demonstrated the analgesic and respiratory benefits of this technique.

Upper abdomen

Thoracic extradural or paravertebral blocks for pain relief in the upper abdomen are theoretically superior to simple intercostal blocks because they interrupt both the somatic pain impulses from the abdominal wall and visceral pathways (Simpson and Parkhouse, 1961); in practice, however, simple intercostal blockade affords satisfactory relief in routine cases in which the peritoneum is not soiled.

Lower abdomen

Intercostal blocks are also valuable in controlling pain in the lower abdomen.

Lumbar extradural analgesia is an easier and less complicated technique than thoracic extradural; it has gained wide acceptance for lower abdominal surgery. If bupivacaine is used for the operation it also provides satisfactory postoperative analgesia.

Inguinal region

A simple ilio-inguinal/ilio-hypogastric block produces good surgical muscular relaxation and satisfactory postoperative analgesia.

A syringe with a 5 cm, 21 gauge needle is inserted through the skin at a point one patient's finger breadth medial to the anterior superior iliac spine. Minimum pressure is required to push the needle through the subcutaneous tissue but the tip meets with resistance at the external oblique aponeurosis. The needle is now pushed through the aponeurosis and, after an aspiration test to avoid intravascular injection, about 0.3 ml/kg of 0.5% bupivacaine with adrenaline is injected to spread out in the fascial plane beneath the external oblique.

Perineum

Single injection caudal analgesia with a 5 cm, 21 gauge needle is a simple, rapid and reliable technique. This can be used to provide analgesia and relaxation during surgery and postoperative analgesia for haemorrhoidectomy and other operations on the anus and on the vulva. The volume of the sacral extradural space is approximately 0.5 ml/kg up to a maximum of 30 ml; this also happens to be the maximum safe dose of 0.5% bupivacaine.

Circumcision

Both Davenport (1953) and Kay (1974) have emphasised the value of caudal analgesia for pain relief in small boys undergoing circumcision. It is, however, the present author's opinion that caudal block should not be used for this operation after the age of 10 years, nor in the adult. Just before and after puberty, caudal block causes the penis to dilate and, although it remains flaccid, it becomes vascular and bleeds freely at surgery. A simple root block of the penis can however, provide great relief for the older patient who has to undergo this operation. Bupivacaine *without* adrenaline should be used to avoid dangerous constriction of the blood supply of the tip of the organ.

Orchidopexy

The combination of the ilio-inguinal/hypogastric and caudal blocks is useful during and after the operation of orchidopexy. The bupivacaine is diluted so that the maximum safe dose of the equivalent of 0.5 ml of 0.5% per kg is not exceeded. The penis dilates in older boys but the tiresome complication of true priapism, quite often seen during this operation, is largely avoided.

DISCUSSION

Single injection regional blockade with bupivacaine is thus a useful technique for up to 12 hr after operation, which is the period when most analgesia is required. It must be realised however, that, since under normal conditions many patients do not require analgesia (over 50% in the case of inguinal herniotomy for example) (Parkhouse et al., 1961), the routine prospective use of nerve block with bupivacaine may be unnecessary in many cases. It is therefore wise to confine the use of the more complicated techniques of local analgesia like thoracic epidural analgesia, which have an appreciable complication rate, to those procedures in which pain can reasonably be anticipated or in which the particular regional technique forms an accepted part of the anaesthetic. The simpler techniques which have virtually no complications should be used for less major operations. The observation that these simpler techniques like intercostal nerve block are effective in the abdomen confirms that, in routine cases, most postoperative pain originates in muscle in the abdominal wall rather than from the viscera (Zollinger, 1941; Ablondi et al., 1966).

SUMMARY

The aetiology and incidence of postoperative pain and its control have been discussed. The value of single injection postoperative pain relief using various regional techniques with bupivacaine has been emphasised.

REFERENCES

Ablondi, M. A., Ryan, J. F., O'Connell, C. T. and Haley, R. W. (1966): *Anesth. Analg. Curr. Res.*, *45*, 185.

Allen, C. W. (1918): *Local and Regional Anaesthesia*, 2nd ed., p. 205. W. B. Saunders Co., Philadelphia, Pa.

Atherley, D. W. (1961): *Anaesthesia*, *16*, 503.

Beecher, H. K. (1962): *Practitioner*, *189*, 141.

Bickham, W. S. (1924): *Operative Surgery*, *Vol. 1*, p. 176. W. B. Saunders Co., Philadelphia, Pa.

Bonica, J. J. (1953): *The Management of Pain*, *1st ed.*, Henry Kimpton, London.

Blades, B. and Ford, W. B. (1950): *Surg. Gynec. Obstet.*, *91*, 525.

Bryce-Smith, R. (1960): *Lancet*, *1*, 1039.

Capelle, W. (1935): *Dtsch. Z. Chir.*, *246*, 466.

Cole, P. V. (1964): *Anaesthesia*, *19*, 562.

Comroe, J. H. and Dripps, R. D. (1948): *Surg. Gynec. Obstet.*, *87*, 221.

Cottingham, J. W. (1964): *Med. Ann. D.C.*, *33*, 495.

Davenport, H. T. (1973): *Paediatric Anaesthesia*, 2nd ed., p. 143. William Heinemann Medical Books Ltd., London.

Dawkins, C. J. M. and Steele, G. C. (1971): *Anaesthesia*, *26*, 41.

De Clive-Lowe, S. G., Gray, P. W. S. and North, J. (1954): *Anaesthesia*, *12*, 426.

Delikan, A. E., Lee, C. K., Yong, N. K. and Ganendran, A. (1973): *Anaesthesia*, *28*, 561.

Editorial (1953): *Brit. med. J.*, *2*, 385.

Editorial (1964): *Lancet*, *1*, 751.

Ellis, M. W. and Bryce-Smith, R. (1965): *Brit. med. J.*, *2*, 1412.

Foster, C. A. (1969): *Lancet*, *1*, 528.

Gius, J. A. (1940): *Surgery*, *8*, 832.

Gerwig, W. H., Thompson, C. W. and Blades, B. (1951): *Arch. Surg.*, *62*, 678.

Green, R. and Dawkins, M. (1966): *Anaesthesia*, *21*, 372.

Hingston, R. A. and Edwards, W. B. (1943): *J. Amer. med. Ass.*, *121*, 225.

Hovell, B. C., Masson, A. H. B. and Wilson, J. (1967): *Anaesthesia*, *22*, 284.

Ito, Y. and Ichiyanagi (1974): *Anaesthesia*, *29*, 222.

Jaggard, R. S., Zager, L. L. and Wilkins, D. S. (1950): *Arch. Surg.*, *61*, 1073.

Kay, B. (1974): *Anaesthesia*, *29*, 611.

Keats, A. S. (1956): *J. chronic Dis.*, *4*, 72.

Keats, A. S. and Beecher, H. H. (1950): *J. Pharm. Pharmacol.*, *100*, 1.

Krogh, L. (1970): *S. Afr. med. J.*, *44*, 847.

Labat, G. (1930): *Surg. Gynec. Obstet.*, *50*, 74.

Lewis, D. L. and Thompson, W. A. L. (1953): *Brit. med. J.*, *1*, 973.

Loder, R. E. (1962): *Thorax*, *17*, 375.

Lowenstein, E., Hallowell, P., Levine, E. H., Daggett, W. M., Austen, W. G. and Laver, M. B. (1969): *New Eng. J. Med.*, *281*, 1389.

McLachlin, J. A. (1945): *Canad. med. Ass. J.*, *52*, 383.

Morgan, C. N. (1935): *Brit. med. J.*, *2*, 938.

Muneyuki, M., Veda, Y., Urabe, N., Takash Ita, H. and Inamoto, A. (1968): *Anesthesiology*, *29*, 304.

Papper, E. M., Brodie, B. B. and Rovenstein, E. A. (1952): *Surgery*, *32*, 107.

Parbrook, G. D., Rees, G. A. D. and Robertson, G. S. (1964): *Brit. med. J.*, *2*, 480.

Parkhouse, J., Lambrechts, W. and Simpson, B. R. J. (1961): *Brit. J. Anaesth.*, *23*, 345.

Pooler, H. E. (1949): *Brit. med. J.*, *2*, 1200.

Roe, B. B. (1963): *Arch. Surg.*, *87*, 912.

Roualle, H. L. M. (1952): *Brit. med. J.*, *2*, 1418.

Roualle, H. L. M. (1953): *Brit. med. J.*, *2*, 830.

Rutter, A. G. (1952): *Brit. med. J.*, *2*, 1418.

Samaraji, W. N. and Clarke, A. D. (1973): In: *Proceedings, Fifth World Congress of Anaesthesiologists, Kyoto, 1972*, p. 468. Editors: M. Miyazaki, K. Iwatzuki, M. Fujita and J. N. Lunn. Excerpta Medica, Amsterdam.

Simpson, B. R. J. and Parkhouse, J. (1961): *Brit. J. Anaesth.*, *23*, 336.

Simpson, B. R. J., Parkhouse, J., Marshall, R. and Lambrechts, W. (1961): *Brit. J. Anaesth.*, *23*, 628.

Simpson, B. R. J. and Salt, R. H. (1961): *Brit. J. Anaesth.*, *23*, 664.

Smith, C. (1969): *Lancet*, *1*, 426.

Smith, M. P. (1964): *Northw. Med. (Seattle)*, *63*, 698.

Spence, A. A. and Smith, G. (1971): *Brit. J. Anaesth.*, *43*, 144.

Telivuo, L. (1963): *Ann. Chir. Gynaec. Fenn.*, *52*, 513.

Yakaitis, R. W., Cooke, J. E. and Redding, J. S. (1972): *Anesth. Analg. Curr. Res.*, *51*, 208.

Yeomans, F. C., Gorsch, R. V. and Mathesheimer, J. L. (1928): *Med. J. Rec.*, *127*, 19.

Zollinger, R. (1941): *Surgery*, *10*, 27.

The place of brachial plexus analgesia in modern anesthetic practice

V. BURKHARDT

Central Anesthesia Section, Regional Hospital, Karl-Marx-Stadt, German Democratic Republic

In consequence of chronic shortage of nurses, the applications of regional anesthesia in modern anesthesia in relation to their costs in instruments and personnel have been examined. Adequate premedication is essential since general anesthesia can always become necessary due to complications during the operation or anesthetic. Diazepam and droperidol have both proved useful.

The supraclavicular route is used, according to the Kulenkampff method for brachial plexus block, for operations on the hand and forearm. This is always restricted to one side. The contraindications are septic processes in the region of the neck, severe dyspnea, cardiac decompensation, and contralateral pneumonectcmy.

During 5 years, 1054 plexus anesthesias were performed. The puncture was made above the clavicle under aseptic conditions and with a 10 ml syringe armed with a 25–40 mm long fine-caliber cannula, immediately lateral to the subclavian artery with the head turned to the contralateral side. Before the first rib is reached, the cannula strikes the brachial plexus so that the patient can clearly describe the presence and the location of paresthesiae. With some experience, a minor change in the placement of the cannula makes it possible to reach each region of the brachial plexus. The injection is of 20 ml 2% lignocaine with a vasoconstrictor.

Anesthesia of the brachial plexus with the upper arm abducted to 90° is an easier method. This axillary route, close to the axillary artery is used with the same instruments and agents. Local paresthesiae allow the location of the position of the cannula, and with a slight change it is possible to reach all the nerves of the arm. The only contraindication is a septic process in the axillary region of the upper arm.

Forty-seven cases were done during the first year. 41% patients complained about considerable pain in the upper arm at the point of the tourniquet. Additional measures, such as circumferential local injections of the upper arm or general anesthesia, were required. This technique was not preferred to the supraclavicular route. Generally, a failure rate between 2–3% is reported with both methods; this rate depends on the technique and the experience of the anesthetist.

The percentage failure rate was slightly lower than 1% in this series since a general anesthesia was used in those cases where technical complications were anticipated, such as cicatrices in the region of injection, or a short, thickset and inflexible neck. Insufficient anesthesia was observed in 3.8% so that an experienced anesthetist made a second injection or changed to general anesthesia. In a training centre, it is not possible to avoid this occasionally. Pneumothorax, verified by X-ray examination, occurred in 0.6% of cases and immediate aspiration was required in 0.1%. All the patients had no complaints within 3 days and the pneumothorax had disappeared after 10 days. Temporary phrenic paresis was seldom observed. Horner's syndrome occurred in 35% cases. The most disagreeable complication in our patients was local neuritis caused by the mechanical damage to the nerve fibres accompanied by paresthesiae. In 14 cases this disappeared within 3 weeks, in 1 case after 5 weeks and in 1 case after 8 weeks. Permanent damage was not observed.

The method of supraclavicular plexus anesthesia according to Kulenkampff has given satisfactory results for operations on the hand and forearm. The risk of complications is low and decreases with increasing experience. Conditions for the elimination of the complications must exist.

Pain and the autonomic system

M. D. CHURCHER

Anaesthetic Department, Plymouth General Hospital (Freedom Fields), Plymouth, United Kingdom

Pain relief is produced in certain conditions by blocking autonomic pathways. Diagnostic and therapeutic blocks can be done in the following sites: (1) stellate ganglion; (2) thoracic paravertebral; (3) coeliac plexus; and (4) lumbar paravertebral.

Local anaesthetics, phenol or alcohol are used. Surgical sympathectomy is performed when necessary. I would like to discuss pain relief by sympathetic blocks in certain diseases illustrated by cases seen at a Pain Clinic.

CANCER

Head and neck

Some patients with glands in the neck have severe burning pain radiating up the line of the carotid sheath. Recumbency produces vascular congestion and exacerbates the pain. A stellate chemical sympathectomy gives relief. Other patients develop a stiff immobile neck following radiotherapy. Mobility is increased by stellate injections.

Upper limbs

The swollen painful postmastectomy arm is now less often seen, but a deep aching pain felt in the arm and relieved by nocturnal elevation is sometimes described by patients with spreading carcinoma of the bronchus. Sympathetic block is again effective.

Abdomen

The deep epigastric backache and referred back pain in abdominal cancer is relieved by coeliac plexus alcohol injections (Bridenbaugh et al., 1964). They also cure the pain of hepatic distension and intestinal obstruction. This visceral pain is poorly controlled by narcotics and an early injection enables some patients to have many active months.

The complications of this injection are sometimes overemphasized. Coeliac plexus block with 30 ml of 45% alcohol was done on 25 patients. 3 patients had complications.

One sedated ill patient developed hypotension immediately after injection. A further patient had significant postural hypotension. A neuritis of the subcostal nerve lasting 3 days was present in the third patient.

Pelvis

Deep pelvic pain is sometimes helped by injecting the sympathetic fibres as they cross the pelvic brim (Bonica, 1968).

Lower limbs

Patients with spreading carcinoma in the pelvis may develop lower limb pain which responds to sympathetic injection. Pain described as burning or bursting in nature due to venous or lymphatic obstruction can be cured by chemical sympathectomy. One other type of leg pain is sometimes found probably in association with metastatic para-aortic nodes.

These patients have a dull aching pain in the lower limb, often confined to a small area and associated with a cold sensation. Skin temperature may be reduced and an increase in sensitivity to touch is sometimes present. When a sympathetic block is done abnormal tissue is felt with the needle at the lateral side of the vertebral body. This syndrome may be due to metastatic masses infiltrating the sympathetic chain.

ISCHAEMIC DISEASE

The beneficial effects of sympathectomy on early skin lesions and rest pain are well known. The place of sympathectomy in claudication has been more contentious. A few clinicians in the British Isles have been doing chemical sympathectomies for 25 years (Haxton, 1949; Reid et al., 1970).

Various techniques for chemical sympathectomy have been described but the results are much the same. More than half the patients have an improvement lasting for over 6 months. Recently sympathetic injections have been shown to give an increase in calf muscle blood flow on exercise in patients with isolated segmental arterial obstruction (Lofstrom and Zetterquist, 1969). Patients unsuitable for surgery exercise after a para-vertebral injection with local anaesthetics.

Over half the patients so treated have a significant increase in their exercise tolerance.

MINOR CAUSALGIA

Acute causalgia is well known but rarely seen.

Following the report of Homans in 1940, there has been increased recognition that this classic form of causalgia represents only one part of a spectrum of painful conditions involving reflexes mediated in part by the sympathetic nervous system. More often one finds in civilian practice a similar but less severe pain where there is no obvious nerve injury. This has been labelled 'minor causalgia' or 'reflex sympathetic dystrophy'. Wirth and Rutherford (1970) noted an average delay of 2 years in their cases before a correct diagnosis was made.

The following criteria are used for making the diagnosis: History of injury, signs of autonomic dysfunction, hyperaesthesia, and pain relief by sympathetic block.

The following observations have been made in the past:

1.   Certain patients with sympathetic overactivity are more likely to develop minor causalgia.

2.   The liability of patients affected to be labelled neurotic.

3.   The assumption that they are 'after' compensation and that a financial settlement will relieve the pain.

4.   The precipitation of the syndrome by phlebitis.

Minor causalgia cases (5-year period)

Injury	*No.*
Fracture	8
Sprain	3
Crush injury	3
Surgery	2
Penetrating injury	1
Blunt trauma	1

Mrs. R, a heavily built lady slipped on a rug and twisted her left ankle. She was seen 3 months later with severe pain; unable to walk more than a few steps. A series of sympathetic blocks cured her. Six months later she had a minor injury to the other ankle. She again developed a minor causalgia or sympathetic reflex dystrophy which responded to treatment.

Mr. B, aged 42, had not worked for 4 years. He had been hit by a ladder and treated for a mild head injury. He gave a history of right sided lumbar and lower limb pain. After full investigations he even spent 2 months in a mental hospital. When seen the right foot was found to be one degree cooler than the left. His wife confirmed that the right side of his body below the waist had been cooler than the left since the accident. Diagnostic and placebo blocks confirmed suspicions and a surgical sympathectomy cured him.

Acute pain was precipitated in the next case by phlebitis following trauma. Mr. D, aged 46, fell off a building scaffold and landed on his hands and feet. Two years later he had aching pains and tenderness in all four limbs. Three months before seeing him he developed severe pain in both legs and evidence of venous thrombosis. He was very agitated when seen, shuffling along with both feet wrapped in bandages. He had cold hyperaesthetic feet with trophic changes. His painful feet were cured by left chemical and right surgical sympathectomies.

HERPES ZOSTER AND POSTAMPUTATION PAIN

Regional sympathetic blocks will permanently relieve the pain in the acute phase of herpes in many patients (Colding, 1973). They are not so effective in postherpetic neuralgia.

Should burning pain and hyperaesthesia predominate, however, sympathetic blocks are worth a trial.

The place of sympathetic block in postamputation pain is well reviewed by Mandl in his book *Paravertebral Block* (Mandl, 1947). I have at the present time an interesting patient who illustrates two points: (1) the efficacy of sympathetic block in certain patients, and (2) the length of action of 6% aqueous phenol.

An elderly diabetic patient has had six chemical sympathectomies at 7–8 monthly intervals for severe phantom limb pain. Good relief lasts for about 6 months following each injection.

SUMMARY

The autonomic nervous system is involved in a variety of painful conditions. Correct diagnosis and treatment presents a challenge to those interested in treating patients with pain.

REFERENCES

Bonica, J. J. (1968): *Anaesthesiology*, *29*, 793.
Bridenbaugh, L. D., Moore, D. C. and Campbell, D. D. (1964): *J. Amer. med. Ass.*, *190*, 877.
Colding, A. (1973): *Proc. roy. Soc. Med.*, *66*, 541.
Haxton, H. A. (1949): *Brit. med. J.*, *1*, 1026.
Homans, J. (1940): *New Engl. J. Med.*, *222*, 870.
Lofstrom, B. and Zetterquist, S. (1969): *Int. Anaesthesiol. Clin.*, *7*, 423.
Mandl, F. (1947): In: *Paravertebral Block*, Chapter 7, p. 244. William Heinemann Medical Books, Ltd., London.
Reid, W., Watt, J. K. and Gray, T. (1970): *Brit. J. Surg.*, *57*, 45.
Wirth, F. and Rutherford, R. (1970): *Arch. Surg.*, *100*, 633.

Continuous dorsal epidural analgesia with long-acting local anesthetic agents for pain relief after upper abdominal surgery

H. RENCK, H. EDSTRÖM, B. KINNBERGER, G. BRANDT and J.-Å. ZELL

Departments of Anesthesiology, Intensive Care and Clinical Chemistry,
Centrallasarettet, Halmstad, and Medical Department, Astra Läkemedel, Södertälje, Sweden

As has been stated earlier (Holmdahl and Renck, 1974), nerve blocking techniques deserve greater attention than at present for relief of postoperative pain. Continuous dorsal epidural analgesia has been proposed for this purpose by several authors (Green and Dawkins, 1966; Spoerel et al., 1970; Dawkins and Steel, 1971; Spence and Smith, 1971; Holmdahl et al., 1972; Brandt and Kvisselgaard, 1972). In the present paper the use of long-acting local anesthetic agents in continuous dorsal epidural analgesia for postoperative pain relief is discussed.

MATERIAL AND METHODS

Nerve blocking techniques have been used on a routine basis on patients after upper abdominal surgery in our hospital for 2 years. Patients randomly selected for continuous dorsal epidural analgesia had an epidural catheter inserted in one of the vertebral interspaces T5–T8. After the initial dose analgesia was prolonged by either (*a*) drip infusion of 0.1% bupivacaine, or (*b*) intermittent injections of 3–5 ml of 1.0% etidocaine with adrenaline 1:200,000, or (*c*) continuous injection of 1.0% bupivacaine. The analgesia was evaluated by the pin prick test, the subjective pain relief of the patients and their expiratory efforts (peak expiratory flow = PEF).

RESULTS

Continuous drip infusion of 0.1% bupivacaine

This method had several practical problems, especially fluctuations of the drip rate necessitating frequent top-up doses and extremely close supervision. A closer evaluation of the method was therefore considered of no practical value. Only the plasma concentrations at different intervals after the start of the drip infusion are reported (Table 1).

Intermittent injections of etidocaine

Repeated doses of 3–5 ml of 1.0% etidocaine with adrenaline 1:200,000 were given to patients after upper abdominal surgery at 3-hr intervals. Figure 1 shows the number of

Table 1.   *Plasma concentrations of bupivacaine at different intervals after start of continuous drip infusion of 0.1% bupivacaine for continuous thoracic epidural analgesia*

Hr	6	12	18	24	30
M	0.69	0.80	0.97	1.11	2.88
SD	0.62	0.38	0.60	–	–
n	17	19	13	4	1

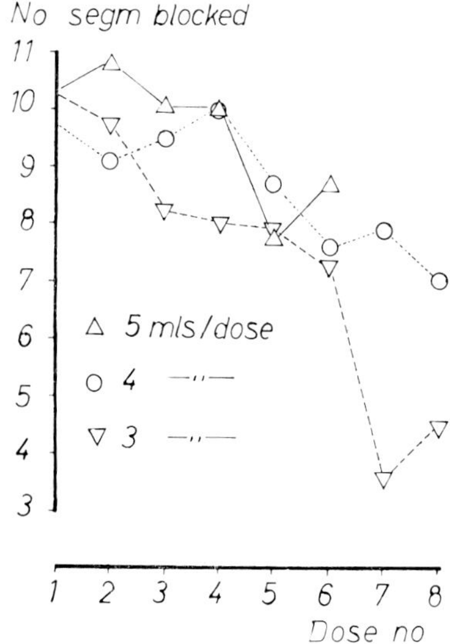

Fig. 1.   *No. of segments blocked after repeated doses of 3, 4 and 5 ml respectively of 1.0% etidocaine with adrenaline 1 : 200,000.*

segments blocked after repeated doses. In Table 2 the number of 3–5 ml doses, the incidences of inadequate analgesia and urinary retention are given. A significantly higher number of segments were blocked when adequate analgesia was achieved than when inadequate analgesia occurred. On the other hand, no difference could be found between the number of segments blocked when urinary retention occurred and when the patients could micturate freely.

Table 2.   *Effects of repeated doses of 3, 4 and 5 ml of etidocaine*

	3 ml	4 ml	5 ml
Total no. of doses administered	75	138	21
No. of doses resulting in inadequate analgesia	13	9	0
No. of doses followed by urinary retention	9	14	4

Five milliliters of etidocaine was followed by pronounced falls in arterial blood pressure (Figure 2) while doses of 3 and 4 ml resulted in smaller changes mainly after the first doses. The plasma concentrations of etidocaine after consecutive injections are shown in Figure 3. Major falls in blood pressure were treated with plasma expanders and vasopressors. No neurological side effects occurred.

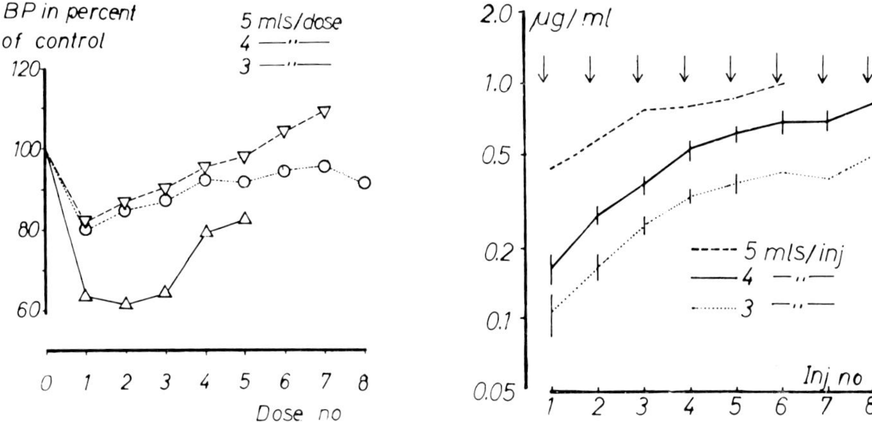

Fig. 2. *Systolic arterial blood pressure – in relation to control – after repeated doses of 3, 4 and 5 ml of etidocaine.*

Fig. 3. *Plasma concentrations of etidocaine – in µg/ml – after repeated doses of 3, 4 and 5 ml of etidocaine.*

Continuous injection of 1.0% bupivacaine

Measures of the sensory block achieved after injection of 2 ml of 1.0% bupivacaine at T5–T6 are given in Table 3. This dose did not affect the patients' expiratory efforts (Table 4). The arbitrarily chosen, initial injection rates used to prolong the analgesia resulted in a decreasing number of segments blocked, so the injection rates were adjusted in each individual case in attempts to provide optimal analgesia (Figure 4). However, the quality of the postoperative analgesia was not ideal (Table 5) and the study was terminated. The patients' expiratory efforts postoperatively – in relation to control – are given in Table 6. The plasma concentrations of bupivacaine at different intervals after the start of the continuous injection are given in Table 7. No neurological or major hemodynamic complications occurred.

Table 3. *Measures of sensory block obtained with 2 ml of 1.0% bupivacaine at T5–T6*

Latency of initial onset (min)	2
Latency of complete spread (min)	11.1 ± 4.4
No. of segments blocked	14.3 ± 4.4

Table 4. *PEF, in relation to control*

		At min					
	Pre	5	10	15	20	25	30
Mean	100	99.3	98.8	101.0	100.1	99.5	101.8
SD	–	6.6	8.4	8.8	13.1	11.3	9.0
n	16	16	16	15	13	13	13

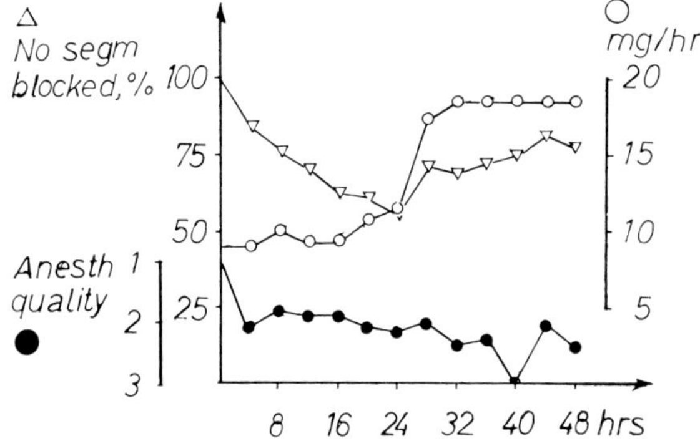

Fig. 4.   *No. of segments blocked, injection rates and quality of analgesia in continuous injection dorsal epidural analgesia with 1.0% bupivacaine.*

Table 5.   *Quality of postoperative analgesia obtained with 1.0% bupivacaine*

	Time interval (hours)											
	4	8	12	16	20	24	28	32	36	40	44	48
M	2.1	1.9	1.9	1.9	2.1	2.2	2.0	2.3	2.3	3.0	2.0	2.4
SD	0.5	0.4	0.5	0.5	0.5	0.4	–	–	–	–	–	–
n	11	13	12	12	12	11	6	3	4	1	2	3

1=painfree at PEF, coughing and moving around in bed; 2=obvious but moderate pain-inhibition at PEF, coughing etc.; 3=PEF, coughing severely inhibited by pain/patient asks for supplementary pain medication.

Table 6.   *PEF postoperatively, in relation to control*

	Hours							
	Pre	0.5	2	4	8	12–16	20–24	48
M	100	31.4	46.2	53.6	53.3	44.6	60.3	55.2
SD	–	12.4	18.2	11.5	21.0	–	21.4	–
n	12	12	12	10	9	5	11	3

Table 7.   *Plasma concentrations of bupivacaine (µg/ml) at different intervals (in hr) after start of continuous injection dorsal epidural analgesia with 1.0% bupivacaine*

	Time interval (hours)							
	6	12	18	24	30	36	42	48
M	0.25	0.49	0.55	0.65	0.90	1.01	1.34	1.26
SD	0.13	0.32	0.33	0.39	0.57	0.54	0.70	0.73
n	14	13	13	13	6	6	5	5

DISCUSSION

Efficacy

In our experience only intermittent injections will provide complete freedom from pain postoperatively. The duration of complete analgesia is most often less than 3 hr. Unfortunately, no systematic evaluation of the duration was performed.

Continuous injection of bupivacaine leads to incomplete analgesia. Increments of the injection rates were followed by an increased spread but not by increased intensity of the blockade. With this technique major reductions of the patients' expiratory efforts were noticed and the PEF values did not significantly differ from those performed by unblocked postoperative patients.

Side-effects

Hypotension was seen chiefly after intermittent injections of the largest dose (5 ml) of etidocaine while it occurred briefly in only one of the patients given continuous injection. There was no apparent relation between the magnitude of the blood pressure drop and the number of segments blocked. Urinary retention occurred in 21, 20 and 50% of the patients given intermittent doses of 3, 4 and 5 ml respectively of etidocaine. During continuous injection dorsal epidural analgesia 62% of the patients sustained urinary retention. Orthostatic reactions limiting the mobilization of the patients occurred only exceptionally.

Tachyphylaxis

Tachyphylaxis was evident in most cases and resulted in a narrower segmental spread and consequently poorer quality of the blockade after intermittent doses and during continuous injection. In the Holmdahl et al. (1972) study there were no obvious signs of tachyphylaxis to lidocaine. Tachyphylaxis to long-acting agents in epidural analgesia has not been well-described.

Accumulation

Accumulation of bupivacaine and etidocaine was noticed regularly. The highest plasma levels were reached under continuous drip infusions. Consequently, too lengthy a prolongation of dorsal epidural analgesia can result in potentially toxic plasma concentrations.

CLINICAL IMPLICATIONS

According to our experience 24 hr of intermittent or continuous nerve blocking is sufficient for pain relief after upper abdominal surgery in routine cases. In patients with chronic obstructive lung disease considerably longer periods of treatment are necessary. Dorsal epidural analgesia with long-acting local anesthetic agents can provide adequate analgesia during sufficient time if prolonged by means of intermittent injections at less than 3-hr intervals. Continuous injection results in partial analgesia.

Both repeated injections and continuous injection lead to side-effects in the form of arterial hypotension and/or urinary retention which necessitate close supervision of the patients. Considering these side-effects, the tachyphylaxis which necessitates consecutive increments of the dosages and the danger of toxic reactions due to accumulation, post-operative pain-relief with continuous dorsal epidural analgesia using long-acting local anesthetic agents can be recommended provided that the patients are extremely closely supervised by personnel familiar with the method, preferably in a recovery or intensive care area. The regular occurrence of accumulation denotes a limit to the duration of the procedure. For general use, the method is not recommended. Intermittent intercostal blocks with these agents offer a safer and more reliable alternative in routine cases.

REFERENCES

Brandt, M. and Kvisselgaard, N. (1972): *Dan. med. Bull.*, *134*, 2378.
Dawkins, M. and Steel, G. C. (1971): *Anaesthesia*, *26*, 41.
Green, R. and Dawkins, M. (1966): *Anaesthesia*, *21*, 372.
Holmdahl, M. H:son, Sjögren, S., Ström, G. and Wright, B. (1972): *Uppsala J. med. Sci.*, *77*, 47.
Holmdahl, M. H:son and Renck, H. (1974): In: *Anesthésiques Locaux en Anesthésie et Réanimation (Anesthésies Loco-Régionales)*, p. 317. Editors: J. Montagne, G.-G. Nahas, J.-C. Salamagne, P. Viars and G. Vourc'h. Librairie Arnette, Paris.
Spence, A. A. and Smith, G. (1971): *Brit. J. Anaesth.*, *43*, 144.
Spoerel, W. E., Thomas, A. and Gerula, G. R. (1970): *Canad. Anaesth. Soc. J.*, *17*, 37.

Mathematical model of pain

SPERANTZA STRATULAT

Hospital No. 2, Jassy, Rumania

There is, at the present time, no objective test to determine the degree of pain which individuals can tolerate. In order to construct a mathematical model of the components of pain and anaesthesia it is essential to start from the basis of normal physiology. Many modifying factors have, therefore, to be ignored. This is the basis on which any mathematical model is applied to biological science when the quantitative aspects are to be studied.

Weber and Flechner's law states that the variation of sensation (S) produced by a physical stimulus is proportional to the difference between the intensity of the stimulus and the level of initial stimulus.

$S = ds$ sensation, is of the same value as pain

$Ds =$ measured subjectively

$E =$ excitability $= DE =$ variations of excitability measured objectively.

$$ds = K \frac{dE}{E}$$

In this study one individual is considered, without taking into consideration the variation of the stimulus.

In this way the general law of Weber and Flechner is applied:

$$(1) \quad dD = K \frac{dE}{E} = (2) \quad D = K \ln E + C \quad \text{where:}$$

$dD =$ the differential of pain

$K =$ individual constant which is calculated

$dE =$ the differential of excitability

$C =$ constant of integration.

The constant C results from integration of the equation where,

$E = 1$ and this is medium excitability (normal).

$D_0 = D$ (1) the corresponding pain is D_0

$D_0 = K \ln 1 + C$

$\ln 1 = 0$ substituting this into equation (1).

$D_0 = C$ we substitute this in equation (2).

$$(3) \quad D - D_0 = K \ln E$$

$$(3') \quad D = D_0 + K \ln E.$$

The pain sensation is defined by the relationship in equation (3') and the graphic representation of the D function is shown in Figure 1.

THE DEVIATION OF AN INDIVIDUAL CONSTANT (K)

If excitability $E = e$, then De, the corresponding sensation of pain under the same conditions, from (3')

$$De = D_0 + K \ln e \Rightarrow De = D_0 + K \text{ because:}$$
$$\ln e = 1$$
and thus:
$$(4)\ K = De - D_0$$
K is the difference between the corresponding sensation of pain at an excitability of the same value as e and the corresponding pain of an excitability equals 1.

Replacing (4) in equation (3′) results
$$(5)\ D = D_0 + (De - D_0) \ln E.$$

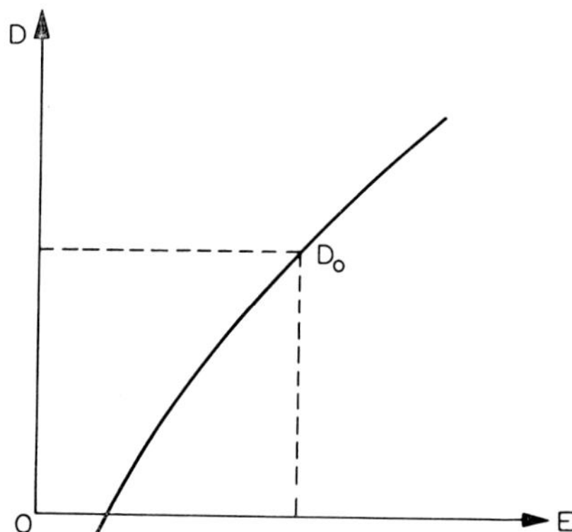

Fig. 1.   *Graphic representation of function D.*

This function can be represented graphically giving values to function E.

$$(6)\ Ep = e^{-\frac{D_0}{D_e - D_0}}$$

This E value (of E) we call threshold of sensation
$$D\,(Ep) = 0 \text{ (see Fig. 2).}$$
$$E = e$$
For studying the influence of anaesthetic upon pain sensation the same law of Weber and Flechner which is modified as follows:

$$(7)\ \frac{dD}{dt} = K \frac{1}{E} \frac{dE}{dt} - f\,(A)$$

$$\frac{dD}{dt} = \text{differential of painful sensation in comparison with time.}$$

f (A) = function of anaesthetic which tends to reduce dD, is a positive function and equals 0 when:
$$A = 0$$
$$(8)\ f\,(A) = 0, \text{ thus}$$
$$f\,(0) = 0$$
in the absence of an anaesthetic f(0) = 0. Equation (7) is reduced to equation (2). The mathematical model represented by differential equation (7) may have 3 interpretations:

1. Equation (7) is a differential equation for the determination of the anaesthetic function

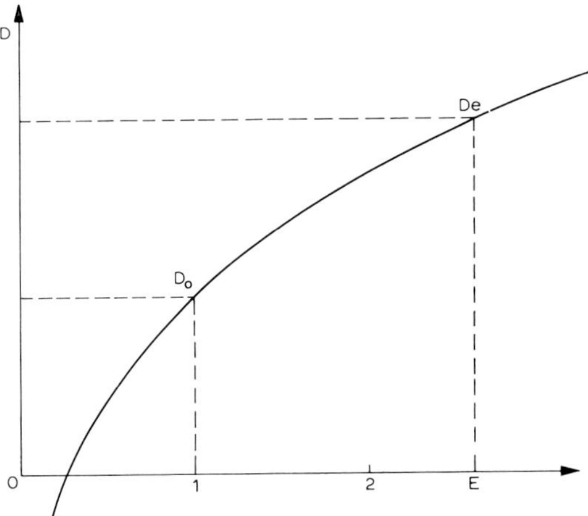

Fig. 2.   *Graphic representation giving values to function* $E = e^{-\dfrac{D_0}{D_e - D_0}}$

if we assume that the variation of excitability for the anaesthetic is known, that is $E = E\,(A)$ when a particular modification of pain sensation is required, for example:

1^0 $D = D_0\,e^{-f\,(A)}$.

The diminution of pain is exponential without ever attaining the *zero line*, but coming close to it,

2^0 $D = D_0 - k_1\,f\,(A)$.

The linear diminution of pain which rapidly approaches the zero line is necessary for surgical operations.

2. Knowing the function of anaesthetic, $f\,(A)$ and the variation of excitability in comparison with anaesthetic, $E = E\,(A)$, equation (7) shows the way in which the pain sensation is modified in relation to the anaesthetic action.

3. Equation (7) becomes a differential equation for the determination of the individual's excitability, if we propose as being known the function of anaesthetic $f\,(A)$ and the modification of pain sensation under anaesthesia, that is $D = D\,(A)$.

The problems which derive from the model have a mathematical solution and research continues.

The solution of these problems and their analysis by a computer will provide important data regarding the optimum method of administration of an anaesthetic in particular individuals.

REFERENCES

Laborit, H. (1967): *Agressologie, 8/2*, 93.
Rashevski, N. (1960): *Mathematical Biophysics Physico-Mathematical foundations of Biology.* Dover Publications, New York, N.Y.
Sato, K. (1969): *Kybernetik, 6/4*, 146.
Sato, K. (1971): *Kybernetik, 9/2*, 45.

The effect of naloxone on the depression of the early respiratory activity of neonates produced by maternal pethidine analgesia

J. M. EVANS, M. I. J. HOGG and M. ROSEN

Department of Anaesthetics, Welsh National School of Medicine, Cardiff, United Kingdom

Maternally administered pethidine has been associated with depression of respiratory activity in the neonate. Koch and Wendel (1968) have shown that in the first hours of life the arterial P_{CO_2} is higher in neonates born to mothers who have received pethidine than in those who have not. Naloxone is a narcotic antagonist which, in contrast to levallorphan and nalorphine, has no agonist activity and which it is believed could be safely given at birth to prevent the depressant effect of pethidine (Evans et al., 1974a, b).

METHOD

22 neonates, all of whose mothers had received pethidine analgesia during labour, were studied. Half of the neonates were given 40 μg of naloxone HCl into the umbilical vein one min after birth.

The time at which the first breath (TFB) was taken and the time to onset of sustained spontaneous ventilation (TSSV) were recorded together with the Apgar score at one and 5 min. At 10 and 30 min the respiratory rate, alveolar carbon dioxide concentration and alveolar ventilation were measured using infrared gas analysis techniques.

RESULTS

Table 1 shows the mean Apgar scores, TFB and TSSV for the naloxone treated group and the control group. Table 2 shows the mean respiratory rate, alveolar carbon dioxide concentration (given as $P_{A_{CO_2}}$) and alveolar ventilation (V_A) at 10 and 30 min.

Table 1. *Mean Apgar scores, TFB and TSSV for the naloxone treated group and the control group*

	Apgar score		TFB (sec)	TSSV (sec)
	1 min	5 min		
Naloxone group	8.99	9.91	45	73
Control group	7.55	9.64	32	85

At one and 5 min after birth there was no statistically significant difference between the Apgar score, TFB or TSSV of the 2 groups. This suggests that initially the general

Table 2. *Mean respiratory rate, alveolar carbon dioxide concentration (given as P_{ACO_2}) and alveolar ventilation ($\dot{V}_A$) at 10 and 30 min*

		Respiratory rate (per min)	P_{ACO_2} (mm Hg)	$\dot{V}_A$ (BTPS) (ml/min/kg)
Naloxone group	10 min	40.0	42.5	125
	30 min	45.1	39.0	123
Control group	10 min	38.1	48.3	123
	30 min	36.7	46.3	111

condition of the neonates in the 2 groups was similar. Ten minutes after birth the respiratory rate and alveolar ventilation were similar in the 2 groups; the mean value of P_{ACO_2}, however, was 5.8 mm Hg lower in the treated group than in the untreated group. At 30 min the P_{ACO_2} had fallen in both groups but the difference between the 2 groups had increased to 7.2 mm Hg. The fall in P_{ACO_2} between 10 and 30 min in the treated group was statistically significant ($P < 0.001$) as was the difference in P_{ACO_2} between the 2 groups at 30 min ($P < 0.05$). The changes in alveolar ventilation were less marked but a trend towards higher values in the treated group was evident.

CONCLUSION

The effect of naloxone upon the early respiratory depressant effect of pethidine is evident; the group treated with naloxone had a lower P_{ACO_2}. It seems probable that more extensive investigation will confirm the value of naloxone in preventing respiratory depression from pethidine shortly after birth.

REFERENCES

Koch, G. and Wendel, H. (1968): *Acta obstet. gynec. scand.*, *47*, 27.
Evans, J. M., Hogg, M. I. J., Lunn, J. N. and Rosen, M. (1974a): *Brit. med. J.*, *2*, 589.
Evans, J. M., Hogg, M. I. J., Lunn, J. N. and Rosen, M. (1974b): *Anaesthesia*, *29*, 721.

Chapter III

New agents in intravenous anaesthesia

Classification of intravenous anaesthetics

J. W. DUNDEE

Department of Anaesthetics, Queen's University of Belfast,
Institute of Clinical Science, Belfast, United Kingdom

The terms 'ultra-short' and 'short' acting are applied indiscriminately to many intravenous anaesthetics and are not only confusing, but may be misleading and have serious consequences for those not aware of the pharmacology of the drugs. These should be reserved for drugs which are rapidly broken down in the body and from which full recovery occurs without redistribution to non-nervous tissues. On this criticism the only applicable drugs are:

Ultra-short acting	– propanidid (Epontol, Fabontal)
Short acting	– Althesin (Alfatésine, CT-1341)

Return of consciousness with the barbiturates occurs with a large amount of active drug in the body and there is a tendency for patients to lapse back to sleep, and drugs given in the early postoperative period can lead to re-induction of anaesthesia.

It is desirable for induction agents to be rapid acting and cause sleep in one arm brain-circulation time, so that dosage can be titrated against the patients' requirements. Other drugs with a slower onset are essentially basal hypnotics which should be used when specifically indicated because of their unique properties.

Rapidly acting
Induction agents

– thiobarbiturates, methybarbiturates
– eugenols
– new steroid (Althesin)

Slower acting
Basal hypnotics

– phencyclidines (ketamine)
– tranquillisers (diazepam)
– neuroleptic drug combinations
– others: gamma OH, hydroxydione, Chlormethiazole (Heminevrine)

Thus a meaningful classification embraces both the rate of onset and duration of action of drugs.

Finally, the intravenous barbiturate anaesthetics can be classified;
a. according to their chemistry:

Thiobarbiturates

– thiopentone, thiamylal, thiobutobarbitone
buthalitone, methitural, thialbarbitone

Methybarbiturates

– hexobarbitone, methohexitone, Narkotal (enibomal);

"

b. according to their clinical acceptability:
Very satisfactory
Equally acceptable   – thiopentone, thiamylal, Inactin, thialbarbitone

Unsatisfactory
Too high an incidence
of side effects   – buthalitone, methitural, hexobarbitone

Compromise
Between side effects
and unique advantages – methohexitone, Narkotal.

The disadvantages of the barbiturates as induction agents

D. W. BARRON

Belfast City Hospital, Belfast, United Kingdom

Almost exactly half a century has elapsed since the introduction of the first intravenous barbiturate; and it is fitting that the compounds which are comprised within this group should be examined critically in order to establish their place in modern anaesthesia.

While it is true that thiopentone is still the most commonly used induction agent in the British Isles, it must be admitted that it owes much of its popularity to the fact that anaesthetists have been familiar with its characteristics for several decades. Attempts to oust it from its favoured position have, until recently, been singularly unsuccessful, only methohexitone, a shorter acting member of the same group, being able to achieve some degree of acceptance as an alternative.

With certain exceptions such as Narcodorm, barbiturates are issued in powder form and have to be dissolved in water to form solutions, which are generally unstable and must be used within a few hours. A notable exception is the solution of methohexitone which remains stable for about 6 weeks.

Cumulative effects vary from compound to compound and are generally observed when a second injection is administered within 30 hours of the first, the prolongation of narcosis being particularly marked when the time interval is less than 6 hours. These drugs are almost completely metabolised, the liver being the principal site of detoxication. The rate at which this occurs depends on such variables as dosage, chemical structure, various pathological processes, etc.

Much has been written about the convulsant properties of this group and their relationship with such factors as the chemical structure of various side chains. Tremors and spontaneous involuntary muscle movements occur with a frequency which varies from drug to drug and the incidence of such movements is related to dosage, the nature of the drugs used in preanaesthetic medication and the rate of administration as shown by Barron (1964). Respiratory side effects such as coughing, hiccoughing and laryngospasm may also be a feature of anaesthesia with some members of this group.

The barbiturates cause myocardial depression leading to hypotension of varying degrees, the more potent members such as methohexitone causing less than the weaker such as hexobarbitone, while thiopentone occupies an intermediate position. This property is not a disadvantage where deliberate hypotensive anaesthesia is required and the response can be modified by such factors as the nature of the premedicants, dosage, posture, rate of injection and preoperative blood pressure levels. Cardiac irregularities, which have been reported, have usually been associated with mild hypoxia and hypercarbia as a result of depression of the respiratory centre.

Barbiturates pass rapidly across the placental barrier, equilibrium between mother and foetus being established within 5 minutes. This aspect has been extensively investigated by many workers such as Crawford and Rudofsky (1965) and requires no elaboration here.

The effects of these compounds on the liver and kidneys are also well known. Hepatic dysfunction can occur and there is evidence that the degree is directly related to the dosage employed. There is depression of urinary excretion but factors other than the induction agent, such as renal blood flow and antidiuretic hormone excretion have to be taken into consideration.

Body metabolism is altered by these agents. There is usually some degree of hyperglycaemia, reduced oxygen consumption in brain, liver and kidney, reduced liver glycogen and alterations in both carbohydrate and protein katabolism. The effects of barbiturate anaesthesia on patients suffering from such conditions as porphyria and dystrophia myotonia have been well documented.

Intravenous injection of these drugs leads to haemolysis and thrombophlebitis or venous thrombosis can occur. Extra venous injection may produce tissue necrosis while the effects of intra-arterial thiopentone may be the cause of nightmares in the tyro anaesthetist.

One of the great disadvantages of the barbiturates is their ability to neutralise the effects of analgesics. This so-called ant-analgesic action, elaborated by Dundee (1960) and Clutton-Brock (1960) is now a well recognised phenomenon producing postoperative restlessness and the need for early administration of strong analgesic drugs.

In circumstances where rapid recovery from anaesthesia is required, as in out-patient or domiciliary dental surgery, the barbiturates compare unfavourably with some other intravenous induction agents. Doenicke et al. (1966) have demonstrated by means of electroencephalography that these agents are not short acting in the true sense of the term and that their actions are potentiated by small amounts of alcohol for a period of up to 24 hours.

I have tried, in the brief time at my disposal, to outline some of the characteristics of this group of drugs and to draw attention to their disadvantages in certain situations. With such a wide variety of agents now available it should be possible for anaesthetists to select the best drug for a particular set of circumstances.

REFERENCES

Barron, D. W. (1964): *Int. Anaesth. Clin.*, *2/4*, 743.
Clutton-Brock, J. (1960): *Anaesthesia*, *15*, 71.
Crawford, J. S. and Rudofsky, S. (1965): *Brit. J. Anaesth.*, *37*, 303.
Doenicke, A., Kugler, F., Schellenberger, A. and Gurtner, Th. (1966): *Brit. J. Anaesth.*, *38*, 580.
Dundee, J. W. (1960): *Brit. J. Anaesth.*, *32*, 407.
Additional reading
Dundee, J. W. (1956): *Thiopentone and Other Thiobarbiturates*. E. and S. Livingstone, Ltd., Edinburgh–London.

Ketamine: Special indications and controversial aspects

D. LANGREHR, R. NEUHAUS and G. SINGBARTL

Department of Anesthesiology, Central Hospital Bremen-North, Bremen,
Federal Republic of Germany

Ketamine, introduced by Chen, Domino and Corssen, is a potent analgesic-cataleptic substance. It is used both intravenously and intramuscularly. The cardiovascular sytem is stimulated. The protective reflexes are better sustained than with other intravenous substances. There is adequate spontaneous ventilation when ketamine is used as a sole anesthetic and if, for special reasons, spontaneous ventilation is at all desirable. The therapeutic range is broad-expressed as the ratio of undesirable effects dose (UED) to anesthetic threshold dose (ATD) (McCarthy).

GENERAL USE

The pharmacological effects are well known and there are more than 500 publications about the drug. From clinical experience of ketamine the following are indications for this drug:

1. Brief ophthalmological and otological procedures lasting less than 30 min, emergency facial surgery, skin grafting for burns, immediate emergency surgery following accidents, septic surgery in the diabetic patient, especially in children, old patients and poor-risk patients.

2. Diagnostic procedures such as bronchoscopy, bronchography, other endoscopic procedures, pneumoencephalography, cardioangiography and so on. This applies especially in children and in the aged in difficult environmental and postural situations from the viewpoint of anesthesiology.

3. Induction of balanced anesthesia of longer duration. Drug interactions between ketamine and the routinely used intravenous or inhalation anesthetics have not yet been described.

Table 1 shows the overall statistics for the type of use in our personal experience with 15,000 cases, including 1,750 cases of ASA risk Groups III, IV and V. The application as a sole anesthetic concerns about 20%. In the majority of cases ketamine was used for induction, where the advantageous effects are evident, while the undesirable side-effects, such as psychomimetic emergence reactions or long-lasting recovery, are minimized.

For this short review we would like to consider some controversial aspects.

OBSTETRICS

There has been a growing interest in the use of ketamine in obstetrics. Despite rapid placental transmission, depression of the newborn is almost negligible, as could be anticipated from

Table 1. *Use of ketamine as a sole anesthetic or in combination*

Type of intervention		Ketamine (sole)	Ketamine +relaxant +O₂	Ketamine induction N₂O : O₂ : fluothane
Minor surgery, ophthalmology	1980	1290	–	690
Minor gynecological surgery	670	32	–	638
Endoscopy, neuro-radiology	2021	82	1757	182
Obstetrics	770	59		711
Induction for major surgery	9559	–	–	9559
ASA risk groups III, IV, V	Σ	1463	1757	11,780
	Σ	3220 (21.5%)		
1750 cases	←Σ	15,000		

the main effects of the drug. Three hundred patients undergoing spontaneous delivery received 0.8–3 mg/kg ketamine 1–6 min before clamping of the cord. This resulted in a mean Apgar score for the neonates of 9.7 at 1 min, while in 1,000 spontaneous deliveries without any anesthesia the mean score was found to be 9.67 in our cases.

Postpartal uterine contractility is excellent and the blood loss is within the normal range. Tocometric recordings show that the antepartum uterine contractions after ketamine are not depressed. A slight increase in the product of frequency and amplitude (Montevideo units) occurs in cases of dystocia of the cervix (Dick et al.).

Ketamine is not normally suitable for spontaneous delivery because of its long-lasting after-effects but it has a remarkable advantage in cases of obstetric surgery.

The distribution of the use of ketamine in 770 deliveries is given in Figure 1. Our present

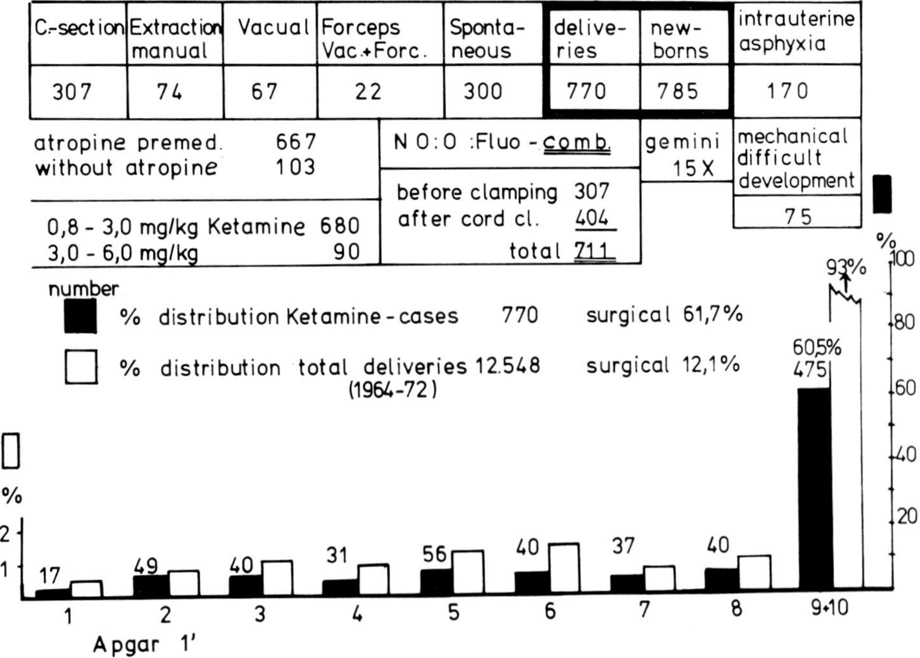

Fig. 1. *Ketamine in obstetrics. Overall statistics of author's material.*

practice is to use the lower dosage (0.8–1.5 mg/kg) and to go on with a combination inhalation anesthesia after the cord has been clamped (404 cases). For cesarean section we use ketamine as the induction agent immediately followed by 50% $N_2O:O_2$ and less than 0.5 Vol% halothane before and after cord clamping (307 cases). Ketamine induction for similar anesthetic procedures also results in neonates in good condition compared to those following barbiturate induction of anesthesia.

The distribution of lower Apgar scores at 1 min in the ketamine group (black columns) shows approximately the same relative percentage of depressed newborns, or even lower, as in the total number of deliveries (white columns), although the part of obstetric emergency surgery (61.7%) is much higher in the ketamine group.

In the case of emergency cesarean section with increased uterine activity and need for immediate tocolysis, ketamine should be used only in combination with halothane which is the most efficient tocolytic drug in obstetric anesthesia. It acts more rapidly and is more suitable for the special circumstances than any other intravenous tocolytic drug.

POOR-RISK PATIENTS

In our experience the poor-risk patient and the cardiovascular poor-risk patient are true indications for ketamine and in this we are in agreement with a number of other investigators.

The main criticism of this indication arose from the cardiostimulatory effects resulting in increased myocardial work (about 30–40% as a maximum) and increased oxygen consumption in patients with relative or absolute coronary insufficiency.

These patients present problems for anesthetists, and our personal opinion is that a familiar anesthesiological technique is more important in poor-risk anesthesia than the choice of drugs.

In animal or isolated organ experiments it has been found by several investigators that:

1. Myocardial contractility is not depressed by dosages equivalent to clinical dosage up to 8–10 mg/kg ketamine i.v. Figure 2 shows, on the left, the known human serum levels, in the middle the homogeneous tissue distribution, making the derivation of myocardial concentration from serum levels possible and, on the right, the finding of dose-related myocardial depression. Increased myocardial depression was found when ketamine was added i.v. to steady state $N_2O:O_2$:halothane anesthesia in the same low range as with ketamine alone, i.e. about 10% depression by 2 mg/kg (Singbartl et al., in press). Considering the fact that in poor-risk or shock patients the dose of ketamine is normally reduced to about 0.5–0.8 mg/kg, the therapeutic ratio remains in the same range as for patients with normal myocardial function at a normal induction dose of 1.0–1.5 mg/kg.

2. The increase in cardiac work after ketamine is accompanied by adequate coronary perfusion; the increased myocardial oxygen consumption is therefore supported. The oxygen utilisation is undisturbed (Spieckermann) and the cardiostimulatory effect of the drug is only effective if ketamine is used as a sole anesthetic and if the myocardium is capable of performing the increased work. No increase in blood pressure, heart rate and cardiac index was found after ketamine, when it was given in addition to a steady state inhalation anesthesia, or after diazepam (Singbartl et al., unpublished data). This applies also to patients in cardiac failure and in the aged patient.

3. Brückner et al. concluded from extreme animal shock experiments that ketamine as a single anesthetic was not satisfactory compared with NLA or morphine-like drugs and $N_2O:O_2$. However, when low-dose ketamine was used in combination (with N_2O or phenoxybenzamine) in the same shock model, these investigators found ketamine to be the best agent in treating cardiac insufficiency, following prolonged hemorrhagic shock. Obviously, this use of ketamine is comparable to clinical technique.

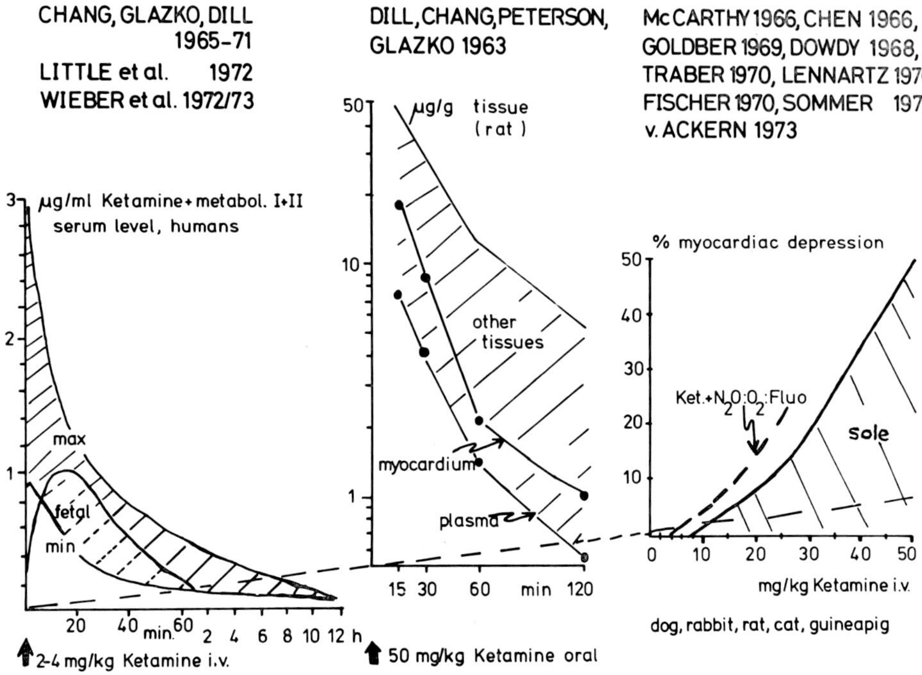

Fig. 2.   *Human serum levels (left), tissue distribution (middle) and myocardial depression (right) after ketamine.*

4. Catecholamine liberation is not believed to be the cause of the cardiostimulatory effect of ketamine. Many experiments including those with adrenergic receptor blocking have shown the importance of sympathetic pathways. However, the exact point of action: central nervous system, ganglionic transmission, nervous and organ catecholamine liberation or membrane receptor interaction, is unknown. Chen emphasized the increase of central nervous sympathetic efferents. However, Montel et al. concluded from isolated organ experiments that ketamine affects the excitable membranes directly in a cocaine-like manner, i.e. the susceptibility of pharmacoreceptors is increased by slowing down the otherwise rapid metabolism and redistribution of endogenous adrenaline from sympathetic nerve terminals.

To evaluate these findings, one should consider the following: The dosage used to obtain these effects was somewhat high on the one hand, i.e. equivalent to clinical i.v. dosage of 10–70 mg/kg. After findings of Ivankovic et al. (1974) centrally administered ketamine to the unanesthetized goat on the other hand caused cardiostimulatory effects 5–7 sec after administration into the temporal artery. This is much sooner than the substance can reach peripheral membranes. Therefore, it is concluded that the cardiostimulatory effects of ketamine are, at least in part, due to a stimulatory effect on the central nervous system.

The complete picture of the cardiovascular effects of ketamine does not support the opinion that ketamine is contraindicated in cardiovascular poor-risk patients. In contrast we advise the use of ketamine, after critical evaluation of the patient with reduced dosage and high inspired O_2, assisted or controlled ventilation in combination with other agents, and careful monitoring for these severely ill patients. In our opinion, ketamine offers several advantages without being miraculous.

NEUROPHYSIOLOGY

Based on neurophysiological findings with various agents, Winters et al. (1964) proposed a multidirectional scheme of progression of the stages of CNS excitation to replace the unidirectional scheme of Guedel (1937). This scheme is given in Figure 3. It is stated that several anesthetics and CNS excitants induce an initial excitation (Stage I), characterized by increased motor activity. Some anesthetics then induce surgical anesthesia (Stage III), characterized by a loss of responsiveness to stimuli and CNS depression. Other anesthetics induce Stage II prior to Stage III. Stage II is characterized by hallucinatory (A, B), then cataleptoid (C) behavior, while the subject is likewise relatively unresponsive to stimuli and without memory. Many anesthetics do not induce Stage III following Stage II, but either induce only Stage II or progress to higher levels of CNS excitation, i.e. myoclonic jerking followed by generalized seizures. All these stages show characteristic patterns of EEG.

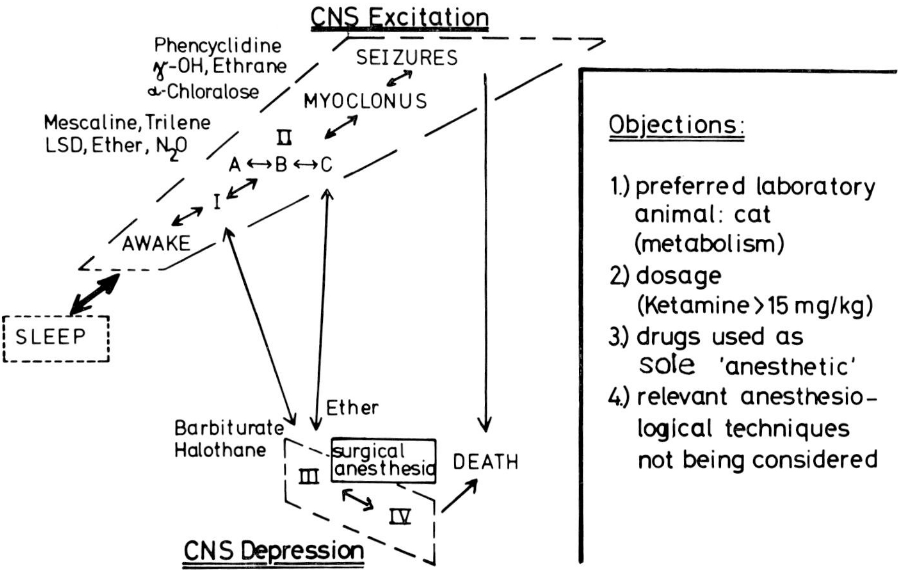

Fig. 3. *Winters' schema of 'multidirectional progression of stages of CNS excitation'. Objections as far as ketamine is concerned.*

As a matter of fact, this scheme seems to cover drug effects observed with the anesthetic agents in present-day use better than the Guedel scheme, which was poorly based on neurophysiological findings.

However, with regard to ketamine there are some objections: (1) The animal preferred here was the cat; however, its metabolism differs from humans (Glazko); (2) since more than 15 mg/kg of ketamine was used, leading to the relevant excitation, this was a serious dose; (3) all the drugs were used as sole anesthetics with subsequently increased dosages; (4) clinically relevant anesthesiological techniques are not considered.

In other words, from the basic pharmacological viewpoint of drug effects the Winters' schema may be of relevance. However, in reality using combinations of drugs, normally Stage III should be reached and levels of higher excitation are always avoided. The classification of most of anesthetics (for instance N₂O) as 'purely hallucinatory and epileptoid agents' seems to be hypothetical.

Ketamine added to 1% enflurane and 50% N₂O:O₂ steady state anesthesia alters the EEG hypersynchronisation pattern in the same direction as 3% enflurane. On the other hand, as shown in Figure 4, after 1 mg/kg ketamine induction the typical 'ketamine induced periodic patterns' precede (higher voltage groups superimposed to ϑ-waves) (B) the normal unaltered development of Ethrane hypersynchronisation (C, D) with rapid reversibility, when the dosage is lowered to 1% (E).

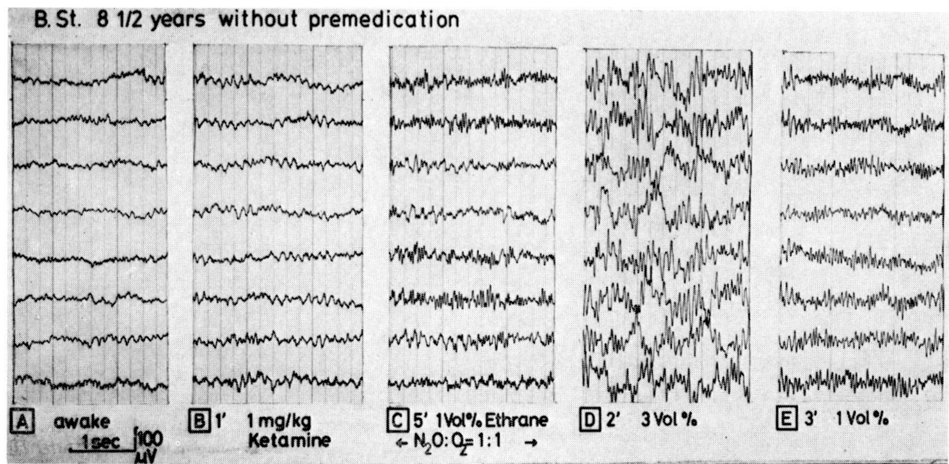

Fig. 4.   *EEG tracings after ketamine induction for N₂O : O₂ : Ethrane anesthesia.*

This is a demonstration of the fact that the effect of anesthetic drug combinations, as normally used in clinical anesthesiology, do not fit well in the Winters' schema.

With regard to the question whether ketamine should be used in subjects with developing cerebral structures (young children, newborns in obstetrics) our own experience, the work of Corssen (20 epileptic volunteers, ketamine as a sole anesthetic, San Francisco, 1974) and the personality evaluation studies (Wilson, Albin and Dressner), show that at this time there is no objection to the use of ketamine in this group of patients, provided the usual and recommended dosages are given and adequate technique is used.

REFERENCES

Available on request from the author.

Alfatesin: Animal pharmacology in relation to clinical anaesthesia

J. A. SUTTON

Medical Department, Glaxo Laboratories Ltd., Greenford, Middlesex, United Kingdom

In this paper I intend to describe results from pharmacological experiments that were done with Alfatesin steroids, the reasons for doing those experiments, and the way in which the human clinical results compare with the pharmacological findings.

Hydroxydione was the starting point since it provided remarkably good quality of recovery and so few side effects that many considered it to be the anaesthetic choice for the elderly and the infirm (Galley and Rooms, 1956; Robertson and Wynn-Williams, 1961). However, it was not an ideal induction agent because the onset of anaesthesia was delayed and the rather alkaline solution was irritant to veins (Robertson, 1963). Tests of Alfatesin in animals soon showed that it produced immediate anaesthesia. Moreover it proved possible to dissolve the two steroids, alphaxalone and alphadolone acetate, in solutions of neutral pH which were remarkably non-irritant (Fig. 1). When it appeared that such solutions could be made concentrated enough to provide conveniently small dose-volumes in animals, a series of experiments was begun. The solution was initially known as CT-1341 but it is now called Althesin in Britain and Alfatesin elsewhere.

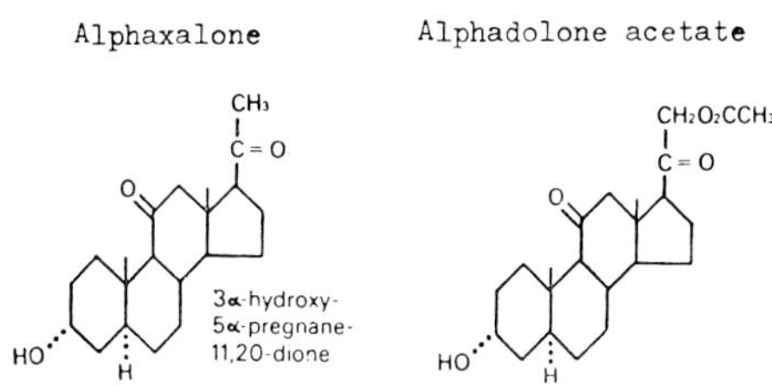

Induction immediate
Potency high
Safety margin high
Thrombophlebitis absent
Insoluble in water
Soluble in Cremophor EL

Potentiates Cremophor
solubility of alphaxalone
Activity similar to alphaxalone
Half as potent as alphaxalone
Additive with alphaxalone

Fig. 1. *The components of Alfatesin.*

LOCAL IRRITANT EFFECT

Alfatesin was injected into the central artery of rabbits' ears and the effects were compared with those of similar injections of 2.5% and 5% thiopentone. Child et al. (1971) reported the following: 'Deliberate intra-arterial injection of CT-1341 into the centre artery of the rabbit ear during occlusion of the marginal ear veins, produced no macroscopic arterial damage whereas similar injections of thiopentone sodium (5%) produced oedema and necrosis . . . . . Thiopentone sodium (2.5%) produced less severe damage which gradually resolved on successive days. No necrotic areas were seen in the ears of rabbits which received CT-1341 and histologically there was no haemorrhage, oedema or arterial damage.' Intravenous injection in animals produced no signs of venous or tissue damage. This work had a clinical parallel in the findings of Carson et al. (1972) who showed that the total amount of venous sequelae with Alfatesin was less than after propanidid, thiopentone 5% and methohexitone 2%. There was no significant difference between Alfatesin and barbiturates at half these concentrations so it is possible that there is a certain minimal incidence of local thrombosis, phlebitis and more extensive thrombophlebitis involved in venepuncture (e.g. Briscoe and Taylor, 1974).

CARDIORESPIRATORY EFFECTS

In animals, respiratory depression was slight compared with other intravenous anaesthetics. Child et al. (1972a) reported that CT-1341 produced the least respiratory depression of the anaesthetics examined and that in 3 of 7 cats respiration became shallow, irregular or slow for a few minutes after induction with the maximum dose (1.6 ml/kg). Considerably greater respiratory depression was seen after all doses of thiopentone, methohexitone and pentobarbitone. Brief hyperventilation, also common clinically, was seen in cats given propanidid (8–32 mg/kg).

This result with CT-1341 has something of a clinical counterpart in the report of Morgan et al. (1973) who showed no significant increase in apnoea when doubling the dose in man from 0.05–0.1 ml/kg. However, it appears that in humans the majority exhibit apnoea of brief duration.

Tomlin (1972) gave a large dose (8 ml) to a 61-year-old female patient and reported that after a very short period of apnoea ventilation returned, albeit slightly depressed, but over the next 3 min there was 'a rapid return towards control values and the slope of the (spirometer) graph shows that half a litre of lung volume had been restored in 3 min and oxygen uptake rapidly returned to pre-induction levels'. In the 30 patients studied he found no change in airway resistance or lung compliance. Some contradictory evidence that Alfatesin does produce considerable apnoea has come from France and was reported by Jones et al. (1972) from London. However, this appears to have been associated with diazepam premedication and possibly, as in combination with other intravenous anaesthetics, this premedication produces more apnoea than otherwise expected.

Cardiocirculatory depression was likewise conspicuous by its transient nature in cats. Child et al. (1972a) showed that CT-1341 0.4 and 1.6 ml/kg produced on average a 20% fall of blood pressure in conscious, unrestrained cats. This is similar to that reported in man at lower doses (Savege et al., 1971, 1972) and has proved to be similar to the hypotensive effect of thiopentone and methohexitone. Thus it appears that man is more susceptible to Alfatesin than animals in both anaesthetic and unwanted effects.

None of this work predicted more serious cardiovascular depression or sudden, severe alterations of respiration such as bronchospasm. Several of these have now been reported (e.g.: Avery and Evans, 1973; Hester, 1973; Notcutt, 1973; Dundee et al., 1974a) but the available evidence indicates that no intravenous anaesthetic is immune from such complications (Dundee et al., 1974; Clarke et al., 1975) and that they are more frequent after some established drugs such as penicillin (Goodman and Gillman, 1970) and propanidid (Kay, 1972).

Changes in cardiac rhythm or ECG were not observed in animals, and Dodds and Twissell (1972) showed that the dysrhythmic threshold to adrenaline in the presence of halothane was raised by CT-1341. They showed a marked protective effect against adrenaline induced dysrhythmias when infusions of Alfatesin were used instead of halothane anaesthesia or even thiopentone infusions. This has a clinical parallel in dental anaesthesia where dysrhythmias have been found to be associated with halothane (Thurlow, 1972; Ryder, 1970) but not found when Alfatesin has been used (Warren, 1972; Rollason et al., 1974). In fact, an *anti*dysrhythmic effect is reported by Cundy (1973) where Alfatesin abolished a dysrhythmia resistant to methohexitone. However, other intravenous anaesthetics are known to have similar properties and Alfatesin may not differ from other intravenous agents in this respect.

THERAPEUTIC RATIO

Child et al. (1971) found that the therapeutic ratio of CT-1341 in mice was about 4 times greater than that of barbiturates, ketamine and propanidid (Table 1). This has been borne out by several clinical studies in which many times a minimal induction dose has been given without irreversible sequelae or, indeed, undue prolongation of anaesthesia. For example, Takahashi (1972) gave 104 ml to a 65 kg man in 5.75 hr when he repeated a fairly large induction dose 16 times at 20 min intervals. Simpson and his colleagues at the London Hospital have infused several litres of Alfatesin into patients in intensive care when using slow infusions to provide continuous sedation (Ramsay et al., 1974). In the first reported study in obstetrics, Downing et al. (1973) gave up to 17 ml of Alfatesin to mothers having either elective or emergency caesarian section and this was enough to depress foetal respiration to the extent that intubation was necessary in 4 out of 31 patients. This must all be compared with the fact that a generous induction dose is 5 ml, so the 17 ml given during the 10 min induction delivery interval is more than 4-times the usual induction dose (0.5 ml/10 kg body weight). It is encouraging that such a relatively large dose may be given without permanent, serious sequelae, though this still does not mean that unnecessarily large doses may ever be justified, nor will they improve the conditions of induction and recovery.

Table 1. *Anaesthetic and lethal doses of CT-1341 and some other anaesthetics by the intravenous route in male CD* mice*

Anaesthetic agent	AD_{50} (mg/kg)	LD_{50} (mg/kg)	Therapeutic index (LD_{50}/AD_{50})
CT-1341	1.79	54.7	30.6
Hydroxydione	18.0	311.0	17.3
Thiopentone sodium	13.2	90.5	6.9
Methohexitone sodium	5.35	39.4	7.4
Propanidid	22.9	184.7	8.1
Ketamine hydrochloride	12.7	108.3	8.5

* Charles River CD 1 strain.

CUMULATION

The safe use of large amounts by increments or infusions depends upon both the therapeutic ratio and the lack of cumulation. Davis and Pearce (1972) showed how little Alfatesin accumulates in mice when they compared the duration of loss of righting reflexes in groups of 5 mice given equal, repeat doses of anaesthetics. As each animal recovered its balance, they repeated the anaesthetic up to 10 times. Thiopentone was so cumulative that a dose which initially lasted 5.7 min (40 mg/kg) lasted 101 min on the 3rd occasion. Methohexitone

(28 mg/kg) increased from 4.9–10.4 min by the 3rd dose (112% increase) and to 17.3 min duration at the 10th dose (249% increase). On the other hand, Alfatesin (1 ml/kg) increased from 6.5 min duration initially to 8.1 min at the 3rd dose (25% increase) and to 9.9 min at the 10th dose (52% increase). Their results are summarised in Figure 2 and this shows that the steroid and eugenol anaesthetics accumulate very little, that methohexitone and ketamine are moderately cumulative and thiopentone is most cumulative.

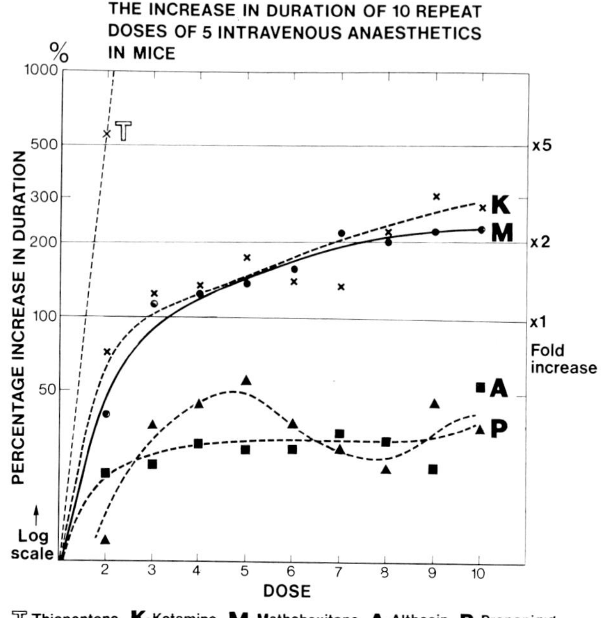

Fig. 2.   *The increase of duration following 10 equal doses of 5 intravenous anaesthetics given to mice immediately they regained their righting reflexes. (After Davis and Pearce, 1972.)*

This has been translated into clinical terms by obtaining prolonged anaesthesia by increments or infusions. The London Hospital use of infusions for sedation (Ramsay et al., 1974) is interesting in this respect for several reasons: firstly, the sedation has lasted 2–3 weeks in some patients and secondly, because the level of sedation was closely monitored, the system was sensitive enough to discern any cumulation or tolerance that might have developed. That the rates of infusion required remained constant for up to 3 weeks was testimony to the lack of cumulation and, incidentally, to the lack of induction of metabolising enzymes.

Although propanidid appears to be equally non-cumulative, its duration is so short that maintenance of anaesthesia requires too frequent increments or too fast infusions for convenience. In addition, it is rather more irritant to veins and tissues than Alfatesin (Carson et al., 1972).

METABOLISM

The lack of cumulation appears to be due to rapid inactivation of Alfatesin steroids by the liver. It would appear that both steroids and eugenols are molecules for which the liver has a large reserve of metabolic enzymes, possibly because such enzymes are constantly in use to assimilate normal food. Steroids are present in much plant tissue as well as meat, and eugenols include oil of cloves, so there is no contrary evidence against this speculation. Barbiturates, on the other hand, are not normal constituents of the diet and the enzyme inducing effects of repeat doses of phenobarbitone, for example, are well known. Brandt et al. (1963) demonstrated that the relatively short duration of barbiturate anaesthetics is due to redistribution in the tissues. Their plasma level decay curves showed that the biotransformation (metabolism) of thiopentone is 15%/hr and they say it is 'quite slow' for methohexitone at 15–19%/hr. When tissues are saturated repeat amounts no longer leave the blood so rapidly and prolongation of effect with higher blood levels results.

With this in mind, pharmacologists at Glaxo injected carbon-14 labelled alphaxalone into rats and then, by autoradiography, investigated the distribution of the anaesthetic at different times postinduction (Card et al., 1972). Figure 3 shows this 10 min post-injection, when the rat was regaining consciousness. The head of the animal is to the left, the eye area being evident near the upper, dorsal surface. The liver is the large, granular dark area in the centre of the rat, its convex, diaphragmatic surface to the left. The rounded, densely black areas are cross-sections of small intestine containing labelled metabolites.

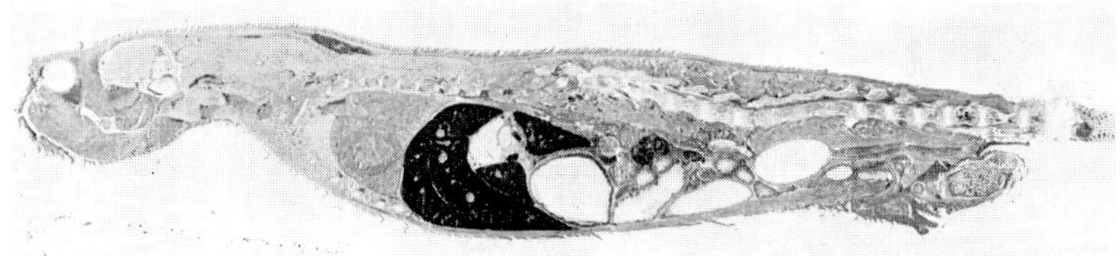

Fig. 3.   *The distribution of radioactive (^{14}C) labelled alphaxalone 10 min after injection into a male rat.*

In serial autoradiographs the radioactivity collects in the liver from the first minute onwards and then passes through the bile ducts, where it becomes very concentrated, out into the gut by 10 min. At one hour, little radioactivity is left in the liver and it has passed down to the lower small intestine.

In these rats the main metabolite in bile has been identified by Child et al. (1972b) as the 2α-hydroxylated derivative of alphaxalone and this has no anaesthetic activity (Phillipps, 1974). The important point to note in Figure 3 is that redistribution to other tissues, in particular fat, is virtually absent and there is almost no radioactivity in the brain at all.

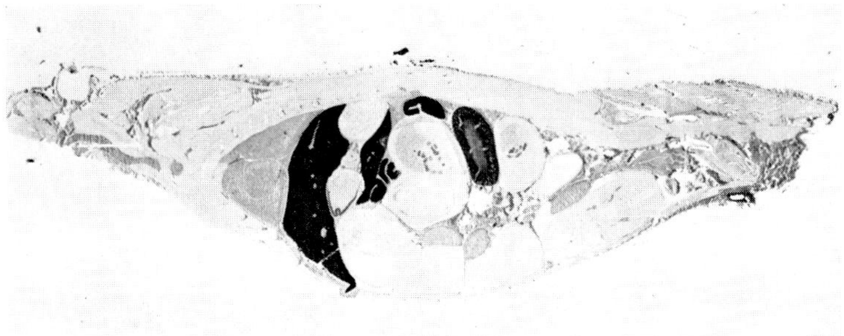

Fig. 4.   *The distribution of radioactive (^{14}C) labelled alphaxalone 10 min after injection into a pregnant rat.*

The rapid uptake by the liver indicates a short half-life for levels in the blood and this has recently been confirmed in man by Strunin and his colleagues at King's College Hospital (Strunin et al., 1974). They report some of their findings at this meeting. Thus, autoradiography has confirmed the absence of significant redistribution in animals and this correlates well with recovery times in man from repeat doses and infusions.

Additional autoradiographs were made from pregnant rats in order to see how much labelled steroid would cross the placenta. Card et al. (1972) showed that small amounts crossed the rat placenta and that the metabolites were to be found in the lumen of the foetal gut within 10 min (Fig. 4). This indicates that the foetus can metabolise Alfatesin, which is perhaps not surprising since the foetus encounters considerable amounts of steroids in utero, and it contrasts with barbiturates, since the foetal liver will not be exposed to barbiturates. Some clinical confirmation of this somewhat theoretical approach is beginning to appear in that early Apgar scores in newborns seem to be lower than in comparable cases given thiopentone (Carson, 1974).

In summary, it appears that most of the clinical characteristics of Althesin were apparent in animals. As in animals it is the most potent of all intravenous anaesthetics, of rapid onset, non-irritant and compatible with all other likely combinations of anaesthetic or medical drugs. The exceptions were that slightly greater depression of respiration has occurred in man than in animals and man requires lower doses. However, since the dose decreases as the phylogenetic scale of the animals is ascended, this latter effect was predicted. The sleep time in both man and animals proved to be similar to thiopentone and longer than methohexitone. The rapid inactivation has been discovered to provide better quality of recovery clinically (Clarke et al., 1971) and greater facility for repeat doses or infusions. The general lack of toxicity of steroids, shown by the high therapeutic ratios in animals, appears to be reflected in the high doses that are tolerated in such techniques without any apparent ill effect. It would seem therefore that the pharmacological testing of new anaesthetics can provide useful comparisons between anaesthetics for extrapolation into man.

ACKNOWLEDGEMENTS

I am grateful for assistance with the manuscript to Mr. B. Davies of Glaxo Research, and to the Editor of the *Postgraduate Medical Journal* for Figures 3 and 4 from the June Supplement, 1972.

REFERENCES

Avery, A. F. and Evans, A. (1973): *Brit. J. Anaesth.*, 45, 301.
Brandt, L., Mark, L. C., Snell, M. McM., Vrindten, P. and Dayton, P. G. (1963): *Anesthesiology*, 24/3, 331.
Briscoe, C. E. and Taylor, P. A. (1974): *Anaesthesia*, 29, 290.
Card, B., McCulloch, R. J. and Pratt, D. A. H. (1972): *Postgrad. med. J. (Suppl. 2)*, 48, 34.
Carson, I. W. (1974): *Clinical Pharmacological Aspects of Althesin.* M.D. Thesis, Belfast.
Carson, I. W., Alexander, J. P., Hewitt, J. C. and Dundee, J. W. (1972): *Brit. J. Anaesth.*, 44, 1311.
Child, K. J., Currie, J. P., Davis, B., Dodds, M. G., Pearce, D. R. and Twissell, D. J. (1971): *Brit. J. Anaesth.*, 43, 2.
Child, K. J., Davis, B., Dodds, M. G. and Twissell, D. J. (1972a): *Brit. J. Pharmacol.*, 46/2, 189.
Child, K. J., Gibson, W., Harnby, G. and Hart, J. W. (1972b): *Postgrad. med. J. (Suppl. 2)*, 48, 37.
Clarke, R. S. J., Dundee, J. W., Garrett, R. T., McArdle, G. and Sutton, J. A. (1975): *Brit. J. Anaesth.*, in press.
Clarke, R. S. J., Montgomery, S. J., Dundee, J. W. and Bovill, J. G. (1971): *Brit. J. Anaesth.*, 43, 947
Cundy, J. M. (1973): *Anaesthesia*, 28, 544.
Davis, B. and Pearce, D. R. (1972): *Postgrad. med. J. (Suppl. 2)*, 48, 13.
Dodds, M. G. and Twissell, D. J. (1972): *Postgrad. med. J. (Suppl. 2)*, 48, 17.

Downing, J. W., Coleman, A. J. and Meer, F. M. (1973): *Brit. J. Anaesth.*, *45*, 381.

Dundee, J. W., Assem, E. S. K., Gaston, J. M., Keilty, S. R., Sutton, J. A., Clarke, R. S. J. and Grainger, D. (1974): *Brit. med. J.*, *1*, 63.

Galley, A. H. and Rooms, M. (1956): *Lancet*, *1*, 990.

Goodman, L. S. and Gillman, A. (1970): In: *The Pharmacological Basis of Therapeutics, 4th ed.*, p. 1228. Editors: L. S. Goodman and A. Gillman. The Macmillan Press Ltd., New York – Melbourne – London.

Hester, J. B. (1973): *Brit. J. Anaesth.*, *45*, 303.

Jones, J., Payne, J. P. and Perry, I. R. (1972): *Brit. J. Pharmacol.*, *46/3*, 553P.

Kay, B. (1972): *Das Ultrakurznarcoticum Methohexital*, p. 149. Editor: C. Lehmann. Springer-Verlag, Berlin.

Morgan, M., Whitwam, J. G. and Page, P. (1973): *Brit. J. Anaesth.*, *45*, 481.

Notcutt, W. G. (1973): *Anaesthesia*, *28*, 673.

Phillipps, G. (1974): In: *Molecular Mechanisms in General Anaesthesia*, p. 35. Editors: M. J. Halsey, R. A. Millar and J. A. Sutton. Churchill Livingstone, Edinburgh.

Ramsey, M. A. E., Simpson, B. R. J., Savege, T. M. and Goodwin, R. (1974): *Brit. med. J.*, *2*, 656.

Robertson, J. D. (1963): *Recent Advances in Anaesthesia and Analgesia, 9th ed.* J. and A. Churchill Ltd., London.

Robertson, J. D. and Wynn-Williams, A. (1961): *Anaesthesia*, *16/4*, 389.

Rollason, W. M., Hough, J. M. and Fidler, K. (1974): *Brit. J. Anaesth.*, *46/2*, 881.

Ryder, W. (1970): *Anaesthesia*, *25*, 46.

Savege, T. M., Foley, E. I., Coutlas, R. J., Walton, B., Strunin, L., Simpson, B. R. and Scott, D. F. (1971): *Anaesthesia*, *26*, 402.

Savege, T. M., Foley, E. I., Ross, L. and Maxwell, M. D. (1972): *Postgrad. med. J. (Suppl. 2)*, *48*, 66.

Strunin, L., Strunin, J. M., Knights, K. and Ward, M. E. (1974): *Brit. J. Anaesth.*, *46*, 319.

Takahashi, T. (1972): *Postgrad. med. J. (Suppl. 2)*, *48*, 96.

Thurlow, A. C. (1972): *Anaesthesia*, *27*, 429.

Tomlin, P. J. (1972): *Postgrad. med. J. (Suppl. 2)*, *48*, 85.

Warren, J. B. (1972): *Postgrad. med. J. (Suppl. 2)*, *48*, 130.

Hemodynamic effects immediately following the induction of anesthesia with Althesin (CT-1341, Glaxo)

FERNANDO AVELLO GARCÍA, JOSÉ MARÍA FERNANDEZ DE MIGUEL,
PEDRO PERAL AGREDA, ALFONSO ASCORVE DOMINGUEZ and
RICARDO PINTADO OTERO

Clínica Puerta de Hierro, Madrid, Spain

The steroid agent Althesin (CT-1341, Glaxo) is a combination of pregnanediones with anesthetic activities, with Cremophor as a solvent. Its effects in animals have been studied by Child et al. (1971, 1972) and others; since 1971 it has been studied clinically by various authors, including Campbell et al. (1971), Savege et al. (1971) and Campbell (1972).

In this work the hemodynamic effects of Althesin have been analyzed in 2 groups of patients who received a dose of 0.075 ml/kg.

MATERIAL AND METHODS

The first group was composed of 32 patients scheduled for general surgery and not pre-medicated. The procedures to which they would be subjected were explained to them, and they voluntarily accepted them.

The criteria of selection were: (1) consent; (2) absence of history of cardiovascular or allergic events; (3) good veins. The group was composed of 16 men and 16 women with a mean age of 42 years (standard deviation (s.d.) $\pm$ 11.5), a mean weight of 61.7 kg (s.d. $\pm$ 10.7) and a mean body surface area of 1.64 m^2 (s.d. $\pm$ 0.1). When classified according to the guidelines of the American Society of Anesthesiology (ASA), 6 patients were placed in Group 1, 20 in Group 2 and 7 in Group 3.

The following determinations were made on these patients initially and at 1, 3 and 9 min: electrocardiogram (ECG); heart rate (HR); cardiac output (CO); cardiac index (CI); stroke index (SI); systolic arterial pressure (SAP); diastolic arterial pressure (DAP); mean arterial pressure (MAP); total peripheral resistance (TPR); pulmonary artery systolic pressure (PASP); pulmonary artery diastolic pressure (PADP); pulmonary artery mean pressure (PAMP); pulmonary capillary pressure (PCP); central venous pressure (CVP); pulmonary vascular resistance (PVR); partial pressure of arterial oxygen (Pa$_{O2}$); partial pressure of arterial carbon dioxide (Pa$_{CO2}$); pH; standard bicarbonate (SB); injection time (IT); sleeping time (ST); duration of anesthesia (DA).

The ECG trace was taken in the first derivation with a Mark 7 AMP Water's preamplifier. The HR was measured with an Mh-8 Water's cardiotachometer. The CO was determined by the dye dilution technic using an X-302 densitometer, Xc-302 cuvette and a Water's Mc-4A computer for the direct reading of the curves. Indocyanine green (5 mg) was injected rapidly into the pulmonary artery (PA) through a Swan Ganz catheter, and the arterial blood was retrieved through a radial catheter using a Harvard No. 2604 constant extraction pump. The CI was obtained by dividing the CO by the body surface area, and the SI was obtained by dividing the CI by the HR. Arterial pressure was measured through a No. 18 medicut Argyle cannula introduced into the radial artery by percutaneous puncture. The pulmonary arterial pressure (PAP), the PCP and the CVP were obtained through a 7-caliber Swan Ganz catheter, introduced through an antecubital vein using the Seldinger technic. Systemic arterial pressures, PAP, PCP and CVP were measured with a P23 Db Statham transductor. The measurements of systemic arterial pressure, CVP, PCP, PAP, CO and ECG were recorded on a Water's model 100, 12-channel recorder, using ultraviolet light for detection. The TPR and PVR were calculated by the Aperia formulae (Aperia, 1940):

$$TPR = \frac{MAP \ (mm \ Hg)}{CO \ (l/min)} \times 80 \ dynes/sec \ cm^{-5}$$

$$PVR = \frac{PAMP - PCP \ (mm \ Hg)}{CO \ (l/min)} \times 80 \ dynes/sec \ cm^{-5}.$$

Whilst the patients breathed ambient air, the blood gases were determined in a Combi-Analyzer using blood extracted from the radial artery. The Pa_{O2} was measured with a Clark electrode, and the pH with a hydrogen electrode adapted to measure Pa_{CO2}. The SB was derived from the Henderson-Haselbach formula.

The determinations were carried out at the end of the 1st min after the commencement of sleep, and after 3 and 9 min.

The 2nd group of patients consisted of 8 persons, 6 men and 2 women, subjected to cardiac catheterization for the diagnosis of their cardiopathies. These patients were pre-medicated with 50 mg meperidine, 12.5 mg promethazine and 12.5 mg chlorpromazine intramuscularly one hour before the start of the hemodynamic investigation.

The criteria for selection of this group were: (1) they suffered discomfort during the routine procedure and requested additional aid, and (2) catheterization of the left ventricle was necessary. The mean age was 38.8 years (s.d. $\pm$ 13.4), the mean weight was 59.7 kg (s.d. $\pm$ 5.2) and the mean body surface area was 1.62 m^2 (s.d. $\pm$ 0.09). All were classified in the ASA Group 3.

Initially and in the 1st, 3rd, 6th and 9th min of sleep, the following determinations were carried out: ECG; HR; left ventricle systolic pressure (LVSP); left ventricle diastolic pressure (LVDP); PCP; V_{max}; dP/dt; injection time (IT); sleeping time (ST); duration of anesthesia (DA).

The ventricular and pulmonary arterial pressures were recorded through 7F-Lehman catheters, 7F-NIH and 7F-Cournand catheters, with a 1280 c Hewlett Packard-Samborn transducer. The dP/dt was measured with an HP-8802 preamplifier, and was expressed in mm Hg/sec. The V_{max} was calculated from the pressure developed, and was expressed as muscular lengths per second (ML/sec). Graphic registration was achieved with an HP-4560 8-channel, instantaneous photographic recorder. The injection time was taken as the time between the start and the finish of injection. The sleeping time was taken as the time elapsing between the start of the injection and the point at which the patient lost the capacity to answer questions. The duration of anesthesia was considered to run from the start of the injection until the patient started to respond to orders.

In both groups note was taken of the unfavourable reactions, such as apnea, obstruction of the air passages, myoclonia, involuntary movements and hiccough. Side-effects to the veins up to 1 week after anesthesia were also noted. All the patients breathed ambient air. The results obtained were analyzed statistically, using the Student's t-test with paired observations.

RESULTS

The results for the first group are given in Tables 1 and 2, together with any statistical significance between the basal values and later values.

Table 1. *Hemodynamic effects immediately following the induction of anesthesia with Althesin (CT-1341, Glaxo) (mean values; standard deviations; comparisons of the means)*

	Basal		1 min		3 min		9 min	
HR (beats/min)	83	(13)	100**	(13)	96**	(15)	95*	(18)
CO (l/min)	5.33	(0.9)	5.28	(0.7)	5.20	(0.6)	5.28	(0.55)
CI (l/min/m^2)	3.32	(0.7)	3.28	(0.7)	3.21	(0.6)	3.24	(0.55)
SI (ml/min/m^2)	40.7	(10.2)	32.9**	(7.2)	33.6**	(8)	34.5*	(9)
SAP (mm Hg)	124	(17)	106**	(16)	114*	(14.5)	118	(15.2)
DAP (mm Hg)	65	(10.5)	59*	(9.7)	60.8*	(9.5)	61.9	(10.5)
MAP (mm Hg)	85.4	(13)	77*	(11.3)	77.6*	(11.5)	82	(12.4)
PCP (mm Hg)	3.2	(1.6)	2.6*	(1.3)	2.5*	(1.2)	2.3*	(1.2)
CVP (mm Hg)	0.6	(1.5)	0.2	(1.8)	0	(1.8)	0	(1.7)
PASP (mm Hg)	16.2	(4.3)	17	(6.8)	16.9	(5.5)	14.6	(5.2)
PADP (mm Hg)	3.58	(2.27)	3.93	(2.28)	3.84	(3.05)	3.21	(2.16)
PAMP (mm Hg)	9.20	(3.50)	10.38	(4.9)	9.32	(3.75)	8.21	(3.45)
TPR (dyne/sec^{-5})	1315	(348)	1219	(332)	1214	(212)	1266	(309)
PVR (dyne/sec^{-5})	88.87	(46.6)	130.90**	(100.6)	111.6	(76.8)	90.6	(43.2)

No. of patients: 32.
* $p < 0.05$ in comparison with basal values.
** $p < 0.001$ in comparison with basal values.

Table 2. *Hemodynamic effects immediately following the induction of anesthesia with Athesin (CT-1341, Glaxo) (mean values; standard deviations; comparisons of the means)*

	Basal	1 min	3 min	9 min
Pa$_{O_2}$ (mm Hg)	78.4	71	73.4	78.1
	(9.4)	(8.8)	(8.5)	(10.5)
Pa$_{CO_2}$ (mm Hg)	38.5	38.5	38.7	38.1
	(3.8)	(4.4)	(4.4)	(3.9)
pH	7.40	7.38	7.38	7.38
	(0.04)	(0.03)	(0.04)	(0.04)
Standard bicarbonate (mEq/l)	23.9	22.8	23	22.7
	(2.5)	(1.8)	(1.8)	(2)

No. of patients: 32.
There were no statistically significant differences.

The mean injection time was 26 sec (s.d. ± 5), the mean sleeping time was 34 sec (s.d. ± 7), and the mean duration of anesthesia was 12.5 min (s.d. ± 2.4). The ECG traces revealed no changes apart from those related to the increase in heart rate. The HR increased significantly throughout the observation time, with the greatest change occurring in the 1st min (20%). Even in the 9th min the increase in HR was statistically significant with $p < 0.01$. The CI underwent no significant modification, although there was a slight decrease in the absolute values. As expected, the changes in HR were associated with a significant decrease in the SI, with the greatest effect found during the first observation (p < 0.001). The SAP and DAP underwent a significant decrease (p < 0.001) between the determinations at time 0 and at 1 min, corresponding to a numerical drop of 14% and 18 mm/Hg for the systolic pressure. The difference between the basal determination and that at the 3rd min also showed a statistically significant fall, but this was not so for the final determination. The MAP also fell significantly. The TPR was decreased in each of the 3 determinations in comparison with the basal value, but without being statistically significant.

The pressures in the pulmonary circulation did not show significant variation, although the absolute values showed an increase from the basal determination to that of the 1st min, followed by a significant decline (p < 0.05) between the pressure at the 1st min and that at the 9th min. PVR increased significantly in the 1st min and followed the direction of PAP. The PCP decreased significantly; the CVP also decreased, but not significantly. There were no alterations in the blood gases, the pH or the standard bicarbonate.

Of these 32 patients, 7 showed some undesirable effect from the respiratory point of view, 3 had hiccoughs (9.5%), 2 had obstruction of the airway from the tongue (6.2%), and 2 had bouts of coughing (6.2%). Another 7 patients showed muscular movements which were interpreted as myoclonias (21%), and 13 (40.7%) showed some involuntary movement before wakening. These movements appeared at distinct moments during anesthesia, mainly at the end.

The results for the 2nd group of patients can be seen in Table 3. The mean injection time was 36.8 sec (s.d. ± 10.3), the mean sleeping time was 38 sec (s.d. ± 22.4) and the mean duration of anesthesia was 22.1 min (s.d. ± 5.26). The ECG traces showed no detectable alterations. The HR was increased in all the determinations, but not significantly so. The greatest increase was at the 3rd determination, with an increase of 12% over the basal value. LVSP, LVDV and PCP were not significantly modified, although the LVSP did show an appreciable decrease in absolute values, especially in the 2nd determination (16% of the basal value).

Table 3. *Hemodynamic effects immediately following the induction of anesthesia with Althesin (CT-1341, Glaxo) (mean values; standard deviations; comparisons of the means)*

	Basal	1 min	3 min	6 min	9 min
HR (beats/min)	97.5	106.9	95	109.8	93.5
	(25)	(10)	(19)	(26)	(13.6)
LVSP (mm Hg)	143.1	120.8	117	129	122
	(51.7)	(29.6)	(40.8)	(33.6)	(30.4)
LVDP (mm Hg)	16.75	18.7	16.8	21.8	16.1
	(11.3)	(12.5)	(11.2)	(10.8)	(10.4)
PCP (mm Hg)	20.6	22.1	21.8	22.6	20.9
	(7)	(5.1)	(6.2)	(5.8)	(4.5)
V_{max} (ML/sec)	1.85	1.61	1.74	1.72	1.78
	(0.4)	(0.4)	(0.5)	(0.1)	(0.5)
dP/dt (mm Hg/sec)	1681	1298	1294	1354	1450
	(610)	(349)	(379)	(539)	(388)

No. of patients: 8.
There were no statistically significant differences.

The tests of myocardial contractility (V_{max} and dP/dt) showed an absolute decrease in all the determinations, but not statistically significant. In this group of patients, one woman was apneic for 1.5 min. Another 2 patients showed involuntary movements. Any side-effects to the veins were not observed in either of the groups.

DISCUSSION

In the 1st group, our results generally agree with those obtained by others (Campbell et al., 1971; Savege et al., 1971; Coleman et al., 1972; Leary et al., 1972), although the variations in CO were less than normally described and were very slightly negative. However, the decrease in blood pressure was similar to that reported before.

The most salient hemodynamic signs are: the increase in HR (20% above the basal value in the first determination), and the fall in blood pressure (14% below the basal value in the first determination). In contrast with other induction agents Althesin does not have a negative effect on the CO. The mechanism of action for the decrease in the blood pressure is unknown, although Doenicke et al. (1973) have shown that Althesin can liberate histamine. The vasodilation may lead to a decrease of the blood pressure, the CVP and the TPR, but the CO is not affected despite the slightly negative inotropic effect, and this appears to be due to the compensatory increase in the HR.

The alterations observed in pulmonary arterial pressure and PVR are small, and mainly appear at the time of the first determination, completely disappearing by min 9. We think that they are due to slight and transitory alterations in the permeability of the air passages. Campbell et al. (1971) mentioned that there were alterations in pulmonary arterial pressures, and stated that they were conflicting. With regard to the adverse reactions (myoclonic movements, apnea, hiccough, etc.), they have been observed by all investigators, and Samuel and Dundee (1973) particularly found a clear relationship between the speed of injection, the dose and these phenomena. In our cases we believe that the large numbers of involuntary movements observed were often nothing more than signals of the end of anesthesia.

In the patients in the 2nd group, attention is called to the fact that the hemodynamic changes were less marked than in the noncardiopathic patients, which disagrees with other observations (Harrison and Sellick, 1972; Lyons and Clarke, 1972).

Since the dP/dt (and V_{max}) values decreased it can be deduced, with all the limitations that this implies, that Althesin seems to produce a slight and transitory negative inotropic effect. On the other hand, Sonntag et al. (1973) showed that Althesin increases the coronary flow and the consumption of oxygen without changing the rate of oxygen extraction (the arteriovenous oxygen difference) and the oxygen content in the coronary sinus, so that it can be said that there is an increase in coronary blood flow parallel to the tachycardia.

These data may imply that Althesin is contraindicated in those patients with fixed HR and in those where the coronary flow is compromised.

REFERENCES

Aperia, A. (1940): *Skand. Arch. Physiol., Suppl. 16/1.*
Campbell, D., Forrester, A. C., Miller, D. C., Hutton, J., Kennedy, J. A., Lawrie, T. D. V., Lorimer, A. R. and McCall, D. (1971): *Brit. J. Anaesth., 43,14.*
Campbell, D. (1972): *Anaesthetist, 21,* 336.
Child, K. J., Currie, J. P., Davis, B., Dodds, M. G., Pearce, B. R. and Twissell, D. J. (1971): *Brit. J. Anaesth., 46,* 189.
Child, K. J., Davis, B., Dodds, M. G. and Twissell, D. J. (1972): *Brit. J. Pharmacol., 46,* 189.
Clarke, R. S. J., Montgomery, S. J., Dundee, J. W. and Bovill, J. G. (1971): *Brit. J. Anaesth., 43,* 947.
Clarke, R. S. J., Dundee, J. W., Carson, I. W., Arora, M. V. and McCaughey, W. (1972): *Brit. J. Anaesth., 44,* 845.
Coleman, A. J., Downing, J. W., Leary, W. P., Moyes, D. G. and Styles, M. (1972): *Anaesthesia, 27/4,* 373.
Doenicke, A., Lorez, W., Beigl, R., Bezecny, H., Uhlig, G., Kalmar, L., Praetoerius, B. and Mann, G. (1973): *Brit. J. Anaesth., 45,* 1097.

Harrison, B. G. C. and Sellick, B. A. (1972): *Brit. J. Anaesth.*, *44*, 1205.

Leary, W. P., Coleman, A. J., Downing, J. W. and Moyes, D. G. (1972): *S. Afr. med. J.*, *46*, 877.

Lyons, S. M. and Clarke, R. S. J. (1972): *Brit. J. Anaesth.*, *44*, 575.

Samuel, I. O. and Dundee, J. W. (1973): *Brit. J. Anaesth.*, *45*, 1215.

Savege, T. M., Foley, E. I., Coultas, R. J., Walton, B., Strunin, L., Simpson, B. R. and Scott, D. F. (1971): *Anaesthesia*, *26/4*, 402.

Sonntag, H., Schenk, H. D., Regensburger, D., Kettler, D., Kholl, D., Donath, U. and Becker, H. (1973): *Acta anaesth. scand.*, *17*, 218.

Metabolism of ^{14}C-labelled alphaxalone in man

LEO STRUNIN, J. M. STRUNIN, K. M. KNIGHTS and M. E. WARD

Anaesthetic Department, King's College Hospital, London, United Kingdom

Alphaxalone is the major active constituent of the steroid induction agent Althesin (0.9%
alphaxalone, 0.3% alphadalone acetate, 20% polyoxyethylated castor oil, 0.25% NaCl
in water). Studies in the rat (Card et al., 1972; Child et al., 1972) showed that the plasma
half life of ^{14}C-alphaxalone was 6–8 min and the liver was the main site of metabolism.
There was no redistribution in fat and approximately 70% of the radioactivity was excreted
in the bile in the first 3 hr after administration. Further excretion studies over 5 days showed
that 60–70% of the radioactivity appeared in the faeces and only 20–30% in the urine.

The present study reports on the metabolism in man of alphaxalone (3α-hydroxy-5α-
pregnane-11,20-dione) labelled with ^{14}C in the 21 position, made up as Althesin with a
specific activity of approximately 5 μCi/ml.

PATIENTS

Three groups of patients were studied. All gave informed consent for the insertion of a
central venous cannula and administration of ^{14}C-Althesin as part of their anaesthetic.
There were 5 patients with normal hepatic and renal function in the first group. The second
group consisted of 5 further patients who required the insertion of a T-tube into the common
bile duct as part of their surgical procedure. In the third group there were 4 further patients
with chronic renal disease who had no appreciable urine output.

METHODS

In Group 1 (controls) anaesthesia was induced with ^{14}C-Althesin (10–20 μCi) and maintained with nitrous oxide, oxygen and pethidine. A central venous cannula was inserted
under local anaesthesia prior to induction and frequent blood samples were taken before,
during and after surgery. In addition all urine up to 5 days after surgery, was collected as
passed.

In Group 2 (T-tubes) anaesthesia was induced with thiopentone. The patients were
paralysed with pancuronium bromide (Pavulon) and anaesthesia maintained with nitrous
oxide, oxygen and either pethidine or fentanyl. ^{14}C-Althesin (10 μCi) was administered
just after the T-tube had been inserted, thereafter blood samples were taken as in Group 1
from a previously inserted central venous cannula, and in addition, bile was collected in
10 min aliquots for an initial hour and thereafter, in hourly aliquots for some 16 hr. Urine
was collected as in Group 1 except that in patients who had a urinary catheter inserted prior
to surgery urine was collected hourly for the first 24 hr and then at either 3, 4 or 6-hourly
intervals according to the regime employed in the ward.

In the third group of patients (renal disease) ^{14}C-Althesin (10–20 μCi) was given for induction and anaesthesia was maintained with oxygen, nitrous oxide and halothane. In these patients, only blood samples were taken as there was no appreciable urine output during the period of study.

All blood samples were taken into heparinised tubes and centrifuged. The separated plasma was diluted 1 in 10 with water and 1 ml of this dilution taken up into 10 ml of Unisolve-1 phosphor (Koch–Light) and counted in a Packard Tricarb liquid scintillation counter. The results were expressed as disintegrations per min (d.p.m.) per ml of plasma.

Aliquots of the bile samples were diluted 1 in 20 with water and 1 ml of this dilution was added to 10 ml of phosphor. The samples were allowed to stand for 10 hr in daylight to bleach out the yellow coloration in the bile and then were kept in the dark for a further

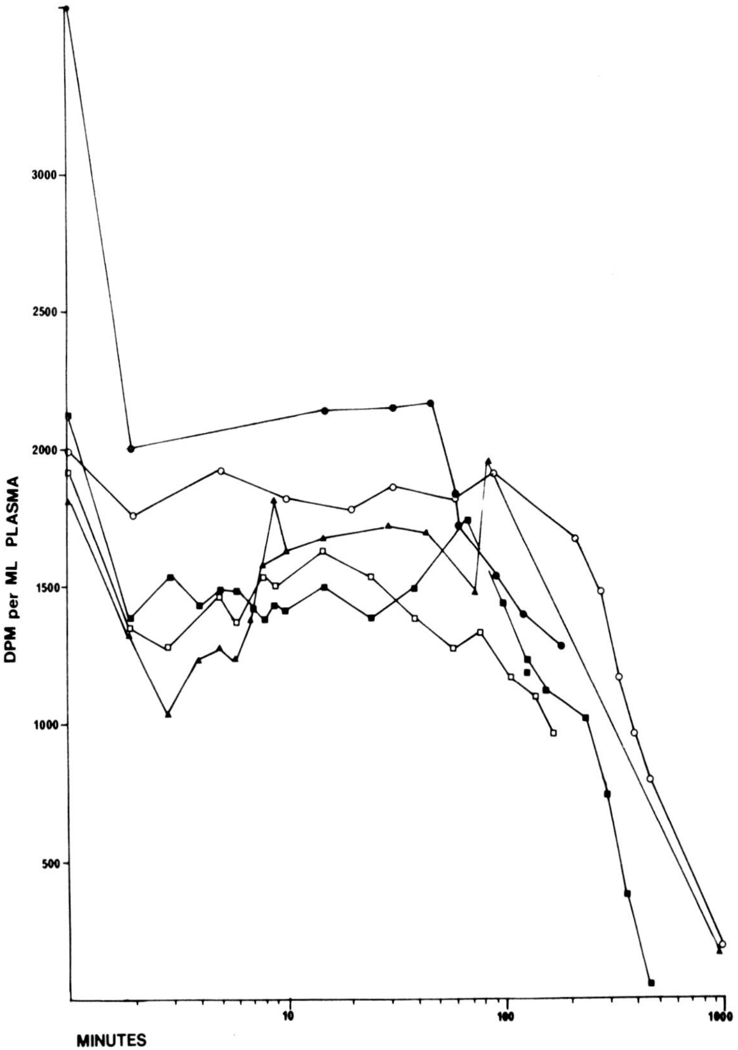

Fig. 1. *Plasma radioactivity in 5 control patients given 10–20 μCi ¹⁴C-alphaxalone.*

12 hr (for phosphor stabilisation) before being counted. The results were expressed as d.p.m. per ml of bile.

Initially 1 ml of each urine aliquot was diluted in 10 ml of phosphor and counted. If quenching due to urine colour exceeded 20%, the samples were further diluted 1 in 10 with water and re-counted.

RESULTS

Figure 1 shows the radioactivity in the plasma of the control patients. It can be seen that there is an initial rapid redistribution followed by a plateau between 10 and 100 min and

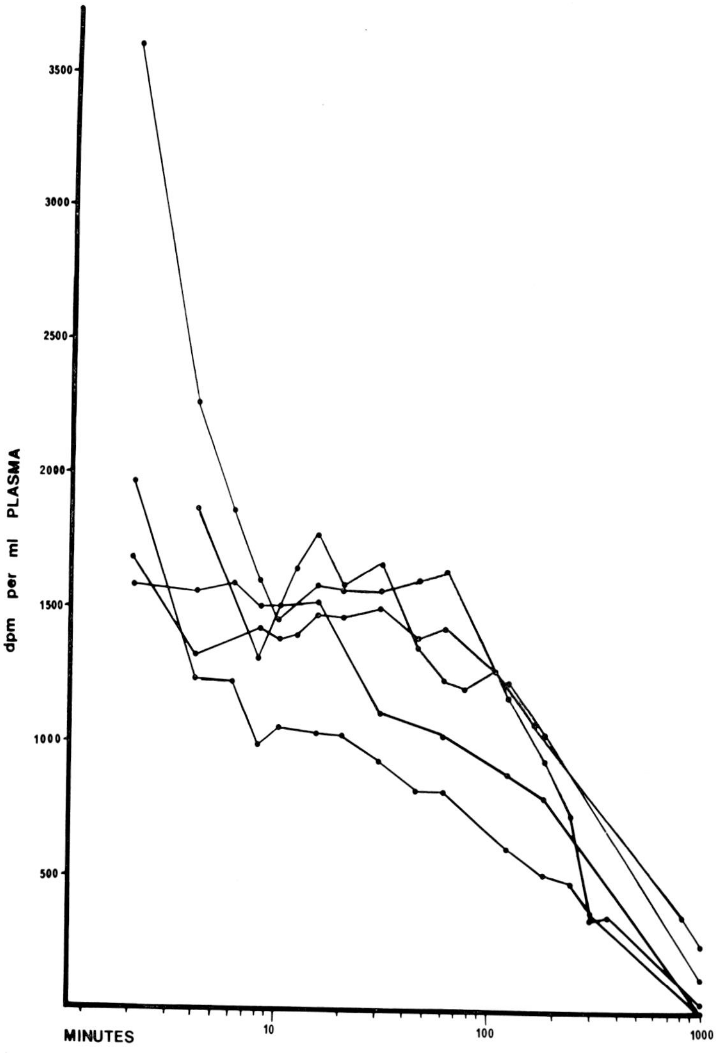

Fig. 2.   *Plasma radioactivity in 5 patients having T-tubes inserted into the common bile duct, given 10 µCi ¹⁴C-alphaxalone.*

then subsequent clearance from the plasma after approximately 1000 min.

Figure 2 shows the radioactivity in the plasma of the patients having T-tubes inserted. These curves are essentially similar to the controls, other than the d.p.m. per ml are lower in value since these patients received only 10 μCi of radioactivity.

Figure 3 shows the radioactivity in the bile samples. Although radioactivity is present in the bile, there is only some 16–24% of the original dose present. In one patient only 0.2% was excreted in the bile.

Figures 4 and 5 represent cumulative output of radioactivity in the urine of the patients in the control and T-tube groups respectively. It can be seen that at 24 hr some 59% and 38% respectively of the injected dose is present in the urine. At 120 hr some 65–84% of

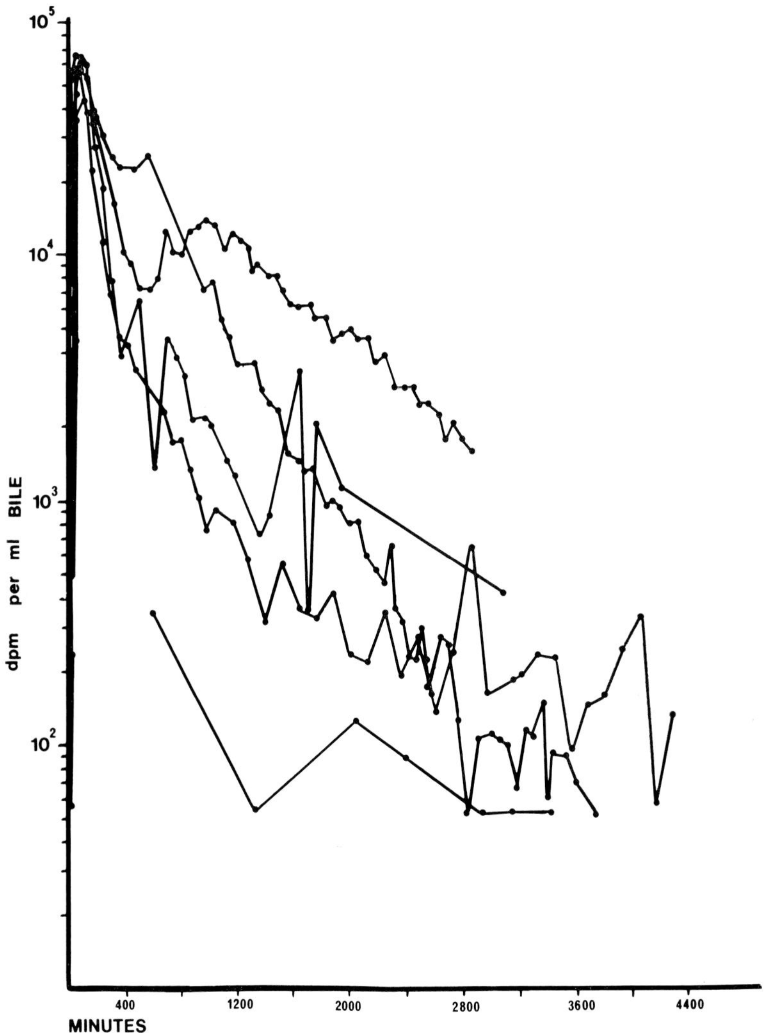

Fig. 3.   *Bile radioactivity in 5 patients having T-tubes inserted into the common bile duct, given 10 μCi ¹⁴C-alphaxalone.*

the total radioactivity had been excreted. In the T-tube group of patients, although the cumulative urine totals are slightly less than the control group (51–70%), if the radioactivity removed in the bile samples is added to this amount then there is no significant difference in the total percent of radioactivity excreted between the T-tube group and the control group.

In Figure 6 is shown the radioactivity in the plasma of the renal disease group. Comparing these curves with those of the control group, redistribution seems equally rapid, but there appears to be a prolongation of the plateau. It did not prove possible to obtain plasma samples beyond 200 min except in one patient. This showed, however, significantly more residual radioactivity than in the control group.

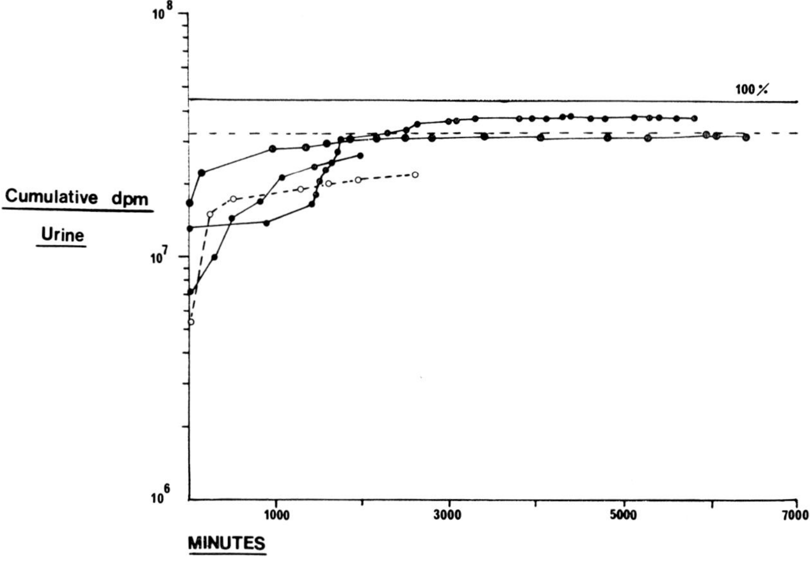

Fig. 4.   *Cumulative urine radioactivity from 4 control patients given 10–20 µCi ¹⁴C-alphaxalone.*

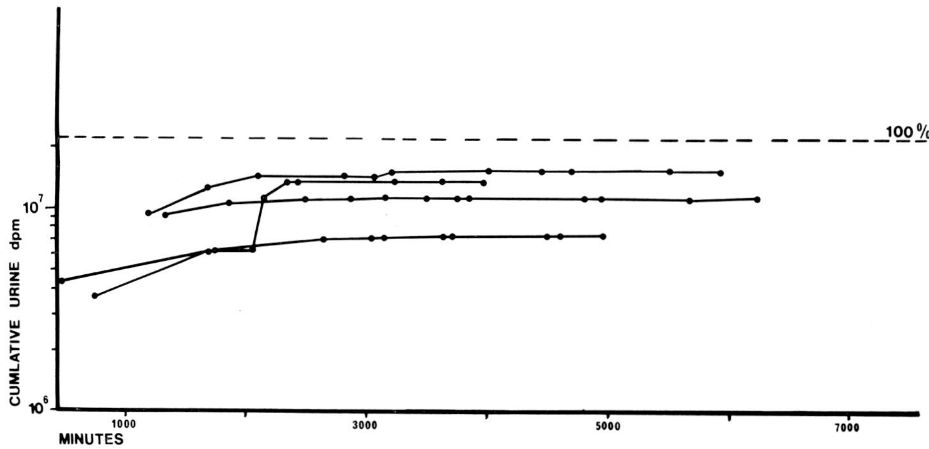

Fig. 5.   *Cumulative urine radioactivity from 4 T-tube patients given 10 µCi ¹⁴C-alphaxalone.*

DISCUSSION

The results show that the injected radioactivity is rapidly redistributed and in the control patients is probably taken up by the liver. There is some excretion of radioactivity into the bile, but since the majority can be recovered from the urine, enterohepatic recirculation must occur. This finding is in contrast to the rat where the majority of injected radioactivity was excreted in the bile in the first 3 hr after administration (Child et al., 1972). It is of interest that the plasma curves for the patients with renal disease are initially identical to those of the patients with normal renal function and this adds weight to the suggestion that the liver is primarily involved in removing the radioactive moiety from the plasma and that excretion via the kidneys is a secondary mechanism.

The nature of the radioactivity in the plasma has yet to be established. It cannot be unchanged alphaxalone since it is present in the plasma long after the patients have recovered

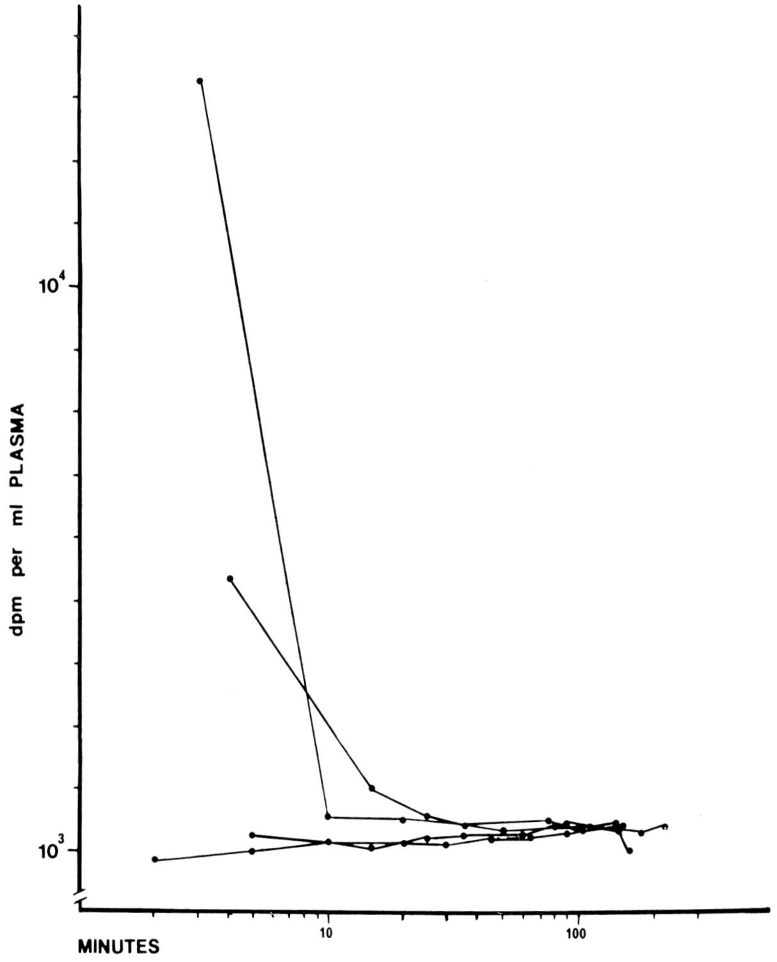

Fig. 6. *Plasma radioactivity in 4 patients with renal disease, having 10–20 µCi ^{14}C-alphaxalone.*

from the effects of anaesthesia. Since this radioactivity is subsequently excreted in the urine, it suggests that the alphaxalone has been metabolised to a more polar compound.

ACKNOWLEDGEMENTS

The authors would like to thank Glaxo Laboratories Limited for kindly supplying the ^{14}C-Althesin used in this study.

REFERENCES

Card, B., McCulloch, P. J. and Pratt, D. A. H. (1972): *Postgrad. med. J.*, *48*, 34.
Child, K. J., Gibson, W., Harnby, G. and Hart, J. W. (1972): *Postgrad. med. J.*, *48*, 37.

Propanidid

A. DOENICKE

Anaesthesiological Service, Department of Surgery, University of Munich,
Munich, Federal Republic of Germany

Ten years ago in São Paulo, the positive advantages of propanidid, that is short duration of action, short postanaesthetic recovery i.e. rapid metabolism, were reported (Doenicke, 1965; Doenicke and Kugler, 1965; Doenicke et al., 1968). The circulatory changes have been confirmed meanwhile by numerous authors using refined methods of investigation. Allergic reactions seemed to be absent or rare in the first few years.

Since 1968 we have been trying, together with Lorenz, to clarify the hypersensitivity reaction after propanidid. The release of histamine is particularly important (Fig. 1) (Lorenz et al., 1969, 1972). Therapy is also important in such incidents (Table 1) (Doenicke and Lorenz, 1970). This is an analysis of the incidence of these reactions.

Two retrospective studies from anaesthesia journals were evaluated and one prospective study was conducted on the manufacturer's initiative (Bayer) (Table 2).

The retrospective evaluation of 3000 anaesthesias showed that 1300 anaesthesias without premedication with an antihistamine, Neclastine, produced an allergic anaphylactic reaction (without bronchospasm) in 4 patients, which is one reaction in 325 anaesthesias.

In 1700 anaesthesias with Neclastine as premedication, 29 allergic reactions were seen. Fifteen were however, after the combination propanidid/suxamethonium, indicating that the relaxant also might have caused the reaction (Table 3). Four patients reacted with a flush after the premedication under continuous infusion of gelatine. After the prednisolone, anaesthesia was induced with propanidid without complications.

The distribution of typical signs may be seen in Table 4. The degree of severity is established according to the degree of hypotension. In 19 patients, whose allergic anaphylactic reactions were considered to be slight, a decrease in blood pressure by 40 mm Hg was recorded, whereas 10 patients showed a severe reaction with an average decrease in blood pressure of 40–60 mm Hg. In 3 of the 10 patients the blood pressure was not measurable. In these 10 patients, propanidid and not suxamethonium was most probably responsible for the reaction (i.e. one reaction in 170 anaesthesias).

In the second retrospective study with 2209 patients who received propanidid repeatedly for the induction anaesthesia, the following questions should be answered: (1) Is there a relation between the amount of propanidid, the frequency and severity of incidents? (2) Is there an increased risk of incidents after repeated use of propanidid? (3) Are allergic persons in greater danger than normal patients? (4) Can prophylactic use of an antihistamine (Neclastine) reduce the incidence and intensity of a reaction?

The total of 5417 anaesthesias with propanidid consisted of 2209 first anaesthesias and 3208 repeat anaesthesias.

1. 500 mg propanidid (Fig. 2) was administered in most cases; 64 incidents were not dose-dependent. This fact is demonstrated even more distinctly by the percentage of incidents (Fig. 3). No severe reaction occurred after the most frequently administered dose of 500 mg. The occurrence rate and the severity of the reactions are not dose-dependent.

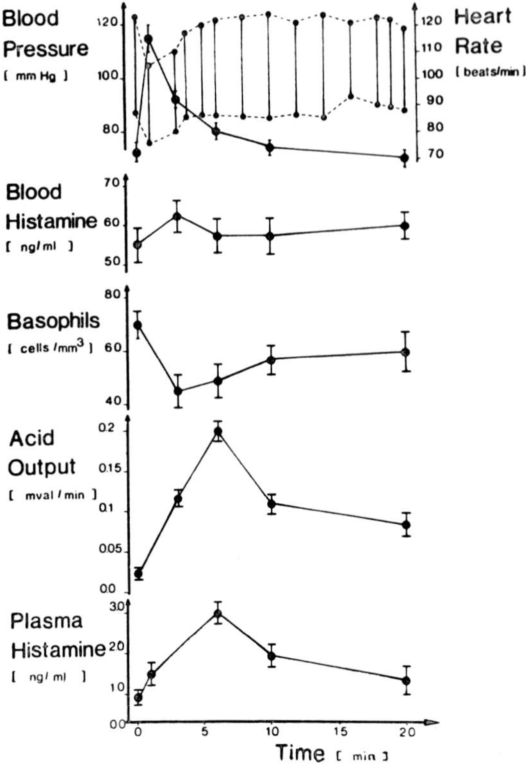

Fig. 1.   *Release of histamine. (From: Lorenz et al., 1972.)*

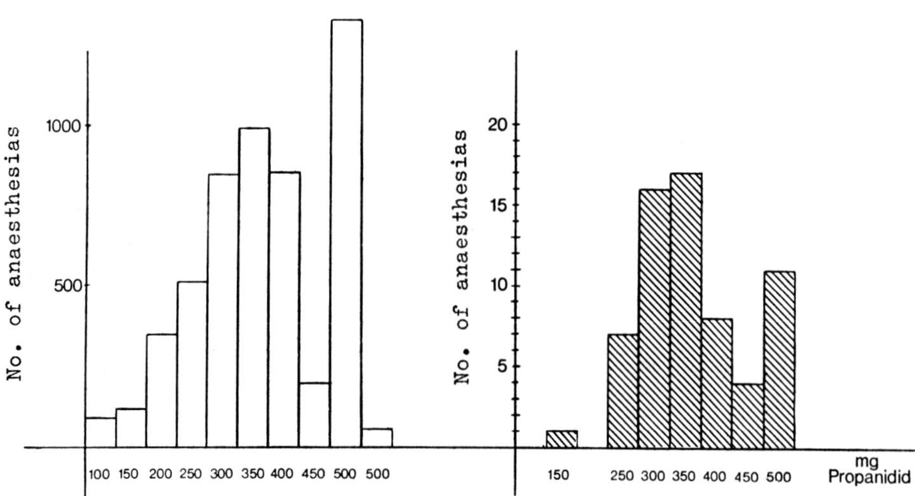

Fig. 2.   *Propanidid anaesthesias (Hospital B.H., Dr Sp.), divided according to dose. (White area=total (n=5417), shaded area=incidents (n=64).)*

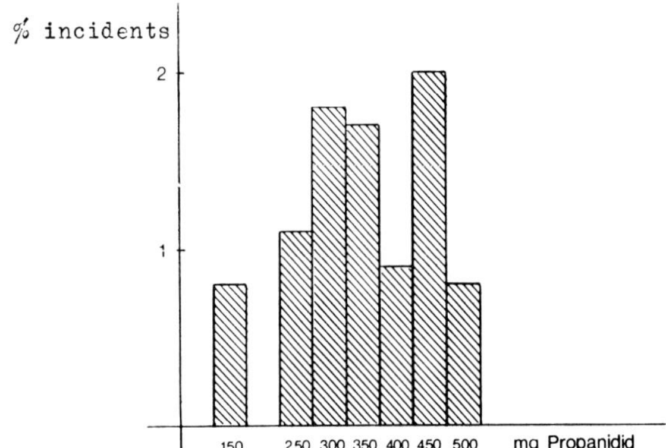

Fig. 3.   *Percentage of incidents after application (n=64).*

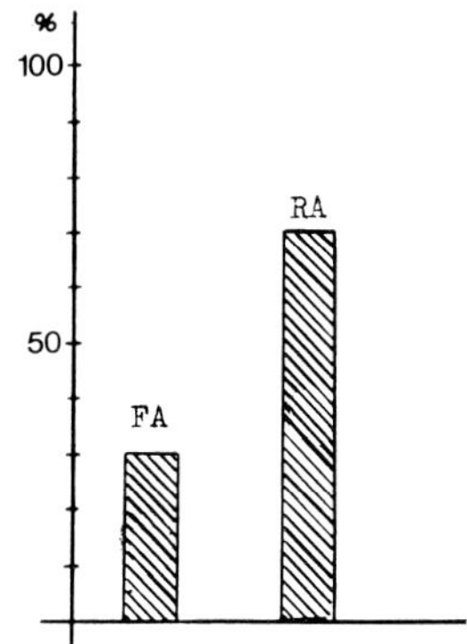

Fig. 4.   *Propanidid anaesthesias – 64 incidents (100%) divided into first anaesthesias (FA – n=14)*
1:157, and repeat anaesthesias (RA – n=50), 1:64.

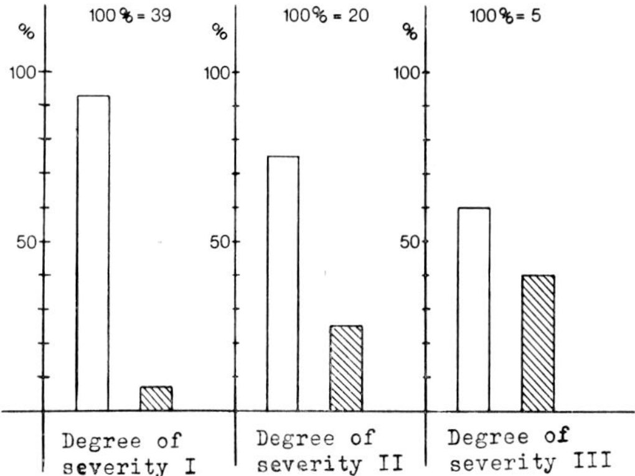

Fig. 5.   *Distribution of 10 allergic persons among the degrees of severity I–III. (I=1 symptom,*
(e.g. erythema), II=at least 2 symptoms, and III=more than 2 symptoms plus distinct
hypotension) out of 5417 propanidid anaesthesias. (White area=nonallergic; shaded
area=allergic.)

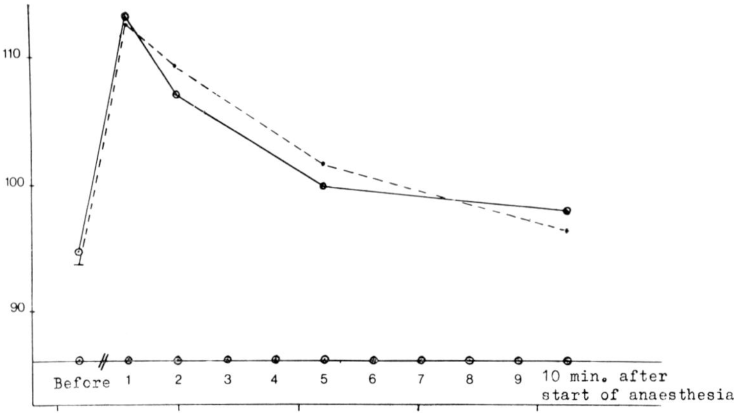

Fig. 6.   *Heart rate (n = 1000). (Solid line = old propanidid, n = 481; broken line = new propanidid, n = 519.)*

2. The risk of a reaction after propanidid is distinctly higher in repeat anaesthesias (Fig. 4), for out of the 64 incidents 14 (21.8%) occurred during first anaesthesias and 50 (78.2%) during repeat anaesthesias.

3. The group of 2209 patients comprised 181 (8.2%) with a history of allergy. Ten patients (15.6%) of the total number with incidents were allergic. The distribution of these 10 allergic persons among the degrees of severity I–III of the incidents (Fig. 5) showed a preponderance of allergic persons in the group having severe reactions, so that out of the 20 incidents of degree II 25% are allergic, whereas the group of severe reactions with a profound fall in blood pressure comprises 40% of allergic persons. The incidence and the severity of the reaction to propanidid are higher for allergic than for normal persons.

Table 1.   *Therapy – according to Doenicke and Lorenz, 1970*

Glucocorticoids	Dexamethasone 15–20 mg or prednisolone 50–100 mg
Antihistamines	e.g. Neclastine i.v. (Tavegil®) 2–3 mg
Infusions	Plasma substitute, sodium bicarbonate
Vasoconstrictors	e.g. Noradrenalin, Norphen® or others
Broncholytics	e.g. Alupent®

Table 2.   *Studies considered*

	No. of anaesthesias with propanidid
1. Retrospective evaluation: Anaesthesiological Department, Out-patient clinic, Munich	3000
2. Retrospective evaluation: Anaesthesiological Department, Bad Hersfeld Hospital	5417
3. Prospective study: A. Doenicke, Munich; H. P. Harrfeldt, Bochum; D. Langrehr, Bremen; H. Lennartz, Dusseldorf; J. Schara, Wuppertal	1000

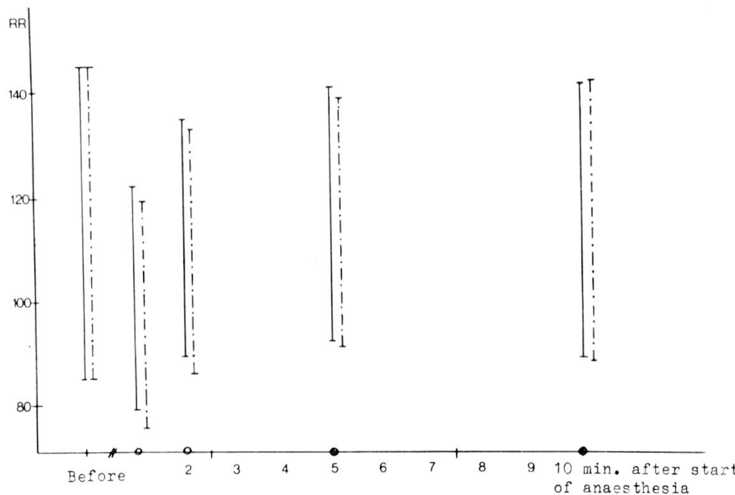

Fig. 7. *Blood pressure (n=1000). (Solid line=old propanidid, n=481; broken line=new propanidid, n=519.)*

4. As already pointed out in the first study, the prophylactic administration of an antihistamine showed the following results: of the 64 patients with reactions 38 (60%) were premedicated with Neclastine. In this group, however, only one severe incident occurred. This one incident in spite of Neclastine contrasts with 4 severe reactions without Neclastine.

The third prospective study was mainly intended to clarify the question whether a reduction of all kinds of side-effects can be obtained by the new solute Cremophor EL. Each of 5 different hospitals performed 200 coded anaesthesias with propanidid, i.e., the anaesthetist did not know whether propanidid had been dissolved in old or new cremophor. An analysis of questionnaires was carried out by the Bayer computer service. There was no significant difference regarding the reaction of the circulatory system – heart rate (Fig. 6), blood pressure (Fig. 7). The results of the increase in the heart rate and the hypotension during the first minute are generally known.

Table 3. *Retrospective evaluation, Dec., 1968–Jan., 1970 (1:170)*

Total No. of anaesthesias with propanidid, premedication with Neclastine	1700
No. of cases with slight allergic anaphylactic reactions (decrease in blood pressure by 40–60 mm Hg)	19
No. of cases with severe allergic anaphylactic reactions (decrease in blood pressure by 40–60 mm Hg; in 3 patients blood pressure was not measurable for a short time)	10

Table 4. *Result of the retrospective evaluation*

Allergic anaphylactic symptoms	No. of symptoms
Quincke's oedema	2
Flush	15
Exanthema (erythema)	8
Bronchospasm	5
Hypotension	5
Total No. of patients	29

Table 5. *Side-effects of propanidid treatment*

	Old propanidid	New propanidid	Total
Uncontrolled muscular reflexes	10	13	23
Hyperventilation	33	34	67
Skin allergy	6	5	11
Circulatory depressions	57	64	121
Peripheral cyanosis	0	3	3
Restlessness	5	4	9
Superficial anaesthesia	7	5	12
Shivering	1	0	1
Total No. of patients	481	519	1000

From: A. Doenicke, H. P. Harrfeldt, D. Langrehr, H. Lennartz, J. Schara.

Table 6. *Side-effects of propanidid treatment*

	Old propanidid	New propanidid	Total
Sneezing	1	0	1
Stridor	0	0	0
Hiccup	2	2	4
Salivation	3	0	3
Circumscribed oedema	0	0	0
Bronchospasm	0	1	1
Coughing	2	1	3
Respiratory depression (Cheyne-Stokes)	1	0	1
Perspiration	0	1	1
Retching	0	0	0
Vomiting	0	0	0
Repeated vomiting	0	0	0
Headache	0	0	0
Short-lasting nausea	0	0	0
Long-lasting nausea	0	0	0
Tiredness	0	0	0
Laryngospasm	0	0	0
Total No. of patients	481	519	1000

From: A. Doenicke, H. P. Harrfeldt, D. Langrehr, H. Lennartz, J. Schara.

The number of allergic reactions (11) (Table 5, see point 3 of the table) showed no difference and corresponded with the results of the 2 retrospective evaluations in respect of frequency. Generally, other side-effects were slight and certainly not more frequent than with other anaesthetic agents (Table 6).

REFERENCES

Doenicke, A. (1965): *Acta anaesth. scand., Suppl. 17*, 95.

Doenicke, A. and Kugler, J. (1965): *Acta anaesth. scand., Suppl. 17*, 99.

Doenicke, A., Krumey, J., Kugler, J. and Klempa, J. (1968): *Brit. J. Anaesth., 40*, 415.

Doenicke, A. and Lorenz, W. (1970): *Anaesthesist, 19*, 413.

Lorenz, W., Doenicke, A., Halbach, S., Krumey, J. and Werle, E. (1969): *Klin. Wschr., 47*, 154.

Lorenz, W., Doenicke, A., Meyer, R., Reimann, H. J., Kusche, J., Barth, H., Gering, H., Hutzel, M. and Weissenbacher, B. (1972): *Brit. J. Anaesth., 44*, 355.

Propanidid (Epontol): Reappraisal of its present position

MARTIN ZINDLER

Department of Anaesthesiology, University of Dusseldorf,
Dusseldorf, Federal Republic of Germany

Since 1963, more than 35 million ampoules of Epontol® have been distributed. The place of this drug has now to be evaluated in relation to its pharmacology and its advantages and disadvantages.

The advantages of ultra-short action with good analgesia which allows the patient to be discharged from the hospital after 20 min to resume daily activities after 2 hr are well-known.

This presentation is a discussion of the *disadvantages*, the main complications and contra-indications. But first, since drug evaluation assumes correct use two common mistakes in administration, overdosage and hypoxaemia must be mentioned.

MISTAKES IN ADMINISTRATION

Dosage

Propanidid has apparently a wider dose-effect variation than other intravenous agents like the barbiturates. Ten mg/kg may fail to produce anaesthesia in husky patients whereas only 2 mg/kg is enough in a cachectic old patient.

In old and dehydrated patients this is due to a decreased extracellular volume with consequently a higher blood level and probably to decreased protein-binding. In old patients the dose must be decreased to $\frac{1}{2}-\frac{1}{4}$ and a 2.5% solution should be used.

Speed of injection, blood level

The effect of any agent given intravenously depends on the blood level. 500 mg given over 10 sec will produce a peak blood level 6-times higher than the same dose given over 60 sec. Therefore, extremely slow administration of propanidid is mandatory, especially in poor-risk patients because all immediate effects on the respiration and particularly the circulation will thus be minimized.

Since the action of propanidid begins after 15–20 sec, very slow injection allows dosage to be regulated according to the effect. About half of the estimated dose is given a little faster and then the remainder is given very slowly – 1 ml in 10–15 sec until the patient is asleep.

Prevention of hypoxaemia

The initial hyperventilation is impressive particularly since this is in contrast to the effect of the barbiturates. Insufficient attention has been paid to the *hypoventilation* which follows.

In normal patients this is not important, but with poor pulmonary function, a low pre-anaesthetic Pa_{O_2} after an initial slight rise, may be reduced to dangerously low levels – 56 and 48 Torr have been measured by Reichel et al., 1965 and Hempelmann et al., 1972, during room air breathing.

Therefore, an increased O_2-concentration has always to be given with propanidid using a mask and assisted respiration just as is routinely done following barbiturates. Usually nitrous oxide is added since the total dose of propanidid, particularly in prolonged cases, can thus be reduced.

COMPLICATIONS

There are 2 different major complications: (1) hypotension without allergic reaction which is an immediate effect, and (2) the rare, allergic-anaphylactoid type which may or may not be associated with hypotension. This is usually delayed for 4–10 min.

Hypotension

In dogs propanidid causes hypotension because of a decrease in total peripheral resistance and a negative inotropic effect of the heart (Dudziak et al., 1973). Similar effects occur in cats (Lennartz and Siepmann, 1973) and in man (Soga et al., 1973; Schenk et al., 1974).

Kreuzer et al. (1973) found less change in patients undergoing cardiac catheterization with slow injection (7 mg/kg over 60 sec) than after rapid injection (over 30 sec) both in the initial increase in heart rate, cardiac output and dP/dt_{max} right ventricle and in the decrease which followed. Control levels were reached after 1–3 min except for dP/dt_{max} which decreased by 15% in the 1st–3rd min and attained the control level by the 8th min. Schenk et al. (1974) in an investigation in 7 patients found that coronary blood flow and myocardial oxygen-consumption increased significantly while coronary venous oxygen-saturation increased only slightly. It is concluded that the use of propanidid in patients with myocardial insufficiency is contraindicated.

Allergic anaphylactoid reactions

Incidence
Severe anaphylactoid reactions of varying degree have been reported. In a completely documented series the frequency varied from 1 : 1,000–1 : 10,000 and was mostly about 1 : 5,000–1 : 6,000. It is remarkable that Harrfeldt (1970, 1973) observed no allergic reaction in the first 35,000 administrations of propanidid and then until 45,000 anaesthetics with propanidid 4 allergic reactions were seen.

Allergic reactions occur more frequently at a second administration after an interval of 2–3 weeks. In the literature 9 cases were found, where anaphylactoid reactions occurred at a second administration of propanidid 1–3 weeks after an uneventful anaesthesia with propanidid. All patients had invasive carcinoma of the cervix and were treated with local administration of radium (Manz and Fank, 1969; Dannemann and Lübke, 1970; Kruger, 1970; Stovner and Endresen, 1971).

Signs
The clinical signs are variable and include flush, exanthema, Quincke-oedema, oedema of the galea, bronchospasm with or without hypotension, tachycardia and eventually respiratory and cardiac arrest; abdominal and chest pain are rare.

Treatment
The treatment depends on the severity of the reaction. But in all reactions corticosteroids

should be given immediately at the first symptoms (prednisolone 50–100 mg, dexamethasone 15–20 mg). It blocks the release of histamine both from endothelial cells and mast cells. At the same time ample fluid (Ringer lactate) should be infused remembering that each millimeter of thickening of the skin by oedema represents one litre of fluid per square metre surface area. Antihistamines, which block the effect of histamine at the H_1-receptors, and calcium have been recommended.

Hypotension is treated by Adrenalin – the functional antagonist of histamine – as drip or with a powered syringe. If bradycardia and bronchospasm are present, isoprenaline (Isuprel®), and orciprenaline (Alupent®) are preferred. Other measures, artificial ventilation with oxygen and external cardiac compression are performed as indicated and infusion of sodium bicarbonate if hypotension is prolonged.

Role of the solvent Cremophor EL

Since adverse reactions to the new intravenous anaesthetic Althesin have been reported which are similar to propanidid reactions, the possibility that the common solvent Cremophor EL is the cause, has been suggested by Horton (1973).

Mehta (1973) described some patients who had an erythematous rash, hypotension and cyanosis after 3 ml of Althesin. Intradermal tests were positive to both Althesin and the pure solvent Cremophor EL, the latter causing a greater reaction.

Another reaction after 5 ml of Althesin was reported by Notcutt (1973) in a girl who had received propanidid previously.

A reaction is possible only to propanidid but not to the solvent or to Althesin (Dundee et al., 1974) – this happened to a consultant anaesthetist who was sensitized to propanidid and showed repeated facial swelling on exposure.

Every patient who has an adverse reaction to propanidid should also have tests with the solvent Cremophor EL.

CONTRAINDICATIONS

Heart failure, coronary insufficiency, marked hypertension, shock and history of allergic reactions are contraindications. Epileptic conditions must be added to the list since the recent publication of Barron (1974). In conditions with high histamine-levels such as burns, sepsis, large abscesses, chronic suppuration, extensive malignancies or after irradiation, propanidid is contraindicated unless a prophylactic premedication with corticosteroids is given. Antihistamines are not always protective (Lorenz et al., 1972).

In patients under treatment with adrenergic β-receptor blockers propanidid may cause a total atrio-ventricular block.

CONCLUSION

The place of any drug has to be evaluated on the basis of careful and correct administration in relation to its pharmacological properties. In propanidd this includes: (1) dose-adjustment according to the tolerance of the patient; (2) avoidance of acute overdose by very slow injection; (3) avoidance of hypoxaemia; and (4) proper indication and observation of contraindications.

If these precautions are observed, it can be said that propanidid continues to be a valuable anaesthetic agent giving excellent amnesia and analgesia for short procedures, especially in out-patients. It has no equal in rapid and complete recovery. The above contraindications should be strictly observed. Anyone who uses propanidid should be prepared and able to cope with the adverse reactions. It is hoped that a new solvent will be found which has no allergic properties.

REFERENCES

Barron, D. W. (1974): *Anaesthesia, 29,* 445.

Dannemann, H. and Lübke, P. (1970): *Z. prakt. Anästh. Wiederbeleb., 5,* 273.

Dudziak, R., Raff, K. W. and Kosche, F. (1973): In: *Anaesthesiologie und Wiederbelebung, Vol. 74,* p. 51. Springer-Verlag, Berlin – Heidelberg – New York.

Dundee, J. W., Assem, E. S. K., Gaston, J. M., Keilty, S. R., Sutton, J. A., Clarke, R. S. J. and Grainger, D. (1974): *Brit. med. J., 1,* 63.

Harrfeldt, H. P. (1970): *Z. prakt. Anästh. Wiederbeleb., 5,* 55.

Harrfeldt, H. P. (1973): In: *Anaesthesiologie und Wiederbelebung, Vol. 74,* p. 234. Springer-Verlag, Berlin – Heidelberg – New York.

Hempelmann, G., Hartmann, W., Reichelt, H. and Hempelmann, W. (1972): *Anaesthesist, 21,* 40.

Horten, J. N. (1973): *Anaesthesia, 28,* 182.

Kreuzer, H., Mertens, H.-M., Spiller, P. and Dudziak, R. (1973): In: *Anaesthesiologie und Wiederbelebung, Vol. 74,* p. 88. Springer-Verlag, Berlin – Heidelberg – New York.

Krüger, H. W. (1970): *Geburtsh. u. Frauenheilk., 30,* 37.

Lennartz, H. and Siepmann, H. P. (1973): In: *Anaesthesiologie und Wiederbelebung, Vol. 74,* p. 40. Springer-Verlag, Berlin – Heidelberg – New York.

Lorenz, W., Doenicke, A., Meyer, R., Reimann, H. J., Kusche, J., Barth, H., Geesing, H., Hutzel, M. and Weissenbacher, B. (1972): *Brit. J. Anaesth., 44,* 355.

Manz, R. and Fank, G. (1969): *Anaesthesist, 18,* 223.

Mehta, S. (1973): *Anaesthesia, 28,* 669.

Notcutt, W. G. (1973): *Anaesthesia, 28,* 673.

Reichel, G., Podlesch, I., Ulmer, W. T. and Zindler, M. (1965): *Anaesthesist, 14,* 184.

Schenk, H.-D., Sonntag, H., Kettler, D., Regensburger, D., Donath, U., Kotseronid, J. and Bretschneider, H. J. (1974): *Anaesthesist, 23,* 105.

Soga, D., Beer, R., Andrae, J. and Bader, B. (1973): In: *Anaesthesiologie und Wiederbelebung, Vol. 74,* p. 27. Springer-Verlag, Berlin – Heidelberg – New York.

Stovner, J. and Endresen, R. (1971): *Brit. J. Anaesth., 43,* 207.

Cardiovascular effects of etomidate

MARTIN ZINDLER

Department of Anaesthesiology, University of Dusseldorf,
Dusseldorf, Federal Republic of Germany

Etomidate has only negligible effects on the heart and the circulation in contrast to all other intravenous anaesthetics. This statement is based on 4 recent investigations which are briefly reviewed.

ANIMAL EXPERIMENTS

Weymar et al. (1974) gave etomidate to dogs consecutively in doses of 0.1 mg/kg (n = 7) 0.2 mg/kg (n=9), 0.4 mg/kg (n=9), 0.8 mg/kg (n=17), 1.6 mg/kg (n=8). The duration of sleep after 0.8 mg/kg etomidate is 5 min, this may be compared with a dose of about 0.3–0.4 mg/kg in humans. No dose-effect relation could be found with the exception of a dose-related slight increase of the pressure in the pulmonary artery (see Fig. 1).

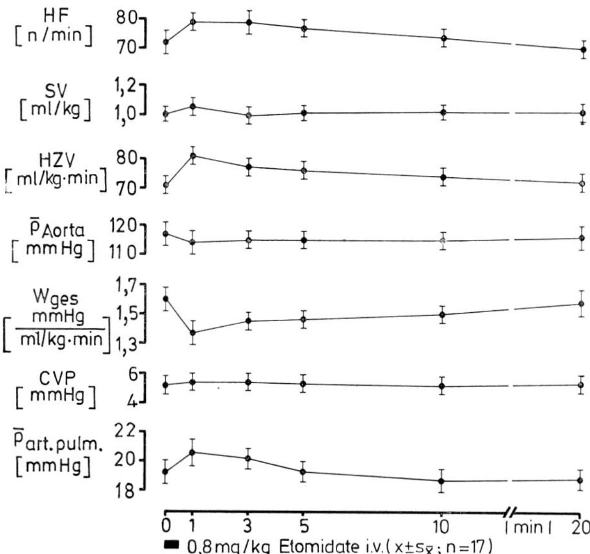

Fig. 1. *Effect of 0.8 mg/kg etomidate in 17 dogs (mean and standard deviation) on heart rate (HF), stroke volume (SV), cardiac output (HZV), mean pressure aorta (P̄ aorta), total peripheral resistance (W ges), central venous pressure (CVP) and mean pulmonary arterial pressure (P̄ art. pulm.). (From Weymar et al., 1974.)*

The dogs were under anaesthesia with 3 mg/kg piritramide (Dipidolor®) – a synthetic opiate – and muscle relaxation with 4 mg/kg diallylnortoxiferine (Alloferin®); controlled ventilation with oxygen was used and anaesthesia was maintained during preparation with 1 mg/kg piritramide and 0.1 mg/kg Alloferin as needed.

Etomidate caused only slight changes: heart rate increased from 72–79 ($p < 0.0125$), a rise of cardiac output from 71–80 ml/kg/min ($p < 0.01$), mean pressure aorta fell from 117–114 mm Hg ($p < 0.025$), both resulting in slight decrease of total peripheral resistance; central venous pressure did not change and the mean pulmonary artery pressure rose slightly from 19–21 mm Hg ($p < 0.01$) (see Fig. 2).

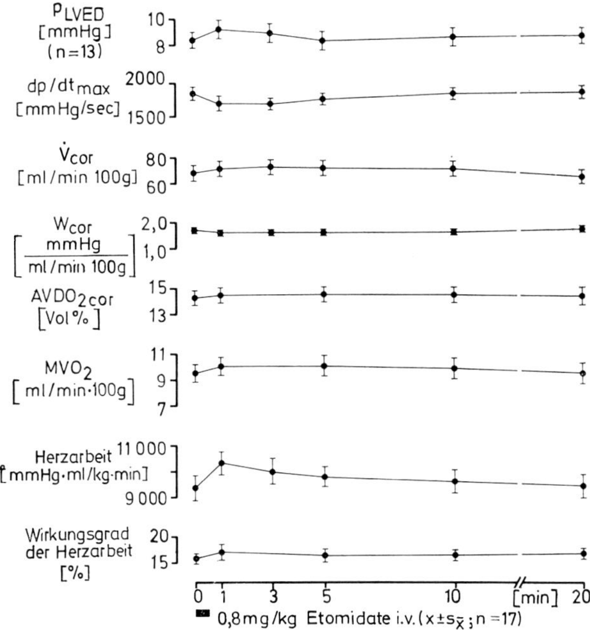

Fig. 2.   *Effect of 0.8 mg/kg etomidate in 17 dogs (mean and standard deviation) of left ventricular end-diastolic pressure (P_{LVED}), dP/dt_{max}, coronary outflow ($\dot{V}_{cor}$), coronary resistance (W_{cor}), arterio-coronary venous oxygen consumption ($M\dot{V}O_2$), external cardiac work (Herzarbeit) and efficiency of cardiac work (Wirkungsgrad der Herzarbeit). (From Weymar et al., 1974.)*

The left ventricular end-diastolic pressure rose from 8–9 mm Hg ($p < 0.05$), dP/dt_{max}, left ventricle decreased slightly by 100–150, mean 130 mm Hg/sec^{-5} ($p < 0.01$).

Coronary perfusion was unchanged and the myocardial oxygen extraction rose from 9.5–10 ml O_2/min $\times$ 100 g ($p < 0.025$). It is remarkable that the external cardiac work increased a little more than the oxygen extraction, so that the efficiency of the heart (calorie energy equivalent) increased slightly from 16–17%.

INVESTIGATION IN HUMANS

This lack of cardiovascular depression was confirmed in 5 patients by the investigation of Kettler et al. (1974). Anaesthesia was induced with 0.3 mg/kg etomidate and maintained for 10 min with additional small doses or by an infusion at a dose of 0.12 mg/kg/min, which is a total dose of 12 mg/kg.

Compared with awake controls without premedication, with the exception of a slight rise in heart rate from 81–88 and in cardiac index from 3.44–3.93 l/min m² (+ 14%) no essential haemodynamic changes were found in mean pressure of aorta, stroke volume, left ventricular end-diastolic pressure, and dP/dt_{max}. Total peripheral resistance was calculated to decrease slightly by 12%.

While coronary perfusion pressure remained unchanged, the coronary perfusion increased by 19% and the coronary arteriovenous difference in O_2-content decreased slightly from 11.8–10.5 vol %.

All changes were statistically significant except the minimal increase in myocardial O_2-consumption from 10.5–11.1 ml/min × 100 g.

Similar results were just published by Brückner et al. (1974). In 8 patients during anaesthesia with nitrous oxide and halothane 0.3%, they also found that 0.3 mg/kg etomidate caused only minimal effects on the cardiovascular system – a slight decrease of the heart rate by 4.2%, but a slight increase of the cardiac index by 4.3% and a decrease of the mean arterial pressure by 14.3%, a decrease of total peripheral resistance by 17.3%, and dP/dt_{max} decreased by 9.4%.

HEART-LUNG PREPARATION

In man and in the intact animal the effects of anaesthetics on the heart are the combination of the direct effect on the myocardium and of compensatory extracardiac effects.

Fischer and Marquort (1974) tested, in a heart-lung preparation of the cat, the direct effect of etomidate on inotropic and chronotropic parameters, thus excluding extracardiac nervous and humoral factors.

The maximal rise of left ventricular pressure with constant preload, afterload and heart rate and ventricular function curves (cardiac index – here aortic flow/kg – versus right atrial filling) with increasing preload, increasing afterload and increasing the heart rate by a pace-maker were investigated.

Inotropic or chronotropic changes were found when doses beyond the clinical range were used. After 3.6 mg/kg etomidate (which is 9-times the sleep-inducing dose) the dP/dt_{max} was depressed by 25% and the heart could deal with increased preload, increased afterload or increased rate more effectively than following similar depression by halothane.

It was concluded that following overdose no depression of cardiac function is to be expected, because the therapeutic index (effective to toxic dose) is 1:20 and is large compared with 1:2–1:4 for barbiturates. In the isolated heart-lung preparation all anaesthetic agents, including ketamine, have significant depressive effect on the heart; the only exceptions are morphine and the opiates. Etomidate has no deleterious effect on the cardiovascular system and slightly improves the energy utilization of the heart.

This is in contrast to all other intravenous agents which are either depressive, like the barbiturates and propanidid or excitatory, like ketamine and Althesin, which increase the O_2-consumption of the heart and decrease its efficiency.

CLINICAL ASPECTS

Etomidate can especially be recommended for high-risk patients with decreased cardiovascular reserve and with coronary insufficiency.

Since it is only a short-acting hypnotic with no analgesic action, etomidate by itself is only suitable for procedures without much pain but combined with a small dose of fentanyl 0.1–0.15 mg and N_2O, can be very useful for short procedures

But it can be argued that the lack of cardiovascular depression has been proven only in dogs and cats and patients in good condition. What really matters is the high-risk patient with severely restricted cardiac reserves, coronary insufficiency or in shock.

During induction of neuroleptanalgesia with etomidate in patients with heart disease for valve replacement, a severe drop in arterial pressure was sometimes observed. It is difficult to prove which of the drugs used, droperidol, fentanyl or etomidate, is responsible for the depression of the arterial pressure and whether the cardiac output is also dangerously decreased.

Using an aortic pulse contour method, where the cardiac output can be monitored *continuously*, with a small computer integrating 5 beats (*This Volume*, p. 631), this problem was investigated. In order to distinguish between the individual drug effects, first 0.3 mg/kg etomidate followed after 10 min by 0.002 mg/kg droperidol and after an interval of 5 min, 0.0015 mg/kg fentanyl, followed 1 min later by 0.3 mg/kg etomidate and succinylcholine, for endotracheal intubation were given.

In 3 patients with valvular heart disease (AHA Class III–IV) and 3 old patients for hip surgery, during the first test run with 0.3 mg/kg etomidate no essential changes in cardiac output, arterial pressure, central venous pressure and mean pressure of the pulmonary artery were observed. Droperidol caused no or only a slight decrease in arterial pressure with no essential change in cardiac output, whereas, when fentanyl caused bradycardia, both arterial pressure and cardiac output decreased. This could be corrected by atropine or if necessary by small doses of orciprenaline (Alupent®). The only marked depression of arterial pressure and of the cardiac output occurred when artificial ventilation had to be started after succinylcholine. This hypotension is only short-lasting, since laryngoscopy and intubation cause, as a rule, tachycardia and a rise in arterial pressure and cardiac output.

It may be concluded that in the induction of anaesthesia, etomidate has less depressing effects than other intravenous anaesthetic agents. It is unknown yet if the combination of etomidate with droperidol, both decreasing the total peripheral resistance, may be unfavourable in high-risk patients.

CONCLUSION

The intravenous hypnotic etomidate has the unusual property that it has no essential adverse effect on the heart and the circulation.

This advantage seems to be particularly valuable for induction of anaesthesia in cardiovascular risk patients. It is especially recommended as the agent of choice in combination with intermittently given fentanyl for the difficult problem of emergency anaesthesia in acute bleeding with haemorrhagic shock. Droperidol should never be given unless it is made absolutely certain that hypovolaemia is more than corrected.

REFERENCES

Brückner, J. B., Gethmann, J. W., Patschke, D., Tarnow, J. and Weymar, A. (1974): *Anaesthesist*, *23/8*, 322.

Fischer, K. J. and Marquort, H. (1974): In: *Probleme der Intravenösen Anaesthesie Symposion, Bremen, 1974*. Schattauer-Verlag, Stuttgart – New York. In press.

Kettler, D., Sonntag, H., Donath, U., Regensburger, D. and Schenk, H. D. (1974): *Anaesthesist*, *23/3*, 116.

Weymar, A., Eigenheer, F., Gethmann, J. W., Reinecke, A., Patschke, D., Tarnow, J. and Brückner, J. B. (1974): *Anaesthesist, 23/3*, 150.

Flunitrazepam (Rohypnol) as the only hypnotic agent during general anaesthesia

R. RIZZI, G. BUTERA and M. L. VENDRAMIN

The Vicenza Regional Hospital, Vicenza, Italy

Any drug employed in clinical anaesthesia, following a more or less prolonged period of clinical experimentation, is later either eliminated from our practise or initial enthusiasm is diminished, inasmuch as it is not possible to ignore the conclusions reached by every anaesthetist. Following the introduction of thiopentone sodium, which represented a remarkable advance in anaesthesiology, there were many research projects with the aim of synthesizing a hypnotic drug showing the same advantages, but with fewer disadvantages.

There is a new benzodiazepine which is a hypnotic, with subcortical action in the limbic system. This aspect, in addition to the cardiocirculatory stability and the assumed absence of hepatorenal toxicity, induced us to perform a thorough clinical evaluation of this new drug in anaesthesia. The pharmacodynamic properties of flunitrazepam are well-known. Contrary to the practise of most authors, we (Rizzi and Butera, 1973*a, b*) administered flunitrazepam to replace barbiturates and the various vapors for induction and maintenance. Our initial trial involved a standard technique of hypnosis with flunitrazepam, analgesia with pentazocine, and muscle relaxation with d-tubocurarine.

933 anaesthesias were studied which lasted between 10 and 320 min. The subsequent stage aimed to study those parameters not examined at first stage, analyzing thoroughly some aspects which were thought to be undecided, but in particular to determine which analgetic (pentazocine or fentanyl), and which muscle relaxant (d-tubocurarine, Alloferine, or pancuronium) was most suitable for combination with flunitrazepam.

From 28th October 1972 to 31st May 1974 we performed 1355 anaesthesias in all fields of surgery, except cardiac with extracorporeal circulation (Table 1). The ages ranged between 15 months and 91 years old. Only long duration anaesthetics were studied – the longest was 455 min (Fig. 1). The premedication given is shown in Table 2 for comparison with our earlier studies and those of other authors.

The data reported are exclusively concerned with the comparison of the use of the 3 drugs in the various combinations. It was not possible to complete the full number of anaesthetics proposed, and therefore a complete statistical analysis was not performed. Data concerning operations lasting more than 50 min in patients over 18 years of age are available and are grouped according to age, duration and type of anaesthesia. Owing to the few cases studied, it was not possible to obtain statistically reliable data for pancuronium with pentazocine or fentanyl, but the results are nevertheless indicated in the tables. A 2-way analysis of variance, a χ^2 test and the orthogonal partition test of Lancaster when appropriate (internal correlation of homogeneous groups) were performed.

In Table 3 two groups according to age, and 3 groups according to the duration of anaesthesia, are shown. The analysis shows an increase ($p < 0.001$) in the doses of flunitrazepam and pentazocine, according to duration, and a reduced average dose of

Table 1. *Distribution of 1,355 cases of anaesthesias according to surgery performed between October, 1972 and May, 1974*

	d-tubocurarine		Alloferine		Pancuronium		No	Total
	Pentazocine	Fentanyl	Pentazocine	Fentanyl	Pentazocine	Fentanyl	curarization	
Neurosurgery	–	–	4	2	5	–	–	11
Maxilofacial surgery	27	37	19	15	13	18	2	131
Neck surgery	33	2	–	2	–	–	–	37
Thoracic surgery	41	1	1	3	1	2	2	51
Abdominal surgery	194	28	5	5	–	2	–	234
Gynaecological surgery	37	21	8	11	1	1	4	83
Urological surgery	6	1	–	1	2	2	–	12
Vascular surgery	30	1	–	–	–	–	–	31
Plastic surgery	32	7	–	3	3	–	6	51
Orthopaedic surgery	21	52	4	1	–	1	28	107
Radiological investigation	–	–	–	–	–	–	168	168
Curettages	–	–	–	–	–	–	411	411
Miscellaneous (ESH, CDV etc.)	–	–	–	–	–	–	28	28
Total	421	150	41	43	25	26	649	1,355

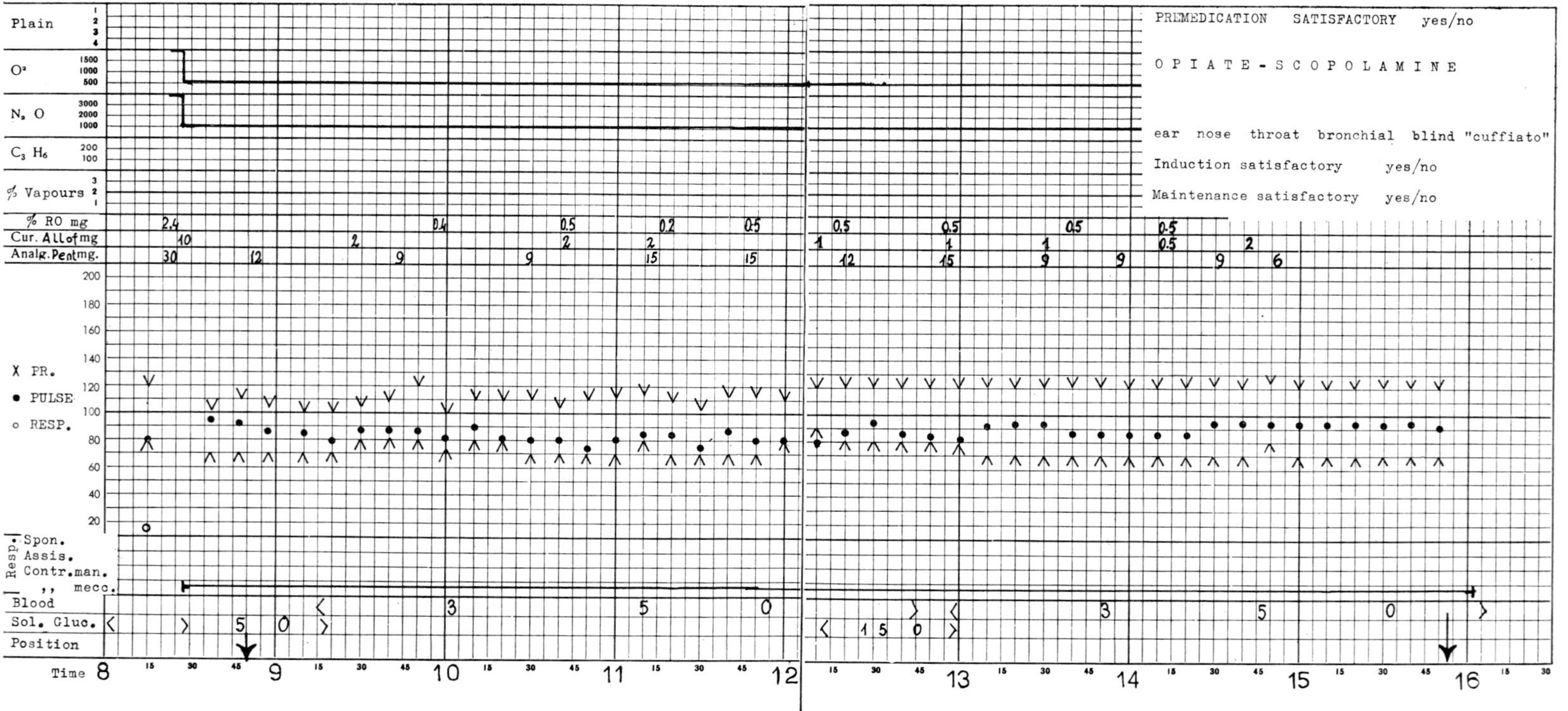

Fig. 1. *Study of long duration anaesthetics.*

Table 2. *Premedication*

No drug	10
Atropine	43
Diazepam or dihydrobenzoperidole-atropine-fentanyl	175
Atropine-morphine	118
Atropine-rectal thiopental	17
Opiate-scopolamine	739
Promethazine-methyl-prednisolone-atropine	145
Meperidine-promethazine-ergotoxine	35
Morphine-atropine-rectal thiopental	31
Promethazine-atropine-meperidine	42
	1,355

Table 3. *Distribution of cases according to age (2 groups) and duration of anaesthesia (3 groups) – using pentazocine*

Age (yr)	No. of cases	Rohypnol (mg)	d-tubocurarine (mg)	Pentazocine (mg)	Duration (min)
< 55	245	2.142 **	19.432 n.s.	41.938 **	
> 55	85	1.817	17.616	38.558	50–150
Total	330	2.058	18.960	41.060	
< 55	21	3.200 **	32.571 n.s.	78.238 *	
> 55	8	2.700	31.500	64.125	151–300
Total	29	3.062 ***	32.275 ***	74.344 ***	
< 55	1	4.300	25.000	80.000	
> 55	–	–	–	–	> 300
Total	1	4.300	25.000	80.000	
Final total	360	2.144	20.047	43.842	

* $P < 0.05$; ** $P < 0.01$; *** $P < 0.001$; n.s. = not significant; n.e. = not evaluated.

both drugs with increasing age ($p < 0.01$). For d-tubocurarine the significance is seen only in relation to the duration ($p < 0.001$) and not to age.

The decreased dosage of flunitrazepam with increasing age is more significant when fentanyl is used in place of pentazocine (see Table 4). Again the dosage of all 3 drugs increased with the increase in duration of anaesthesia; on the other hand, only the dosage of the analgesic and hypnotic decrease with increasing age. On further analysis of these findings in relation to 3 groups of age, it is confirmed that there is always a very striking ($p < 0.001$) difference for flunitrazepam, while for the analgesic the significance is absent or decreased and it never occurs with d-tubocurarine (Table 5).

More or less similar results were obtained for Alloferin with pentazocine (Table 6) or with fentanyl (Table 7) and for pancuronium associated with pentazocine (Table 8) or with fentanyl (Table 9), even though the number of cases is still too small to enable us to come to confident conclusions. It seems however that the tendency is similar.

Table 4. *Distribution of cases according to age (2 groups) and duration of anaesthesia (3 groups) – using fentanyl*

Age (yr)	No. of cases	Rohypnol (mg)	d-tubocurarine (mg)	Fentanyl (mg)	Duration (min)
< 55	72	2.664	21.556	0.183	
		***	n.s.	**	
> 55	17	1.976	20.647	0.159	50–150
Total	89	2.512	21.395	0.176	
< 55	12	3.458	29.250	0.340	
		n.e.	n.e.	n.e.	
> 55	1	3.500	35.000	0.450	151–300
Total	13	3.461 ***	29.692 ***	0.348 ***	
< 55	4	6.175	32.250	0.600	
> 55	–	–	–	–	> 300
Total	4	6.175	32.250	0.600	
Final total	106	2.776	22.734	0.213	

* P< 0.05; ** P< 0.01; *** P< 0.001; n.s. = not significant; n.e. = not evaluated.

Table 5. *Further analysis in relation to 3 groups of age*

Age (yr)	No. of cases	Rohypnol (mg)	d-tubocurarine (mg)	Pentazocine (mg)
17–40	53	2.186	21.905	0.179
		*	n.s.	n.s.
41–60	31	2.324 *	20.789	0.177 *
		*	n.s.	
> 60	12	1.891	20.612	0.158 *
Total	96	2.542	21.395	0.176
17–40	151	2.273	19.761	42.483
		*	n.s.	*
41–60	109	1.926 *	18.706	40.807 *
		*	n.s.	
> 60	71	1.801	17.647	38.422
Total	331	2.058	18.960	41.060

* P< 0.05; ** P< 0.01; *** P< 0.001; n.s. = not significant.

In Table 10 the consumption of the various drugs in relation to the duration of anaesthesia and body surface independent of age is presented. The dosage of flunitrazepam and the analgesic is less when Alloferine is used than where the other 2 muscle relaxants are used, particularly when pentazocine is employed.

None of these findings are significant; examining the consumption of the various drugs, it is clear that there is a remarkable homogeneity (from 0.017–0.023), with a maximum

Table 6. *Results obtained by using Rohypnol in combination with Alloferine and pentazocine, the cases divided according to age (2 groups) and duration of anaesthesia (3 groups)*

Age (yr)	No. of cases	Rohypnol (mg)	Alloferine (mg)	Pentazocine (mg)	Duration (min)
< 55	14	2.435	10.928	54.214	
		***	n.s.	***	
> 55	5	1.720	11.000	26.400	50–150
Total	19	2.247	10.947	46.894	
< 55	5	3.140	17.200	75.400	
		n.s.	n.s.	n.s.	
> 55	6	3.066	18.833	67.500	151–300
Total	11	3.100 ***	18.090 ***	71.090 ***	
< 55	5	5.120	21.800	129.000	
> 55	–	–	–	–	> 300
Total	5	5.120	21.800	129.000	
Final total	35	2.925	14.722	66.228	

*** P < 0.001; n.s. = not significant.

Table 7. *Results obtained by using Rohypnol in combination with Alloferine and fentanyl, the cases divided according to age (2 groups) and duration of anaesthesia (3 groups)*

Age (yr)	No. of cases	Rohypnol (mg)	Alloferine (mg)	Fentanyl (mg)	Duration (min)
< 55	19	2.526	11.842	0.150	
		n.s.	n.s.	n.s.	
> 55	7	2.428	11.000	0.157	50–150
Total	26	2.500	11.615	0.152	
< 55	3	4.233	19.333	0.480	
		n.e.	n.e.	n.e.	
> 55	1	4.000	24.000	0.650	151–300
Total	4	4.175 ***	20.500 ***	0.522 ***	
< 55	3	4.200	21.000	0.500	
> 55	–	–	–	–	> 300
Total	3	4.200	21.000	0.500	
Final total	33	2.857	13.545	0.228	

*** P < 0.001; n.s. = not significant; n.e. = not evaluated.

Table 8. *Results obtained by using Rohypnol in combination with pancuronium and pentazocine, the cases divided according to age (2 groups) and duration of anaesthesia (3 groups)*

Age (yr)	No. of cases	Rohypnol (mg)	Pancuronium (mg)	Pentazocine (mg)	Duration (min)
< 55	9	2.411	6.411	70.222	
		**	n.s.	**	
> 55	4	1.800	5.800	51.000	50–150
Total	13	2.223	6.223	64.307	
< 55	1	5.000	13.000	120.000	
> 55	–	–	–	–	151–300
Total	1	5.000 n.e.	13.000 n.e.	120.000 n.e.	
< 55	1	3.200	10.000	111.000	
> 55	–	–	–	–	> 300
Total	1	3.200	10.000	111.000	
Final total	15	2.473	6.926	71.133	

** $P < 0.01$; n.e. = not evaluated; n.s. = not significant.

Table 9. *Results obtained by using Rohypnol in combination with pancuronium with fentanyl, the cases divided according to age (2 groups) and duration of anaesthesia (3 groups)*

Age (yr)	No. of cases	Rohypnol (mg)	Pancuronium (mg)	Fentanyl (mg)	Duration (min)
< 55	5	3.640	6.800	0.164	
		n.e.	n.e.	n.e.	
> 55	2	1.800	5.100	0.115	50–150
Total	7	2.542	6.314	0.150	
< 55	3	3.866	5.000	0.416	
		n.e.	n.e.	n.e.	
> 55	3	2.760	6.666	0.416	151–300
Total	6	3.316 n.e.	5.850 n.e.	0.416 n.e.	
< 55	2	5.750	9.000	0.875	
> 55	–	–	–	–	> 300
Total	2	5.750	9.000	0.875	
Final total	15	3.273	6.466	0.353	

n.e. = not evaluated.

Table 10. *Consumption of the various drugs in relation to the duration of anaesthesia and body surface independent of age*

(a)

Analysis	No. of cases	Mean time (min)	Rohypnol	Pentazocine	Fentanyl	d-tubocurarine	Alloferine	Pancuronium
Table 3	361	91	0.023560	0.48178	–	0.22029	–	–
Table 4	113	117	0.023726	–	0.0018205	0.19430	–	–
Table 6	35	170	0.017205	0.38957	–	–	0.08671	–
Table 7	33	133	0.021481	–	0.0017142	–	0.10184	–
Table 8	15	140	0.017664	0.50809	–	–	–	0.049471
Table 9	15	181	0.018082	–	0.0019502	–	–	0.035723

(b) Rohypnol

Analysis	Mean body surface	mg/min body surface	Mean age	Range	mg age/min body surface
Table 3	109.35	0.00021545	36	18–61	0.0077563
Table 4	112.33	0.00021116	38	19–65	0.0080241
Table 6	101.59	0.00016930	48	20–81	0.0081267
Table 7	110.81	0.00019384	40	18–68	0.0077538
Table 8	103.59	0.00017047	45	19–69	0.0076715
Table 9	105.71	0.00017103	44	20–91	0.0075254

average difference of 15–16%; these differences are further reduced (to 10–14%) when allowing for surface area differences. Complete homogeneity might be found if the effect of age were included; on the average this is higher in the C–E and F groups.

CONCLUSIONS

On the basis of the above results, the following conclusions may be drawn:
1.   Flunitrazepam can fully substitute for thiopentone and the inhaled anaesthetics in any surgical operation. In 3 cases halogenated hydrocarbons were used: having given 3.5 mg flunitrazepam in 320 min, which was thought to be excessive, the technique was abandoned; secondly, to lower the systolic pressure; and the third case was a child in whom venepuncture was impossible.
2.   Total dosage should be reduced according to the age of the patient, particularly over 60 years.
3.   Weight and body surface area are not determining factors regarding dosage.
4.   Dosage must be reduced when ganglion block is performed (Arfonad).
5.   In this series the analgesic component of the premedication, and the use of the analgetic during maintenance was essential and is in contrast to the practise of Vega (1971). In the few cases where 2–2.5 mg flunitrazepam was not sufficient for hypnosis, this occurred rapidly following 30 mg pentazocine or 0.05–0.10 mg fentanyl. Our highest dosage of flunitrazepam was 8 mg over 355 min and in patients used to psychotropic drugs or in alcoholic subjects.
6.   The synergism between flunitrazepam and central analgetics is confirmed. Muscular relaxation is also evident; this is shown by spirometry before and after the administration of flunitrazepam, with the same curarization, so as to see at once a remarkable decrease in minute volume. Synergism is shown both at the respiratory centre level and at the pain threshold – this could be confirmed by the comparison of these dosages with those of Vega (1971, 1972).
7.   Flunitrazepam has a long duration of action and there are no contraindications, provided that the anaesthetist employs it in suitable dosage in combination with other drugs to constitute a balanced anaesthetic, in order to avoid delayed awakening which might, in some circumstances, be a disadvantage.

REFERENCES

Coleman, A. J., Downing, J. W., Moyes, D. G. and O'Brien, A. (1972): *Paper presented at:* Anaesthetic Congress, Isando, 1972.
De Blasi, S., Dalfano, L., Brienza, A., Fiore, T. and Carreras, B. (1973): *Minerva Anest.*, *39*, 559.
De Castro, J. (1972*a*): *Paper presented at:* Congreso Mundial de Anestesiologia, Japon, Kyoto, 1972.
De Castro, J. (1972*b*): *Ars Med.*, *8*, 1233.
De Castro, J. (1972*c*): *Ars Med.*, *8*, 1286.
De Castro, J. (1972*d*): *Ars Med.*, *8*, 1305.
Del Nero, R. R., Saviano, A., Canneiro, A. P. and Tellini, J. T. C. (1973): *Rev. bras. Anest.*, *23*, 79.
De Oliveira, A. A. M. and Duarte, D. F. (1973): *Rev. bras. Anest.*, *23*, 72.
Dos Santos, C. B. and Goncalves, B. (1973): *Rev. bras. Anest.*, *23*, 61.
Feldman, S. A. and Crawley, B. E. (1970): *Brit. med. J.*, *2*, 336.
Freuchen, I. B. and Ostergaard, J. (1973): In: *Proceedings, XI Congress of the Society of Anesthesiologists, Reykjiavik, 1973.*
Lecron, L., Levy, I., Collard, C., Delville, F. and Toppet, E. (1972): *Ars Med.*, *8, 1269.*
Pizarro Suarez, H. and Torres Larios, C. (1973): *Paper presented at:* Segundo Congreso Europeo de Narco-Odontoestomatologia, Bologna, 1973.

Polisena, A. A. and Sando, O. (1972): *Paper presented at:* XI Jornadas Argentinas de Anestesiologiae, Córdoba, 1972.

Rizzi, R. and Butera, G. (1973*a*): *Minerva Anest.*, *39*, 321.

Rizzi, R. and Butera, G. (1973*b*): *Paper presented at:* XIII Gemeinsame Tagung der Deutschen Schweizerischen und Österreichischen Gesellschaft für Anaesthesiologie und Reanimation, Linz, 1973.

Stovner, J., Endresen, R. and Østerud, A. (1973): *Acta anaesth. scand.*, *17*, 163.

Ungerer, M. J. and Erasmus, F. R. (1972): *Paper presented at:* Anaesthetic Congress, Johannesburg, 1972.

Vega, D. E. (1971): *Rev. urug. Anest.*, *5*, 41.

Vega, D. E. (1972): Tecnica de Anestesia General Andovenosa Utilizando una Nueva Benzodiazepina (RO 5–4200), Succinilcolina y Procaina. *Submitted for publication.*

Neuroleptanesthesia for neonates and infants

B. KAY

Derby Group of Hospitals, Derby, United Kingdom

Anesthesia for very small children has always posed exceptional problems of apparatus, technic, and method. It is an area where anesthesiologists have been traditionally reluctant to apply recent advances and have clung to the obsolete, often to the detriment of the child.

Even the use of ether still persists despite its general toxicity, slow and difficult inductions, and occasional hyperthermia and convulsions. Cyclopropane is similarly dangerous, frequently producing laryngeal spasm, cardiac arrhythmias, vasoconstriction, and poor relaxation. Halothane is generally used now, although the combination of vasodilatation and decreased cardiac output can produce sudden and dangerous hypotension in the neonate. Acute hypotension leading to cardiac arrest is still the major cause of operative mortality in the neonate.

Cardiovascular stability, however, is one of the major features of anesthesia with droperidol and fentanyl (Holderness et al., 1963), and the technic is frequently recommended for use in the poor-risk patient (Corssen et al., 1964). This cardiovascular stability is based on the effectiveness of a large dose of fentanyl in reducing cardiovascular responses to pain, and the maintenance of a constant intravascular space after extensive α-adrenergic blockade by droperidol, which also has an antiarrhythmic effect (Bertolo et al., 1972). Neither drug is cardiotoxic (Zauder et al., 1965; Kreuscher, 1966).

These conditions lead to stabilizing factors not seen in other forms of anesthesia. Prevention of peripheral constriction helps to maintain tissue blood flow and normal blood pH and gas tensions. Renal hemodynamics are unaffected (Gorman and Craythome, 1966), and a diuretic response to excess infusion occurs more readily than under conventional light anesthesia (Kay, 1972). This safety factor allows an aggressive infusion regime, with less chance of underinfusion or overloading. Finally, the technic does not increase cerebro-spinal fluid tension (Miller and Barker, 1969), and the agents are not hepatotoxic (Tornetta and Boger, 1964).

For these reasons I conducted a clinical trial of the use of neuroleptanesthesia in neonates and infants.

METHOD

One hundred children were included in the trial, 31 neonates (under 10 days) with a mean weight of 2.7 kg, of which 14 were premature (under 2.25 kg), the smallest weighing 1.4 kg. The other 69 were under 18 months old and had a mean weight of 7.12 kg. The distribution of operations performed is seen in Table 1. All operations were of a major category, and I would not use the technic on a patient where the operation was expected to last for less than 1 hour.

A similar method was used throughout, varying only in detail. An intravenous infusion was started at operation, except for the few patients already being infused. In infants a

Table 1. *Distribution of operations*

100 children (1.4–9 kg)	Operations performed
31 neonates (under 10 days; mean weight 2.7 kg. Of these 14 premature, under 2.25 kg)	8 intestinal obstruction 6 tracheoesophageal fistula 4 exomphalos 7 meningocele 2 nephrectomy 1 ureteric transplant 3 imperforate anus
69 infants (under 18 months; mean weight 7.12 kg)	Mainly operations on kidney, ureter, or colon pull-through

percutaneous cannula was generally used, in neonates an umbilical catheter or scalp vein needle. No premedication was given.

Induction of anesthesia was preceded by a rapid infusion of lactated Ringer's solution, into which was given rapidly 0.3 mg/kg of droperidol, 0.01 mg/kg of fentanyl, and 0.06–0.2 mg of atropine, according to weight and age. After about 30 sec, when these drugs began to take effect, respiration was assisted for approximately 2 min, using 60% nitrous oxide and 40% oxygen, until the full effect of the induction drugs was apparent, judged by gross constriction of the pupil. In these small children, no chest-wall stiffness was encountered. Pancuronium (0.07 mg/kg) was then given, and after a further 2 min the child was intubated.

Maintenance of anesthesia was by 60% nitrous oxide in oxygen at a rate of 3 l/min humidified by a Bird 500 nebulizer (Kay and Allen, 1971) and delivered into a modified T-piece. Automatic ventilation was maintained by a baby Bird ventilator, or an Air-Shields Ventimeter at 40 breaths/min with equal inspiratory and expiratory periods and a maximum inspiratory pressure of 15 cm water. Additional doses of 0.001 mg/kg of fentanyl were given as indicated by rise in pulse and blood pressure, sweating, movement, or dilating pupils. Additional doses were, however, avoided if the operation would apparently be completed in the next half hour. Further pancuronium was used if required and relaxation reversed after operation by 0.02 mg/kg of atropine and 0.04 mg/kg of neostigmine, except in the cases of tracheoesophageal fistula and exomphalos where automatic ventilation was continued electively.

Monitoring was by thermometer, precordial stethoscope, pulse monitor, and systolic blood pressure.

Intravenous fluids were given in sufficient quantity and rapidity to compensate for the

Table 2. *Approximate mean infusions (ml)*

	Lactated Ringer's	Dextran, 70,000 mol. wt.	Dextrose, 5%	Blood	Mannitol	Estimated blood loss	Time (min.)
31 neonates							
Mean 2.7 kg	50	30	20	16	–	56	121
Per kg	20	12	8	5	–	20	–
			(17 patients)	(9 patients)			
69 infants							
Mean 7.12 kg	140	20	50	10	25	65	118
Per kg	20	3	7	1.5	3.5	9	–
		(29 patients)		(15 patients)	(33 patients)		

existing dehydration in the starved child and the α-blocking effect of droperidol. No child in this series required fluid or electrolyte replacement for abnormal losses. The following regime was adopted in principle:

1. Lactated Ringer's solution. An initial fast infusion with a total of 20 ml/kg, often split into separate infusions between other fluids.

2. Dextran (70,000 mol. wt.) in normal saline for initial blood loss up to 15 ml/kg. Blood loss of less than 5 ml/kg was ignored.

3. Blood for replacement of loss in excess of 15 ml/kg.

4. Dextrose (5%) in water for maintenance, out of the 24-hr allowance of up to 100 ml/kg.

5. Mannitol (10% up to 10 ml/kg) for a specific diuretic effect.

The approximate mean infusions administered are shown in Table 2. Note that mannitol was only used on infants undergoing urinary tract surgery.

RESULTS

The clinical results obtained indicate the excellence of this technic for neonatal and infant anesthesia.

The character of the anesthesia was similar to that of adults under the technic (Kay, 1972). Cardiovascular stability was marked, with little variation in pulse or systolic blood pressure and obviously excellent peripheral perfusion and renal output. Recovery of consciousness, ability to suck, and normal respiration usually followed withdrawal of nitrous oxide in a few minutes, though nalorphine was administered to 5 infants who had a slower respiratory rate than normal.

More than half the patients had Astrup determinations of arterial blood pH and P_{CO_2}, and the normality of these figures is seen in Table 3. The samples were taken between 90 and 120 min postoperatively, the time when Scott and Inkster (1973) found the greatest metabolic acidosis in neonates anesthetized by other methods. Table 4 shows the blood electrolyte state in the period 12–20 hr postoperatively, the high average blood urea levels being due to the number of infants with high blood urea content who had undergone renal tract procedures.

Table 3.   *Arterial blood Astrup results 90–120 min after operation (52 children)*

	pH	P_{CO_2}	Base excess	Buffer base	Standard bicarbonate
Mean	7.39	36.7	—1.6	47	24.4
Range	(7.28–7.51)	(28–43)	(—9–+2)	(33–59)	(18–30)

Table 4.   *Blood electrolytes 12–20 hr after operation (59 children)*

	Sodium	Potassium	Chloride	Urea
Mean	133.1	4.9	99.5	43
Range	(112–152)	(3.3–6.1)	(76–113)	(7–94)

SUMMARY

Anesthesia with droperidol and fentanyl was used on 100 neonates and infants undergoing major operations. The results indicate the safety of the technic when used in small children and demonstrate that the theoretical advantages attributed are evident in clinical use.

REFERENCES

Bertolo, L., Novakovich, L. and Penna, M. (1972): *Anesthesiology, 37*, 529.
Corssen, G., Domino, E. F. and Sweet, R. B. (1964): *Anesth. Analg. Curr. Res., 43*, 748.
Gorman, H. M. and Craythome, N. W. (1966): *Anaesthesiol. scand. (Suppl. 24)*, 111.
Holderness, M. C., Chase, P. E. and Dripps, R. D. (1963): *Anesthesiology, 24*, 336.
Kay, B. (1972): *Advances in Anaesthesiology and Resuscitation*, p. 5. Editor: L. Holder. Medical Press, Prague.
Kay, B. and Allen, T. (1971): *Canad. Anaesth. Soc. J., 18*, 571.
Kreuscher, H. (1966): *Die Neuroleptanalgesie*, p. 66. Editor: W. F. Henschel. Springer-Verlag, Berlin.
Miller, J. D. and Barker, J. (1969): *Brit. J. Anaesth., 41*, 554.
Scott, J. C. and Inkster, J. S. (1973): *Anaesthesia, 28*, 268.
Tornetta, F. J. and Boger, W. P. (1964): *Anesth. Analg. Curr. Res., 43*, 544.
Zauder, H. L., Del Guercio, L. R. M., Feins, N., Barton, N. and Wollman, H. (1965): *Anesthesiology, 26*, 266.

*Atara-analgesia mixtures: Diazepam-ketamine**

E. K. ZSIGMOND, S. P. KOTHARY, A. MATSUKI ** and O. MARTINEZ

Department of Anesthesiology, University of Michigan Medical Center, Ann Arbor, Mich., U.S.A.

Reviews of anesthetic morbidity and mortality indicate that induction of anesthesia by intravenous barbiturates is associated with severe supine arterial hypotension, hypotension in response to head-up tilt and turning of the patient leading to myocardial infarction or cardiac arrest (Edwards et al., 1956; Dinnick, 1964). Indeed, determination of cardiac output and peripheral and pulmonary vascular resistances in cardiac patients, who underwent cardioversion for persistent atrial fibrillation following mitral valve replacement under thiopental anesthesia or diazepam-induced sleep, indicated that diazepam caused lesser depression of stroke index than thiopental (Dundee et al., 1969). Furthermore, Matsuki et al. (1973) demonstrated that during thiamylal anesthesia there was no compensatory increase in plasma free-norepinephrine and pulse rate in response to the hypotension in contrast to the normal rise observed in non-anesthetized healthy volunteers. Therefore, in hypovolemic patients and in those with reduced cardiac output, the intravenous administration of barbiturates may precipitate fatal complications. A depression of sympathetic autoregulation by diazepam was not demonstrated in either healthy volunteers or lung disease patients by Zsigmond (1967).

Moreover, our earlier studies showed that diazepam caused no depression of ventilation in cardiac and lung disease patients and of course, in healthy volunteers and furthermore, caused no potentiation of the narcotic-analgesic induced respiratory depression (Zsigmond, 1967). Because of these advantages of intravenous diazepam as induction agent over barbiturates, we have used it alone and in combination with narcotic-analgesics such as morphine, 14-hydroxydihydromorphinone (Numorphan), and fentanyl for induction and maintenance of atara-analgesia or anesthesia with nitrous oxide. Although ketamine was recommended as an induction and maintenance agent for poor-risk patients (Corssen et al., 1966) the marked sympathetic and central stimulation resulting in tachycardia, hypertension and increase in plasma free-norepinephrine levels (Zsigmond et al., 1972), increased motor activity and hallucinations limit its routine use (Dundee, 1970). Since diazepam depresses the limbic system while ketamine stimulates it, we studied the influence of diazepam on the ketamine-induced circulatory changes and norepinephrine and epinephrine levels in 46 good-risk patients.

In addition, we utilized diazepam-ketamine induction and ketamine or morphine in combination with oxygen or nitrous oxide:oxygen 4:2 l/min for maintenance of anesthesia of over 400 poor-risk surgical patients. A sample of these was analyzed and the circulatory

* The generous support of Hoffman La Roche, Inc. and Parke Davis and Co. made these studies possible.
** Present address: Department of Anesthesia, University of Hirosaki School of Medicine, Hirosaki, Aomori-ken, Japan.

and blood gas changes were compared to halothane anesthesia in cardiac bypass operations, the results of which will be presented.

METHODS

46 patients of ASA physical state No. 1–3 volunteered to the study. Group I, 12 patients, received only 2.0 mg/kg ketamine intravenously, with respiratory assistance with oxygen; Group II, 6 patients, received 2.0 mg/kg ketamine intravenously without oxygenation; Group III, 6 patients, received 0.2 mg/kg diazepam followed by 2.0 mg/kg ketamine 5 min later intravenously without oxygenation; Group IV, 8 patients, received a placebo (5% caramelized dextrose in Ringer's lactate) followed by 2.0 mg/kg ketamine with oxygenation; Group V, 8 patients, received 0.2 mg/kg diazepam followed by 2.0 mg/kg ketamine 5 min later with oxygenation; Group VI, 6 patients, received 2.0 mg/kg ketamine followed by 0.09 mg/kg pancuronium. Arterial and venous norepinephrine and epinephrine were determined by Vendsalu's method, before and 2, 5 and 10 min following ketamine injection. ECG, blood gases and arterial blood pressure were recorded throughout the study.

RESULTS

The results are presented in Table 1.

(1) 2.0 mg/kg i.v. ketamine caused a significant increase in both arterial and venous norepinephrine and epinephrine 2 and 5 min following injection; (2) 0.2 mg/kg diazepam given 5 min before this dose of ketamine prevented its circulatory effects and rise in catecholamines; (3) pancuronium 0.09 mg/kg injected immediately following 2.0 mg/kg ketamine prevented rather than increased, the circulatory changes and rise in epinephrine and norepinephrine induced by ketamine.

Table 1. *Results of study conducted in 46 patients*

Study groups	Norepinephrine levels (ng/ml) following ketamine combinations			
	0 min	2 min	5 min	10 min
Group I (12) *	$0.4 \pm 0.15^{++}$	$0.5 \pm 0.15^{+}$	$0.8 \pm 0.32^{***}$	$0.6 \pm 0.49^{***}$
Group II (6) **	0.3 ± 0.07	0.4 ± 0.19	$0.5 \pm 0.07^{+}$	$0.4 \pm 0.15^{+}$
Group III (6) **	0.3 ± 0.08	0.3 ± 0.08	0.3 ± 0.07	0.3 ± 0.06
Group IV (8) **	0.4 ± 0.08	$0.5 \pm 0.14^{***}$	$0.6 \pm 0.17^{***}$	$0.4 \pm 0.12^{+}$
Group V (8) **	0.3 ± 0.04	0.3 ± 0.03	0.3 ± 0.05	0.3 ± 0.05
Group VI (6) **	0.4 ± 0.07	0.4 ± 0.02	0.4 ± 0.06	0.4 ± 0.05

*   Venous samples.
** Arterial samples.
*** $p < 0.01$ as compared to 0 min level.
+ $p < 0.05$ as compared to 0 min level.
++   S.D.

Comparison of circulatory complications associated with atara-analgesia with diazepam ketamine-succinylcholine-N_2O (N = 25) and thiamylal-succinylcholine-halothane-N_2O (N = 22) sequences in 47 cardiac patients operated for valvular defects in the first 30 min of anesthesia before cardiopulmonary bypass indicated a lower incidence of complications with atara-analgesia, as Table 2 indicates.

Table 2.   *Comparison of circulatory complications associated with atara-analgesia and thiamylal-halothane anesthesia*

Complications	Diazepam-ketamine-morphine-N₂O (%)	Thiamylal-halothane-N₂O (%)
Hypotension	0	14
Bradycardia	4	14
Hypertension	8	10
Tachycardia	16	6

RECOMMENDED TECHNIQUE

Hydroxyzine, 1.5 mg/kg i.m. 2 hr and atropine, 0.007 mg/kg i.v. 2 min before induction, 0.2 mg/kg diazepam intravenously. After 5 min waiting period, 2.0 mg/kg ketamine i.v. followed by 0.05 mg/kg pancuronium. Intubate and titrate patient with the analgesic, ketamine, morphine or fentanyl, etc. intravenously until no response to skin incision is detected. Oxygen for respiratory assistance during induction is mandatory. Analgesics and pancuronium with O₂ for maintenance of the anesthetic and muscle relaxation. After 2 hr or if hypertension or tachycardia develops, repeat diazepam dose. Reversal of muscle relaxant by pyridostigmine and that of narcotic by narcotic-antagonists.

REFERENCES

Corssen, G. (1966): *Sth med. J. (Bgham, Ala.)*, *59*, 801.
Dinnick, O. P. (1964): *Anaesthesia*, *19*, 536.
Dundee, J. W. et al. (1969): *Int. Anesthesiol. Clin.*, *7*, 91.
Dundee, J. W. (1970): *Lancet*, *2*, 106.
Edwards, G. et al. (1956): *Anaesthesia*, *11*, 194.
Matsuki, A. et al. (1973): *Anaesthesist*, *22*, 289.
Zsigmond, E. K. (1967): Paper presented at: *Pan American Medical Association, 42nd Anniversary Congress Buenos Aires, Nov. 21, 1967*, p. 22.
Zsigmond, E. K. et al. (1972): *Rev. bras. Anest.*, *22*, 443.

Modifications of effects of Althesin and of thiobarbiturate as affected by the metabolic activity of the liver

G. P. NOVELLI, M. MARSILI and P. LORENZI

Department of Anaesthesiology and Intensive Therapy, University of Florence, Florence, Italy

One of the main clinical aspects of Althesin is that its action ends completely in a few minutes; the period of hangover following barbiturate anaesthesia is absent. This character of the anaesthetic steroid seems to be related to rapid metabolic breakdown of the drug in the liver.

In this sense Card et al. in 1972 reported that in autoradiographs of rats injected with ^{14}C-labelled alphaxalone the highest concentration of isotope occurred within 3 min and was in the liver and bile ducts. In the same year, Child et al. (1972) attempted to study the breakdown processes involved in the pharmacodynamics of Althesin. Their results indicate that the major metabolite of the drugs in rats is a glucuronide of hydroxyalphaxalone. The same authors also performed experiments on Gunn rats, which are deficient in glucuronyl-transferase – the sleeping-time was twice that in the control rats.

These data have not been confirmed, but it seems to be possible to modify the effects of Althesin by modifying the metabolizing activity of the liver.

In an attempt to examine this hypothesis, Althesin was injected into rats of a single strain whose liver function was normal, increased or decreased – the duration of analgesia, sleeping-time and cardiovascular effects were considered. Each rat was also given thiopentone.

MATERIAL AND METHODS

Male Wistar rats, 250 g weight, uniformly stabilised on a standard commercial diet were used in all experiments after a 12-hr fasting period.

During light ether anaesthesia, the right femoral artery and the left femoral vein were cannulated with thin plastic catheters which were introduced up the aorta and vena cava. The arterial catheter was connected to an electromanometer and the venous line was for injection of drugs. In all experiments a median laparotomy was performed and a plastic catheter was introduced into the portal vein through a branch of the superior mesenteric vein; the abdomen was sutured but the end of the catheter was left outside for injection of drugs in the 2nd group experiments. Needle electrodes for electrocardiographic tracing were applied.

The whole preparation of rats with cholestasis and marked icterus was often lethal (surgical ligation and section of the bile ducts). After complete recovery from ether anaesthesia, the effects of Althesin and of thiopentone were evaluated according to the following parameters:

(*a*) duration of analgesia, considered as time interval between the injection of drugs and the reappearance of a motor response to tail-crushing with a forceps – the tail was crushed every 30 sec;

(*b*) sleeping-time, considered as time interval between the injection of drugs and reappearance of a spontaneous righting reflex;

(*c*) decrease of mean arterial pressure measured by the electromanometer (Statham) connected to the arterial catheter whose tracing was continuously recorded during the whole experiment (OTE-Galileo, Florence). Results are reported as percent of basal values 30, 120 and 180 sec after injection of both drugs;

(*d*) decrease of cardiac rate measured on an electrocardiographic tracing obtained in D_2 (OTE-Galileo, Florence). Results are reported as percentage of basal values measured 30, 120 and 180 sec after injection of both drugs.

1st group (8 animals): Althesin was injected through the femoral vein in normal, non-pretreated rats. This group was the control group. *2nd group* (8 animals): Althesin was injected through the portal system in the same non-pretreated rats. The aim of these experiments was to expose the injected drug immediately to the metabolizing action of the liver and so functionally to increase the activity of the liver. *3rd group* (12 animals which survived in apparently good condition): Althesin was injected through the femoral vein in rats with cholestatic liver damage.

Experiments were performed injecting Althesin (0.25 ml/kg diluted in 0.2 ml of saline) and thiopentone (20 mg/kg diluted in 0.2 ml of saline) according to a randomized sequence. The standard error and mean value were calculated for each group of results and their statistical significance was evaluated according to the Student's t-test, comparing each group with the control.

RESULTS

Results are reported in Tables 1–4. It is evident that all the effects of Althesin are less in Group 2, that is following portal injection. In Group 3 analgesia and sleeping-time are very prolonged but cardiovascular derangements are not different from control values.

Effects of thiopentone are not influenced by the 2 methods of increasing or decreasing liver activity.

Table 1. *Duration of analgesia (min) after injection of Althesin and thiopentone*

Group	Althesin (0.25 ml/kg)		Thiopentone (20 mg/kg)	
1 (control)	$7'00'' \pm 1.31$	–	$8'00'' \pm 2.11$	–
2 (portal injection)	$3'00'' \pm 0.50$	$P < 0.05$	$7'00'' \pm 3.70$	NS
3 (cholestasis)	$15'00'' \pm 2.96$	$P < 0.05$	$8'43'' \pm 2.65$	NS

Table 2. *Sleeping-time (min) after injection of Althesin and of thiopentone*

Group	Althesin (0.25 ml/kg)		Thiopentone (20 mg/kg)	
1 (control)	$23'20'' \pm 4.28$	–	$29'16'' \pm 4.27$	–
2 (portal injection)	$13'00'' \pm 2.42$	$P < 0.05$	$29'40'' \pm 8.90$	NS
3 (cholestasis)	$44'55'' \pm 3.75$	$P < 0.05$	$31'20'' \pm 2.70$	NS

Table 3. *Percentage changes of basal values of arterial mean pressure after injection of Althesin and thiopentone*

Group		Althesin (0.25 ml/kg)		Thiopentone (20 mg/kg)	
1 (control)	30″	—34.84 ± 2.15	–	—43.9 ± 3.10	–
	120″	—44.63 ± 3.36	–	—41.1 ± 2.07	–
	180″	—41.90 ± 4.30	–	—37.4 ± 3.05	–
2 (portal injection)	30″	— 7.82 ± 2.07	$P < 0.01$	—10.73 ± 3.02	$P < 0.01$
	120″	—14.43 ± 1.97	$P < 0.01$	—23.42 ± 2.70	NS
	180″	—15.10 ± 3.50	$P < 0.05$	—32.15 ± 2.51	NS
3 (cholestasis)	30″	—53.33 ± 3.52	$P < 0.01$	—35.60 ± 3.31	NS
	120″	—36.66 ± 3.33	NS	—40.06 ± 2.42	NS
	180″	—31.66 ± 0.33	NS	—42.21 ± 2.15	NS

Table 4. *Percentage changes of basal values of cardiac rate after injection of Althesin and thiopentone*

Group		Althesin (0.25 ml/kg)		Thiopentone (20 mg/kg)	
1 (control)	30″	—13.90 ± 3.10	–	—21.02 ± 2.82	–
	120″	—16.82 ± 2.73	–	—24.04 ± 3.06	–
	180″	—13.06 ± 2.58	–	—27.40 ± 2.66	–
2 (portal injection)	30″	— 3.13 ± 2.02	$P < 0.01$	— 8.07 ± 3.15	$P < 0.01$
	120″	— 7.52 ± 3.00	$P < 0.05$	—17.91 ± 2.81	NS
	180″	— 9.10 ± 2.97	$P < 0.05$	—27.94 ± 3.24	NS
3 (cholestasis)	30″	—27.70 ± 3.65	NS	—14 ± 3.02	NS
	120″	—18.20 ± 3.29	NS	—22 ± 2.77	NS
	180″	—16.06 ± 3.16	NS	—27 ± 2.92	NS

DISCUSSION

It is well known that pharmacological effects of anaesthetic drugs are terminated by redistribution in the whole organism, by elimination or by metabolic breakdown.

In the experiments reported here 2 drugs have been compared. The first one is thiopentone whose action is ended by redistribution; however, there is also delayed and slow metabolism (10–15%/hr according to the classical data of Brodie et al., 1950). There is some doubt about the brief action of Althesin, because the metabolic breakdown by glucuronidation seems to be probable but has not yet been confirmed. In fact, experiments conducted by Child et al. (1972) on rats deficient in glucuronyl-transferase, were performed on 2 different strains of animals and, therefore, results are not strictly comparable.

The results show a clear difference in the relationship between the functional state of the liver and the duration of action of Althesin. The effects of thiopentone are unaffected by the liver because redistribution is not altered. Therefore, it must be accepted that (1) effects of thiopentone and Althesin are terminated by different mechanisms, and (2) the action of Althesin is limited by hepatic breakdown.

In conclusion, these results could have a clinical importance, since it is possible that Althesin anaesthesia could be modified according to the functional state of the liver and to its ability to metabolize Althesin.

REFERENCES

Brodie, B. B., Mark, L. C., Papper, E. M., Lieg, P. A., Bernstein, E. and Rovenstine, E. A. (1950): *J. Pharmacol. exp. Ther.*, *98*, 85.

Card, B., McCulloch, R. G. and Pratt, D. M. (1972): *Postgrad. med. J.*, *48 (Suppl. 2)*, 34.

Child, K. J., Gibson, W., Harnby, G. and Hart, J. W. (1972): *Postgrad. med. J.*, *48 (Suppl. 2)*, 37.

Tetrahydroaminoacridine (THA).
I. Effect on postanesthetic emergence responses and anesthesia sleep-time after ketamine, phencyclidine and thiamylal in animals

MAURICE S. ALBIN, LEONID BUNEGIN, PETER J. JANNETTA
and LEO C. MASSOPUST Jr

Departments of Anesthesiology and Neurological Surgery and the Neuroanesthesia Laboratory,
University of Pittsburgh School of Medicine, Pittsburgh, Pa., and Department of Anatomy,
St. Louis University School of Medicine, St. Louis, Mo., U.S.A.

Ketamine hydrochloride (KH), a phenylcyclohexylamine derivative, is a cataleptoid type of anesthetic (Domino et al., 1965) that has been used in humans for less than 7 years. The effective use of KH as a parenteral anesthetic agent has been limited because of the incidence of postanesthetic emergence reactions. These responses have ranged from pseudo-hallucinations and marked delirium to hypnogogic states and anxiety reactions (Albin et al., 1970; Albin and Dresner, 1970; Albin et al., 1972; Knox et al., 1970; Massopust et al., 1972). Attempts to decrease these responses have involved psychological preparation of the patient, reduction in volume of afferent stimuli during the postanesthetic period, and pharmacologic agents including sedatives, narcotics and major and minor tranquilizers (Fine and Finestone, 1973; Hunter, 1965; Medical Summary, 1970).

In our search for an antagonist to the ketamine hydrochloride side effects, we noted the ability of a potent cholinesterase inhibitor, tetrahydroaminoacridine (1,2,3,4-tetrahydro-5-aminoacridine) to reverse psychotic episodes precipitated by some anticholinergic psychotomimetics (Bell et al., 1964; Bell and Gershon, 1964; Brown, 1971). The other properties of tetrahydroaminoacridine (THA) include mild neuromuscular blocking action, respiratory stimulation and partial antagonism to morphine (Pender, 1972; Shaw and Bentley, 1949; Shaw, 1960).

Because of the high incidence of behavioral side effects, phencyclidine (1-(1-phenyl-cyclohexyl) piperidine hydrochloride) was abandoned as a parenteral analgesic and anesthetic agent for humans and its anesthetic use limited to animal species (especially the subhuman primate). Unfortunately, during the past 5 years phencyclidine has become an important hallucinogenic drug of abuse, with oral ingestion as the primary route of administration. Phencyclidine has been labelled by the drug cult as 'PCP' and the 'peace pill' (Taylor et al., 1970).

Because of the structural relationship between phencyclidine (PC) and ketamine hydrochloride (KH), this study will also test tetrahydroaminoacridine (THA) against PC in the animal model. A review of the literature has revealed conflicting reports concerning the ability of the aminoacridines to affect barbiturate intoxication (Shaw and Bentley, 1949; Shaw, 1960). This study will also evaluate THA against an ultra-short acting barbiturate, thiamylal sodium (ST).

METHODS

The canine was used as the experimental model since prolonged and exaggerated post-anesthetic emergence reactions after ketamine are commonplace in this species. This allowed for developing a model test system similar to that used in evaluating hallucinogens (Bell et al., 1964). Conversely the equivalent postanesthetic behavioral response in the subhuman primate was found to be too weak and inconsistent to make satisfactory observations. Observations were made on 12 dogs averaging 20 kg body weight. Each dog was given intravenous KH (10 mg/kg) or THA (1.0 mg/kg) alone or in combination in a randomized fashion and assigned to the following treatment groups: KH alone (control); THA alone (control); THA followed after 5 min by KH; KH followed after 2 min by THA; KH followed by THA at headlift.

Observations were made as to *anesthesia induction time* (time needed to produce unconsciousness); *duration of anesthesia* (from unconsciousness to first sign of headlift); emergence time was calculated from headlift to maintenance of a *good gait* without ataxia, including ability to *complete stand* (standing on all fours without falling down). Emergence responses included barking, whining, ataxia, agitated pawing, rigidity, disorientation and chasing 'unseen' objects.

Similarly, another group of 7 dogs (averaging 20 kg body weight) was given intravenous PC (1.0 mg/kg) or THA (2.0 mg/kg) alone or in combination (5 min after PC and THA 30 min after PC).

For the barbiturate study 7 additional dogs (averaging 20 kg body weight) were given thiamylal sodium (10 mg/kg intravenously) alone or THA (1.0 mg/kg) was given intravenously 5 min after ST.

RESULTS

The results for KH-THA can be seen in Table 1 and were subjected to analysis of variance on the four treatment groups (THA alone was not included since no anesthetic effects were noted). Multiple contrasts (Dunnett's test) was used on each of the significant factors in order to pinpoint the treatment groups accounting for the difference (Dunnett, 1955).

Table 1.   *Anesthesia induction, anesthesia duration and anesthesia emergence responses to KH and THA*

Factors	Treatment means (min)				F ratio *	Statistical significance **
	K_C	T_2	$T_{H.L.}$	T_5		
Injection						
/Anesthesia induction time	1.67	1.75	1.67	1.67	0.0208	NS
Unconsciousness						
/Duration of anesthesia	9.58	4.75	9.08	7.17	11.7609	S
Headlift						
/Complete stand	25.92	23.92	21.42	24.00	2.2822	NS
/Good gait	8.58	1.83	3.50	1.75	11.9368	S
Emergence						

*   Degrees of freedom were 3 and 11 for each test.
** All tests performed at the 5% level.

K_C=Ketamine alone (control), T_2=THA – 2 min after ketamine, $T_{H.L.}$=THA – at head lift, T_5=THA – 5 min to ketamine, NS=not significant, S=significant.

The responses to THA were statistically significant in the factors concerning *duration of anesthesia* and *good gait* (emergence). THA given 2 min after KH showed a marked decrease in the duration of anesthesia compared to the KH alone (control). All treatment groups employing THA showed a significant narrowing in the emergence reaction time since the animals were able to ambulate much quicker.

THA also appeared to have a statistically significant effect against phencyclidine when given 5 min after PC injection and also after 30 min. The duration of anesthesia was shortened and emergence reaction time decreased. Mean time to *stand* in the control PC group was 112.6 min as compared to 75.7 min when THA was given 5 min after PC and 73.0 min when THA was given 30 min after PC.

This would seem to indicate that it is possible for the first time to report the attenuation or reversal of the anesthetic effects of a parenteral agent. Equally important, THA reduced important components of the postanesthetic emergence response to KH and PC.

As can be seen from Table 2, ST had no effect in attenuating emergence time or emergence reaction.

Table 2. *ST and THA response*

	Control (min) ST 10 mg/kg	Experimental (min) ST 10 mg/kg and THA 1 mg/kg after 5.0 min
Unconscious	1.0	1.0
Head lift	13.0	12.0
Stand	14.0	57.0
Good gait	18.0	–

Central cholinergic mechanisms have been implicated in overt inhibitory behavior which can be modified by drugs having pharmacological actions similar to the tropanes and glycolates. This anticholinergic activity can be identified in some synthetic psychotropics and even in some of the tetrahydrocannabinols. Antagonism by THA probably involves interactions between adrenergic as well as cholinergic receptor sites in brain.

Aside from its reversal effects on KH, it is also possible that THA might be of clinical use in treatment of acute intoxications with drugs of abuse such as phencyclidine and other hallucinogens.

REFERENCES

Albin, M. S. and Dresner, A. J. (1970): *Ars Med. (Gand)*, *1*, 179.
Albin, M. S., Dresner, A. J., Paolino, A. F., Virtue, R. W., Sweet, R. B. and Miller, G. L. (1972): In: *Advances in Anesthesiology and Resuscitation, Proceedings, Third European Congress of Anesthesiology*, p. 627. Medical Press, Prague.
Albin, M. S., McCarthy, D. A. and Dresner, A. J. (1970): *Ars Med. (Gand)*, *1*, 85.
Bell, C. and Gershon, S. (1964): *Med. exp. (Basel)*, *10*, 15.
Bell, C., Gershon, S., Carroll, B. and Holan, G. (1964): *Arch. int. Pharmacodyn.*, *147*, 9.
Brown, H. (1971): *Pharmacol. Clin.*, *21*, 294.
Domino, E. F., Chodoff, P. and Corssen, G. (1965): *J. clin. Pharmacol. Ther.*, *6*, 279.
Dunnett, C. W. (1955): *J. Amer. statist. Ass.*, *50*, 1096.
Fine, J. and Finestone, S. C. (1973): *Anesth. Analg. Curr. Res.*, *62*, 428.
Hunter, A. R. (1965): *Brit. J. Anaesth.*, *37*, 505.
Knox, J. W. D., Bovill, J. G., Clarke, R. S. J. and Dundee, J. (1970): *Brit. J. Anaesth.*, *42*, 875.

Massopust Jr., L. C., Wolin, L. R. and Albin, M. S. (1972): *Anesth. Analg. Curr. Res.*, *53*, 329.
Medical Summary (1970): In: *Ketalar CI-581: A Short Acting Anesthetic*, p. 266. Parke-Davis and Company, Detroit, Mich.
Pender, J. (1972): *J. Amer. med. Ass.*, *215*, 1126.
Shaw, F. H. (1960): *Brit. J. clin. Pract.*, *14*, 23.
Shaw, F. H. and Bentley, G. (1949): *Med. J. Aust.*, *2*, 868.
Stone, V., Moon, W. and Shaw, F. H. (1961): *Brit. med. J.*, *1*, 471.
Taylor, R. L., Maurer, J. I. and Tinklenberg, J. R. (1970): *J. Amer. med. Ass.*, *213*, 422.

Tetrahydroaminoacridine (THA).
II. Modification of postanesthetic emergence responses and anesthesia sleep-time after ketamine hydrochloride (KH) in the human

MAURICE S. ALBIN, EDGAR MARTINEZ AGUIRRE and ROGER L. ALBIN

Departments of Anesthesiology and Neurological Surgery,
University of Pittsburgh School of Medicine, Pittsburgh, Pa., U.S.A., and
Catedra de Anestesiologia, Facultad de Medicina,
Universidad Central de Venezuela, Caracas, Venezuela

Ketamine hydrochloride [2-(o-chlorophenyl)-2-methylaminocyclohexanone hydrochloride], a relatively new parenteral anesthetic, is an analogue of a potent psychotomimetic agent, phencyclidine (Domino et al., 1965).

The effective use of ketamine hydrochloride (KH) as a parenteral anesthetic agent has been limited because of the incidence of postanesthetic emergence reactions. These responses have ranged from pseudohallucinations and marked delirium to hypnogogic states and anxiety reactions. Attempts to decrease these responses have involved psychological preparation of the patient, reduction in volume of afferent stimuli during the postanesthetic period, and pharmacologic agents including sedatives, narcotics and major and minor tranquilizers (Virtue et al., 1967; Winters, 1967; Knox et al., 1970; Pender, 1972; Massopust et al., 1972; Albin et al., 1972; Fine and Finestone, 1973).

In our search for an antagonist to the ketamine hydrochloride side effects we noted the ability of a potent cholinesterase inhibitor, tetrahydroaminoacridine (THA) to reverse psychotic episodes precipitated by some anticholinergic psychotomimetics. The other properties of THA * include mild neuromuscular blocking action, respiratory stimulation and partial antagonism to morphine (Shaw and Bentley, 1955; Stone et al., 1961; Bell et al., 1964; Bell and Gershon, 1964; Clark and Dundee, 1965; Hunter, 1965; Benveniste et al., 1967; Brown, 1971). THA has been used extensively in Europe and Latin America in both oral and parenteral forms in humans for prolongation of muscle relaxation with succinylcholine and to counteract the respiratory depressant effects of morphine.

Because of our findings in the animal model, and because of the fact that THA has been used safely for many years for respiratory stimulation, succinylcholine enhancement and its anticurare effect, it was felt that a study was warranted to evaluate the effect of THA in modifying the anesthetic effects of KH used in a double blind fashion.

METHODS

Subject selection

Pediatric and adult patients (till age 45) undergoing relatively short elective surgical or

---

* Package insert and labeling, Ward Blenkinsop and Co., Ltd., U.K.

diagnostic procedures with ASA status of No. 1 or 2 were selected. All pregnant females were eliminated. Informed consent was obtained from all patients (or their guardians) being notified as to the surgical procedure, anesthetic agent used (KH) and the fact that an approved drug (THA) was being used for a new indication and data as to emergence responses was being obtained.

Study design

All patients were randomly assigned to one of two study groups:

> Group 1 – KH followed by THA
> Group 2 – KH followed by placebo

THA and placebo were coded and blinded at the University Hospital, Caracas, Venezuela. All patients received 0.1–0.2 mg i.m. of sodium glycopyrrolate (Robinul) as a premedicant drying agent 45 min prior to induction of anesthesia. Robinul was chosen as the antisialagogue since in these doses it does not cross the blood-brain barrier.

Patients received either an i.v. induction dose of 2.0 mg/kg of KH or an i.m. induction dose of 10.0 mg/kg. Maintenance was with 1.0 mg/kg i.v. doses every 15 min (or sooner if needed) till the procedure was terminated. KH was the sole anesthetic agent used.

On termination of the procedure, each patient received an i.v. injection from a coded and blinded ampule containing either 1.0 mg/kg THA or an ampule having an equivalent volume of placebo.

Vital signs, postanesthetic emergence responses and other adverse reactions were noted on specially designed reporting forms. After surgery, the patient was moved to the recovery room for further observation.

RESULTS

In this series a total of 100 patients were processed with 3 patients being dropped from the study because of insufficient data, leaving 97 patients for evaluation. Another group of 100 patients has been studied and will be presented on another occasion since the data has not been completely analyzed at this date.

Group 1 (THA) consisted of 31 children and 18 adults and Group 2 (control) had 29 children and 19 adults. *Females* predominated in this study with a total of 66 against 31 males. Both the THA and control group matched very well in terms of *operative procedures, duration of anesthesia, duration of surgical procedure, routes of administration* and *KH dosing*.

The outstanding difference between the THA and control group occurred in 'recovery time' (from moment of injection of either THA or placebo at termination of procedure to time when patient is oriented and can respond to questions and commands). Group 1 (THA) children had a mean recovery time of 20 min as opposed to Group 2 (control) children with a mean recovery time of 63.0 min. Group 1 (THA) adults had a mean recovery time of 47.0 min compared to Group 2 (control) mean recovery time of 75.0 min. These findings are significant at greater than a 95% level.

Intraoperative side effects were similar in Group 1 and 2 and it appears that important emergence response components were greater in the control group than in the THA group.

Vomiting occurred in Group 1 (THA) adults with slightly higher frequency than in Group 2 (control) adults.

Because of space limitation, we have given the highlights of a double blind clinical study of THA–KH interaction, indicating that THA appears to have the capability of attenuating 'recovery time' and postanesthetic 'emergence responses.'

REFERENCES

Albin, M. S., Dresner, A. J., Paolino, A., Virtue, R., Sweet, R. and Miller, G. L. (1972): In: *Proceedings, III European Congress of Anesthesiology, Prague*, p. 942. Medical Press, Prague.

Bell, C. and Gershon, S. (1964): *Med. exp. (Basel), 10*, 15.

Bell, C., Gershon, S., Carroll, B. and Holan, G. (1964): *Arch. int. Pharmacodyn., 147*, 9.

Benveniste, D., Hemmingsen, L. and Juul, P. (1967): *Acta anaesth. scand., 11*, 297.

Brown, H. (1971): *Pharmacol. Clin., 21*, 294.

Clark, R. S. J. and Dundee, J. W. (1965): *Brit. J. Anaesth., 37*, 779.

Domino, E. F., Chodoff, P. and Corssen, G. (1965): *Clin. Pharmacol. Ther., 6*, 279.

Fine, J. and Finestone, S. C. (1973): *Anesth. Analg. Curr. Res., 62*, 428.

Hunter, A. R. (1965): *Brit. J. Anaesth., 37*, 505.

Knox, J. W. D., Bovill, J. G., Clarke, R. S. J. et al. (1970): *Brit. J. Anaesth., 42*, 875.

Massopust Jr., L. C., Wolin, L. R. and Albin, M. S. (1972): *Anesth. Analg. Curr. Res., 51*, 329.

Pender, J. (1972): *J. Amer. med. Ass., 215*, 1126.

Shaw, F. H. and Bentley, G. A. (1955): *Aust. J. exp. Biol. med. Sci., 33*, 143.

Stone, V., Moon, W. and Shaw, F. H. (1961): *Brit. med. J., 1*, 471.

Virtue, R. W., Alanis, J. M., Mori, M. et al. (1967): *Anesthesiology, 28*, 823.

Winters, W. D. (1967): *Anesthesiology, 28*, 65.

Tetrahydroaminoacridine (THA). III. Preliminary report: Attenuation of abstinence syndrome after morphine addiction in the monkey

MAURICE S. ALBIN, MALCOLM D. ORR and LEONID BUNEGIN

Departments of Anesthesiology and Neurological Surgery and the Neuroanesthesia Research Laboratory, University of Pittsburgh School of Medicine, Pittsburgh, Pa., U.S.A.

Morphine antagonism with tetrahydroaminoacridine (THA) has been reported in a number of animal species and in man. This has consisted of rapid arousal, respiratory stimulation, decrease in euphoria and no inhibition of the cough reflex. It has also been reported that the use of THA did not inhibit the analgesic action of morphine. The most significant potential use of THA appears to be in the reduction of addiction liability to morphine in patients with intractable pain. Because of these aforementioned findings, this pilot study is concerned with the role of THA in attenuating physical dependence during chronic morphine administration and withdrawal in the Rhesus monkey.

METHODS

Eight Rhesus monkeys were divided into 2 groups of 4 with Group 1 (control) receiving 3.0 mg/kg morphine sulfate (MS) parenterally every 6 hr for 31 days. Group 2 (THA) received a mixture of 3.0 mg/kg MS and 1.0 mg/kg THA parenterally every 6 hr for 31 days.

Physical dependence was monitored in both groups on the 14th and 28th day of drug dosing by the administration of 2.0 mg/kg nalorphine parenterally to provoke an abstinence syndrome. On day 31 all dosing was terminated and the monkeys observed during the ensuing two weeks. Each animal was evaluated during the entire period according to an 'abstinence syndrome profile' (ASP) which rated symptoms by assigning a '0' for no change, '—1' for moderate change and '—2' for marked change from the norm. This is shown in Table 1. Food and water intake and daily weights were also monitored.

RESULTS

After two weeks of dosing, one animal in the MS group began presenting its buttocks for the daily injection. Both groups exhibited some weight loss, with a higher water and food consumption in the MS group.

Precipitation of withdrawal by nalorphine on Day 14 showed a marked difference between the two groups, with the MS group having an ASP rating twice that of the THA group. This difference became even more marked on Day 28, with the ASP rating still higher in the MS group.

Table 1. *Abstinence syndrome profile*

Behavior	Involuntary somatic	Sympathetic	Parasympathetic
apprehension	muscle rigidity	yawning	rhinorrhea
restlessness	muscle tenderness	perspiration	lacrimation
handling	muscle weakness	piloerection	cough
vocalization	tremor	pallor	miosis
posture	convulsions		abdominal cramps
	dehydration		anorexia
	weight loss		nausea
	strabismus		salivation
			diarrhea
			retching
			vomiting

The most intense reaction differences occurred on Day 34 (3 days after drug cessation) with the ASP rating of the MS group more than double the THA group. On Day 35 a monkey in the MS group died after severe convulsions.

In general the MS group showed more pronounced vocalization, piloerection, cage shaking, restlessness than the THA group. Animals dosed only with MS showed more activity and spent less time floor-sitting in the corner than the THA group.

While this study is in the nature of a preliminary report, it may be possible that THA attenuates the physical dependence to MS and hence decreases its addiction liability. More complete studies using other centrally acting opiates in crossover studies are now in progress.

The cardiovascular pharmacology of etomidate (R-26490), a new, potent and short-acting intravenous hypnotic agent

R. S. RENEMAN, A. H. M. JAGENEAU, R. XHONNEUX and P. LADURON

Cardiovascular Department, Janssen Pharmaceutica, Beerse, Belgium

Etomidate is a new, potent, short-acting and relatively non-toxic intravenous hypnotic agent (Janssen et al., 1971; Doenicke et al., 1973a, b) developed in our laboratories. In the present study the cardiovascular effects of etomidate and the commercially available short-acting hypnotics methohexital and propanidid were compared in unanesthetized dogs

METHODS

The hemodynamic studies were performed on 12 unanesthetized Labradors with chronically implanted devices. The dogs (22–30 kg), who were trained to lie down quietly, were divided into 2 groups of 6 dogs each. Before implantation, the dogs with the lowest heart rates were selected for the fixed rate experiments in Group I.

In *Group I* heart rate was determined from the ECG. Ascending aortic blood pressure was measured through a silastic catheter, implanted according to the technique of Herd and Barger (1964). Left ventricular pressure was measured through the apex with a high fidelity pitran transducer (Van den Bos et al., 1974). The maximum first derivative of left ventricular pressure (dP/dt_{max}) was determined with an analog differentiator (Schaper et al., 1965). Heart rate was kept constant with a stimulator and a bipolar electrode on the right ventricle.

In *Group II* heart rate and ascending aortic blood pressure were measured as in Group I. Electromagnetic flowprobes were placed on the ascending aorta and the left circumflex coronary artery, and distal to the latter a pneumatic cuff for zero flow determination (Jageneau et al., 1969). The diastolic level of the instantaneous aortic blood flow signal was used as a zero reference. The electromagnetic flowmeter used in these experiments was the Transflow 600. Mean flows were obtained by active integration.

The variables were recorded on a mingograph (Elema-Schönander). After a recorded control period of 30 min, the hypnotics were injected into a fore- or hindleg vein over a period of approximately 30 sec. Up to 10 min after the beginning of the injection, the variables were measured at one minute intervals and the average over 5 heart beats determined. The measurements were repeated 15 min after the beginning of the injection. The hypnotics were injected randomly with an interval of at least 2 days.

Comparative doses of the various hypnotics were selected on the basis of sleep duration (Jageneau et al., 1973). Etomidate was used in a solution as described by Xhonneux et al. (*This Volume*, p. 157). Propanidid (Epontol®, Bayer) and methohexital (Brietal®, Lilly) were used as the commercially available solutions.

In 6 unanesthetized beagles (12–15.5 kg) histamine plasma levels were measured before (30 and 15 min) and after administration (3, 5, 15 and 30 min) of the hypnotics according to a modification of the technique of Taylor and Snijder (1971).

Changes in the values of the determined hemodynamic variables during the first 15 min after administration of the hypnotics, compared with the values before compound administration, were evaluated for statistical significance by applying Wilcoxon's matched-pairs signed-ranks test (2-tailed probability).

RESULTS

In the experiments with methohexital and propanidid (Group I), heart rate could not be kept constant because of the pronounced increase in heart rate after the injection of these hypnotics. Therefore, the heart rate and aortic blood pressure values of Group I and II were combined. Three of the 12 dogs temporarily stopped breathing after the injection of methohexital, which was associated with a severe fall in aortic blood pressure. Therefore, these experiments were not included in the aortic pressure analysis. One dog died 7.5 min after administration of propanidid. In the etomidate experiments the aortic blood pressure values of Group I and II were combined since the changes in aortic pressure after the injection of this hypnotic were not significantly different in these groups.

Etomidate, 1.25 and 2.5 mg/kg i.v., slightly, but significantly decreased systolic and diastolic aortic blood pressure, while the higher dose also significantly increased heart rate. Etomidate had no significant effect on dP/dt$_{max}$ (at a constant heart rate of 120 beats/min), and on mean aortic and mean coronary blood flow (Figs. 1 and 2).

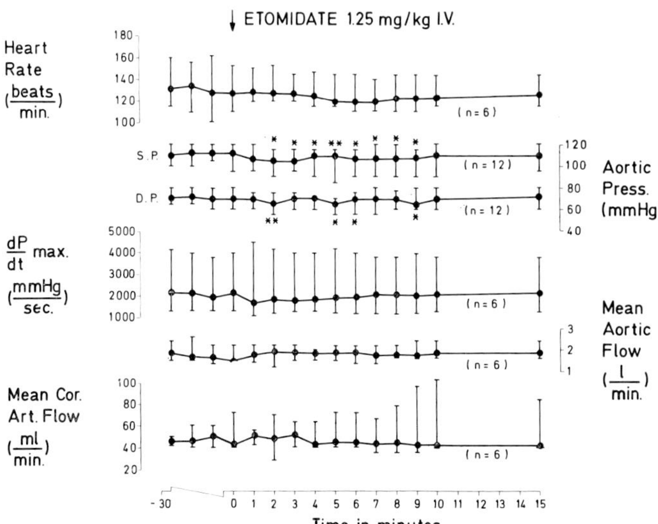

Fig. 1. *The effect of etomidate, 1.25 mg/kg i.v., on various hemodynamic variables in unanesthetized dogs. The median and 95% limits are shown. The dP/dt measurements are performed at a constant heart rate of 120 beats/min. (*=p < 0.05; **=p < 0.01.)*

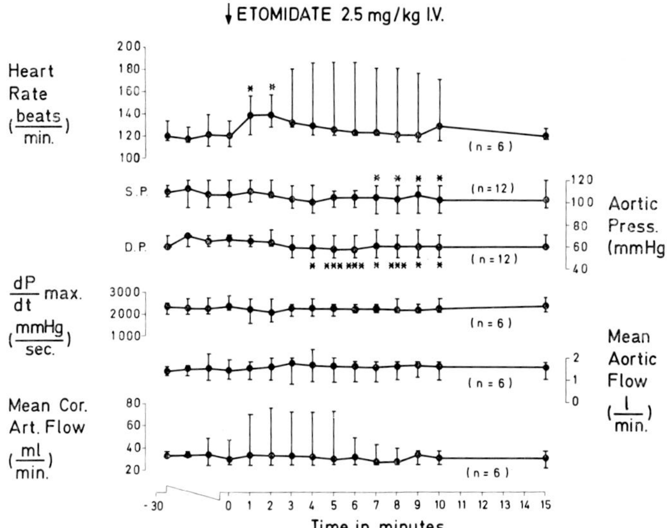

Fig. 2.   *The effect of etomidate, 2.5 mg/kg i.v., on various hemodynamic variables in unanesthetized dogs. The median and 95% limits are shown. The dP/dt measurements are performed at a constant heart rate of 120 beats/min. (*=p < 0.05; ***=p < 0.005.)*

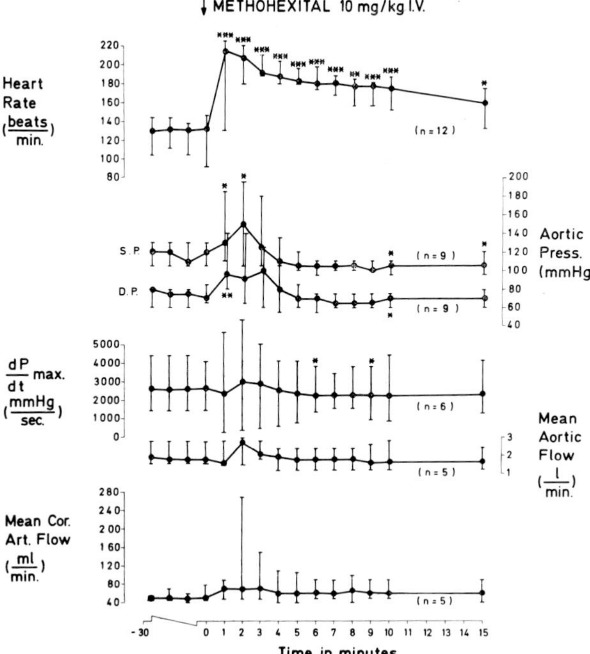

Fig. 3.   *The effect of methohexital, 10 mg/kg i.v., on various hemodynamic variables in unanesthetized dogs. The median and 95% limits are shown. (*=p<0.05; **=p<0.01; ***=p<0.005.)*

Methohexital, 10 mg/kg i.v., significantly increased heart rate and systolic and diastolic aortic blood pressure, and induced in one dog a short-lasting period of ventricular tachycardia. The effect of methohexital on dP/dt_{max} was biphasic: a non-significant initial increase was followed by a significant fall 6 and 9 min after the injection. The increases in mean aortic blood flow and mean coronary blood flow after the administration of methohexital were not significant (Fig. 3). In one dog no flow measurements could be made because of technical failures.

Propanidid, 50 mg/kg i.v., significantly increased heart rate and significantly decreased systolic and diastolic aortic blood pressure, dP/dt_{max} and mean aortic blood flow. The increase in mean coronary blood flow was not significant (Fig. 4). The mean aortic blood flow values were evaluated for statistical significance only up to 4 min after the injection since one animal died and the flow measurements were unreliable in 2 additional experiments because of the poor vessel fit of the electromagnetic flow probe due to the fall in aortic blood pressure. In 2 experiments the increase in heart rate was preceded by extreme bradycardia.

Etomidate and methohexital did not induce histamine release, but propanidid highly increased histamine plasma levels.

DISCUSSION

The present study shows that the cardiovascular effects of etomidate are minimal. The slight decrease in aortic blood pressure is probably the result of a direct vasodilatory property

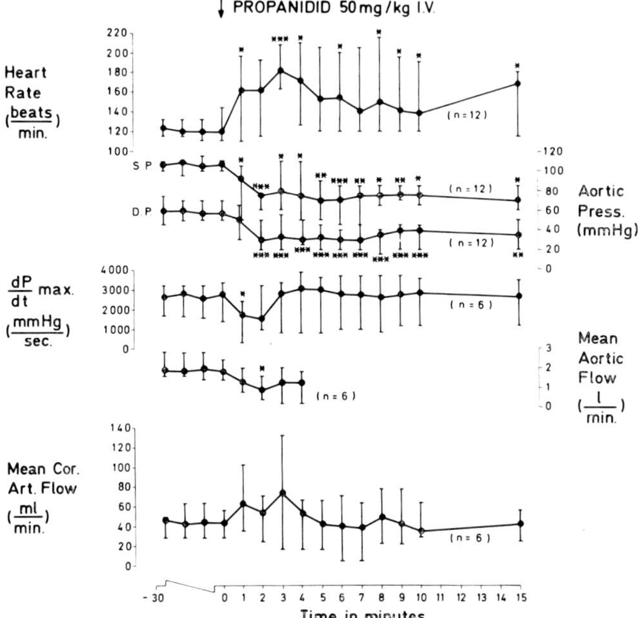

Fig. 4.   *The effect of propanidid, 50 mg/kg i.v., on various hemodynamic variables in unanesthetized dogs. The median and 95% limits are shown. One animal died 7.5 min after injection. Therefore, the number of experiments indicated only hold for the measurements up to 7 min after injection. (*=p < 0.05; **=p < 0.01; ***=p < 0.005.)*

of the compound because etomidate does not induce histamine release. Since etomidate has no effect on the spontaneous activity in auricular muscle (Xhonneux et al., *This Volume*, p. 157), the increase in heart rate is likely to be secondary to the decrease in aortic blood pressure.

Methohexital increases the oxygen demand of the left ventricle since it markedly increases heart rate and systolic blood pressure. The expected increase in mean coronary blood flow, however, was not significant, due to the small number of experiments. The significant fall in dP/dt_{max} 6 and 9 min after the injection, in the presence of a significant increase in heart rate, indicates that methohexital has some negative inotropic properties, either direct or via depression of respiration.

Propanidid has marked negative inotropic properties, as demonstrated by the significant decrease in dP/dt_{max} and mean aortic blood flow, in the presence of a significant increase in heart rate. The decrease in diastolic aortic blood pressure started after the decrease in dP/dt_{max} indicating that the fall in the latter variable does not result from the decrease in diastolic aortic pressure. The fall in diastolic aortic blood pressure and the secondary increase in heart rate result from histamine release. The extreme bradycardia, preceding the increase in heart rate probably in some experiments, is probably due to a direct effect of propanidid since this hypnotic decreases the spontaneous activity in auricular muscle (Xhonneux et al., *This Volume*, p. 157).

The doses of etomidate, methohexital and propanidid, required for adequate sleep durations are respectively about 5, 6 and 10 times higher in dogs than in man.

REFERENCES

Doenicke, A., Kugler, J., Penzel, G., Laub, M., Kalmar, L., Killian, I. and Bezecny, H. (1973*a*): *Anaesthesist*, *22*, 357.

Doenicke, A., Wagner, E. and Beetz, K. H. (1973*b*): *Anaesthesist*, *22*, 353.

Herd, J. A. and Barger, A. C. (1964): *J. appl. Physiol.*, *19*, 791.

Jageneau, A. H. M., Schaper, W. K. A. and Rens, W. (1969): *Pflügers Arch. ges. Physiol.*, *310*, 182.

Jageneau, A. H. M., Xhonneux, R. and Reneman, R. S. (1973): *Biological Research Report 26490/3*. Janssen Research Product Information Service, Beerse, Belgium.

Janssen, P. A. J., Niemegeers, C. J. E., Schellekens, K. H. L. and Lenaerts, F. M. (1971): *Arzneimittel-Forsch.*, *21*, 1234.

Schaper, W. K. A., Lewi, P. and Jageneau, A. H. M. (1965): *Arch. Kreisl.-Forsch.*, *46*, 27.

Taylor, K. M. and Snijder, S. H. (1971): *J. Pharmacol. exp. Ther.*, *179/3*, 619.

Van den Bos, G. C., Dolfing, J., Nassenstein, F., Heerooms, B., Buitenweg, R., Engel, W. and Dijkema, F. K. (1974): *Cardiovasc. Res.*, *8*, 290.

The electrophysiological effects of etomidate (R-26490), a new, short-acting hypnotic, in various cardiac tissues

R. XHONNEUX, E. CARMELIET and R. S. RENEMAN

Cardiovascular Department, Janssen Pharmaceutica, Beerse, and
Department of Physiology, University of Louvain, Louvain, Belgium

Etomidate is a new, potent, short-acting and relatively non-toxic intravenous hypnotic agent (Janssen et al., 1971; Doenicke et al., 1973*a*, *b*) developed in our laboratories. The present study was conducted to compare the influence of etomidate and the commercially available short-acting hypnotics methohexital and propanidid on electrophysiological variables determined in different cardiac tissues.

METHODS

The experiments were performed on guinea-pig auricles, guinea-pig papillary muscles, and Purkinje strands and papillary muscles isolated from dog hearts. The preparations were isolated within 5 min after killing the animals and stored in a warm ($33°$ C), saturated (95% O_2 + 5% CO_2) tyrode solution (pH = 7.4) of the following composition in mmol/l: NaCl 136.9; KCl 5.4; $CaCl_2$ 1.8; $MgCl_2$ 1.8; $NaHCO_3$ 11.9; NaH_2PO_4 0.42 and glucose 5.55.

Transmembrane potentials were recorded between an intracellular and an extracellular microelectrode, and displayed, via a cathode follower stage, on a Tektronix R 5031 dual beam storage oscilloscope. The preparations were stimulated at a basal frequency of 1 Hz, unless spontaneous activity was studied. The effective refractory period, defined as the period in which no propagated action potential can be obtained, and the recovery time, defined as the period needed for the maximum rate of depolarization to recover its full amplitude, were measured by interpolating an extra stimulus at variable times in the regular series of stimuli, using a programmable multipurpose stimulator of our own design (Geivers et al., 1973). Conduction time was measured between 2 intracellular microelectrodes and the conduction velocity calculated. The maximum rate of depolarization (dV/dt) was obtained by electrically differentiating the upstroke of the action potential.

Comparative doses of the hypnotics under investigation, were selected on the basis of sleep duration (Jageneau et al., 1973). Since the sleep duration after 1.25 mg/kg and 2.5 mg/kg i.v. etomidate was not significantly different from the sleep duration after 10 mg/kg i.v. methohexital and 50 mg/kg i.v. propanidid, respectively, the cardiac tissues were incubated with the various compounds in the following concentrations. Etomidate (R-(+)-ethyl 1-(α-methylbenzyl)imidazole-5-carboxylate sulphate) was dissolved in 1.1 mg Na_2HPO_4 12 aqua and 0.9 mg Na_2HPO_4 1 aqua with 4.4% glucose in a concentration of 0.75 mg/ml (pH = 3.4). The preparations were exposed to 2.5 mg etomidate/l tyrode solution. Methohexital (Brietal ® Lilly) and propanidid (Epontol ® Bayer) were used as the commercially available solutions. The preparations were exposed to 10 mg methohexital and 50 mg propanidid/l tyrode solution. Incubation with the hypnotics started at least 20 min after the recorded action potentials had become stable. The duration of this incubation was 15 min for each compound.

Changes in the values of the determined variables after administration of the hypnotics, compared with the values before compound administration, were evaluated for statistical significance by applying Wilcoxon's matched-pairs signed-ranks test (one-tailed probability).

RESULTS

Purkinje strands (dog)

The results obtained on Purkinje strands are shown in Table 1A and in Figures 1 and 2. *Etomidate* had no significant effect on any of the determined variables in Purkinje fibres. *Methohexital* significantly reduced the amplitude of the action potential (P < 0.05), the maximum rate of depolarization (P < 0.001) and the conduction velocity (P < 0.01) in

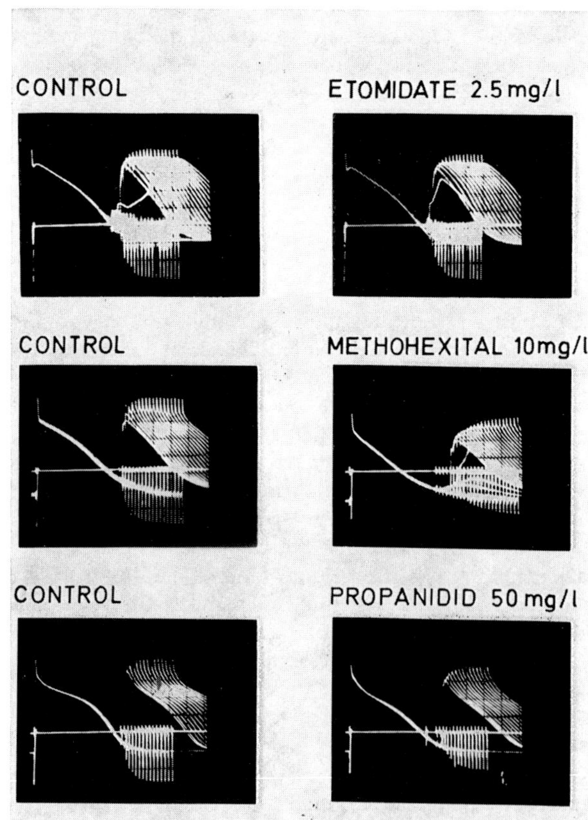

Fig. 1. *The effect of etomidate, methohexital and propanidid on the amplitude, duration and rate of rise (negative deflection at the onset of the action potential), and on the effective refractory period and the recovery time in Purkinje fibres.*

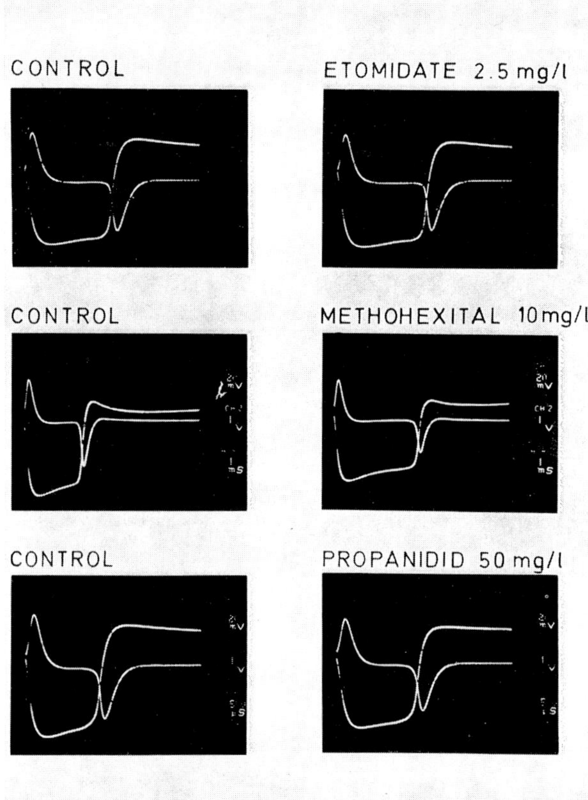

Fig. 2.   *The effect of etomidate, methohexital and propanidid on the conduction velocity in Purkinje fibres. The upstrokes of the two consecutive action potentials and their first derivatives (one positive and one negative) are shown.*

this preparation. Both the effective refractory period and the recovery time were significantly prolonged after incubation with methohexital ($P < 0.05$). *Propanidid* induced in Purkinje fibres a significant decrease in the amplitude of the action potential ($P < 0.01$), the maximum rate of depolarization ($P < 0.001$) and the conduction velocity ($P < 0.01$), and a significant prolongation of the effective refractory period ($P < 0.05$).

Papillary muscles (dog and guinea-pig)

None of the hypnotics under investigation had a significant effect on the variables determined in papillary muscles of the dog (Table 1B) and the guinea-pig.

Auricular muscles (guinea-pig)

Propanidid significantly reduced ($P < 0.01$) the spontaneous activity of guinea-pig auricular muscles (Table 1C). In some cases the spontaneous activity even stopped after incubation with this hypnotic, but the preparations remained electrically excitable. *Etomidate* and *methohexital* had no significant effect on the spontaneous activity of auricular muscles in guinea-pigs (Table 1C).

Table 1. *The effect of etomidate, methohexital and propanidid on dog Purkinje fibres (A), dog papillary muscle (B) and guinea-pig auricular muscle (C)*

Variables	Etomidate (2.5 mg/l)		Methohexital (10 mg/l)		Propanidid (50 mg/l)	
	Control	15 min	Control	15 min	Control	15 min
A. Duration of the	400*	400	400	450	350	350
action potential	(320–700)**	(320–1000)	(300–600)	(300–700)	(300–560)	(300–510)
(msec)	n:9	NS	n:7	NS	n:7	NS
Amplitude of the	110	110	112	106	106	100
action potential (mV)	(108–124)	(108–120)	(104–132)	(88–118)	(84–120)	(76–116)
	n:9	NS	n:7	†	n:7	††
Rate of rise of the	300	290	280	260	300	250
action potential	(200–370)	(140–330)	(230–340)	(60–320)	(230–330)	(120–290)
(V/sec)	n:17	NS	n:23	†††	n:18	†††
Effective refractory	268	268	252	280	270	277
period (msec)	(200–410)	(240–360)	(235–340)	(235–340)	(250–320)	(250–300)
	n:8	NS	n:8	†	n:8	NS
Recovery time	480	470	450	500	415	475
(msec)	(350–660)	(350–620)	(400–540)	(420–610)	(350–540)	(400–640)
	n:8	NS	n:7	†	n:8	†
Conduction velocity	208	200	240	178	222	190
(cm/sec)	(190–242)	(185–228)	(190–266)	(129–238)	(160–243)	(53–222)
	n:7	NS	n:8	††	n:7	††
B. Duration of the	250	260	270	270	230	230
action potential	(250–380)	(250–380)	(160–300)	(160–350)	(210–330)	(230–370)
(msec)	n:9	NS	n:9	NS	n:9	NS
Amplitude of the	100	104	112	104	80	80
action potential (mV)	(72–120)	(72–116)	(84–116)	(88–112)	(68–116)	(72–116)
	n:9	NS	n:9	NS	n:9	NS
Rate of rise of the	200	200	180	170	120	100
action potential	(145–300)	(145–280)	(120–240)	(120–220)	(90–250)	(80–140)
(V/sec)	n:9	NS	n:9	NS	n:9	NS
C. Spontaneous activity	123	120	99	96	114	90
(depol/min)	(90–186)	(96–180)	(48–126)	(41–102)	(50–168)	(0–144)
	n:10	NS	n:6	NS	n:7	††

* Median. ** Range. NS = $P > 0.05$. † $P < 0.05$. †† $P < 0.01$. ††† $P < 0.001$.

DISCUSSION

The present study shows that etomidate is devoid of any significant effect on the electro-physiological variables determined in Purkinje fibres, papillary muscles and auricular muscles. Both methohexital and propanidid depress the fast sodium conductance in Purkinje fibres as demonstrated by the reduction in amplitude and rate of rise of the action potential. These changes also explain the decrease in conduction velocity. Furthermore, the prolongation of the effective refractory period and the recovery time again indicates an interference with the sodium carrying system, namely a slowing of its repriming process (Carmeliet, 1975). That these effects are not seen in papillary muscles is not surprising since this preparation is known to be less sensitive to drugs than Purkinje fibres (Kleinfeld et al., 1964).

A slowing of the time-dependent fall in potassium conductance and/or a fall in background sodium conductance might explain the reduction in spontaneous activity in guinea-pig auricles, seen after the administration of propanidid.

SUMMARY

Intracellular microelectrode techniques were used to study the electrophysiological effects of the new, short-acting hypnotic agent etomidate (2.5 mg/l) in various cardiac tissues isolated from dog and guinea-pig hearts. Methohexital (10 mg/l) and propanidid (50 mg/l) were used as reference substances.

Etomidate was devoid of any significant effect on the electrophysiological variables determined in Purkinje fibres, papillary muscles and auricular muscles. Methohexital and propanidid had no significant effect on the variables determined in papillary muscles but significantly reduced the amplitude and the rate of rise of the action potential and the conduction velocity, and significantly prolonged the effective refractory period in Purkinje fibres. Propanidid significantly decreased the spontaneous activity in auricular muscle.

These findings demonstrate that methohexital and propanidid depress the fast sodium conductance in Purkinje fibres, while etomidate is devoid of this side effect.

REFERENCES

Carmeliet, E. (1975): In: *Recent Advances in Studies on Cardiac Structures and Metabolism.* University Tark Press, Baltimore, Md. In press.

Doenicke, A., Kugler, J., Laub, M., Kalmar, L., Killian, I. and Bezecny, H. (1973*a*): *Anaesthesist*, *22*, 357.

Doenicke, A., Wagner, E. and Beetz, K. H. (1973*b*): *Anaesthesist*, *22*, 353.

Geivers, H., Xhonneux, R., Wauquier, A., Van Nueten, J. and Reneman, R. S. (1973): In: *Proceedings, 4th Annual Meeting of the Biomedical Engineering Society, Los Angeles, Calif.* Paper 3.12.

Jageneau, A. H. M., Xhonneux, R. and Reneman, R. S. (1973): *Biological Research Report 26490/3.* Janssen Research Product Information Service, Beerse, Belgium.

Janssen, P. A. J., Niemegeers, C. J. E., Schellekens, K. H. L. and Lenaerts, F. M. (1971): *Arzneimittel-Forsch.*, *21*, 1232.

Kleinfeld, M., Stein, E. and Murphy, B. (1964): *Amer. J. Physiol.*, *206*, 975.

Evaluation of Ro 5-4200 as the principal narcotic agent in 1017 anesthesias for major surgery

W. K. MARTI, H. GUMPENBERGER, M. LUCAS and J. F. VEGA

Department of Anesthesiology and Resuscitation,
Thurgau Cantonal Hospital, Münsterlingen, Switzerland

INTRODUCTION

Benzodiazepines have been known since 1933. However the interest in these compounds has increased in the last 10 years. Randall et al. (1960) reported investigations of the central depressant, anticonvulsant and sleep inducing properties of these drugs. In 1961 diazepam (Valium®) and chlordiazepoxide (Librium®) were introduced to therapy (Randall et al., 1961; Randall, 1961). Because of their anxiolytic effect, anesthesiologists were soon interested in these substances for premedication and numerous papers report good results. The experience that higher doses of diazepam could produce unconsciousness led to the use of these substances for short surgical procedures, where no specific analgesia was required, because benzodiazepines are not analgetics. This form of light anesthesia was especially useful for out-patients and the limited indications for this technique are wellknown. Whilst diazepam and chlordiazepoxide have almost no hypnotic properties – which allows their use as daytime sedatives – another compound, called nitrazepam (Mogadon®) was found to be an excellent hypnotic. Again nitrazepam has been used extensively in premedication and produces sleep and freedom from anxiety in the preoperative phase. Since no injectable form is available, nitrazepam cannot be used for premedication immediately prior to surgery. By introducing a fluorine atom into the nitrazepam molecule, flunitrazepam was obtained. The purpose of the present paper is to demonstrate that this compound alone, which is about 15 times more potent than nitrazepam, is capable of producing profound sleep and long-acting amnesia, which, with certain technical precautions, makes prolonged general anesthesia possible. This substance has already been investigated by a number of anesthesiologists (Ungerer and Erasmus, 1972; Colemann et al., 1972; Martins de Oliveira et al., 1972; Vega, 1971; De Castro, 1972a, b, c; Lecron et al., 1972; Stovner et al., in press) who all agree that besides the general properties of the benzodiazepines this is a very potent hypnotic. It has therefore been used for induction of anesthesia, either in combination with intravenous cocaine, with neuroleptanalgesia or with ketamine or simply to replace thiopentone.

Apart from local irritation at the injection site, the clinical absence of toxicity of the new compound is noteworthy. Based on the general pharmacology of the benzodiazepines and the specific hypnotic action of flunitrazepam, its use as a sole hypnotic agent for general anesthesia is investigated. Amnesia should last into the postoperative phase, due to the slow elimination, which could also produce postoperative sedation. The anticonvulsant and slight muscle relaxant properties of the substance are also of interest in general anesthesia. In particular the possible use of this drug from the day before surgery through the actual premedication, the general anesthesia and the postoperative phase is of interest.

The number of cases was set from the beginning to a minimum of 1,000 since only a large number would allow accurate evaluation.

METHOD

In the first phase different indications for this anesthesia were examined. Because of the lack of analgesia, the drug could only be used in minor surgery, for endoscopy, cardioversion and reduction of dislocated joints. In surgical procedures for out-patients it became clear that the drug had no advantage, because of the prolonged sleepiness and muscular weakness. After a few dozen cases it was clear that anesthesia with Ro 5–4200 was indicated in those cases where intubation and controlled respiration with muscle relaxants was to be used. General anesthesia with Ro 5–4200 has been used for 1,017 cases having the following type of operations: general surgery 55%; orthopedics 5%; traumatology 14%; urology 9%; neurosurgery 1%; gynecology 16%, and a few obstetrical cases.

The technique was always as follows: In spite of frequent use of benzodiazepines no clinical signs of tolerance were found. The night before surgery the patient received 2 mg of flunitrazepam by mouth, which produced in 78% cases profound sleep which lasted more than 6 hr and from which the patients recovered relaxed and free from hangover. 45–60 min prior to surgery all the patients received 0.5 mg of atropine and 2 mg of flunitrazepam i.m. Usually this again produced sleep after 5–10 min and the majority of the patients were sufficiently amnesic so as to recall neither the transport to the operating room nor the transfer to the operating table. After measuring the blood pressure, heart and respiratory rate, venepuncture was performed, using a butterfly-needle (Abbott) on the back of the left hand. Then, depending on the state of somnolence, up to 2 mg of flunitrazepam was rapidly injected intravenously, which produced some pain in 58% cases. Patients who were completely asleep after the premedication received no further drug. The average dose was 2 mg, but in poor-risk cases, and also for older patients this dose was reduced to 1 mg. At the beginning of the study up to 4 and 5 mg were given because it was uncertain if the drug would produce sufficient anesthesia. Once the patient became drowsy, 0.3 mg/kg of alcuronium chloride (Alloferin®) was given, and artificial ventilation with 30% oxygen and 70% nitrous oxide was started at first with an open system and later with a rebreathing system. After intubation, the Engström ER 311-ventilator with a rebreathing system was used with a fixed rate of 18 and an average of 10 l/min. A central venous pressure line was inserted, using the brachial approach with a drum-cartridge catheter (Abbott). All patients were monitored completely. In a few cases only the ECG and heart rate were monitored but in 75% cases the left femoral artery was cannulated with a catheter (Arteriocath), in about 10% cases the left radial approach was used, and arterial and venous pressure were monitored continuously, using Statham-transducers and Liechti-Medicath electro-manometers. Mean arterial pressure was also measured. This direct monitoring of arterial pressure, which is a standard procedure in our hospital, allowed also frequent investigations of arterial blood-gases which were checked at least at the end of every anesthesia. In a few cases central body temperature and EEG were also monitored; all the data were displayed on a 2-channel oscilloscope and in some cases permanently recorded on a 3-channel recorder. Since the respiratory volume and frequency were given by the Engström respirator, there was no need for specific monitoring of these parameters. It was only necessary to maintain muscular relaxation by injections of an average of 2 mg alcuronium chloride every 30 min; no other drugs were used in these 1,017 anesthesias. The duration of the operation was of no concern, since even operations lasting over 8 hr (Whipple's procedure) were performed with the initial dose of 2 mg Ro 5–4200. Initially 1 mg flunitrazepam was given after 4 hr of anesthesia but this is not necessary. In contrast to other investigators the patients needed larger doses of alcuronium chloride and not less but different techniques were used by the other workers. At the end of the operation, the muscle relaxant was reversed in the usual way, using atropine and neostigmine, and as soon as adequate spontaneous respiration returned, the endotracheal tube was removed. Most cases were sleepy but could be awakened at the end of the operation. If unstimulated, the patients went back to sleep, but nevertheless all had protective reflexes. Only in one case was reintubation necessary, and this patient was in very poor general condition and was amongst the first 10 cases, and had consequently received too much flunitrazepam. At the end of every anesthesia, arterial blood was withdrawn for arterial blood-gas analysis and then the catheter was removed, except if the patient went to the ICU, where the femoral catheter was required for further arterial blood pressure monitoring.

Using this technique 1,017 patients were anesthetised. The age distribution was similar to that for the surgical diseases treated in a general hospital. The youngest patient was 2.5 years old and the oldest 99. In both these cases anesthesia was completely uneventful. The type of operation tended to be major or prolonged, because this type of anesthesia was restricted to patients who required intubation and muscle relaxation. But flunitrazepam has also been used for short procedures, especially endoscopy, curettage and cardioversion. Those patients received nitrous oxide and oxygen with spontaneous respiration. The average duration of anesthesia was slightly over 2 hr.

DISCUSSION

Evaluation was on the basis of the patients' opinion and the opinion of the anesthesiologist and the operating team including the nursing staff.

Except for one patient, who had been benzodiazepine addict for 7 years and in whom even 6 mg flunitrazepam did not cause sleep and who, therefore, was anesthetised with a different method, there was no case with incomplete amnesia for the operating procedure. Since the patients became relaxed following the premedication and often had complete amnesia until the day after surgery, this type of anesthesia was usually appreciated. It was not unusual for a patient to ask on the day after the operation, why no operation had been performed. The drug clearly produces complete and prolonged amnesia.

This type of anesthesia has become standard in our hospital. In all new procedures the stability of circulation is stressed to a point, where it seems doubtful if this is actually a valuable criterion for assessment. Nevertheless, the complete stability of the circulation under flunitrazepam anesthesia was very impressive. Usually a slight increase in arterial pressure and mean arterial pressure at the beginning of the operation is observed, which might be due to peripheral vasoconstriction with increased peripheral resistance because of lack of analgesia. This so-called stability of the circulation might therefore be a hemodynamic disadvantage. About 60% cases had a slight metabolic acidosis which could be further evidence of an increase in peripheral resistance with lower tissue perfusion. However, in some cases, in which the increase in blood pressure seemed significant, analgesia with 0.1 mg of fentanyl did not produce a fall in blood pressure. It is not known if this rise in blood pressure is due to pain with a subsequent increase in catecholamines. In these cases with a significant rise of blood pressure, there was usually no increase in heart rate. The patients reacted neither to the incision nor to the manipulation, which, with other forms of anesthesia, are known to produce tachycardia. By measuring the circulating volume with the RIHSA method, it was possible to prove that the hypertension was not due to overtransfusion. Another interesting observation under flunitrazepam anesthesia was the decrease in number of ectopic beats in patients with ventricular arrhythmia prior to anesthesia. Some patients with frequent ectopic beats returned to sinus rhythm during the operation. In some cases with auricular fibrillation, a partial or complete return to sinus rhythm occurred, but only in cases with tachycardia. In some cases where a cardioversion was scheduled, the patient returned spontaneously to sinus rhythm under flunitrazepam premedication. Especially in poor-risk cases (intestinal occlusion, peritonitis, perforated gastric ulcer) who had, prior to anesthesia, very poor peripheral circulation, there was an increase in mean arterial pressure and reduction of heart rate shortly after injection of flunitrazepam and controlled respiration. Since the skin of the patients feels warm and has a rosy appearance, it seems improbable that the increase in mean arterial pressure is only due to peripheral vascular constriction. This is a simple technique. As soon as the patient is asleep and intubated the anesthetic management is limited to the maintenance of curarisation and fluid balance even in very long procedures. Some patients showed mydriasis and in a very few cases there was also slight sweating, signs which are attributed normally to light anesthesia. These cases had complete amnesia also and it is unnecessary to combine the technique with halothane (10 cases) or fentanyl (7 cases), because this does often not result in the disappearance of these symptoms. In the last 600 cases these signs of too light anesthesia were ignored and in none of the cases did the patient recall his operation, or show autonomic circulatory reflexes other than those usually observed.

The end of the anesthetic is also uneventful and consists only of reversal of neuromuscular block. Immediately the patient recovers his reflexes back and only one case of postoperative vomiting has occurred. There is therefore no worry about the immediate postoperative period provided that there is adequate spontaneous ventilation. In patients with intestinal obstruction intubation was either during spontaneous ventilation or with succinylcholine, to prevent passage of air into the stomach due to prolonged ventilation. Further anesthesia was then administered according to the standard procedure.

The new method was less widely accepted by the nursing staff. After a rather bad start, due to overdosage in the early cases, the technique has now generally been accepted on the surgical wards. The nurses considered positively the circulatory stability and the fact that, due to amnesia, the patients needed less analgetics. There were usually fewer problems in postoperative care with patients following flunitrazepam anesthesia. However, there were a few cases of severe excitation after 2 mg of flunitrazepam (orally) during the night before anesthesia. These patients had usually advanced arteriosclerosis and were also poor-risk cases. In similar cases therefore the dose of the hypnotic has been reduced to half a tablet (1 mg) or nothing.

The main objection to flunitrazepam anesthesia was because of the prolonged somnolence and the lack of cooperation of some patients in the postoperative period. For 20 years anesthesiologists have told nurses, that a good anesthetic was when a patient returned to the ward completely awake. Under flunitrazepam anesthesia patients remain somnolent for a number of hours. They can be awoken, but usually return to the somnolent state, as soon as stimulation is discontinued. Since early mobilisation of the patient immediately after surgery is the rule (prophylaxis of thromboembolism), this somnolent state increased the nurses' workload. Thus, especially on the gynecological ward, there was an outright hostility towards flunitrazepam anesthesia. By increasing education and by stressing the advantages for the patient, it was finally accepted. On the gynecological ward the nurses felt that the patients were in worse condition after surgery than after halothane anesthesia particularly because gynecological patients usually have an uncomplicated recovery. With these exceptions, flunitrazepam anesthesia has finally been accepted by the nursing staff.

COMPLICATIONS

Among the first 10 cases an old lady for total replacement of the hip joint had postoperative respiratory failure, which necessitated reintubation and ventilation for about one hour. This was due to severe overdosage because this lady, weighing only 40 kg, had received 5 mg of flunitrazepam with a very long recovery period. Three patients showed a skin rash for about 30 min immediately after injection of flunitrazepam, similar to that after thiopentone. There was one case of ventricular arrhythmia during anesthesia, which coincided with severe blood loss. In 2 further cases there was slight postoperative respiratory depression, which did not require reintubation or respirator treatment. One patient with multiple intestinal perforations and severe peritonitis died during the operation; necropsy showed that this was due to extensive myocardial infarction. No other complications have been observed.

FLUNITRAZEPAM AND METABOLISM

In all cases very extensive studies in blood-chemistry were performed, but apart from metabolic acidosis no other significant changes could be found. Among the first 100 cases there were different patients with postoperative hyperbilirubinemia, which led the surgeons to claim that the new drug was responsible for this complication. However, there was always a satisfactory explanation available, and a few cases have been reoperated upon for different reasons under flunitrazepam anesthesia without recurrence of icterus.

CONCLUSION

Flunitrazepam anesthesia has proved in over a 1000 cases to be a very safe technique which, if properly performed, assures, without any apparent toxicity, an almost perfect anesthesia for the patient, the operating team and, last but not least, for the anesthesiologist. It allows general anesthesia to be given serenely in poor-risk cases, where all the other forms of anesthesia would be considered as potentially dangerous.

The slight disadvantage of a long recovery period with some muscular weakness, limiting the mobilisation in the first 24 hr, must be weighed against the apparent advantages as described in this paper.

REFERENCES

Colemann, A. J., Downing, J. W., Moyes, D. G. and O'Brien, A. (1972): Paper presented at: Anaesthetic Congress, Johannesburg, 1972.

Castro, J. de (1972*a*): *Ars Med. (Gand)*, *27/8*, 1286.

Castro, J. de (1972*b*): *Paper presented at:* Congreso Mundial de Anestesiologia, Kyoto, 1972.

Castro, J. de (1972*c*): *Ars Med. (Gand)*, *27/8*, 1233.

Kurka, P. (1973): Paper presented at: XIII Gemeinsame Tagung der Deutschen, Schweizerischen und Oesterreichischen Gesellschaft für Anästhesiologie und Reanimation, Linz, 1973.

Lecron, L., Levy, D., Collard, C., Delville, F. and Toppet, E. (1972): *Ars Med. (Gand)*, *27/8*, 1269.

Martins de Oliveira, A. A., Duarte, D. F., Gesser, N. and Linhares, S. (1972): Paper presented at: Brazilian Congress on Anaesthesiology, Fortaleza, 1972.

Randall, L. O. (1961): *Dis. nerv. Syst.*, *22*, 7.

Randall, L. O., Heise, G. A., Schallek, W., Bagdon, R. E., Banziger, R., Boris, A., Moe, R. A. and Abrams, W. B. (1961): *Curr. ther. Res.*, *3*, 405.

Randall, L. O., Schallek, W., Heise, G. A., Keith, E. F. and Bagdon, R. E. (1960): *J. Pharmacol. exp. Ther.*, *129*, 163.

Randall, L. O., Schallek, W., Scheckel, C., Bagdon, R. E. and Rieder, J. (1965): *Schweiz. med. Wschr.*, *95*, 334.

Stovner, J., Endresen, R. and Østerud, A. (1975): Intravenous Anaesthesia with a new benzdiazepine, Ro 5–4200. In press.

Ungerer, M. J. and Erasmus, F. R. (1972): Paper presented at: Anaesthetic Congress, Johannesburg, 1972.

Vega, D. E. (1971): Paper presented at: Sociedad de Anestesiologia del Uruguay, 1971.

The 0.5 MAC equivalent of thiopental

RICHARD L. FRAIOLI, LEE A. SHEFFER and JOHN L. STEFFENSON

Medical Corps, Naval Regional Medical Center, United States Navy, Oakland, Calif., U.S.A.

Thiopental is a very popular barbiturate for intravenous induction of anesthesia. Because of its lack of analgesic effect, it is used for maintenance of anesthesia in conjunction with nitrous oxide, a narcotic or both. Since little information is available relating serum levels of thiopental with maintenance of adequate surgical anesthesia, it is given empirically.

In this study, we have defined the serum thiopental level equal to 0.5 MAC with the hope that this information will allow a more precise administration of the drug.

Eighteen healthy patients ranging in age from 18–41 years undergoing elective surgery were studied. Following an induction dose of thiopental of 4 mg/kg, given as a bolus, patients were paralyzed with succinylcholine 1.5 mg/kg. Laryngotracheal anesthesia was obtained with 2% lidocaine and endotracheal intubation performed. Sixty per cent nitrous oxide, a concentration which has been shown to produce 0.5 MAC, 40% oxygen, and an infusion of sodium thiopental were started upon completion of the induction dose of thiopental. The infusion was administered via a Harvard infusion pump with doses of 0.2 mg/kg/min (5 patients), 0.3 mg/kg/min (9 patients), and 0.4 mg/kg/min (4 patients). Ventilation was assisted to maintain normal end-tidal CO_2.

Thiopental infusion was discontinued at 30 min at the time the skin incision was made. Patients were observed for movement or no movement at the time of incision. Other observations included changes in heart rate, blood pressure, respiratory rate, pupillary dilitation and the time at which those patients not moving at skin incision, did move in response to the surgical procedure.

Arterial blood samples were taken from a radial artery catheter before the induction dose and at 5, 10, 15, 20, 25, 30, 40, 50, and 60 min after, and serum thiopental levels measured. A 30-min specimen was also analyzed for pH, Po_2, Pco_2, and base excess.

The blood samples were centrifuged to obtain the serum and the serum extracted with chloroform and analyzed in duplicate for thiopental levels using the spectrophotometric method described by Brodie in 1950.

Postoperatively the patients were interviewed and any unfavorable response to the anesthetic noted.

Significant differences between the various groups were done using the Student's t-test with scores of 0.05 being accepted as showing statistical significance. All variability is reported as standard error of the mean.

Since all patients received 4 mg/kg thiopental as a bolus for induction, any differences seen in arterial serum thiopental levels are due to differences in the infusion rates after the induction bolus.

Figure 1 describes the arterial serum levels of thiopental from 5–60 min. Remember that the infusion was discontinued at 30 min.

It can be seen that the 0.2 mg/kg/min infusion rate produced arterial serum levels that were essentially unchanging during the first 25 min with only a slight elevation of 3 μg/ml at 30 min. This suggests that at 0.2 mg/kg/min, the rate of uptake of the thiopental by the

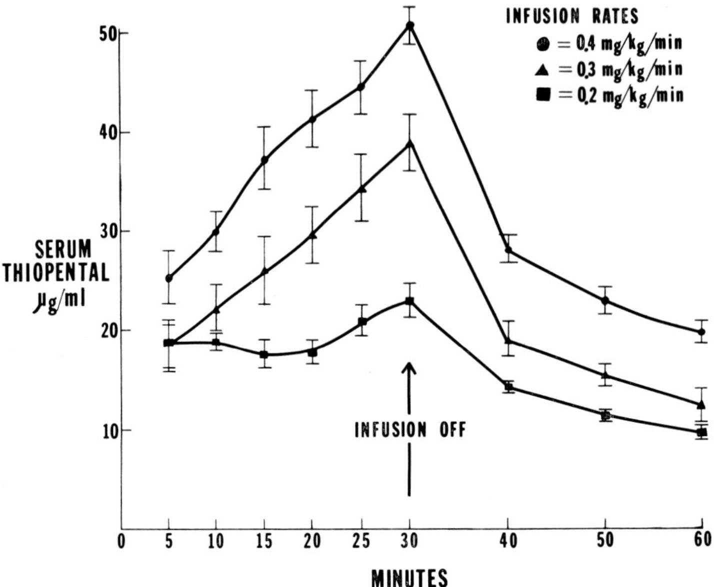

Fig. 1.   *The arterial serum levels of thiopental from 5–60 min.*

tissues essentially equals the infusion rate and only when the lean tissue mass approaches saturation does the serum level begin rising. The two higher infusion rates both showed steadily increasing serum levels until the 30-min point. With discontinuation of the infusion at 30 min, all serum levels fell in a similar fashion.

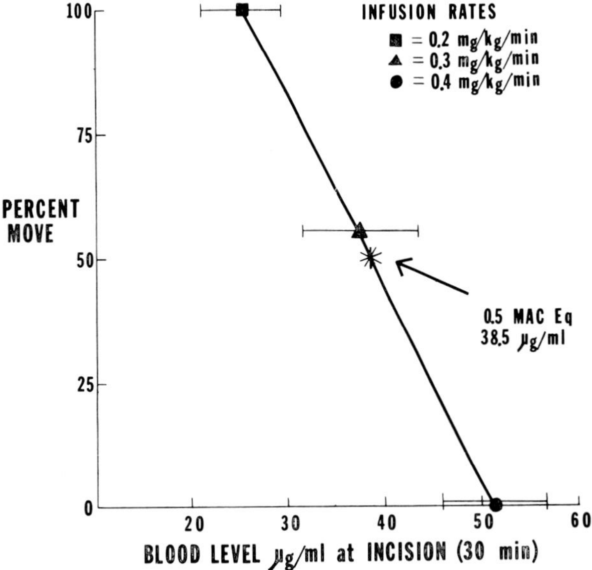

Fig. 2.   *Patients' responses to skin incision at 30 min, according to dose and serum levels.*

Patients' responses to skin incision at 30 min fell into three distinct groups according to dose and serum levels. In Figure 2, we see that an infusion rate of 0.4 mg/kg/min produced a mean serum level of 51.27 ± 2.67 µg/ml at 30 min, and none of the patients moved with skin incision. Therefore, these patients were at levels of anesthesia greater than 1.0 MAC. An infusion rate of 0.2 mg/kg/min produced a mean serum level of 25.34 ± 4.33 µg/ml and all patients moved at skin incision. These patients were below 1.0 MAC. The 0.3 mg/kg/min group had a mean serum level of 37.36 ± 1.97 µg/ml and 55% of patients moved with skin incision. By plotting these data we determined the 50% movement or 1.0 MAC point. We found that a serum thiopental level of 38.50 µg/ml is the 0.5 MAC equivalent for thiopental.

In analyzing our results there are several points that should be made. First, in the 0.4 mg/kg/min group, the 0.5 MAC equivalent was achieved at 17 min and higher levels were maintained until 36 min. Second, these patients moved in response to the surgical procedure at a mean of 46 min at which time the mean thiopental level fell to 25 µg/ml. Third, all of the non-moving 0.3 mg/kg/min patients moved at a mean time of 37 min, a point at which the serum level was 25 µg/ml. It is not surprising that these patients did not move until the serum levels fell well below the 0.5 MAC equivalent point since it is generally recognized that the skin incision is the most stimulating part of superficial surgical procedures. Fourth, all of the non-moving 0.3 mg/kg/min patients exhibited increases in systolic blood pressure, respiratory rate and pupillary dilatation at the time of incision. Those patients in the higher dose groups showed less of these changes. Fifth, none of the patients, including those in the 0.2 mg/kg/min group had any recollection of intra-anesthetic events. Sixth, none of the three dose groups had excessive somnolence postoperatively. Therefore, except for muscle relaxation, all the criteria of true anesthesia are obtained with 60% N_2O and a serum level of 38.5 µg/ml of thiopental. We believe that the determination of 0.5 MAC equivalency of intravenous agents results in better balanced anesthesia technique by assuring adequate anesthesia while avoiding drug overdose.

Barbiturate metabolism by the liver microsomal fraction in sensitive and resistant mice*

S. HALEVY [1], S. ROSENTHAL [2] and W. G. LEVINE [3]

[1] Department of Anesthesiology, Columbia University College of Physicians and Surgeons, and
[2] Departments of Anesthesiology and [3] Pharmacology,
Albert Einstein College of Medicine, New York, N.Y., U.S.A.

The species-related variations in response to short-acting barbiturates and other drugs have been attributed in the past to differences in the tissue distribution of the drug (Butler, 1951; Mark et al., 1958). This view has recently been under scrutiny since, in some strains and species, these variations can be attributed to differences in receptor sites sensitivity and drug metabolism (Brodie, 1964; Saidman and Eger, 1966; Conney, 1967; Catz and Yaffe, 1967; Noordhoek, 1968; Goldstein et al., 1968).

We have studied hexobarbital (H) metabolism by liver microsomal fractions prepared from adult mice of two inbred paired genotypes obtained by selective breeding. These strains exhibit contrasting differences in sensitivity to a variety of stresses such as murine salmonellosis, experimental allergic encephalomyelitis and St. Louis encephalitis (Lee et al., 1954; Böhme et al., 1959; Lee, 1964; Wajda et al., 1967). The two strains have been designated as BSVS (bacterial susceptible viral susceptible) and BRVR (bacterial resistant viral resistant).

We have shown that the BSVS strain is sensitive and the BRVR strain resistant to the hypnotic effects of pentobarbital and hexobarbital injected intraperitoneally (i.p.) (Halevy and Frumin, 1973). Sensitivity and resistance to these barbiturates has been established utilizing the frequency and duration of the loss of righting reflex (LRR) (Figs. 1 and 2). We have also noted that males of both strains were more sensitive than the corresponding females. In a separate study we have measured brain and serum H concentrations at 5 or 10 min following i.p. administration and we have found an apparent lack of correlation between drug concentrations and (a) pharmacologic response (LRR), (b) strain, (c) sex, and (d) time intervals after injection (Halevy et al., 1974).

In view of these findings, we decided to investigate whether these strains of mice differ in microsomal liver metabolism, a major factor in the recovery from short-acting barbiturate anesthesia.

METHODS

Liver microsomal H metabolism (H-oxidase) was measured in 55 mice, using at least

---

* The study was supported in part by a grant from the Albert Einstein College of Medicine (NIH) General Research Support Grant funds to Simon Halevy and a United States Public Health Service Research Grant No. 1 ROI CA 14231 from the National Cancer Institute to Walter G. Levine.

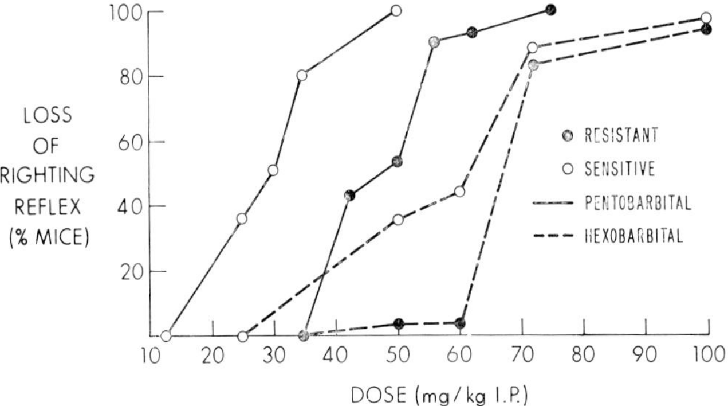

Fig. 1. *Frequency of loss of righting reflex after pentobarbital and hexobarbital. Reproduced from Halevy and Frumin (1973) by courtesy of the Editor, British Journal of Anaesthesia.*

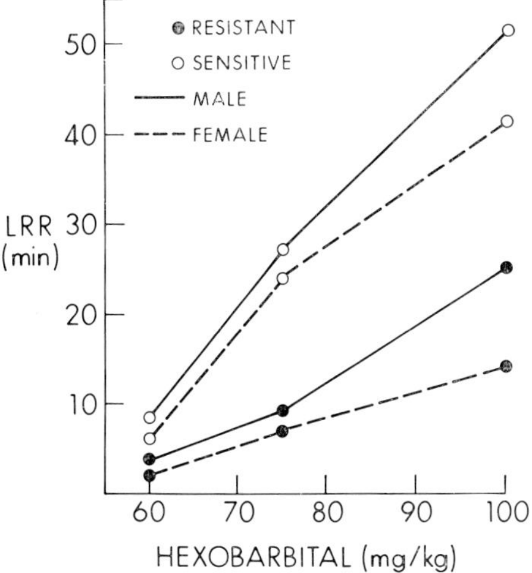

Fig. 2. *Duration of loss of righting reflex after intraperitoneal hexobarbital. Reproduced from Halevy and Frumin (1973) by courtesy of the Editor, British Journal of Anaesthesia.*

10 mice of either sex for each test. H metabolism was estimated from the rate of disappearance of the drug from an incubation mixture. The animals were sacrificed by cervical dislocation, exsanguinated and livers removed and weighed. Liver homogenates were prepared in cold 1.15% KCl in a Potter-Elvehjem homogenizer. Homogenates were centrifuged at $10,000 \times g$ for 10 min at 5° C. The supernatant which contained the microsomal fraction was retained for the metabolism studies. The incubation mixture contained: phosphate buffer (48 mM) pH 7.4, NADP (0.05 mM), isocitrate (10 mM), magnesium sulphate (6.6 mM), sodium H solution in water (0.2 mM) and $10,000 \times g$ supernatant (enzyme) in a total volume of 5 ml. Standards and blanks (without supernatant) were also used. The mixture described was first preincubated for 5 min without H at 37° C in a Dubnoff incubator. The reaction started by addition of H (time 0 min). Two ml of mixture was removed at 0 min and after 15 min of incubation and H was determined spectrophotometrically by a modified technique used for oxybarbiturates (Brodie et al., 1953; Cooper and Brodie, 1955). H

was extracted with n-heptane from the incubation mixture in a citric acid solution (0.5 M). After centrifugation the organic phase was extracted with phosphate buffer (0.8 M) pH 11 and the aqueous phase retained. The optical densities of this solution were determined at 245 and 290 nm. The standards and blanks were treated in a similar manner. The specificity of H extraction as unchanged drug by n-heptane with this method has been previously established (Brodie and Udenfriend, 1945; Brodie et al., 1953; Cooper and Brodie, 1955). We also confirmed this using ^{14}C-labelled hexobarbital (*a*) injected to mice, and (*b*) added to tissues in vitro, followed by thin layer chromatography and determination of radioactivity.

The differences between the amount of H found at 0 min and that found at 15 min represented the H metabolized. The results were expressed as nmoles of H metabolized/g liver/min. In a preliminary study, the enzyme activity was found to be proportional to concentrations with 1, 2 and 3 ml of $10,000 \times g$ supernatant added to incubation mixture and the reaction was linear within the 15 min incubation interval used.

Student's t-test for independent samples was used for statistical evaluation of data and significance established at 5% level.

RESULTS

The results are depicted in Figure 3. H metabolism by the liver microsomal fraction in the strains studied was virtually identical with the exception of resistant females. These mice showed significantly lower metabolic activity ($P < 0.05$) compared with other groups. BRVR males showed higher mean values of H metabolized by the liver than the other mice. However, these differences were not significant ($P < 0.05$).

DISCUSSION

An important number of factors could influence drug metabolism by the liver. Environmental

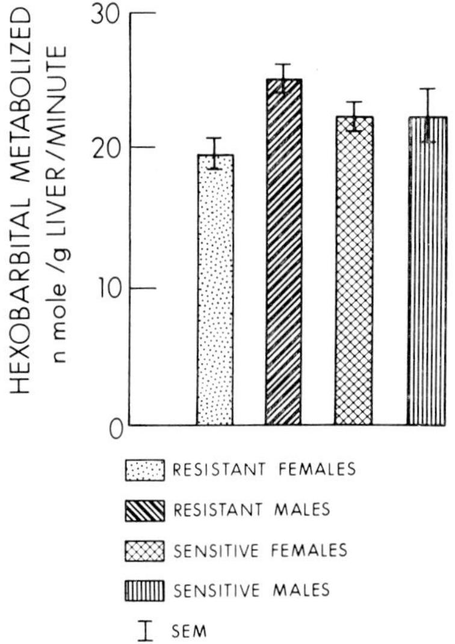

Fig. 3.   *Hexobarbital metabolism by hepatic microsomes in 'resistant' and 'sensitive' mice. Reproduced from Halevy et al. (1974) by courtesy of the Editor, British Journal of Anaesthesia.*

factors are among the most common conditions which influence drug metabolism in laboratory animals (McLaren and Michie, 1956; Killam et al., 1958; Irwin, 1964; Vesell, 1968; Sotaniemi, 1967). We were aware of these factors and we have attempted to minimize their influence by: maintaining constant environmental temperature, avoiding crowding, performing the experiments at the same hour of the day and using uniform caging, bedding and diet for all animals.

The major findings in the present study are: (*a*) the differentiation between strains, i.e. sensitive or resistant, with respect to pharmacologic responses (LRR) could not be explained by differences in liver metabolism, and (*b*) H oxidase activity was uncorrelated with the behavioral response in both strains and sexes. Furthermore, the resistant females, which slept less than all other subjects, following the i.p. injection of H (Fig. 2) displayed the lowest liver microsomal activity (Fig. 3).

In a previous study we measured serum ^{14}C-labelled H concentrations in these strains of mice 5 or 10 min following i.p. administration of the drug (unpublished data). We have also found that serum H concentrations did not correlate with the behavioral responses in either strain or sex or at any time interval considered. It is commonly assumed that the concentration of the drug in plasma or serum will determine the amount of drug at the receptor sites and thereby the intensity of the pharmacologic response. A number of factors could have influenced serum concentrations of the drug. Metabolism is one major possibility but our present study showed no difference in the groups in their capacity to metabolize H which could explain variations in serum levels. Furthermore, it is obvious from this study that both variations in CNS receptor sensitivity and H metabolism by the liver depend upon a sex related genetic mechanism since these strains were obtained by selective breeding.

In conclusion, such lack of correlations between drug metabolism and pharmacologic responses to H (narcosis) within and between these two inbred strains, as well as serum and regional brain distribution data, suggest that there are genetically related differences in sensitivity of receptors to barbiturates.

REFERENCES

Böhme, D. H., Schneider, H. A. and Lee, J. M. (1959): *J. exp. Med., 110*, 9.

Brodie, B. B. (1964): In: *Animal and Clinical Pharmacologic Techniques in Drug Evaluation, Vol. 1,* Chapter 6, p. 69. Editors: J. H. Nodine and P. E. Siegler. Year Book Medical Publishers, Chicago, Ill.

Brodie, B. B., Burns, J. J., Mark, L. C., Lief, P. A., Bernstein, E. and Papper, E. M. (1953): *J. Pharmacol. exp. Ther., 109/1*, 26.

Brodie, B. B. and Udenfriend, S. (1945): *J. biol. Chem., 158/3*, 705.

Butler, T. C. (1951): *J. Pharmacol. exp. Ther., 100/2*, 219.

Catz, C. and Yaffe, S. J. (1967): *J. Pharmacol. exp. Ther., 155/1*, 152.

Conney, A. H. (1967): *Pharmacol. Rev., 19/3*, 317.

Cooper, J. R. and Brodie, B. B. (1955): *J. Pharmacol. exp. Ther., 114/4*, 409.

Goldstein, A., Aronow, L. and Kalman, S. M. (1968): *Principles of Drug Action, 1st ed.* Harper and Row, New York, N.Y.

Halevy, S. and Frumin, M. J. (1973): *Brit. J. Anaesth., 45/10*, 999.

Halevy, S., Frumin, M. J., Rosenthal, S. and Levine, W. G. (1974): *Brit. J. Anaesth., 46/1*, 43.

Irwin, S. (1964): In: *Animal and Clinical Pharmacologic Techniques in Drug Evaluation, Vol. 1,* Chapter 21, p. 15. Editors: J. H. Nodine and P. E. Siegler. Year Book Medical Publishers, Chicago, Ill.

Killam, K. F., Brody, T. B. and Bain, J. A. (1958): *Proc. Soc. exp. Biol. (N.Y.) 97/4*, 744.

Lee, J. M. (1964): *Z. Immun. Allergie-Forsch., 126/1*, 14.

Lee, J. M., Olitsky, P. K., Schneider, H. A. and Zinder, N. D. (1954): *Proc. Soc. exp. Biol. (N.Y.), 85/3*, 430.

Mark, L. C., Burns, J. J., Brand, L., Campomanes, C. I., Trousof, N., Papper, E. M. and Brodie, B. B. (1958): *J. Pharmacol. exp. Ther.*, *123/1*, 70.
McLaren, A. and Michie, D. (1956): *J. Genet.*, *54/3*, 440.
Noordhoek, J. (1968): *Europ. J. Pharmacol.*, *3*, 242.
Saidman, L. J. and Eger II, E. J. (1966): *Anesthesiology*, *27/2*, 118.
Sotaniemi, E. (1967): *Acta pharmacol. (Kbh.)*, *25*, Suppl. 5.
Vesell, E. S. (1968): *Ann. N.Y. Acad. Sci.*, *151*, 900.
Wajda, I. J., Lee, J. M. and Waelsch, H. (1967): *J. Neurochem.*, *14/4*, 389.

Chapter IV

New agents in inhalation anaesthesia

Pharmacological development of the fluorocarbon anaesthetic agents

P. DE TEMMERMAN

Department of Anaesthesiology, University of Louvain, Louvain, Belgium

After the discovery of the 3 first general anaesthetic agents between 1846 and 1850, 80 years passed before a real advance occurred with the discovery of cyclopropane (Lucas Henderson and Waters, 1926) and propyl methyl, isopropenyl vinyl and ethyl vinyl ethers (Krantz, 1930–40) (Fig. 1).

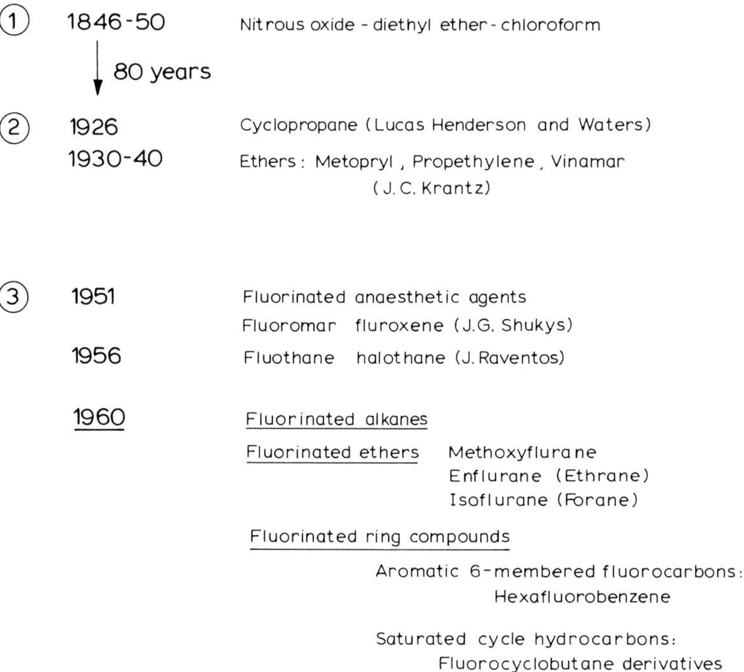

Fig. 1. *Discovery of general anaesthetic agents.*

A definite forward step has been the introduction of the present-day fluorinated anaesthetic agents. This 3rd state originated with the atomic bomb, in an entirely new technology of fluorine compounds. The first fluorinated anaesthetic was fluroxene (Shukys, 1951), flammable and rapidly supplanted by halothane (Raventos, 1956). The immediate and striking success of the latter discouraged further investigations.

But halothane itself had limitations and research for a better anaesthetic (nonflammable, chemically and biologically stable with fewer possibly toxic metabolites, without myocardial sensitization to catecholamines, harmless to the liver and kidney, providing good muscular relaxation, cheap to produce, etc.) was revived. Chemically, and as a general rule, halogenation is very important for nonflammability, chemical stability, boiling point and potency of the fluorinated anaesthetics. Totally fluorine-substituted agents have no anaesthetic properties. The iodine and bromine substituted are often unstable. The most interesting ones are the chlorinated compounds.

1960 seems to have been a milestone: In England and in the U.S.A. several fluoroalcohols, alkanes, ethers and some new cyclic derivatives, fluorinated 6-membered ring compounds, were investigated.

1. The *fluorinated alkanes* with 'in-line' molecules and directly bounded and saturated carbons have as a salient feature a definite tendency to arrhythmogenic properties (Fig. 2).

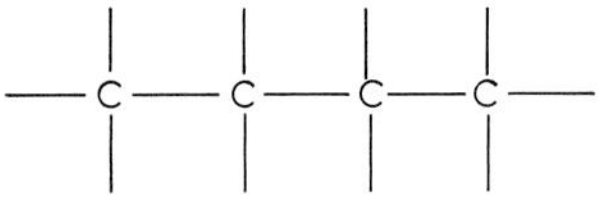

Propensity to arrhythmogenic properties

halopropane
teflurane·
norflurane
] = arrhythmias !

Fig. 2. *Fluorinated alkanes.*

Halopropane, teflurane and norflurane appeared in succession and practically vanished on account of cardiac arrhythmias.

2. *Fluorinated ethers* were most promising and interesting anaesthetics. The 2 radicals bounded by oxygen induce less cardiorespiratory depression. Muscular relaxation is generally better and no arrhythmia problems arise with or without catecholamines. All the ether series did not prove to be equally interesting. The dimethyl derivatives are hard

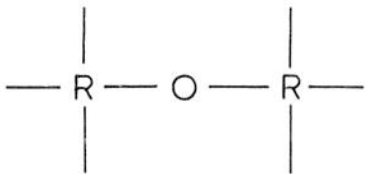

Less cardiorespiratory depression
Better muscular relaxation
No arrhythmia problem with catecholamines

Dimetyl	hard to synthesize - unstable
Isopropyl methyl	unstable
Isopropyl ethyl	unstable
Diethyl	convulsions , gasping , death (animals)
Many others	flammability - toxicity - synthesis !
Methyl ethyl	

Methoxyflurane
C-347 (enflurane) 1963 } (R.C. Terrell)
C-469 (isoflurane) 1965 }

Fig. 3. *Fluorinated ethers.*

to synthesize and unstable, as are the isopropyl methyl and isopropyl ethyl derivatives. Surprisingly, the diethyl ethers are quite different and proved to be very toxic. In animals convulsions are induced followed by gasping respiration and immediate or delayed death (Fig. 3). There are many others which proved impossible to use on account of their flammability, toxicity or difficult synthesis. The methyl-ethyl derivatives are the most promising and useful anaesthetics. Methoxyflurane is a fluorinated methyl-ethyl ether but its limitations, high boiling point and incidental renal toxicity, are known.

In 1963, Terrell discovered the compound 347 (enflurane or Ethrane) and in 1965, the compound 469 (Isoflurane or Forane). The latter is the isomer of enflurane which is easier to synthesize and especially easier to purify.

The lower blood solubility of Isoflurane accounts for a rapid induction. The striking interest in these 2 new compounds is the fact that they are chemically stable. This property is reflected in biological stability and less detoxification which means that there is less risk of the production of potentially toxic metabolites.

3. The *fluorinated cyclic derivatives* are quite a recent development. In England Burns et al. (1961*a, b*) about 14 years ago, investigated 83 original compounds and, amongst aromatic 6-membered fluorocarbons, hexafluorobenzene alone offered any pharmacological advantage over halothane – it appeared to stimulate breathing, maintain blood pressure and did not appear to sensitize the heart to epinephrine (Garmer and Leigh, 1967). Extensive tests have been carried out in the University of Cambridge Veterinary School by Hall and Jackson (1973). Hexafluorobenzene is a very attractive new anaesthetic but has an unexpected disadvantage – the anaesthetic concentrations are close to the lower limits of flammability (6% in oxygen) (Fig. 4).

Recently a new concept has been introduced which utilizes the simplicity of the saturated cyclic hydrocarbons. In an attempt to eliminate the explosive and arrhythmogenic properties of cyclopropane, some work has been done with other low molecular weight cyclic

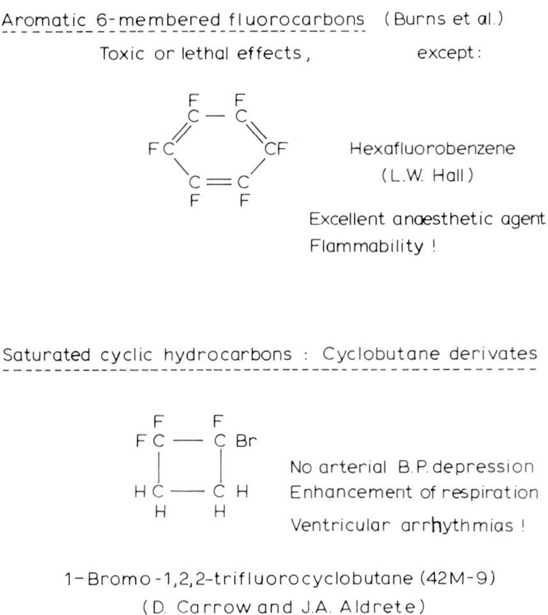

Fig. 4. *Fluorinated ring compounds.*

hydrocarbons, especially cyclobutane. Out of the 50–60 new compounds, about 10 possess anaesthetic properties.

Carrow et al. (*This volume*, p. 205) evaluated clinically 1-bromo-1,2,2-trifluorocyclobutane (42M-9). With anaesthetic and physical characteristics similar to that of methoxyflurane and halothane, there is an apparent absence of hypotension and stimulation of respiration. Simple modification of the molecule might eliminate the arrhythmogenic component.

A variety of methods of evaluation of anaesthetic properties of chemical compounds have been described. The investigation of new anaesthetics is still very much a matter of trial and error (Burns and Bracken, 1973).

Indeed, after summarizing all the generally accepted ideas of the structure-activity relationship, we find ourselves in the same position as Krantz, who says 'there are exceptions to each of these statements' (Krantz and Rudo, 1966, quoted in: Burns and Bracken, 1973).

REFERENCES

Burns, T. H. and Bracken, A. (1973): In: *Modern Inhalation Anesthetics*, p. 409. Editor: M. B. Chenoweth. Springer-Verlag, Berlin.

Burns, T. H., Hall, J. M., Bracken, A. and Gouldstone, G. (1961*a*): *Anaesthesia, 16/3*, 333.

Burns, T. H., Hall, J. M., Bracken, A., Gouldstone, G. and Newland, D. S. (1961*b*): *Anaesthesia, 16/1*, 3.

Carrow, D. J., Aldrete, J. A., Shoemaker, D. A. and Nicholson, J. A. (1974): *Rev. bras. Anest., 24/2*, 206.

Downing, A. C. (1966): In: *History of Organic Fluorine Industry, Kirk-Othmer Encyclopedia of Chemical Technology, 2nd ed., Vol. 9*, p. 704. Interscience, New York, N.Y.

Fabian, L. W., Carnes, M. A. and Dewitt, H. (1960): *Anesth. Analg. Curr. Res., 39/5*, 456.

Garmer, N. L. and Leigh, J. M. (1967): *Brit. J. Pharmacol., 37*, 345.

Hall, L. W. and Jackson, S. A. (1973): *Anaesthesia, 28/2*, 155.

Lucas, G. H. W. and Henderson, V. E. (1929): *Canad. med. Ass. J., 21*, 173.

Temmerman, P. de (1974): *Acta anaesth. belg., 25/2*, 169.

Vitcha, J. F. (1971): *Anesthesiology, 35/1*, 4.

Presentation of enflurane

ÅKE WÅHLIN

Department of Anaesthesiology, Huddinge Hospital, Huddinge, Sweden

Enflurane is a halogenated inhalation anaesthetic agent, and, consequently, non-explosive and non-flammable. Chemically the agent is very similar to ether as demonstrated in Figure 1. The substance is also remarkably stable and does not attack anaesthetic equipment.

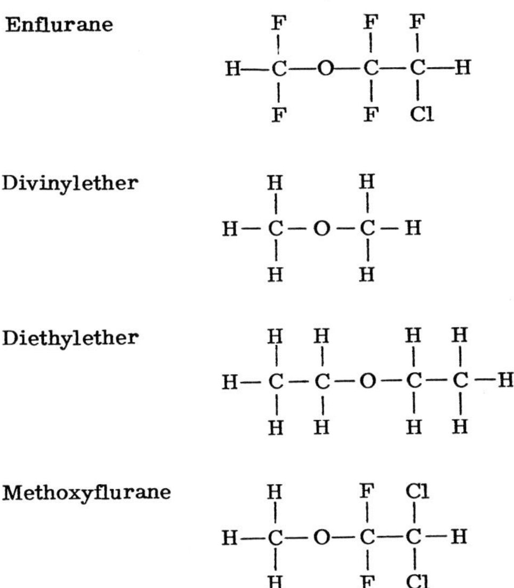

Fig. 1.   *Chemical comparison of enflurane and ether.*

The synthesis of enflurane was performed by Ohio Medical Products and the substance was studied in animal experimentation first by Krantz (unpublished data). The first clinical investigations were carried out by Virtue et al. (1966) and 2 years later by Dobkin et al. (1968). Since then clinical studies have been carried out extensively (at a conservative estimation of about 50,000 cases) and more than half a million anaesthetics have been given in the U.S. alone. Enflurane is registered in 19 countries under different names such as Efrane and Ethrane. Enflurane is recommended to be used in concentrations between 0.5 and 3%. For induction concentrations up to 3% may be needed but maintenance of anaesthesia is generally achieved with concentrations below 2%.

To give a rough idea about enflurane, its properties with general anaesthetics in common use, are compared. Chemically it is closely related to methoxyflurane but clinically it behaves more like halothane. Enflurane has, however, been compared with halothane, its own particular features, such as especially its short induction time, quick recovery, cardiac stability and low biotransformation rate, and relatively good muscle relaxant action, good hypnotic effect with minimal or no stimulation of salivary and bronchial secretions.

Further, enflurane does not alter the blood picture nor does it affect blood coagulation. The agent can be combined with all commonly used muscle relaxants. Non-depolarizing relaxants are markedly potentiated. Its ethereal odour is pleasant.

EFFECTS ON THE RESPIRATORY SYSTEM

The induction time is low, because the alveolar concentration rises quickly to the inspired concentration and the alveolar tension increases rapidly and consequently also the cerebral tension.

The minimum alveolar concentration (MAC) is about twice that of halothane. Torri (1973) showed that in the first few minutes, enflurane uptake was more rapid than that of halothane. After 15 min the 2 curves were similar. According to Gion and Saidman (1971) 70% N_2O reduce MAC for enflurane to about one third (1.90 to about 0.56%).

In the presentation of enflurane it is often emphasized that the respiratory rate remains essentially unchanged in general anaesthesia. This may be an argument to allow spontaneous breathing in enflurane anaesthesia. The most significant contribution to modern anaesthetic technique, however, is systematically assisted or controlled ventilation. During surgery and anaesthesia it is not only a question of depression of the respiration caused by the anaesthetic, but also respiratory depression because of surgical operation, the position of the patient during surgery, and, last but not least, the threat to the airway due to unconsciousness and loss of protective reflexes. Therefore, there will never exist an anaesthetic that, because of its inherent qualities, can compensate for all the possible non-pharmacological influences on respiration. Consequently, this irrelevant argument for spontaneous respiration in general anaesthesia and surgery will not be considered further.

It is obvious that Hanquet (1973) and other enflurane investigators (Linde et al., 1970; Lebowitz et al., 1970) have arrived at this conclusion. For its own interest it may be worth mentioning that the sigh mechanism is maintained intact during enflurane anaesthesia (Linde et al., 1970; Lebowitz et al., 1970).

The mechanism causing short induction time is also responsible for the quick elimination of enflurane and consequently a quick recovery. The rapid elimination is combined with an early need for analgetics postoperatively.

EFFECTS ON THE CARDIOVASCULAR SYSTEM

Heart rhythm is remarkably stable during anaesthesia with enflurane and this has been pointed out by many investigators (Dobkin et al., 1969; Linde et al., 1970; Hanquet, 1973). Together they represent clinical experience from about 2000 cases. I would like to quote from Hanquet's paper: 'Cardiac stability under Ethrane anaesthesia is probably the fact which has most impressed us'.

To analyse the effect on blood pressure accurately is difficult because general anaesthesia is often induced with barbiturates intravenously and barbiturates cause hypotension. It is a common description by investigators that the arterial blood pressure decreases during induction and that surgical stimulation reestablishes the control values. It should be remembered, however, that the circumstances involved in routine anaesthesia and surgery do not reflect the pure effect of the anaesthetic agent on the arterial blood pressure. Tables 2 and 3 (Wåhlin, 1974) demonstrate the changes in arterial blood pressure and pulse rate in a small series during induction and surgery expressed as per cent of control values with the effect of intubation excluded. The depth of anaesthesia provided abdominal surgery without muscle relaxants. The effect on the blood pressure seems to be less than for equivalent concentrations of halothane. The effect on pulse rate is remarkably small and it can be seen that the bradycardia of halothane anaesthesia does not occur.

Table 1. *Changes in mean systolic blood pressure during induction of anaesthesia and surgical procedure as per cent of control level (n = 24)*

Mean systolic blood pressure			
Induction		Operation	
Highest	Lowest	Highest	Lowest
81	60	88	69

From: Heyner and Wåhlin, 1973.

Table 2. *Changes in mean pulse rate during induction of anaesthesia and surgical procedure as per cent of control level (n = 24)*

Mean pulse rate			
Induction		Operation	
Highest	Lowest	Highest	Lowest
116	96	122	103

From: Heyner and Wåhlin, 1973.

Some investigators have tried to evaluate the effect of enflurane on myocardial contractility. Shimosato et al. (1969) have demonstrated in preparations that enflurane is less depressant to myocardial contractility than methoxyflurane or halothane. In a clinical study Marshall et al. (1971) have shown that cardiac output is well sustained during enflurane anaesthesia at different carbon dioxide tensions. The authors have, however, not made clear the depth of anaesthesia used during the studies.

BIOTRANSFORMATION

Much attention has been paid to the statement that the biotransformation (Van Dyke, 1973) of enflurane is lower than halothane and much lower than that of methoxyflurane. This observation is of course of great interest and seems to be a positive feature.

LIVER AND KIDNEY

On the presentation of a new halogenated inhalation anaesthetic agent, most interest is focussed on its effect on parenchymatous tissues such as the liver and kidney. Objections are usually raised against the first few studies on account of the small sizes of the series. Carefully studied material is needed from thousands of cases for accurate conclusions. From another point of view this may be an indication that the pharmacological status of the halogenated anaesthetics is fairly high.

In the normal liver and kidney, effects of the halogenated agents are rare. When the liver and kidney are diseased it seems reasonable to be careful with halogenated anaesthetics.

In an animal study Rietbrook (1973) has shown in a convincing way under various experimental conditions that enflurane is less liver-toxic than halothane.

The effect on renal function has been evaluated by Granberg and Wåhlin (1973) and Dvoracek et al. (1973) and these studies have not revealed any effect on renal function.

There are many investigations on liver and kidney functions, but in this presentation at least the European studies may be summarized with a reference to the work by Foitzik (1973), who made a statistical evaluation of GOT, GPT, LDH, alkaline phosphatases, creatinine and nitrogen in serum from about 2000 patients before operation, and 24 and 72 hr after anaesthesia. The partly significant changes in these parameters did not exceed normal limits. In this study, side-effects such as shivering, nausea, vomiting, muscular twitching and convulsions appeared very rarely.

Recently a report of one case of possible nephrotoxicity from enflurane has been published (Loehning and Mazze, 1974). The patient in question had chronic renal dysfunction leading to transplantation of a cadaver kidney with episodes of rejection and secondary complications such as aseptic necrosis of a femoral head. Deterioration of the renal function was assumed to be due to enflurane anaesthesia.

These patients are exposed to pharmacological depression of defence mechanisms, to antibiotics and to hormone control. Under such circumstances articles based on assumption that enflurane, combined with a diverse group of pharmacological agents, is responsible for deterioration of renal function in an individual in whom renal function is nearly zero do not contribute to our knowledge. The same may be said about descriptions of liver damage in single cases where liver function is affected by advanced failure and disturbed environmental metabolism (Van der Reis et al., 1974) before anaesthesia and surgery. They can only serve as guidelines and contraindications in these particular cases.

SYMPTOMS FROM THE NERVOUS SYSTEM

In anaesthesiological routine during the last few decades convulsions occurred during the era of ether especially during induction of anaesthesia particularly in children suffering from high fever. During the current halothane era there is the condition characterized by general rigidity during the early recovery stage. All these neurological phenomena have not been explained to us and scientific interest has never been focussed on them. These phenomena, however, have one feature in common, they are completely reversible.

EEG-changes have been reported but these have been reversible without harm to the patients. These EEG-changes have caused exceptional interest amongst anaesthesiologists and the authorities responsible for the approval of enflurane. Possibly this interest may be interpreted as a desire to understand what really is going on in the brain during anaesthesia.

Bimar et al. (1973) and Lebowitz et al. (1972) have described the EEG-changes under enflurane anaesthesia. Joas et al. (1971) and Kavan et al. (1972) have compared the EEG-pattern of enflurane with other volatile anaesthetic agents. Enflurane seems to have a special type of EEG-pattern. There is still no explanation of the cerebral activity, but it has been fully shown that the changes are reversible.

GERIATRIC CASES AND MYASTHENIA GRAVIS

Enflurane has been used on 2 very delicate groups of patients, one geriatric group and another group suffering from myasthenia gravis (Wåhlin, 1974), and both groups have sustained anaesthesia and surgery remarkably well.

Finally, because of the smooth and rapid induction, quick recovery and cardiac stability, enflurane is a new useful addition to our routine anaesthetic agents.

REFERENCES

Bimar, J., Masse-Bergier, M. and Emperaire, N. (1973): *Anaesthesiol. Resuscitat.*, *84*, 62.

Dobkin, A. B., Heinrich, R. G., Israel, J. S., Levy, A. A., Neville Jr, J. F. and Ounkasem, K. (1968): *Anesthesiology*, *29/2*, 275.

Dobkin, A. B., Nishioka, K., Gengaje, D. B., Kim, D. S., Evers, W. and Israel, J. S. (1969): *Anesth. Analg. Curr. Res.*, *48/3*, 477.

Dvoracek, B., Ducardus, R., Van Haelst, U. J. M., Kubat, K., Lip, H. and Van den Pluijm, W. J. M. (1973): *Anaesthesiol. Resuscitat.*, *84*, 158.

Foitzik, H. (1973): *Anaesthesiol. Resuscitat.*, *84*, 338.

Gion, H. and Saidman, L. J. (1971): *Anesthesiology*, *35*, 361.

Granberg, P.-O. and Wåhlin, Å. (1973): *Acta anaesth. scand.*, *17*, 41.

Hanquet, M. (1973): *Anaesthesiol. Resuscitat.*, *84*, 6.

Joas, T. A., Stevens, W. C. and Eger, E. I. (1971): *Brit. J. Anaesth.*, *43*, 739.

Kavan, E. M., Julien, R. M. and Lucero, J. J. (1972): *Brit. J. Anaesth.*, *44*, 1234.

Lebowitz, M. H., Blitt, C. D. and Dillon, J. D. (1970): *Anesth. Analg. Curr. Res.*, *49/1*, 1.

Lebowitz, M. H., Blitt, C. D. and Dillon, J. D. (1972): *Anesth. Analg. Curr. Res.*, *51*, 355.

Linde, H. W., Lamb, V. E., Quimby Jr, C. W., Homi, J. and Eckenhoff, J. E. (1970): *Anesthesiology*, *32*, 555.

Loehning, R. W. and Mazze, R. I. (1974): *Anesthesiology*, *40/2*, 203.

Marshall, B. E., Cohen, P. J., Klingenmaier, C. H., Neigh, J. L. and Pender, J. W. (1971): *Brit. J. Anaesth.*, *43*, 996.

Rietbrock, I. (1973): *Anaesthesiol. Resuscitat.*, *84*, 42.

Shimosato, S., Sugai, N., Iwatsuki, N. and Etsten, B. E. (1969): *Anesthesiology*, *30/5*, 513.

Torri, G. (1973): *Anaesthesiol. Resuscitat.*, *84*, 18.

Van der Reis, L., Askin, S. J., Frecker, G. N. and Fitzgerald, W. (1974): *J. Amer. med. Ass.*, *227/1*, 76.

Van Dyke, R. A. (1973): *Canad. Anaesth. Soc. J.*, *20/1*, 21.

Virtue, R. W., Lund, L. O., Phleps Jr, M., Vogel, J. H. K., Beckwitt, H. and Heron, M. (1966): *Canad. Anaesth. Soc. J.*, *13/3*, 233.

Wåhlin, Å. (1974): *Acta anaesth. belg.*, *25*, 215 and 220.

Effect of enflurane on the liver

M. A. NALDA

Department of Anesthesiology, University of Salamanca Faculty of Medicine, Salamanca, Spain

Since Enflurane is a halogenated compound it may affect the liver; this is a study on the effects of this anesthetic agent on liver function. There are 25 cases in this report which can be regarded as a pilot study.

Serum transaminases: GOT and GPT, aldolase (ALD), alkaline phosphatase (AP) and γ-glutamyl transpeptidase (GGTP or γ-GT), have been studied in samples obtained on the day prior to anesthesia from patients. Enflurane was used as the sole anesthetic and samples were taken at 24 and 48 hr after anesthesia. No patient with hepatic dysfunction was included. The results obtained after analysis are shown in Tables 1–5.

Table 1. *G O T*

Before	At 24 hr	At 48 hr
N 25	25	25
Ex 104.00	124.00	157.00
$\bar{x}$ 20.80	24.80	31.40
σ^2 17.70	72.70	229.80
σ 4.20	8.52	15.15
$\sigma\bar{x}$ 1.88	3.81	6.77

Before 24 hr: $T = 1.545$; P not significant.
24 hr–48 hr: $T = 1.165$; P not significant.
Before 48 hr: $T = 1.883$; P not significant.

Table 2. *G P T*

Before	At 24 hr	At 48 hr
N 25	25	25
Ex 105.00	147.00	185.00
$\bar{x}$ 21.00	29.40	37.00
σ^2 22.00	17.30	592.00
σ 4.69	4.15	24.33
$\sigma\bar{x}$ 2.09	1.86	10.88

Before 24 hr: $T = 1.832$; P not significant.
24 hr-48 hr: $T = 0.676$; P not significant.
Before 48 hr: $T = 1.492$; P not significant.

Table 3. *A L D*

Before		At 24 hr	At 48 hr
N	25	25	25
Ex	23.50	27	88.00
$\bar{x}$	4.70	5.40	17.60
σ^2	6.70	28.92	429.80
σ	2.58	5.37	20.73
$\sigma\bar{x}$	1.15	2.40	9.27

Before 24 hr: $T = 0.268$; P not significant.
24 hr–48 hr: $T = 1.195$; P not significant.
Before 48 hr: $T = 1.558$; P not significant.

Table 4. *A P*

Before		At 24 hr	At 48 hr
N	25	25	25
Ex	11.00	12.00	14.50
$\bar{x}$	2.20	2.40	2.90
σ^2	0.57	0.17	0.42
σ	0.75	0.41	0.65
$\sigma\bar{x}$	0.33	0.18	0.29

Before 24 hr: $T = 1.000$; P not significant.
24 hr–48 hr: $T = 3.162$; $P < 0.05$.
Before 48 hr: $T = 5.715$; $P < 0.05$.

Table 5. *G G T P*

Before		At 24 hr	At 48 hr
N	25	25	25
Ex	46.00	126.00	111.00
$\bar{x}$	9.20	25.20	22.20
σ^2	19.70	128.70	165.70
σ	4.43	11.34	12.87
$\sigma\bar{x}$	1.98	5.07	5.75

Before 24 hr: $T = 3.073$; $P < 0.05$.
24 hr–48 hr: $T = 0.508$; P not significant.
Before 48 hr: $T = 1.832$; P not significant.

Those enzymes whose elevation is indicative of hepatic cell damage (GOT, GPT, and ALD) showed no significant change from the control value while those in whom an elevation reveals a compromise in permeability (or patency) of the biliary tree (AP and GGTP), show a significant rise during the postanesthetic period. It is concluded that, contrary to previous reports, enflurane has a deleterious effect on the secretory function of the liver.

In order to conclude this study, ultrastructural analysis and BSP-loading tests, to study the plasma clearance of the dye at short intervals, are being performed in order to locate the exact level at which liver function is altered.

Liver function tests in patients under enflurane anaesthesia

E. LOPES SOARES * and MORTÓ DESSAI *

Hospitais Civis, and Instituto Português de Oncologia de Francisco Gentil, Lisbon, Portugal

The results of an earlier study, reported elsewhere (Soares and Dessai, 1973; Soares et al., unpublished data) may be summarised as follows: determinations made for SGOT, SGPT, LDH and γ–GT in patients anaesthetized with enflurane up to the 7th day after surgery revealed no changes suggesting the existence of an immediate toxic effect on the liver cell. Another group of 40 patients anaesthetized with enflurane has been studied.

MATERIAL AND METHODS

There were 25 males and 15 females whose ages ranged between 31 and 75 years; physical status was ASA I, II and III. Many patients in this series had undergone upper abdominal, particularly biliary tract surgery (Table 1). Two of them had preoperative obstructive jaundice. Premedication consisted for almost all of the patients of diazepam, promethazine and atropine according to the patients' weight and physical condition.

Table 1. *Types of surgery*

Gastrectomy	9
Cholecystectomy	5
Biliary digestive anastomosis	2
Colectomy	1
Splenectomy	2
Exploratory laparotomy	3
Total hyterectomy	3
Thyroidectomy	1
Inguinal herniorraphy	4
Mastectomy	2
Lumbar sympathectomy	6
Amputation of the thigh	2

Induction was with thiopentone (150–400 mg) followed by pancuronium (4–6 mg). Succinylcholine (50–100 mg) was used in some cases. The patients were ventilated with oxygen, and an orotracheal cuffed tube was inserted. Anaesthesia was maintained with 50% N_2O/O_2 and enflurane (0.5–3%) from a vaporiser calibrated for enflurane, put outside

---

* The authors were assisted by Professor J. M. Quadros e Costa of the 'Academia Militar'.

a semi-closed circle absorption system. In some cases a non-rebreathing technique was used. Most of the patients were ventilated with a Manley ventilator. During operation, Ringer's lactate solution was given to all patients, and blood when necessary.

Laboratory

Venous blood samples were drawn before anaesthesia (A), 24 hr after surgery (B), and on the 7th postoperative day (C) for the following serum enzymes: SGOT, SGPT, LDH, LAP (leucine-amine-peptidase) and γ-GT. The normal values in our laboratory are shown in Table 2. For SGOT and SGPT we considered as borderline values between 12 and 20 mU/ml. Only values above this are rated as abnormal.

Table 2. *Normal values*

SGOT		up to	12	mU/ml
SGPT		up to	12	mU/ml
LDH		up to	195	mU/ml
LAP		8 to	22	mU/ml
γ-GT	Males	5 to	28	mU/ml
	Females	4 to	18	mU/ml

RESULTS

The results are estimated from samples of 40 patients for collections A and B, and 38 for C (Table 3). The overall evaluation of these results shows that there were no significant changes above the normal limit. Of the 5 enzymes the greatest fluctuations were found with SGOT. For the other 4 the values found in samples A, B and C do not deviate from normal.

Table 3. *Results*

		A	B	C
SGOT	$\bar{x}$	10.950	17.825	17.333
	Sx	8.165	14.818	18.746
	S$\bar{x}$	1.291	2.343	3.002
SGPT	$\bar{x}$	4.525	8.447	6.459
	Sx	4.432	9.788	3.694
	S$\bar{x}$	0.700	1.588	0.607
LDH	$\bar{x}$	94.340	122.720	105.550
	Sx	47.340	112.840	56.508
	S$\bar{x}$	7.780	18.807	9.290
LAP	$\bar{x}$	6.293	7.376	7.882
	Sx	2.985	3.128	3.604
	S$\bar{x}$	0.466	0.507	0.584
γ-GT	$\bar{x}$	8.184	7.575	9.307
	Sx	5.187	3.241	10.829
	S$\bar{x}$	0.841	0.512	1.734

$\bar{x}$ = Mean; Sx = Standard deviation; S$\bar{x}$ = Standard error.

SGOT

In Table 4 the cases considered as normal (up to 12), borderline (12–20) and abnormal (> 20) are grouped together. It is seen that of the 36 cases which at A are in the normal and borderline groups, 30 remain in this group at B and C.

Considering now the transition from A to C a contingency table (Table 5) was constructed. The χ^2 test was used to test the hypothesis of independence of classes N, BL and ABN in the transition A–C, the conclusion being arrived at that $\chi^2 = 7.9$. At the 10% level, the hypothesis of independence must be rejected. This shows that the transition to *abnormal* at C is not statistically independent of the patients being in N or BL, possibly depending on the fact of their being in BL.

Table 4. *Cases considered as normal (N), borderline (BL), and abnormal (ABN)*

	A	B	C
N	33	15	19
BL	3	15	11
ABN	4	10	8
Total	40	40	38

Table 5. *Contingency (A–C)*

	Sample C			Total
	N	BL	ABN	
Sample A				
N	17	8	6	31
BL	2	0	1	3
ABN	0	3	1	4
Total	19	11	8	38

Table 6. *Contingency*

	Sample C		
	N + BL	ABN	Total
Sample A			
N + BL	27	7	34
ABN	3	1	4
Total	30	8	38

From the preceding table the contingency table was obtained (Table 6). Thus, in these 38 patients: 27 passed over from N + BL to N + BL; 3 passed over from ABN to N + BL; 7 passed over from N + BL to ABN; and 1 passed over from ABN to N.

From the χ^2 test the hypothesis of independence is one to be accepted, which shows that normal or borderline values tend to stay within their group and that the same happens with regard to abnormal values.

SGPT

Only 2 patients with normal values at A rose to values > 20 at B, but both with values < 20 at C. Two patients with values > 20 at A remained raised at B, but both with values < 20 at C. Two patients with values > 20 at A remained raised at B, but at C, 1 dropped to less than 20, and the values for the other were > 20.

LAP

All the patients presented normal values at samples A, B and C.

γ-GT

All the patients presented normal values at A and B. Two patients had $>$ normal values at C.

Special cases

The details of 3 special cases are given in Table 7.

Table 7. *Special cases*

No. 306: Preoperative obstructive jaundice.

	A	B	C
SGOT	20	22	16

All other enzyme values were normal in A, B and C.

No. 308: Carcinoma of the stomach with liver metastases

	A	B	C	D
SGOT	16	56	46	24
SGPT	6	45	16	13
LDH	122	460	122	191
LAP	5	10	10	10
γ-GT	10	16	5	10

D = Sample taken 16 days after surgery; onset of jaundice 5 days after surgery.

No. 312: Preoperative jaundice (carcinoma of the biliary tract)

	A	B	C	D
SGOT	56	80	36	16
SGPT	30	45	16	6
γ-GT	19	10	68	16

LDH and LAP normal. D = Sample taken 11 days after surgery; clinically jaundice remained unchanged.

Patients with more than one anaesthesia

One patient (No. 301) was anaesthetized thrice and another patient (No. 325) was anaesthetized twice with enflurane. Neither of these patients had any clinical problem in the post-surgery period, and in both patients all the values for the 5 enzymes at A, B and C were normal.

CONCLUSION

The statistical analysis of the data supports previously published clinical observations and strengthens the view that enflurane produces no significant changes in liver function.

REFERENCES

Soares, E. L. and Dessai, M. (1973): In: *Ethrane Proceedings, I European Symposium on Modern Anaesthetic Agents, Hamburg, 1973*, p. 150. Editors: P. Lawin and R. Beer. Springer-Verlag, Berlin.

Renal tubular changes following anaesthesia in pigs: A comparison of nitrous oxide and enflurane

B. DVORACEK, W. C. DE BRUIJN, A. P. R. BLOK,
N. S. FAITHFULL and R. DUCARDUS

Department and Laboratory of Anaesthesiology, and Department of Clinical Pathology I,
University Hospital Dijkzigt and Faculty of Medicine,
Erasmus University, Rotterdam, The Netherlands

It has been suggested that renal tubular changes following prolonged methoxyflurane or enflurane anaesthesia in pigs may be significantly affected by circulatory disturbances or hypoxia (Dvoracek et al., 1974). Therefore we decided to stress animals under enflurane with hypoxia using a series of animals under nitrous oxide-relaxant techniques as controls.

TECHNIQUES

We used 24 female Yorkshire pigs (average weight 11001 g), divided into 4 groups of 6 each as follows: Group A, nitrous oxide-oxygen-muscle relaxant anaesthesia; Group B, nitrous oxide-oxygen-muscle relaxant-enflurane anaesthesia; Group C, nitrous oxide-oxygen-muscle relaxant anaesthesia, stressed with hypoxia; Group D, nitrous oxide-oxygen-muscle relaxant-enflurane anaesthesia, stressed with hypoxia.

The experiments lasted 24 hr. Induction was achieved with 10 mg/kg metomidate (Hypnodil®, Janssen, Breerse) intraperitoneally and 2 mg/kg azaperone (Stresnil®, Janssen) by intramuscular injection. Twenty minutes later the animals were intubated and ventilated with a Bennett ventilator in a semi-closed absorber system. A urinary catheter was inserted. Femoral arterial and venous pressures and the ECG were displayed continuously on a Grass Polygraph. The temperature was measured continuously with an Ellma thermometer inserted into the oesophagus.

The pigs lay on a warmed mattress but, if the temperature rose above $39°$ C, cooling with ice bags was instituted for short periods. All animals received infusions of glucose/saline (approximately 5 ml/kg/hr). Ventilation was controlled during the experiments. The oxygen concentration was $30\% - 10\%$ during hypoxic periods. Expired carbon dioxide was held at between 5 and 6 vol% by adjusting soda lime absorption. Blood pH, Po_2 and Pco_2 were periodically measured in arterial blood samples.

Relaxation was achieved with d-tubocurarine, injected intramuscularly at the rate of 3 mg every hr in the non-enflurane groups, or 3 mg every 3 hr in the enflurane groups. In the enflurane groups $1-1.5$ vol% enflurane was added; the concentration was checked by gas chromatography. The length of the hypoxic periods was determined by the circulatory state of the pigs – when blood pressure fell and cardiac irregularities occurred, hypoxia was stopped and the previous oxygen rich mixture was administered. The next hypoxic period was started as soon as the circulation appeared stable.

194   *B. Dvoracek et al.*

Table 1 shows the duration and frequency of the hypoxic periods. The hypoxic periods were instituted approximately 4 hr after the beginning of anaesthesia (after the first renal biopsy) and were all completed during the first 8 hr of anaesthesia (before the 2nd biopsy). Stable anaesthesia was then continued till the end of the experimental period in order to allow possible tissue changes to occur in the hypoxically stressed kidneys.

Table 1.   *Duration and frequency of hypoxic periods*

Group	Pig No.	Length of hypoxic periods (min)	Total length of hypoxia (min)
C	13, 14	22, 62, 8, 12, 12	116
	15, 16	110, 100	210
	17, 18	210, 13	223
D	19, 20	27, 95	122
	21, 22	65, 15, 26	106
	23, 24	54, 5	59

Four hours after the start of anaesthesia a unilateral lumbotomy was performed and a needle biopsy was obtained from the exposed kidney using the Travenol disposable biopsy needle (2N2702, 1.65 mm). The lumbotomy was then provisionally closed and 4 hr later reopened and a 2nd biopsy performed. At the end of the experiment (24 hr) a 3rd sample from this kidney was taken and another obtained from the other previously undisturbed kidney. Biopsy specimens were prepared and mounted using techniques described by De Bruijn (1973). After polymerisation sections were cut on a LKB Ultrotome with glass-knives, either 1 nm or 50 nm thick. The semi-thin sections were stained with methylene blue, the ultrathin sections were collected on carbon-coated Formvar films and were used either unstained or stained by lead citrate following the method of Venable and Cogge-shall (1965).

RESULTS

In Group A (nitrous oxide-relaxant) only 4 pigs of the 6 survived for the whole of the 24-hr period; one died 7 hr and the second 20 hr after the start of the anaesthesia. This was caused by failure of the ventilators. In Group C (nitrous oxide-relaxant-hypoxia) 5 animals of the 6 survived for the 24-hr period, one died 19 hr after the start of anaesthesia of heart failure in the presence of severe bronchopneumonia, which developed during the course of anaesthesia.

All other animals survived the whole period in a good condition. The partial pressures of oxygen in the arterial blood fell significantly during hypoxic periods and the hydrogen ion concentration rose. This 'metabolic acidosis' was not corrected and was still observable at the end of the experiments. During the hypoxia the partial pressure of carbon dioxide was significantly lower than in the controls – probably due to poor tissue perfusion in the presence of a depressed cardiovascular system.

In spite of institution of active cooling the body temperature of the pigs under nitrous oxide was markedly higher than those under enflurane – due, no doubt, to vascular dilatation in the skin under enflurane. The ratio of administered intravenous fluids to urine output was not significantly different in the 4 groups. There were no significant differences either in weight or in the ventilatory patterns between the different groups of animals.

MICROSCOPY

The 4 experimental sets of pigs may be taken as homogeneous groups, there being no significant differences between them.

Group A (N_2O plus relaxant; Fig. 1)

Light-microscopic observations
All animals appeared to have normal glomeruli, the proximal tubules were distinct; in some places the epithelial cells were slightly separated from each other. The distal tubules were more or less open.

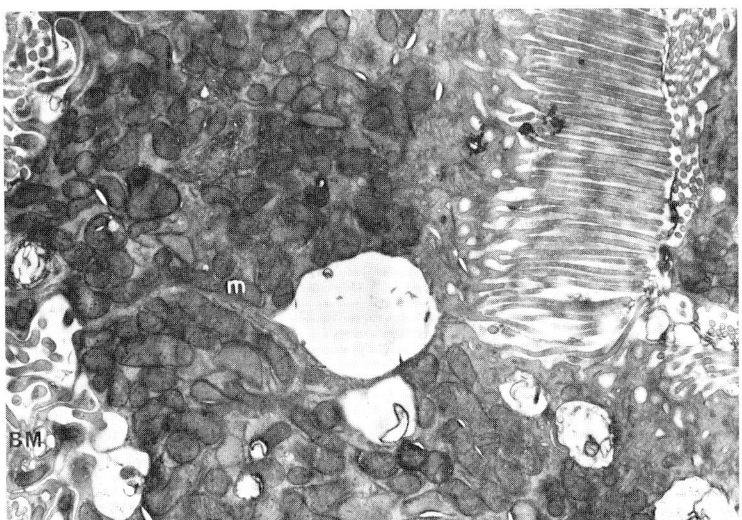

Fig. 1. *Proximal tubule cell from a control animal after 4 hr anaesthesia with nitrous oxide-relaxants. No striking abnormalities are observable. The basement membrane and the mitochondria are clearly seen; abnormal vacuoles are absent. ×7,800. (BM = basement membrane; m = mitochondria).*

Electron-microscopic observations
The endothelial cells of the glomeruli were normal and neatly covered the basement membrane, with distinct pores. The epithelial cells were normal and covered the outside of the basement membrane with small podocytic processes. The proximal tubules consisted of neatly arranged cells with nicely orientated villi at the apex. At the basal site the peculiarly arranged cell membrane processes were present with normal mitochondria present in between. The basement membranes were normal, as were the endothelial cells covering the intertubular capillaries.

Group B (N_2O plus relaxant plus enflurane; Fig. 2)

Light-microscopic observations
All animals had normal appearing glomeruli, the proximal tubules showed marked dilatation of the inter-epithelial cell spaces, suggesting distortion by some (crystalline ?) material,

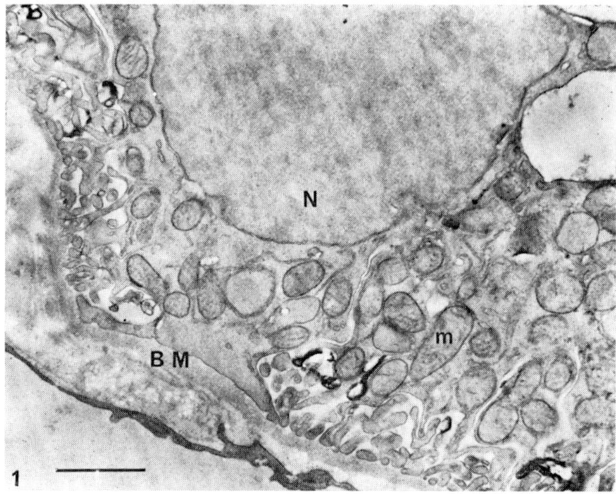

Fig. 2.   *A proximal tubular cell of the kidney of a pig anaesthetised with enflurane. The basal parts of the cell are normal. $\times$ 11,520. (N = nucleus; BM = basement membrane; m = mitochondria; magnification: bar = 1 μm).*

although the presence of such material under polarised light was not confirmed. The distal tubules appeared normal, without such distortions.

Electron-microscopic observations

The endothelial cells covering the glomeruli were apparently normal, the basement membranes were good and the epithelial cells showed the normal arrangements of the podocytic processes with no signs of confluent changes. In the proximal tubules the enlargement of the intercellular spaces was clearly observed and at some places the presence of hard material was deduced from rather frequent damage of the sections by square-angled non-electron dense vacuolar structures at these places. These structures were present both in the apex of the tubular cell spaces as well as at the base, in between the fine filamentous cellular cell processes, that mark the cell membranes of the proximal tubular cells. Inside these cells the vacuoles frequently observed at the apex, were present. These consisted of a fine granular electron dense material. The mitochondria appeared to be normal with rather prominent electron dense granules in the mitochondrial matrix. There was little or no difference between the biopsies taken following 4, 8 or 24 hr of anaesthesia.

Group C (N₂O plus relaxant plus hypoxia; Fig. 3)

Light-microscopic observations

The glomeruli of the kidneys appeared to be normal, as were the proximal and distal tubules. Separation of the tubular cells in the proximal tubules was not observed. There was a slight tendency for oedematous swelling to occur around the tubules and between the capillaries.

Electron-microscopic observations

Both endothelium and epithelium covering the basement membranes of the glomeruli were apparently normal. The perikarya contained normal-looking mitochondria. In the proximal tubules the cells were normally arranged and the spaces between the epithelial cells were not markedly widened. Hard material was not observed in between the spaces.

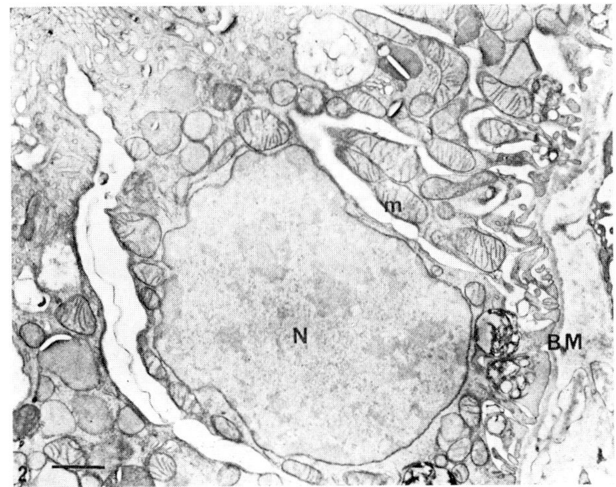

Fig. 3. *Undamaged proximal tubular cells from the kidneys of pigs anaesthetised by nitrous oxide in the presence of severe hypoxia. × 7,200. (N=nucleus; BM=basement membrane; m=mitochondria; magnification: bar=1 μm).*

In the proximal tubular cells the normal cell organelles were present. Only a few large vacuoles were present at the apex of the cells between the villi. The mitochondria were quite normal looking, although the presence of the electron dense granules in the mitochondrial matrix was reduced in quantity and intensity. The typical cell processes at the base of the proximal cells appeared to be normal. There was a slight impression, that the biopsies taken at 8-hr interval were more changed as compared to those taken at 4 and 24 hr.

Group D (N₂O plus enflurane plus hypoxia; Figs. 4, 5)

Light-microscopic observations
Tubular changes were clearly observed in these animals, all proximal tubular cells appeared to be separated by large vacuoles both at the apex of the cells and at the base. Cellular necrosis and desquamation was observed in some tubules especially in the biopsies taken at 8 hr. Recovery was observable to some extent in biopsies taken at 24 hr. Slight oedematous swelling was present in the spaces between the tubules and the inter-tubular capillaries.

Electron-microscopic observations
The endothelial and epithelial coverings of the basement membranes of the glomeruli were apparently normal, the cristae of the mitochondria were in good shape although the amount and the intensity of the electron dense granules in the mitochondrial matrix was reduced. In the proximal tubules severely damaged, necrotic cells were observed. Swollen mitochondria and myelin like changes inside the cytoplasm were observed. At the bases of the proximal tubular cells the typical cell processes were mostly lost or rounded up. Desquamation was observed. At the apex of the proximal cells the villi were irregular and shortened. In the lumen swollen parts of cellular elements and mitochondrial fragments were present. Although desquamation of tubules was observable in the 24-hr biopsies and irregular spaces in between the cells suggested the presence of hard crystal-like material, these cellular changes were minimal in the remaining cells. Thus recovery from the damage had apparently occurred.

The oedematous swelling of the connective tissue elements between the proximal tubules

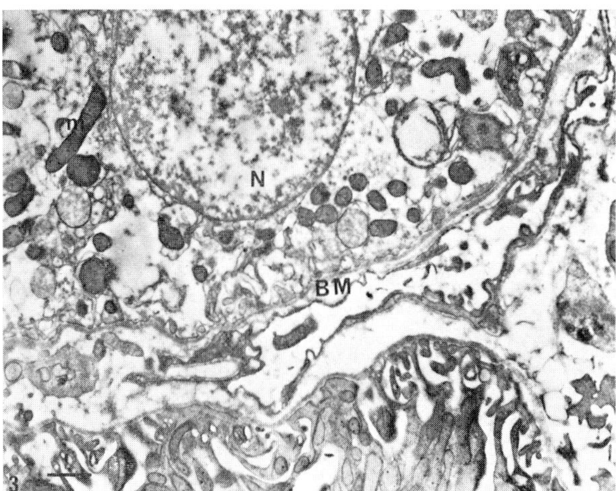

Fig. 4.   *Severely damaged cells of the proximal tubules following hypoxia under enflurane. Desquamation and necrosis are demonstrated. × 5,820.   N= nucleus; BM= basement membrane; m= mitochondria; magnification: bar= 1 μm).*

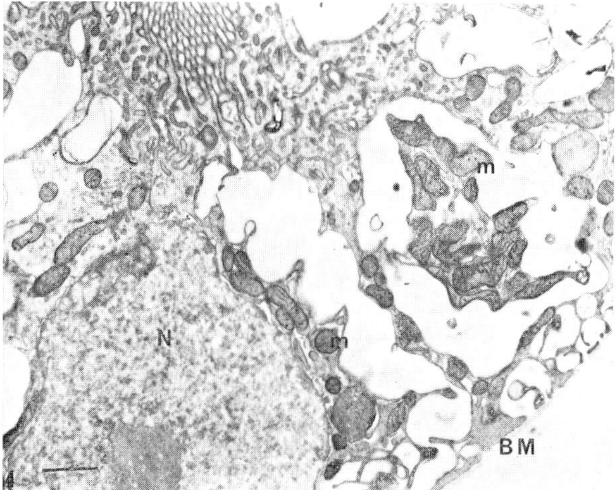

Fig. 5.   *In those areas where the proximal tubules are not necrotic the intercellular spaces are distorted following enflurane and hypoxia. × 7,200. (N= nucleus; BM= basement membrane; m= mitochondria; magnification: bar= 1 μm).*

and the peritubular capillaries was present in all cases although rather minimal in the 24-hr biopsies.

DISCUSSION

Cystic degeneration of the cells of proximal tubules of the kidneys in different experimental animals was mentioned by Raventós (1956) presenting his first experiences with Fluothane. He did not think this to be of great clinical importance, because in no case was renal necrosis to be seen such as that described by Eschenbrenner and Miller (1945) in rats treated with chloroform.

Raventós and Lemon (1956) have found impurities in Fluothane, of which Buthene was the most nephrotoxic, but they did not consider them to be important in a clinical situation due to their extreme dilution under these circumstances. Fratello (1964) studied the Fluothane effect in kidneys of guinea pigs. Using high concentrations (4 vol%) he found cystic degeneration of the proximal tubules. He was obliged to stop the experiments after 90 min due to the poor condition of the animals and he thought that the changes were caused by hypoxia.

It seems that in none of these experiments were the animals ventilated and it may be postulated that hypoxia could have occurred. Renal damage following methoxyflurane anaesthesia started investigations which resulted in evidence of biotransformation of all inhalation anaesthetics. In the case of fluorinated agents inorganic fluoride has been identified as an end product of metabolism. Chase et al. (1971) have demonstrated this in studies on enflurane and similar results have been obtained by Hitt et al. (1974) working with isoflurane.

Inorganic fluoride, in addition to its marked bone changes in chronic fluorosis, was shown by Bond and Murray (1952) to cause renal damage, in which tubular function was affected more than that of the glomeruli. Withford and Toves (1973) in Sprague-Dawley rats and Kosek et al. (1972), Mazze et al. (1972) and Mazze and Cousins (1973) in 344 Fischer rats demonstrated cystic degeneration of the proximal tubules following administration of sodium fluoride in doses necessary to achieve blood fluoride concentrations similar to those occurring during deep methoxyflurane anaesthesia. There seems little doubt, that cystic degeneration of the proximal tubules, seen in our previous experiments (Dvoracek et al., 1974) and those here presented (Groups B and D) is related to inorganic fluoride. Nevertheless the role of hypoxia seems to be demonstrated to be of spectacular importance.

Low biotransformation of enflurane has been demonstrated by Chase et al. (1971) and Halsey (1972). Because of this it is postulated that enflurane anaesthesia resulted in low inorganic fluoride levels in the blood. These low levels only caused minimal changes during normal oxygenation. Under hypoxia the same levels produced tubular changes progressing in some cases to necrosis. If anaesthesia with enflurane is continued after the hypoxic period (Group C) the renal changes do not tend to progress, on the contrary they improve. The negligible changes in the cells of proximal tubules after hypoxia in pigs anaesthetised with nitrous oxide only (Group C) tend to support our conclusions.

For technical reasons the hard crystal-like material seen in the renal histology from both enflurane groups (Groups B and D) has not been identified. During fixation of the biopsy materials calcium chloride was added and it is suggested that the material may be crystalline calcium oxalate. Further investigation of this point is needed.

CONCLUSIONS

1. Twenty-four hours' anaesthesia with 1–1.5 vol% enflurane in the absence of hypoxia does not damage the proximal tubular cells of pigs to any great extent. Although the presence of hard crystal-like material was suggested as a cause for the dilatation of the cells, the presence of such material needs further proof.

2. Nitrous oxide anaesthesia with hypoxia changes the appearance of the proximal tubular cells, the granules in the mitochondrial matrix being especially affected. Hypoxia does not, as judged by the 8-hr biopsies, markedly affect the morphological appearance of the mitochondria.

3. The combination enflurane plus hypoxia clearly damages the proximal tubular cells causing gross cellular changes. The cellular changes were, however, to some extent reversed after about 16 hr of further enflurane anaesthesia under normal oxygen tensions.

4. The noxious factor in kidney damage seems to us the combination hypoxia plus inorganic fluoride, occurring as a result of biotransformation of any fluorinated anaesthetic agent.

REFERENCES

Bond, A. M. and Murray, M. M. (1952): *Brit. J. exp. Path.*, *33/2*, 168.

Chase, R. E., Holaday, D. A., Fiserova-Bergerova, V., Saidman, L. J. and Mack, F. E. (1971): *Anesthesiology*, *35/3*, 262.

De Bruijn, W. C. (1973): *J. Ultrastruct. Res.*, *42*, 29.

Dvoracek, B., Ducardus, R., Van Haelst, U. J. M., Kubat, K. and Van der Pluijm, W. J. M. (1974): In: *Ethrane*, p. 158. Editors: P. Lawin and R. Beer. Springer-Verlag, Berlin – Heidelberg – New York.

Eschenbrenner, A. B. and Miller, E. (1945): *Science*, *102/2647*, 302.

Fratello, U. (1964): *G. ital. Chir.*, *20*, 527.

Halsey, M. J. (1972): Paper presented at: Symposium on Controversial Thoughts in Modern Anesthesiology, Department of Anesthesiology, Rijksuniversiteit, Ghent, 1972.

Hitt, B. A., Mazze, R. I., Cousins, M. J., Edmunds, H. N., Barr, G. A. and Trudell, J. R. (1974): *Anesthesiology*, *40/1*, 62.

Kosek, J. C., Mazze, R. I. and Cousins, M. J. (1972): *Lab. Invest.*, *27/6*, 575.

Mazze, R. I. and Cousins, M. J. (1973): *Canad. Anaesth. Soc. J.*, *20/1*, 64.

Mazze, R. I., Cousins, M. J. and Kosek, L. C. (1972): *Anesthesiology*, *36/6*, 571.

Raventós, J. (1956): *Brit. J. Pharmacol.*, *11*, 394.

Raventós, J. and Lemon, P. G. (1956): *Brit. J. Anaesth.*, *37*, 716.

Venable, J. H. and Coggeshall, R. (1965): *J. Cell Biol.*, *25/2*, 2.

Withford, G. M. and Toves, D. R. (1973): *Anesthesiology*, *39/4*, 416.

Hexafluorobenzene in veterinary anaesthesia*

L. W. HALL, SUSAN R. K. JACKSON** and GILLIAN M. MASSEY

School of Veterinary Medicine, University of Cambridge, Cambridge, United Kingdom

About 14 years ago it was shown that relatively low concentrations of hexafluorobenzene would anaesthetize mice (Burns et al., 1961), and that this agent did not react with hot soda-lime.

The pharmacological properties of hexafluorobenzene in cats were studied by Garmer and Leigh (1967) who demonstrated that it caused less hypotension and respiratory depression than did halothane. Induction of anaesthesia was often associated with salivation and retching and both induction and recovery were slower than with halothane. However, no cardiac irregularities were observed even when catecholamines were injected intravenously in anaesthetized animals.

More recently the actions of hexafluorobenzene in other species of animal have been studied (Hall and Jackson, 1973), while Massey (1973) has described its use for clinical anaesthesia in dogs. A review of these two articles from the University of Cambridge Veterinary School, together with observations made since their publication, will be presented in this paper.

PHYSICAL PROPERTIES OF HEXAFLUOROBENZENE

The hexafluorobenzene used in all the trials was supplied by ISC Chemicals, was guaranteed 99% pure, and according to the manufacturers had a molecular weight of 186, a boiling point of 80° C, a vapour pressure at 20° C of 66 mm Hg and an oil/water solubility coefficient of 470.

ADMINISTRATION

Hexafluorobenzene was always vapourized from the smaller (Trilene) bottle of a Boyle's apparatus in a mixture of nitrous oxide/oxygen. The vapour concentration emerging from this bottle at several gas flow rates and temperatures was determined by gas chromatography and shown to be reasonably stable at any given temperature and flow rate. For all small animals the Magill circuit, Ayre's T-piece, Water's circuit or Boyle Mark II circle absorber were used and for horses special circle or to-and-fro absorption systems were used as semi-closed circuits.

---

* The work was facilitated by grants from the Horserace Betting Levy Board, the Wellcome Trust and the Royal Society.

** Mrs S. R. K. Jackson received a grant from the British Oxygen Co. Ltd.

ANAESTHESIA IN HORSES

After premedication with either acepromazine * (0.05 mg/kg by intramuscular injection) or xylazine ** (2 mg/kg by intramuscular injection) anaesthesia was induced with thiopentone sodium (approximately 8–9 mg/kg) injected into the jugular vein. After oral endotracheal intubation with a cuffed tube, anaesthesia was maintained with 4% hexafluorobenzene.

Hexafluorobenzene inhalation appeared to stimulate breathing for at least the first 5 min of anaesthesia. Arterial carbon dioxide tension (Pa_{CO_2}) declined from pre-anaesthetic values of 36–40 mm Hg to between 30 and 35 mm Hg and both the rate and depth of breathing were increased. This contrasted sharply with the fairly rapid rise to Pa_{CO_2} values of 55–60 mm Hg seen in horses anaesthetized with halothane.

The arterial blood pressure fell rapidly to 50–60% of the standing, conscious, level when hexafluorobenzene was inhaled and the heart rate increased to nearly twice that of the animal standing quietly at rest. No change in cardiac rhythm was recorded on a lead II electrocardiogram but during very deep anaesthesia there was an increase in height, and in some instances inversion, of the T-wave. Cardiac output under hexafluorobenzene anaesthesia was generally double the conscious resting value. These findings again contrast with those under halothane anaesthesia where similar levels of arterial hypotension are encountered with a decrease in cardiac output and no increase in heart rate.

The recovery period was similar in duration to that after halothane anaesthesia and was completely free from excitement.

ANAESTHESIA IN SHEEP

The inhalation of 5–6% hexafluorobenzene vapour induced anaesthesia in sheep within 5–7 min. Administration of the vapour through a face-mask caused no obvious resentment, and once anaesthetized endotracheal intubation presented no difficulties. Hexafluorobenzene anaesthesia was associated with arterial hypotension, an increase in heart rate and an increase in cardiac output. Halothane anaesthesia in sheep produces similar hypotension, a slower heart rate and a decreased cardiac output.

Recovery from hexafluorobenzene anaesthesia was similar in type and duration to that after halothane anaesthesia.

ANAESTHESIA IN PIGS

In pigs the inhalation of hexafluorobenzene at a concentration of 5% through a face-mask produced an uneventful induction of anaesthesia. Anaesthesia was associated with initial respiratory stimulation followed by respiratory depression after 5–6 min, and an initial fall in arterial blood pressure was followed by a slow rise. Similar levels of hypotension and similar degrees of respiratory depression occur in pigs anaesthetized with halothane. Recovery, after periods of anaesthesia of up to 30 min duration, was as rapid as after halothane.

---

*   'Acetylpromazine', Boots Drug Co., United Kingdom.
** 'Rompun', Bayer, Federal Republic of Germany.

ANAESTHESIA IN DOGS

Dogs premedicated with atropine and acepromazine or pethidine were anaesthetized by the intravenous injection of thiopentone sodium (approximately 10 mg/kg) or methohexitone sodium (4 mg/kg). After endotracheal intubation with a cuffed tube, anaesthesia was maintained with hexafluorobenzene, given first at a concentration of 3–6% and reducing to 0.3–1% as surgical anaesthesia was obtained. Induction of anaesthesia with hexafluorobenzene in premedicated dogs required the administration of 6% vapour through a close-fitting face-mask for 7–9 min and after some initial breath holding, inhalation of the vapour was not resented. It was difficult to ensure an absence of response to surgical stimulation and two dogs undergoing aural resection shook their heads persistently throughout the operation. Muscular tremor was seen during anaesthesia in 3 of 60 dogs given hexafluorobenzene.

Respiration was not depressed under hexafluorobenzene anaesthesia and blood gas values remained within normal limits. Tachypnoea was often seen in response to surgical stimulation. Pulse rates remained within the normal range and were comparable with those recorded in dogs anaesthetized with halothane. Any sudden increase in inhaled vapour concentration produced a transient marked fall in arterial blood pressure, but no cardiac irregularities were seen in the electrocardiogram. Six of the 60 dogs shivered during the recovery period and one dog became excited. There was no vomiting either at induction or recovery, no post-anaesthesia complications and no deaths in this series of dogs. Limited studies failed to show any evidence of liver damage due to hexafluorobenzene anaesthesia.

ANAESTHESIA IN CATS

In cats anaesthesia was induced with 4% hexafluorobenzene vapour and maintained with 1.5–2%. The excessive salivation during induction noted by Garmer and Leigh (1967) was abolished by premedication with 0.3 mg atropine, but 4 of 8 cats induced using a face-mask developed conjunctival congestion although their eyes were never beneath the mask. Respiratory depression and hypotension were less marked than with halothane anaesthesia but recovery was more prolonged.

DISCUSSION

Hexafluorobenzene appeared to be a safe anaesthetic agent and, compared with halothane, produced less respiratory depression and arterial hypotension in horses, sheep, pigs, dogs and cats. In most animals, unlike halothane, this agent was apparently capable of producing a marked rise in cardiac output unrelated to an increase in arterial carbon dioxide tension. In dogs, however, during intermittent positive pressure ventilation at normocapnia hexafluorobenzene caused a decrease in cardiac output (Hall and Jackson, 1973). No cardiac arrhythmias were observed during the clinical or experimental use of hexafluorobenzene and very limited trials failed to show evidence of liver damage due to this agent. The vapour appeared to be irritant to the conjunctiva but the facial oedema reported in a cat by Garmer and Leigh (1967) was not encountered in clinical cases.

It was clear, as found by Burns et al. (1961), that hexafluorobenzene is an acceptable anaesthetic free from the toxic or lethal effects these workers demonstrated with other fluorinated 6-membered ring compounds. Nevertheless, it seems unlikely that it will ever find a place in clinical anaesthesia because the advantages it offers over anaesthetics such as halothane and methoxyflurane are probably not sufficiently great to offset the disadvantage that it needs to be used close to its flammability limits.

SUMMARY

Hexafluorobenzene was administered in known concentrations from standard anaesthetic equipment to spontaneously breathing horses, dogs, cats, sheep and pigs undergoing a variety of surgical procedures. In general the course of anaesthesia appeared to be similar in all species of animal included in the trials. The effects observed were compared with those seen in animals subjected to similar procedures under halothane anaesthesia and there was less evidence of cardiovascular and respiratory depression. No signs of hepatic or renal toxicity were observed with either agent. The inspired concentrations of hexafluorobenzene needed to induce anaesthesia were close to the lower limits of flammability for this compound.

ACKNOWLEDGEMENTS

Hexafluorobenzene was kindly provided by ISC Chemicals. Miss K. W. Clarke, M.R.C.V.S., D.V.A., very kindly carried out the cardiac output determinations and technical assistance was given by Miss C. Donovan and Miss J. R. Tiplady.

REFERENCES

Burns, T. H. S., Hall, J. M., Bracken, A. and Gouldstone, G. (1961): *Anaesthesia, 16,* 333.
Garmer, N. L. and Leigh, J. M. (1967): *Brit. J. Pharmacol., 31,* 345.
Hall, L. W. and Jackson, S. R. K. (1973): *Anaesthesia, 28,* 155.
Massey, G. M. (1973): *Anaesthesia, 28,* 327.

Clinical evaluation of a new inhalational anesthetic: 1-bromo-1,2,2-trifluorocyclobutane (42M-9)

DONALD J. CARROW, J. ANTONIO ALDRETE,
DONALD R. SHOEMAKER and JOHN A. NICHOLSON

Department of Anesthesiology, University of Louisville
School of Medicine, Louisville, Ky., U.S.A.

Although it had long been established that the presence of halogens on low molecular weight hydrocarbons enhanced their anesthetic value, it was not until 1951, with Skuky's synthesis of fluroxene, that this concept was fully appreciated. Since then many low molecular weight halogenated hydrocarbons and ethers have been evaluated as anesthetics on the premise that fluoride enhances potency, that flammability is hampered by bromide and chloride, and that ethers contribute to cardiovascular stability.

Two agents, halothane and methoxyflurane, have been used more frequently. However, clinical and experimental evidence has attributed hepatic and renal complications, respectively, to these agents. Thus the search for safer and more potent anesthetics was renewed, resulting in two agents with chemical structures similar to halothane and methoxyflurane.

The anesthetic properties of Ethrane, a fluorinated compound similar in structure to methoxyflurane, have been documented by Dobkin et al. (1969), Botty et al. (1968) and Lebowitz et al. (1970), and it is now marketed commercially. Forane, another compound, although still under clinical investigation, appears very promising, as reported by Stevens et al. (1971).

A variety of methods to evaluate anesthetic properties in chemical compounds have been described. Recently a new concept has been introduced which utilizes not only the advantages of the halogens and ethers but also the simplicity of the saturated cyclic hydrocarbons as anesthetic agents (Grace and Co., 1972).

In 1929 Lucas and Henderson proposed cyclopropane as an anesthetic agent. Owing to its potency and the rapid onset and emergence, it became a valuable agent in clinical anesthesia. Unfortunately, it was also found to be explosive and arrhythmogenic. Consequently, limited work has been done with other low molecular cyclic hydrocarbons, specifically cyclobutane, in an attempt to eliminate the undesirable effects of cyclopropane. Krantz et al. (1948) and Vandam and Dripps (1955), demonstrated that cyclobutane was similar to cyclopropane as an anesthetic, although somewhat less potent.

With the concept of a halogenated or alkylated cyclobutane in mind, it was easy to envision the advent of numerous agents (Fig. 1). Thus far the substituted cyclobutane structure has yielded 50–60 new compounds, of which 6–12 have been found to possess anesthetic properties.

This report describes the preliminary evaluation of one of these compounds, 1-bromo-1,2,2-trifluorocyclobutane (42M-9) (Fig. 2), undertaken on the basis of previous laboratory and animal studies (Grace and Co., 1972) which indicated that it has anesthetic properties and physical characteristics similar to those of methoxyflurane and halothane (Table 1).

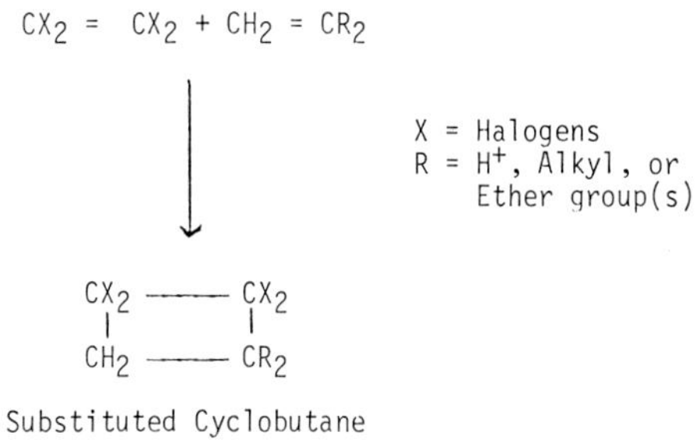

$$CX_2 = CX_2 + CH_2 = CR_2$$

X = Halogens
R = H⁺, Alkyl, or Ether group(s)

Substituted Cyclobutane

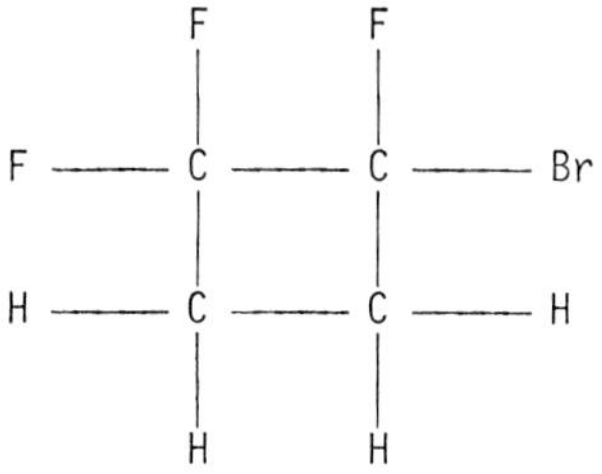

Fig. 1.   *General reaction equation for cyclobutane derivatives.*

Fig. 2.   *1-bromo-1, 2, 2-trifluorocyclobutane (42M-9).*

Table 1. *Selected physical properties of 42M-9*

	42M-9	Halothane	Methoxyflurane
Molecular weight	189	197	164
Density d_4^{25}	1.704		
Boiling point	99.5° C	50.2° C	104.6° C
Vapor pressure			
at 25° C	33 mm	300 mm	30 mm
at 37° C	63 mm	478 mm	55 mm
Heat of vaporization	48 cal/g	36 cal/g	55 cal/g
Partition coefficients			
(tentative) at 37° C			
oil/gas	560	140	820
blood/gas	8	2.3	13
oil/blood	38	60	63
Molar refractivity	26.5 ml	23.9 ml	27.3 ml

OUTLINE OF STUDY

Sixteen young, informed, male volunteers, 21–31 years of age, were subjected to the inhalation of 42M-9 vapor in 100% oxygen. All were found to be in excellent health by physical examination, including EKG and chest X-ray. None was currently on any medications and all appeared to have a negative past history of serious illness. After fasting for 8 hr, each subject was taken to the operating room where venous and arterial (radial) cannulas were inserted under local anesthesia. Numerous blood chemistry studies, including arterial blood gases (on room air), were made. Control values of respiratory rate, tidal volume (V_T) and minute volume ($\dot{V}$) were measured utilizing a Wright respirometer in a semiclosed anesthesia circuit with a carbon dioxide absorber under tight fitting mask. Six of the 16 volunteers were premedicated 45 min before being brought to the operating room with intramuscular atropine (0.01 mg/kg) and either Innovar ® (1 ml/30 kg) or hydroxazine (1 mg/kg). Regardless of premedication, each subject was then exposed to a predetermined vapor concentration of 42M-9 (from 0.50–1.25%) with a total flow ranging from 2–6 l/min of 100% oxygen. The 42M-9 was vaporized into the circuit with a flow and temperature compensated (Pentamatic) vaporizer, which vaporized closely to 1.25 concentrations (see calibration curve, Fig. 3). This vaporizer was chosen because of the vapor pressure of 42M-9, which is essentially the same as that of methoxyflurane.

Each subject was exposed to the vapor for 60 min or until such time as an unusual occurrence made it necessary to discontinue the experiment. Throughout the entire exposure, and up to 15 min afterward, blood pressure, pulse rate and electrocardiograph were continuously monitored. Every 15 min arterial blood gases and respiratory function were determined.

After completion of the exposure time, each of the subjects remained in the operating room at least 30 min, during which time he was given 100% oxygen by mask. In addition, blood and urine samples were obtained for chemical analysis. Upon returning to the recovery room, they were under close observation until completely recovered from all anesthetic effects. A regular diet was given 2–3 hr post-anesthesia and 6 hr post-anesthesia additional samples of blood and urine were obtained for study. The volunteers were again thoroughly evaluated and then discharged from the recovery room to the care of a relative or friend.

Subsequently, each subject was seen 24 and 48 hr later for questioning, evaluation, when blood and urine studies were repeated.

RESULTS

Induction and emergence

Of the 16 subjects, 9 were considered to have reached discernible levels of anesthesia. It appeared that a concentration of 0.75% of 42M-9 was required to produce unconsciousness, while greater than 0.75% resulted in surgical anesthesia levels (Table 2).

All subjects complained at the onset that the vapor of 42M-9 smelled like paint remover, but felt it was not intolerable. Consistently 5–10 min after the beginning of exposure and regardless of the concentration, they developed peripheral tingling, followed immediately

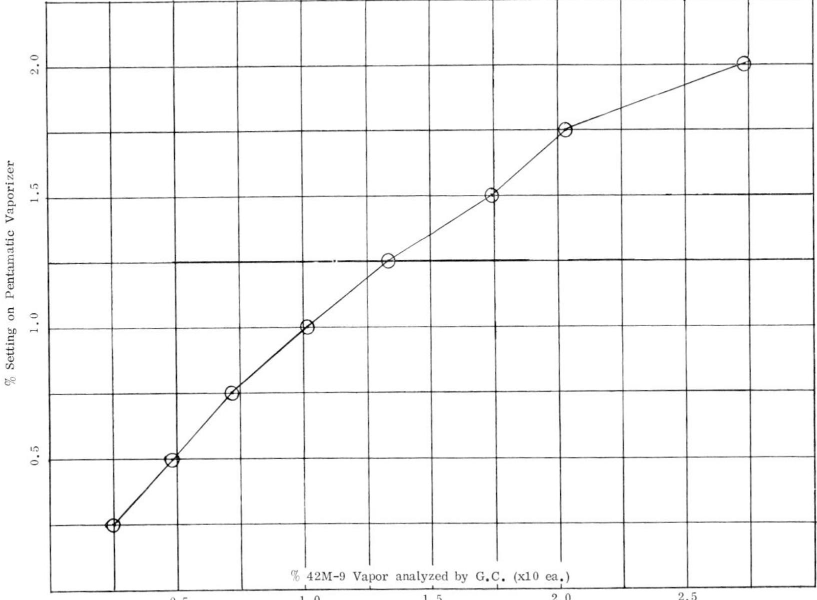

Fig. 3. *Calibration curve of Pentamatic vaporizer with 42M-9 anesthetic.*

by slurring of speech. Within 20 min, all volunteers experienced dizziness and felt sleepy even at the lowest concentration of vapors. For all subjects exposed to less than 1.0% vapor, recovery was rapid, lasting about 10–15 min. At concentrations greater than 1.0%, recovery was prolonged 15–30 min.

Cardiovascular effects

Of the first four experiments at a 42M-9 concentration of 0.50%, only one subject appeared to have reached Stage I level of anesthesia, as described by Artusio (1955). The following four studies were carried out at 0.75%, which placed them between Stages II and III level. After 15 min exposure to this concentration, one of these subjects developed a ventricular bigeminy rhythm (Fig. 4). He was immediately given 100 mg of lidocaine intravenously and the anesthetic was discontinued. This arrhythmia subsided immediately with prompt return to a sinus rhythm. Subsequent evaluations of the patient revealed no changes from his pre-exposure physical or mental status.

Another subject was then exposed to 0.5% 42M-9 without untoward effects. The next 2 subjects inhaled concentrations of 1.0% without the occurrence of arrhythmias. Only one of these subjects reached a Stage III level. After reconfirming the purity of the agent and the concentration at which it was being administered, a volunteer was exposed to 1.25%. He reached a Stage III level after 20 min of exposure, but after 44 min ventricular bigeminy rhythm was noted, which again subsided after intravenous lidocaine was given and the agent discontinued.

Three of the next 4 patients were exposed to 42M-9 vapor in a stepwise progressive manner, starting at 0.5% concentration for 15 min followed by 0.75% concentration for an equal period. In each case, the concentration was increased up to 1%; within 5–10 min of exposure, a ventricular bigeminy rhythm occurred in both instances, which terminated the experiment. The fourth patient was exposed to 1.25% for 12 min; a ventricular bigeminy rhythm developed which subsided after the concentration of 42M-9 was decreased to 0.75%. Consequently, the experiment was pursued again advancing the concentration gradually to 1.25% for the remaining 45 min of the study without the recurrence of arrhythmias. Three of the 4 subjects appeared to have reached Stage III plane III level of anesthesia, while only one remained at a Stage III plane I level.

At no time in any of the experiments, regardless of the concentration, or time, were any significant changes noted in the arterial blood pressure (Fig. 5). Even at concentrations between 0.75%–1.25% only a 6–8 mm decrease in mean arterial pressure was noted while heart rate increased 20–30 beats/min. Even in those cases in which an arrhythmia occurred, blood pressure levels were maintained near normal values. In every instance, around 30 sec prior to the onset of the arrhythmias, there was tachycardia in the order of 130–160 beats/min, which eventually was considered to be an ominous sign.

Respiratory effects

The inhalation of 0.25 and 0.5% of 42M-9 resulted in an increase in $\dot{V}$ of 79.7%, and V_T of 20.3%, while the number of respirations per minute increased only 5.0% (Fig. 6).

When the anesthetic concentration was augmented to 0.75% it produced average increases in $\dot{V}$ of 59.0%, V_T 3.5% and respiratory frequency per minute of 96.0% (Fig. 6).

The most obvious increase in ventilation from control values was seen in the 5 subjects exposed to 1.0%, who averaged a $\dot{V}$ of 122.5%, a V_T of 43.0%, and a respiratory rate of 136% (Fig. 6). In contrast, for the 2 subjects exposed to 1.25% the average increase in $\dot{V}$ was only 73.5%, while V_T fell 20.0%, and respiratory frequency rose 148.0% (Table 3).

Table 2. *Summary of observations during 42M-9 project I*

Subject	Date	Total O_2 flow	42M-9 lot No. used	Total experimental time (min)	Experimental time at specific concentration in minutes (%)				42M-9 concentration at which arrhythmia occurred	Stage I	Stage II	Stage III
					0.50	0.75	1.00	1.25				
513306	8–16	2	14944P	60	60				–			
514335	8–21	2	14944P	60	60				–			
484335	8–22	2	14944P	60		60			–			
468106	8–23	2	14944P	60		60			–			
467859	8–24	2	14944P	60			60		–	×		
514606	8–28	2	14944P	60			60		–			
514642	8–29	2	14944P	44				44	1.25		×	
484272	8–30	3	14944P	60	60				–			
484295	8–31	3	14944P	60		60			–	×		
484314	9–6	6	14944P 14956P	8			8		1.00			
514024	9–7	6	14944P 14956P	60	60				–	×		
506815	9–28	6	14944P 14956P	15		15			0.75	×		
516362	10–3	6	14944P 14956P	57		17		40	1.25			×
516026	10–4	6	14944P 14956P	60	50		10		1.00		×	
495495	10–9	6	14944P 14956P	35	15	15	5		1.00			×
484275	10–11	6	14959P	35	15	15	5		1.00			×

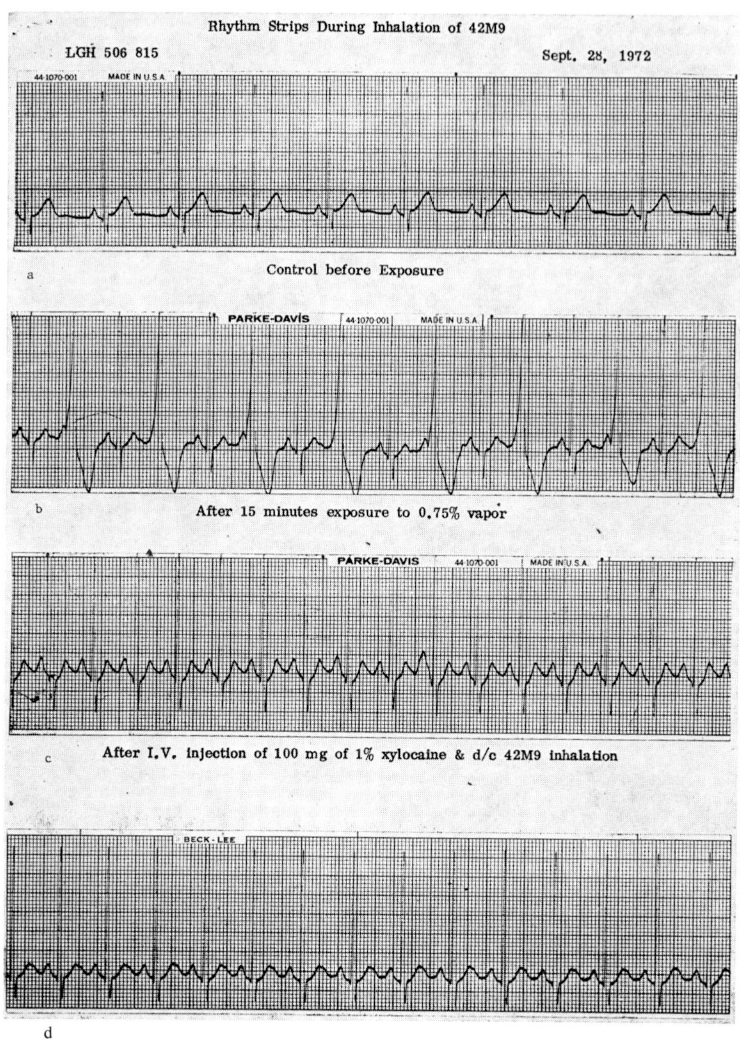

Fig. 4.   *Rhythm strips during inhalation of 42M-9. (a) Control before exposure; (b) after 15 min exposure to 0.75% vapor; (c) after i.v. injection of 100 mg of 1% xylocaine and d/c 42M-9 inhalation; (d) 15 min after d/c of 42M-9 inhalation.*

Laboratory studies

In 13 subjects Pa_{CO_2} decreased an average of 6.1 Torr. These changes were based on the lowest values obtained from arterial sampling at 15-min intervals throughout each study.

No significant change was observed in the serial results of blood and urine laboratory determinations during the anesthetic exposure or through the 48-hr following observation period, as listed in Table 4.

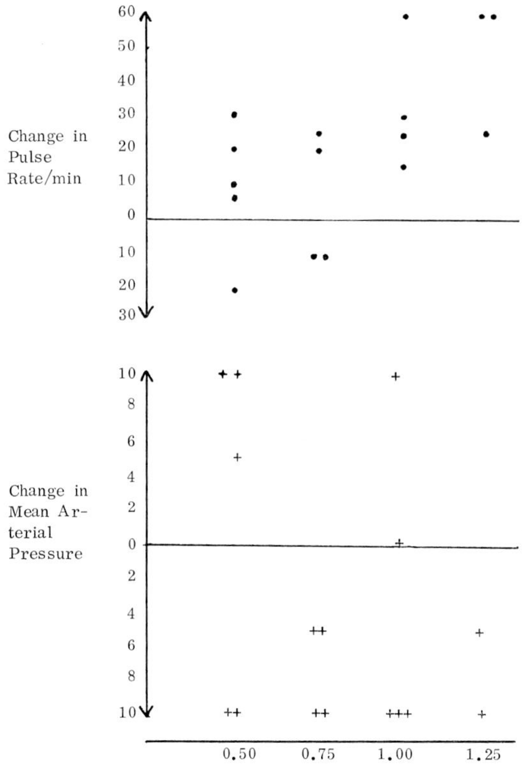

Fig. 5. *Effect of 42M-9 exposure on mean arterial pressure and pulse rate in 16 subjects.*

DISCUSSION

From this study, it appeared that direct exposure of human subjects to the inhalation anesthetic and subanesthetic concentrations of 42M-9 vapor in oxygen was not an undesirable experience to the volunteers. This conclusion was based on careful observations and questioning of the 16 subjects in the study. In general, below 1.0% the acceptability of 42M-9 vapor inhalation was comparable to that experienced by patients given halothane or fluroxene under similar conditions (Stephen et al., 1957; Burns et al., 1957). Upon initial exposure to the highest concentrations used (1.0–1.25%), all 7 subjects complained that the first few breaths were somewhat irritating, though this feeling appeared to subside in each case after about 1 or 2 min.

At low concentrations emergence was also found to be similar to that from halothane. In fact neither the investigators nor the recovery room nurses were able to detect any appreciable differences. It was noted, however, that after inhalation of 1.0% concentrations or higher, the recovery time, as determined by Aldrete's recovery scoring method, was prolonged up to 15–30 min (Aldrete and Kroulik, 1970).

In similarity with cyclopropane, arterial blood pressure was maintained stable in all subjects throughout the entire 42M-9 exposure time. The maximum variation was not greater than ±8 mm Hg in mean arterial pressure (Fig. 5). This apparent advantage of

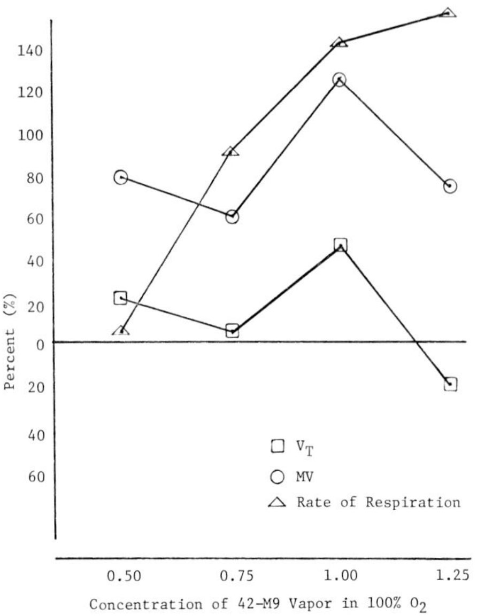

Fig. 6.   *Average change (%) in pulmonary functions of 16 subjects exposed to increasing concentrations of 42M-9 vapor in 100% O₂.*

Table 3.   *Changes in ventilatory volumes in subjects exposed to 42M-9*

Subject	Exposure (min)	Concentration of vapor (%)	MV (ml) C	MV (ml) △	V_T (ml) C	V_T (ml) △	Rate/min C	Rate/min △	Blood gases (△) pH	Blood gases (△) P_CO₂ (mm)
1	60	0.50	9,600	400	600	100	16	4	0.070	5.2
2	60	0.50	5,100	3,100	800	1,300	6	2	0.035	6.0
3	60	0.50	6,500	600	600	100	12	2	0.063	7.9
4	60	0.50	4,200	4,400	375	100	12	5	0.044	4.0
5	60	0.50	7,500	5,500	700	NC	11	5	0.037	1.7
6	60	0.75	3,600	1,200	400	100	10	2	0.014	4.3
7	15	0.75	4,200	9,800	250	200	16	16	0.059	5.0
8	60	0.75	5,100	2,700	500	150	11	13	0.022	3.1
9	60	0.75	4,800	4,350	600	50	12	2	0.015	6.6
10	60	1.00	6,000	9,200	450	50	14	16	0.020	2.1
11	60	1.00	6,500	350	600	100	12	13	0.029	3.4
12	8	1.00	4,600	–	250	–	18	–	0.027	11.1
13	35	1.00	3,900	3,600	300	350	12	NC	0.016	2.9
14	35	1.00	7,000	650	1,000	300	7	13	0.062	8.9
15	44	1.25	8,800	5,200	1,100	300	8	12	0.048	8.5
16	57	1.25	6,400	5,600	800	100	8	11	0.013	5.3

C=control, △=maximum change. Underlined figures indicate decrease in numerical value.

Table 4. *Laboratory studies performed*

Blood

Red blood cell count	Albumin/globulin ratio	Calcium
Hemoglobin	SGOT	Magnesium
Hematocrit	SGPT	pH
White blood cell count	LDH	Carbon dioxide pressure
Platelets	LDH isoenzymes	Oxygen pressure
Reticulocytes	OCT	Bicarbonate
Blood urea nitrogen	ICD	Base excess
Creatinine	Cholinesterase	Total carbon dioxide
Glucose	CPK	Bromsulphalein
Prothrombin time	Sodium	Free fatty acids
Partial prothrombin time	Potassium	Triglycerides
Bilirubin 1 min	Chloride	Cholesterol
Bilirubin 5 min	Carbon dioxide	Uric acid
Total protein	Phosphorus	Alkaline phosphatase

Urine

Specific gravity	Potassium	Phosphorus
Creatine	Chloride	Magnesium
Sodium	Calcium	

Blood and urine studies obtained from each subject involved in the 42M-9 study at the following intervals: Control (before exposure), immediately at the end and 6, 24 and 48 hr post-exposure.

42M-9 as an anesthetic agent was outweighed by the occurrence of ventricular arrhythmias in some of the subjects exposed to it.

Of the 16 subjects exposed to 42M-9 vapor, 7 (43%) developed ventricular arrhythmias. From Table 2 it is apparent that arrhythmias occurred predominantly at concentrations ranging from 1.0%–1.25%; in one instance, however, premature ventricular beats were noted after only 15 min of exposure to a concentration of 0.75%, thus suggesting that exposure time was not necessarily related to the appearance of arrhythmias.

Premedication did not prevent occurrence of arrhythmias, since 5 out of the 7 volunteers who experienced arrhythmias were premedicated with atropine, and Innovar® or hydroxazine.

Measurements of ventilation in all 16 subjects (Table 3) indicated stimulation with a limited dose-effect relationship. These values were higher at 1.0% for minute and tidal volumes, when elevations of 122.5% and 43.0% respectively were seen. The respiratory frequency followed a similar trend, although of less magnitude (Fig. 6). The inhalation of 42M-9, independent of its concentration produced an average $\dot{V}$ elevation of 70.9% although only 10 subjects showed V_T rises averaging 46.4%. Eleven subjects exhibited a mean rise of 125.0% in respiratory rate. Arterial blood gas measurements showed no essential changes in arterial P_{O_2}, though 13 of the subjects were found to have a mean decrease in Pa_{CO_2} of 6.1 Torr.

CONCLUSIONS

The experimental inhalational compound 42M-9 was found to have anesthetic properties in 16 healthy young male volunteers as had been predicted from previous animal studies. Its use in human subjects, however, did result in an unusually high percent of ventricular arrhythmias, which would certainly interfere with its acceptance as a commercial anesthetic agent at this time.

In view of the apparent absence of arterial blood pressure depression and the enhancement of respiratory function, more detailed investigation may be justified.

Perhaps a simple modification in the substituted cyclobutane molecule should be made in an attempt to eliminate what appears to be an arrhythmogenic component of 1-bromo-1,2,2-trifluorocyclobutane (42M-9). In fact, any structural change in this molecule likely would also have the circulatory stabilizing effect of the etheral type linkage.

If further studies are to be undertaken with this agent, we would propose to utilize routine induction and maintenance techniques such as: intravenous sodium thiopental and nitrous oxide/oxygen mixtures for maintenance. The purpose of this change in the experimental protocol would be to suppress the release of endogenous catecholamines, frequently associated with direct induction under bag and mask when using oxygen and anesthetic vapor only. Furthermore, to confirm its lack of toxicity, blood and urine chemistries would also be in order.

REFERENCES

Aldrete, J. A. and Kroulik, D. (1970): *Anesth. Analg. Curr. Res., 49,* 6.

Artusio, J. F. (1955): *J. Amer. med. Ass., 157,* 33.

Botty, C. et al. (1968): *Anesth. Analg. Curr. Res., 47,* 499.

Burns, T. H. S. et al. (1957): *Brit. med. J., 2,* 483.

Dobkin, A. B. et al. (1969): *Anesth. Analg. Curr. Res., 48,* 477.

Grace and Co. (1972): *Notice of Claimed Investigational Exemption For a New Drug.* Dewey and Almy Chemical Division, W. R. Grace and Co., Cambridge, Mass., U.S.A.

Krantz Jr., J. et al. (1948): *Anesthesiology, 9,* 594.

Lebowitz, M. H., Blitt, C. D. and Dillon, J. B. (1970): *Anesth. Analg. Curr. Res., 49,* 1.

Lucas, G. H. W. and Henderson, V. E. (1929): *Canad. med. Ass. J., 21,* 173.

Stephen, C. R. et al. (1957): *Canad. Anaesth. Soc. J., 4,* 246.

Stevens, W. C. et al. (1971): *Anesthesiology, 35,* 8.

Vandam, L. D. and Dripps, R. D. (1955): *Anesthesiology, 16,* 48.

Pulmonary morbidity in patients unconscious from drug overdose

CHRISTOPHER G. MALE*, J. ANTONIO ALDRETE and DONALD J. CARROW

Department of Anesthesiology, School of Medicine,
University of Louisville, Louisville, Ky, U.S.A.

Pulmonary complications remain a major avoidable factor in the morbidity of patients unconscious from drug overdose. This study reviews aspects of such morbidity in consecutive overdose admissions to the University of Louisville General Hospital over a 30-month period following the establishment of a protocol for their management.

METHOD

Awareness of the high risk of aspiration in this group of patients prompted the training of all emergency room doctors in early endotracheal intubation by both oral and blind nasal routes. Gastric lavage was not practised routinely but restricted to specific overdoses such as salicylates, glutethimide and iron tablets. Baseline values for white blood cell count, body temperature and chest X-ray were obtained within 3 hr of admission. Ventilatory support was started early if tolerated by the patient. Assisted ventilation with at least 40% inspired oxygen delivered from the Bennett MA-I ventilator was preferred to controlled ventilation throughout the study. The effective heated cascade humidifier maintained inspired gas temperature between 95 and 100° F. The staff in the intensive care unit were taught aseptic techniques for endotracheal suction which was performed every 2 hr or more frequently as indicated. Nearly all comatose patients received a forced diuresis with mannitol (12.5+12.5 g) and 0.5 N saline intravenously. The positive fluid balance was limited to 2000 ml with urine production measured by aseptic bladder catheter drainage. The antibiotic policy restricted the prescription of ampicillin to those patients with a radiological pulmonary infiltrate, abnormal physical signs on chest auscultation and a pyrexia exceeding 102° F. Other antibiotics were used as indicated by the sensitivity reports of daily sputum cultures. In the first 15 months of the study, moderate doses of steroids were given for suspected aspiration, but since February 1973 steroids have been avoided except for those cases with severe bronchospasm, tachycardia and hypotension following aspiration (Mendelson's syndrome) (Mendelson, 1946).

RESULTS

The age of the patients ranged from 10–84 years with a peak early in the 3rd decade. Although female patients represented two-thirds of all overdose admissions, pulmonary complications were more frequently seen in the male patients in whom 7 of the 9 deaths occurred.

* Present address: Department of Anaesthesia, Plymouth General Hospital (Freedom Fields), Plymouth, United Kingdom.

The 9 deaths in the series of 1481 cases give a mortality rate of 0.6%. Six patients died primarily from respiratory complications such as bilateral diffuse lobular and broncho-pneumonia. Three of these 6 patients were conscious from the time of admission and yet were without a documented history of aspiration. A young narcotic addict took an overdose of morphine and died of bacteraemia from staphylococcal pneumonia which developed 8 days after admission. A 63-year-old patient with painful venous stasis ulceration of the legs ingested an excess of aspirin tablets and was admitted with a blood salicylate level of 62 mg/100 ml. He developed respiratory insufficiency after 36 hr followed by pneumococcal lobar pneumonia, renal and hepatic failure succumbing 9 days later. A 67-year-old man drank some lye and subsequently suffered oesophageal strictures and tracheo-oesophageal fistula whereon numerous episodes of spill-over led to recurrent pneumonitis. The patient died of overwhelming sepsis 8 months after admission. A 4th patient who was conscious from the time of admission died from cardiac asystole and convulsions 4 hr after taking Roach powder containing fluorine salts.

The other 5 fatalities all suffered prolonged unconsciousness requiring at least 48 hr intensive care. Phenobarbitone was the major drug taken in 3 patients who died after 2, 10 and 16 days respectively from bilateral diffuse pneumonia. Klebsiella enterobacter was the prominent growth in 2 cases, and *Staphylococcus aureus* in the 3rd. Two unconscious patients both died after 5 days without cerebral electrocortical activity – an 18-year-old with overdose of heroin developed pulmonary and cerebral oedema resistant to all treatment and a 20-year-old suffered brain damage secondary to cardiac arrest after intravenous injection of phencyclidine and other hallucinogens.

The pulmonary morbidity rate for the whole study (N=1481) was 2.2% with 33 patients demonstrating radiological lung lesions. The chest X-rays of the non-infective group of 24 patients demonstrated infiltrates (19), lung (3) and lobar (9) atelectasis, pulmonary oedema (6) and congestion (3), pleural effusion (1), pneumothorax (5) and fractured ribs (2) or combinations thereof. All were intubated on admission and required at least 48 hr intensive care for prolonged unconsciousness. The infective group developed significant pneumonitis diagnosed by strict criteria described below. Six out of 9 cases suffered prolonged unconsciousness, and the other 3 who were conscious from the time of admission all developed fatal septicaemia secondary to staphylococcal, pneumococcal and gram-negative pneumonias respectively.

Three positive findings within 3 hr of admission were considered specific of aspiration – a rectal temperature of 100° F or greater, a white blood cell count exceeding 10,000/mm^3 and an infiltrate on chest X-ray. The findings for the 56 cases of prolonged unconsciousness are shown in Table 1. The association of the 3 factors has a very significant chi-square value of 15.9 and a probability value of $p < 0.001$. Surprisingly the results of chest auscultation correlated poorly with these 3 findings and were not considered diagnostic of aspiration.

Table 1.   *Criteria for aspiration on admission*

Temperature	WBC ($\geqslant$ 10,000) +chest X-ray	WBC ($\geqslant$ 10,000) only	Positive chest X-ray only	Neither	Total
$\geqslant$ 100° F	6*	3	1	2	12
$<$ 100° F	2	5	4	33	44
Total	8	8	5	35	56

* $\chi^2 = 15.9$ (1° freedom); $p < 0.001$.

Only one of the 6 patients satisfying the criteria for aspiration died; this morphine overdose developed significant pneumonitis during recovery and died of cerebral and pulmonary oedema.

The criteria for significant pneumonitis developing during recovery were more difficult to define. An infiltrate on chest X-ray was an absolute prerequisite. The peak value of daily white blood cell counts and of 2-hourly rectal temperature readings during recovery were analysed in 56 cases of prolonged unconsciousness. Seven cases had a temperature rise to as high as 102.8° F without a leucocytosis (WBC $> 10,000/\text{mm}^3$). On the other hand, of 18 patients with a peak temperature over 103° F, only half showed a leucocytosis greater than $20,000/\text{mm}^3$. With these figures, a rectal temperature of 103° F or higher and WBC exceeding $20,000/\text{mm}^3$ were selected as the other two criteria for diagnosing significant pneumonitis. A table of these findings (Table 2) in patients suffering prolonged unconsciousness shows an abnormally large number with three positive criteria. The association of these three factors is highly significant with an exact value of p = 0.0011 (Fisher's test) (Fisher, 1958).

Table 2. *Criteria for significant pneumonitis during recovery*

Temperature	WBC ($\geqslant$ 20,000) +chest X-ray	WBC ($\geqslant$ 20,000) only	Positive chest X-ray only	Neither	Total
$\geqslant$ 103° F	6*	2	5	5	18
$<$ 103° F	2	3	13	20	38
Total	8	5	18	25	56

* From Fisher, 1958. Exact significance p=0.0011.

Four of the 6 patients who demonstrated significant pneumonitis during recovery eventually died; in 3 of these the respiratory complications were the primary cause of death.

Steroids were given within 3 hr of admission to 12 of the 56 cases of prolonged unconsciousness. In a comparison of admission and recovery findings (Table 3) 3 of the 6 cases with positive criteria aspiration developed significant pneumonitis during recovery, but all 3 patients had received steroids. The number is too small for statistical analysis but is highly suggestive that steroids may not prevent significant pneumonitis during recovery.

Table 3. *Correlation of positive criteria for aspiration, significant pneumonitis and steroid therapy*

Steroids	Admission +recovery	Admission only	Recovery only	Neither	Total
Given	3	0	2	7	12
Not given	0	3	1	40	44
Total	3	3	3	47	56

Gram-negative organisms were cultured from daily endotracheal sputum specimens in 23 of 38 patients who received antibiotics, but only in 2 of the 18 patients who did not. These included Klebsiella enterobacter (16), Pseudomonas (13), *Escherichia coli* (9), Proteus (6), *Serratia marcescens* (5) *Haemophilus influenzae* (5) and Neisseria (4) in 56 cases of prolonged unconsciousness. Gram-positive organisms were cultured on twice as many occasions as gram-negative organisms with *Staphylococcus aureus* (23), *Streptococcus viridans* (19) and pneumoniae (14) being the predominant bacteria.

Review of the antibiotic therapy in 56 cases of prolonged unconsciousness was interesting. No antibiotics were prescribed for 18 cases, and there was one death from hypoxic brain damage secondary to cardiac arrest prior to admission. In 19 cases, the correct antibiotic was given according to sensitivity reports of the aerobic organisms cultured, but one patient died of bronchopneumonia and pulmonary abscesses involving mixed gram-negative and staphylococcal organisms, and another died of cerebral oedema secondary to heroin self-medication. In the other 19 cases, antibiotic cover was inadequate for the aerobic organisms identified and 2 deaths were attributed to pulmonary candidiasis and Klebsiella pneumonia.

A comparison of the clinical course with the routes of endotracheal intubation showed that all 6 patients who developed significant pneumonitis during recovery underwent nasotracheal intubation. Again the numbers were too few to draw any firm conclusions. The organisms cultured from the lower respiratory tract during recovery did not differ between the patients and the chosen route of intubation.

Tranquillisers (295), barbiturates (175), non-barbiturate hypnotics and sedatives (220), analgesics (166), central nervous system stimulants (132) were the predominant drugs taken by history and identification but of specific drugs, diazepam (200) and pheno-barbitone (68) were the most popular amongst the 1481 cases. In the group of 56 patients suffering prolonged unconsciousness, phenobarbitone, glutethimide, salicylates, heroin and phencyclidine were proportionately over-represented, as were phenobarbitone and heroin among the 9 deaths (Table 4).

Table 4.   *Some drugs taken by overdose admissions*

Drug taken	Study (N = 1481)	Prolonged unconsciousness (N = 56)	Deaths (N = 9)
Phenobarbitone	68	15	3
Diazepam	200	12	1
Glutethimide	5	4	0
Salicylates	80	13	1
Heroin	11	3	2
Phencyclidine	14	4	1

DISCUSSION

Overdose patients are particularly susceptible to pulmonary aspiration because pharyngo-laryngeal reflexes are impaired by the diminished level of consciousness. Gastric regurgitation may occur during transport to hospital with aspiration more likely in the dangerous supine posture. Therapeutic measures such as the administration of an emetic or gastric washout may leave a residue which can be regurgitated later.

Early endotracheal intubation should be performed to isolate the tracheobronchial tree from the pharynx thereby reducing the risk of aspiration thereafter. The method of intubation should not, however, induce vomiting. Blind nasal intubation stimulates vomiting or gag reflex to a lesser degree than orotracheal intubation under direct laryngoscopic vision, but it may require repeated attempts especially if respirations are not deep and the cords not widely abducted. Nasotracheal intubation requires both expertise and practice and qualified personnel may not be available at the time of admission. With the nasotracheal route, there is an increased risk of transferring upper respiratory tract organisms into the tracheobronchial tree where they may become pathogenic. The results of our study suggest that there is a greater risk of significant pneumonitis during recovery with the nasal route, but an analysis of more cases is needed to determine statistical significance.

The diagnosis of pulmonary aspiration is not easy to make in overdose patients. The usual reaction with coughing, increased respiratory rate and cyanosis may be impaired by central nervous system depression or stimulation by the drugs taken, and the patient may be cyanosed from secondary hypoventilation. A review of the results of chest auscultation on admission shows a poor correlation with the subsequent course. Infection is not thought to play much of a role in the early phases of aspiration (Olsen, 1970), and yet we have chosen leucocytosis (WBC $> 10,000/mm^3$) and pyrexia (rectal temperature $\geq 100^\circ$ F) as two criteria for aspiration. However, the former can arise from acute hypoxia and stress, and the latter from atelectases. An infiltrate on chest X-ray is the 3rd criterion and confirms the intensity of the lesion as macroscopic. It is difficult to exclude pre-existing infection as a differential diagnosis except from the history.

The choice of a temperature exceeding 103° F and a WBC greater than $20,000/mm^3$ as two criteria of significant pneumonitis during recovery may be controversial. Both prolonged endotracheal intubation and atelectasis can cause pyrexia and leucocytosis, but analysis of the cases in this study shows these values to be of a lesser degree.

A comparison of our experience with steroid therapy for aspiration and the results of other studies is difficult. The small number of 3 cases with evidence of aspiration who were given steroids and subsequently developed significant pneumonitis suggested that the anti-inflammatory, capillary membrane-stabilising effects (Dudley and Marshall, 1974) of the drug may not prevent the development of significant pneumonitis. Animal studies (Hamelberg and Bosomworth, 1964) describe the benefits of steroids in reducing morbidity when the pH of the aspirated material is less than 1.5, but other animal (Chapman et al., 1974; Downs et al., 1974) and human (Cameron et al., 1973) studies fail to confirm this therapeutic effect. None of our overdose admissions developed Mendelson's syndrome (Mendelson, 1946) which suggests that such patients do not produce excessively acidic gastric secretions, despite starvation. This being so, steroids may be contraindicated in aspiration following drug overdose because of undesirable side-effects, particularly suppression of immunological defence mechanisms in the fight against infection.

A prospective study of 54 cases of pulmonary infection following aspiration by Bartlett et al. (1974) revealed a very high rate of anaerobic infection (93%). The mean peak temperature of 102.5° F and mean peak WBC of $17,500/mm^3$ are criteria of pulmonary infection similar, but slightly less strict, than ours though their group may have included patients not intubated. In our series of 56 cases, an unidentified anaerobic chest infection could explain one death despite adequate antibiotic cover of the aerobic organism cultured. The significance of anaerobes in the pathogenesis of pneumonia following aspiration is that these micro-organisms dominate the upper respiratory tract flora.

The appearance of gram-negative organisms in endotracheal sputum cultures of patients in our study, was strongly associated with the exhibition of broad-spectrum antibiotics; this reaffirms the conclusions of others (Downs et al., 1974; Stoddart, 1974). In view of the results of our study, it is likely that antibiotic therapy will be withheld at our hospital until the three criteria of significant pneumonitis are satisfied. Anaerobic organisms are now sought for daily in endotracheal sputum cultures.

SUMMARY

Various aspects of pulmonary morbidity in a select group of patients susceptible to aspiration have been discussed. The incidence of radiological lesions in 2.2% of 1481 consecutive overdose admissions, and 53.6% of 56 patients suffering prolonged unconsciousness reflects the importance of central nervous system depression in the aetiology of pulmonary complications.

The establishment of a protocol for the management of overdose admissions and careful attention to detail can reduce pulmonary morbidity in those who are likely to be unconscious for more than 48 hr. Future review of the next 30-month period of this on-going study should reveal the wisdom of our decisions by providing more significant statistical analysis.

REFERENCES

Bartlett, J. G. et al. (1974): *Amer. J. Med., 56*, 202.

Cameron, J. L. et al. (1973): *Arch. Surg., 106*, 49.

Chapman, R. L., Modell, J. H., Ruiz, B. C., Calderwood, H. W., Hood, C. I. and Graves, S. A. (1974): *Anesth. Analg. Curr. Res., 53*, 556.

Downs, J. B. et al. (1974): *Anesthesiology, 40*, 129.

Dudley, W. and Marshall, B. (1974): *Anesthesiology, 40*, 136.

Fisher, R. A. (1958): *Statistical Methods for Research Workers, 13th ed.* Oliver and Boyd, London – Edinburgh.

Hamelberg, W. and Bosomworth, P. P. (1964): *Anesth. Analg. Curr. Res., 43*, 669.

Mendelson, C. L. (1946): *Amer. J. Obstet. Gynec., 52*, 191.

Olsen, A. (1970): *Ann. Otol. (St. Louis), 79*, 875.

Stoddart, J. C. (1974): *Crit. Care Med., 2*, 17.

Influence of inhalation anaesthetics on sympathoadrenal catecholamine release: Comparison of enflurane (Ethrane) and halothane

M. GÖTHERT

Institute of Pharmacology, University of Hamburg, Hamburg, Federal Republic of Germany

At least part of the cardiovascular depression observed during anaesthesia with enflurane or halothane may result from a reduction in catecholamine release from the adrenal medulla and postganglionic sympathetic nerves. Therefore, the effect of enflurane on sympathoadrenal catecholamine output was investigated and was compared to the results previously obtained for halothane (Göthert and Dreyer, 1973; Göthert et al., 1974*a*).

The effect of inhalation anaesthetics on spontaneous catecholamine release from the adrenal medulla and on the secretion evoked by splanchnic nerve stimulation was studied in cats which had received pentobarbital (30 mg/kg) for basal anaesthesia. The left adrenolumbar vein was cannulated in a retrograde direction and blood samples were drawn before, during and after inhalation of enflurane or halothane. The concentrations of adrenaline and noradrenaline in adrenolumbar venous blood were measured spectrofluorometrically according to the trihydroxyindole method of Häggendal (1963). Further details of all methods used were described in previous papers (Göthert and Dreyer, 1973; Dreyer et al., 1974). Each concentration of the anaesthetics was inspired for 35 min. In control cats (N = 5) which had received only pentobarbital for anaesthesia no significant changes in spontaneous adrenaline or noradrenaline output were observed as a function of time (195 min). Both enflurane (1.2% and 2.2% in inspired air) and halothane (0.7%, 1.0%, and 1.5% in inspired air) caused a concentration-dependent decrease in spontaneous adrenaline and noradrenaline release. Quantitatively, differences between the effects of enflurane and halothane can be evaluated when equieffective concentrations are administered. In the cat MAC values for enflurane and halothane are 1.2% and 0.82%, respectively (Brown and Crout, 1971). Since multiples of MAC values may also be regarded as equieffective, the inhibitory action of 2.2% enflurane was compared to that of 1.5% halothane (1.83 MAC). As shown in Table 1, enflurane inhibited the spontaneous adrenaline secretion (expressed as per cent of the preanaesthetic output) to about the same extent as halothane; however, the decrease in noradrenaline secretion caused by enflurane was less pronounced than that caused by halothane. During both enflurane and halothane anaesthesia the blood pressure and pulse rate fell parallel to the inhibition of catecholamine release.

In addition the inhibition of catecholamine secretion from the adrenal medulla evoked by splanchnic nerve stimulation by the inhalation anaesthetics was studied. For this purpose a platinum electrode was fixed to the left splanchnic nerve 1.0–1.5 cm cephalad to the left adrenal gland, and the nerve was stimulated for 5 min with 4 V, 1 msec, and 10 Hz. In control cats (N = 5) which had only received pentobarbital (30 mg/kg) for basal

Table 1. *Effects of 2.2% enflurane (1.83 MAC; N=5) and 1.5% halothane (1.83 MAC; N=8) on the spontaneous catecholamine secretion from the cat adrenal medulla in vivo*

	Adrenaline (ng/kg/min)		Noradrenaline (ng/kg/min)	
	Enflurane	Halothane	Enflurane	Halothane
Before anaesthesia	4.40 ± 1.30	2.28 ± 0.34	3.50 ± 1.10	2.10 ± 0.29
During anaesthesia	0.86* ± 0.38	0.60** ± 0.07	1.00* ± 0.54	0.26** ± 0.10
(1.83 MAC, 35 min)	(20%)	(26%)	(29%)	(12%)

The data for halothane are taken from Göthert and Dreyer (1973). Means ± SEM are given.
* $p < 0.05$; ** $p < 0.001$.

anaesthesia the catecholamine release evoked by splanchnic nerve stimulation was measured 4 times at intervals of 35 min. The values obtained did not differ significantly from each other. However, during anaesthesia with enflurane (1.2% and 2.2% in inspired air) or halothane (1.0 and 1.5% in inspired air) the adrenaline and noradrenaline output from the stimulated gland was inhibited in a concentration-dependent fashion. Table 2 shows that at equieffective concentrations, halothane decreased the catecholamine secretion evoked by splanchnic nerve stimulation to a higher extent than enflurane. Obviously the decrease in adrenal medullary catecholamine output evoked by splanchnic nerve stimulation is a common effect of all inhalation anaesthetics since it was also observed during anaesthesia with methoxyflurane (Dreyer et al., 1974), chloroform and diethyl ether (Göthert et al., unpublished observations).

Table 2. *Effects of 2.2% enflurane (1.83 MAC; N=6) and 1.5% halothane (1.83 MAC; N=7) on the catecholamine secretion from the cat adrenal medulla evoked by splanchnic nerve stimulation*

	Adrenaline (ng/kg/min)		Noradrenaline (ng/kg/min)	
	Enflurane	Halothane	Enflurane	Halothane
Before anaesthesia	69.7 ± 14.9	77.8 ± 10.8	106.1 ± 28.0	89.7 ± 21.4
During anaesthesia	21.1* ± 5.6	11.4** ± 1.1	21.1* ± 9.3	6.1** ± 1.2
(1.83 MAC; 35 min)	(30%)	(15%)	(20%)	(7%)

The data for halothane are taken from Göthert and Dreyer (1973). Means ± SEM are given.
* $p < 0.02$; ** $p < 0.005$.

In order to investigate whether the decrease in catecholamine output is due to an inhibition of the effect of acetylcholine released from splanchnic nerve endings, isolated bovine adrenal glands were perfused in a retrograde fashion with Locke solution at a rate of 2 ml/min. The concentrations of catecholamines in the perfusates were measured spectrofluoro-metrically (for details of the method used see Göthert, 1972; Göthert et al., 1974b). Figure 1 shows that acetylcholine added to the Locke solution evoked an increase in catecholamine secretion by about 200%. The basal release of catecholamines was not altered by enflurane; however, in the presence of the same enflurane concentration, the stimulating effect of acetylcholine was inhibited by 67.3% ($p < 0.01$) as compared to the control effect without anaesthetic. Similar results were obtained with halothane (2.7×10^{-4} g/ml) which decreased the effect of acetylcholine by 81% ($p < 0.001$).

It is concluded from the experiments in cats and in isolated bovine adrenals that the

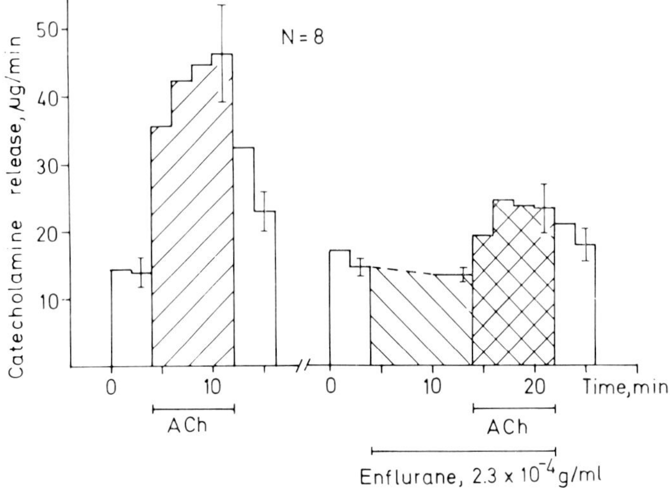

Fig. 1.   *Inhibitory effect of enflurane on the catecholamine secretion evoked by acetylcholine (ACh, 10^{-5} g/ml) from isolated bovine adrenal glands. 4 adrenals were first stimulated without enflurane and were again stimulated in the presence of enflurane after 32 min. In 4 adrenals the order was reversed.*

decrease in adrenal medullary catecholamine secretion observed during enflurane and halothane anaesthesia is due to the inhibition of the stimulating effect of acetylcholine released from splanchnic nerve endings. In addition to this mechanism, spontaneous catecholamine output may be decreased by central nervous inhibition of the sympatho-adrenal system which was observed for both enflurane (Millar et al., 1970; Skovsted and Price, 1972) and halothane (Millar et al., 1969, Skovsted et al., 1969). It can be supposed that the considerable decrease in catecholamine secretion contributes to the depressant effect of these anaesthetics on the blood pressure and to their negative inotropic and chronotropic effects.

In isolated rabbit hearts perfused at $33°$ C with a constant volume of Tyrode solution the effect of halothane and enflurane on the release of noradrenaline from postganglionic sympathetic nerves was studied. In hearts with an intact postganglionic sympathetic nerve supply (preparation according to Huković and Muscholl, 1962) halothane at concentrations of 7.5×10^{-5} and 2.24×10^{-4} g/ml did not alter the noradrenaline release in response to submaximal electrical stimulation of the nerves. Halothane (2.24×10^{-4} g/ml) and enflurane (2.28×10^{-4} g/ml) caused a significant decrease in noradrenaline output evoked by stimulation of nicotinic receptors in sympathetic nerve terminals by acetylcholine (3×10^{-5} g/ml; in the presence of atropine, 10^{-6} g/ml) or by nicotine (6.5×10^{-6} g/ml). Thus, inhalation anaesthetics cause a depression of the peripheral sympathetic nervous system at any site where nicotinic receptors are involved in stimulation, i.e. at sympathetic ganglia (Alper et al., 1969), at the chromaffin cells of the adrenal medulla and at sympathetic nerve terminals.

ACKNOWLEDGEMENT

The author is indebted to Mrs. G. Thielecke for skilful technical assistance and to the Deutsche Abbott (Ingelheim, Rhein) for the gift of Ethrane.

REFERENCES

Alper, M. H., Fleisch, J. H. and Flacke, W. (1969): *Anesthesiology, 31*, 429.
Brown, B. R. and Crout, J. R. (1971): *Anesthesiology, 34*, 236.
Dreyer, C., Bischoff, D. and Göthert, M. (1974): *Anesthesiology, 41*, 18.
Göthert, M. (1972): *Anaesthesiologie und Wiederbelebung, Vol. 70.* Springer Verlag, Berlin – Heidelberg – New York.
Göthert, M. and Dreyer, C. (1973): *Naunyn-Schmiedeberg's Arch. exp. Path. Pharmak., 277*, 253.
Göthert, M., Guth, M. and Bille, U. (1974a): *Naunyn-Schmiedeberg's Arch. exp. Path. Pharmak., 282*, R 26.
Göthert, M., Schmoldt, A. and Thielecke, G. (1974b): *Anaesthesist, 23*, 137.
Häggendal, J. (1963): *Acta physiol. scand., 59*, 242.
Huković, S. and Muscholl, E. (1962): *Naunyn-Schmiedeberg's Arch. exp. Path. Pharmak., 241*, 81.
Millar, R. A., Warden, J. C., Cooperman, L. H. and Price, H. L. (1969): *Brit. J. Anaesth., 41*, 918.
Millar, R. A., Warden, J. C., Cooperman, L. H. and Price, H. L. (1970): *Brit. J. Anaesth., 42*, 366.
Skovsted, P. and Price, H. L. (1972): *Anesthesiology, 36*, 257.
Skovsted, P., Price, M. L. and Price, H. L. (1969): *Anesthesiology, 31*, 507.

Chapter V

Advances in neuromuscular transmission and new blocking drugs

Affinity constant and neuromuscular block

STANLEY A. FELDMAN

Magill Department of Anaesthetics, Westminster Hospital, London, United Kingdom

Paton (1961) in his rate theory of action of drugs, proposed that a biological response would occur during the association of an agonist agent with a receptor site. The amount of activity produced by such a drug would coincide with its maximum concentration at the receptor site. The concentration of drug at the receptor site will be influenced by the rate at which the drug associates and dissociates with the receptor. The more rapid the dissociation, relative to the rate of association, the greater will be the 'turnover' of drug and the more active it will appear as a biological agonist.

Thus if association rate $= K_1$, dissociation rate $= K_2$

$$D + R \underset{K_2}{\overset{K_1}{\rightleftharpoons}} DR$$

$$\frac{K_1}{K_2} = \text{affinity constant } K_D \quad (D = \text{drug}; \ R = \text{receptor})$$

The lower the affinity constant K_D the more active the agonist.

Conversely, should a drug possess a high affinity constant with the rate of dissociation less rapid than that of association it will possess a weak agonist effect. Any agonist activity which will depend upon the intrinsic activity manifest in its initial reaction with the receptor (Ariens, 1954). Because of its high affinity constant, it will be released too slowly from the receptor to be available to produce a continuing biological effect.

It has been suggested (Feldman and Tyrrell, 1970) that a drug with a high affinity constant will act as an antagonist as it will actually occupy receptor sites until the moment of dissociation, rendering them unavailable to the normal biological transmitter. This theory suggests that only drugs with a high affinity constant are capable of acting as antagonist agents like curare. In order to be an effective agonist agent, like suxamethonium or C_{10}, it is necessary that the drug possesses both intrinsic activity and a low affinity constant.

This theory renders the concept of a dynamic competition theory, based on the Law of Mass Action, inappropriate to describe the antagonism of a drug with a high affinity constant, such as curare and a drug as protean in its action as acetylcholine. If the competition theory did correctly describe the relationship between curare-like drugs and acetylcholine, then the amount of drug activity (y) would be proportional to the concentration of drug at the receptor (C) relative to the concentration of acetylcholine (ACh):

$$y \propto \frac{(C)}{(ACh)}.$$

This does not accord with the observations using an isolated arm technique (Feldman, 1973). In this technique doses of antagonist drug (d-tubocurarine 3 mg, gallamine 8 mg,

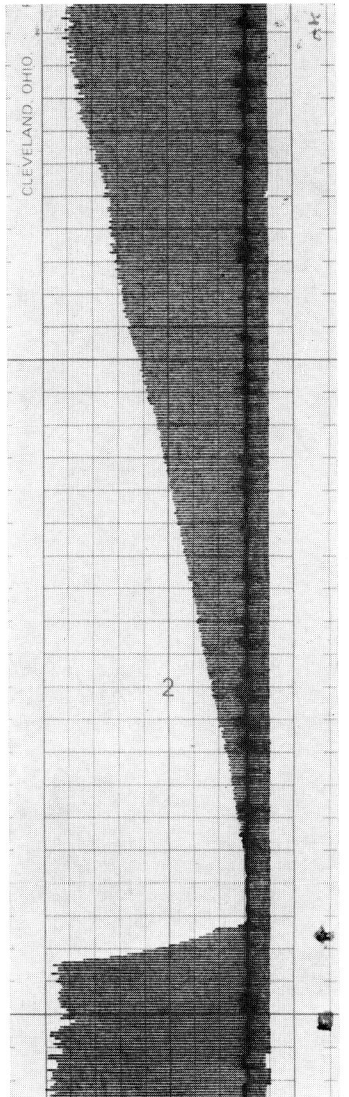

Fig. 1a. Slow recovery of neuromuscular transmission after plasma level of gallamine reduced to zero (↑). Recovery index 9.8 min. (Scale: 1 square = 1 min.)

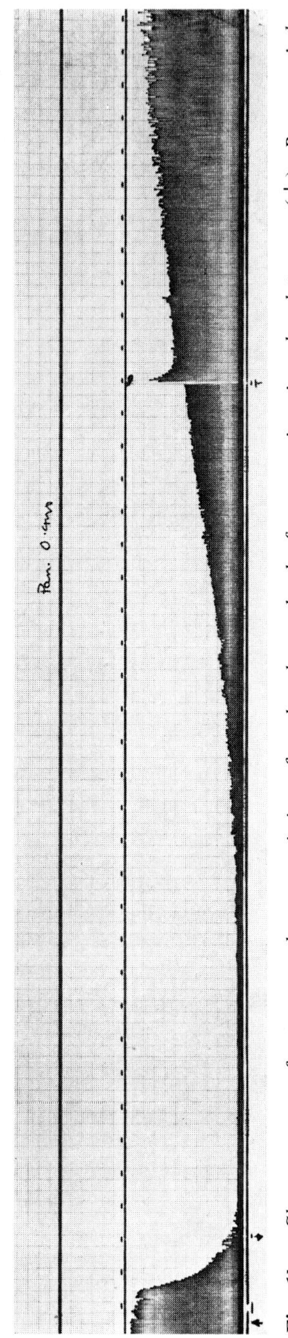

Fig. 1b. Slow recovery of neuromuscular transmission after the plasma level of pancuronium is reduced to zero (↓). Recovery index 12.5 min.

pancuronium 0.4 mg diluted in 30 ml saline) are injected into a vein on the back of the hand whilst the circulation to the limb is temporarily obstructed by a tourniquet. With this technique the drug passes passively from the distended veins, in a retrograde manner into the tissues, producing paralysis within 3 min. The cuff is then released. On release of the tourniquet the circulation to the arm is re-established and the concentration of drug in the arm falls to virtually zero. If the competition theory were an adequate explanation of the action of these drugs the neuromuscular block should be reversed as the drug is washed out of the biophase. Figure 1 (*a*, *b*) shows that duration of block is not greatly affected by reducing the plasma level of drug to virtually zero. This demonstrates the affinity of these drugs with the receptor sites. It can be seen that gallamine has a shorter duration of action (recovery index (Feldman, 1974) 9.8 min) than pancuronium (recovery index 12.5 min) probably because it has a lower affinity constant with the receptor.

With this technique it can be demonstrated that agonist drugs like C_{10} have a low affinity constant (Fig. 2). As soon as the blood level of C_{10} is reduced, by releasing the tourniquet, recovery follows the 'washout' from the biophase (recovery index 2.2 min).

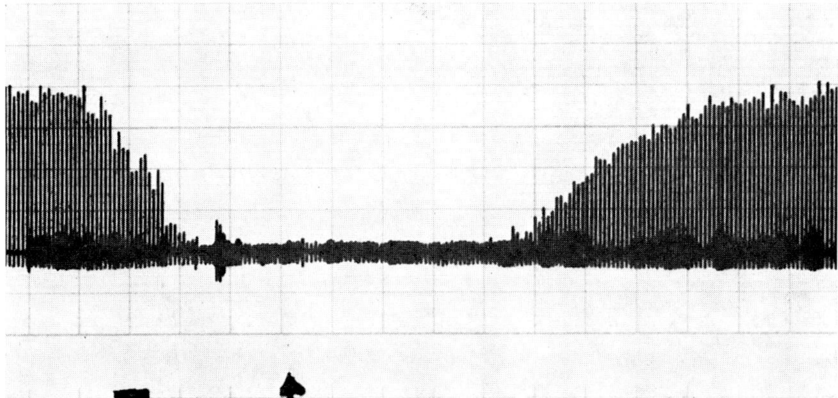

Fig. 2. *Rapid recovery of neuromuscular conduction after block by* C_{10} *when the drug concentration is reduced;* (↑) *tourniquet released.* (*Scale: 1 square = 1 min.*)

It is proposed that acetylcholine normally displaces the antagonist drug from the receptor site. During a normal anaesthetic the acetylcholine release is minimal, less if the patient is more deeply anaesthetised. If acetylcholine release is increased at the motor nerve endings, as by repeated tetanic discharge, then recovery will be accelerated. We have demonstrated this by observing the recovery of neuromuscular conduction in both arms of patients who had received d-tubocurarine and in whom one ulnar nerve was tetanized at 30 Hz every 1–2 min. It can be seen from Figure 3 that recovery in the tetanized arm is more rapid than in the control arm.

It is proposed that a depolarizing neuromuscular blocking agent is a drug with high intrinsic activity and low affinity constant. A non-depolarizing antagonist drug is one with high affinity constant for the receptor (Feldman, 1973). Factors that affect acetylcholine release will affect the recovery from neuromuscular block produced by non-depolarizing drugs.

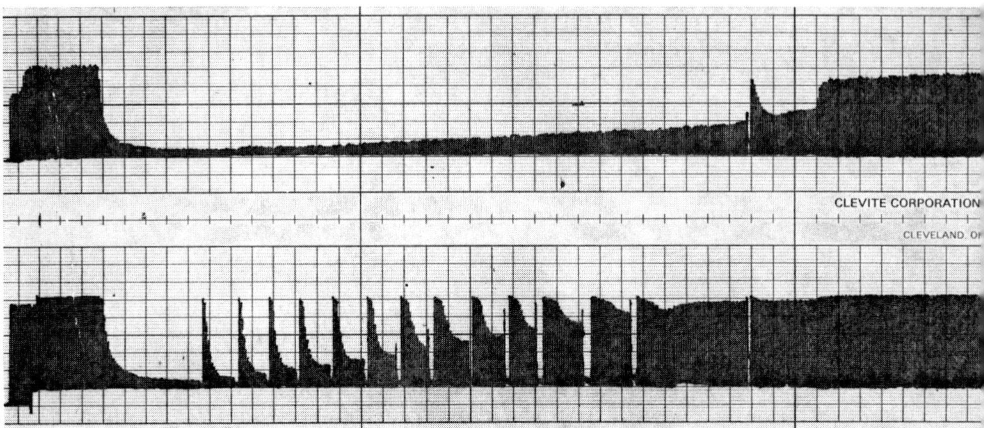

Fig. 3.   *The effect of repeated tetany at 30 Hz upon recovery from neuromuscular block by d-tubocurarine. Upper trace – stimulation 1/5 sec; lower trace – in addition to faradic stimulation, tetanic stimuli at 30 Hz (scale: 1 square = 1 min).*

REFERENCES

Ariens, E. J. (1954): *Arch. int. Pharmacodyn.*, *99*, 32.

Feldman, S. A. (1973): *Muscle Relaxants – Major Problems in Anaesthesia.* W. B. Saunders, Ltd., London.

Feldman, S. A. (1974): In: *Measurement of Neuromuscular Block – Measurement in Anaesthesia*, p. 43. Editors: Feldman, S. A., Leigh, J. M. and Spierdijk, J. University of Leiden Press, Leiden.

Feldman, S. A. and Tyrrell, M. F. (1970): *Proc. roy. Soc. Med.*, *63*, 692.

Paton, W.D.M. (1961): *Proc. roy. Soc. B*, *154*, 21.

Dual block with depolarizing relaxants*

ANIBAL GALINDO ** and ROSS D. KENNEDY

Department of Anesthesiology and Anesthesia Research Center,
University of Washington School of Medicine, Seattle, Wash., U.S.A.

Under some clinical circumstances the administration of succinylcholine (SCh) or deca-methonium (C 10) induces a neuromuscular depression with characteristics commonly observed during the administration of d-tubocurarine. This type of depression is associated with marked fatigue during tetanic stimulation followed by post-tetanic potentiation (PTP) of muscle contractions, and may occasionally be reversed by neostigmine. Since these characteristics are not seen during the initial administration of depolarizing agents in most patients, it has been postulated that the neuromuscular blockade has entered a different 'phase' or is acting in double manner – 'dual block'.

The above clinical observation has been readily compared to laboratory findings in which a constant concentration of decamethonium induces first a muscle paralysis which spontaneously recovers to later appear without further recovery (Jenden et al., 1954). The first muscle paralysis had been called 'phase I block' and the second 'phase II block'. Two types of blockade have also been described in different experiments in frog muscles, an initial depression of neuromuscular transmission apparently caused by depolarization and a secondary blockade caused by desensitization of the end-plate membrane to acetyl-choline (Katz and Thesleff, 1957).

Not surprisingly, results from these two different series of experiments were incorporated into a single explanation and extrapolated to clinical findings. Thus phase I was considered a 'depolarizing block' and phase II a 'desensitization block' or dual block (Churchill-Davidson and Katz, 1966). Unfortunately, this simple interpretation of clinical observations has not been proven and may be inaccurate.

In the first place not all 'depolarizing agents' are alike. Second, their mode of action greatly depends on the speed of administration (Galindo and Kennedy, 1974). And third, it is difficult to extrapolate to man observations made in vitro, especially from experiments in frog muscles at low temperatures.

Dual block, or phase II block, appears as a single event in old patients, states of malnutrition, deficient and/or abnormal pseudocholinesterase levels, and in patients with myasthenia gravis or myasthenic syndrome (Galindo, unpublished observations). It appears as a late type of neuromuscular depression following continuous administration of large doses of succinylcholine or decamethonium in normal patients. Actually, there is a period of tachyphylaxis between the initial paralysis induced by a bolus SCh or C 10 (e.g., doses for intubation) and the development of the persistent depression known as 'dual block' or phase II. However, one must be careful in identifying the sequence of neuromuscular

* Supported by USPHS Grant GM 15991-04 from the National Institute of General Medical Sciences, National Institutes of Health.
** *Also of:* Instituto Neurologico de Colombia, Bogota, Colombia.

depression observed clinically with in vitro experimental results. Moreover, the mode of action and the changing pattern of depression is different for SCh and C 10 (Galindo and Kennedy, 1974). The kinetics of drug penetration into synaptic structures and the muscle itself, notwithstanding the disposal of the drug and the anesthetic agent being administered to the patient, may account for this changing mode of action presently classified in two phases.

In describing the mode of action of depolarizing muscle relaxants, it must be understood that changes in the resting membrane potential at the end-plate should not be associated with their mechanism of action (Galindo, 1971, 1972) and that it is more accurate referring to a specific changing mode of action for each drug rather than to a fixed phasic response for 'depolarizing agents' in general.

REFERENCES

Churchill-Davidson, H. C. and Katz, R. L. (1966): *Anesthesiology*, *27*, 536.
Galindo, A. (1971): *J. Pharmacol. exp. Ther.*, *178*, 339.
Galindo, A. (1972): *Anesthesiology*, *36*, 598.
Galindo, A. and Kennedy, R. (1974): *Brit. J. Anaesth.*, *46*, 405.
Jenden, D. J., Kamijo, K. and Taylor, D. B. (1954): *J. Pharmacol. exp. Ther.*, *111*, 229.
Katz, B. and Thesleff, S. (1957): *J. Physiol. (Lond.)*, *138*, 63.

Factors affecting muscle relaxants.
I. Volatile anaesthetics

R. HUGHES

Pharmacology Laboratory, Wellcome Research Laboratories, Beckenham, Kent, United Kingdom

Volatile and other general anaesthetics relax voluntary muscle tone by depression of the central nervous system. In addition many synergise with skeletal muscle relaxants at neuromuscular junctions.

ETHER

The concentration of inhaled ether required for anaesthesia in cats, dogs and man approximates 3–15%, depending on the depth of anaesthesia required. Anaesthetic concentrations cause muscle relaxation by actions on the central nervous system. Depression of spinal reflexes has been demonstrated by Austin and Pask (1952) in cats. Higher concentrations are required to cause neuromuscular paralysis. For example, whereas only 6% ether was needed to abolish spinal, corneal and masseter reflexes in decerebrate and spinal cats, concentrations as high as 10–25% were required to significantly decrease the twitch response of the tibialis muscle to indirect stimulation (Ngai et al., 1965). Similarly, whereas inhalation of 5–9% ether relaxed the abdomen and markedly depressed electromyographic activity in cats and man, concentrations of even 15% only occasionally caused some reduction in neuromuscular transmission (Katz, 1966).

The mechanism of action of ether on neuromuscular transmission has been studied in isolated frog sciatic nerve – sartorius muscle preparations (Karis et al., 1966). Blockade by diethyl ether in contrast to that by non-depolarising muscle relaxants, was not effectively antagonised by edrophonium or suxamethonium. Ether reduced the amplitude and prolonged the time course of both the end-plate potentials and the miniature end-plate potentials and diminished the sensitivity of the muscle postjunctional membrane to the depolarising effect of acetylcholine and other quaternary ammonium compounds. It was postulated that the reduction in the sensitivity of the postjunctional membrane to acetylcholine caused by ether could become of importance when neuromuscular transmission is impaired by skeletal muscle relaxants (Karis et al., 1967).

Anaesthetic concentrations of ether potentiate neuromuscular blockade by tubocurarine and to a lesser extent by suxamethonium in animals and man (Gross and Cullen, 1943; Cullen, 1944; Watland et al., 1957; Katz, 1966). The interpretation of these interactions is discussed above.

HALOTHANE

Muscular relaxation during halothane anaesthesia is well known and it has been concluded that this results primarily from depression of the central nervous system. This conclusion is based on several studies in experimental animals and man. Inhalation of 0.4–1 % halothane abolished the spinal, corneal and masseter reflexes, whereas concentrations of 1–2% did not decrease the twitch response of the tibialis muscle in spinal and decerebrate cats (Ngai et al., 1965). Studies in man have shown that the tone and electromyographic activity of the abdominal muscles were reduced by 1–2% halothane without depression of the twitch responses of the thumb (Katz and Gissen, 1967). Similarly, impairment of twitch responses was not observed with 1–4.4% halothane (Burn et al., 1957; Watland et al., 1957; Katz and Gissen, 1967; Baraka, 1968). Neuromuscular transmission in isolated nerve muscle preparations is however blocked by high concentrations of halothane. This has been demonstrated with 4–8% halothane in human intercostal muscle (Sabawala and Dillon, 1958) and with 4% halothane in the frog sciatic nerve sartorius muscle preparation (Gissen et al., 1966). The effect in the frog preparation was ascribed to desensitisation of the post-junctional membrane to acetylcholine (Karis et al., 1967).

Studies in my laboratory have also shown that the effects of halothane on neuromuscular transmission are weak in cats. In the experiments reported here cats were lightly anaesthetised with chloralose, prepared as described previously and ventilated with oxygen using a Starling pump (Hughes, 1970). Chloralose has no peripheral action at anaesthetic doses according to Secher (1951). The inspired concentration of halothane was limited to approximately 0.5%, this being just less than that found to cause severe hypotension. The responses of the gastrocnemius muscle to indirect stimulation every 10 sec were not affected but the responses of the contralateral muscle to tetanic bursts of 30 Hz were slightly reduced in 9 of 17 experiments (mean reduction 8%, SE 4%) (Fig. 1). The inhibition of tetanic concentrations was not necessarily due to neuromuscular paralysis. It may be in part attributable to the associated hypotension and reduced muscle blood flow with halothane (Schweitzer, 1945; Lindgren et al., 1964).

Interactions between halothane and neuromuscular blocking agents are also known. There have been numerous reports that inhalation of 1–3 % halothane potentiates paralysis

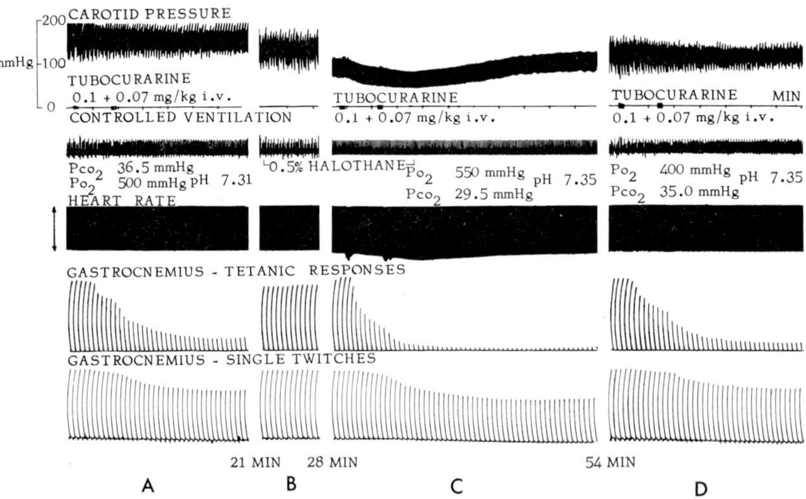

Fig. 1.   *Records from a cat 3.1 kg lightly anaesthetised with chloralose. (A) Control dose of tubocurarine, 0.17 mg/kg i.v. depressed the tetanic contractions of the gastrocnemius muscle stimulated at 30 Hz every 10 sec and partially reduced the single twitches of the contralateral muscle; (B) ventilation with ca 0.5% halothane lowered blood pressure; (C) paralysis by tubocurarine, 0.17 mg/kg i.v. was increased during treatment with halothane; marked hypotension and bradycardia occurred; (D) further control dose of tubocurarine, 0.17 mg/kg i.v. Intervals of 60 min were allowed between doses.*

by tubocurarine, gallamine and pancuronium but not suxamethonium in man (Burns et al., 1957; Katz and Gissen, 1967; Baraka, 1968; Katz, 1971; Miller et al., 1971a, b; 1972) and in cats (Burn et al., 1957). Results of comparable studies using groups of 4 cats anaesthetised with chloralose are presented in Table 1. Ventilation with halothane significantly intensified blockade of the twitch and tetanic responses by tubocurarine (Fig. 2) and delayed recovery (Fig. 3) in comparison with control tests carried out before and after exposure to halothane. In similar experiments with gallamine paralysis of the twitch and tetanic responses tended to be intensified and prolonged (Fig. 3) by halothane, but not significantly. The paralysing action of suxamethonium during ventilation with halothane was virtually unaltered (Figs. 2 and 3).

Table 1. *Effects of halothane: Mean values in groups of 4 cats*

Drug standard dose i.v. (mg/kg)	Procedure	Blood pressure (mm Hg)	Single shock stimulation		Tetanic stimulation, sustained response	
			Paralysis (%)	Recovery time (min)	Paralysis (%)	Recovery time (min)
Tubocurarine	Pre-control	139**	28*	18**	94**	47*
0.15	0.5% halothane	74	51	37	100	78
	Post-control	124**	27**	19**	94*	54
Gallamine	Pre-control	150	20	10	94	33
0.62	0.5% halothane	101	33	15	98	44
	Post-control	145	18	9	93	28
Suxamethonium	Pre-control	121**	40	7.5	93	9
0.04	0.5% halothane	60	46	8	96	12
	Post-control	111*	43	7.5	94	9

Effects in cats, lightly anaesthetised with chloralose, of ventilation with 0.5% halothane on arterial blood pressure and on neuromuscular paralysis by tubocurarine, gallamine and suxamethonium. Paralysis was determined on both gastrocnemius muscles stimulated indirectly every 10 sec, one with single shocks and the other with tetanic shocks at 30 Hz. Mean values for groups of 4 cats are shown for before (pre-control), during, and after (post-control) the treatment period. Asterisks denote differences between control and treatment values significant at the 5% (*) and 1% (**) levels respectively.

Statistical examination of the results revealed a significant negative correlation between the mean arterial blood pressure at the time of administration of the neuromuscular blocking agents and the ensuing intensity and duration of paralysis. A lower arterial blood pressure and presumably a reduced blood flow during exposure to halothane was associated with a more intense and prolonged paralysis.

Halothane also increased the hypotensive action of tubocurarine (Fig. 1). In contrast, gallamine and, at high doses, pancuronium, because of their vagolytic properties may oppose the bradycardia and hypotension produced by halothane. Some anaesthetists consider that the combination of halothane with tubocurarine to produce controllable hypotension and bradycardia may be desirable but that in other clinical situations it may be advantageous to avoid such effects by using halothane with gallamine or pancuronium.

METHOXYFLURANE

Methoxyflurane in anaesthetic concentrations abolishes the electrical activity of the ab-

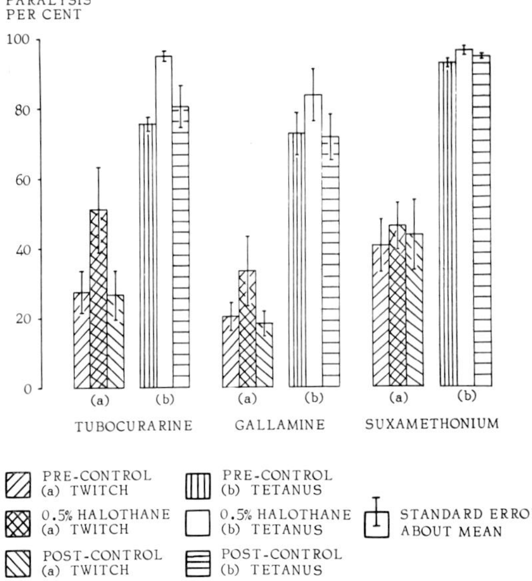

Fig. 2.   *Effects of ventilation with ca 0.5% halothane on the intensity of neuromuscular paralysis in groups of 4 cats lightly anaesthetised with chloralose: (a) The twitch responses of the gastrocnemius muscle to single shocks every 10 sec; and (b) the tetanic responses of the contralateral muscle stimulated indirectly at 30 Hz every 10 sec. Percentage paralysis for controls and treatments were taken from Table 1.*

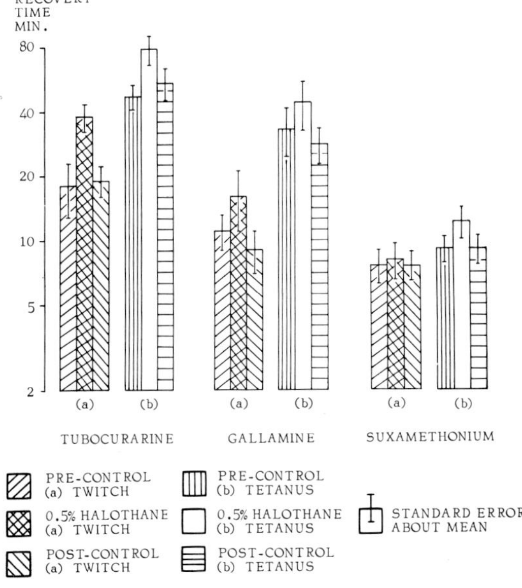

Fig. 3.   *Effects of ventilation with ca 0.5% halothane on recovery from neuromuscular paralysis in cats lightly anaesthetised with chloralose: (a) The twitch responses of one gastrocnemius muscle to single shocks every 10 sec; and (b) the tetanic responses of the contralateral muscle stimulated indirectly at 30 Hz every 10 sec. Recovery times for controls and treatments were taken from Table 1.*

dominal muscles without affecting the twitch responses of the hypothenar muscles to electrical stimulation of the ulnar nerve (Ngai and Hanks, 1962). In decerebrate and spinal cats, inhalation of 4% methoxyflurane did not significantly reduce the tibialis twitch response to peroneal nerve stimulation but 0.2–0.5% abolished the reflex contraction of the quadriceps femoris to central stimulation of the ligated sciatic nerve (Ngai et al., 1965). This concentration was less than that required for surgical anaesthesia (0.5–1.5%). It was concluded that methoxyflurane also produces muscular relaxation principally through its depressant action on the spinal cord.

TRICHLOROFLUOROMETHANE (FORANE)

Clinical investigations of trichlorofluoromethane have shown that, although the twitch responses of the thumb were unaffected by anaesthetic concentrations, the ability to sustain a tetanus was reduced (Miller et al., 1971*a*). Neuromuscular blockade by tubocurarine, gallamine and pancuronium was increased to a greater extent than by halothane (Miller et al., 1971 *a, b*). Further studies, (Miller et al., 1972) showed that the intensity of paralysis by tubocurarine or pancuronium was directly related to the alveolar concentration of trichlorofluoromethane or halothane. Miller and his colleagues (1971*b*) also found that only about two thirds of the dose of suxamethonium was required for neuromuscular paralysis during anaesthesia with trichlorofluoromethane than with halothane. The reason for this difference is uncertain but the authors pointed out that both trichlorofluoromethane and diethyl ether increased muscle blood flow and that both potentiate paralysis by suxamethonium.

REFERENCES

Austin, G. M. and Pask, E. A. (1952): *J. Physiol. (Lond.), 118*, 405.
Baraka, A. (1968): *Brit. J. Anaesth., 40*, 602.
Burn, J. H., Epstein, H. G., Feigan, G. A. and Paton, W. D. M. (1957): *Brit. med. J., 2*, 479.
Burns, T. H. S., Mushin, W. W., Organe, G. S. W. and Robertson, J. D. (1957): *Brit. med. J., 2*, 483.
Cullen, S. C. (1944): *Anesthesiology, 5*, 166.
Gissen, A. J., Karis, J. H. and Nastuk, W. L. (1966): *J. Amer. med. Ass., 197*, 770.
Gross, E. G. and Cullen, S. C. (1943): *J. Pharmacol. exp. Ther., 78*, 358.
Hughes, R. (1970): *Brit. J. Anaesth., 42*, 826.
Karis, J. H., Gissen, A. J. and Nastuk, W. L. (1966): *Anesthesiology, 27*, 42.
Karis, J. H., Gissen, A. J. and Nastuk, W. L. (1967): *Anesthesiology, 28*, 128.
Katz, R. L. (1966): *Anesthesiology, 27*, 52.
Katz, R. L. (1971): *Anesthesiology, 35*, 602.
Katz, R. L. and Gissen, A. J. (1967): *Anesthesiology, 28*, 564.
Lindgren, P., Westermark, L. and Wåhlin, Å. (1964): *Acta anaesth. scand., 9*, 83.
Miller, R. D., Eger Jr., E. I., Way, W. L., Stevens, W. C. and Dolan, W. M. (1971*a*): *Anesthesiology, 35*, 38.
Miller, R. D., Way, W. L., Dolan, W. M., Stevens, W. C. and Eger Jr., E. I. (1971*b*): *Anesthesiology, 35*, 509.
Miller, R. D., Way, W. L., Dolan, W. M., Stevens, W. C. and Eger Jr., E. I. (1972): *Anesthesiology, 37*, 573.
Ngai, S. H. and Hanks, E. C. (1962): *Anesthesiology, 23*, 158.
Ngai, S. H., Hanks, E. C. and Farhie, S. E. (1965): *Anesthesiology, 26*, 162.
Sabawala, P. B. and Dillon, J. B. (1958): *Anesthesiology, 19*, 587.
Secher, O. (1951): *Acta pharmacol. (Kbh.), 7*, 231.
Schweitzer, A. (1945): *J. Physiol. (Lond.), 104*, 21.
Watland, D. C., Long, J. P., Pittinger, C. B. and Cullen, C. S. (1957): *Anesthesiology, 18*, 883.

Protein binding

J. STOVNER

Rikshospitalet, Oslo, Norway

The neuromuscular blocking agents are water-soluble and highly ionized substances with strong electrostatic charges on the quaternary N groups. This makes them lipid-insoluble so they do not generally penetrate cell membranes or the blood-brain barrier during the course of an ordinary clinical anaesthetic. From this it follows that the relaxants are distributed in the extracellular fluid space. To achieve a standardized effect they should therefore be given, not as a dose/kg body weight or as a dose/m² body surface, but rather as a dose/litre extracellular fluid. An intravenous dose to an adult would be expected to be redistributed from the 3 l of plasma to the 15 l of extracellular fluid with a rapid fall of the peak plasma level to one fifth of the total dose injected. Studies using ^{3}H-labelled curare have shown that the plasma level falls well below this anticipated 20% in 5 min. As it is unlikely that any significant amount of drug is metabolized or excreted during this short time, we are forced to conclude that a certain amount of drug is lost through binding to proteins and there is now good evidence that the plasma proteins represent such unspecific receptor sites for the muscle relaxants. Exact figures for the amount of relaxants that are bound by the various fractions of plasma proteins are not available. It would be expected, however, that if the concentration of a certain plasma protein fraction rises, more drug bound to this fraction would be required to cause a certain degree of block. It now seems that this simple working hypothesis cannot be sustained, although it has formed the basis of a number of observations and investigations which are briefly summarized in the following section.

More than 20 years ago Dundee and Gray (1953) observed that patients with liver disease required greater than average doses of tubocurarine. This finding was confirmed 10 years later in patients with bilharzial cirrhosis by El-Hakim and Baraka (1963). Furthermore, it was suggested that such patients had high γ-globulin levels and a binding to this fraction could be the explanation. Since then a positive correlation between the γ-globulin concentration and the requirement of tubocurarine in series of patients has been demonstrated by 4 different studies in 4 different countries (Stout, 1963; Baraka and Gabali, 1968; Stovner et al., 1971*a*; Shanks and Penny, 1972). Figure 1 shows the scatter diagram obtained for 50 gynaecological laparotomies performed with a standard technique. The anaesthetics were all performed by the author who also determined the requirement of tubocurarine. A pathologist took the blood samples and determined the plasma protein fractions and a statistician calculated the correlations which were significant at a 5% level. Our finding was supported by the result of Aladjemoff et al. (1958) who had shown that, in vitro, tubocurarine moves with the γ-globulins during electrophoresis. Other workers, however, have shown that tubocurarine in vitro is bound to an equal extent by the other plasma protein fractions (Cohen et al., 1965). Increased binding does not occur in vitro with plasma from patients with high γ-globulin levels (Ghoneim et al., 1973). These facts have raised the alternative possibility that perhaps the γ-globulin levels are secondary to some other factors. Attention has recently been focussed on the ability of the liver cells to trap and excrete tubocurarine and pancuronium. Hypergammaglobulinaemia is usually associated with an enlarged liver or altered hepatic metabolism and the following factors may influence the requirement of tubocurarine: (1) The liver cells may sequestrate an increased quantity of tubocurarine. (2) Arteriovenous shunting may occur with a resulting high output state and increased plasma and extracellular fluid volume (Feldman, 1973). The first factor would affect those relaxants that can be excreted by the liver cells and therefore enter these cells during the time of an ordinary anaesthetic. Such is the case with tubocurarine and pancuronium in contrast to gallamine and alcuronium. Pancuronium has recently been shown to be sequestrated in appreciable amounts by the liver (Agoston et al., 1973). This explains the increased requirements of pancuronium in patients with liver disease reported by Nana et al. (1972). The second factor would be expected to increase the requirements of all relaxants because the distribution volume is increased. As increased

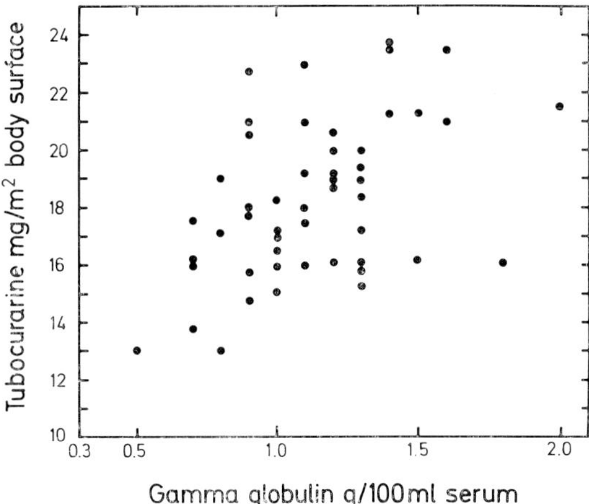

Fig. 1. *Scatter diagram showing correlation between tubocurarine (mg/m² body surface) and the serum level of γ-globulin (g/100 ml) (r = 0.48). Fifty women undergoing radical hysterectomies.*

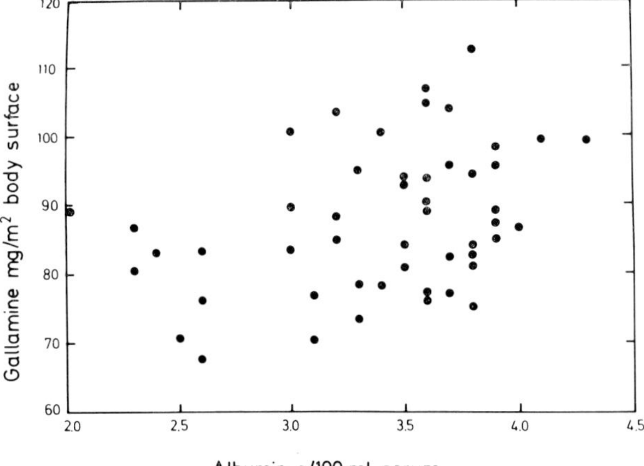

Fig. 2. *Scatter diagram showing correlation between gallamine (mg/m² body surface) and the serum level of albumin (g/100 ml) (r = 0.34). Fifty women undergoing radical hysterectomies.*

resistance has only been found for tubocurarine and pancuronium in liver disease, it appears that both factors must be involved for such resistance to be detected clinically.

The requirements of gallamine and alcuronium were found in our studies to be correlated to the albumin level in plasma (Stovner et al., 1971*a, b*). Figure 2 shows the scatter diagram for gallamine and plasma albumin level. The correlation is just significant at the 5% level.

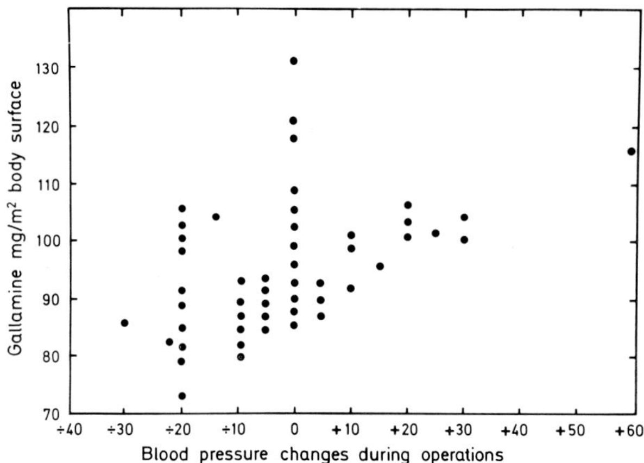

Fig. 3.   *Scatter diagram showing correlation between gallamine (mg/m² body surface) and blood pressure changes during operation (r=0.40). Fifty women undergoing radical hysterectomies.*

The result does not agree with reported findings in vitro by Skivington (1972) who has shown that gallamine is bound to the globulins. On going through the anaesthetic records, I noticed that the patients with low albumin levels frequently sustained blood pressure falls during the operation probably due to hypovolaemia. When we correlated the blood pressure changes during the observation period with the gallamine requirements for the same period we obtained a linear association which is shown on a scatter diagram in Figure 3. The linear association between these two variables appeared to be just as strong as between gallamine and albumin. It appears that the primary factor is a tendency to blood pressure fall in response to anaesthesia and surgery in patients with low albumin levels. The reduced perfusion of the skeletal muscles prolongs the action of the relaxants. This finding has taught me that I should not believe everything I read in the *British Journal of Anaesthesia* even when I have written it myself!

REFERENCES

Agoston, S., Kersten, U. W. and Meijer, D. K. F. (1973): *Acta anaesth. scand., 17*, 129.
Aladjemoff, L., Dickstein, S. and Shafrir, E. (1958): *J. Pharmacol. exp. Ther., 123*, 43.
Baraka, A. and Gabali, F. (1968): *Brit. J. Anaesth., 40*, 89.
Cohen, E. N., Corbascio, A. and Fleischli, G. (1965): *J. Pharmacol. exp. Ther., 147*, 120.
Dundee, J. W. and Gray, T. C. (1953): *Lancet, 2*, 16.
El-Hakim, M. and Baraka, A. (1963): *Kasr-El-Aini J. Surg., 4*, 99.
Feldman, S. A. (1973): *Muscle Relaxants*, p. 132. W. B. Saunders Co. Ltd., London.
Ghoneim, M. M., Kramer, S. E., Bannow, R., Pandya, R. and Routh, J. J. (1973): *Anesthesiology, 39*, 410.
Nana, A., Cardan, E. and Leitersdorfer, T. (1972): *Anaesthesia, 27*, 154.
Shanks, C. A. and Penny, R. (1972): *Anaesth. Intensive Care, 1*, 62.
Skivington, M. A. (1972): *Brit. J. Anaesth., 44*, 1030.
Stout, R. J. (1963): *W. Indian med. J., 12*, 256.
Stovner, J., Theodorsen, L. and Bjelke, E. (1971*a*): *Brit. J. Anaesth., 43*, 385.
Stovner, J., Theodorsen, L. and Bjelke, E. (1971*b*): *Brit. J. Anaesth., 43*, 953.

Blood flow and muscle relaxants

STANLEY A. FELDMAN

Magill Department of Anaesthetics, Westminster Hospital, London, United Kingdom

Considering the great differences in cardiac output and regional blood flow that occur in patients presenting for anaesthesia and the changes that may be induced by anaesthesia itself, it is remarkable how little we know about the effects of alterations in flow upon the action of the muscle relaxants. Indeed, as Hughes (1970) and Stovner (*This Volume*, p. 238) have pointed out, some of the findings they have recorded when studying the relationship between the activity of the muscle relaxants and one or other physiological change, may have been in part due to concomitant changes in blood flow. We wished to study the effect of alterations in temperature upon neuromuscular conduction in the intact animal and realized that it would first be necessary to exclude the effects of possible changes in blood flow that may result from cooling a muscle. As a result we made a preliminary investigation into the effects of alteration in flow at normal temperature and with a controlled environment.

If one accepts that a non-depolarizing muscle relaxant is a drug with high affinity constant then it is possible to predict that as the recovery of neuromuscular transmission is independent of the plasma concentration, it should not be greatly affected by changes in blood flow. However, the activity of depolarizing drugs parallels the plasma concentration and therefore, increasing the blood flow to a muscle paralysed by means of one of these agents should increase the washout and hence promote a more rapid recovery. Churchill-Davidson and Richardson (1952) elegantly demonstrated that increasing the blood flow through one

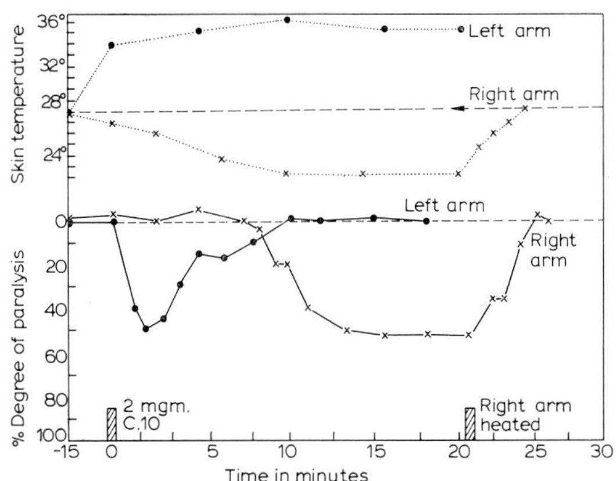

Fig. 1(a). *Effect of blood flow upon recovery from C 10; blood flow increased by warming arm. (From Churchill-Davidson and Richardson, 1952, by courtesy of the Editor, Proceedings of the Royal Society of Medicine).*

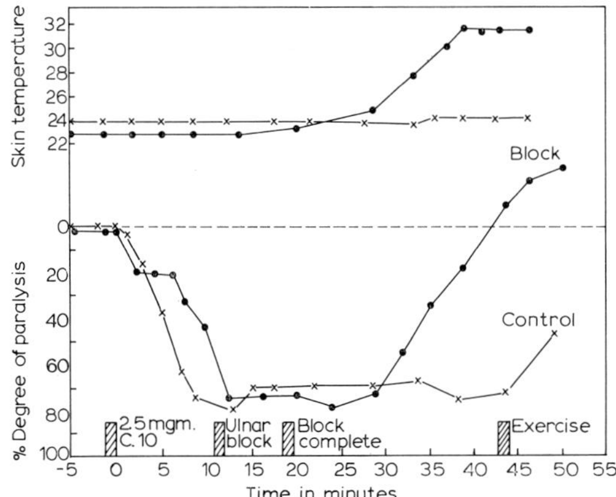

Fig. 1(b). *Effect of increased blood flow upon recovery from C 10; blood flow increased by ulnar block. (From Churchill-Davidson and Richardson, 1952, by courtesy of the Editor, Proceedings of the Royal Society of Medicine.)*

arm, either by warming the arm, or by ulnar nerve block, increased the rate of recovery from the paretic effect of a small dose of decamethonium (Fig. 1*a*, *b*).

In order to study the effect of alteration in blood flow on the recovery from non-depolarizing agents in dogs we have used an extracorporeal circuit from the carotid artery to the femoral artery, incorporating a roller pump, so that the precise blood flow to the hind limb could be controlled (Goat, 1974). It was found that the recovery index (time taken for recovery of twitch height from 25–75%) for the muscle paralysis induced with gallamine, was unaffected (Fig. 2).

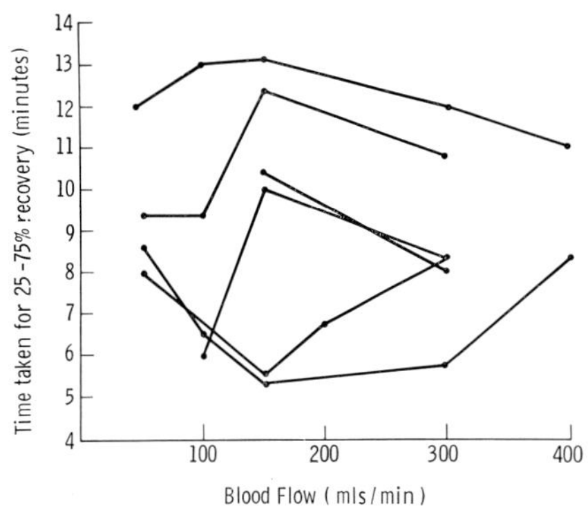

Fig. 2. *Effect of alteration in blood flow upon recovery from gallamine neuromuscular block. (From Goat, 1974).*

The next problem was to study the effect of blood flow on the distribution of the drug in the hind limb. If a drug is given slowly then it is usual to require a greater quantity of drug to produce the desired effect. If, however, it is given rapidly as a 'bolus', a smaller dose is effective. As the muscle relaxants, as used in Europe, are in small volumes, they are always given rapidly; however, if the circulation is slow, then the resulting effect on the distribution of the drug will be similar to giving the drug slowly into a rapid circulation. This was borne out by our results (Fig. 3).

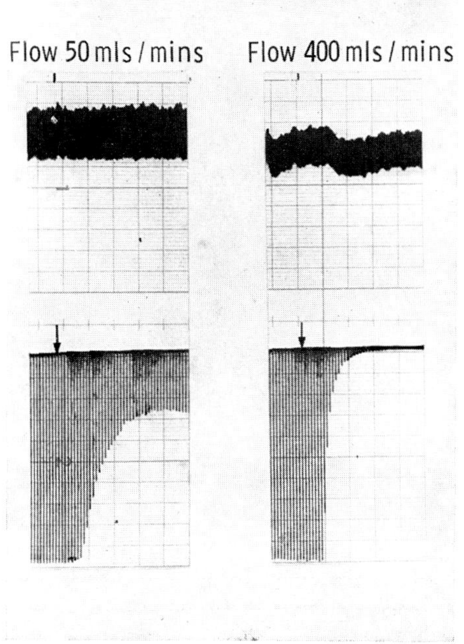

Fig. 3.   *Effect of alteration in blood flow to hind limb of dog, from 50 ml/min to 400 ml/min, upon rate of onset and amount of paralysis produced by a given dose of gallamine. (Upper section: B.P.; lower section: anterior tibialis muscle twitch).*

The clinical implication of this finding is important. It explains the commonly observed phenomena that old patients and patients with a low cardiac output state, frequently require a much larger dose of muscle relaxant than would be anticipated on the basis of their lean body weight and physical condition; it also illustrates the futility of using repeated injections of minute doses of non-depolarizing relaxants in these ill patients.

REFERENCES

Churchill-Davidson, H. C. and Richardson, A. T. (1952): *Proc. roy. Soc. Med.*, *45*, 179.
Goat, V. A. (1974): In: *Abstracts, IV European Congress of Anaesthesiology, Madrid, 1974*, p. 124, Editors: A. Arias, R. Llaurado, M. A. Nalda and J. N. Lunn. Excerpta Medica, Amsterdam.
Hughes, R. (1970): *Brit. J. Anaesth.*, *42*, 658.

Pharmacological concepts

R. HUGHES and D. J. CHAPPLE

Pharmacology Laboratory, Wellcome Research Laboratories, Beckenham, United Kingdom

Neuromuscular blocking agents can be divided into depolarizing and non-depolarizing, the distinction reflecting differences in the nature of their competition with the acetylcholine released at the muscle end-plate. Depolarizing agents include decamethonium and suxamethonium. The latter is popular because of the brevity of its effect due to its rapid hydrolysis by plasma cholinesterase, but as a result of its depolarizing action, it can cause post-operative muscle pains and cramps. Non-depolarizing drugs include tubocurarine (now known to be a monoquaternary salt), dimethyltubocurarine, gallamine, pancuronium and 1,1′-azobis-[3-methyl-2-phenyl-1H-imidazo (1,2-a) pyridinium] dibromide (AH 8165). None approaches suxamethonium in brevity of effect though their time courses do differ sufficiently to affect their relative merits in different clinical situations.

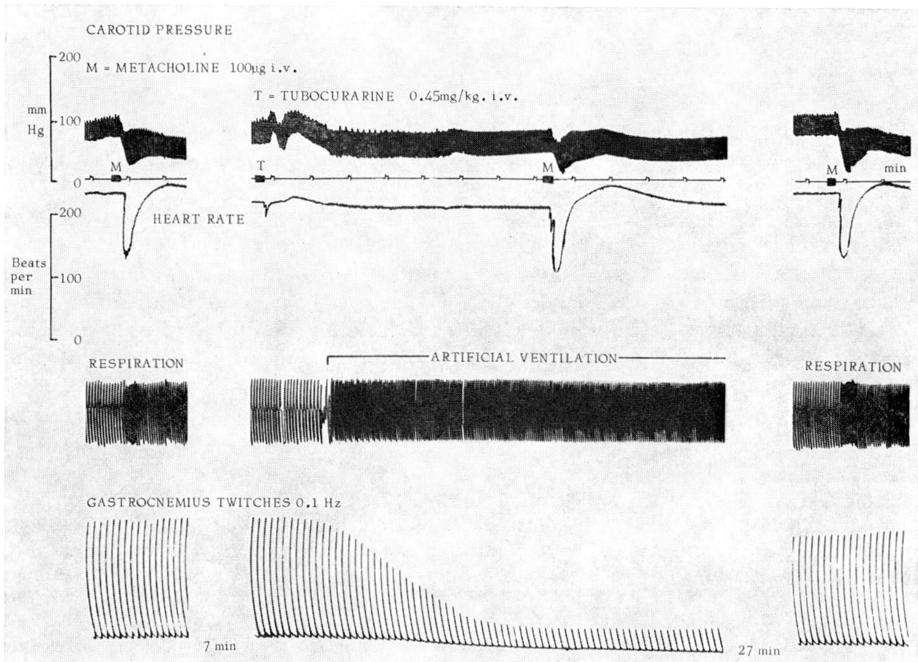

Fig. 1. *Record from a cat, 3.5 kg; chloralose anaesthesia. An intravenous dose of 0.45 mg/kg tubocurarine reduced carotid blood pressure and heart rate, arrested breathing and greatly diminished the twitches of the gastrocnemius muscle to indirect stimulation. The bradycardia induced by 100 μg methacholine i.v. was unimpaired.*

Another factor influencing clinical usefulness depends on the degree of separation between their neuromuscular effects and their inhibitory actions on autonomic mechanisms. A comparison has therefore been made, using cats under chloralose anaesthesia, of the relative doses of each of several muscle relaxants for inhibition of (*a*) responses of the gastrocnemius muscle to indirect stimulation, and (*b*) autonomic nerve function.

METHODS

Cats were anaesthetized with chloralose (60–80 mg/kg i.v.) and the trachea and left carotid artery were cannulated for recording respiration and blood pressure and the jugular vein for the administration of drugs. The sciatic nerve was stimulated supramaximally at 0.1 Hz and the contractions of the gastrocnemius muscle recorded. Effects on autonomic mechanisms were investigated in the same animal by measuring the bradycardia caused by stimulating the peripheral stump of the cut right cervical vagus periodically for 10 sec at 10–20 Hz and by recording contractions of the nictitating membrane caused by stimulating the cranial end of the cut right preganglionic cervical sympathetic nerve periodically for 60 sec at 10–20 Hz. In each case supramaximal voltage was applied. Body temperature was maintained at 36–37° C.

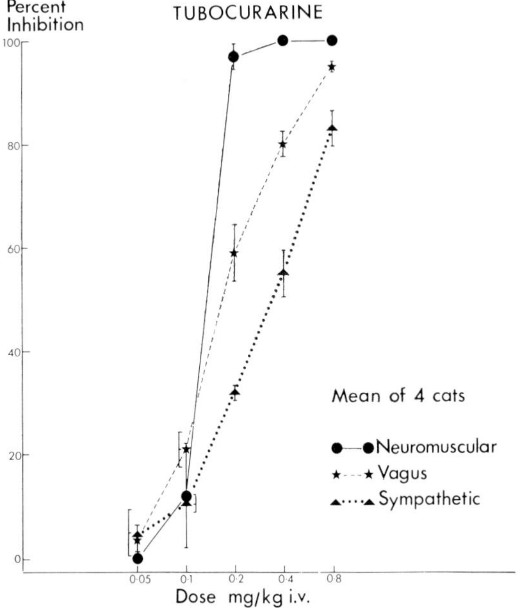

Fig. 2. *Dose-response relationships for tubocurarine given intravenously to cats anaesthetized with chloralose: (●——●) Percentage inhibition of the twitch response of the gastrocnemius muscle to indirect stimulation at 0.1 Hz. (★---★) Percentage inhibition of the bradycardia response to vagal stimulation at 10–20 Hz per 10 sec. (▲···▲) Percentage inhibition of the response of the nictitating membrane to sympathetic nerve stimulation at 10–20 Hz for 60 sec. Vertical lines indicate standard errors. Neuromuscular paralysis of the gastrocnemius muscle was accompanied by impairment of the vagal-induced bradycardia and of the contractions of the nictitating membrane caused by sympathetic nerve stimulation.*

RESULTS

Tubocurarine

Neuromuscular paralyzing doses reduced the vagal-induced bradycardia and the contraction of the nictitating membrane caused by sympathetic nerve stimulation. Arterial blood pressure and heart rate were slightly reduced. The vagal blockade was directed at the parasympathetic ganglion because the bradycardia induced by methacholine was unimpaired during neuromuscular paralysis by tubocurarine (Fig. 1). The dose-response relationships show concomitant vagal and sympathetic blockade at neuromuscular paralyzing doses (Fig. 2).

Dimethyltubocurarine

Changes in arterial blood pressure, heart rate and the responses to vagal and sympathetic nerve stimulation were minimal during neuromuscular paralysis by dimethyltubocurarine. The bradycardia response induced by methacholine was also maintained which confirmed the absence of atropinic effects on the cardiac vagus. The dose-response relationships show the selective action of dimethyltubocurarine at the neuromuscular junction as vagal and sympathetic function was unimpaired (Fig. 3).

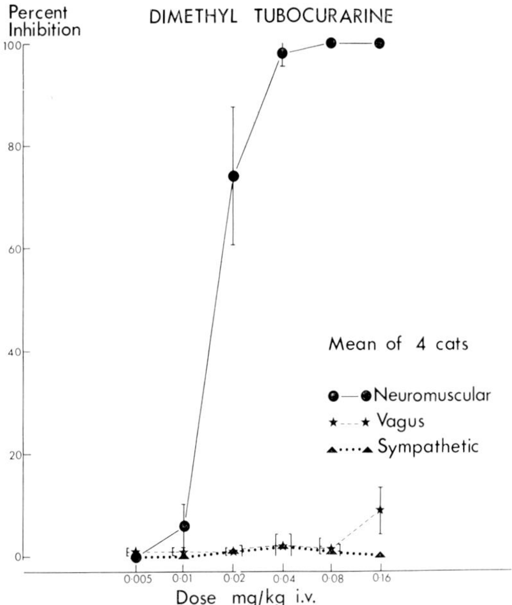

Fig. 3.   *Dose-response relationships for dimethyltubocurarine given intravenously to cats anaesthetized with chloralose. (For other details see legend, Figure 2). Impairment of the vagal-induced bradycardia and of the contractions of the nictitating membrane, caused by sympathetic nerve stimulation, was minimal at the neuromuscular paralyzing doses employed.*

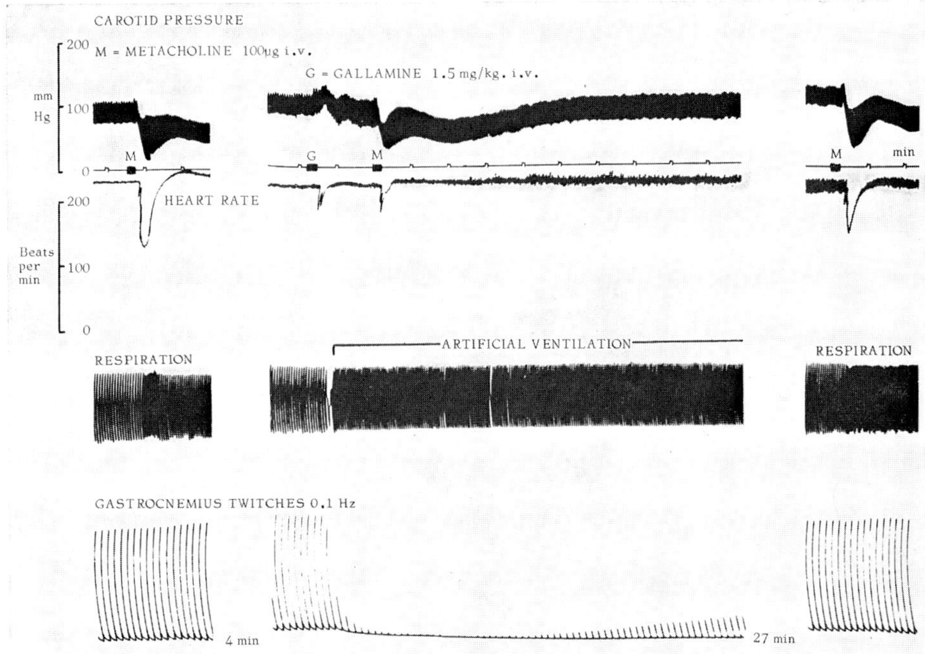

Fig. 4. *Record from a cat, 3.5 kg; chloralose anaesthesia. An intravenous dose of 1.5 mg/kg gallamine transiently increased carotid blood pressure; heart rate was unchanged. Breathing was arrested and the twitches of the gastrocnemius muscle to indirect stimulation and the bradycardia induced by 100 µg methacholine i.v. were abolished.*

Gallamine

The known vagolytic effect by neuromuscular paralyzing doses of gallamine and the absence of sympathetic blockade were demonstrated; increases in blood pressure and heart rate were small. The vagal block was directed at the parasympathetic nerve endings in the heart (i.e. atropinic) because the bradycardia induced by methacholine was abolished (Fig. 4). The dose-response relationships show that the atropinic action occurred at doses below those required to cause neuromuscular paralysis (Fig. 5). Sympathetic impairment was minimal even at doses more than sufficient to cause complete neuromuscular paralysis.

Pancuronium

Neuromuscular paralysis by pancuronium was accompanied by vagal blockade but no disturbance of arterial blood pressure, heart rate or sympathetic mechanisms occurred. The vagolytic effect was atropinic, the bradycardia induced by methacholine being suppressed. The dose-response relationships confirmed that the vagal blockade was appreciable at doses sufficient to cause complete paralysis whereas sympathetic impairment was minimal (Fig. 6).

AH 8165

Neuromuscular paralyzing doses of AH 8165 caused some hypotension and slight brady-cardia. Sympathetic blockade was only evident with high dosage but a powerful atropinic effect occurred at doses below those producing neuromuscular paralysis (Fig. 7).

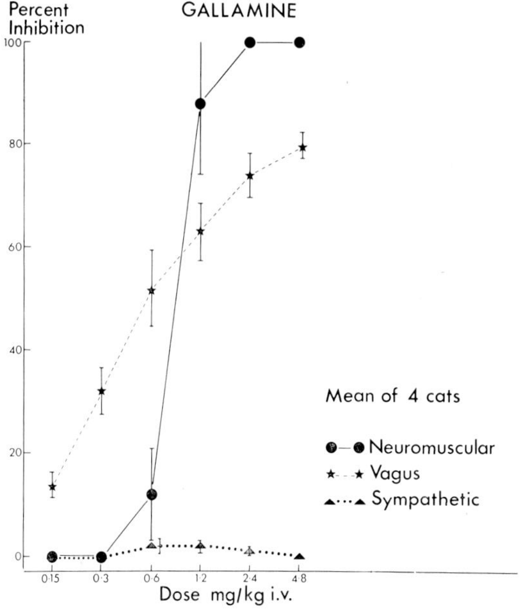

Fig. 5.   *Dose-response relationships for gallamine given intravenously to cats anaesthetized with chloralose. (For other details see legend, Figure 2). Neuromuscular paralysis was accompanied by impairment of the vagal-induced bradycardia. Effects on the contractions of the nictitating membrane, caused by sympathetic nerve stimulation, were minimal at the doses employed.*

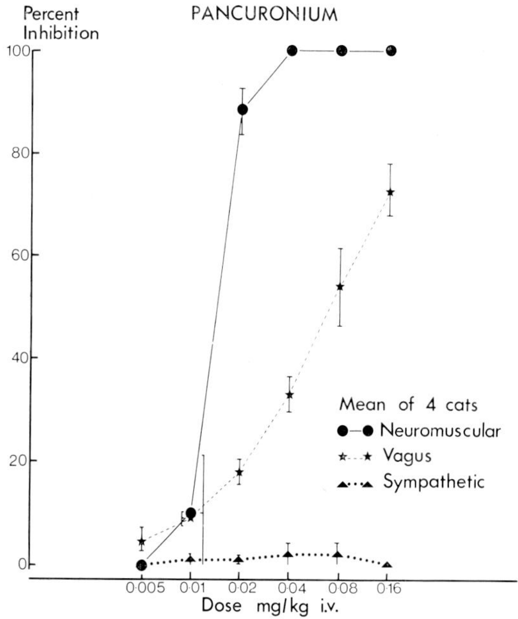

Fig. 6.   *Dose-response relationships for pancuronium given intravenously to cats anaesthetized with chloralose. (For other details see legend, Figure 2). Neuromuscular paralysis was accompanied by some impairment of the vagal-induced bradycardia. Effects on the contractions of the nictitating membrane, caused by sympathetic nerve stimulation, were minimal at the doses employed.*

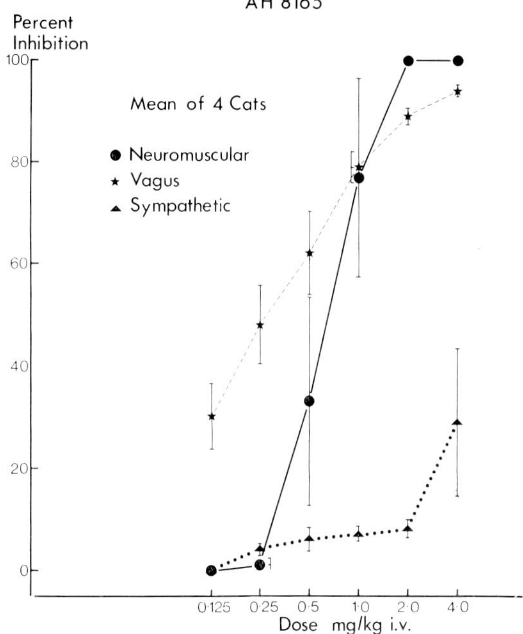

Fig. 7. *Dose-response relationships for AH 8165 given intravenously to cats anaesthetized with chloralose. (For other details see legend, Figure 2). Neuromuscular paralysis was accompanied by impairment of the vagal-induced bradycardia. Effects on the contractions of the nictitating membrane caused by sympathetic nerve stimulation, were slight at the doses employed.*

DISCUSSION

Neuromuscular paralyzing doses of many non-depolarizing skeletal muscle relaxants have atropinic effects on responses to vagal nerve stimulation in cats. Such vagolytic effects in man can explain why these drugs can cause hypertension and tachycardia in anaesthetic practice. The results reported here for gallamine, pancuronium, and AH 8165 in this respect are in keeping with previous findings both in experimental animals and in man (Riker and Wescoe, 1951; Foldes, 1960, 1972; Smith and Whitcher, 1967; Kennedy and Farman, 1968; Kelman and Kennedy, 1970; Saxena and Bonta, 1970; Blogg et al., 1973; Brittain and Tyers, 1973; Marshall, 1973; Savege et al., 1973). Experimental and clinical evidence suggests that a parallel can be drawn between vagolytic (atropinic) activity relative to neuromuscular blocking activity in cats and liability to cause hypertension and tachycardia in man. Humans may be more inclined than cats to show hypertension and tachycardia when atropinic drugs are given because the influence of the parasympathetic system on heart rate may be dominant in man (Glick and Braunwald, 1965; Higgins et al., 1973).

The blockade by tubocurarine of responses to preganglionic stimulation of sympathetic and parasympathetic nerves is attributable to ganglion blockade (Guyton and Reeder, 1950; Randall, 1951). Dimethyltubocurarine, at multiples of the full neuromuscular paralyzing dose, was devoid of effects on autonomic mechanisms – the ideal non-depolarizing muscle relaxant would be short-acting.

REFERENCES

Blogg, C. E., Savege, T. M., Simpson, J. C., Ross, L. A. and Simpson, B. R. (1973): *Proc. roy. Soc. Med.*, *66*, 1023.
Brittain, R. T. and Tyers, M. B. (1973): *Brit. J. Anaesth.*, *45*, 837.
Foldes, F. F. (1960): *Clin. Pharmacol. Ther.*, *1*, 345.
Foldes, F. F. (1972): *Drugs*, *4*, 153.
Glick, G. and Braunwald, E. (1965): *Circulat. Res.*, *16*, 363.
Guyton, A. C. and Reeder, R. C. (1950): *J. Pharmacol. exp. Ther.*, *98*, 188.
Higgins, B. C., Vatner, S. F. and Braunwald, E. (1973): *Pharmacol. Rev.*, *25*, 119.
Kelman, G. R. and Kennedy, B. R. (1970): *Brit. J. Pharmacol.*, *40*, 567P.
Kennedy, B. R. and Farman, J. V. (1968): *Brit. J. Anaesth.*, *40*, 773.
Marshall, I. G. (1973): *J. Pharm. Pharmacol.*, *25*, 530.
Randall, L. O. (1951): *Ann. N.Y. Acad. Sci.*, *54*, 460.
Riker, W. F. and Wescoe, W. C. (1951): *Ann. N.Y. Acad. Sci.*, *54*, 373.
Savege, T. M., Blogg, C. E., Ross, L., Lang, M. and Simpson, B. R. (1973): *Anaesthesia*, *28*, 253.
Saxena, P. R. and Bonta, I. L. (1970): *Europ. J. Pharmacol.*, *11*, 332.
Smith, N. T. and Whitcher, C. E. (1967): *J. Amer. med. Ass.*, *199*, 114.

Other relaxants and the ideal relaxant

J. STOVNER

Rikshospitalet, Oslo, Norway

From originally being pharmacological curiosities the preparations of curare became routine drugs in anaesthesia about 25 years ago. Although these drugs today are included in most of the general anaesthetics given in Europe, an enormous literature deals with the drawbacks, complications and side effects of these drugs. What then are all these shortcomings of the relaxants and what requirements would we like to see fulfilled in a future ideal relaxant?

REQUIREMENTS OF THE IDEAL RELAXANT

(1) Nondepolarization; (2) distribution in the extracellular compartment; (3) selective neuromuscular action; (4) decomposition to inactive compounds; (5) minimal interaction with other compounds; (6) rapid onset of action; and (7) rapid and complete reversal.

Nondepolarization

Succinylcholine is the only depolarizing relaxant extensively used today. Although it has been used for more than 20 years, its many drawbacks have only been realized during the last 10 years. These are hyperkalaemia with cardiac arrest, myoglobinuria, rise in serum creatine phosphokinase, muscle stiffness with occasional malignant hyperthermia, increased intragastric and intraocular pressure. The side effects are all caused by the process of depolarization and would therefore occur with any depolarizing agent. These complications occur more frequently and excessively in patients after trauma and burns, in tetanus uraemia or spastic disorders. If excessive muscle stiffness occurs after a single dose of succinylcholine, the anaesthetic should be cancelled as malignant hyperthermia may ensue. In addition to all these shortcomings no antagonist is available against depolarization block. To avoid all these dangers a nondepolarizing agent would be preferable.

Distribution in the extracellular compartment

All the relaxants are water soluble ionized compounds which are distributed in the extracellular compartment and do not cross the blood-brain barrier or the placenta. It is so wisely ordained that the synaptic cleft communicates with the extracellular fluid. Tubocurarine and pancuronium are exceptional in their ability to penetrate liver cells and are also to a certain extent excreted in the bile.

However, accumulation in the liver cells and excretion in the bile might not be synonymous. Some of the newer steroid relaxants accumulate rapidly in the liver cells after injection into cats but are not rapidly excreted into the bile. With a change in homeostasis such potent drugs could again be liberated into the systemic circulation and cause recurarization.

Tertiary relaxant compounds would penetrate cell membranes and barriers readily and be likely to cause unwanted side effects. The same would hold for a gaseous relaxant agent which has also been suggested (Karis and Gissen, 1971). At present it seems that an ionized compound limited to the extracellular compartment would be preferable.

Selective neuromuscular action

A highly selective blocking of the nicotinic receptors at the neuromuscular junction is desirable in the ideal relaxant. The muscarinic receptors especially in the heart are blocked by at least two relaxants in common use, namely gallamine and pancuronium. In 1950, Ord and Thompson showed that the serumcholinesterase was present in excess at the muscarinic receptors while acetylcholinesterase was present at the nicotinic receptors. Todrick (1954) postulated therefore that the muscarinic receptors resembled serumcholinesterase because vagolytic agents like atropine showed affinity to serumcholinesterase. This hypothesis agrees with the finding that gallamine and pancuronium are selective inhibitors of serumcholinesterase (Stovner et al., 1975). Admittedly a slight vagolytic action is sometimes desirable during halothane anaesthesia but can be produced at will with atropine independent of the relaxant.

Decomposition to inactive compounds

Chemical decomposition in the body would be preferable providing that the breakdown products did not produce neuromuscular block or other unwanted effects. The model is succinylcholine which is hydrolysed by serumcholinesterase. In Boston new choline esters are being developed which are nondepolarizing and susceptible to rapid hydrolysis by serumcholinesterase (Ginsburg et al., 1971). Rapid hydrolysis, however, might only shorten their action to a certain extent. The affinity with the receptors which depends on the dissociation rate from these structures decides the duration of action. Further prolongation of action might occur in patients with low or atypical serumcholinesterase. Being nondepolarizers, however, neostigmine reversal can be obtained with these compounds.

The profile of relaxants that will come in the future is unknown. For short action an agent with a built-in self-destructive button has been suggested.

Minimal interaction with other compounds

Agents which reduce the liberation of acetylcholine from the nerve endings will potentiate the action of any relaxant. I can think of two such conditions occurring in clinical practice. One is the parenteral use of more than one gram of certain antibiotics. The other is a high level of plasma magnesium. Hypermagnesaemia might occur as a result of renal insufficiency, after administration of magnesium salts for eclamptic patients or by overcorrection of magnesium deficiency. Recently, we had a patient on a ventilator for 30 hr after resection of a small bowel segment. Only 22 mg alcuronium had been used during the operation resulting in prolonged neostigmine-resistant block. The patient suffered from ileitis (Mb. Crohn) and had been admitted to the medical ward with convulsions due to magnesium deficiency. This had been overcorrected before surgery. Plasma magnesium level in normal individuals is 1.5–2 mEq/l while our patient was found to have 4.7 mEq/l (Aune, unpublished case report).

Rapid onset of action

This is desirable for 'crash induction' of patients with a full stomach. The nondepolarizing agent AH 8165 which is at present undergoing trial in Europe is said to have an onset of action more rapid than succinylcholine but without all the drawbacks connected with depolarization (Simpson et al., 1972). It is not, however, short acting and depends on renal elimination.

Rapid and complete reversal: Dimethyltubocurarine

It has been postulated that a nondepolarizing relaxant cannot have both high potency and short duration of action at the same time (Feldman, 1973). The high potency means slow dissociation from the receptors limiting the speed of recovery independent of the blood level of the drug. We should therefore seek a drug which can be rapidly and completely reversed with neostigmine rather than a short acting compound. Dimethyltubocurarine seems to fulfil this requirement as it has proved easier to reverse than any of 5 other nondepolarizing relaxants. The study is based on 60 patients of which 10 each received

Table 1. *Reversal as C_4/C_1 increase*

No. of patients	Relaxants	C_4/C_1 ratio increase (%) after neostigmine
10	Tubocurarine	37 ± 3.7
10	Dimethyltubocurarine	60 ± 4.0
10	Alcuronium	31 ± 5.0
10	Gallamine	44 ± 4.0
10	Pancuronium	46 ± 5.0
10	Toxiferine	37 ± 2.4

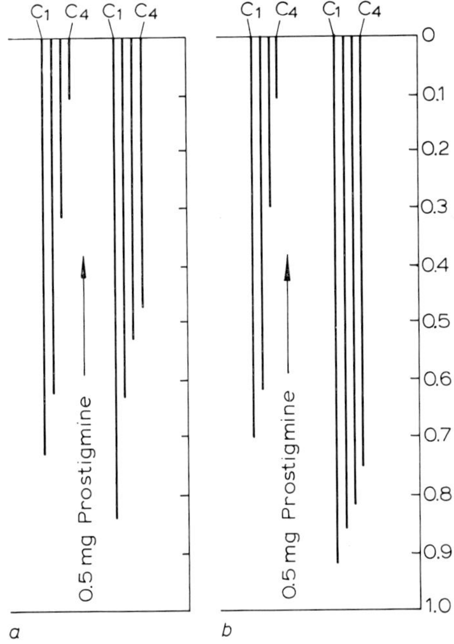

Fig. 1. *(a) Patient partly relaxed with tubocurarine. (b) Patient with dimethyltubocurarine. Tracings taken before and 4 min after 0.5 mg prostigmine i.v. In tracing (a) the C_4/C_1 ratio increased 37%; in tracing (b) the C_4/C_1 ratio increased 60%.*

tubocurarine, dimethyltubocurarine, alcuronium, gallamine, pancuronium and toxiferine. Using the method of Ali et al. (1970) we recorded the responses to a train of 4 single stimuli with half second intervals. At a state where the C_4 contractions were just visible we gave 0.5 mg neostigmine and recorded the increase in C_4/C_1 over the next 4 min. The results are shown in Table 1 and a typical recording in Figure 1. Only dimethyl-tubocurarine showed significantly better reversal with this method than any of the other relaxants. There were no significant differences between the other relaxants. In addition to this, dimethyltubocurarine has been shown to be more potent as well as shorter acting than tubocurarine and has no histamine-releasing or ganglion-blocking action (Wilson et al., 1950). From the point of view of the patient, the surgeon and the anaesthetist, this drug fulfils a number of requirements for the ideal relaxant. However, the manufacturer also has to be considered and he finds this drug difficult to prepare and it is not marketed in Europe.

REFERENCES

Ali, H. H., Utting, J. E. and Gray, T. C. (1970): *Brit. J. Anaesth.*, *42*, 967.

Feldman, S. A. (1973): *Muscle Relaxants*, p. 158. W. B. Saunders Co., Philadelphia, Pa.

Ginsburg, S., Kitz, R. J. and Savarese, J. J. (1971): *Brit. J. Pharmacol.*, *43*, 107.

Karis, J. H. and Gissen, A. J. (1971): *Anaesthesiology*, *35*, 149.

Ord, M. G. and Thompson, R. H. S. (1950): *Biochem. J.*, *46*, 346.

Simpson, B. R., Savage, T. M., Blogg, C. E., Maxwell, M. P., Strunin, L., Walton, B., Foley, E. I. and Ross, L. A. (1972): *Lancet*, *1*, 516.

Stovner, J., Oftedal, N. and Holmboe, J. (1975): *Brit. J. Anaesth.*, *47*, in press.

Todrick, A. (1954): *Brit. J. Pharmacol.*, *9*, 76.

Wilson. H. W., Gordon, H. E. and Raffan, A. W. (1950): *Brit. med. J.*, *1*, 1296.

Neuromuscular effects of galanthamine versus neostigmine and hexafluorenium

ANIS BARAKA

Department of Anesthesiology, American University of Beirut, Beirut, Lebanon

Galanthamine is a natural anticholinesterase (Paskov et al., 1962), which is extracted from the blossom and leaves of the Snowdrop flower *Galanthus nivalis*. In vitro experiments have shown that galanthamine inhibits both muscle and plasma cholinesterases (Irwin and Smith, 1960).

The present investigation demonstrates the neuromuscular effects of galanthamine versus two other anticholinesterases (neostigmine and hexafluorenium). The report also compares their interaction with the nondepolarizing block of tubocurarine, and the depolarizing block of suxamethonium.

MATERIALS AND METHODS

Thirty-three healthy adults undergoing inguinal herniorrhaphies were studied. Their body weight ranged from 65–70 kg. Patients were premedicated with pethidine 100 mg and atropine 0.6 mg injected intramuscularly, 30 min before operation. Anesthesia was induced with thiopentone 250–300 mg and maintained with 0.5–1 % halothane in nitrous oxide-oxygen (3:2).

The ulnar nerve was supramaximally stimulated by a Block-Aid monitor at 4-sec intervals. The resultant adduction of the thumb was measured by a modified Grass model FT-03 force displacement transducer, recording on a Grass polygraph at a speed of 0.5 mm/sec.

When a steady twitch response was obtained, the effect of galanthamine and hexafluorenium 20–40 mg (about 0.3–0.6 mg/kg) on the twitch response was investigated and compared to that produced by neostigmine 1–2 mg (about 0.015–0.03 mg/kg).

In a second group of patients, neuromuscular block was produced by 10–15 mg tubocurarine. The interaction of the three anticholinesterases with the block was compared.

In a third group of patients, suxamethonium 10 mg was injected intravenously and its effect on the twitch response was observed. After complete recovery of neuromuscular transmission, one of the three anticholinesterases was injected. Five minutes later the same dose of suxamethonium was repeated. The effect of the second dose of suxamethonium on the muscle response and heart rate was observed.

In all patients, the heart rate was continuously observed by a Hewlett-Packard pulse monitor.

RESULTS

Effect on neuromuscular transmission

The injection of neostigmine 1–2 mg (about 0.015–0.03 mg/kg), or galanthamine 20–40 mg

"

(about 0.3–0.6 mg/kg) did not affect the twitch response. On the other hand, the injection of hexafluorenium 20–40 mg (about 0.3–0.6 mg/kg) was followed by depression of neuromuscular transmission. Hexafluorenium block was proportional to the dose used. The block was not preceded by muscle fasciculation. Tetanic stimulation was maintained, but was not followed by post-tetanic facilitation. Recovery was not markedly affected by neostigmine (Fig. 1).

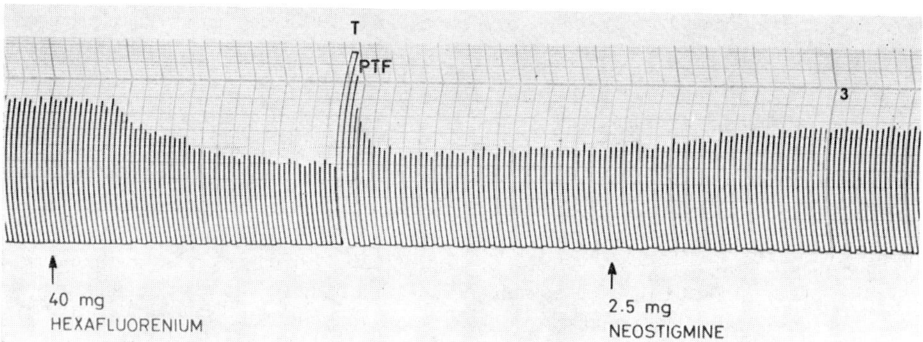

Fig. 1.   *Tracing of the twitch response to ulnar nerve stimulation at 4-sec intervals showing the neuromuscular block produced by 40 mg hexafluorenium. The block was characterized by a sustained response to tetanus (T) and post-tetanic facilitation (PTF). The rate of recovery was not significantly affected by 2–5 mg neostigmine.*

Interaction with tubocurarine block

In all patients, hexafluorenium 20 mg (about 0.3 mg/kg) delayed recovery of the neuromuscular block achieved by tubocurarine 10 mg, while neostigmine 1 mg (about 0.015 mg/kg), or galanthamine 20 mg (about 0.3 mg/kg), could reverse the block (Fig. 2).

When 1.5-times the blocking dose of tubocurarine was used, the resultant block could not be reversed by up to 40 mg of galanthamine (about 0.6 mg/kg), while neostigmine 2–3 mg (about 0.03–0.05 mg/kg) achieved reversal (Fig. 3).

Interaction with suxamethonium block

The injection of suxamethonium 10 mg after neostigmine 1 mg, or galanthamine 20 mg was followed by muscle fasciculation. The heart rate slowed in most patients to 20–60/min. The duration of suxamethonium block after neostigmine or galanthamine was only about 1.5–2 times that produced by the control dose of suxamethonium (Fig. 4).

On the other hand, the injection of suxamethonium 10 mg after hexafluorenium 20 mg was not associated with fasciculation or bradycardia. Five- to ten-fold prolongation of the block was observed. The block was characterized by tetanic fade and post-tetanic facilitation, and was partially reversed by neostigmine (Fig. 5).

DISCUSSION

The present report shows that clinical doses of neostigmine or galanthamine do not depress neuromuscular transmission, while hexafluorenium can produce a significant neuromuscular

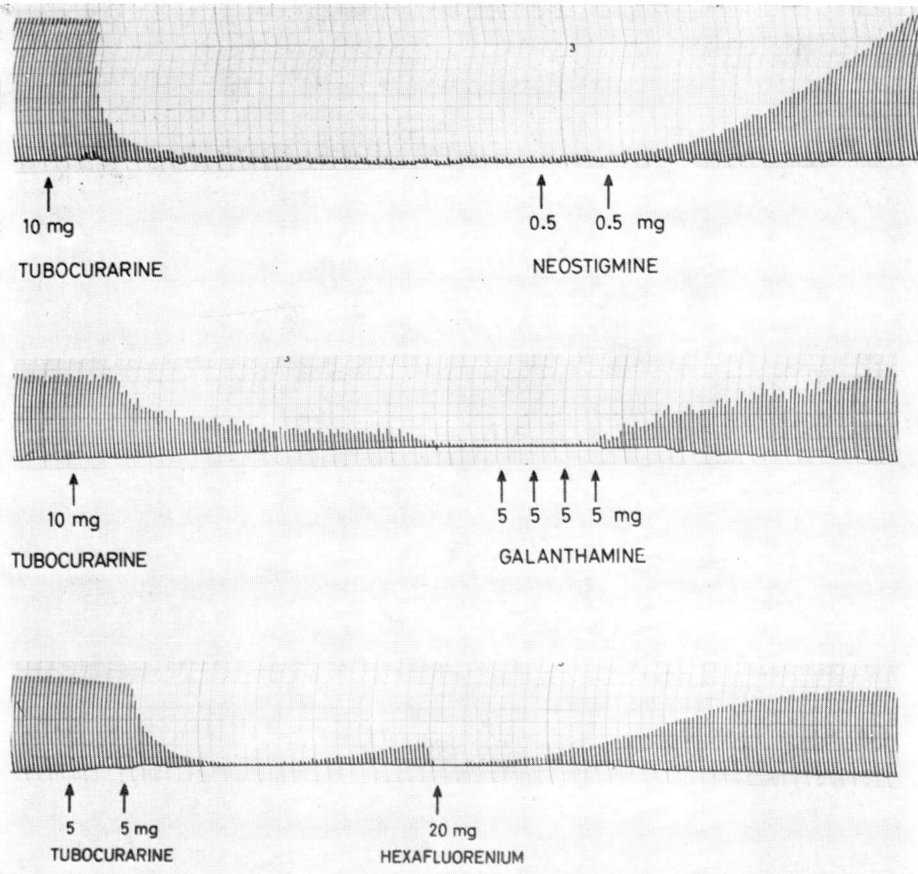

Fig. 2.   *Tracings of the twitch response to ulnar nerve stimulation at 4-sec intervals, showing reversal of the neuromuscular block of tubocurarine (10 mg) by neostigmine and galanthamine, as contrasted with potentiation by hexafluorenium. The reversal dose of galanthamine is 20 times that of neostigmine.*

block. The neuromuscular block of hexafluorenium is typical neither of depolarizing nor of nondepolarizing mechanisms, and has been described by Nastuk and Karis (1964) as antidepolarizing. Such an effect can potentiate the neuromuscular block of tubocurarine.

In contrast with hexafluorenium, the two other anticholinesterases (neostigmine and galanthamine) can reverse a blocking dose of tubocurarine. However, the reversal activity of galanthamine is only 1/10 (De Angelis and Walts, 1972) to 1/20 that of neostigmine (Baraka and Cozanitis, 1973). It has been reported that the muscarinic effects of galanthamine are much less than those of neostigmine, and therefore it may be given for reversal without atropine (Mayrhofer, 1966; Cozanitis, 1971). However, this conclusion is not based on comparison of equipotent doses of the two drugs. Many of the patients given galanthamine without atropine can develop arrhythmias of a vagal type (Cozanitis et al., 1973).

The reversal of the nondepolarizing block of tubocurarine depends on both the plasma level of tubocurarine and on the degree of block at the time of reversal (Baraka, 1967). With moderate overdosage of tubocurarine, galanthamine in increasing dosage cannot

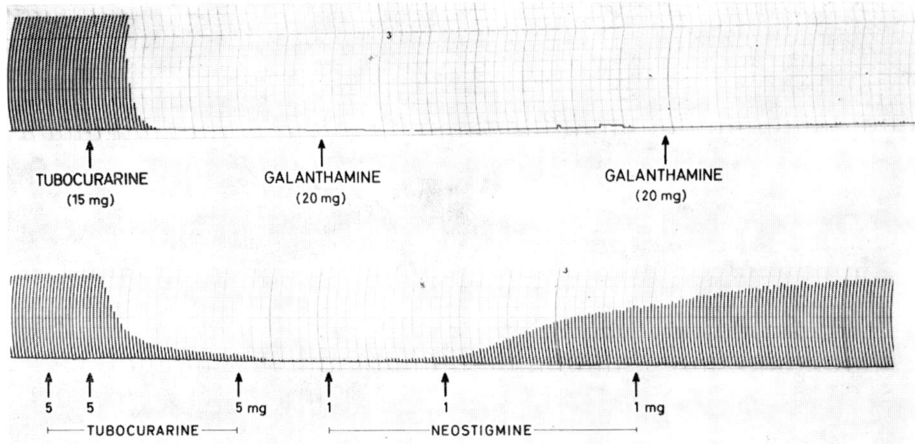

Fig. 3.   *Tracings of the twitch response to ulnar nerve stimulation showing the neuromuscular block of tubocurarine 15 mg. Galanthamine up to 40 mg could not reverse the block, while neostigmine 3 mg achieved reversal.*

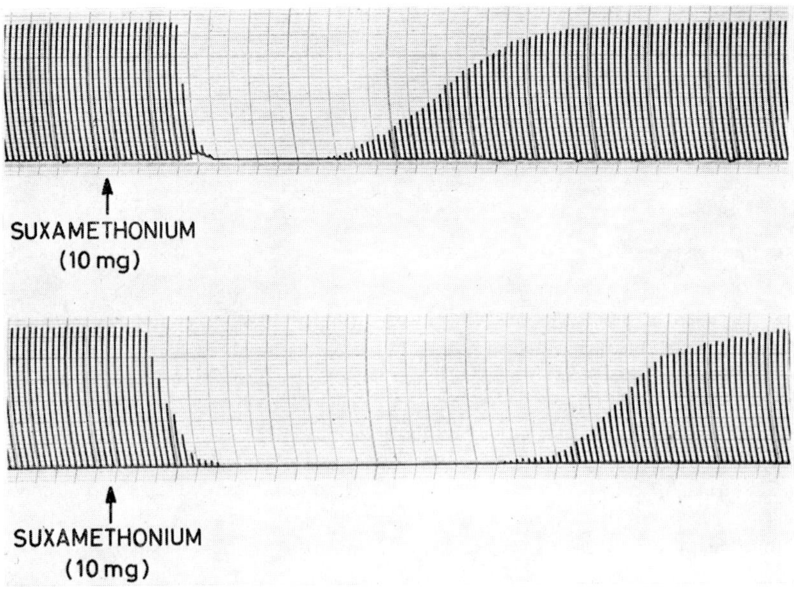

Fig. 4.   *Tracings of the twitch response to ulnar nerve stimulation at 4-sec intervals. Injection of suxamethonium 10 mg after galanthamine 20 mg (lower tracing) prolonged the duration of block 1.5 times as compared to that produced by a control dose of suxamethonium (upper tracing). A comparable response has been achieved by the interaction of suxamethonium with neostigmine 1 mg.*

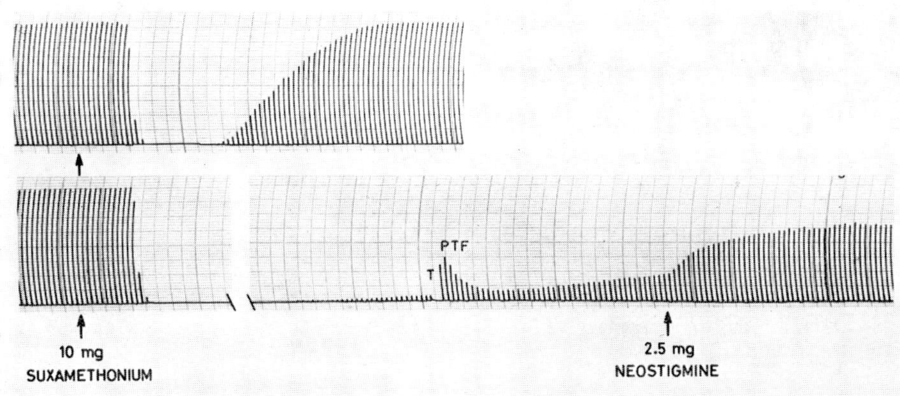

Fig. 5. *Tracings of the twitch response to ulnar nerve stimulation at 4-sec intervals. Injection of suxamethonium 10 mg after hexafluorenium 20 mg (lower tracing) markedly prolonged the duration of the block as compared to that produced by a control dose of suxamethonium (upper tracing). The potentiated block was characterized by tetanic fade (T) and post-tetanic facilitation (PTF), and the rate of recovery was enhanced by 2.5 mg neostigmine.*

reverse the block, while neostigmine can still achieve reversal. It is probable that neostigmine is not only more potent than galanthamine, but also has a wider decurarizing range.

In vitro experiments by Irwin and Smith (1960) have shown that galanthamine, like neostigmine (Barrow and Johnson, 1966), inhibits not only acetylcholinesterase but also plasma cholinesterase. This can explain the potentiated neuromuscular block and the marked bradycardia of suxamethonium following these two anticholinesterases. Thesleff (1952) has shown that the use of neostigmine to potentiate suxamethonium block can produce severe muscarinic side effects that make it unsuitable for clinical application.

On the other hand, hexafluorenium is a selective plasma cholinesterase inhibitor which has been used clinically to delay the hydrolysis of suxamethonium (Foldes et al., 1960a, b). Injection of suxamethonium after hexafluorenium is not associated with bradycardia and results in a markedly prolonged block. The block is not initiated by fasciculation and is characterized by tetanic fade and post-tetanic facilitation denoting a qualitative change in the type of suxamethonium block. Karis et al. (1966) have shown in vitro that hexafluorenium prevents the depolarization of the post-junctional membrane by suxamethonium; the resulting block, though potentiated is essentially nondepolarizing in nature.

Such a qualitative change in the mechanism of action of suxamethonium after hexafluorenium might occur in other post-junctional membranes, e.g., the heart. This can explain the absence of bradycardia when repeated doses of suxamethonium follow hexafluorenium. A similar protection against suxamethonium bradycardia has been achieved by other antidepolarizing agents such as tubocurarine both in vivo (Mathias et al., 1970) and in the isolated mammalian heart (Goat, 1972). This suggests that the negative chronotropic effect of succinylcholine, similar to acetylcholine, may result from a direct agonistic action on the cholinergic receptors of the heart (Goat and Feldman, 1972a, b). Therefore, it can be blocked by agents that antagonize such cholinergic activity and exaggerated by vagotonic agents.

The chief advantage of suxamethonium is essentially its rapid hydrolysis by the plasma cholinesterase. The use of different anticholinesterases to delay hydrolysis is inadvisable since neostigmine and galanthamine exaggerate the muscarinic side effects of suxamethonium while hexafluorenium markedly prolongs its action and modifies its blocking activity.

REFERENCES

Baraka, A. (1967): *Brit. J. Anaesth.*, *39*, 891.
Baraka, A. and Cozanitis, D. (1973): *Anesth. Analg. Curr. Res.*, *52*, 832.
Barrow, M. E. and Johnson, J. K. (1966): *Brit. J. Anaesth.*, *38*, 420.
Cozanitis, D. A. (1971): *Anaesthesist*, *6*, 226.
Cozanitis, D., Nuuttila, K., Karhunen, P. and Baraka, A. (1973): *Anaesthesist*, *22*, 457.
De Angelis, J. and Walts, L. F. (1972): *Anesth. Analg. Curr. Res.*, *51*, 196.
Foldes, F. F., Hillmer, N. R., Molloy, R. E. and Monte, A. P. (1960a): *Anesthesiology*, *21*, 50.
Foldes, F. F., Molloy, R. E., Zsigmond, E. K. and Zwortz, J. A. (1960b): *J. Pharmacol. exp. Ther.*, *120*, 400.
Goat, V. (1972): *Proc. roy. Soc. Med.*, *65/2*, 149.
Goat, V. and Feldman, S. (1972a): *Anaesthesia*, *27/2*, 143.
Goat, V. and Feldman, S. (1972b): *Anaesthesia*, *27/2*, 149.
Irwin, R. L. and Smith III, H. J. (1960): *Biochem. Pharmacol.*, *3*, 147.
Karis, J. H., Nastuk, W. L. and Katz, R. L. (1966): *Brit. J. Anaesth.*, *38*, 762.
Mathias, J., Evans-Prosser, C. and Churchill-Davidson, H. (1970): *Brit. J. Anaesth.*, *42*, 609.
Mayrhofer, O. (1966): *Sth. med. J. (Bgham, Ala.)*, *59*, 1364.
Nastuk, W. L. and Karis, J. H. (1964): *J. Pharmacol. exp. Ther.*, *144*, 236.
Paskov, D. S., Stojanov, E. A. and Saev, S. K. et al. (1962): *Cult. med.*, *30*, 219.
Thesleff, S. (1952): *Acta physiol. scand.*, *25*, 348.

The fate of pancuronium in man

W. BUZELLO

Institut für Anaesthesiologie der Universitätskliniken, Freiburg, Federal Republic of Germany

Pancuronium is now used widely in clinical anaesthesiology. The metabolism of the drug in man was, however, obscure until some Dutch authors published a detailed study on this subject at the end of 1973 (Agoston et al., 1973). At the same time we concluded our own clinical investigations (Buzello, 1974, 1975), which will be summarized in this paper.

The chemical structure of pancuronium is characterized by an esterification of the hydroxylated steran-system with acetic acid both in position 3 and 17 (Buckett et al., 1968). These 2 ester linkages are broken in the metabolism producing the 3 metabolites 3-desacetyl-, 17-desacetyl-, and 3,17-desacetyl-pancuronium. Our analytical procedure is different from that of Agoston et al. (1973) and easier to perform. The principle is to form a pancuronium-complex which is blue with the acid dye bromophenol blue in an alkaline solution. The diacetylated derivatives give the same reaction as pancuronium itself. The complexes are extracted into chloroform and evaluated colorimetrically. After evaporation of the chloroform the desacetylated derivatives are separated from the parent compound by thin layer chromatography using a modified (Buzello, 1975) system of Kersten et al. (1973).

Figure 1 shows the concentration curve of pancuronium in human serum. During the first 5 min after the intravenous injection there is a strikingly steep drop to half of the initial value which is followed by a more shallow section of about 40 min duration leading to a 3rd phase which asymptomatically approaches zero concentration within a number of hours. The maximum muscle relaxation is achieved about 2 min after the injection and successively weakens during the intermediate phase of the curve. The complete termination

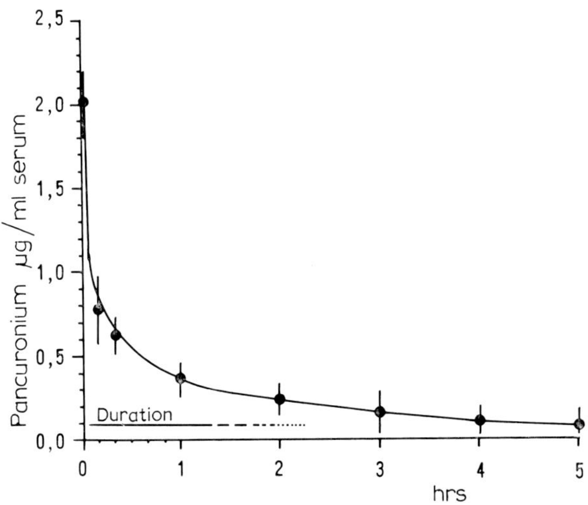

Fig. 1.   *The concentration of pancuronium in human serum ($\overline{X} \pm s$; n = 7; 6 mg pro dosi).*

of action is situated in the 3rd section of the curve and coincides with a concentration of 0.2–0.5 µg of pancuronium/ml serum.

Regarding the renal elimination of the total pancuronium base (Fig. 2) the following remarkable features should be noticed:

1. 6 mg of pancuronium may produce muscular paralysis for 1–1.5 hr. After 2 hr however the urine does not contain more than 15–35% of the injected dose.
2. The renal elimination of pancuronium takes at least 12 hr.
3. On the average not more of half of the injected dose is recovered from the urine, and
4. this rate ranges from 20–90% of the injected dose.

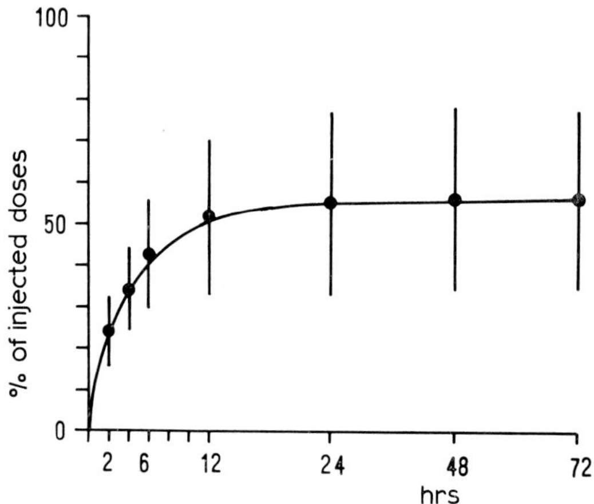

Fig. 2.   *Cumulative renal elimination of pancuronium* ($\overline{X} \pm s$; *n = 8; 6 mg pro dosi*).

Three fractions of derivatives of pancuronium were isolated by thin layer chromatography of the urinary extracts. About 80% of the renally excreted total base is unchanged pancuronium, about 15% is monodesacetylated, and 5% is completely desacetylated derivatives. This pattern changes slightly with time with wide individual variations. The incubation of urine samples with glucuronidase and sulphatase did not yield any evidence for glucuronide or sulphate formation with pancuronium.

Pancuronium was also demonstrated in the bile, but this pathway does not play an important part in patients without renal failure. Nothing is known about the compensatory significance of biliary elimination in patients suffering from renal failure.

CONCLUSION

Our experimental data agree with those of Agoston et al. (1973).

Pancuronium is a non-depolarizing muscle relaxant which may be inactivated principally by metabolic breakdown. In man this mechanism is quantitatively negligible and does not determine the termination of the neuromuscular block.

In man the termination of neuromuscular block from pancuronium mainly is based on the redistribution of the drug from specific receptor sites to non-specific compartments. Renal elimination of the drug is of secondary importance. There is no evidence that pancuronium is superior to other nondepolarizing agents in patients with renal failure. Impaired renal function is still a problem for the anaesthesiologist.

REFERENCES

Agoston, S., Vermeer, G. A., Kersten, U. W. and Meijer, D. K. F. (1973): *Acta anaesth. scand.*, *17*, 267.
Buzello, W. (1974): *Anaesthesist*, *23*, 443.
Buzello, W. (1975): *Anaesthesist*, *23*, 13.
Buckett, W. R., Christine, E. B., Majoribanks, C. E. B., Marwick, F. A. and Norton, M. B. (1968): *Brit. J. Pharmacol.*, *32*, 671.
Kersten, U. W., Meijer, D. K. F. and Agoston, S. (1973): *Clin. chim. Acta*, *44*, 59.

The safety of pancuronium in renal failure

F. Y. DALAL and E. J. BENNETT

Department of Anesthesiology, Loyola University Stritch School of Medicine, Maywood, and
Department of Anesthesiology, University of Illinois Hospitals, Chicago, Ill., U.S.A.

Renal transplant surgery has to have a technique that will do least harm or none at all to the kidney by having minimal effect on renal function. This will present the results of the use of pancuronium bromide in: (1) normal donors, (2) patients in renal failure before and after transplants, with functioning and rejected kidneys.

METHOD

All patients, both normal donors and the recipients on whom the effects of pancuronium were to be studied, were premedicated with 2.5–10 mg of droperidol intramuscularly. Anesthesia was induced with sleep dose of thiopentone followed by 120 μg/kg of pancuronium. This sequence was changed in emergency when a full stomach was suspected. In these cases pancuronium was given 30 sec prior to thiopentone and intubation carried out immediately, using the Sellick maneuver.

Maintenance of anesthesia was with 70% nitrous oxide in oxygen supplemented by increments of fentanyl 0.05 mg as required. Ventilation was controlled using a Cape ventilator (V_T 15 ml/kg, f 10–15/min). Subsequent incremental doses of pancuronium were 1/5 of the initial dose. The residual effects of the relaxant were antagonized by a mixture of 0.02 mg/kg of atropine and 0.08 mg/kg of neostigmine given intravenously.

Vital signs, CVP, EKG, temperature, and urine output (where possible) were monitored. Also, for the majority of the patients, a Block-Aid monitor was used to assess the time taken for 90% and 100% twitch depression. Intubating conditions were judged good, fair, or poor after 2–3 min.

RESULTS

As can be seen from Table 1, 124 anesthetics were administered to 70 patients, 20 of whom were normal donors. Of the 50 who received a transplant kidney, 16 had been performed prior to this study. However, they returned for some of the repeat operations mentioned in the table along with the present recipients.

Statistical analysis was performed on the 6 groups mentioned in Table 1 using 15 variables by Duncan's new multiple range test (Sokol and Rohlf, 1969). The duration of the first dose was calculated from the time of initial injection to the time when an incremental dose was necessary, or to that when adequate reversal was achieved. Hence those patients who could not be reversed satisfactorily were excluded from the analysis (4 out of 34). The requirements were calculated from the number and timing of incremental doses. It therefore does not include the initial dose. These results can be seen in Table 1.

Table 1. *Results from 124 anesthetic administrations to 70 patients*

Parameter		Normals	Siblings	Recipients	Nephrectomy	Working transplants	Rejection
Requirement	n	20	16	34*	24	34** (30)	12
(μg/kg/hr)	$\overline{m}$	40.29	29.85	31.87	32.92	60.88	68.75
	SD	18.42	8.03	17.00	8.58	25.84	22.85
	SEM	4.22	2.08	2.95	1.79	4.79	6.89
Duration	$\overline{m}$	131.5	194.69	179.59	172.5	112.0	112.08
	SD	60.41	55.58	97.55	87.34	43.2	48.06
	SEM	13.86	24.67	16.98	18.21	8.02	14.49

* Includes 16 siblings.
** Of these 34, 4 who failed to reverse at the conclusion of surgery were not considered for the calculation of the requirement and duration of the relaxant.
SD = 1 standard deviation $\pm$; SEM = standard error of mean.

In comparing the different categories of patients by analysis of variance, 2 homogenous groups could be discerned for both the requirements as well as the duration of action of the initial dose.

REQUIREMENTS

From Table 2 it is evident that there was no statistical difference in the requirements of pancuronium in the normal siblings, recipients, or those in whom bilateral nephrectomies were performed (Group A). Similarly, patients with either working transplants or rejected kidneys (Group B) showed no statistical difference in the dose requirements. However, there was a statistical difference for the requirements if any of the subdivisions from Group A was compared to that from Group B.

Table 2. *Statistical analysis*

	Requirements		μg/kg/hr	
Group A	No $\varDelta$ Normals Siblings Recipients Nephrectomy	$-\varDelta-$ $P < 0.05$	No $\varDelta$ Working transplants Rejects	Group B

There is no statistical difference between any of the groups in the left hand column, or between the 2 in the right hand column. There is a statistical difference between any from the left and any from the right.

DURATION

For the duration of action, there was no statistical difference between normals, patients with working transplants, and those who had rejected the kidneys (Group C). Similarly there was no significant difference in the duration of action between siblings, recipients, or patients with bilateral nephrectomies (Group D). However, there was a statistical difference in the duration of action between any of the subdivisions of Group C when compared to that from any one of Group D with the exception of the comparison between normals and those who had bilateral nephrectomies.

Other observations of interest were: (*a*) With the initial dose of 120 μg/kg and using this protocol, the time to 90% twitch depression was a mean of 45 sec and for 100% depression, 75 sec elapsed. In the presence of full stomach, it was possible to rapidly intubate the patient by injecting pancuronium 30 sec prior to the thiopentone. Cricoid pressure was applied to prevent regurgitation. Twenty-seven of the 124 patients were intubated by this rapid method because of a full stomach without any problems. In the remaining 97 patients, the intubating condition at 2–3 min was good in 82, fair in 12, and poor in 3. (*b*) Reversal was good in 111, fair in 9, and poor in 2. Of the patients in whom the reversal was less than satisfactory, 2 had received 400 μg/kg by error and 4 were on azothioprine. Of these 4, 2 had received cadaveric kidneys, which do not excrete this drug well, also 3 were rejecting the kidneys. In these types of patients azothioprine tends to accumulate and it is known to have a neuromuscular blocking action. Two other patients required postoperative mechanical ventilation. They had unsuspected pneumothorax from the faulty insertion of the CVP catheters via the subclavian route. The condition was diagnosed only in the recovery room. (*c*) Pulse varied $\pm$ 20 beats/min. (*d*) Blood pressure showed a mean increase of 12 mm Hg with a range of $+$ 20–10 Torr. Arrhythmia or tachycardia was not observed in any group.

DISCUSSION

The problems associated with patients in renal failure are well documented in the literature (Monks and Lumley, 1972; Aldrete et al., 1971) and will only be enumerated here. They are: (1) anemia, (2) electrolyte imbalance, (3) high BUN, NPN, and creatinine, (4) hypertension, (5) bleeding tendency, (6) the possibility of a drug interaction or enzyme induction, (7) risk of infection, (8) care of the A-V fistula, (9) an increased risk of contracting hepatitis by the patient and personnel, (10) hypertension due to release of renin after the anastamosis of renal vessels, and (11) a full stomach, especially with cadaveric transplants.

Practically every technique has been used for anesthetizing these patients, but the trend is N$_2$O/narcotic/relaxant technique as this causes a minimal amount of physiological disturbance.

Pancuronium bromide is a bisquaternary ammonium salt. The literature indicates that it is excreted by the kidney, some taken up by the liver and some appears in the bile. It has a steroid nucleus with two esteratic sites and it has been shown recently that breakdown occurs by de-esterification at the 3 and 17 carbon atom sites (Avery, 1972). Lubke et al. (1971) demonstrated that while in dogs 33–65% is excreted by kidneys, this accounts for only 3% in man, the remainder being metabolized probably to the 3-oxo and tetrahydro forms in the liver. Strunin et al. (1972), using canine liver slices, have suggested that metabolic breakdown is a distinct possibility. Further support has come from the work of Agoston et al. (1973) who studied the urinary as well as biliary excretion of unchanged pancuronium and its 3-hydroxy derivative. They found that after 30 hr the proportion of unchanged to 3-hydroxy derivative in urine was 40 : 60 and 60 : 40 in bile as percentage of amount excreted. Even though they mention that only a small proportion undergoes biotransformation, they postulate that further biotransformation is not excluded since the total recovery of the bisquaternary compounds in the investigated excreta by the end of the observation period amounted to 55% of the injected dose.

This study seems to give additional support to the concept of metabolic degradation of pancuronium, at least in patients in renal failure. It becomes apparent when Tables 2 and 3 are analyzed in depth. It can be seen that there is a significant difference if the duration of action of the first dose between patients who had bilateral nephrectomies and those who had a functioning transplant, the total requirement being more in the former. Also it can be seen that there was no statistical difference in the total requirements between normal donors and their siblings who were in renal failure. Of particular interest is the fact that patients who were rejecting the kidneys required more pancuronium and the duration of the first dose was less when compared to the whole group of recipients. The explanation could be an enhanced metabolism because of enzyme induction or drug interaction. There was statistically no difference between normal patients and patients undergoing bilateral nephrectomies when requirements and the duration of the first dose was considered. This suggests that alternate routes for metabolism are available.

Table 3. *Statistical analysis*

	Duration	1st Dose	Minutes	
	No $\varDelta$		No $\varDelta$	
	Normals		Siblings	
Group C	Working transplants	$-\varDelta-$ $P < 0.05$	Recipients	Group D
	Rejection		Nephrectomies	

But no $\varDelta$ between normals and nephrectomies.

There is no statistical difference between any of the 3 in the left hand column, or between any of the 3 in the right hand column. There is a statistical difference between any from the left and any from the right, with the exception when normal patients and bilateral nephrectomies are compared.

The drug has other advantages in having a faster onset of action, more profound blockade for equivalent doses, stable blood pressure, and easier reversal. Because of these facts, it appeared that pancuronium may have an advantage over curare in patients for transplant surgery.

There was no evidence of a cumulative action or tachyphylaxis. Some of the recipients who were operated almost immediately after the first operation because of various complications were given the same dose of pancuronium for the next anesthetic without any obvious cumulative effect.

In conclusion, it can be said that in spite of the degree of illness exhibited by these patients, their response to pancuronium was remarkably normal and because of the advantages of pancuronium it may be the relaxant of choice in these patients. Renal excretion is not necessary for the termination of its action and its response was predictable. The differences in duration and requirements in these patients in renal failure and in other series could be due to the differences in technique either for dialysis or anesthesia.

REFERENCES

Agoston, S., Vermeer, G. A., Kersten, U. W. and Meijer, D. K. F. (1973): *Acta anaesth. scand., 17,* 267.
Aldrete, J. A., Daniel, W., O'Higgins, J. W. et al. (1971): *Anesth. Analg. Curr. Res., 50,* 321.
Avery, G. S. (1972): *Drugs, 4,* 163.
Lubke, P., Wilhelm, G. and Behler, K. (1971): *Anaesthesist, 20,* 221.
Miller, R. D., Stevens, W. C. and Way, W. L. (1973): *Anesth. Analg. Curr. Res., 52,* 661.
Monks, P. S. and Lumley, J. (1972): *Ann. roy. Coll. Surg. Engl., 50,* 354.
Sokol, P. R. and Rohlf, J. J. (1969): *Biometry 1969.* W. H. Freeman and Company, San Francisco, Calif.
Strunin, L., Strunin, J. M., Layten, J., Sim, A. W. and Simpson, B. R. (1972): *Brit. J. Anaesth., 44,* 624.

Rapid termination of prolonged neuromuscular block after suxamethonium in 8 patients by administration of serum cholinesterase

K. L. SCHOLLER and H. W. GOEDDE

Institute of Anaesthesiology, Freiburg University, Freiburg/Br., and
Institute of Human Genetics, Hamburg University, Hamburg, Federal Republic of Germany

The depolarizing muscle relaxant suxamethonium (succinyldicholine) is reversed by the hydrolytic action of serum cholinesterase. After a normal dose of 1 mg/kg suxamethonium the paralysis disappears within 8 min. A prolonged paralysis of several hours' duration is a rare and unexpected event. After frequently observing the occurrence of this phenomenon in blood relatives, Kalow et al. (1957) detected a genetic variant of serum cholinesterase which cannot hydrolyse suxamethonium. In approximately 2/3 of the patients who have shown prolonged apnoea after administration of suxamethonium, variants of serum cholinesterase have been found. The most common variant, homozygotes for the dibucaine resistant or atypical allele, showed a much reduced affinity for suxamethonium (Goedde et al., 1968). The incidence of this anomaly in the European population is about 1 : 2800 (Goedde et al., 1967b). In cases of liver disease the activity of normal serum cholinesterase may be markedly reduced. However, there are hardly any liver diseases in which the synthesis of serum cholinesterase is so strongly depressed that a paralysis of more than an hour's duration results following 1 mg/kg suxamethonium. If an overdose of suxamethonium has been given to such a patient, the resulting clinical signs are the same as found in patients with atypical serum cholinesterase and the treatment is also the same.

A highly purified human serum cholinesterase has recently been marketed in ampoules containing 45 mg of dry substance (Serum Cholinesterase Behringwerke). The contents of one ampoule are equal to the amount of serum cholinesterase in 500 ml of human plasma. As the enzyme preparation is expensive it should only be used if certain criteria are fulfilled, which make it highly probable that the respiratory disturbance is the result of an atypical variant.

CLINICAL SIGNS OF PROLONGED ACTION OF SUXAMETHONIUM

Biochemical tests to detect genetically determined variants of serum cholinesterase are not carried out routinely in most clinical laboratories because they are time-consuming and unreliable.

A dissociation in the triggering of reflexes in the smooth and striated muscle can be taken as a clinical demonstration of the presence of an atypical variant serum cholinesterase. This observation is only valid if the central nervous system is not depressed by anaesthetics, i.e. the degree of anaesthesia must be only minimal, and the motor action of the pupils

Table 1. *Data of 8 patients with prolonged neuromuscular block after suxamethonium and treatment with serum cholinesterase (Behringwerke)*

Patient		Operation	Suxa-methonium (mg)	Block duration (hr)	Serum cholinesterase (mg*)	Recovery time (min)	Phenotype	DN**	Family investigation
Age	Sex								
46	F	Excision of lymph nodes	100	3	110	10	A	27	Not performed
6	M	Strabismus surgery	30	1.5	70	18***	A	23	Refused
60	M	Palatal graft	70	1.5	135	8	A	24	Positive
43	M	Bronchoscopy	100	1.5	90	8	AF	56	Positive
10	F	Appendectomy	70	3	90	10	A	26	Refused
34	F	Bronchography	160	1	90	9	A	20	Not performed
39	F	Jaw cavity surgery	80	1.5	90	9	A	22	Positive
55	M	Bronchoscopy	120	1	90	12	A	23	No relatives

All patients showed a positive pupillary reflex and had no cough reflex before injection of the enzyme.
* Commercial product currently 1 Amp=45 mg. ** Normal: dibucaine No. DN=80. *** Delayed injection.

must not be depressed by drugs of the morphine family, ganglion blockers or miotics. In order to test the patient's pupillary reaction, anaesthesia is with nitrous oxide and oxygen alone. The patient must not be allowed to regain consciousness during this procedure, since inability to move combined with the presence of a tube in the trachea is extremely unpleasant and hearing would be possible. If the patient's pupils react promptly to light while under nitrous oxide anaesthesia, in the absence of response of the diaphragm when the bronchial mucosa is touched with a suction catheter (cough reflex), dissociation of reflex triggering between smooth muscle and striated muscle arouses the suspicion of a delay in the destruction of suxamethonium. If almost an hour has elapsed since the last administration of suxamethonium, if no other muscle relaxants or cholinesterase inhibitors have been given in the meantime, and if gross disturbances in gas exchange and electrolyte balance can be excluded, it is probable that the patient has a genetically determined protein variant of serum cholinesterase (see also Goedde et al., 1967*a*).

DOSAGE OF SERUM CHOLINESTERASE

In the last 6 years 8 patients with prolonged apnoea after suxamethonium have been treated with serum cholinesterase (Table 1). These were 4 female patients and 4 male patients of ages ranging from 6–60 years. In the 8 patients the paralysis after a dose of 1–1.5 mg/kg suxamethonium lasted from 1–3 hr before serum cholinesterase was injected.

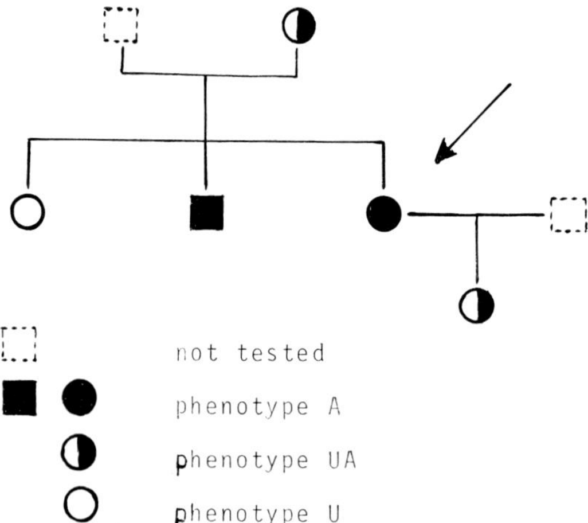

Fig. 1.   *Distribution of the dibucaine resistant enzyme variant in the living members of the family of patient No. 7 (arrow) in Table 1. The investigation of the patient's siblings revealed one additional carrier of phenotype A.*

The pupillary reaction to light was positive under light N_2O-O_2 anaesthesia and the cough reflex was negative to suction with a catheter in the bronchus. The average recovery time for the restoration of normal respiration in the 8 patients, to whom we gave a minimum of 90 mg dry substance of Behringwerke serum cholinesterase intravenously, was 10.5 min. The enzymatic analysis of the patients' serum, withdrawn before injection, confirmed the presence of a genetic variant of serum cholinesterase, in most cases the phenotype A (homozygous) with a low dibucaine number. Since the activity of the injected serum cholinesterase fades away after several days the previous sensitivity to suxamethonium subsequently reappears. An examination of the family of patient No. 7 revealed the following pedigree (Fig. 1). Patients, and the members of their families who exhibit a genetically determined variant of serum cholinesterase, are given a medical certificate stating that should they ever require anaesthesia with suxamethonium, prolonged apnoea is to be expected, due to their atypical serum cholinesterase.

Serum cholinesterase is a stable protein. Preparations kept in a refrigerator for 3 years at $+ 8°$ C do not lose efficacy. The danger of infection with homologous serum hepatitis is practically nonexistent because of the manufacturing procedure used by the Behring industry.

REFERENCES

Kalow, W., Genest, K. and Staron, N. (1957): *Canad. J. Biochem.*, *35*, 339.
Goedde, H. W., Altland, K. and Scholler, K. L. (1967*a*): *Med. Klin.*, *62*, 1631.
Goedde, H. W., Doenicke, A. and Altland, K. (1967*b*): *Pseudocholinesterasen, Pharmakogenetik, Biochemie, Klinik*. Springer Verlag, Berlin – Heidelberg – New York.
Goedde, H. W., Held, K. and Altland, K. (1968): *Molec. Pharm.*, *4*, 274.

The influence of repeated relaxation on muscular strength

M. KJELLBERG and T. TAMMISTO

Department of Anaesthesia, Helsinki University Central Hospital, Helsinki, Finland

Occasionally patients must be anaesthetized for a reoperation shortly after reversal of a neuromuscular block with anticholinesterases. If muscle relaxants are to be used in the second anaesthesia as well, their action is probably altered through the residual effects of anticholinesterases and muscle relaxants given during the first operation. Since information on this complex interaction seems to be scanty, we studied muscle relaxation in patients recurarized 15 min after reversing the first block with various doses of neostigmine.

METHODS

The series comprised 15 healthy women who were operated on for varicose veins under N_2O/O_2-relaxant-analgesic anaesthesia. Atropine (0.01 mg/kg), pethidine (1 mg/kg) and promethazine (25–50 mg) were given for premedication. Anaesthesia was induced with 200–300 mg of thiopental and maintained with N_2O/O_2 (70/30%) using frequent doses of fentanyl (0.05–0.1 mg) for analgesia. In some patients thiopental and droperidol were also given for supplementation. Muscle relaxation was monitored by measuring the force of thumb adduction caused by indirect stimulation of the ulnar nerve. The ulnar nerve was stimulated through bare needles placed subcutaneously on the ulnar nerve at the elbow and wrist. Supramaximal square wave stimuli of 0.1 msec duration were delivered at a rate of 0.25 Hz from a specially built stimulator. In addition the fade in the train of 4 twitches at 1 Hz was used as an indicator of muscle paralysis. The interval between single stimuli and the train of 4 was at least 10 sec. The force of the twitches was measured with a Grass FT-03 force transducer and recorded on a Sanborn 322 dual amplifier.

Care was taken to ensure that the adduction occurred in the axis of movement of the transducer. A slight preload was applied to the transducer.

The mode of administration of drugs is shown in Figure 1. After ascertaining the stability

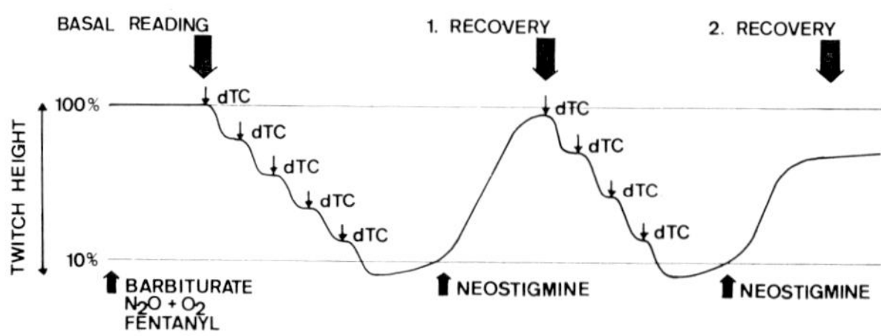

Fig. 1. *The mode of administration of drugs.*

of the control readings (usually observed during 2–3 min) dTC was given in 5 mg doses at 5-min intervals until the twitch height was less than 10% of the control. The patients were then intubated and connected to an infrared CO_2 analyzer. The end-tidal CO_2 values were kept around 5%.

When the twitch height again reached the 10% level neostigmine together with atropine was given. The procedure was repeated 15 min after the neostigmine dose. The patients were divided into 3 homogenous groups of 5 each (Table 1) and given neostigmine, 0.75 mg, 1.5 mg or 3.0 mg on both occasions.

Table 1. *Characteristics of the patients in the 3 groups (mean ± SE)*

Neostigmine (mg)	Age (yrs)	Weight (kg)	Length (cm)
0.75	42 ± 3.9	63 ± 4.5	167 ± 3.6
1.5	43 ± 5.8	63 ± 4.2	161 ± 4.0
3.0	38 ± 8.6	66 ± 5.8	168 ± 1.3

RESULTS

The amount of dTC needed to reduce the twitch height to less than 10% of control values varied from 15–30 mg. In the 1.5 mg group slightly more dTC had to be used – on an average 23 mg, as against 20 mg in the other 2 groups (Table 2). The first reversal with neostigmine was fairly effective in all groups, the muscular strength being above 50% of control in every patient 15 min after neostigmine. The efficacy of the reversal was clearly dose-dependent (Table 3).

Table 2. *The amount of d-tubocurarine needed to cause a 90% reduction in the twitch tension before and after neostigmine*

Neostigmine (mg)	dTC (mg) needed	
	Before neostigmine	After neostigmine
0.75	20 (15–30)	15 (10–20)
1.5	23 (20–30)	20 (15–25)
3.0	20 (15–25)	21 (15–25)

Table 3. *Muscular strength, 15 min after 3 doses of i.v. neostigmine, given in percentages when assessed by using single twitches or fade in the train of 4 twitches*

Mode of assessment	0.75 mg	1.5 mg	3.0 mg
Twitch tension	77 ± 4.6	86 ± 8.6	99 ± 5.3
Train of 4	60 ± 3.0	70 ± 6.4	87 ± 5.7

The reversal seemed to be about 15% less effective when fade in the train of 4 stimuli was used as an indicator. This is in accordance with the findings of others that the registered degree of muscle blockage depends upon the frequency of stimulation, a tetanic stimulation at 200 Hz being the most sensitive indicator of muscle relaxation. In our study the available force transducer, Grass FT-03 did not, however, allow a reliable registration of forces caused by tetanic stimulation. The presented values therefore serve only as a relative indicator of the degree of muscle relaxation. Since the fade in the train of 4 is a more sensitive indicator, it will be used hereafter.

Less dTC was needed for re-relaxation after 0.75 mg and 1.5 mg of neostigmine, whereas after 3.0 mg rather more dTC was needed than for the first relaxation (see Table 2).

When the need for dTC for recurarization was plotted against the efficacy of the first reversal, no clear correlation was found (Fig. 2). It therefore seems that the greater demand for dTC after 3.0 mg neostigmine depends upon the antagonism between neostigmine and dTC rather than upon the better recovery after the first relaxation in this group.

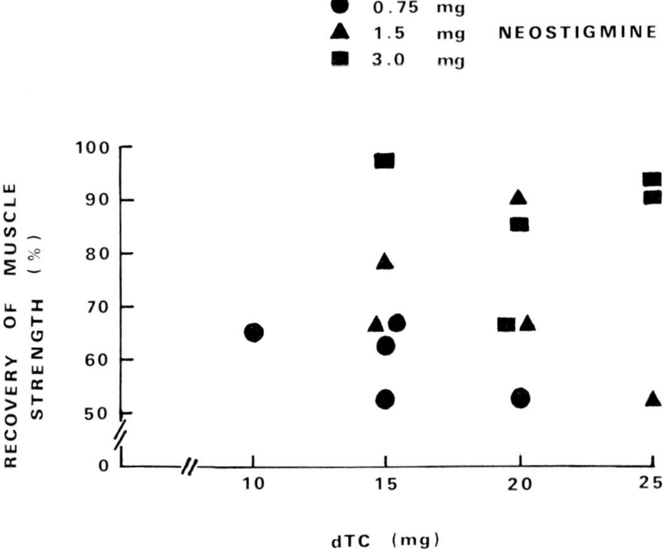

Fig. 2.   *Amount of d-tubocurarine needed for recurarization plotted against the muscular strength after the first reversal.*

The second reversal was less effective in all groups than the first one (Table 4). There was no dose-dependence; on the contrary the reversal seemed to be least effective after 3.0 mg of neostigmine. In this group the lowest individual value was 17%. This probably depends upon the increase in the total dose of dTC and thus upon increased plasma levels and retarded redistribution from the synaptic cleft. Additional administration of neostigmine (1.0–1.5) in the 0.75 mg neostigmine group increased the muscular strength to 68% in 5 min. On the other hand, the poor reversal in the 3.0 mg neostigmine group is in

Table 4.   *Muscular strength, assessed by using fade in the train of 4 twitches, 15 min after the first and second dose of i.v. neostigmine*

Neostigmine (mg)	Muscular strength (%) 15 min after	
	Neostigmine (1st dose)	Neostigmine (2nd dose)
0.75	60 ± 3.0	44 ± 3.8
1.5	70 ± 6.4	49 ± 10.0
3.0	87 ± 5.7	39 ± 5.6

accordance with the general concept that the total dose of neostigmine should not exceed 5 mg. Two patients – one after 1.5 mg and one after 3.0 mg neostigmine – showed clear signs of residual curarization in the recovery room.

The results thus indicate that under these circumstances reversal of re-relaxation may be difficult, especially if high doses of neostigmine have been used after the first operation.

In a real clinical situation it is probably more common for the interval between reversal and re-relaxation to be longer than in the present study. Consequently the effect of the first neostigmine dose has time to wear off. This probably reduces the amount of dTC needed for recurarization and makes the second reversal more effective.

Neuromuscular transmission and gentamicin

P. J. DRURY and T. E. J. HEALY

University Department of Surgery, and Department of Anaesthetic Studies,
Nottingham General Hospital, Nottingham, United Kingdom

Streptomycin, neomycin and colomycin have been shown to interfere with neuromuscular transmission in animals and in man (Pridgen, 1956; Brazil and Corrado, 1957; Perkins, 1964). Gentamicin has a similar structure to these 3 drugs and it has been suggested (Finland, 1969) that it might also affect neuromuscular transmission. Barnett and Ackerman (1969) demonstrated the potentiation of low doses of tubocurarine by gentamicin and the reversal of this effect by neostigmine. High concentrations of gentamicin have been shown to produce neuromuscular blockade in the isolated rat phrenic nerve-diaphragm preparation (Brazil and Prado-Franceschi, 1969), and furthermore, respiratory failure in rats treated with gentamicin (15.62–59.15 mg/kg) was antagonised by calcium and neostigmine. Gentamicin is frequently used in patients with a low serum calcium level associated with impaired renal function. If respiratory failure occurs in these patients it may be due to accumulation of the drug and the lowered serum calcium level (Warner and Sanders, 1971).

This study reports the effect of therapeutic concentrations of gentamicin and streptomycin on the neuromuscular junction using an isolated rat phrenic nerve-diaphragm preparation.

METHOD

The phrenic nerve and diaphragm of an adult male Sprague Dawley rat weighing 300–400 g was dissected and mounted in Krebs' solution (Bulbring, 1946). Isometric tension, developed by the muscle in response to phrenic nerve stimulation, was measured and recorded using a force transducer (Scientific Research Instrumentation) and a pen recorder (Vitatron). The phrenic nerve was stimulated with a frequency of 6 impulses/min. A voltage within the range 1.5–3.0 V was selected to produce a maximal contraction response. The temperature was maintained at 37° C by a thermocirculator (Churchill). Drugs were introduced to the preparation at 15-min intervals, and allowed to remain in contact with the preparation for 3 min and then removed by washing with Krebs' solution for 12 min.

A series of 6 investigations was carried out using the following combinations and concentrations of the drugs:

(1) gentamicin only: $5 \times 10^{-9} - 3.2 \times 10^{-4}$M (0.002 μg/ml — 0.14 mg/ml);
(2) gentamicin: $5 \times 10^{-9} - 3.2 \times 10^{-4}$M + neostigmine: 6.4×10^{-7}M (0.19 μg/ml);
(3) gentamicin: $5 \times 10^{-9} - 3.2 \times 10^{-4}$M + tubocurarine: 5.2×10^{-6}M (4.09 μg/ml);
(4) streptomycin only: $5 \times 10^{-9} - 3.2 \times 10^{-4}$M (0.003 μg/ml — 4.7 mg/ml);
(5) streptomycin: $5 \times 10^{-9} - 3.2 \times 10^{-4}$M + neostigmine: 6.4×10^{-7}M (0.19 μg/ml);
(6) streptomycin: $5 \times 10^{-9} - 3.2 \times 10^{-4}$M + tubocurarine: 5.2×10^{-6}M (4.09 μg/ml).

Each investigation was repeated using 5 preparations and a mean dose-response curve for each drug was determined. In separate experiments, the response of the preparation to either neostigmine or to tubocurarine was also determined.

The concentration of neostigmine which when used alone produced a peak increase in muscle response was used in investigations 2 and 5, and the concentration of tubocurarine which when used alone produced approximately 40% reduction in muscle response was used in investigations 3 and 6.

RESULTS

A progressive increase in the contraction response of the diaphragm was shown with increasing doses of neostigmine until a maximum response occurred with a concentration of 6.4×10^{-7}M (0.19 μg/ml) solution (p = < 0.001). High concentrations produced a progressive decrease in muscle response until no muscle contraction could be elicited in the presence of 6.6×10^{-4}M (0.2 mg/ml) neostigmine. Gentamicin produced little alteration in the muscle response at both a low dose of 5×10^{-9}M (0.002 μg/ml) and even at higher doses of 3.2×10^{-4}M (0.14 mg/ml) (Fig. 1). On the other hand streptomycin reduced the muscle response approximately 30% at the highest dose used 3.2×10^{-4}M (p = < 0.001) (Fig. 1).

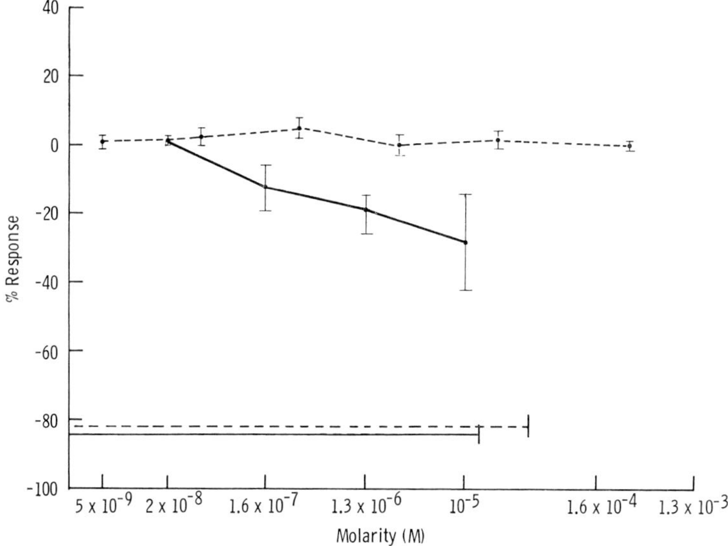

Fig. 1. *The effect of streptomycin and gentamicin on the rat diaphragm response to phrenic nerve stimulation. The accepted blood therapeutic concentrations of these drugs are indicated by the horizontal bars. (Solid line: streptomycin only; broken line: gentamicin only).*

Gentamicin in the normal clinical concentration had little effect on the muscle response to a fixed dose of 6.4×10^{-7}M neostigmine (p = > 0.9) but the increase in muscle response produced by 6.4×10^{-7}M neostigmine was reduced by streptomycin (p = < 0.01) (Fig. 2).

The reduction produced in the response of the diaphragm by tubocurarine was unaffected by gentamicin in doses which ranged from 0.002 μg/ml to 69.66 μg/ml (p = > 0.2) (Fig. 3). However, streptomycin potentiated the effect of tubocurarine (p = < 0.01) (Fig. 3).

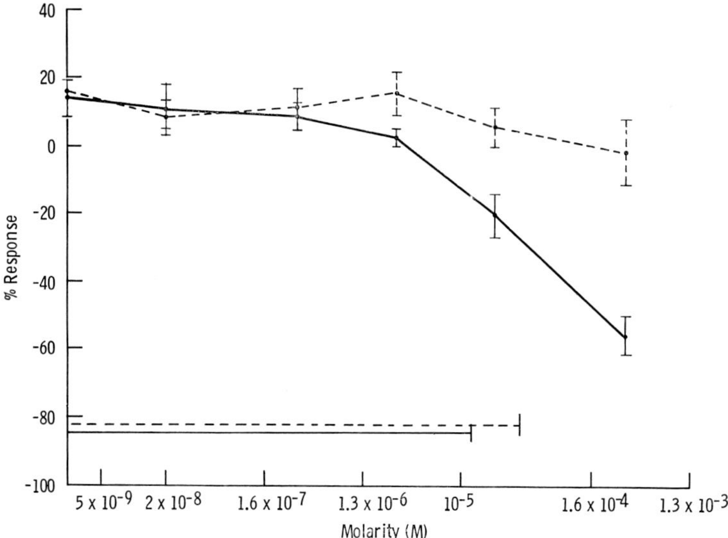

Fig. 2.   *The effect of streptomycin and gentamicin on the rat diaphragm response to phrenic nerve stimulation, in the presence of neostigmine (6.4× 10⁻⁷ M). The accepted blood therapeutic concentrations of these antibiotics are indicated by the horizontal bars. (Solid line: 6.4× 10⁻⁷ M neostigmine+streptomycin; broken line: 6.4× 10⁻⁷ M neostigmine+ gentamicin).*

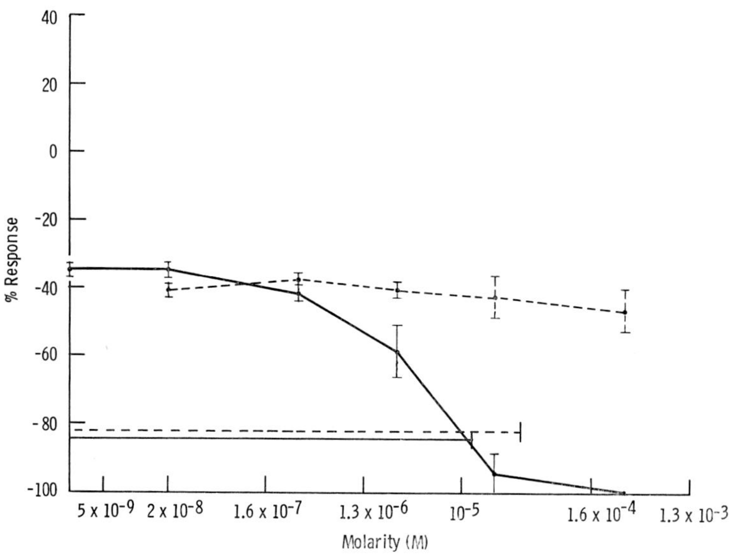

Fig. 3.   *The effect of streptomycin and gentamicin on the rat diaphragm response to phrenic nerve stimulation, in the presence of a concentration of tubocurarine that alone produced approximately 40% reduction in response. The accepted blood therapeutic concentrations of antibiotics are indicated by horizontal bars. (Solid line: tubocurarine+streptomycin; broken line: tubocurarine+gentamicin).*

DISCUSSION

In patients with renal failure, accumulation of tubocurarine and lignocaine administered at the same time as gentamicin, or of gentamicin given alone has been reported to cause prolonged neuromuscular blockade leading to respiratory failure and high concentrations of these drugs alone or interaction between them may cause blockade of neuromuscular transmission (Hall et al., 1972). However, the clinical importance of any reduction in neuromuscular transmission due to gentamicin, must be related to the concentration required for its effective action as an antibiotic.

Consequently, the isolated rat phrenic nerve-diaphragm preparation which allows the effect of known concentrations of drugs individually, or in combinations, to be studied, was selected to investigate the action of these drugs.

Brazil and Prado-Franceschi (1969), using a similar preparation, demonstrated a 20–50% inhibition of muscle response with pharmacological concentrations of gentamicin (300–500 μg/ml).

In the present study as in that of Brazil and Prado-Franceschi (1969) the higher concentrations of gentamicin (0.002 μg/ml–140 μg/ml) used greatly exceeded the accepted blood level concentrations (0–15.6 μg/ml) recommended for clinical use (Martindale, 1972).

In this study using gentamicin alone we have not detected a change in neuromuscular transmission. Neostigmine at low concentrations enhanced the muscle response to nerve stimulation and the maximum increase in muscle response was consistently produced by a concentration of 6.4×10^{-7}M.

Gentamicin did not affect the muscle response to neostigmine, nor did gentamicin potentiate the action of tubocurarine. A 6% reduction in the effect of tubocurarine by gentamicin was, however, not significant (p $= > 0.2$).

The results obtained using antibiotic concentrations of streptomycin suggest a distinct effect on neuromuscular transmission and agree with other published work (Pridgen, 1956; Brazil and Corrado, 1957; Perkins, 1964). However, the results reported using gentamicin are at variance with the literature (Barnett and Ackerman, 1969; Brazil and Prado-Franceschi, 1969; Hall et al., 1972). Nevertheless we obtained no effect using concentrations up to 9-times greater than the nephrotoxic concentration of gentamicin (15.6 μg/ml; Martindale, 1972) and up to 12-times greater than the ototoxic concentration (12 μg/ml; Wersall et al., 1969). It is recommended that the effective antibiotic concentration of gentamicin need not exceed these levels (Martindale, 1972).

These results suggest, therefore, that when gentamicin is used in effective antibiotic concentrations it has no detectable effect on neuromuscular transmission, and therefore prolonged neuromuscular blockade should not occur when tubocurarine is administered to patients already receiving gentamicin therapy.

SUMMARY

Gentamicin, in effective antibiotic concentrations, produced no detectable change in neuromuscular transmission.

REFERENCES

Barnett, A. and Ackerman, E. (1969): *Arch. int. Pharmacodyn., 181*, 109.
Brazil, O. V. and Corrado, A. P. (1957): *J. Pharmacol. exp. Ther., 120*, 452.
Brazil, O. V. and Prado-Franceschi, J. (1969): *Arch. int. Pharmacodyn., 179*, 65.
Bulbring, E. (1946): *Brit. J. Pharmacol., 1*, 38.

Finland, M. (1969): *J. infect. Dis.*, *119*, 537.
Hall, D. R., McGibbon, D. H., Evans, C. C. and Meadows, G. A. (1972): *Brit. J. Anaesth.*, *44*, 1329.
Martindale (1972): *The Extra Pharmacopoeia, 26th ed.* Editor: N. W. Blacow. Pharmaceutical Press.
Perkins, R. L. (1964): *J. Amer. med. Ass.*, *190*, 421.
Pridgen, J. E. (1956): *Surgery*, *40*, 571.
Warner, W. A. and Sanders, E. (1971): *J. Amer. med. Ass.*, *215*, 1153.
Wersall, J., Lundquist, P. G. and Bjorkroth, B. (1969): *J. infect. Dis.*, *119*, 410.

Chapter VI

Pharmacological incompatibilities and medicinal interferences in anaesthesia and resuscitation

Fundamental considerations of drug interactions

FRANCIS F. FOLDES and ANDREW F. FORBAT

Departments of Anesthesiology, Montefiore Hospital and Medical Center, and Albert Einstein College of Medicine, New York, N.Y., U.S.A.

The interaction of drugs may be based on: (1) physical, physicochemical, chemical; (2) pharmacokinetic; and (3) pharmacological reactions.

PHYSICAL, PHYSICOCHEMICAL AND CHEMICAL DRUG INTERACTIONS

The simplest form of physical drug interaction is the adsorption of drugs, for example, that of insulin to the glass container. Another not uncommon drug interaction is complex formation between multivalent cations (e.g., Ca^{++}, Mg^{++}, Al^{++}) and chelating agents (e.g., tetracycline). Mixing of alkaline and acid solutions may result in precipitation or rapid alkaline or acidic hydrolysis of certain drugs. Thus, for example, if meperidine hydrochloride which has an acid pH is mixed with thiopental sodium which has an alkaline pH, precipitation occurs. The mixing of succinylcholine chloride with thiopental sodium results in the rapid alkaline hydrolysis and inactivity of the former. Salt formation may also occur between an acidic drug, such as heparin, and a basic drug, such as protamine. All these reactions may result in the partial or total inactivation of drugs.

PHARMACOKINETIC DRUG INTERACTIONS

Various pharmacokinetic drug interactions may result in the alteration of: (1) the absorption of drugs from various sites of administration; (2) the plasma binding of agents; (3) the membrane permeability of compounds; (4) the urinary excretion of drugs; and (5) the metabolism of compounds.

DRUG INTERACTIONS AFFECTING ABSORPTION FROM SITES OF ADMINISTRATION

Agents causing changes in the ionization and thereby in the membrane permeability of the drugs may increase or decrease the rate of absorption. Thus, for example, acidic drugs like salicylates are more completely ionized if the pH is elevated and therefore they are absorbed less well from the stomach in the presence than in the absence of antacids when they are less well ionized. Ionization, however, is not necessarily the most important determinant of the rate of absorption. Other factors, such as water or lipid solubility of the drug and surface area of the site of absorption, are also important.

Agents which delay or facilitate the emptying time of the stomach and the motility of the gastrointestinal tract also have a profound effect on the absorption of orally administered drugs. Thus for example, narcotic analgesics or antimuscarinic drugs (e.g., atropine) which slow the emptying of the stomach, will delay the absorption and development of the therapeutic effect of compounds that are absorbed from the intestines. Cathartics, by causing a rapid elimination of the orally administered drug will also result in decreased rate of absorption. For example, unless their muscarinic effect is controlled by atropine or similar compounds, orally administered anticholinesterases used in the therapy of myasthenia gravis may interfere with their own absorption and therapeutic efficacy. Compounds with high lipid solubility may be eliminated almost completely in the presence of paraffin-type laxatives.

Drug interactions may increase or decrease the rate of absorption of drugs after parenteral administration. For example, the rate of absorption of insulin can be delayed, and thereby its action can be prolonged, by adding Zn^{++} and protamine to its solution. At the pH of the tissue, a fine precipitate is formed and the absorption of insulin from this precipitate is delayed. Similarly, adding 0.1% $ZnCl_2$ to a solution of Pitressin after injection will result in the formation of a complex consisting of ZnO, tissue protein and Pitressin after injection (Foldes, 1943). The absorption of Pitressin from this complex is so slow that diabetes insipidus patients may be controlled for 24–48 hr with a single injection. Conversely, the admixture of glucose will markedly facilitate the speed of onset and intensity of action of local anesthetic agents injected intrathecally (Foldes, 1954). The absorption of parenterally injected local anesthetic agents can also be delayed and thereby their duration of action prolonged and their systemic toxicity decreased by the admixture of low concentrations of vasopressors.

Various agents can increase or decrease the rate of absorption of other agents administered through the lung. Thus, for example, narcotics and sedatives which depress alveolar ventilation rate will diminish, and CO_2 which increases alveolar ventilation rate will facilitate the absorption of inhalation anesthetic agents. Similarly, agents causing bronchiolar constriction (e.g., histamine, anticholinesterases, β-adrenergic blocking agents) will inhibit, and those causing bronchial dilatation (e.g., isoproterenol) will increase absorption from the lung. An interesting aspect of drug interaction affecting absorption from the alveoli is the second gas effect. It was demonstrated that when an anesthetic agent, for example, halothane, is administered together with a rapidly absorbing gas such as N_2O, the rate of absorption of the former is accelerated. The increased rate of absorption was attributed to an increased rate of inflow of gases from the trachea due to the subatmospheric pressure created in the alveoli (Epstein et al., 1964) and also to the increase in the concentration of the first gas (e.g., halothane) by the rapid absorption of the second gas (Stoelting and Eger, 1969).

Interactions affecting plasma binding

Drugs absorbed into the circulation are partly adsorbed to plasma proteins and partly are present in free form. As much as 95% of neostigmine present in the plasma may be bound to serum albumin (Foldes and Smith, 1966). The reversible binding of drugs to plasma proteins is important because only the free drug is capable of reaching its site of action, and therefore the intensity of drug action of reversibly acting drugs depends primarily on the concentration of its free form in the plasma. The gradual release of the bound fraction is important from the point of view of the duration of action of drugs. Plasma binding depends on: (*a*) the number of binding sites and (*b*) the relative affinity of the drug to the binding site. With low drug concentrations, the affinity, and at high concentrations, the drug concentration is the primary determining factor of protein binding. The pH of the drug is also important. In general, drugs which are weak bases, are bound to numerous low affinity sites and their displacement by other drugs is relatively unimportant. Weak acids, however, are usually bound to less numerous high affinity sites which are easily saturated and thereby can be displaced by other drugs with higher affinity to these sites. Thus, for example, the oral antidiuretic tolbutamide can be displaced by the anticoagulant bishydroxycoumarin; thus, combined administration of the two drugs may result in severe hypoglycemia. Conversely, tolbutamide may displace bishydroxycoumarin and the increased anticoagulant activity may cause severe internal bleeding. In general, decreased concentration of serum albumin (e.g., malnutrition, liver disease, nephrosis) increases the concentration of the free plasma level and thereby the toxicity of high affinity drugs.

Interactions affecting membrane permeability

Decreased pH causes hypercapnia or ammonium chloride decreases ionization and thereby increases the blood-brain permeability of weak acids, such as barbiturates, and thereby increases their effect. Hyperventilation or alkalinization has the opposite effect. Conversely, the absorption of weak bases is influenced in the opposite direction by pH changes. Local anesthetics which are weak bases are less well ionized in alkaline media and thereby penetrate nerve membranes better than in acid solutions. After penetrating the membranes, at the prevailing neutral pH of the interior of the nerve fiber, they become more ionized and exert their activity in their cationic form (Ritchie and Ritchie, 1968).

Interactions affecting urinary excretion

Urinary excretion of drugs is influenced by: (*a*) renal blood flow and glomerular filtration; (*b*) tubular absorption; (*c*) tubular excretion; and (*d*) urinary pH and the pKa of the drug in question. In general, water soluble polar compounds are excreted primarily by glomerular filtration, lipid soluble non-polar compounds primarily by active tubular transport. Polar compounds are less likely to be reabsorbed into the tubules than lipid soluble compounds. High urinary pH increases the ionization and thereby decreases the reabsorption and facilitates the excretion of weak acids. In contradistinction, low pH increases ionization and decreases reabsorption of weak bases. Consequently, alkalinization will increase the excretion of weak acids like barbiturates or salicylates and acidification of the urine will increase the excretion of basic drugs such as amphetamines. These considerations are useful in the treatment of intoxication with acid or alkaline compounds.

Since most general anesthetic agents decrease renal blood flow and/or glomerular filtration rate, the urinary excretion of drugs is usually decreased during and after general anesthesia. Urinary excretion of drugs can be increased by diuretics which increase the glomerular filtration (e.g., mannitol) or interfere with tubular reabsorption (e.g., mercurial diuretics or benzothiazides). Blocking of tubular transport by specific drugs (e.g., probenecid) may interfere with the excretion of certain other compounds (e.g., penicillin).

Interactions affecting drug metabolism

Various drugs can accelerate or inhibit the metabolism of other drugs and also their own metabolism. Acceleration of the activity of the microsomal enzymes of the liver has great clinical significance. Drugs such as phenobarbital, aminopyrine, tranquillizers, antihistamines, antidiabetics, antiinflammatory drugs and even such commonly used agents as nicotine, alcohol and coffee increase the metabolism of other compounds. This phenomenon is commonly referred to as 'enzyme induction'. Thus, for example, induction of the microsomal enzyme activity of the liver by pentobarbital increases the rate of metabolic transformation of bishydroxycoumarin and this in turn will cause a decrease of the prothrombin time toward normal levels.

Increased rate of metabolic transformation of drugs usually decreases pharmacological activity and increases urinary excretion rate of the compound. The reason for this is that the metabolic breakdown products of drugs are usually more polar than the parent compound and thereby filtered more rapidly through the glomeruli and reabsorbed to a lesser extent through kidney tubules. On occasion, however, drug metabolism may result in the production of pharmacologically more active (e.g., demethylation of codeine to morphine) or more toxic (e.g., oxidation of parathion to paraoxon) metabolites. The toxic metabolic breakdown products of halogenated inhalation anesthetic agents have considerable clinical significance.

The hydrolysis of the aromatic substrates of plasma cholinesterases (e.g., procaine) can also be accelerated by tertiary amines (e.g., narcotic analgesics) and simple quaternary ammonium compounds (Erdös et al., 1959). This, however, has little or no clinical significance.

The activity of drug metabolizing enzymes can also be inhibited by certain drugs. SKF-525 (β-diethylamino-ethyl-diphenylpropylacetate) is an experimentally widely used enzyme inhibitor. Clinically used compounds such as morphine, meperidine, diethyl ether and chloramphenicol may also have significant inhibitory effects on the microsomal enzymes of the liver.

Deliberate inhibition of plasma cholinesterase activity by hexafluorenium has been utilized to potentiate and prolong the desired neuromuscular blocking activity, and minimize the unwanted side effects of succinylcholine (Foldes et al., 1960a, b). Irreversible inhibition of this enzyme in patients with irreversible organophosphorus type cholinesterase inhibitors may result in marked prolongation of the desired and undesired effect of succinylcholine (Pantuck, 1966).

Monoamine oxidase inhibitors may interfere with the metabolism of sympathomimetic amines, narcotic analgesics and barbiturates and cause an increase in the desired pharmacological and especially the undesired toxic effects of these compounds.

PHARMACOLOGICAL INTERACTIONS

To obtain a pharmacological effect, it is necessary to reach an effective drug concentration at specific receptors, usually large protein molecules, and thereby stimulate or depress physiological mechanisms dependent on the action of physiological transmitters. The site of action of these drugs may be the active centers of the receptor, at which the physiological substances act, or they may be absorbed to other sites on the receptor, to so-called allosteric sites. Interaction at such allosteric sites may change the configuration of the receptor in a way that changes the absorption of the physiological transmitters to the receptor. Such changes are usually referred to as conformational changes.

Drugs acting at the same receptor sites as the physiological transmitter may form reversible or irreversible complexes with the receptor. Compounds forming reversible complexes with the receptor may mimic the effect of the physiological transmitter. An example of this mechanism is the interaction of succinylcholine or decamethonium with the cholinergic receptor of the end-plate. Other compounds which become adsorbed to the same receptor site as the physiological transmitter, may be inert and their pharmacological effect is due to prevention of the adsorption of the physiological transmitter to the receptor. This mechanism is called 'competitive inhibition' (e.g., the adsorption of d-tubocurarine to cholinergic receptors). Some drugs form irreversible complexes with the receptor and permanently destroy it (e.g., irreversible organophosphate type cholinergic inhibitors). Yet another group of compounds acting at the same site of the same receptor may have partial intrinsic, agonistic and partial competitive, antagonistic effects. These compounds are called agonist-antagonists. A good example of these are the agonist-antagonist type narcotic antagonists in some of which the antagonistic (e.g., nalorphine) and in some the agonistic (e.g., pentazocine) effect predominates.

The effect of different drugs acting on physiological functions dependent on more than one transmitter mechanism may be additive or greater than additive (potentiation). Thus, for example, the combined effect of atropine and β-adrenergic stimulants on the heart rate, or the combined effect of certain antibiotics or inhalation anesthetic agents and nonpolarizing relaxants may be greater than the sum of the individual effects of these drugs.

Certain drugs influence the pharmacological effect of other drugs by changing the physiological 'milieu intérieur.' Thus, for example, anticholinesterases may increase the acetylcholine concentration and monoamine oxidase inhibitors, the catecholamine concentration at their respective receptor sites. Conversely, serotonin acts by decreasing the available concentration of sympathomimetic amines. Other drugs may act by lowering the concentration of essential ions. A good example of this is the potassium depletion caused by diuretics and mineralocorticoids.

CONCLUSIONS

The number of different drugs administered to surgical patients before and during hospitalization and in the course of anesthesia and surgery is steadily increasing. Therefore it is essential that the anesthesiologist be familiar not only with the pharmacological actions, but also with the desirable and undesirable interactions of drugs. It is one of the most important functions of the anesthesiologist to obtain an accurate 'drug history' at the time of the preoperative visit and to plan the anesthetic management and base the choice of anesthesia on the information obtained. In the choice of agents to be used for the production of anesthesia he should not only attempt to avoid unfavorable drug interactions, but whenever possible try to take advantage of drug combinations with desirable interactions. While many technical details of anesthetic management may be safely delegated to well-trained and supervised technicians, the supervision of preanesthetic preparation and the choice of anesthesia must remain the domain of the knowledgeable anesthesiologist.

Addendum

Limitations of time and space did not permit a more thorough discussion of this important topic. Those interested in obtaining further information on various aspects of drug interactions are referred to review articles and monographs by Goldstein (1949), Albert (1952), Veldstra (1956), Ariëns (1957), Brodie and Erdös (1962), Ariëns and Simons (1963), Binns (1964), Furchgott (1964), Remmer (1962), MacGregor et al. (1965), Milne (1965), Pletscher (1966), Morelli and Melmon (1968), Gravenstein (1968), Jenkins (1968), Ward (1968), Prescott (1969), Goldstein et al. (1969), Hunninghake (1970), Weiner (1970), Ghoneim (1971), LaDu et al. (1971), Hansten (1971), Viars and Seebacher (1971).

REFERENCES

Albert, A. (1952): *Pharmacol. Rev., 412*, 136.
Ariëns, E. J. and Simonis, A. M. (1963): *Arch. int. Pharmacodyn., 141/1*, 309.
Ariëns, E. J. et al. (1957): *Pharmacol. Rev., 9/2*, 218.
Binns, T. B. (1964): *Absorption and Distribution of Drugs.* Williams and Wilkins Co., Baltimore, Md.
Brodie, B. B. and Erdös, E. G. (Eds.) (1962): *Proceedings, First International Pharmacological Meeting, Stockholm, 1961, Vol. 6.* Pergamon Press, London – Oxford – New York – Toronto.
Epstein, R. M. et al. (1964): *Anesthesiology, 25/3*, 364.

Erdös, E. G. et al. (1959): *Biochem. Pharmacol.*, *2/1*, 97.

Foldes, F. F. (1943): *J. clin. Invest.*, *22/4*, 499.

Foldes, F. F. (1955): In: *Proceedings, Third Congress of the Scandinavian Society of Anesthesiologists, Copenhagen, 1954*, p. 143. Aarhus Stiftsbogtrykkerie AIS, Aarhus.

Foldes, F. F. and Smith, C. J. (1966): *Ann. N.Y. Acad. Sci.*, *135/1*, 287.

Foldes, F. F. et al. (1960a): *J. Pharmacol. exp. Ther.*, *129/4*, 400.

Foldes, F. F. et al. (1960b): *Anesthesiology*, *21/1*, 50.

Furchgott, R. F. (1964): *Ann. Rev. Pharmacol.*, *4/1*, 21.

Ghoneim, M. M. (1971): *Canad. Anaesth. Soc. J.*, *18/4*, 353.

Goldstein, A. (1949): *Pharmacol. Rev.*, *1/1*, 102.

Goldstein, A. et al. (1969): *Principles of Drug Action. The Basis of Pharmacology.* Harper and Row, New York, N.Y.

Gravenstein, J. S. (1968): *Int. Anesthesiol. Clin.*, *6*, 33.

Hansten, P. D. (1971): *Drug Interactions.* Lea and Febiger, Philadelphia, Pa.

Hunninghake, D. B. (1970): *Postgrad. Med.*, *47/1*, 71.

Jenkins, L. C. (1968): *Canad. Anaesth. Soc. J.*, *15/2*, 111.

La Du, B. N. et al. (1971): *Fundamentals of Drug Metabolism and Drug Disposition.* Williams and Wilkins Co., Baltimore, Md.

MacGregor, A. G. et al. (1965): *Proc. roy. Soc. Med.*, *58* (*Suppl.*), 943.

Milne, M. D. (1965): *Proc. roy. Soc. Med.*, *58* (*Suppl.*), 961.

Morelli, H. F. and Melmon, K. L. (1968): *Calif. Med.*, *109/5*, 380.

Pantuck, E. J. (1966): *Brit. J. Anaesth.*, *38/5*, 406.

Pletscher, A. (1966): *Pharmacol. Rev.*, *18/1*, 121.

Prescott, L. F. (1969): *Lancet*, *2*, 1239.

Remmer, H. (1962): In: *Proceedings, First International Pharmacological Meeting, Stockholm, 1961, Vol. 6*, p. 235. Pergamon Press, London – Oxford – New York – Toronto.

Ritchie, J. M. and Ritchie, B. R. (1968): *Science*, *162/20*, 1394.

Stoelting, R. K. and Eger II, E. I. (1969): *Anesthesiology*, *30/3*, 273.

Veldstra, H. (1956): *Pharmacol. Rev.*, *8/3*, 339.

Viars, P. and Seerbacher, J. (1971): *Les Interférences Médicamenteuses.* Librairie Arnette, Paris.

Waud, D. R. (1968): *Pharmacol. Rev.*, *20/1*, 49.

Weiner, M. (1970): *New Engl. J. Med.*, *283/16*, 871.

Advantages and disadvantages of drug interaction in anesthesia

J. S. GRAVENSTEIN

Department of Anesthesiology, University Hospitals, Cleveland, Ohio, U.S.A.

Many drugs used in anesthesia are weak acids (e.g. barbiturates) and weak bases (e.g. local anesthetics and vasopressors). These drugs ionize, are bound to proteins, and are broken down by enzymes. Hence, changes in ionization, protein binding, and enzymatic breakdown can alter their effectiveness. Advertently or inadvertently the physician can modify these physicochemical characteristics, and thus alter the effects of such drugs. A hypothetical case may illuminate the principles involved.

CHANGE OF DRUG EFFECT THROUGH A CHANGE IN pH

A patient in diabetic ketoacidosis is admitted to the emergency room with an arterial pH of 7.0, a P_{CO_2} of 40 Torr, and a standard bicarbonate of 9.6 mEq/l. The patient is known to have taken secobarbital daily and recently a suicidal overdose. This explains his inadequate respiratory response to metabolic acidosis and his profound somnolence. On the electro-cardiogram, frequent multifocal ventricular extrasystoles are seen.

The treatment plan includes: (*a*) Respiratory support with oxygen. (*b*) Insulin and fluids as dictated by blood glucose and electrolyte measurements. (*c*) Intravenous lidocaine to combat the potentially dangerous arrhythmias. (*d*) Diuresis and alkalinization of the urine to accelerate the excretion of secobarbital.

Let us now examine the effect of the change in pH on the action of lidocaine, secobarbital, and their renal excretion. We will have to examine three facets of this problem, namely:
1. The hydrogen ion concentration.
2. pH effect on ionization of weak acids and bases.
3. The pH effect on protein binding.

Hydrogen ion concentration

Hydrogen ions are usually expressed in terms of pH values, an awkward system because it forces us to use a logarithmic scale which expresses the hydrogen ion concentration so that high pH values reflect low hydrogen ion concentrations and low pH values are indicative of a high hydrogen ion concentration. We need to dwell on this so that we can deal with these issues easily.

The following scale shows pH values in the upper and the concentration of hydrogen ions in nanomoles per liter in the lower scale.

pH	4	5	6	7	8	9	10
$[H^+]$ nmol	100,000	10,000	1000	100	10	1	0.1

One nanomole (nmol) equals 1×10^{-9} or 0.000000001 moles. As is true for all logarithmic scales each step on the pH scale is associated with a 10-fold change on the hydrogen ion scale. The patient with an arterial pH of 7.0 therefore has 100 nmol of hydrogen ions per liter of plasma, while at pH 8.0 it would be 10 nmol $[H^+]$.

pH effects on ionization of weak acids and bases

Without deriving the formula, we can write the Henderson-Hasselbalch equation which is commonly used to discuss acid-base balance. It states:

$$pH = pK_{(acid)} + \log \frac{\text{ionized weak acid}}{\text{unionized weak acid}}$$

Anesthesiologists are familiar with this expression for the carbonic acid system where certain assumptions permit the following formulation:

$$7.4 = 6.1 + \log \frac{24 \text{ mEq/l bicarbonate } (= \text{ionized weak acid})}{40 \text{ Torr } P_{CO_2} \times 0.03 \ (= \text{unionized weak acid})} .$$

When pH equals pK, i.e. when

$$6.1 = 6.1 + \log \frac{\text{bicarbonate}}{P_{CO_2} \times 0.03} ,$$

the logarithmic expression on the right must become zero. This occurs when there is as much ionized as unionized weak acid present, or:

$$6.1 = 6.1 + \log \frac{1}{1} ,$$

i.e. the pK is that pH at which 50% of a weak acid is ionized.

What we have said for weak acids also applies to weak bases, except that the formula now reads

$$pH = pK_{(base)} + \log \frac{\text{unionized weak base}}{\text{ionized weak base}} .$$

As we shall see, all of this becomes quite important for the discussion of our patient since:

(*a*)   Many drugs are weak acids (secobarbital) or weak bases (lidocaine).

(*b*)   Changing the pH and with it the degree of ionization can alter the effectiveness of such drugs by:

(i) Affecting the ease with which the drug can penetrate into a cell or across a lipid membrane. Highly ionized drugs cannot readily cross lipid membranes.

(ii) Affecting the rate of its renal excretion which increases with ionization.

(iii) Affecting the degree of its protein binding.

The pH effect on ionization is particularly pronounced when the pK of the compound lies close to the physiologic pH. This can easily be shown in the following tabulation where pH is changed and the pK of two different weak acids are 7.4 and 9.2, respectively. Note that the log expression is actually a ratio term so that units of concentration would cancel out.

These examples demonstrate vividly that:

(*a*) Every time we change pH by 0.3 units (e.g. from 7.4 to 7.1) we also alter by 0.3 units the logarithmic expression on the right:

$$\log \frac{\text{ionized weak acid}}{\text{unionized weak acid}} .$$

Table 1. *Weak acid*

[H$^+$] in nmoles	pH $=$ pK$_a$ $+$ log $\dfrac{\text{ionized}}{\text{unionized}}$	pH $=$ pK$_a$ $+$ log $\dfrac{\text{ionized}}{\text{unionized}}$
160	$6.8 = 7.4 + \log \dfrac{0.25}{1}$	$6.8 = 9.2 + \log \dfrac{0.004}{1}$
80	$7.1 = 7.4 + \log \dfrac{0.5}{1}$	$7.1 = 9.2 + \log \dfrac{0.008}{1}$
40	$7.4 = 7.4 + \log \dfrac{1}{1}$	$7.4 = 9.2 + \log \dfrac{0.016}{1}$
20	$7.7 = 7.4 + \log \dfrac{2}{1}$	$7.7 = 9.2 + \log \dfrac{0.03}{1}$
10	$8.0 = 7.4 + \log \dfrac{4}{1}$	$8.0 = 9.2 + \log \dfrac{0.06}{1}$
5	$8.3 = 7.4 + \log \dfrac{8}{1}$	$8.3 = 9.2 + \log \dfrac{0.125}{1}$
2.5	$8.6 = 7.4 + \log \dfrac{16}{1}$	$8.6 = 9.2 + \log \dfrac{0.25}{1}$
1.25	$8.9 = 7.4 + \log \dfrac{32}{1}$	$8.9 = 9.2 + \log \dfrac{0.5}{1}$
0.6	$9.2 = 7.4 + \log \dfrac{63}{1}$	$9.2 = 9.2 + \log \dfrac{1}{1}$
0.5	$9.3 = 7.4 + \log \dfrac{80}{1}$	$9.3 = 9.2 + \log \dfrac{1.25}{1}$

(*b*) With every change of 0.3 units, we change the represented quantity by a factor of 2: [H$^+$] ion concentration falls by half from 80–40 as pH rises from 7.1–7.4 while the ratio ionized/unionized doubles from $\dfrac{0.004}{1}$ to $\dfrac{0.008}{1}$ as the logarithmic expression $6.8 = 9.2 - 2.4$ is changed to $7.1 = 9.2 - 2.1$.

(*c*) A full unit change on the logarithmic scale represents a 10-fold change in the quantity expressed, e.g.,

$$\text{pH } 8.3 = 5 \text{ nmol [H}^+\text{]}$$
$$\text{pH } 9.3 = 0.5 \text{ nmol [H}^+\text{]}.$$

(*d*) While any given change of pH will cause a proportional change in the ratio of ionized/unionized weak acids, the overall change is large if the pH change occurs close to the pK value of the weak acid; it is small if the pH change is far removed from the pK. Consider two examples from Table 1 for pK$_a$ 7.4, and pK$_a$ 9.2. At pH 7.4 the former is 50% ionized, the latter 1.6%. Raising pH from 7.4 to 7.7 will change this to 67% and 2.9% respectively. While the absolute amount of the ionized fraction was approximately doubled in both instances, in one instance (50% → 67%) much more drug was converted from unionized to ionized than in the other (1.6% → 2.9%).,

(*e*) Until now, we have discussed only weak acids. However, the same principles apply to weak bases, except that the ratio ionized/unionized is reversed.

$$\text{pH} = \text{pK}_{\text{(base)}} + \log \frac{\text{unionized weak base}}{\text{ionized weak base}} .$$

When we increase the pH of solutions containing weak bases the ionized fraction will decrease, whereas it will increase in the case of weak acids.

We can now return to our patient. As we treat him and his arterial pH moves from 7.0 to 7.4 both lidocaine and secobarbital will change in their degree of ionization. For lidocaine, a weak base with a pK of 7.9, we can calculate (compare with Table 1):

$$\text{pH } 7.0_{\text{(pH pat. blood)}} = 7.9_{\text{(pK lidocaine)}} + \log \frac{0.125 \text{ lid. units unionized}}{1 \text{ lid. units ionized}}$$

$$\downarrow \qquad\qquad\qquad\qquad\qquad\qquad \downarrow$$

$$7.4 \qquad\qquad = 7.9 \qquad\qquad + \log \frac{0.32 \text{ unionized}}{1 \text{ ionized}} \; .$$

Thus, with alkalinization by 0.4 pH units we have increased the *unionized* fraction of lidocaine from 11% to 24%, a significant change.

For secobarbital the opposite change would occur, since it is a weak acid with a pK of 7.9! Here, the *ionized* fraction will have increased from 11% to 24%!

These changes are significant because the unionized fraction is usually more lipid soluble and penetrates membranes more readily than the ionized, charged fraction. The clinical effect of this feature can be demonstrated in a schematic presentation of our patient (assuming a much simplified picture) as follows:

For secobarbital (pK$_a$ 7.9) at equilibrium of the unionized fraction:

	brain		blood		urine
pH	7.0		7.0		6.7
ionized	11		11		5.6
unionized	89	→	89	→	89.0
Total	100		100		94.6

After alkalinization to arterial pH 7.4 and prior to new equilibrium:

	brain		blood		urine
pH	7.3		7.4		7.7
ionized	20		24		36.6
unionized	80	→	76	→	58.0
Total	100		100		94.6

Now the unionized fraction of secobarbital can move from brain to blood and into urine, where it becomes ionized (the urinary pH being higher than blood as bicarbonate is excreted). The ionized fraction is not reabsorbed and barbiturate is removed. For lidocaine the opposite would be true.

For lidocaine (pK 7.9) and assuming equilibrium of the unionized fraction:

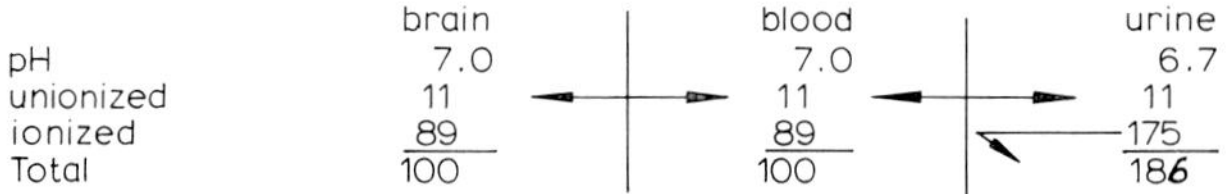

	brain		blood		urine
pH	7.0		7.0		6.7
unionized	11		11		11
ionized	89		89		175
Total	100		100		186

After alkalinization and before new equilibrium:

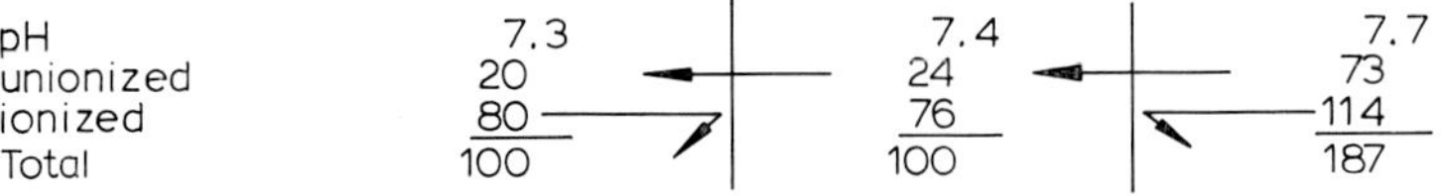

	brain		blood		urine
pH	7.3		7.4		7.7
unionized	20		24		73
ionized	80		76		114
Total	100		100		187

Thus, alkalinization would not favor the removal of the weak base, lidocaine, via the urine. Indeed, it would, in our example, facilitate the movement of lidocaine into the central nervous system and into cells!

In addition to the consideration of the distribution of the ionized and the unionized drug, we have to consider their effectiveness. Barbiturates are effective in their unionized form. For local anesthetics much evidence suggests that it is the ionized form that is pharmacologically active, but it is the unionized form that reaches the effector site. Thus, alkalinization would favor a decrease in drug effect at the effector site for both of these agents. It would facilitate renal excretion of the weak acid, secobarbital, while working against renal excretion of lidocaine, a weak base.

Lidocaine (and other local anesthetics) in the unionized form might more easily diffuse to the effector site where some part of the drug, depending on the pH, ionizes and exerts its action.

The pH effect on protein binding

One additional feature of drug disposition may be influenced by the $[H^+]$ ion concentration. This is the degree of binding of the drug to proteins. For secobarbital (as incidentally also for d-tubocurarine) binding is said to increase as pH is raised (Eger, 1974). The protein bound fraction of the drug is not available for diffusion to the effector site. It constitutes a silent and pharmacologically inactive depot. Any enhancement of binding would reduce the drug effect for secobarbital. Conversely, giving another drug that is also highly bound might displace some of the barbiturate from its binding site and increase toxicity. Many examples of these mechanisms have been reported in the literature, admittedly not as yet related to anesthesia.

SUMMARY

In summary, as we begin appropriate treatment and reverse the acidosis, this patient will show interesting pharmacologic effects. Alkalinization will cause the barbiturates to be ionized in urine and to be excreted more rapidly in this form. The ionized barbiturate will be pharmacologically less active. If we institute a diuresis along with this alkalinization of urine, removal of the barbiturate from the patient will be hastened.

Protein binding of the barbiturate may also increase as pH is raised so that another mechanism will remove barbiturate from the central nervous system by binding it to silent receptors in the plasma and possibly to other proteins.

Increasing the pH will have different effects for the action of lidocaine. The renal excretion of lidocaine will be slowed but the pharmacologically effective ionized form will decrease with increasing pH. On the other hand, the drug will penetrate tissue more readily.

Alkalinization of course also causes a shift of sodium and potassium across the cell membrane of the heart and may thus contribute to a decrease in irritability concurrent with a decrease in sympathetic activity. The arrhythmias may therefore disappear not only because of the administration of lidocaine, decreased effectiveness of barbiturates, a redistribution of potassium across the membrane but also because of a reduction in sympathetic overactivity.

ENZYME INDUCTION

The final factor in this complex picture deals with enzyme induction. The patient has been taking secobarbital for weeks. He can be assumed to have an increased activity of his P_{450} system and hence metabolize many different agents more rapidly than comparable patients not exposed to enzyme inducers. In the acute situation described here, enzyme induction may not be of clinical significance. Many cases, however, have been described where drugs and hormones were less effective in the patient with an actively induced microsomal enzyme system.

Microsomal enzymes are quite nonspecific and this may lead to different problems. Thus, unexpected toxic reactions have been observed in diabetic patients who were receiving tolbutamide and dicumarol simultaneously. Both of these drugs are metabolized by liver microsomes and hence the two drugs may interfere with each other if they happen to be substrates for the same enzyme. The hypoglycemic action of tolbutamide, in the specific example, was increased when dicumarol was given. At the same time the effect of dicumarol would be enhanced because of competition from tolbutamide for metabolism by the microsomal enzyme system.

CONCLUSION

Anesthesiologists frequently administer many drugs and many of their patients already are under the influence of several different pharmacologic agents when they come to the operating room. In the preceding pages, I have attempted to show how a simple shift in pH can cause a significant alteration in the effectiveness, distribution and excretion of such common drugs as barbiturates and local anesthetics. It is easily imagined how such an interaction between sodium bicarbonate and these agents can be employed advantageously or how it may work out to the disadvantage of the patient. We know relatively little about the effects of protein binding in the anesthetic circumstances but begin to realize that some local anesthetics, such as bupivacaine, are highly bound. Because they are potentially displaceable from their protein binding sites in plasma, they can become toxic unexpectedly. Enzyme induction is now well recognized and we must appreciate that many of our patients have a certain degree of microsomal stimulation due to exposure to insecticides, many other drugs, and contaminants in our industrialized society.

We must be alert and can anticipate many new problems as well as potential advantages which the interaction of drugs will bring for our patients.

REFERENCES

Eger II, E. I. (1974): *Anesthetic Uptake and Action*. Williams and Wilkins Co., Baltimore, Md.
Gravenstein, J. S. (1974): In: *ASA Refresher Courses in Anesthesiology, 1974, Vol. 2*, p. 97. Editor: S. G. Hershey. J. B. Lippincott Co., Philadelphia, Pa.
Gravenstein, J. S. and Anton, A. H. (1971): In: *Clinical Anesthesia, Vol. 3*, p. 199. Editor: L. W. Fabian. F. A. Davis Co., Philadelphia, Pa.

The interactions of neuromuscular blocking agents with anesthetic and adjuvant drugs

FRANCIS F. FOLDES and ANDREW F. FORBAT

Departments of Anesthesiology, Montefiore Hospital and Medical Center, and
Albert Einstein College of Medicine, New York, N.Y., U.S.A.

The interactions of anesthetic and adjuvant drugs with neuromuscular blocking agents (muscle relaxants; MR) has great clinical significance. Because of this, the understanding of the biochemical and pharmacological basis of these interactions is essential for the safe conduct of anesthesia. Limitations of space do not allow the in-depth coverage of this important topic. For this reason the ensuing discussion will be primarily concerned with those aspects of the interactions of MR and anesthetic and adjuvant drugs which have practical clinical importance.

THE INTERACTION OF DEPOLARIZING AND NONDEPOLARIZING MUSCLE RELAXANTS

The different types of depolarizing and nondepolarizing MR have additive effects (Foldes, 1957). The combined use of different depolarizing MR may be indicated when decamethonium bromide (Syncurine) or hexamethylene-1,6-bis-carbamoylcholine bromide (Imbretil) are used for the maintenance of muscular relaxation during abdominal surgery. On these occasions SCh (Anectine) may be used to facilitate peritoneal closure. Different nondepolarizing MR may be employed if the side effects of either the muscle relaxant or the anesthetic agents used make this advisable. Thus, for example, if the administration of d-Tc (Tubarine) causes histamine release or severe ganglionic blockade, the maintenance of muscular relaxation may be continued with corresponding doses of gallamine triethiodide (Flaxedil) or pancuronium bromide (Pavulon). Conversely, if gallamine or pancuronium causes tachycardia, then the maintenance of muscular relaxation may be continued with d-Tc.

The interaction of depolarizing and nondepolarizing MR depends on the sequence and duration of administration and the relative dosage of the two types of agents. In general, single doses of depolarizing and nondepolarizing MR will mutually antagonize each other (Torda et al., 1967). Thus, for example, small, subparalytic doses of nondepolarizing MR will prevent the rapid depolarization caused by neuromuscular (NM) blocking doses of depolarizing agents (Foldes et al., 1957). The intravenous administration of 3 mg of d-Tc, 20 mg of gallamine, 2 mg of diallylnortoxiferine or 0.6 mg of pancuronium 2–3 min before the intravenous injection of SCh used for the facilitation of endotracheal intubation had been recommended for the prevention of fasciculations and muscular twitching, potassium loss (Mayrhofer, 1958) and the postanesthetic muscle pain (Katz and Katz, 1966) encountered after the intravenous administration of SCh. Under these circumstances, however, 2–3 times larger doses of SCh are required to produce comparable conditions for endotracheal intubation. Rapid depolarization of the NM junction and its consequences can usually be eliminated by the slow intravenous administration of moderate doses of SCh (0.6 mg/kg injected over 30 sec). Consequently, the minor advantages that may be obtained by the preliminary administration of nondepolarizing MR do not warrant the assumption of the risks associated with this technique. If it is essential to avoid rapid depolarization of the endplate and the use of long-acting nondepolarizing MR is contraindicated, then the combined administration of 0.3 mg/kg hexafluorenium bromide (Mylaxen) and small (0.2 mg/kg) doses of SCh (Foldes et al., 1960) is the technique of choice.

The use of SCh to facilitate peritoneal closure in patients in whom relaxation was maintained with nondepolarizing MR, is seldom indicated. The very large doses of SCh required to produce muscular relaxation in the presence of seemingly noneffective doses of nondepolarizing MR (Foldes et al., 1957) may cause serious complications. This technique should not be employed unless the last dose of a nondepolarizing agent had been administered at least 90–120 min earlier.

The prolonged administration of depolarizing MR, for example SCh in continuous intravenous infusion, may cause tachyphylaxis, necessitating the continuous increase of the rate of administration of SCh. At the same time when tachyphylaxis develops to depolarizing MR, there is increased sensitivity to nondepolarizing compounds. The decreased sensitivity to depolarizers and the increased sensitivity to nondepolarizers is characteristic of the development of a phase II block (Foldes et al., 1957). The development of the phase II block may lead to desensitization of the endplate (Thesleff, 1955) that may cause prolonged NM block at the termination of surgery (Foldes, 1966). When, in the course of anesthesia, increasing requirements of depolarizing agents indicate the development of endplate desensitization, it is advisable to stop the administration of the depolarizing agents and continue the maintenance of anesthesia with nondepolarizing MR.

INTERACTION OF NEUROMUSCULAR BLOCKING AGENTS AND ANTICHOLINESTERASES

Anticholinesterases antagonize the NM effects of nondepolarizing MR; potentiate the phase I block caused by depolarizing agents (Castillo and DeBeer, 1950); may or may not antagonize the phase II depolarization block (Foldes, 1959); and consistently increase the intensity and duration of action of MR hydrolyzed by plasma cholinesterase (e.g., SCh) (Foldes et al., 1960).

Antagonism of the NM effects of nondepolarizing MR depends primarily on the inhibition of the hydrolysis of ACh at the NM junction. The accumulated ACh will competitively displace the nondepolarizing MR from the endplate receptors. The displaced MR is carried away by the circulation and thereby NM transmission is reestablished. Because of the competitive nature of the reaction the NM block is more easily reversed, at lower concentrations of MR at the NM junction (Baraka, 1967). For this reason the reversal of residual curarization should be delayed as long as possible, preferably until the start of the suturing of the skin. In addition to their inhibitory effect on the hydrolysis of ACh, anticholinesterases, especially edrophonium, also have a direct depolarizing effect on the postjunctional membrane. This may also contribute to the reversal of the residual nondepolarization block.

Although many of the characteristics of phase II block are similar to those of nondepolarization block (Foldes et al., 1957), their residual effect cannot be reliably terminated in all instances by anticholinesterases. A possible explanation for the failure of the reversibility of phase II block by anticholinesterases is end-plate desensitization (Thesleff, 1955).

The inhibitory effect of anticholinesterases on the hydrolysis of SCh by plasma cholinesterase has been utilized for the maintenance of prolonged muscular relaxation by the combination of small doses of SCh and hexafluorenium bromide (Mylaxen) (Foldes et al.,

1960). This technique has the following advantages: (*a*) because of the slight curare-like action of hexafluorenium (Foldes et al., 1960) and the small doses of SCh required, there is no rapid depolarization of the end-plate, no muscular fasciculation or twitching, the release of potassium is inhibited and the incidence and severity of postoperative muscle pain is significantly decreased; (*b*) tachyphylaxis to SCh and end-plate desensitization do not develop; (*c*) since the total amount of SCh used (30–60 mg/hr) is small, there is no danger of prolonged apnea due to the accumulation of succinylmonocholine (Foldes et al., 1956). The small initial dose of SCh also prevents the development of excessively prolonged apnea in patients who have atypical plasma cholinesterase (Foldes et al., 1963). At the termination of anesthesia, the NM block will wear off reliably, in most cases within 15–25 min after the administration of the last dose of SCh without the need for any antagonist. This technique was found to be especially useful for the maintenance of muscular relaxation during surgery in patients with end-stage kidney disease (e.g., removal of kidneys before renal transplant).

INTERACTIONS OF NEUROMUSCULAR BLOCKING AGENTS AND ANESTHETIC DRUGS

Inhalation anesthetic agents

Many inhalation anesthetic agents increase the NM blocking action of nondepolarizing and occasionally also that of depolarizing MR. The mechanism of this potentiation is complex, not completely clarified and often controversial. The degree of potentiation depends on the type and concentration of the inhalation anesthetic agent. Because of differences in experimental conditions (e.g., the concentration and the duration of inhalation of the agent) evaluation of the relative potentiating effects of the various inhalation anesthetic agents is difficult from published data. It seems that of the clinically used inhalation anesthetic agents, ether, enflurane (Ethrane) and isoflurane (Forane) are the most effective. After 30–60 min inhalation of 5–9% ether in oxygen or in nitrous oxide/oxygen, both the intensity and duration of action of 0.05–0.1 mg/kg d-Tc was doubled (Katz, 1966). The potentiating effect of ether on the NM effects of SCh was less and variable in different subjects. One to 2% halothane (Fluothane) also increased the intensity and duration of the d-Tc induced NM block (Katz and Gissen, 1967). Other studies (Lebowitz et al., 1970; Walts and Dillon, 1970) indicate that during the inhalation of less than 2% enflurane or about 5% ether, 8 mg/m² body surface d-Tc caused complete NM block in 95 and 65% of patients respectively. Five to 10% recovery occurred in 66 ± 29 min in the enflurane and in 30 ± 11 min in the ether group. During the inhalation of equipotent concentrations (1.25 MAC) of enflurane and halothane, 1.7 mg/m² and 5.6 mg/m² d-Tc respectively, caused a 50% decrease of twitch tension. In other words, the potentiating effect of enflurane was about 3.3 times greater than that of halothane (Miller et al., 1971).

It appears from the available experimental data and clinical experience that in comparable anesthetic concentrations, ether enflurane and isoflurane have the greatest potentiating effect on nondepolarizing MR. Fluroxene (Fluoromar), methoxyflurane (Penthrane), halothane, cyclopropane and trichloroethylene also potentiate the effects of nondepolarizing relaxants especially that of d-Tc. Few controlled studies have been reported on the potentiating effect of inhalation anesthetic agents on other nondepolarizing relaxants (e.g., gallamine (Foldes et al., 1961) or pancuronium (Katz, 1971)). Clinical experience, however, indicates that inhalation anesthetic agents also depress the NM effects of other nondepolarizing MR, although to a lesser extent.

Because of the potentiation of MR by most inhalation anesthetic agents, with the exception of nitrous oxide/oxygen, the dose of MR must be appropriately reduced when used with these agents. The degrees of reduction will depend on the potentiating effect of the inhalation anesthetic agent in question. As already mentioned, the potentiating effect of ether, enflurane and isoflurane is the greatest and even in moderately deep planes of anesthesia induced with these agents the dose of d-Tc should be reduced to one third to one half of the amount used with various forms of balanced anesthesia. Since the potentiating effect of inhalation anesthetic agents depends on their partial pressure, the degree of relaxation can be regulated by deepening or lightening the plane of anesthesia. If the level of anesthesia is lightened immediately after peritoneal closure, then usually no antagonist will be required at the end of anesthesia for the reversal of residual curarization. With inhalation agents that potentiate nondepolarizing MR to a lesser extent (e.g., halothane, fluorexene, methoxyflurane, cyclopropane and trichloroethylene) and/or are excreted more slowly (e.g., methoxyflurane) it is usually necessary to reverse residual NM block at the termination of surgery. Because of the smaller doses of muscle relaxants required with inhalation anesthetic agents, not only is it necessary to use little or no antagonist at the termination of surgery, but the side-effects (e.g., histamine release, bradycardia, tachycardia, hypotension, hypertension), that may be associated with the use of muscle relaxants, will also be diminished.

When inhalation anesthetic agents and nondepolarizing MR are to be used together, they should be so selected that the side-effects of one should counteract those of the other. For example, with halothane, which has a tendency to produce bradycardia, the MR of choice is gallamine (Foldes et al., 1961) or pancuronium (Foldes et al., 1971) which have a tendency to produce tachycardia. In contrast, with ether which frequently produces tachycardia, the agent of choice is d-Tc. Ether, by its catecholamine releasing effect will also tend to antagonize the pharmacological effects of the histamine liberated by d-Tc.

Ganglionic blocking agents

Hexamethonium bromide (Bistrium) increases the effect of nondepolarizing MR and antagonizes the effects of depolarizing MR (Paton and Zaimis, 1949); trimethaphan (Arfonad) potentiates most depolarizing and nondepolarizing MR (Eckenhoff, 1955). In view of this, the dose of both depolarizing and nondepolarizing MR should be reduced when trimethaphan is used for the production of controlled hypotension.

Antibiotics

Streptomycin (Brazil and Corrado, 1957), neomycin (Mycifradin) (Pittinger et al., 1958), kanamycin (Kantrex) (Mullet and Keats, 1961), and other antibiotics (Pittinger, 1966) have NM blocking activity. The NM blocking activity of antibiotics is potentiated by ether (Sabawala and Dillon, 1959). The intraperitoneal or intravenous administration of antibiotics with NM activity at the end of surgery, at the time when the clinically discernible residual effects of NM have worn off, may cause recurarization and prolonged respiratory depression (Benz et al., 1961).

The NM effects of most, but not all (e.g., polymyxin B (Adamson et al., 1960)) antibiotics are antagonized by Ca^{++} (Corrado, 1963) and/or neostigmine (Brazil and Corrado, 1957). The NM effect of antibiotics have been attributed to the inhibition of the ACh releasing effect of Ca^{++} (Brazil and Corrado, 1957). Because of this, for the reversal of the NM effects of antibiotics Ca^{++} (0.5–1.0 g calcium chloride or 1.0–2.0 g calcium gluconate intravenously) should precede the administration of a neostigmine-atropine mixture. Occasionally larger doses of Ca^{++} may be required. Because of its potentially dangerous cardiac effects Ca^{++} must be administered slowly, preferably under continuous EKG monitoring. If reasonable doses of Ca^{++} and neostigmine fail to reverse the NM block, patients should be mechanically ventilated and, if necessary, the effects of these compounds on the residual NM block, be tested several hours later.

SUMMARY AND CONCLUSION

Numerous drugs used before, during, and/or after anesthesia may influence both the desired and undesired effects of muscle relaxants. For this reason, it is essential that the anesthesiologist be aware of the effects of these compounds and their combinations with neuromuscular blocking agents on neuromuscular transmission. Knowledge of the interaction of these drugs with neuromuscular blocking agents is essential for the selection and the optimal administration of the most suitable muscle relaxant.

REFERENCES

Adamson, R. H. et al. (1960): *Proc. Soc. exp. Biol. (N.Y.)*, *105/3*, 494.
Baraka, A. (1967): *Brit. J. Anaesth.*, *39/11*, 891.
Benz, H. G. et al. (1961): *Brit. med. J.*, 2, 241.
Brazil, O. V. and Corrado, A. P. (1957): *J. Pharmacol. exp. Ther.*, *120/4*, 452.
Castillo, J. C. and DeBeer, E. J. (1950): *J. Pharmacol. exp. Ther.*, *99/4*, 458.
Corrado, A. P. (1963): *Anesth. Analg. Curr. Res.*, *42/1*, 1.
Eckenhoff, J. E. (1955): *Surg. Clin. N. Amer.*, *35/6*, 1579.
Foldes, F. F. (1957): *Muscle Relaxants in Anesthesiology*, p. 40. Charles C. Thomas, Springfield, Ill.
Foldes, F. F. (1959): *Anesthesiology*, *20/4*, 464.
Foldes, F. F. (1966): In: *Clinical Anesthesia: Muscle Relaxants*, Vol. 2, Chapter 1, p. 1. Editor:
  F. F. Foldes. F. A. Davis Co., Philadelphia, Pa.
Foldes, F. F. et al. (1956): *Anesth. Analg. Curr. Res.*, *36/6*, 609.
Foldes, F. F. et al. (1957): *Anesth. Analg. Curr. Res.*, *36/5*, 23.
Foldes, F. F. et al. (1960): *Anesthesiology*, *21/1*, 50.
Foldes, F. F. et al. (1961): *Anesth. Analg. Curr. Res.*, *40/6*, 629.
Foldes, F. F. et al. (1963): *Anesthesiology*, *24/2*, 208.
Foldes, F. F. et al. (1971): *Anesthesiology*, *35/5*, 496.
Katz, R. L. (1966): *Anesthesiology*, *27/1*, 52.
Katz, R. L. (1971): *Anesthesiology*, *35/6*, 602.
Katz, R. L. and Gissen, A. J. (1967): *Anesthesiology*, *28/3*, 564.
Katz, R. L. and Katz, G. J. (1966): In: *Clinical Anesthesia: Muscle Relaxants*, Vol. 2, Chapter 7,
  p. 121. Editor: F. F. Foldes. F. A. Davis Co., Philadelphia, Pa.
Lebowitz, M. H. et al. (1970): *Anesthesiology*, *33/1*, 52.
Mayrhofer, O. (1959): In: *Proceedings, I International Symposium on Curare-like Agents, Venice,
  1958*, p. 376. Istituto Tipografico Editoriale S. Nicolo, Lido-Venice.
Miller, R. D. et al. (1971): *Anesthesiology*, *35/1*, 38.
Mullett, R. D. and Keats, A. S. (1961): *Surgery*, *49/4*, 530.
Paton, W. D. M. and Zaimis, E. J. (1949): *Brit. J. Pharmacol.*, 4, 381.
Pittinger, C. B. et al. (1958): *Anesth. Analg. Curr. Res.*, *37/5*, 276.
Pittinger, C. B. (1966): In: *Clinical Anesthesia: Muscle Relaxants*, Vol. 2, Chapter 6, p. 95. Editor:
  F. F. Foldes. F. A. Davis Co., Philadelphia, Pa.
Sabawala, P. B. and Dillon, J. B. (1959): *Anesthesiology*, *20/5*, 659.
Thesleff, S. (1955): *Acta physiol. scand.*, *34/2 and 3*, 218.
Torda, T. A. G. et al. (1967): *Anesthesiology*, *28/6*, 1010.
Walts, L. F. and Dillon, J. B. (1970): *Anesth. Analg. Curr. Res.*, *49/1*, 17.

Biological and pharmacological changes and the actions of digitalis and antiarrhythmic drugs

F. NICOLAS

Département d'Anesthésie-Réanimation, UER de Médecine, Nantes, France

I. BIOLOGICAL AND PHARMACOLOGICAL CHANGES OF DIGITALIS ACTIVITY

There are several practical applications of this information with which it is useful for anesthetists to be familiar. The treatment of acute digitalis poisoning, the control of digitalis therapy, the anesthetic management of the digitalized patient and in discussion about prophylactic digitalization are examples.

BIOLOGICAL CHANGES

Digitalis and electrolytes

The part played by potassium, sodium and calcium shifts in myocardial automaticity, conduction and contractility and the part played by magnesium in membrane ATPase activity explain the effects of alterations of electrolytes. Cardiac glycosides have an action on myocardial properties by means of changes in the ATPase activity and cellular permeability. Digitalis activity may be modified by ionic alterations.

Potassium
Depletion of body potassium stores sensitizes the myocardium to the toxic action of digitalis (Lown et al., 1960). When 5–10% of a dog's total body potassium has been removed and when the serum concentration has been lowered to 2 mEq/l, only 40% of the normal toxic dose of digitalis is required to produce severe ventricular arrhythmias. A rise in extracellular potassium restores the activity of the enzymatic transfer of the cationic pump which is altered by digitalis and reduces the digitalis-induced hyperautomaticity of the myocardium. The changes in the effects of digitalis due to corticoids and diuretics result mainly from potassium depletion.

Calcium
Calcium and digitalis act synergistically to increase contractility (Lown, 1960). This synergism is not used practically to induce cardiotonic effects of digitalis because of the fear of enhancing its toxic effects (Lown, 1960). Intravenous calcium infusions were a cause of digitalized patients' death (Somylo, 1960). EDTA chelation may be useful in the treatment of digitalis intoxication (Soffer et al., 1960; Somylo, 1960).

Magnesium
Magnesium depletion decreases the dose of digitalis required to induce ventricular arrhythmia. Magnesium administration restores the situation.

Digitalis and acid-base balance

Acidosis increases tolerance to digitalis and alkalosis decreases it (Schaffer et al., 1960; Bliss et al., 1963). It is agreed that alterations of tolerance to digitalis due to acidifying of alkalizing drugs are linked to potassium and particularly to variations of serum potassium concentration more than to the changes of pH.

Digitalis and hypoxia

Hypoxia increases cardiac automaticity and sensitizes the myocardium to digitalis toxicity (Williams et al., 1968; Harrison et al., 1968).

Digitalis and hypothermia

Hypothermia increases tolerance to digitalis. This has been demonstrated by Crismon and Elliot (1947) in the rat, Angelakos et al. (1958) in the dog, Szekely and Wynne (1960) and Akhtar et al. (1971) in the cat. The positive inotropic effects of digitalis are decreased under hypothermia (Szekely and Wynne, 1960).

PHARMACOLOGICAL INTERACTIONS

Among the numerous interactions which occur between digitalis and drugs used for anesthesia or intensive care, some are beneficial, others are not. The problem is complex for a given combination since it can be beneficial from one point of view (for instance, heart muscle contraction) and noxious from another (for example, ventricular fibrillation).

General anesthetics

Several works indicate that digitalis toxicity is reduced by halothane (Morrow and Townley 1964; Morrow, 1967*b*), by methoxyflurane (Ivankovic, 1972) as well as by ketamine and Innovar (Ivankovic, 1972). On the other hand, digitalis toxicity is increased by cyclopropane (Morrow, 1967*b*, 1970) and not altered by pento- and penthiobarbital (Morrow, 1970).

Muscle relaxants

Succinylcholine
Dowdy and Fabian (1963) indicate that in fully digitalized patients having electrocardiographic evidence of digitalization, succinylcholine can induce serious ventricular arrhythmias with a frequency higher than in nondigitalized patients. These manifestations were reproduced experimentally in the dog (Dowdy et al., 1965; Dowdy and Fabian, 1963). In man and in the dog, serious arrhythmias caused by the combination of digitalis and succinylcholine can be efficiently treated with large doses of d-tubocurarine (15–30 mg for an adult patient) However, some authors claim that statistically significant clinical differences do not exist between the incidence of arrhythmias after succinylcholine administration in digitalized and nondigitalized patients.

d-Tubocurarine
According to Dowdy et al. (1965) d-tubocurarine in normal dosage can prevent arrhythmias due to cardiac glycosides and increases myocardial tolerance to digitalis. In practice it seems reasonable to avoid using succinylcholine and to prefer d-tubocurarine in the

preoperative period. The new muscle relaxant drugs have not been studied from this point of view.

Anticholinesterase drugs

Edrophonium injection in digitalized patients produces more or less serious arrhythmias (Pitt and Kurland, 1966). Ivankovic et al. (1971), in dogs receiving normal doses of ouabain, showed a decrease of auriculoventricular conduction greater than in control dogs; but the doses of succinylcholine used in this experiment (0.15 mg/kg) are different from those used in anesthetic practice.

Sympathomimetic drugs

The additive effect of digitalis and catecholamines on automaticity and positive inotropism are well-known (Becker et al., 1962; Morrow, 1967*a*).

Glucagon

Recently some authors stressed the modifications of digitalis toxicity under the influence of glucagon (Cohn et al., 1970; Einzig et al., 1971). With glucagon it is possible to prevent arrhythmias produced by toxic doses of digitalis without reducing contractility. This is a drug of great promise for the treatment of the digitalis induced arrhythmias.

Digitalis effect on the action of anesthetics

For the anesthetist, alterations caused by digitalis on the action of general anesthetics are not less important than those on the action of digitalis during anesthesia. Digitalis can prevent cardiac failure induced by pentobarbital in the dog or in a heart lung preparation (Boniface and Brown, 1953; Vick et al., 1957). Goldberg et al. (1962) emphasized the beneficial effect of previous digitalization with digoxin on myocardial depression due to thiopental (45–60 mg/kg) in the dog. Goldberg et al. (1962) and Shimosato and Etsten (1963) demonstrated the increase of the heart contractile force during halothane anesthesia in digitalized dogs compared to control dogs.

In conclusion, in spite of much work the interaction between digitalis therapy and drugs used for anesthesia and intensive care is not very clearly defined. Many theoretical expectations or experimental results are waiting for clinical confirmation. It is sometimes difficult to discern what is really important among all the data. However it seems that the increase of digitalis toxicity under the influence of succinylcholine, anticholinesterase drugs, sympathomimetic drugs, hypokalemia and calcium infusions are important and the potentiation of conduction changes due to digitalis by antiarrhythmic drugs may also be important. Evidence for beneficial effects of interaction between digitalis and drugs used for anesthesia and intensive care is rare and their practical utilization is limited.

II. INTERACTIONS BETWEEN ANTIFIBRILLATORY AGENTS AND DRUGS USED FOR ANESTHESIA AND INTENSIVE CARE

CARDIOVASCULAR SYSTEM

All the antifibrillatory drugs have an antidepressive action on the heart contractile force and on conduction. Every anesthetic drug with identical properties increases these effects.

Interactions between β-blocking drugs and anesthetics have been studied recently. β-blocking drugs were found to be effective in preventing myocardial hyperexcitability provoked by increased endogenous and exogenous catecholamines during anesthesia. Potentiation exists between bradycardia due to propranolol and neostigmine and it is essential not to give neostigmine before atropine to a patient treated with propranolol (Johnstone, 1966). Indeed reciprocal antagonism exists between bradycardia produced by β-blocking drugs and tachycardia induced by atropine and gallamine. Cardiac arrest can result from the association between β-blocking agents and halothane. More often this combination provokes marked hypotension due to the decrease of cardiac output essentially linked to bradycardia. The decrease of systolic blood flow is not very important in the patient with a normal heart (Iwatsuki et al., 1966; Sharma, 1967; Stephen et al., 1971). Previous atropinization largely prevents excessive hypotension. The hypotension obtained by associating halothane and propranolol may be used for controlled hypotension (Johnstone, 1966). This technic must be used very carefully since it is based upon a decrease of cardiac output associated with peripheral vasoconstriction from which some organs can suffer. In pathological hearts, the potentiation of myocardial depressive effects of propranolol by anesthetics can lead to disaster (Merin, 1972). Interaction between barbiturates and β-blocking drugs also leads to bradycardia and decrease in arterial pressure, cardiac output and myocardial contractile force (Shanks, 1966). This occurs despite previous atropinization (Nayler et al., 1969; Shanks, 1966) and seems to be due to sympathetic blockade and lack of catecholamine release during anesthesia.

OTHER SYSTEMS

Quinidine potentiates the neuromuscular blocking effects of some muscle relaxants. Several workers (Grogogno, 1963; Schmidt et al., 1963; Boere, 1964; Way et al., 1967; Cuthbert, 1966; Miller et al., 1967) have demonstrated the return of neuromuscular paralysis after the injection of quinidine in patients previously paralysed with suxamethonium or d-tubocurarine but not with gallamine. The prolongation of paralysis with d-tubocurarine also occurred following other antifibrillatory drugs. β-blocking agents are the most important for useful and noxious interactions with drugs used during anesthesia and intensive care. Sleep caused by barbiturates is longer with concomitant administration of β-blocking drugs. Interactions between β-blocking agents and inhalation anesthetics are of great interest. Boissier et al. (1968) demonstrated that every inhalational anesthetic provoked bronchospasm in guinea pigs previously treated with propranolol (1 mg/kg). According to the authors this bronchospasm is due to direct action of the anesthetic drug on the bronchial muscle previously sensitized by β-adrenergic blockade.

Pharmacologically an interaction between central analgesic drugs and β-blocking agents with regard to the bronchoconstrictive effects can be foreseen, since the bronchoconstrictive effects of narcotic analgesics are due to β-blocking effects (Roquebert et al., 1966) as well as to cholinergic effects, histamine release or to direct effects on bronchial muscles (Viars and Guidicelli, 1968). This theoretical interaction was confirmed in a personal case (Nicolas et al., 1972). Finally, among the most interesting interactions of β-blocking drugs is the potentiation of hypoglycemic effects of insulin by β-blocking agents so that hypoglycemia is possible if a β-blocking agent is given in an emergency to a patient receiving insulin therapy.

To sum up, interactions between antifibrillatory drugs and anesthetics cause more harmful effects than benefit especially if the antifibrillatory drug is a β-blocking agent. Antifibrillatory drugs should be reserved for emergency use in anesthesia, that is for severe arrhythmias due to ventricular hyperautomaticity due to the increased catecholamines which occur mainly under halogenated anesthesia. In patients who received β-blocking drugs preoperatively, several authors (Shand et al., 1970; Connolly et al., 1970) suggest that this therapy should be stopped 24–36 hr before operation.

REFERENCES

Akhtar, M., Chakravarti, A. N., Sarkar, A. K. and Wahi, P. L. (1971): *Indian J. med. Res.*, *59/1*, 58
Angelakos, E. T., Torres, J. and Driscoll, M. S. (1958): *Amer. Heart J.*, *56/3*, 458.
Aroesty, J. M. and Cohen, J. (1966): *Amer. Heart J.*, *71/4*, 503.
Becker, D. J., Nonkin, P. M., Bennett, L. D., Kimball, S. G., Sternberg, M. S. and Wasserman, F. (1962): *Amer. J. Cardiol.*, *10/2*, 242.
Bliss, H. A., Fishman, W. E. and Smith, P. M. (1963): *J. Lab. clin. Med.*, *62/1*, 53.
Boniface, K. J. and Brown, J. M. (1953): *Anesthesiology*, *14/1*, 23.
Boere, L. A. (1964): *Anaesthesist*, *13/11*, 368.
Boissier, J. A., Giudicelli, J. F., Viars, P. and Larno, S. (1968): *Thérapie*, *23/4*, 827.
Butler, V. P. (1972): *Acquis. nouv. Path. Cardiovasc.*, *14/6*, 631.
Cohn, K. E., Agmon, J. and Gamble, O. W. (1970): *Amer. J. Cardiol.*, *25/6*, 683.
Connolly, M. E., Paterson, J. T. and Dolley, C. T. (1970): *Clin. Sci.*, *38*, 10.
Crismon, J. M. and Elliott, H. W. (1947): *Amer. J. Physiol.*, *151*, 221.
Cuthbert, M. F. (1966): *Brit. J. Anaesth.*, *38/10*, 775.
Dowdy, E. G., Duggar, P. N. and Fabian, L. W. (1965): *Anesth. Analg. Curr. Res.*, *44/5*, 608.
Dowdy, E. G. and Fabian, L. W. (1963): *Anesth. Analg. Curr. Res.*, *42/4*, 501.
Einzig, J., Todd, E. P. and Nicoloff, D. M. (1971): *Circulat. Res.*, *29*, 88.
Erlig, D. and Mendez, A. (1963): *Fed. Proc.*, *22*, 184.
Faulkner, S. L. and Hopkins, J. T. (1973): *New Engl. J. Med.*, *289/12*, 607.
Goldberg, A. H., Maling, H. M. and Gaffney, T. E. (1961): *Anesthesiology*, *22/6*, 974.
Goldberg, A. H., Maling, H. M. and Gaffney, T. E. (1962): *Anesthesiology*, *23/2*, 207.
Grogogno, A. W. (1963): *Lancet*, *2*, 1039.
Harrah, M. D., Way, W. L. and Katzung, B. G. (1970): *Anesthesiology*, *33/4*, 406.
Harrison, D. C., Robinson, M. D. and Kleiger, A. E. (1968): *Amer. J. med. Sci.*, *256/6*, 352.
Hilmi, K. I. and Regan, T. J. (1968): *Amer. Heart. J.*, *76/3*, 365.
Ivankovic, A. D. (1972): *Anesth. Analg. Curr. Res.*, *51/4*, 607.
Ivankovic, A. D., Ruggiero, R. P., El-Etr, A. A. and Kaye, M. P. (1971): *Anesth. Analg. Curr Res.*, *50/6*, 1079.
Iwatsuki, K., Yusa, T., Yasuda, I., Hashimoto, Y., Takahasi, K. and Iwatsuki, N. (1966): *J. exp. Med.*, *88*, 263.
Johnstone, M. (1966): *Brit. J. Anaesth.*, *38/7*, 516.
Johnstone, M. and Horsfall, B. (1966): *Acta anaesth. scand.*, *10/Suppl. 23*, 248.
Lown, B., Black, H. and Moore, F. D. (1960): *Amer. J. Cardiol.*, *6/2*, 309.
Merin, R. G. (1972): *Anesth. Analg. Curr. Res.*, *51/4*, 617.
Miller, R. D., Nay, W. L. and Katzung, B. G. (1967): *Anesthesiology*, *28/6*, 1036.
Morrow, D. H. (1967a): *Anesth. Analg. Curr. Res.*, *46/3*, 319.
Morrow, D. H. (1967b): *Anesth. Analg. Curr. Res.*, *46/6*, 675.
Morrow, D. H. (1970): *Anesth. Analg. Curr. Res.*, *49/2*, 305.
Morrow, D. H. and Townley, N. T. (1964): *Anesth. Analg. Curr. Res.*, *43/5*, 510.
Murmann, W., Almirante, L. and Saccani-Guelfi, M. (1966): *J. Pharm. Pharmacol.*, *18*, 692.
Nayler, W. G., McInnes, I., Carson, V., Swann, J. and Lowe, T. E. (1969): *Amer. Heart J.*, *77/2*, 346.
Nicolas, F. and Nicolas, G. (1973): In: *Proceedings, XXIII Congrès Français d'Anesthésie Réanimation*, *Vol. 1*, p. 209. Editor: P. Stieglitz, Masson et Cie, Paris.
Nicolas, F., Verdier, M., Baron, D. and Souron, R. (1972): *Anesth. Analg. Réanim.*, *29/2*, 253.
Perez, H. R. (1970): *Anesth. Analg. Curr. Res.*, *49/1*, 33.
Peters, M. A. (1972), *J. Pharmacol. exp. Ther.*, *181/3*, 417.
Pitt, B. and Kurland, G. S. (1966): *Amer. J. Cardiol.*, *18/4*, 557.
Roquebert, J., Canellas, J., Dumartin, A and Quintard, D. (1966): *C.R. Soc. Biol. (Paris)*, *160/8–9*, 1560.
Schafer, H. H., Whithan, H. C. and Burns, J. H. (1960): *Amer. Heart J.*, *60/3*, 388.
Schmidt, J. L., Vick, N. A. and Sadove, M. S. (1963): *J. Amer. med. Ass.*, *183/8*, 669.
Shand, D. G., Nuckolls, E. M. and Oates, J. A. (1970): *Clin. Pharmacol. Ther.*, *11/1*, 112.
Shanks, R. G. (1966): *Brit. J. Pharmacol.*, *26/3*, 322.
Sharma, P. L. (1967): *Brit. J. Anaesth.*, *39/3*, 215.
Shimosato, S. and Etsten, B. (1963): *Anesthesiology*, *24/1*, 41.

Soffer, A., Toribara, T., Moore-Jones, D. and Weber, D. (1960): *Arch. intern. Med., 106/6,* 824.

Somylo, A. P. (1960): *Amer. J. Cardiol., 5/4,* 523.

Stephen, G. W., Davie, I. T. and Scott, D. B. (1971): *Brit. J. Anaesth., 43/4,* 320.

Szekely, P. and Wynne, N. A. (1960): *Brit. Heart J., 22/5,* 647.

Talso, P. J., Remenchik, A. P. and Cutilleta, A. (1962): *Circulation, 26/4,* 794.

Vaugnan-Williams, E. M. and Sekiya, A. (1963): *Lancet, 1,* 420.

Viars, P. and Giudicelli, J. F. (1968): In: *Proceedings, XVIII Congrès Français d'Anesthésie-Réanimation, Vol. 1,* p. 74. Editor: Sfaar. Masson et Cie, Paris.

Vick, R. L., Kahn, J. B. and Acheson, G. H. (1957): *J. Pharmacol. exp Ther., 121/3,* 330.

Viljoen, J. F. and Estafanous, F. G. (1972): *J. thorac. cardiovasc. Surg.s 64/5,* 826.

Way, W. L., Katzung, B. G. and Larson Jr., C. P. (1967): *J. Amer. med. Ass., 200/2,* 153.

Williams Jr., J. F., Boyd, D. L. and Border, J. F. (1968): *J. clin. Invest., 47/8,* 1885.

Interaction of psychotropic agents with other drugs used during anaesthesia

J. W. DUNDEE

Department of Anaesthetics, The Queen's University of Belfast,
Institute of Clinical Science, Belfast, United Kingdom

Psychotropic drugs are very widely used in most countries in the world and since, like anaesthetics, they act on the brain, it is not surprising that there is a danger of their interaction with drugs used during anaesthesia. Two things increase the problem:

(*a*) Patients may have been taking tranquillisers or antidepressants for many years at home (e.g. a morning and evening tablet of diazepam) and no longer consider these worthy of mention when they come into hospital, particularly for an emergency operation. They have become part of their life-style and are not looked on as being important.

(*b*) Even today there appears to be some stigmata attached to taking psychotropic drugs and patients may deliberately withhold such information. It is not uncommon for patients to get tranquillisers or antidepressants from doctors who are not their regular medical attendants.

It is well-known that many patients collect large quantities of 'nerve tablets' and these may be taken in suicide attempts, either alone or with other sedatives or alcohol. Patients have been known to obtain tablets from relatives or neighbours for this purpose.

TYPES OF INTERACTIONS

The types of interactions which can occur between drugs given before and during anaesthesia have already been discussed and have been fully documented by Dundee and McCaughey (1972) and it is sufficient to mention that as far as an additive effect is concerned, summation, synergism and potentiation may all occur. One is not likely to encounter chemical or competitive antagonism, but both non-competitive and functional antagonism may occur.

RESISTANCE

The prolonged administration of most cerebral depressants leads to cross tolerance to other depressants and this can be induced by long-term administration of most psychotropic drugs. It is shown by the need of a larger induction dose of barbiturate and frequent injections of narcotics during balanced anaesthesia. This is very similar to what occurs in chronic alcoholics and, as in these latter patients, cerebral tolerance is not accompanied by tolerance of the cardiovascular system and large induction doses can lead to prolonged hypotension and/or respiratory depression. Perhaps enzyme induction may play a role here, particularly as far as repeated doses of drugs are concerned. Barbiturates certainly can increase the activity of hepatic microsomal or other enzymes which metabolise drugs, and not only anaesthetics but others used in the care of the surgical patient may be involved.

The prolonged administration of barbiturates decreases the action of coumarin derivatives, diphenylhydantoin, zoxazolamine and griseofulvin, while chlorcyclizine and chlorpromazine shorten the action of certain barbiturates. Barbitone, chlordiazepoxide, meprobamate, methyprylon, nitrazepam and Mandrax (methaqualone and diphenhydramine) stimulate drug metabolism but ethanol, morphine and amphetamine are inactive in this respect (Jenkins and Graves, 1965; Ballinger et al., 1971). The situation as regards the widely used diazepam is not clear, but the available evidence suggests that it is not an enzyme inducer, or if it has this property it is of no clinical importance.

The time between taking the last dose of the psychotropic drugs and the induction of anaesthesia is an important factor in determining whether resistance or sensitivity occurs. One does not always encounter tolerance in patients who are known to be taking large doses of psychoactive drugs and this may be the explanation.

INDIVIDUAL DRUGS

Historically the phenothiazines were the first effective tranquillisers and their preoperative use makes patients more susceptible to the hypotensive effect of induction agents and blood loss. They may increase the frequency of excitatory effects occurring with methohexitone and this is of particular importance in outpatient anaesthesia where depressant premedication is best avoided. Some phenothiazines, particularly perphenazine, fluphenazine and prochlorperazine may produce extrapyramidal side effects and this should be remembered when they are used as antiemetics.

The tricyclic antidepressants are chemically similar to the phenothiazines and are generally considered to be fairly safe. A leading article in the *British Medical Journal* (1971) has drawn attention to cases of EKG changes and myocardial infarction during prolonged therapy with the tricyclic antidepressants and phenothiazines. There may also be an increase in circulating catecholamines in some patients who are hypotensive and this is thought to be the main cause of these disturbances. No specific interactions with anaesthetics have been reported, but caution in the use of potentially hypotensive techniques is essential.

The monoamine oxidase inhibitor (MAOI) group of drugs are widely used as antidepressants and Jenkins and Graves (1965) estimated that in 1963 half a million people in Canada and three and a half million in the U.S.A. would have taken tranylcypromine. Their effectiveness is thought to be due to their ability to inhibit brain monoamine oxidase with a resultant increase in brain serotonin and/or noradrenaline. Their main interaction is with sympathomimetic amines – the so-called 'cheese reaction' of hypertension following ingestion of tyramine-rich cheeses. A similar effect can occur when amphetamine or ephedrine is injected and the implications of this are obvious in anaesthetic practice and should be remembered when local anaesthetics containing vasopressors are injected. This is particularly important in outpatient dental surgery. If in doubt felypressin should be used in preference to adrenaline. Another cardiovascular effect is an enhancement of the hypotensive action of thiazides and ganglion-blocking drugs.

There are a few isolated reports of prolongation of the action of pethidine in patients receiving MAOIs, and this is thought to be due to a non-specific inhibition of liver microsomal enzymes.

Iproniazid is a toxic drug and the overaction of pethidine was first described after its use (Hunter et al., 1970). It may also potentiate general anaesthetics. Tranylcypromine (which has been withdrawn from sale in some countries) is the drug most likely to augment the action of vasopressors although this could theoretically occur after phenelzine and isocarboxazid.

The enzyme inhibition by MAOIs is irreversible and their effects persist for several weeks. Cousins and Maltby (1971) have reported a hypertensive crisis occurring three weeks after stopping pargyline. When there is any doubt anaesthetists should avoid drugs which may overact in the presence of MAOIs. In an emergency small increments of pethidine can be given intravenously and the total dose estimated on the response to these.

In clinical practice MAOIs can have a very significant toxicity and may not infrequently present a threat to the life of the patient. As with many psychotherapeutic drugs it is difficult to assess their effectiveness, but it is probably not greater than that of other antidepressant drugs. For this reason current opinion is that these drugs should never be given as treatment of first choice, and probably they should be confined to treatment of hospital inpatients. There are many compounds marketed today which contain MAOIs in a mixture with other drugs and these have a variety of trade names. If in doubt, one must find their exact content before inducing anaesthesia.

The use of lithium in psychiatric practice is increasing, but it is too soon to assess its ability to interact with other drugs. However, a case is reported when there may have been an association of cyanosis and flaccidity in the newborn and the fact that the mother was being treated with lithium (Willbanks et al., 1970).

What of diazepam? It is now the most widely prescribed psychotropic drug and yet, despite this, there have been remarkably few interactions described following its use. One cannot say that it is 'trouble free' but at least it has the best record of any available drug in this respect.

REFERENCES

Ballinger, B., O'Malley, K., Stevenson, I. H. and Turnbull, M. J. (1971): *Brit. J. Pharmacol.*, *41*, 383.
Cousins, M. J. and Maltby, J. R. (1971): *Brit. J. Anaesth.*, *43*, 803.
Dundee, J. W. and McCaughey, W. (1972): In: *Recent Advances in Anaesthesia and Analgesia*, *11th ed.*, Chapter 3, p. 41. Editor: C. L. Hewer. Churchill-Livingstone, Edinburgh – London.
Hunter, K. R., Boakes, A. J., Laurence, D. R. and Stern, G. M. (1970): *Brit. med. J.*, *3*, 388.
Jenkins, L. C. and Graves, H. B. (1965): *Canad. Anaesth. Soc. J.*, *12*, 121.
Leading Article (1971): *Brit. med. J.*, *1*, 3.
Willbanks, G. D., Bressler, B., Peele, C. H., Cherny, W. B. and London, W. L. (1970): *J. Amer. med. Ass.*, *213*, 865.

The blocking action of dextromoramide on β-adrenergic receptors

J. A. GONZALEZ BERNALDEZ,[1] R. MONTERO BENZO,[1] R. ALEGRE [2] and E. TRULL BORRAS [1]

[1] Department of Anaesthesia and Reanimation, and [2] Department of Clinical Biopathology, Ciudad Sanitaria 'La Fe', Valencia, Spain

Dextromoramide is widely used in a variety of anaesthetic techniques (Bergmann, 1962; Du Cailar et al., 1959; De Castro, 1962; Mundeleer and De Castro, 1962; Kapferer, 1961; Sabathie and Danter, 1959, 1960; Sabathie, 1962a, b). It has been in use in our clinic for a long time as an ataralgesic agent and dextromoramide occupies a very important place in the field of general anaesthesia and as a sedative. Bradycardia and arterial hypotension are constant features of its use and appear to be dose-related.

Chronotropism and inotropism are inhibited by dextromoramide, which suggests that the drug has β-adrenergic effects on the myocardium.

This is a study of clinical data and electrocardiographs together with determinations of sugar and fat metabolism in order to demonstrate possible β-blocking effects. The patients had varied pathology and were pretreated only with atropine 0.5 mg i.m. an hour before operation. Venous blood samples were obtained prior to induction for blood glucose, triglycerides, glycerol, free fatty acids and cholesterol. Pulse rate, systolic and diastolic blood pressure and the ECG were recorded. These observations were repeated 10–15 min after the administration of dextromoramide 0.1 mg/kg i.v. β-adrenergic effects on the myocardium are chronotropic, dromotropic and bathmotropic, and are reversed by the action of dextromoramide. So clinically and electrocardiographically, significant slowing of the cardiac rate occurred constantly. The decrease of nervous conduction (dromotropism) is real and is seen as a slight increase of the refractory period, and electrocardiographically as a slight decrease in A-V conduction with a very slight increase in the PR interval. Systolic blood pressure is decreased after dextromoramide, indicating a negative inotropic effect and probably an antiadrenergic action to extrinsic stimulation. It is not known whether dextromoramide has inhibitory action on intrinsic contraction, i.e., a direct membrane effect.

No inhibition of the response to nervous stimulation (bathmotropism) has been observed but dextromoramide was not used in cases or disorders of myocardial conduction.

4,8 (free fatty acids – FFA) are continuously released into the circulation from adipose tissue by the action of catecholamines which is a fast reaction which involves the enzyme adenylcyclase system, identified with a β-adrenergic receptor, by increasing the 3,5 cyclic-AMP and transforming the inactive lipase into the active form, which aids lipolysis of the triglyceride (TG) in the FFA. By the same method, the inactive phosphorylase is converted into the active form, which assists the transformation of glycogen into glucose. These reactions are blocked by the adrenergic β-blockers.

Under the action of the dextromoramide there is a lipogenetic effect, and an increase of the TG. The total cholesterol and the FFA decrease. It is believed that these transformations of inactive lipase and phosphorylase into active forms, are prevented by dextromoramide which is a β-adrenergic blocking effect. The sympathetic hyperactivity in surgery (Coward and Smith, 1966; Franksson et al., 1954; Halme et al., 1957) is well known and under anaesthesia it has frequently been proposed that β-adrenergic blocking drugs should be used, for example, to prevent the cardiac effects of halothane (Johnstone, 1969; Sharma, 1969). The relationship between Pa_{CO_2} and catecholamine discharge is well known (Prys-Roberts, 1971). The use of adrenergic β-blockers has been suggested in shock (Berk et al., 1967, 1969), and used in tetanus (Nicolas, 1973).

REFERENCES

Bergmann, H. (1962): *Anaesthesist, 11*, 109.

Berk, J. L., Hagen, J. F., Beger, W. H., Dochat, G. R. and La Pointe, R. (1967): *Surg. Gynec. Obstet., 125*, 311.

Berk, J. L., Hagen, J. F., Beger, W. H. and Dochat, G. R. (1969): *Ann. Surg., 169*, 74.

Björntorp, P., Olson, E. L. and Schröder, G. (1967): *Acta pharmacol. (Kbh.), 25 (Suppl. II)*, 51.

Coward, R. F. and Smith, P. (1966): *Clin. chim. Acta, 14*, 832.

Castro, J. de (1962): In: *Proceedings, I Congress of Anaesthesiology, Vienna, 1962.*

Cailar, J. du, Vernette-Durand, M., Herail, J. and Rioux, J. (1 59): *Anesth. Analg. Curr. Res., 16*, 797.

Fingers, K. F., Page, J. G. and Feller, D. R. (1966): *Biochem. Pharmacol., 15*, 1020.

Franksson, C., Gemzell, C. A. and Enler, V. S. von (1954): *J. clin. Endocr., 14*, 608.

Halme, A., Pekkarinen, A. and Turumen, M. (1957): *Acta endocr. (Kbh.), Suppl. 32*, 5.

Johnstone, M. (1969): *Brit. J. Anaesth., 41*, 130.

Kapferer, J. M. (1961): *Anaesthesist, 10*, 101.

Mundeleer, P. and J. De Castro (1962): In: *Proceedings, I Congress of Anaesthesiology, Vienna, 1962.*

Nicolas, F. (1973): *Anesth. Analg Réanim , 30*, 1.

Prys-Roberts, C. (1971): In: *Hypercapnia. General Anaesthesia, Vol. 1*, p. 171. Editors: Gray and Nunn. Butterworths, London – Sydney – Washington.

Sabathie, M. (1962*a*): *Anaesthesist, 11*, 20.

Sabathie, M. (1962*b*): *Anaesthesist, 11*, 20.

Sabathie, M. and Danter, A. (1959): *Bordeaux chir.*, April, 1959.

Sabathie, M. and Danter, A. (1960): *Anesth. Analg. Curr. Res., 17*, 186.

Sharma, P. L. (1969): *Brit. J. Anaesth., 41*, 481.

Contraceptives and pseudocholinesterase medicamental interference

J. PUENTE, M. ANIBARRO, J. BERNAT, J. CAMARASA,
J. COSTA, A. PAYA and E. PUERTO

Department of Anaesthesia-Reanimation-Maternity Centre,
Ciudad Sanitaria 'La Fe', Valencia, Spain

Eighty-six women of different ages who were taking contraceptive pills have been studied. Thirty-six had been taking them for less than a year, 26 less than 2 years and 13 less than 3 years and 9 more than 3 years. They were all having combined contraceptives with both progesterones and oestrogens. Pseudocholinesterase levels were measured and compared with a control group of 40 women. Four patients received single doses (of 1 mg/kg) of succinylcholine. Prolonged apnoea occurred in 2 patients – 25 and 65 min respectively.

The duration of contraceptive administration and the depression of pseudocholinesterase levels are related. The depression starts from the first month and continues until the third year by which time there was a very significant fall in the pseudocholinesterase level.

There was no relation between the age and the pseudocholinesterase level. The greater the body surface, the higher was the pseudocholinesterase level. In the control group there was no relationship between age and pseudocholinesterase level but the pseudocholinesterase level was lower in relation to the surface area than in the group taking contraceptives.

The indirect bilirubin varies between 3 and 10 mg/100 ml; transaminases were discretely elevated; the alkaline phosphatase was raised in a third of the cases studied; bromsulphthalein retention was increased to 21% in 80% of the cases. The 2 women with prolonged apnoea had pseudocholinesterase levels of 62 and 24; they had been taking contraceptives for 3 and 15 months respectively.

Manual ventilation was used to avoid hyperventilation or inhibition of the Hering-Breuer reflex. Premedication did not include large amounts of morphine or chlorpromazine, nor any respiratory depressant. During the apnoea which lasted 65 min nallylnormorphine was used without effect.

Haemaglobin, haematocrit and total protein were normal. Both patients had reduced serum albumin, with 'α' decreased, 'α_2' increased, 'β' decreased, 'γ' increased, and the albumin-globulin ratio almost normal. Oxygenation acid base state and serum electrolytes were all normal.

Another patient whom we anaesthetized, was an obese woman who had been taking contraceptives for 4 years but whose pseudocholinesterase level was 125. She metabolized the succinylcholine in a few seconds and it was necessary to repeat the dose in order to obtain sufficient relaxation for intubation. The apnoea may in many cases have no relation to pseudocholinesterase level. Sometimes to explain an apnoea without a full genetic study, the presence of a normal homozygote, a heterozygote with normal pseudocholinesterase or atypical or abnormal homozygote with atypical pseudocholinesterases, is deduced. The woman who metabolized the succinylcholine quickly, could have had a pseudo-cholinesterase type C_5 which metabolizes succinylcholine 30% more rapidly than normal.

The decrease in pseudocholinesterase is probably a hepatic lesion produced by the contraceptives.

Pseudocholinesterase is a mucoprotein which is closely related to the serum albumin which is produced in the liver; when there is a lesion in the liver which affects the production of proteins there is also a reduction in pseudocholinesterase.

Forges (1970), Pujot Amat (1970) and others have observed anovulatories, cholestatic jaundice or derangements of hepatic function in women taking contraceptives. It is believed that contraceptives act as hepatotoxic agents, which interfere in the synthesis of proteins and in the energy exchange in the mitochondria of hepatic cells. The explanation of this activity could be in the substitution of the 17th carbon of the alkali group in the α-position, giving this structure apparent hepato-toxicity.

These substances could interfere with the secretory mechanisms of the bile, reducing the capacity of the hepatic cell to excrete conjugated bilirubin or bromsulphthalein, and by producing an alteration in the biliary canaliculus. Tyler found that in women who were taking contraceptives, there was an increase in retention of bromsulphthalein of 27%. The 2 components of the contraceptives may potentiate the hepato-toxic effect but this was not demonstrated.

Intrahepatic cholestasis has been demonstrated by intrahepatic biopsy and during the period of administration of the contraceptives there was an increased risk of parenchymatous damage.

REFERENCES

Miguel Martines, J. (1974): *Rev. Esp. Anest. Reanim.*
Miguen, J. (1971): *Cah. Anesth.*, 19/7,
Millgerodt, H. et al. (1971): *Zbl. Gynäk.*,
Moren Forgas (1970): *Efectos Secundarios de los Anovulatories.*
Pujol Amat (1970): *Progestagenos de Sintesis y Funcion Ovarica.*
Robertson, D. G. (1967): *Lancet, 1,*
Redderson, Cl. (1973): *Int. J. clin. Pharmacol.*
Rozenbaum, H. (1970): *Los Anticonceptivos Orales.*
Whittaker, M. et al. (1971): *J. Reprod. Fertil.*

Recovery room analgesia: A comparison of preoperative and intraoperative drug effects

LEE A. SHEFFER, JOHN L. STEFFENSON, RICHARD L. FRAIOLI
and HAROLD N. DEAN

Medical Corps, United States Navy, Naval Regional Medical Center, Oakland, Calif., U.S.A.

This study was designed to compare the effects of various drug treatment methods on the preparation, induction, and emergence from anesthesia in pediatric tonsillectomy patients. This group was chosen because of the high incidence of emergence excitement they manifest.

Two hundred and eighty-eight healthy patients ranging in age from 3–12 years were studied. All patients received 60% nitrous oxide, 1% halothane anesthesia following inhalation induction. Ventilation was spontaneous and end-tidal carbon dioxide concentrations were measured with an infrared analyzer. All patients were intubated without muscle relaxants.

Assignment of patients to the 17 treatment groups (Table 1) was according to a randomized

Table 1. *Total study material as divided into 17 treatment groups*

Group	Preoperative drug	Intraoperative drug	Meperidine for emergence excitement (%)	Incidence of emesis (%)
1	None	Saline	71	29 (Control)
2	None	Hydroxyzine 1 mg/kg	64	36
3	None	Diazepam 140 μg/kg	53	41
4	(Meperidine 0.5 mg/kg { Nembutal 1 mg/kg (Atropine 0.01 mg/kg	Saline	47	47
5	None	Meperidine 0.5 mg/kg	40	47
6	None	Meperidine 0.5 mg/kg Diazepam 140 μg/kg	33	27
7	None	Ketamine 2 mg/kg	25	58
8	Nembutal 3 mg/kg (p.o.)	Meperidine 1 mg/kg	21	21
9	None	Methadone 80 μg/kg	20	33
10	None	Meperidine 1 mg/kg	20	20
11	None	Fentanyl 1.25 μg/kg	20	60
12	Meperidine 1 mg/kg Atropine 0.01 mg/kg	Saline	20	27
13	Atropine 0.01 mg/kg	Droperidol 62.5 μg/kg Meperidine 0.5 mg/kg	19	6
14	None	Morphine 0.1 mg/kg	13	40
15	Innovar 0.025 ml/kg	Saline	6	13
16	None	Innovar 0.025 ml/kg	3	10
17	None	Ketamine 4 mg/kg	0	39

""

list and the study conducted in a double-blind fashion. Preoperative medicines, given 60 min prior to induction, included atropine, a central depressant, or a combination of atropine with a depressant.

The resident anesthesiologist evaluated the patients prior to induction. Sedation, tranquility, and the overall preanesthetic condition were judged to be either adequate or inadequate. The induction was rated overall as excellent, good, fair, or poor. Airway secretions were reported as minimal or excessive. Ten minutes before the anticipated end of the anesthetic, an intramuscular injection was made consisting of either saline or an active drug. The unpremedicated group receiving saline intraoperatively served as the control group.

Following the anesthetic, patients were observed in the recovery room by a staff anesthesiologist. Scoring on a 1–4 scale for alertness and tranquility was performed (Fig. 1), higher scores indicating a higher degree of alertness and tranquility. Scoring was done on arrival in the recovery room (zero time), and every 5 min thereafter for 30 min and at 45 and 60 min after arrival.

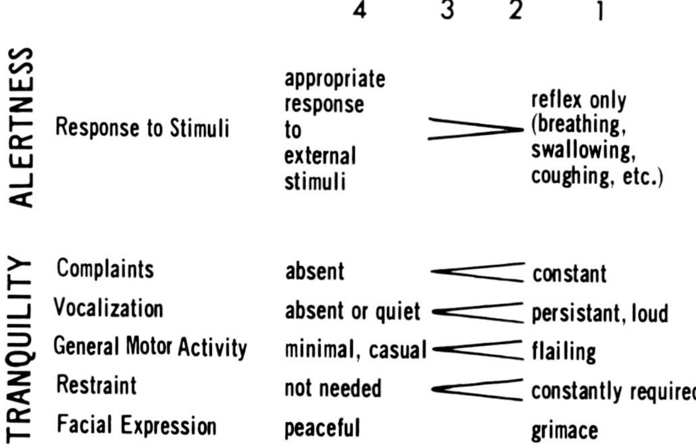

Fig. 1.   *Scale scoring (1–4) for alertness and tranquility.*

Agitated patients, defined as those given tranquility scores of 2 or less over a 10-minute interval, were given meperidine 1 mg/kg intramuscularly. The occurrence of undesirable events such as airway obstruction and emesis were recorded. Blood pressure and heart rate were obtained immediately prior to the recording of alertness and tranquility scores.

The evaluation of the patients on arrival in the operating room produced the following information: First, sedation scores for patients receiving depressant premedicant drugs preoperatively and those not receiving depressants showed no significant difference. Second, significant differences were found in scores for tranquility and scores for overall adequacy of the patient's preanesthetic state. Administration of depressant drugs preoperatively produced greater patient tranquility and a more satisfactory overall patient status than was seen in the patients not receiving depressants ($p < 0.02$). Correlation of the tranquility scores with the 'overall adequacy' score suggests that anesthetists equate patient tranquility, more than sedation, with a well medicated patient.

Innovar® * pretreated patients were rated the most sedate, tranquil and best premedicated

---

* Fentanyl 1.25 μg/ml with droperidol 62.5 μg/ml.

overall. The incidence of good to excellent inductions was 94% when depressant premedication was given and 73% when those drugs were withheld (p < 0.05). No patient receiving atropine preoperatively was said to have excessive secretions though those not receiving atropine were found to have an incidence of excessive secretions of 28% (p < 0.005).

The mean end-tidal carbon dioxide concentration at the time of injection of drug during the anesthetic was 5.6%. There were no significant differences between groups. Administration of narcotics preoperatively did not result in higher end-tidal CO_2 values during the anesthetic. However, injection of narcotic during the anesthetic produced a significant elevation of end-tidal CO_2 within 4 min. End-tidal CO_2 reached 6% by 10 min. No significant change in end-tidal CO_2 followed injection of saline.

Recovery of alertness, defined as reaching a score of 3, was found to occur at a mean time of 23 min after arrival in the recovery room in the control group. Administration of narcotics either preoperatively or intraoperatively prolonged awakening to an average of 36.5 min which was considered acceptable. Only two treatment methods prolonged awakening to more than 40 min. Recovery of alertness was not attained by 60 min for patients treated with ketamine 4 mg/kg or the pentobarbital-meperidine sequence. Scores for tranquility in the recovery room were good (a score of 3 or better) at all scoring intervals except for the following:

Intraoperative saline (control)
Intraoperative tranquilizers (hydroxyzine and diazepam)
Intraoperative fentanyl
Intraoperative meperidine 0.5 mg/kg
Intraoperative meperidine with diazepam

The other methods produced good to excellent tranquility scores during recovery. It is of interest that though diazepam failed to improve the tranquility scores when combined with the low dose of meperidine, the use of droperidol did (p < 0.05).

The incidence of administration of meperidine to agitated patients during emergence ranged from 71% in the control group to zero in the excessively depressed patients treated with ketamine 4 mg/kg (Table 1). Innovar given either preoperatively or intraoperatively produced the next lowest rates of excited patients.

Emesis was by far the most frequent complication seen in the recovery room (Table 1). Emesis occurred in 29% of the control group. Fentanyl intraoperatively produced an incidence of emesis of 60%, the highest seen in the study. Marked reduction of vomiting followed the addition of droperidol to both fentanyl and meperidine (p < 0.05). Emesis occurred in only 10% of patients treated with droperidol compared to 36% in patients not receiving droperidol (p < 0.02).

We conclude that atropine given preoperatively does prevent excessive secretions and that this effect is discernible by the anesthetist. Central depressants given preoperatively do improve inhalation induction in pediatric patients. Narcotics can be administered to prevent emergence excitement without prolonging recovery of alertness excessively. Finally, emesis on emergence can be prevented by the use of droperidol.

To achieve these benefits, the preoperative administration of atropine 0.01 mg/kg with Innovar 0.025 ml/kg is recommended.

Competitive action of acidosis and endogenous catecholamines

E. TRULL BORRAS,[1] G. RODRIGUEZ ARGENTE,[1] R. MONTERO BENZO,[1]
B. ALEGRE[2] and J. AZNAR[2]

[1] Department of Anaesthesia and Reanimation, and [2] Department of Clinical Biopathology,
Ciudad Sanitaria 'La Fe', Valencia, Spain

It is widely asserted that catecholamines are inactive in acidotic patients. Lipolysis involves the transformation of inactive lipase into active lipase, using the adenyl-cyclase system whose second messenger (cyclic-AMP) is associated with catecholamine receptors. This liberation of free fatty acids into the circulation is in sufficient concentrations to enable easy identification. However, the average life of the FFA in the circulation is only a few minutes and almost all tissues, apart from nervous tissue, use them readily.

A series of patients has been studied in whom different pathogenic mechanisms (hypovolaemic shock, operations under extracorporeal circulation, septic shock, etc.) were presumed to have activated adrenergic mechanisms with the liberation of circulating catecholamines. Acidosis was also present.

METHOD

Determinations of pH, Pa_{CO_2}, bicarbonate and base excess were made on samples of arterial blood. Neutralization of any metabolic acidosis was with 8.4% bicarbonate. Blood pressure, heart rate and body temperature were recorded. Free fatty acids (FFA) and free glycerol were measured.

RESULTS

The patients were not under the influence of other substances which could influence lipolysis such as ACTH, glucocorticoids or insulin etc.

In all patients, after correcting the acidosis, there was significant increase of systolic and diastolic blood pressure. The heart rate decreased in all patients (except one with severe tachycardia) to normal following correction of the acidosis.

Body temperature was increased in almost all the patients, although this effect was delayed until the peripheral perfusion had become normal.

The glycerides (AGL) and the free glycerol levels did not vary in a uniform manner; although the number studied was not sufficient for statistical significance, it is possible to distinguish clearly different groups. Those patients with metabolic acidosis and respiratory compensation so that the pH was nearly normal, had some values of AGL within normal limits and the correction of the metabolic acidosis was not followed by an increase in circulating FFA. There was, however, a decrease of the free glycerol when the pH became more alkaline.

In the group with inadequately compensated metabolic acidosis, the pH was less than 7.10 and when the acidosis was corrected, there was an increase of AGL and free glycerol.

A third group of patients with metabolic and respiratory acidosis (about 7) showed a large increase of AGL and free glycerol to twice normal levels.

In these patients, after correction of the acidosis with bicarbonate and mechanical ventilation, there was a slight decrease of AGL and free glycerol but the pH was kept higher than normal.

Patients with respiratory acidosis only were not studied.

CONCLUSIONS

It is likely that those patients with a combined acidosis have the highest levels of circulating catecholamines and all these cases had high levels of glycerides and free glycerol. It also seems likely that the reduction in these levels occurs on correction of the acidosis because of a reduction in the release of catecholamines rather than because these compounds are inactive.

Chapter VII

Anaesthesia and the endocrine glands

The value of cortisol plasma levels in intensive care and coronary patients

F. J. DE ELÍO, A. ORIOL BOSCH and MARTIN SANTOS

Intensive Care and Coronary Unit, Clinical Hospital of the Medical Faculty, Madrid, Spain

The plasma 11-hydroxycorticosteroids (cortisol) are a valuable index for determining the state of adrenal function. In patients admitted to intensive care and coronary units (I.C. and C.U.) it might be useful to have at one's disposal a prognostic index at the moment of admission. Plasma cortisol levels have been studied by the fluorimetric method of Mattingly (1962) in 135 nonselected patients on admission to the I.C. and C.U. and at 8 a.m. the following day. These patients were divided into the following groups: myocardial infarction 40 (without cardiac failure 15, with cardiac failure 20, died 5); angina pectoris 7; cardiac failure without infarction 12; arrhythmias not included in the previous groups 25; chronic bronchopneumopathy during acute exacerbation 30; cerebral vascular accidents 12; drug poisoning 9. A group of 29 normal subjects was used as controls.

The statistical analysis between groups and subgroups was carried out in the following way: Student's t-test comparing the means with Cochrane's modification for the presence of distinct variances, and line of regression of least squares with calculation of the correlation coefficient (r).

RESULTS

The results (Table 1) obtained at 8 a.m. show raised plasma cortisol levels in all patient groups, compared with the controls, with the exception of the group of patients with angina pectoris.

In the infarction group the cortisol values on admission were correlated with the hour at which infarction occurred, since there was a disturbance of the normal daily rhythm. For this purpose, results obtained in patients admitted before and after 8 p.m. were compared, but no significant difference could be found between the 2 groups. Correlation between values on admission and at 8 a.m. gave a value of $r = 0.482$, which is different from 0 ($p < 0.01$), and indicates interdependence. The dependence of the 8 a.m. cortisol values on the time of admission to the I.C. and C.U. was studied, but none was found, either in absolute values or in their decrease relative to the value on admission. The values of creatine phosphokinase and cortisol on admission were compared, and no significant correlation was established. At no time was there significant difference between the survivors following infarction, due to the presence or absence of cardiac failure. On the other hand, both these groups showed statistically lower values than the patients with fatal infarction. However, there is no difference between cortisol values on admission and at 8 a.m., which indicates that no major information can be derived from the measurement of cortisol values other than those obtained on admission. Those patients over 60 years old with infarction had higher values on admission than younger patients, but there was no difference at 8 a.m.

Table 1. *Plasma cortisol levels in each of the groups and subgroups on admission and at 8 a.m.*

Groups	No. of patients	Plasma cortisol levels (μg/100 ml)	
		On admission	At 8 a.m.
1. Infarction	40	33.7 ± 17.4	24.5 ± 12.6
(a) infarction without failure	(15)	29.6 ± 14.1	25.9 ± 11.6
(b) infarction with failure	(20)	33.0 ± 16.5	21.3 ± 11.1
(c) deceased infarction cases	(5)	57.6 ± 21.2	44.4 ± 22.7
2. Angina pectoris	7	10.9 ± 5.5	19.1 ± 8.4
3. Failure without infarction	12	74.3 ± 54.4	50.1 ± 39.9
4. Arrhythmia	25	19.0 ± 13.3	22.7 ± 14.1
5. Bronchopneumopathy	30	52.3 ± 39.1	35.2 ± 17.6
6. Vascular accidents	12	56.9 ± 28.6	45.4 ± 29.6
7. Drug poisoning	9	23.3 ± 16.9	24.9 ± 20.2
8. Controls	29		16.7 ± 5.8
Total	164		

Mean values ± deviation.

Patients with angina pectoris have relatively low cortisol values which suggests that the daily rhythm is not affected. On the other hand, patients with cardiac failure without infarction show higher values than those in cardiac failure after infarction. The group of patients with disorders of rhythm (Group 4) show no cortisol decrease at 8 a.m. as compared with the values obtained on admission.

In patients with acute exacerbations of chronic bronchopneumopathies a correlation between pH, P_{CO_2} and cortisol on admission and at 8 a.m. was sought, but no significant correlation was found. Patients with cerebrovascular accidents showed raised values on admission, but there was no significant decrease at 8 a.m. Finally, a similar phenomenon occurs in drug poisoning, though the cortisol values on admission are rather lower.

The highest cortisol values occur in cardiac failure (without infarction) and in chronic bronchopneumopathies; also cerebrovascular accidents have very high values on admission. It should be emphasized that among infarction cases those who died showed the highest values.

DISCUSSION

The disturbance of the daily cycle in myocardial infarction patients has been described before (Logan and Murdoch, 1966; Bailey and Abernethy, 1967). It has also been reported that infarction patients who develop complications have higher cortisol values (Prakash et al., 1972). This fact has been confirmed in our study for those patients who died, but not for those with cardiac failure. From the correlation between the cortisol values on admission and at 8 a.m. and from the fact that their changes do not depend on the time interval, it is concluded that in infarction the information given by cortisol values does not depend on the moment at which the sample is taken, since serial determinations do not supply any additional information. Chopra et al. (1972) did not gain any more information from serial cortisol determinations. The lack of correlation between CPK and cortisol on admission may be due to a temporary reduction of the increase of this enzyme, though Prakash et al. (1972) also did not find any relation between this and other enzymes as the development of the infarction continues. The differences related to age of the infarction patients could be attributed to the diminution of the steroid metabolism which takes place with advancing age, although it is not easy to understand why at 8 a.m. the differences have disappeared. Kaalund and Blichert-Toft (1971) did not find any significant variations of cortisol plasma levels at 8 a.m. related to age, and in normal volunteers. The modest rises observed in patients with angina pectoris or with arrhythmia suggest that the hypothalamo-pituitary-adrenal axis responds more intensively to demonstrable somatic 'stress' situations, as shown by Korpassy et al. (1972) in prolonged organic stress' situations, than to those of psychological 'stress'.

Chronic respiratory failure in the acute phase is associated with marked rises, as described previously by Sadoul and Laxenaire (1970) and Voisin et al. (1970). However, in this study these changes in relation to acidosis have not been found. In patients with chronic broncho-pneumopathy and in cardiac failure without infarction, it is probable that the high levels are due to the maintenance of the continued stimulus by the pathological process. Conolly and Wills (1967) and Knapp (1967), also found raised plasma cortisol values in cardiac failure. In cerebrovascular accidents with raised values of plasma cortisol there is a suggestion that the hypophyseal hypothalamic zone is not affected, and that there is an alteration of inhibitory systems of this zone. On the other hand, drug poisoning associated with inhibition of the central nervous system is accompanied by only slight stimulation of the hypothalamo-pituitary-adrenal axis.

CONCLUSIONS

The determination of cortisol in patients admitted to the I.C. and C.U. is thought to be of value. In myocardial infarction patients it has a prognostic value. In chronic broncho-pneumopathy and cardiac failure without infarction it may help to decide which therapeutic course to take.

REFERENCES

Bailey, R. R. and Abernethy, M. H. (1967): *Lancet, 1*, 970.
Connolly, C. K. and Wills, M. R. (1967): *Brit. med. J., 2*, 25.
Chopra, M. P., Thadani, U., Clive, P. A., Portal, R. W. and Parkes, J. (1972): *Brit. Heart J., 34*, 992.
Kaalund, J. H. and Blichert-Toft, M. (1971): *Acta endocr. scand., 66*, 25.
Knapp, M. S., Keane, P. M. and Wright, J. G. (1967): *Brit. med. J., 2*, 27.
Korpassy, A., Stoeckel, H. and Vecsei, P. (1972): *Acta anaesth. scand., 16*, 161.
Logan, R. W. and Murdoch, W. R. (1966): *Lancet, 2*, 521.
Mattingly, D. (1962): *J. clin. Path., 15*, 374.
Prakash, R., Parmley, W. W., Horvat, M. and Swan, H. J. C. (1972): *Circulation, 45*, 736.
Sadoul, P. and Laxenaire, M. C. (1970): *Bull. Physiopath. Resp., 6*, 681.
Voisin, C., Fossat, P., Wattel, F., Lefebvre, J., Racadot, M., Tonnel, A., Leleu, J. C. and Linquette, M. (1970): *Lille méd., 10*, 1367.

Anaesthetic management of patients with myasthenia gravis

E. LOPES SOARES

Hospitais Civis, Lisbon, Portugal

Myasthenia gravis is a rare disease (1 : 20,000 to 1 : 40,000), being more frequent in females than in males (ratio 3:1 among young adults); the onset appears, on the average, between the age of 20 and 30 years. Clinically, it is defined by excessive fatigue of the voluntary muscles, with rapid recovery at rest.

The muscular fatigue of myasthenia gravis is characterized by weakness, varied in location but always affecting muscles of the head and neck; there is variation in the severity during the day and from day to day, with periods of exacerbation and remission; there are no signs of a neural lesion, and there is consistent and reproducible improvement after the administration of cholinergic drugs (Rowland et al., 1956).

Dysphagia, dysarthria, difficulty in chewing and limb weakness are frequent. The signs of muscular fatigue are more marked at night than in the morning, and the symptoms may become worse with effort, fever, menstruation, pregnancy, etc.

DIAGNOSIS

The diagnosis is made from the history, clinical examination and various tests. Amongst the latter, the most commonly used are:
1. Neostigmine test: i.m. injection of 1–2 mg.
2. Edrophonium test: i.v. injection of 10 mg.
Both neostigmine and edrophonium act by inhibiting cholinesterase, thereby causing a rise in the concentration of acetylcholine (ACh) at the motor end-plates, and a clinical improvement of the tired muscles. Muscle power and its response to an anticholinesterase may be evaluated by means of a dynamometer or an ergograph.
3. Decamethonium test (Churchill-Davidson and Richardson, 1953): i.v. injection of 2.5 mg in separate doses. In myasthenic patients there is first a resistance to block, and finally a dual block.
4. Tubocurarine test (Foldes and McNall, 1962): i.v. injection of 0.5–1 mg at 3 min intervals up to a maximum of 4 mg. A decrease in muscular contraction and in vital capacity is found to occur.
5. Electromyographic test and muscle biopsy.

PHYSIOPATHOLOGY

Myasthenia gravis is due to a defect of neuromuscular transmission. Four different theories exist of its aetiology:

1. Decreased synthesis or release of acetylcholine. This prejunctional theory is based on investigations made by Dahlback et al. (1961) and Elmqvist et al. (1964).

2. Altered response of the motor end-plate. This postjunctional theory is based on investigations made by Churchill-Davidson and Richardson (1953).

3. Circulating neuromuscular blocking agent.

4. An auto-immune response (Nastuk et al., 1960; Simpson, 1960). The role of the thymus in the development of immune capacity is now known. In myasthenia gravis histological lesions have been found in the thymus (presence of germinal centres and plasma cells) suggesting an immune response. The nature of the antigen, however, is unknown. The associations of myasthenia gravis with auto-immune diseases are frequent: thyrotoxicosis, lupus erythematosus, auto-immune haemolytic anaemia (Albahary et al., 1972), erythroblastopenia (Lenormand et al., 1972), etc.

It is now considered possible that, in fact, there is a presynaptic failure of ACh, dependent on mechanisms proper to auto-immune disease.

TREATMENT

Since the fundamental alteration in myasthenia gravis is a defect in neuromuscular transmission, the basic treatment rests on the administration of anticholinesterase drugs, in association, if necessary, with atropine to counteract the muscarinic effects of the drugs. The administration of anticholinesterase drugs increases the duration of life of ACh and, therefore, its concentration. An overdose of anticholinesterase drugs leads to the non-destruction of ACh, the presence of which maintains the depolarisation of the end-plate and renders it refractory to subsequent excitation. The block then produced results in the symptoms of the disease reappearing; in an exaggerated form this is called a cholinergic crisis. Therapy with anticholinesterase drugs has 2 aims: to determine the optimum dose and to avoid the occurrence of the cholinergic crisis arising from over-therapy.

The drugs now used are: (1) neostigmine (Prostigmine): 15 mg tablets, 1–3 tablets every 2–6 hr; duration of action, about 4 hr; (2) pyridostigmine (Mestinon): 60 mg tablets, 3–15 tablets/day; duration, about 4 hr; (3) ambenonium (Mytelase): 10 mg tablets, 3–10 tablets/day; duration, 5–6 hr; (4) edrophonium (Tensilon) has a very quick and brief action. More used as a diagnostic tool, i.v. injection of 10 mg produces a rapid improvement immediately followed by a return to the basic condition.

Besides the anticholinesterase drugs, drugs which exert influence on the release of ACh have been tried: Ca, K, and Guanethidine. In severe forms of myasthenia gravis which respond badly to anticholinesterase drugs, ACTH has been used, its effect may be due to its immunosuppressive properties or to the fact that it produces a postsynaptic potassium shift. Doses of 100 U of ACTH over a period of 10 days together with a non-salt diet and associated with anti-acids and potassium replacement are recommended.

The use of prednisolone (100 mg every other day) has also been recommended. Both ACTH and corticosteroids should only be given to patients admitted to Intensive Care Units (ICU). Some drugs must not be administered to myasthenic patients. Among these prohibited drugs are muscle relaxants, benzodiazepines, neuroleptics, quinine and some antibiotics, like streptomycin, kanamycin, polymyxin, colomycin, neomycin, etc.

ANAESTHETIC MANAGEMENT

The anaesthetist may be called upon to co-operate in the treatment of a myasthenic patient in 3 different situations: (1) respiratory care of patients in a myasthenic crisis or in a cholinergic crisis; (2) anaesthesia for operations on the thymus; and (3) anaesthesia for incidental operations.

Respiratory care

Alterations in swallowing, weak cough or difficulty in speaking are alarm signals which should lead to the admission of the patient into an ICU unless there is quick improvement after the administration of an anticholinesterase drug. The inability to take deep breaths and to cough may lead to atelectasis and to the retention of secretions. Airway obstruction and hypoventilation are almost always found in association with this. Airway obstruction is caused by saliva, food or vomitus collecting in the oropharynx due to weakness of the muscles of swallowing. Muscular weakness in myasthenic patients invariably leads to respiratory failure.

The assessment of respiratory capacity should be accurately made. It is necessary to check the tidal volume and respiratory rate, the force of coughing and the possibility of swallowing. Spirometry is very important. If the vital capacity has fallen to about one third or one fourth of normal, this is an immediate indication for artificial respiration with nasotracheal intubation or tracheotomy. Blood gas values have to be measured frequently.

Besides anticholinesterase therapy, acute respiratory failure should be treated by the usual measures: postural drainage, aspiration of secretions, physiotherapy of the chest and nasotracheal intubation and/or tracheotomy and mechanical ventilation – controlled or assisted. Nasotracheal intubation should always precede tracheotomy. Tracheal intubation in itself may suffice if the crisis is brought under control in a few days' time. If the situation, is not resolved until the 5th or 7th day it is preferable to perform tracheotomy. If the patient is connected to a ventilator and kept under controlled ventilation, therapy with anticholinesterase drugs should be interrupted, which makes it easier for the patient to become adapted to the machine and obviates the dangers of the cholinergic crisis.

When the patient recovers sufficient spontaneous ventilation, he is given intermittent ventilation, being always however, left connected with the ventilator during the night. Anticholinesterase medication – starting always with low doses which are gradually increased – may be recommenced.

When the myasthenic crisis is resolved, the nasotracheal or the tracheotomy tube is left in position for a further 2 days, though artificial ventilation is stopped. If there is no relapse, the tracheal or the tracheotomy tube is removed, and the stoma is allowed to close. As a safety measure, one can start by replacing the tracheotomy cannula by a fenestrated plastic tube with an obturator, which will allow the patient to breathe in the ordinary manner while maintaining the facilities for aspiration of the secretions and for connecting the patient to the ventilator should the need arise.

All the usual care is taken, such as humidification of room air or dry gas from cylinders, prevention of infections, change of posture in bed, antibiotherapy, etc. The patient must be fed through an intragastric tube.

The results of the resuscitation of patients in a myasthenic or a cholinergic crisis have greatly improved since treatment was transferred to an ICU (Bryan-Brown, 1971).

Anaesthesia for thymectomy

Though the myasthenic patient is not a good surgical risk, the surgical treatment by thymectomy has progressed greatly in these last years, thanks mostly to the advances in respiratory care, which has reduced postsurgical complications and mortality.

It being admitted that myasthenia gravis is an auto-immune thymopathy where the thymus segregates myasthenizing substances or pathological lymphocytes, thymectomy should be viewed as an essential treatment when there is a thymoma and in myasthenic cases which have progressed beyond the ocular stage and are not amenable to medical treatment.

Several statistical studies like those of Perlo et al. (1966) and Mulder et al. (1972) show the superiority of surgical treatment as reflected in improvement following thymectomy in about 80% of patients without a thymic tumour, and in 45% of those with a neoplasm.

Patients should be hospitalized a few days before operation so that a careful pre-surgery preparation may be made, including the study of respiratory function, blood gas determination, X-ray of the chest, thyroid function, psychological preparation and respiratory physiotherapy. The patient should be in the best possible physical state. Oral cholinergic medication is reduced to the level required to keep the patient just comfortable. A few hours before operation, anticholinesterase drugs are stopped; this will contribute to muscular relaxation (Bendixen et al., 1965). Premedication should be minimal, respiratory depressants (morphinomimetics, narcotics and barbiturates) being avoided. The use of atropine or scopolamine is imperative, though high doses which tend to thicken the secretions, should be avoided.

The anaesthetics should encourage rapid induction and recovery, should not increase secretions and should not produce neuromuscular block. The anaesthetics frequently used are: thiopentone, N_2O, halothane and enflurane. Muscle relaxants should be strictly avoided; the action of succinylcholine is unpredictable and there is no antagonist to it (Foldes, 1962). The observed resistance may lead to the use of high doses and produce dual block. In, addition, myasthenic patients are very sensitive to non-depolarising relaxants (tubocurarine gallamine, Alloferine and pancuronium), wherefore, if these are used, the doses should be reduced to 1/10 or 1/20 of the normal (Foldes, 1957). Tracheal intubation, if it proves necessary, should be performed under local anaesthesia. Controlled ventilation – manual or mechanical – is absolutely necessary. Certain antibiotics should not be used topically such as neomycin, streptomycin, colomycin, etc.

If tracheotomy has been performed on the patient before surgery, mechanical ventilation should be maintained through the tracheotomy after surgery. If no tracheotomy has been performed, a nasotracheal tube should be kept in place for 6–8 days, up to a maximum of about 20 days.

At the end of 48 hr anticholinesterase treatment is resumed, but with much lower doses than formerly. A test with edrophonium will be useful. If the result is positive, low doses of cholinergics should be given intravenously. Pyridostigmine in doses of 1 mg every 6 hr up to 8 mg every 4 hr may be used. If these doses are insufficient or if the patients begin to have abundant secretions or abdominal cramp, the cholinergics should be interrupted and the patients should again be ventilated. Atropine should not be used after surgery. The patients should stay in the ICU to ensure proper respiratory care.

Anaesthesia for incidental operations

The general principles of anaesthesia under these circumstances are the same as those described for thymectomy.

Whenever possible, local or loco-regional anaesthesia techniques should be resorted to. Local anaesthetics of the ester group (cocaine, procaine, amethocaine), being hydrolysed by non-specific cholinesterases, should not be used. Local anaesthetics of the amide group, metabolised in the liver (lignocaine, prilocaine, mepivacaine and bupivacaine) should be resorted to instead.

If it proves necessary to use general anaesthesia, the patients should be hospitalized in advance for study and preparation. Premedication should be minimal (atropine or scopolamine) and the most adequate anaesthetics are those ensuring very quick induction and recovery, no increase in secretions and no muscular relaxation. These conditions are met by barbiturates, N_2O, halothane and enflurane.

Muscle relaxants, whatever their type, are contraindicated, and tracheal intubation should be performed under local anaesthesia.

At the end of anaesthesia, ventilation should be repeatedly measured (with a Wright respirometer). If ventilation is inadequate, the tracheal tube should not be removed; aspiration of tracheal secretions and eventual connection to a ventilator are both readily achieved.

Anticholinesterase medication is resumed as described above.

MYASTHENIC SYNDROME

A myasthenic syndrome has been described in patients suffering from bronchial carcinoma, with histories of muscle weakness and fatigue. Incidentally, the same syndrome has been reported in connection with tumours of the bowels and elsewhere.

The anaesthetic problems of these patients are the same as for myasthenic patients. It sometimes happens that the syndrome is not diagnosed during the preoperative period and that the anaesthetist is the first to suspect it when he finds that the patient has a greatly increased sensitivity to muscle relaxants or to respiratory depressants.

CONCLUSION

The chief alteration met with in myasthenia gravis is a defect in neuromuscular transmission, probably due to presynaptic failure of ACh, dependent on mechanisms proper to auto-immune disease in which the thymus is likely to play an important role.

The basic therapy consists in the administration of anticholinesterase drugs. During the myasthenic crisis and cholinergic crisis the patients often require respiratory care, wherefore they should be admitted in ICU's.

Myasthenia gravis patients are not good surgical risks. Loco-regional techniques are recommended whenever possible. Muscle relaxants and respiratory depressants are counter-indicated. Barbiturates, N_2O and halothane are the most currently used anaesthetics.

REFERENCES

Albahary, C., Homberg, J. C., Guillaume, J., Martin, S. and Boulangiez, J. P. (1972): *Nouv. Presse Méd.*, 29, 1931.

Bendixen, H. H., Egbert, L. D., Hedley-White, J., Laver, M. B. and Pontoppidan, H. (1965): In: *Respiratory Care*, 1st ed., Chapter 17, p. 173. C. V. Mosby Co., St. Louis, Mo.

Bryan-Brown, C. W. (1971): *Mt Sinai J. Med.*, 38, 573.

Churchill-Davidson, H. C. and Richardson, A. N. (1953): *J. Physiol. (Lond.)*, 122, 252.

Dahlback, O., Elmqvist, D., Johnst, T. R., Radners, S. and Thesleff, S. (1961): *J. Physiol. (Lond.)*, 156, 336.

Elmqvist, D., Hofmann, W. W., Kugelberg, J. and Quastel, D. M. J. (1964): *J. Physiol. (Lond.)*, 174, 417.

Foldes, F. F. (1957): In: *Muscle Relaxants in Anesthesiology*, 1st ed., Chapter 11, p. 141. Editor: John Adriani. Charles C. Thomas, Springfield, Ill.

Foldes, F. F. and McNall, P. G. (1962): *Anesthesiology*, 23, 837.

Lenormand, Y., Sterin, D., Barge, J. and Boivin, P. (1972): *Sem. Hôp. Paris, 48*, 13.

Mulder, D. G., Braitman, H., Li, W. and Herrmann Jr, C. (1972): *J. thorac. cardiovasc. Surg.*, 63, 105.

Nastuk, W. L., Plescia, O. J. and Osserman, K. E. (1960): *Proc. Soc. exp. Biol. (N.Y.)*, 105, 177.

Perlo, V. P., Poskanzer, D. C., Schwab, R. S., Viets, H. R., Osserman, K. E. and Genkins, G. (1966): *Neurology (Minneap.)*, 16, 131.

Rowland, L. P., Hoffer, P. F. A., Aranow, H. J. R. and Merrit, H. H. (1956): *Neurology (Minneap.)*, 6, 306.

Simpson, J. A. (1960): *Scot. med. J.*, 5, 419.

Anaesthesia and postoperative management of patients with diseases of the pituitary gland

EMERIC GORDON

Department of Neuroanaesthesia, Karolinska Hospital, Stockholm, Sweden

THE ROLE OF HORMONES IN TRAUMA: THE ANTERIOR PITUITARY GLAND

The fundamental importance of hormones in trauma has been known since the observations of Cannon (1932) and the well-known studies of Selye (1947) on the stress-phenomenon. It became evident from these studies that the adrenal cortex by secreting cortisol plays a decisive role in the maintenance of normal homeostasis and metabolic balance. Further studies have shown, however, that there are several hormones involved in this regulation, and that all hormones are directly or indirectly involved in traumatic or stress situations.

Recent observations (McCann and Porter, 1969) have made it clear that hormonal regulation is a complex mechanism interrelated through the hypothalamus-pituitary gland – peripheral endocrine organs – peripheral tissues. Thus hypothalamic centres direct the secretion of pituitary hormones called corticotrophin releasing factor (CRF) which on its part regulates, amongst others, ACTH-secretion, TRF (thyrotropin releasing factor) for TSH-secretion, GRF (growth hormone releasing factor) for GH-secretion. According to detailed studies (Chowers et al., 1967; Davidson and Feldman, 1967) stimulation of the peripheral endocrine glands can also hamper hormonal secretion from the pituitary (negative feedback) on different levels: (*a*) cortisol or GH can stop secretion of both hypothalamic factors and pituitary hormones (direct feedback); (*b*) cortisol can inhibit other pituitary hormones than ACTH, such as GH and TSH (cross feedback); (*c*) some metabolites (calcium or glucose) can influence the ability of the hormone-producing organ to respond to stimuli.

Secretion of ACTH and GH can be stimulated during stress, but these 2 hormones are not necessarily bound to respond always in a same manner. Yalow et al. (1969) have shown in human experiments how these dissociations can appear (Table 1). ACTH-secretion is stimulated by all forms of stress, while the response of GH-secretion is more difficult to

Table 1. *Responses of ACTH and GH (growth hormone) to stress*

Stressor	Effect
Moderate hypoglycaemia	Prompt effect on GH, no effect on ACTH
Electroconvulsive shock	No effect on GH, prompt effect on ACTH
Histalog	Delayed effect on GH, prompt effect on ACTH
Vasopressin	No effect on GH, prompt effect on ACTH
Major surgery in general anaesthesia (5 patients)	Response of GH in 2, response of ACTH in 4, no response in 1

After Yalow et al., 1969.

predict. It is also interesting that GH-secretion is extremely sensitive to hypoglycaemia as a stress factor (Luft et al., 1966).

Hormones can influence important metabolic processes during stress situations even without an increased concentration by a permissive action. For example, in Addison's disease not even a noradrenaline infusion can result in a blood pressure increase because of a lowered sensitivity to sympathomimetic amines. After the administration of corticosteroids normal blood pressure is restored (Luft et al., 1970).

Another vital function of hormones is emphasized by the fact that the central nervous system, unlike all other organs in the body, is unable to make use of free fatty acids as a source of energy, and is totally dependent on glucose and oxygen. In order to provide the central nervous system with its requirements for glucose, the glucose uptake in other tissues is restrained by 2, hormonally controlled, mechanisms: (1) depression of insulin secretion, and (2) increase in the concentration of free fatty acids in plasma, which directly depress glucose uptake (Randle, 1966). In other words, hormones distribute the required metabolites in such a manner that the body can meet stress effectively.

POSTERIOR PITUITARY GLAND

Of the 2 posterior pituitary hormones, vasopressin (ADH) and oxytocin, ADH is by far the most important during surgery, anaesthesia and intensive care. ADH exerts its influence on the distal renal rubuli which results in water resorption, thereby regulating the osmotic pressure of the extracellular fluid.

Preoperative psychic stress stimulates ADH secretion, which emphasizes the importance of adequate premedication. Anaesthesia usually diminishes urinary secretion of water and electrolytes. A great amount of clinical research has shown (Oyama and Kimura, 1970; Oyama and Sato, 1970; Oyama et al., 1971) that anaesthetic agents stimulate ADH secretion and the level of plasma ADH is elevated during anaesthesia. The same is valid for surgical interventions (Moran et al., 1964).

THE EFFECT OF ANAESTHESIA AND SURGERY ON HORMONE SECRETION

ACTH in plasma shows significant and sudden increases during all types of anaesthesia including halothane and neuroleptanaesthesia, while the level of cortisol increases more gradually. A significant increase of GH is also recorded during surgery and anaesthesia with diethyl ether and neuroleptanaesthesia, while halothane, thiopentone and Ethrane do not alter plasma levels of GH (Oyama et al., 1970). The reasons for this difference are not known. No significant changes in TSH levels in plasma are recorded during anaesthesia (Charters et al., 1969; Oyama et al., 1972) but ether and halothane increase serum thyroxine levels. The effect of anaesthetic agents on hormone secretion is shown in Table 2.

ANAESTHESIA AND INTENSIVE CARE

It is sufficiently clear from the previous data that operative trauma have a profound influence on the complex hormonal balance in the human organism. In cases of patients with disease of the pituitary gland these fine mechanisms can be more or less seriously disturbed. It is therefore of utmost importance for the successful outcome of an operation that such patients should undergo extensive preoperative endocrinological investigation. Cooperation with an endocrinological department is thus an absolute necessity.

Table 2. *The effect of anaesthetic agents and surgery on hormone secretion*

| | ACTH | Cortisol | Aldosterone | Catecholamine | | GH | TSH | ADH |
				Adrenaline	Noradrenaline			
Induction + surgery	+++	+++	++			+++	0	+++
Premedication		—						0
Halothane	+++	—		0	0	+	0	++
Methoxyflurane		0	++	0	0	+++	0	++
Enflurane		+				0		
Ether	++		++	+	++	++	0	++
Cycloprane					++	+		+
Thiopentone		0—	++	0	0	0	0	0
Muscle relaxant		0—						
Ketamine		++						
Pethidine		0				+++		0
Droperidol	++	0		+	—	+++		
Pentazocine	++	+		+		+++		
Fentanyl	++	0		+	—			
Spinal anaesthesia	0			0	0	0	0	

O = no change; + = insignificant increase; ++ = significant increase; +++ = marked increase.
After Oyama, 1973.

It is impossible to go into a detailed description of routine endocrinological procedures within the framework of this symposium. Only the most relevant points which have direct implication to anaesthetic practice will be discussed.

INDICATIONS FOR PITUITARY GLAND SURGERY

Operations on and around the pituitary gland are performed in our clinic almost exclusively for cases of pituitary tumour. Previous indications for hypophysectomy, for carcinoma of the breast, diabetic retinopathy, malignant essential hypertension are almost completely abandoned for reasons which are outside the scope of this paper. In rare cases trans-sphenoidal resection of the pituitary gland is performed. Operations for craniopharyngeomas have also disappeared from the operative schedule of this clinic, and these patients are treated now with stereotaxic puncture of the cystic part of the tumour and the injection of radioisotopes' into the cystic cavity (Backlund, 1972). This treatment has almost totally eliminated the severe complications of water and electrolyte disturbances, hyperthermia, blood pressure irregularities which were often seen after classic operations, which also had an extremely high mortality rate.

PREOPERATIVE MANAGEMENT

Irrespective of the operative technique used, preoperative routine endocrinological examinations are performed in every case. These include: plasma cortisol, T_4, T_3, cholesterol, calcium, and urinary output of 17-ketosteroids and corticosteroids. Substitution is then started according to the result of this screening. The scheme for the substitution of cortisol is seen in Table 3 and is used not only in connection with operations but also with neuro-radiological examinations under either local or general anaesthesia. It must be emphasized

Table 3. *Substitution of patients with primary or secondary adrenocortical insufficiency during operation*

Day of operation

(a)   30 min before operation 100 mg cortisone acetate i.m.
(b)   Slow i.v. drop-infusion of isotonic glucose containing 80 mEq sodium and 100 mg hydrocortisone
(c)   Following this infusion: 50 mg cortisone acetate every 4 hr

Postoperatively

Day 1: 50 mg cortisone acetate × 4 i.m.
Day 2: 25 mg cortisone acetate × 5 i.m. or p.o.
Day 3: 25 mg cortisone acetate × 3 p.o.
Day 4: 12.5 mg cortisone acetate × 4 p.o.
Thereafter: 12.5 mg cortisone acetate × 3 under 'normal' conditions.

In cases of blood pressure fall an additional dose of 100 mg hydrocortisone is administered i.v. In cases of postoperative complications (e.g. hyperthermia) higher doses of cortisone should be given. In difficult cases the endocrinologist should be consulted.

here that normal endocrinological status does not necessarily guarantee an uncomplicated course, as many of the patients can develop more or less severe shock during pneumo-encephalography or surgical operation. The reason for these complications could be latent insufficiency, which becomes manifest during stress situations. It is therefore of vital importance, that even in these cases adequate emergency equipment is maintained so that rapid action is possible and serious irreversible damage is avoided.

PREMEDICATION AND ANAESTHESIA

Premedication and anaesthesia in patients undergoing neuroradiological examinations or operations for diseases of the pituitary gland do not differ essentially from techniques used in other patients. For premedication a combination of atropine or scopolamine is given together with droperidol and diazepam in appropriate doses. Induction is started with small doses of thiopentone followed by pancuronium and endotracheal intubation. Controlled ventilation is maintained thereafter during the whole anaesthesia with gas mixtures containing 40% oxygen and 60% nitrous oxide. Moderate hyperventilation is achieved keeping Pa_{CO_2} around 25–30 mm Hg. Anaesthesia is maintained with incremental doses of fentanyl or phenoperidine to which small doses of pancuronium are added when necessary.

The surgical approach is largely facilitated by a decrease of intracranial pressure. This is partly achieved by the moderate hyperventilation, to which lumbar drainage through a plastic catheter is added. These 2 techniques have usually such a good effect, that further decompressive methods, e.g. the intravenous administration of osmotic diuretics, are seldom necessary. If this is required 20% mannitol in a dose of 1–1.5 g/kg is used. Half this dose is, administered during a period of 10–15 min, the other half during the following 1–2 hr.

Apart from the substitution indicated in Table 3, usually no additional cortisone is necessary during operation. If complications ensue (profuse bleeding, hypotension) additional doses of 100 mg hydrocortisone are given intravenously.

Toward the end of the operation ventilation is decreased to normal volume to obtain a normal Pa_{CO_2} level and a rapid return of normal spontaneous ventilation. Pancuronium is reversed in the usual way, but neuroleptic drugs very seldom need antidotes. With experienced anaesthesia personnel the last dose of these drugs can be given at a time which permits the return of normal ventilation after the last suture. In other case the analgesic drug is reversed by a small dose of naloxone (0.1 mg intravenously for an adult).

The patient is most often awake after extubation and responds willingly to questions. If this is not the case for one reason or another, the endotracheal tube is left in place and controlled ventilation is continued in the immediate postoperative period. Unconsciousness and/or respiratory troubles are seldom encountered after these operations. If these complications occur because of postoperative oedema, haematoma or a hypothalamic or brain-stem lesion, controlled ventilation is instituted until the patient's condition improves.

POSTOPERATIVE CARE

Usually there is no major difficulty in starting normal nutrition on the first or second postoperative day. Until then parenteral nutrition is achieved with isotonic glucose to which 80 mEq sodium is added, in a dose of about 1500–2000 ml/24 hr. The cortisol substitution scheme is, of course, followed as given in Table 3. Daily determinations of electrolyte and water balance studies are made rigorously until the patient's condition is firmly stabilized. As after many other intracranial interventions, a polyuric phase is often observed in these patients, when the urinary output is somewhat greater than expected, i.e. around 3000 ml/day. If oral nutrition is maintained, intake corresponding to loss is allowed. However, in patients supported parenterally, a more restricted regime is applied with no more than 2000–2500 ml/24 hr, to avoid the risk of postoperative cerebral oedema. These minor disturbances disappear, however, after about a week, without any treatment. More serious complications of water balance with signs of diabetes insipidus are treated with small doses of Pitressin in close cooperation with the endocrinologists.

REFERENCES

Backlund, E.-O. (1972): *Acta chir. scand., 139,* 237.

Cannon, W. B. (1932): *The Wisdom of Body.* W. W. Norton and Co., New York, N.Y.

Charters, A. C., Odell, W. D. and Thompson, J. C. (1969): *J. clin. Invest., 29,* 63.

Chowers, J., Conforti, N. and Feldman, S. (1967): *Neuroendocrinology, 2,* 193.

Davidson, J. M. and Feldman, S. (1967): *Acta endocrin. (Kbh.), 55,* 240.

Luft, R., Cerasi, E., Madison, L. L., Euler, U. S. von, Della Casa, L. and Roovete, A. (1966): *Lancet, 2,* 254.

Luft, R., Efendić, S. and Cerasi, E. (1970): *Nord. Med., 84/40,* 1257.

McCann, S. M. and Porter, J. C. (1969): *Physiol. Rev., 49,* 240.

Moran Jr, W. H., Miltenberger, F. W., Shuayb, W. A. and Zimmermann, B. (1964): *Surgery, 56,* 99.

Oyama, T. (1973): *Anesthetic Management of Endocrine Disease.* Springer-Verlag, Berlin – Heidelberg – New York.

Oyama, T. and Kimura, K. (1970): *Canad. Anaesth. Soc. J., 17,* 495.

Oyama, T. and Sato, K. (1970): *Anaesthesia, 25,* 500.

Oyama, T., Sato, K. and Kimura, K. (1970): *Canad. Anaesth. Soc. J., 18,* 614.

Oyama, T., Kimura, K. and Sato, K. (1971): *Med. J. Osaka Univ., 21,* 113.

Oyama, T., Matsuki, A. and Kudo, T. (1972): *Brit. J. Anaesth., 44,* 841.

Randle, P. J. (1966): *Diabetologia, 2,* 237.

Selye, H. (1947): *Acta endocr. (Montreal).*

Yalow, R. S., Varsano-Aharon, N., Echemendia, E. and Berson, S. A. (1969): *Hormone Metab. Res., 1,* 3.

Adrenal glands and anesthesia

I. Effects of general anesthesia, spinal anesthesia and surgery on plasma aldosterone levels in man

T. OYAMA *, T. JIN, T. SATONE and T. KUDO

II. Effects of new steroid anesthetic, Althesin, on endocrine function

T. OYAMA *, A. MAEDA and T. KUDO

Department of Anesthesiology, University of Hirosaki, School of Medicine, Hirosaki, Japan

I. Aldosterone, a mineral corticoid of adrenal cortex, is an important hormone which influences electrolyte metabolism. Aldosterone causes increased tubular reabsorption of sodium and excretion of potassium, which decreases urinary Na and Cl and increases K, and expands extracellular fluid compartment.

Aldosterone secretion is increased by ACTH, sodium depletion, potassium increase, a fall in the plasma sodium to potassium ratio and by reduction in the extracellular fluid or blood volume. A fall in blood volume, a fall in blood pressure or vasoconstriction of the renal arteries produces a decrease in pressure in the afferent arteriole leading to a release of renin from the juxtaglomerular cells of kidney. The renin converts angiotensinogen manufactured in the liver to angiotensin I. This substance is further converted in the blood stream by an enzyme to angiotensin II which stimulates the adrenal cortex to release aldosterone. Aldosterone, in turn, leads to sodium retention and a rise in blood pressure, which acts as a feedback mechanism to shut off the further release of renin.

Effects of ether-N_2O anesthesia (16 patients), halothane-N_2O (15 patients), methoxyflurane-N_2O (15 patients), spinal anesthesia (7 patients) and surgery on plasma aldosterone concentrations were determined in 53 surgical patients by means of radioimmunoassay. Anesthesia alone was kept for 45 min before the start of surgery. Serum sodium and potassium concentrations were measured simultaneously in all cases and urinary Na/K ratios were determined in all general anesthesia groups, and plasma renin activity (PRA) was measured in 4 cases from each of the ether-N_2O and halothane-N_2O anesthesia groups, respectively. Plasma ACTH levels were measured in 10 patients who underwent halothane-N_2O anesthesia.

Plasma aldosterone concentrations were markedly elevated during ether-N_2O anesthesia alone (2.5-fold), halothane-N_2O or methoxyflurane-N_2O anesthesia alone (1.5- or 1.6-fold) compared with the control preinduction level. The further increase (3-fold) in plasma levels of aldosterone was noted 0.5–2 hr after the start of the operation. Elevated concen-

---

* Present address: Department of Anesthesiology, The Medical College of Wisconsin, Milwaukee-Wood, Wis., U.S.A.

trations of the plasma aldosterone were observed on the first postoperative day. It returned to preanesthetic control values on the 7th postoperative day. A significant decrease in urinary Na/K ratio was associated with the increase in plasma aldosterone levels. Plasma ACTH levels remarkably increased during halothane-N_2O anesthesia and surgery but they decreased on the first postoperative day. Renin activity in the plasma elevated slightly during ether-N_2O and halothane-N_2O anesthesia and surgery; however, no significant changes were observed in serum sodium and potassium concentrations. No significant changes in plasma aldosterone levels or serum sodium or potassium concentrations were observed during spinal anesthesia. These findings indicate that general anesthesia with ether, halothane or methoxyflurane stimulates aldosterone secretions from the adrenal cortex, but spinal anesthesia does not stimulate aldosterone secretion in man. The marked increase in ACTH secretion and/or elevated plasma renin activity appeared to play an important role in the increase of plasma aldosterone levels.

II. Plasma concentrations of luteinizing hormone increased markedly during Althesin-N_2O anesthesia alone for 45 min (2–2.5 times) compared with control value in 10 male patients. The peak level lasted for 30 min after the start of surgery, followed by decreasing tendency to decrease, although it was still significantly higher than the control level.

Plasma cortisol level did not change during anesthesia alone, but it rose significantly during surgery and in the recovery room. Plasma testosterone level decreased slightly but significantly during both anesthesia alone and surgery, and the lowest concentration was noted on the first postoperative day.

Clinical evaluation of the use of corticosteroids in orthopaedics and traumatic surgery

RICARDO VELA

Department of Anaesthesia and Resuscitation 'La Paz', Madrid, Spain

The indications for corticosteroids in traumatology are based upon their haemodynamic and metabolic effects which, directly or indirectly, effectively contribute to the restoration of homeostasis, together with macromolecular solutions, vasodilators, alkalinizing solutions, glucose solutions, protease inhibitors and other factors that form part of the therapeutic procedure. The standard indications – anti-inflammatory and anti-exudative – retain their current importance.

Trauma to the skull and brain, whether or not surgery is involved, constitutes one of the fundamental indications for glucocorticoid therapy. Traumatic cerebral oedema, and the presence of contused areas, cause ischaemic phenomena which are more or less prolonged and aggravate the clinical picture and its subsequent development. Since the oedema is a functional alteration of water metabolism, it is logical to act to reduce the volume of water in the body and consequently the cerebral volume by a rapid and profound diuresis.

Urea is no longer used because of rebound; 20% mannitol and furosemide are used, by means of which 300 ml of urine is produced for each 100 ml infused. Methylprednisolone, 200 mg, is given for the first 3 days, and then progressively reduced during subsequent days, and stopped after 15 days. This dose is doubled in serious cases.

Glucocorticoids have diuretic action in that they increase the renal flow, which results in an increase in glomerular filtration. Glucocorticoids also inhibit the antidiuretic hormone and seem to have specific diuretic effect, at the level of the collecting tubules, by impeding the reabsorption of water.

The therapeutic sequence in unconscious patients, whether or not they are receiving artificial ventilation, has been as follows: (a) fluid therapy: from 1000–1500 ml in 24 hr; (b) methylprednisolone: 200 mg in 24 hr; (c) furosemide: 80 mg in 24 hr.

pH, fluid and electrolyte monitoring is essential.

Corticosteroids are to some extent contraindicated in the delirious states of posttraumatic acute psychoses, since they may aggravate these mental conditions.

Glucocorticoids are very effective in *thoracic injuries*. Both inspiration and expiration may be inadequate; retention of secretions and progressive alveolar-capillary block interfere with gaseous exchange; artificial ventilatory devices are sometimes required.

The corticosteroids have anti-inflammatory effects, by reducing the increased permeability and diminishing exudation. The improvement in the circulation reduces peri-alveolar oedema which is otherwise inevitable. Bronchial diameter is increased so that distribution to terminal airways is improved.

Thoracic trauma accounts for 24% of all the injured patients during the past 7 years, and apart from rare exceptions methylprednisolone has always been used in these cases, 100–200 mg daily at first.

Prolonged therapy with glucocorticoids has not been required since after the 3rd week general improvement occurred and the fractures were stable so that effective thoracic movement was possible. There was therefore no need for steroids after the end of the 3rd week or the start of the 4th.

Spinal injuries and injuries of the legs result in large haematomas which may cause ischaemic compression phenomena. These are susceptible to glucocorticoid therapy combined with macromolecular solutions of dextran (40 and 70). The latter have rheological effects due to the associated vasodilation, and ostensibly improve the microcirculation and increase the number of active capillaries in the affected area. Reabsorption of haematomas may thus be facilitated.

In vertebral trauma with medullary involvement, the use of glucocorticoids in addition to anatomical alignment of the vertebrae reduces the medullary compression by the peri-medullary haematoma and hastens its reabsorption.

When the medullary lesion is irreversible, corticosteroids may shorten the time that elapses until the lesion becomes delineated. Many vertebral lesions, above the 7th thoracic vertebra, may also involve the respiratory musculature, so that the patient has to undergo temporary artificial ventilation. In these cases the use of corticosteroids limits the duration of artificial ventilation.

Orthopaedic operation for hip-joint replacement by a total prosthesis involves specific anaesthesiological problems, and there are also those caused by previous prolonged glucocorticoid therapy for the pathological condition itself.

The incidence of suprarenal insufficiency due to this therapy is not as great as might have been expected from the considerable increase in joint disease which has been observed recently in young and old people.

There is also a considerable increase in osteoporotic lesions secondary to glucocorticoid treatment in patients who also have chronic bronchopneumonic conditions.

Methylprednisolone is used for suprarenal insufficiency, as outlined below.

The day before operation: 80 mg intramuscularly every 12 hr. The day of operation: before inducing anaesthesia: 120 mg i.m., on terminating anaesthesia: 120 mg i.m., continuing with 80 mg every 12 hr. On subsequent days: 40 mg i.m. every 12 hr on the 1st day, 20 mg i.m. every 12 hr on the 2nd day, 10 mg i.m. every 12 hr on the 3rd day, 10 mg i.m. on the 4th day, 5 mg i.m. on the 5th day, 5 mg i.m. on the 6th day.

The intravenous route is reserved for emergency treatment when a double dose is used.

The use of corticosteroids in acute cardiovascular collapse and serious clinical situations was initially justified by the existence of functional depletion of the suprarenal glands, but since there is a physiological increase in response to stress this is now no longer justified.

In states of progressive shock, particularly those of cardiogenic aetiology and those of septic origin, Bloch et al. (1966), Dietzman et al. (1967) and Lillehei et al. (1967) advise the use of hydrocortisone and methylprednisolone in large doses in order to mobilize the blood volume that has accumulated due to microcirculatory stasis. Corticosteroids in appropriate doses have important vasodilator effects due to a direct action on the smooth muscle of the vessels in the postcapillary venules, and trapped red cells are returned to the circulation.

The improvement in the microcirculation is shown by the progressive disappearance of metabolic acidosis and the subsequent diminution of lactacidaemia. This improvement is due to the conversion of lactic acid (accumulated in anaerobiosis) to pyruvic acid by dehydrogenation due to nicotinamide adenine dinucleotide (NAD) which is reduced by the 2 hydrogen ions from the lactic acid.

Glucocorticoids also help to induce the entry of the aminoacids and fatty acids into the Krebs cycle, directly, and by means of decarboxylation of pyruvic acid, which passes into the most active form of acetic acid, acetyl-coenzyme A. All this presupposes marked general stimulation of gluconeogenesis and a considerable increase in the cellular reserves of adenosine triphosphate (ATP), which had been exhausted by increased consumption which occurs in these pathological situations.

Glucocorticoids, at the cellular level, protect the lipoprotein membranes which enclose the cellular granules formed by acid hydrolases and which are biochemically inert and are constituents of the lysosomes. The lysosomal and cellular rupture allows polypeptide products such as histamine, 5-hydroxytryptamine or serotonin, and the so-called 'vasoactive kinins' to escape. The vasodilator effects of histamine at the arteriolocapillary level are well known; there is also an increase in capillary permeability. Serotonin, for its part, is liberated by the platelets during platelet lysis; this initiates blood coagulation and a vasoconstrictor effect is produced. The precursors of the vasoactive kinins, such as trypsin and kallikrein, have to be combined with the α-2 globulins in order to be activated. The latter only appear in the blood as a result of trauma, haemorrhage, septicaemia, etc., and generally in response to any aggression.

There is a progressive induction of a state of hypercoagulability, which increases the viscosity of the blood and may initiate a change in haemostasis, which is facilitated by increases in factors, I, V, VI, VIII and IX, activated by the contact factors and especially by factor XII (Hageman's factor). This state of hypercoagulability may in its turn initiate a widespread intravascular coagulation; fibrinolytic activation by factor XII may contribute to this.

Clinically, the use of large doses of glucocorticoids, combined with the restoration of blood volume by dextran and blood transfusion, has given good results. When 30 mg/kg was administered intravenously (sometimes repeated after 6 hr), the vasoconstrictor phenomena receded, venous stasis disappeared and the trapped blood was again incorporated in the circulation. Plethysmographic recording of the capillary circulation in the lobe of the ear clearly showed an improvement in the microcirculation, the waves being amplified and their frequency diminished.

Recently Dietzman et al. (1973) have advised the use of corticosteroids in the treatment of cardiogenic shock, combined with mechanical devices designed to aid the pumping action of the heart. These devices in series diminish the pressure of the contractile effort, and in parallel reduce the volume expelled by the left ventricle.

The devices arranged in series act as a counter-pulse, increasing the diastolic pressure. The devices arranged in parallel imply that a shunt is set up, preventing the blood that has to be expelled from passing into the left ventricle. In both cases these devices reduce the work of the heart and its energy expenditure, while at the same time there is recovery of the ischaemic process.

Finally, glucocorticoids have positive inotropic action, which may contribute to the improvement of the acute cardiovascular syndrome.

The vasodilator effect of large doses of glucocorticoids is undoubtedly due to a direct action upon the capillary and postcapillary region. Whether the benefit is due to a direct action or an indirect consequence of the improvement in the microcirculation, is a problem yet to be resolved.

Surgical shock, including traumatic and posthaemorrhagic shock, is no longer a problem due to the rational, ordered and sequential use of regulated therapy, whose fundamental crux is the restoration of blood volume.

REFERENCES

Bloch, J. H., Dietzman, R. H., Pierce, C. H. and Lillehei, R. C. (1966): *Brit. J. Anaesth.*, *38*, 234.
Dietzman, R. C., Beckman, C. B. and Lillehei, R. C. (1973): *Geriatrics*, *28*, 69.
Dietzman, R. C., Bloch, J. H. and Lillehei, R. C. (1967): *Amer. Acad. Gen. Prac.*, *36*, 135.
Lillehei, R. C., Dietzman, R. H., Mousas, S. and Bloch, J. H. (1967): *Mod. Treatm.*, *4*, 321.

Anesthesia and reanimation in thyroid and parathyroid surgery

JOSE MARIA GUTIERREZ GOICOECHEA

Department of Anesthesia and Reanimation, Virgen del Rocio Hospital, Seville, Spain

The thyroid and parathyroid glands may undergo pathological changes which require surgery. The close anatomical relations and physiological integration of the glands pose problems in anesthesia and necessitate adequate and efficient reanimation.

The thyroid gland produces the hormones thyroxine (T_4), discovered in 1927 by Harrington and Barker, and triiodothyronine (T_3), named in 1952 by Gross and Pitt. These hormones are produced with the metabolism of iodine, are mobilized under hypothalamo-hypophyseal control, with probable storage in the liver, are utilized in the tissues by means of cyclic AMP, and are finally eliminated in the urine and feces (Fig. 1).

Briefly, their functions relate to: regulation of oxygen consumption and basal metabolism ($37\ cal/m^2/hr$); stimulation of growth and cellular maturation; stimulation of carbohydrate, fats and protein metabolism; excitability tone of the nervous and muscular systems; inter-

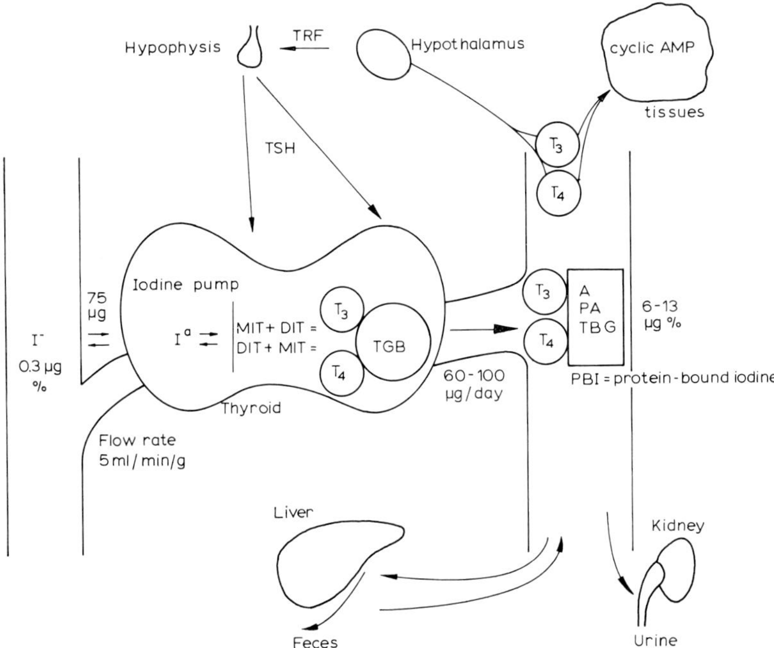

Fig. 1. *Metabolic cycle of the thyroid hormones.*

vention in muscular metabolism of ions and vitamins A and B; effects on the cardiovascular system and on catecholamines; synthesis of hemoglobin; digestive and gonadal effects.

Of especial interest is the direct action of thyroxine on the heart and blood vessels, particularly in the case of hyperfunction or thyrotoxicosis, with sensitization of the α- and β-adrenergic receptors, the production of hypertension with tachycardia, palpitations and arrhythmias, increases in the cardiac debit and cardiac oxygen consumption, and slight peripheral action of a vascular type.

Various groups of patients can be distinguished from the surgical point of view: (*a*) Hyper- or hypothyroid patients who undergo normal or emergency surgery for other conditions, with the possible combination of shock, infection, etc. (*b*) Thyroidectomy for simple or diffuse goiter without severe metabolic repercussions or with mechanical compression e.g., endothoracic goiter. (*c*) Extirpation of the gland for toxic goiter with severe metabolic disturbances (thyrotoxicosis) of a nodular (Plummer) or diffuse (Graves or Basedow) type, in which case adequate preoperative preparation is required. (*d*) The presence of primary or metastatic cancer, with the possible association of pheochromocytoma or paraneoplastic myasthenia, which may involve extensive surgery, with profuse hemorrhage, etc.

PREPARATION OF THE PATIENT

This can be summarized as: Hygienic-dietetic treatment; protein diet; ionic and emotional equilibrium; administration of iodine as Lugol's solution (10–20 drops/day). *Antithyroid drugs*: methylthiouracil (Athyroid – 300 mg/day); propylthiouracil (Prothiural – 400 mg/day); methimazole (Tomizol – 30 mg/day); carbimazole (Neo-Tomizol – 20 mg/day); salts of lithium and ^{131}I (4-8 mCi). *Circulatory drugs*: Reserpine, β-blockers, glycosides, etc., which must be evaluated and used carefully with due consideration of possible deleterious interactions with drugs which will be used at the time of the operation or postoperatively. Hematic protection and normalization of blood constants (Hb, proteins, ions, etc.) is also required.

PREMEDICATION

Basically, preoperative fear and excitement mobilizes the secretion of catecholamines and thyroxine, which potentiate and aggravate the preexistent circulatory condition. It is therefore necessary to achieve adequate and potent sedation to impede hormone secretion. Barbiturates are used orally, with diazepoxides and the combination of pethidine-promethazine and haloperidol or diazepam, together with Thalamonal; on occasions a rise in thyroxine cannot be avoided.

In emergency cases without preoperative warning, induction can be performed in the patient's bed with transfer later to the operating theatre.

The use of vagolytics is not routine. A test dose of atropine may be tried if there has been prior bradycardia (reserpine), or if halothane is to be used; scopolamine is preferable.

ANESTHESIA

The Lawen technique for local anesthesia has been described, with or without low doses of adrenaline (1/500,000), but techniques of general anesthesia are preferred, with intubation for improved control of airway. Combination is possible with local anesthesia to avoid dangerous reflexes and to allow a reduction in the depth of general anesthesia. The position should be semi-seated with 20° head-up tilt to facilitate venous drainage and to avoid swallowing of the gland with the throat extended.

Dilute thiopentone induces sleep and reduces thyroxine levels; succinylcholine ensures good relaxation of the vocal cords, which can be anesthetized with Xylocaine to avoid 'bucking' during the operation. Cuffed endotracheal tubes, of the hooped Woodbridge type or with a lateral hole, are used for intubation in order to avoid obstruction due to tracheal deviation and to allow constant control of pulmonary ventilation.

Anesthesia must be maintained with slight relaxation and with adequate analgesia. Coughing and vomiting, which increase bleeding, must be avoided. From the recent studies of Oyama it is known that the TSH level hardly varies with different anesthetics, but that the thyroxine level is increased by ether and by halothane, but is not affected by N_2O or the morphine-like drugs (Fig. 2). Enflurane has given ambiguous results but it is useful because of its circulatory stability, combined with pancuronium if relaxation is needed (and without which the cardiac rhythm and arterial pressure are affected at low halothane concentrations of 0.5–1 %), and which can be reinforced by small doses of pethidine or morphine-mimetics.

	TSH	thyroxin	catecholamines
Halothane	O	↑↑	O↑
Penthrane	O	↑	O↑
Ethrane	O	↑↓	O↑
Thiobarbital	O	↓↓	O
Ether	O	↑↑↑	↑↑↑
Halothane N_2O	O	↑↑	↑
Morphia derivs N_2O	O	O	O

Fig. 2.

Hypoxia and hypercapnia must always be avoided, and a clear airway and mild hyperventilation are needed. Negative expiratory pressure is a debatable practice, but it can be useful to diminish capillary or venous bleeding at the site of the operation without controlled hypotension. Naturally, it is useful and convenient to monitor the patient for ECG, arterial and venous blood pressures, temperature, diuresis, etc., and to prepare the venous lines for sera and transfusions.

COMPLICATIONS

As the methods of preparation and anesthesia and of surgery have improved, so the incidence of complications has fallen. These can be summarized as: (1) Compression of the eyes (in exophthalmos) by the anesthetic mask. (2) Respiratory: Obstruction of the endotracheal tube (secretions, compression); surgical manipulations, compression and tracheomalacia; hyperventilation; pneumothorax; tracheal rupture; emphysema. (3) Circulatory: Profuse hemorrhage; air embolism; severe ventricular or paroxysmal dysrhythmias; alteration of the cardiac output and venous return; surgical reflexes; hypertension or shock; hyperthermia; sweating; signs of sympathetic stimulation; carotid stimulation syndrome (Turner).

With early and firm diagnosis, these can be treated etiologically.

POSTOPERATIVE CARE

There seems to be an average mortality of 0.5%, so that a strict vigilance is required in the first few hours after extubation. A nonobstructive compression bandage allows secondary bleeding to be detected. The biological constants quoted previously are monitored, and the effort involved in coughing and vomiting is avoided. It is convenient to administer aerosols and to keep the air humid, together with the careful use of antibiotics, mild analgesics, and liquid diet or fluid therapy if there is dysphagia.

The most frequent complication is the appearance of a thyroid crisis with acute and intense thyrotoxicosis. This is favoured by poor preoperative preparation, by emotional stress, infection, pregnancy, acidosis, etc., and appears in 1–3% of cases, although it was previously more frequent and of poor prognosis. It develops with hyperthermia (over 39°C), hypertension or collapse, severe tachycardia, cardiac insufficiency and possible fibrillation, excitation with later coma, abdominal pains, nausea, and vomiting.

Its treatment must be rapid and intensive, with oxygen, abundant fluids, cardiotonic drugs, large doses of corticoids, intravenous iodine, β-blockers, reserpine, lithic cocktail, phentolamine, cooling, spinal anesthesia to the D_4 level, and sympathetic block to combat the intense thyrotoxicosis and the circulatory condition.

RESPIRATORY COMPLICATIONS

The following may be observed: airway obstruction by hematoma, edema or laryngeo-tracheal spasm; stridor; paralysis of the vocal cords or diaphragm; nerve lesion; retention of bronchial mucus – increased secretion; overdoses of analgesics and relaxants; para-thyroid tetany.

There may also be a delayed crisis of hypothyroidism, which is treated with triiodo-thyronine, but it must be remembered that hypothyroid patients are more sensitive to sedatives, analgesics, anesthetics and vasoactive drugs. There is a danger of hypotension, hypothermia and hypocapnia.

PARATHYROIDS

Their main function is the control of ionic metabolism, especially of calcium and phosphorus, via Parathormone, discovered by Collip in 1925 and having a hypercalcemic action. Calcitonin, produced by the thyroids and named by Copp in 1961, acts to decrease blood calcium levels. Both functions are related to vitamin D.

Pathologically, their hyperfunction initiates the clinical state of hyperparathyroidism, and occurs through hyperplasia or neoplasm, or by chronic renal insufficiency and repeated hemodialysis. This condition is complicated by gastric ulcers, pancreatic syndrome, articular and osseous pain, renal calculi, hypercalcemia (from 12 mg or 6 mEq%) and hyperphosphatemia (from 2.5 mg or 1.5 mEq%).

Preanesthetic evaluation basically consists of: determination of the adequacy of renal function, diuresis and drug elimination; recognition of the presence of states of asthenia and hypo-excitability of muscles and neuromotor plates; a study of cardiovascular function – the high calcium level gives short Q-T values and a reduction or absence of ST; the presence of hypercalcemic crisis (asthenia, drowsiness, vomiting, etc.).

Preparation consists of dialysis if necessary, the use of calcium EDTA or sodium citrate, ethacrynic acid as a diuretic, and the use of alkalis and gastric vagolytics etc. Premedication need not be so potent as in the case of thyroid patients, especially since there is not the anxiety which leads to elevated catecholamine levels. This is followed by the preoperative infusion of 1 % toluidine or methylene blue solutions which concentrate in the parathyroid gland to give it colour and thus aid in its detection and excision. Relaxants should be used cautiously because of their slow renal elimination, and maintenance of anesthesia is similar to that suggested for thyroid patients.

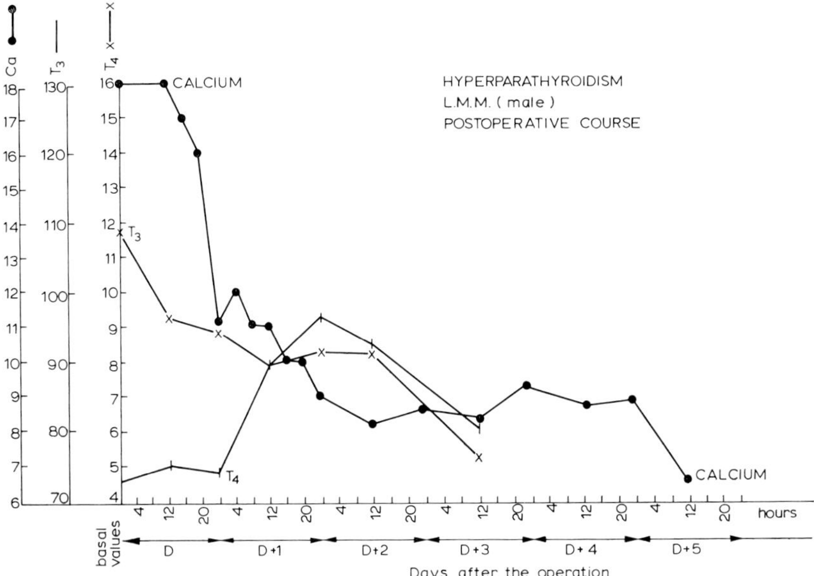

Fig. 3.   *Evolution of calcium-T₃ and T₄ in postoperative period.*

Vigilance is necessary in the postoperative period to detect any fall in calcium level, which can be rapid, using laboratory assays and clinical observation of the Trouseau sign with sphygmometry. This detects the early signs of tetany, which is treated with calcium salts (gluconate or the more active chloride). Also, vitamin D should be given (50,000–150,000 units). The phosphorus content of the diet should be reduced, and a watch kept on the behaviour of Mg^{2+}, an inseparable companion of calcium. Emotional stress and anxiety are to be avoided since they induce hyperventilation, which in turn aids in the appearance of tetany (Fig. 3).

A rational approach to the management of the glucocorticoid-treated surgical patient

HENRIK KEHLET

Hvidøre Hospital, Klampenborg, Denmark

The aim of this study was to establish a scheme of rational management of supplementary glucocorticoid-replacement therapy (steroid cover) for glucocorticoid-treated patients undergoing surgery. The following points were investigated: (1) The risk of stress-induced adrenocortical insufficiency in unsupplemented glucocorticoid-treated patients; (2) glucocorticoid-preparation and dosage of the steroid cover; and (3) a simple test for preoperative assessment of hypothalamic-pituitary-adrenocortical (HPA) function in glucocorticoid-treated patients.

1. The prophylactic use of steroids has resulted in ignorance about the risk involved in omitting supplementary glucocorticoids, since early reports claiming stress-induced adrenocortical insufficiency in unsupplemented glucocorticoid-treated patients are inconclusive (Roberts, 1970). In a recent study in 104 unsupplemented glucocorticoid-treated surgical patients the occurrence of hypotension could not be correlated to the plasma cortisol measured at the same time (Kehlet and Binder, 1973*a*), an observation made previously in a smaller group of patients (Jasani et al., 1968; Oyama and Takiguchi, 1972). Hypotension did not require administration of glucocorticoids, but responded to usual fluid therapy (Kehlet and Binder, 1973*a*). Additional studies of postoperative changes in plasma volume (Kehlet et al., 1974*a*) and plasma catecholamines (Kehlet et al., 1974*b*) further emphasized that hypotension is not related to adrenocortical insufficiency. In summary, it is concluded that adrenocortical insufficiency is not a significant risk in unsupplemented glucocorticoid-treated surgical patients, but, on the contrary, it must be rare.

2. The glucocorticoid preparations usually recommended for parenteral substitution therapy are cortisone acetate or a water-soluble cortisol (hydrocortisone) preparation. However, cortisone acetate in usually recommended dosage may be incapable of raising plasma cortisol sufficiently (Plumpton et al., 1969*b*; Kehlet et al., 1974*c*) and therefore, only the water-soluble cortisol preparations should be used for steroid cover. A physiological approach to the dosage of the supplementary glucocorticoid-replacement therapy would be to recommend the amount of glucocorticoid secreted during surgery in normal patients, thereby imitating the HPA response to surgery even in the occasional glucocorticoid-treated patient with no HPA function. The amount of cortisol secreted during surgery in normal patients has been estimated at 75–150 mg/24 hr during major surgery and about 50 mg/24 hr during minor surgery (Kehlet, 1974). This amount of glucocorticoid is administered (see below), every 24 hr, postoperatively until gastrointestinal function is normal, since normal function excludes serious postoperative complications and removes the indication for continued supplements and also allows the normal dosage of oral glucocorticoid to be given safely. Preoperative supplementary glucocorticoid is not indicated,

since plasma cortisol level is not elevated preoperatively in normal patients. There is no indication for an increased dosage of the steroid cover during acute surgery since cortisol secretion is similar during elective and acute surgery in normal patients. Supplementary glucocorticoids during surgery in patients previously under treatment with glucocorticoids is indicated if glucocorticoid treatment has been stopped less than 2 months before surgery (Plumpton et al., 1969*a*).

3. Preoperative assessment of HPA function can be made using the insulin hypoglycemia test, the lysine-vasopressin test, the metyrapone test (Jasani et al., 1968) or the pyrogen test. However, these tests are either time-consuming, uncomfortable for the patient or have certain contraindications. Recently, it has been demonstrated (Kehlet and Binder, 1973*b*) that the simple 30 min ACTH stimulation test is reliable in predicting the HPA response to surgery in glucocorticoid-treated patients, and therefore is recommended when preoperative assessment of HPA function is desirable. This approach requires careful observation for signs of adrenocortical insufficiency; immediate therapy for adrenocortical insufficiency must be available.

The following regime is recommended.

SUPPLEMENTARY GLUCOCORTICOIDS TO GLUCOCORTICOID-TREATED SURGICAL PATIENTS

1. Patients under treatment with glucocorticoids

25 mg cortisol intravenously with induction of anaesthesia in all patients. Following *major surgery* (abdominal, thoracic, major orthopedic) 100 mg cortisol dissolved in saline or glucose is given by continuous intravenous infusion every 24 hr, until gastrointestinal function permits oral intake of usual glucocorticoid treatment. If an infusion of cortisol is undesirable, 25 mg cortisol is given intravenously every 4 hr. Following *minor surgery* (hand surgery, herniotomy, uterine curettage) the usual glucocorticoid therapy is started immediately after operation.

2. Patients previously treated with glucocorticoids

(*a*) Glucocorticoids received less than 2 months previously: supplementary glucocorticoids are given as above (1). (*b*) Glucocorticoid treatment stopped more than 2 months previously: no indication for supplementary glucocorticoids.

3. Preoperative assessment

If supplementary glucocorticoids are undesirable, preoperative assessment of the hypothalamic-pituitary-adrenocortical function is made using the 30 min ACTH stimulation test. In selected patients supplementary glucocorticoids may be omitted. However, this approach requires careful observation for adrenocortical insufficiency; immediate therapy for adrenocortical insufficiency must be available.

REFERENCES

Jasani, M. K., Freeman, P. A., Boyle, J. A., Reid, A. M., Driver, M. J. and Buchanan, W. W. (1968): *Quart. J. Med.*, *37*, 407.
Kehlet, H. (1974): *Acta anaesth. scand.*, in press.

Kehlet, H. and Binder, C. (1973*a*): *Brit. J. Anaesth.*, *45*, 1043.
Kehlet, H. and Binder, C. (1973*b*): *Brit. med. J.*, *2*, 147.
Kehlet, H., Engquist, A. and Greibe, J. (1974*a*): *Brit. J. Anaesth.*, *46*, 452.
Kehlet, H., Nikki, P., Jäättela, A. and Takki, S. (1974*b*): *Brit. J. Anaesth.*, *46*, 73.
Kehlet, H., Nistrup Madsen, S. and Binder, C. (1974*c*): *Acta med. scand.*, *195*, 421.
Oyama, T. and Takiguchi, M. (1972): *Canad. Anaesth. Soc. J.*, *19*, 239.
Plumpton, F. S., Besser, G. M. and Cole, P. V. (1969*a*): *Anaesthesia*, *24*, 3.
Plumpton, F. S., Besser, G. M. and Cole, P. V. (1969*b*): *Anaesthesia*, *24*, 12.
Roberts, J. C. (1970): *Surg. Clin. N. Amer.*, *50*, 363.

Anesthesia mechanisms and endocrine action: The effects of morphine, halothane, and ketamine on brain cyclic AMP and cerebral metabolism

JULIEN F. BIEBUYCK, DANIEL F. DEDRICK and YVETTE D. SCHERER

Department of Anesthesia, Harvard Medical School,
Massachusetts General Hospital, Boston, Mass., U.S.A.

Cyclic AMP (adenosine 3',5'-monophosphate) has been implicated as an intracellular mediator in the actions of a variety of hormones on their target tissues (Sutherland, 1972). The mechanism of action of certain neural transmitters is thought to be similar. Both these groups of substances act at membranes of specific receptor cells to cause intracellular release of an active molecule (cyclic AMP) which, in turn, modifies cellular function. Cyclic AMP in brain may function post-synaptically in interneural transmission, particularly at adrenergic synapses (Greengard and Costa, 1970). We have examined in vivo brain levels of cyclic AMP and other intermediates reflecting the energy reserves and cytoplasmic redox state during exposure of animals to three anesthetic agents with differing chemical structure. The use of a newly-developed method of rapid brain tissue sampling and freezing has enabled the known effects of anoxia on labile intermediates to be eliminated. In addition, careful monitoring and control of physiological parameters has avoided neurochemical alterations (Miller et al., 1972) associated with hypercarbia and hypothermia.

METHODS

Brain sampling

Male rats (Wistar strain, 200 g body weight) were used for this study. The technic for rapid brain sampling and freezing has been previously described in detail (Biebuyck and Hawkins, 1972; Veech et al., 1973; Lust et al., 1973). The apparatus (Fig. 1) consists of two hollow stainless steel probes which are driven into the cranial cavity of a rat immobilized in a special restraining cage. When in position, air under pressure (26 lb/sq. inch) enters through one probe and the supratentorial portion of the brain is displaced through the other probe into an aluminum chamber pre-cooled to the temperature of liquid N_2 ($-196°$ C). Samples of 0.7–1.0 g of brain tissue are obtained from animals weighing approximately 200 g. The technic is equally applicable to awake or anesthetized animals.

Physiological monitoring

In all anesthetized animals, blood pressure, blood gases, and temperature were maintained in a constant range. A 22-gauge cannula was inserted into a tail vein for intravenous injections. The femoral artery was cannulated with a 22-gauge catheter, connected through a sampling stopcock to a strain gauge pressure transducer. The blood pressure was

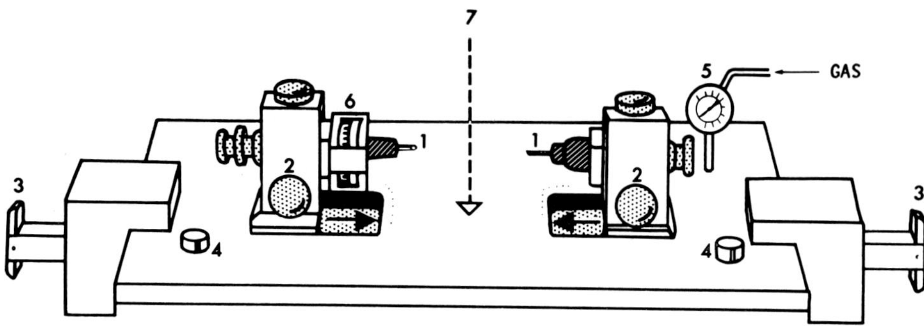

Fig. 1.   *Diagram of apparatus used for rapid freezing of brain tissue. (1) Hollow stainless steel probes. (2) Movable blocks. (3) Solenoids. (4) Actuating buttons. (5) Entry point of gas under pressure (communicating with probe on right). (6) Aluminium plates (pre-cooled in liquid N₂). (7) Position of rat on restraining platform.*

displayed on an oscilloscope. Systolic blood pressure was always above 100 mm Hg at the time of brain sampling. A rectal thermistor probe was used to monitor temperature (maintained at 37–38° C). Ventilation was controlled with a volume-cycled small animal ventilator, connected to an endotracheal tube inserted by direct laryngoscopy (see Table 1).

Table 1.   *Arterial blood gases prior to brain sampling*

	Halothane	Morphine	Ketamine
P_{O_2}	213.9 $\pm$ 21.7 (16)	268.9 $\pm$ 21.2 (17)	324.9 $\pm$ 32.5 (15)
P_{CO_2}	37.27 $\pm$ 1.37 (16)	40.23 $\pm$ 0.80 (17)	37.79 $\pm$ 0.16 (15)

Samples were obtained from the femoral artery cannula. Details of drug dosage appear in Methods section. Results expressed in mm Hg (means $\pm$ standard error of the mean (S.E.M.) with the number of observations in parenthesis).

Anesthesia

Halothane in O₂ (1.5% v/v) was used for maintenance following induction of anesthesia. The second group received morphine 20 mg/kg body weight intravenously. A second dose of 10 mg/kg was given at 30 min. The third group received ketamine (10 mg/kg body wt) at 5–10 min intervals as indicated by the minimal anesthetic concentration requirements. Brain sampling was at 60 min following induction of anesthesia. Control samples were obtained from awake animals unanesthetized.

Metabolite assays

These were performed on extracts of the frozen brain tissue by enzymatic methods (see Biebuyck et al., 1972; Miller et al., 1972; Biebuyck et al., 1974). Substrate concentrations are expressed per gram wet weight of brain tissue as sampled, and are *not* corrected for theoretical or presumed contents of blood, cerebral spinal fluid (CSF) and extracellular fluid (ECF).

RESULTS

No decrease in brain energy stores occurred with any of the agents tested (Fig. 2). In fact, a statistically significant increase in brain phosphocreatine concentration occurred during halothane exposure. A highly significant increase in brain cyclic AMP concentrations occurred with each of the anesthetic drugs (Table 2). This was associated with a similar increase (approximately 2-fold) of brain glucose concentrations. The calculated redox state (free [NAD$^+$]/free [NADH]) of the brain tissue cytoplasm was unaltered (halothane and ketamine) or significantly raised (morphine) during anesthesia (Table 3).

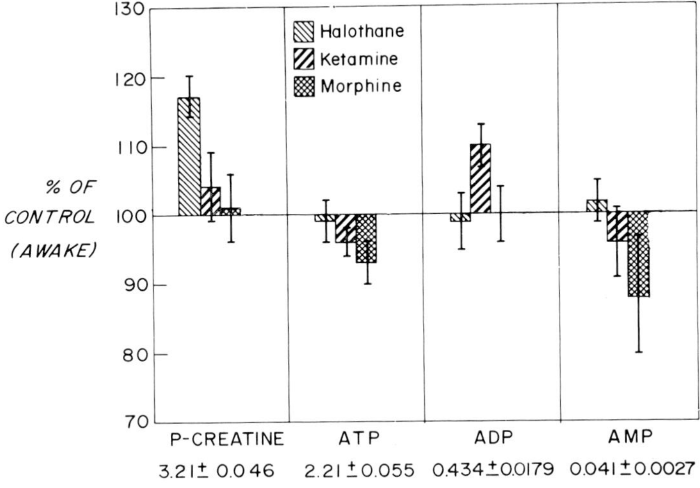

Fig. 2.   *Brain energy intermediates during anesthesia. Results are expressed as a percentage of the control awake values. (The latter values in μmol/g wet weight ± S.E.M. appear below). The vertical bars on the histogram refer to the S.E.M. of the experimental groups.*

Table 2.   *Brain cyclic AMP and glucose concentrations*

	Awake	Halothane	Morphine	Ketamine
Glucose	1.20 ± 0.031 (12)	2.66 ± 0.198 * (13)	2.71 ± 0.190 * (13)	2.02 ± 0.146 * (14)
Cyclic AMP	1.29 ± 0.100 (11)	2.50 ± 0.130 * (8)	2.65 ± 0.154 * (8)	2.33 ± 0.308 * (8)

* P < 0.01.
Brain tissue was rapidly sampled and frozen as described in the Methods section. Results expressed as nmol/g wet weight (cyclic AMP) or μmol/g wet weight (glucose). Means ± S.E.M. (number of observations in parenthesis).

DISCUSSION

The finding of unaltered brain energy stores and a normal redox state in the tissue cytoplasm, during anesthesia with these diverse agents, is in general agreement with the concept of a reduced demand for ATP during anesthesia and coma (Quastel, 1939; Stone,

Table 3.   *Brain tissue cytoplasmic redox state during anesthesia*

Awake	699 ± 43 (20)
Halothane	796 ± 74 (7)
Morphine	849 ± 59 (8)*
Ketamine	804 ± 24 (7)

* $P < 0.05$.

The free NAD^+/free NADH ratio was calculated as described in the Discussion section, from the lactate dehydrogenase reaction. Results expressed as mean of ratios $\pm$ S.E.M. (number of observations in parenthesis).

1938; Lowry et al., 1964; Richter and Dawson, 1948; Van den Noort et al., 1970; Derr and Zieve, 1973). The ratio of the concentrations of free NAD^+ and NADH at the site of oxido-reductions is of importance because it bears on the metabolic behavior of the cell. This ratio may be obtained by measuring the ratio of the concentrations of the oxidized and reduced metabolites of suitable NAD-linked dehydrogenase systems that are located in different cell compartments; and, on account of their high activity, are in equilibrium or near-equilibrium with the nucleotides. The equation used for the cytoplasmic redox state in these experiments (lactate dehydrogenase (LDH) system) was:

$$\frac{[NAD^+]}{[NADH]} = \frac{[Pyruvate]}{[Lactate]} \times \frac{1}{K}$$

(where K is the equilibrium constant of the LDH reaction: 1.11×10^{-4} at pH 7.0) (Williamson et al., 1967; Miller et al., 1973).

Norepinephrine increases the levels of cyclic AMP (Shimuzu et al., 1970) in the brain. The physiological significance of the regulation of cyclic AMP levels by hormones and neuro-transmitters during anesthesia is still open to question. We have correlated the present findings with measurements of levels of four putative neuro-transmitter substances (GABA, glutamate, glutamine, aspartate) during anesthesia (Biebuyck et al., 1974). Our present work is involved with comparison of these results with the neurochemical changes induced by hepatic coma.

REFERENCES

Biebuyck, J. F., Dedrick, D. F. and Scherer, Y. D. (1975): In: *Molecular Mechanisms of Anesthesia*, p. 451. Editor: B. R. Fink. Raven Press, New York, N.Y.
Biebuyck, J. F. and Hawkins, R. A. (1972): *Brit. J. Anaesth., 44*, 226.
Biebuyck, J. F., Lund, P. and Krebs, H. A. (1972): *Biochem. J., 128*, 700.
Derr, R. F. and Zieve, L. (1973): *J. Neurochem., 72*, 1555.
Greengard, P. and Costa, E. (1970): In: *Advances in Biochemical Psychopharmacology, Vol. III.* Editors: E. Costa and E. Gracobini. Raven Press, New York, N.Y.
Lowry, O. H., Passonneau, J. V., Hasselberger, F. X. and Schulz, D. W. (1964): *J. biol. Chem., 239*, 18.
Lust, W. D., Passonneau, J. V. and Veech, R. L. (1973): *Science, 181*, 280.
Miller, A. L., Hawkins, R. A., Harris, R. L. and Veech, R. L. (1972): *Biochem. J., 129*, 463.
Miller, A. L., Hawkins, R. A. and Veech, R. L. (1973): *J. Neurochem., 20*, 1393.
Quastel, J. H. (1939): *Physiol. Rev., 19*, 135.
Richter, D. and Dawson, R. M. C. (1948): *Amer. J. Physiol., 154*, 73.
Stone, W. E. (1938): *Biochem. J., 32*, 1908.
Shimuzu, H., Creveling, C. R. and Daly, J. (1970): *Proc. nat. Acad. Sci. (Wash.), 65*, 1033.
Sutherland, E. W. (1972): *Science, 177*, 401.
Van den Noort, S., Eckel, R. E., Brine, K. L. and Hrldlicka, J. (1970): *Arch. intern. Med., 126*, 831.
Veech, R. L., Harris, R. L., Veloso, D. and Veech, E. H. (1973): *J. Neurochem., 20*, 183.
Williamson, D. H., Lund, P. and Krebs, H. A. (1967): *Biochem. J., 103*, 514.

Effect of epidural anaesthesia on the endocrine response to surgery

M. R. BRANDT [1], H. KEHLET [2], C. BINDER [2], C. HAGEN [3]
and A. S. McNEILLY [3]

[1] Department of Anaesthesiology, Gentofte Hospital, and
[2] Hvidøre Hospital, Copenhagen, Denmark; and
[3] Department of Chemical Pathology, St. Bartholomew's Hospital, London, United Kingdom

It has been suggested that epidural anaesthesia may inhibit the endocrine-metabolic response to surgical stress as expressed by changes in plasma cortisol and plasma glucose (Bromage et al., 1971; Lush et al., 1972; Gordon et al., 1973). The present study considers changes in plasma concentrations of glucose, cortisol, growth hormone, prolactin, insulin and glucagon during surgery using epidural anaesthesia and compared to the changes during general anaesthesia.

Ten otherwise healthy females were studied during abdominal hysterectomy. None had received any medication previously. All patients were anaesthetized with atropine, promethazine for premedication, thiopentone and suxamethonium for induction and enflurane, pancuronium and $N_2O + O_2$ for maintenance of anaesthesia. Five of the patients in addition received continuous epidural analgesia effective before the skin incision and for the following 26 hr. Bupivacaine without adrenaline was used. Fourteen blood samples for hormonal measurements were taken before, during and after anaesthesia and surgery as indicated in Table 1. Glucose concentration was determined by a glucose oxidase method, cortisol concentration by a competitive protein-binding technique and concentrations of growth hormone, prolactin, insulin and glucagon by specific radioimmunoassays.

The results (Table 1) showed a postoperative increase in plasma concentration of glucose after general anaesthesia, while epidural analgesia almost blocked this increase. Plasma concentration of cortisol increased per- and postoperatively, with a tendency to lower values during epidural analgesia. Growth hormone showed an insignificant increase during surgery only under general anaesthesia. Prolactin showed a pronounced increase immediately after induction and in both groups. Insulin and glucagon were unchanged during and after surgery in both groups.

Thus, epidural analgesia inhibited the hyperglycaemic response to surgical stress, but this could not uniformly be correlated to a single component in the endocrine response to surgery as expressed by changes in concentrations of cortisol, growth hormone, prolactin, insulin and glucagon in peripheral plasma.

REFERENCES

Bromage, P. R., Shibata, H. R. and Willoughby, H. W. (1971): *Surg. Gynec. Obstet., 132,* 1051.
Gordon, N. H., Scott, D. B. and Percy Robb, I. W. (1973): *Brit. med. J., 1,* 581.
Lush, D., Thorpe, J. N., Richardson, D. J. and Bowen, D. J. (1972): *Brit. J. Anaesth., 44,* 1169

Table 1.   *Blood samples for hormonal measurements taken before, during and after anaesthesia and surgery*

	Preanaesthetic control		Period after skin incision (hr)											
			0	1/3	2/3	1	2	3	4	6	9	14	24	26
Glucose *(a)*	78 ± 7	79 ± 9	86 ± 9	102 ± 12	105 ± 11	108 ± 11	119 ± 10	136 ± 4	144 ± 7	147 ± 6	139 ± 6	131 ± 12	121 ± 12	103 ± 6
(mg/100 ml) *(b)*	79 ± 3	75 ± 3	77 ± 4	80 ± 7	84 ± 7	90 ± 6	97 ± 2	105 ± 5	102 ± 5	97 ± 1	97 ± 3	98 ± 5	88 ± 4	89 ± 4
Cortisol	17 ± 4	15 ± 4	22 ± 4	30 ± 3	37 ± 2	40 ± 4	41 ± 3	48 ± 4	52 ± 3	54 ± 3	58 ± 5	37 ± 8	25 ± 2	19 ± 1
(μg/100 ml)	10 ± 2	9 ± 2	17 ± 3	21 ± 2	25 ± 1	29 ± 2	32 ± 2	39 ± 4	43 ± 4	46 ± 3	49 ± 3	35 ± 3	26 ± 2	20 ± 2
Growth hormone	8 ± 4	7 ± 3	6 ± 2	12 ± 2	13 ± 2	11 ± 1	13 ± 5	8 ± 1	7 ± 2	8 ± 1	8 ± 1	6 ± 2	13 ± 5	6 ± 1
(ng/ml)	6 ± 1	7 ± 1	5 ± 1	7 ± 2	9 ± 2	5 ± 1	5 ± 1	4 ± 1	6 ± 1	10 ± 2	8 ± 1	7 ± 2	9 ± 2	5 ± 1
Prolactin	14 ± 4	17 ± 7	80 ± 6	61 ± 6	75 ± 6	67 ± 6	67 ± 9	54 ± 12	23 ± 6	13 ± 3	15 ± 6	15 ± 4	8 ± 1	14 ± 4
(ng/ml)	9 ± 1	8 ± 1	57 ± 12	79 ± 7	75 ± 8	68 ± 9	61 ± 6	44 ± 12	14 ± 3	8 ± 1	7 ± 5	6 ± 1	10 ± 3	12 ± 2
Insulin	12 ± 2	7 ± 2	8 ± 1	8 ± 2	10 ± 1	9 ± 2	9 ± 1	9 ± 2	7 ± 1	8 ± 1	10 ± 1	12 ± 2	21 ± 5	15 ± 4
(μU/ml)	8 ± 2	7 ± 1	6 ± 1	5 ± 1	5 ± 1	6 ± 1	6 ± 1	4 ± 1	7 ± 2	5 ± 1	7 ± 1	9 ± 1	14 ± 3	9 ± 2
Glucagon	230 ± 20	224 ± 17	226 ± 17	236 ± 22	214 ± 14	252 ± 17	250 ± 17	254 ± 33	286 ± 32	282 ± 42	268 ± 28	292 ± 41	260 ± 24	268 ± 22
(pg/ml)	250 ± 0	240 ± 0	234 ± 14	234 ± 14	242 ± 10	228 ± 10	248 ± 17	264 ± 22	274 ± 14	302 ± 26	268 ± 48	258 ± 37	333 ± 47	340 ± 45

(a)   General anaesthesia (mean $\pm$ SEM).
(b)   General anaesthesia+epidural analgesia (mean $\pm$ SEM).

Variations of thyroxine (T_3 and T_4) during thyroid surgery

J. L. GARCIA PERLA, J. M. GUTIERREZ GOICOECHEA and L. TORRADO RUIZ

Department of Anesthesia and Reanimation, Virgen del Rocio Hospital, Seville, Spain

The serum levels of the thyroid hormones T_3, T_4 and the FT_4I fraction were studied during various thyroid operations in order to determine the effects of premedication, the basic anesthetic used, and pre- and postoperative stress. The original technique of Hamolsky was considered, but the Murphy technique and the Mallinckrodt test are routinely used by the Isotopes Department of this Hospital.

The accepted normal values for these techniques are: T_4 between 5 and 13, FT_4I between 5 and 13.7 and T_3 between 87 and 113. Twelve cases have been studied. These were:

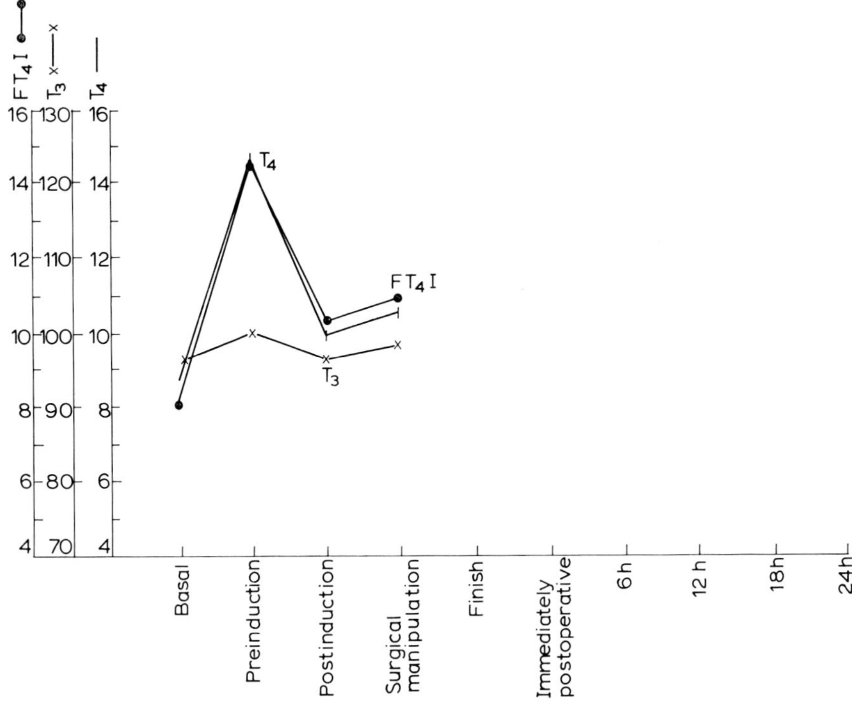

Fig. 1. *Endothoracic goiter. E.G.C., female, 67 years. Premedication with diazepam 10 mg; maintenance with enflurane.*

thyroid cancer (2), multinodular goiter (1), Plummer syndrome (2), hypertrophic thyroids with inactive lingual thyroid (1), hyperparathyroidism (1), colloidal nodular goiter (4), and intrathoracic goiter (1).

Various combinations of the following sedative drugs were used: pethidine, promethazine, haloperidol, diazepam and Thalamonal.

The maintenance anesthetic was: N_2O+Palfium in 6 cases, halothane alone in 2 cases, supplemented with N_2O in 2 cases and enflurane in 2 cases.

The results obtained for T_3, T_4 and FT_4I after premedication, after the induction of anesthesia, during surgical manipulation of the thyroid gland, on awakening of the patient in the theater, and during the immediate postoperative period (6, 12 and 24 hr) were compared with the values in the serum extracted on the day before surgery (see Figs. 1 and 2).

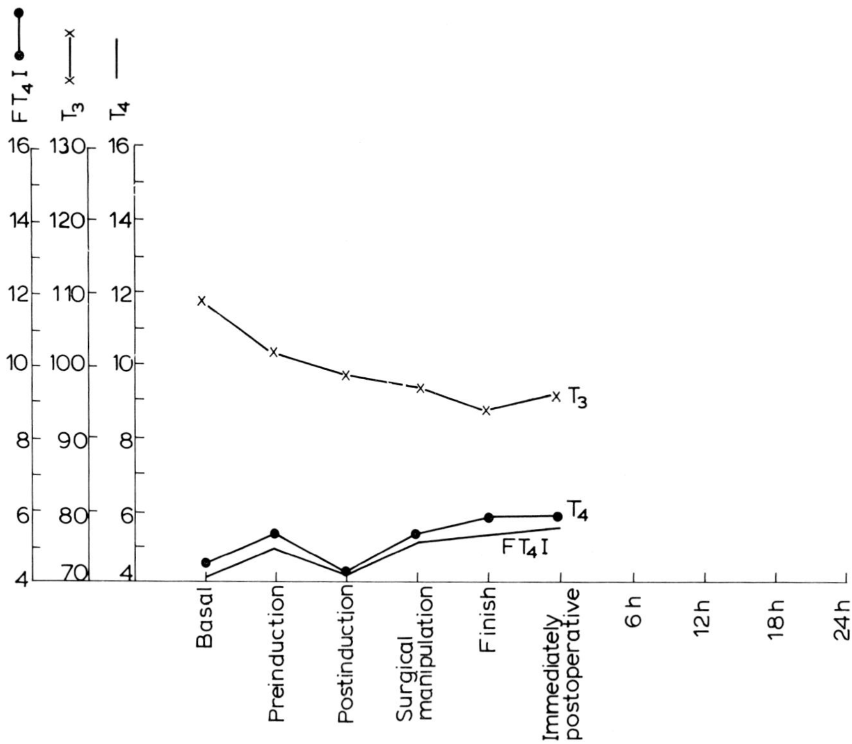

Fig. 2.   *Hyperparathyroidism. L.M.M., male. Premedication with haloperidol 5 mg, pethidine 50 mg, and promethazine 25 mg; maintenance with halothane.*

These conclusions refer solely to variations in the T_4 level; this is because only this parameter gives a direct measure of total circulating thyroxine, being the sum of free thyroxine and protein-bound thyroxine, and so it is the one parameter which is of interest in the evaluation of the effects which the type of premedication, the type of anesthetic and the pre-, per- and postoperative stress may have on the liberation of thyroid hormones. The values are always within the normal limits and scarcely enter into the zones of extreme upper or lower normal limits. This seems to indicate that the surgical-anesthetic procedure and the concomitant stress have hardly any effect on the release of thyroxine.

In the postoperative period, the changes were also minor and always within normal

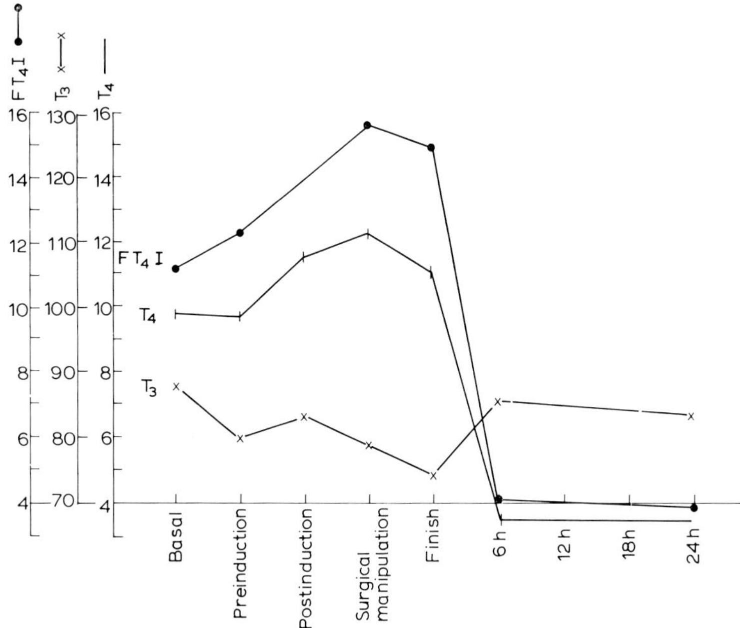

Fig. 3. *Plummer syndrome. A.R., female. Premedication with diazepam 20 mg, Thalamonal 2 ml; maintenance with $N_2O+O_2+halothane$.*

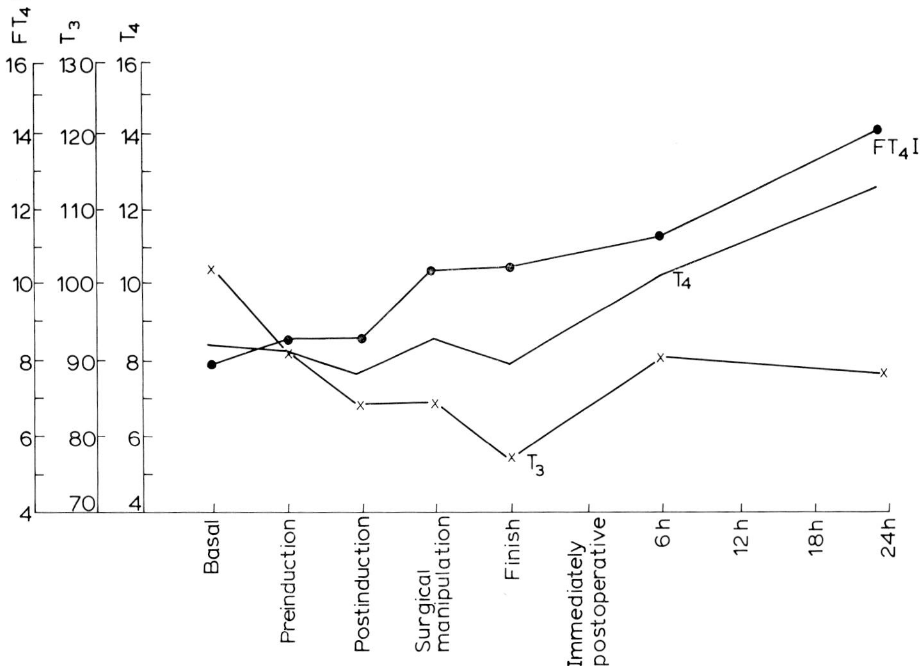

Fig. 4. *Multinodular goiter. R.P.G., female, 31 years. Premedication with pethidine 50 mg, promethazine 25 mg, haloperidol 25 mg; maintenance with $N_2O+O_2+dextromoramide$.*

limits. Note should be taken of the sharp and immediate fall in the T$_4$ level in one case of Plummer syndrome, as well as the rise in T$_4$ found in another case despite the thyroidectomy and which can be attributed to the thyroxine stored in the liver (see Figs. 3 and 4).

REFERENCES

Hamolsky, M. W. (1971): *Tests on Thyroid Function.* (In Spanish). Toray-Masson, Barcelona.
Oyama, T. (1973): *Anesthetic Management of Endocrine Disease.* Springer-Verlag, Berlin – Göttingen
  – Heidelberg – New York.

Endocrine aspects of malignant hyperthermia in Pietrain pigs

G. M. HALL * and DAVID LISTER

Department of Anaesthesia, Royal Postgraduate Medical School
Hammersmith Hospital, London, and
Meat Research Institute, Langford, Bristol, United Kingdom

Malignant hyperthermia (M.H.) is one of the most perplexing complications of modern anaesthesia. Its sudden occurrence during an otherwise uneventful anaesthetic makes the prevention and treatment of this syndrome very difficult. Fourteen years after the first description of M.H. (Denborough and Lovell, 1960) the mortality rate is still 60–70%. Investigation of survivors of M.H. has generally been limited to serum enzyme studies and the structural and pharmacological assessment of muscle biopsies.

Hall et al. (1966) described the development of M.H. in Landrace pigs and subsequently Pietrain (Sybesma and Eikelenboom, 1969) and Poland China pigs (Nelson et al., 1972) were also shown to be susceptible to suxamethonium and/or halothane. The incidence of M.H. in certain breeds of pig is but one facet of their generalised 'stress susceptibility'. These pigs are also characterised morphologically by their mesomorphism which is caused not by an increase in protein synthesis but by increased lipolysis, fatty acid utilisation and decreased lipogenesis (Wood and Lister, 1973).

It has been suggested that some hormonal imbalance is responsible for the characteristics of the 'stress-susceptible' breeds of pigs (Lister, 1970). Investigation of the hypothalmic-pituitary-adrenal axis in Pietrain pigs showed no consistently significant difference between these animals and Large White (control) pigs. (Lister et al., 1972). A fall in the serum free thyroxine index was found to accompany the development of hyperthermia following the administration of suxamethonium to Pietrain pigs (Lister, 1973). Furthermore the otherwise fatal outcome in the suxamethonium-triggered pigs could be prevented by the rapid administration of large doses of triiodothyronine (T-3). We have therefore investigated the role of the thyroid in M.H.-susceptible Pietrain pigs.

Two doses of 50 mg suxamethonium are a reliable stimulus for the triggering of M.H. in Pietrain pigs anaesthetised with thiopentone and ventilated with nitrous oxide and oxygen. However, thyroidectomy in 4 Pietrain pigs, 21 days before challenge with suxamethonium, abolished their susceptibility to this drug. The subsequent administration of maintenance doses of L-thyroxine for 3–4 weeks restored the sensitivity to suxamethonium. In an additional 6 Pietrain pigs the administration of large doses of the thiourea derivative, carbimazole, for 21 days was sufficient to reduce the serum free thyroxine index to very low levels and also abolished the susceptibility to suxamethonium. Withdrawal of the goitrogen for 4 weeks restored the sensitivity of the pigs to suxamethonium and was associated with a rise in the serum free thyroxine index to low-normal levels. Although all the pigs in which thyroid function had been abolished survived the suxamethonium

* G. M. H. received support from the Muscular Dystrophy Group of Great Britain.

challenge, a small response was still present as indicated by changes in the arterial pH, Pa_{CO_2} and serum potassium values.

The administration of triiodothyronine to a thyroidectomised pig immediately before suxamethonium challenge would not precipitate hyperthermia, nor could hyperthermia be prevented by thyroidectomy just prior to suxamethonium. This indicated that the effect of thyroid hormone was a conditioning one and not directly related to the circulating level of hormone at the time of challenge. Indeed a time-lag of at least 12 hr is usually present before an effect of thyroid hormones is detectable on a hormone-sensitive process such as protein synthesis.

The serum free thyroxine indices of Pietrain pigs were similar to those of control Large White animals when measured under anaesthesia. A comparison of the rates of thyroidal iodine release between the two breeds was made using the method of Nicoloff (1970). This involved labelling of the thyroid with ^{131}I and the use of ^{125}I-thyroxine as a constant reference source. The ratio values of $^{131}I/^{125}I$ were then determined for successive 24 hr urine collections for a period of 14 days. No difference was found in the urinary $^{131}I/^{125}I$ ratio between the Large White and Pietrain pigs but the total amount of radioactivity excreted in the 'release phase' was greater in the Pietrain pigs. In 8 pigs with a mean body weight of 26 kg the amount of labelled iodide excreted was 40% greater in the 4 Pietrain animals than in the 4 Large White breed. In a further 8 pigs of mean body weight 55 kg the Pietrain group again excreted 15% more labelled iodide. This result indicated that the rate of peripheral utilisation of thyroid hormone was increased in susceptible pigs, particularly in younger animals. Romack et al. (1964) recorded raised secretion rates of thyroxine in susceptible breeds of pigs which would be necessary to maintain normal serum levels in the presence of increased hormonal utilisation.

An increase in thyroid hormone turnover in Pietrain pigs may be responsible for their abnormal muscle metabolism and susceptibility to develop hyperthermia following suxamethonium. Ash et al. (1972) and Suko (1973) have demonstrated that alterations in thyroid function in experimental animals influenced the calcium-accumulating ability of the sarcoplasmic reticulum and the behaviour of the contractile proteins in skeletal muscle.

Although we have shown that thyroid hormones play a major role in the development of M.H. in Pietrain pigs other hormones may be involved. Thyroid-catecholamine interactions have been established for over a hundred years and yet remain poorly understood (Melander et al., 1974). Preliminary experiments have shown the importance of catecholamines in M.H. and this aspect of the problem is at present under investigation (Lister et al., 1974).

REFERENCES

Ash, A. S. F., Besch, H. R., Harigaya, S. and Zaimis, E. (1972): *J. Physiol. (Lond.)*, *224*, 1.
Denborough, M. A. and Lovell, R. R. H. (1960): *Lancet*, *1*, 45.
Hall, L. W., Woolf, N., Bradley, J. W. P. and Jolly, D. W. (1966): *Brit. med. J.*, *4*, 1305.
Lister, D. (1970): In: *Physiology and Biochemistry of Muscle as a Food. Vol. II*, Chapter 34, p. 705. Editors: E. J. Briskey, R. G. Cassens and B. B. Marsh. University of Wisconsin Press, Madison, Wis.
Lister, D. (1973): *Brit. med. J. 1*, 208.
Lister, D., Hall, G. M. and Lucke, J. N. (1974): *Brit. J. Anaesth.*, *46*, 803.
Lister, D., Lucke, J. N. and Perry, B. N. (1972): *J. Endocr.*, *53*, 505.
Melander, A., Ericsson, L. E. and Sundler, F. (1974): *Life Sci.*, *14*, 237.
Nelson, T. E., Jones, E. W., Venable, J. H. and Kerr, D. D. (1972): *Anesthesiology*, *36/1*, 52.
Nicoloff, J. T. (1970): *J. clin. Invest.*, *49*, 1912.
Romack, F. D., Turner, C. W., Lesley, J. F. and Day, B. N. (1964): *J. Animal Sci.*, *23*, 1143.
Suko, J. (1973): *J. Physiol. (Lond.)*, *228*, 53.
Sybesma, W. and Eikelenboom, G. (1969): *Neth. J. vet. Sci.*, *2/2*, 155.
Wood. J. and Lister, D. (1973): *J. Sci. Food Agric.*, *24*, 1449.

Plasma renin activity in surgical patients

H. D. JAKUBOWSKI and H. D. TAUBE

Departments of General Surgery and Anaesthesiology,
University of Essen, Essen, Federal Republic of Germany

Braun-Menendez et al. (1947) reported high renin levels in dogs during intraabdominal operations. This increase of plasma renin activity (PRA) was thought to be partly responsible for the 4-fold elevation of aldosterone in anaesthetized dogs during laparotomy (Davis et al., 1964). According to these findings McKenzie et al. (1967) showed a 3-fold increase of PRA in rabbits by opening the peritoneum. Moore and Ball (1952) and Le Quesne and Lewis (1953) interpreted the postoperative retention of sodium and fluid to be induced by stimulation of the renin-angiotensin-aldosterone system. Robertson and Michelakis (1972) investigated the effect of anaesthesia and surgery on PRA in man. PRA levels increased 3-fold at the midpoint of the surgical procedures.

In the present study 3 questions were posed: (1) How do operations in the upper abdomen alter the PRA in man? (2) Is the surgical manipulation or the anaesthesia responsible for the alterations? (3) Do various anaesthetic procedures influence the PRA differently?

MATERIAL AND METHODS

Twenty-five patients for operation in the upper abdomen were studied. The operations performed in 13 men, aged 22–59 years (average 38.1 years) were proximal selective vagotomy (8), cholecystectomy (2), splenectomy for lymphogranulomatosis (1) and truncal vagotomy with excision of a gastric ulcer (2). The 12 female patients, aged 16–61 years (average 43.6 years) were submitted to proximal selective vagotomy (2), cholecystectomy (5), splenectomy (4) and gastric resection (1). No patient suffered from arterial hypertension, cardiovascular or metabolic diseases. No drugs had been given in recent weeks. Fourteen patients received, 30 min before starting neurolept anaesthesia (NLA), 0.25 mg atropine and 5 mg droperidol i.m. Eleven patients for halothane anaesthesia (HA) were premedicated with 0.25 mg atropine plus 50 mg meperidine plus 25 mg promethazine i.m. Three ml of oxygelatine solution/kg were administered to each patient before anaesthesia. NLA was induced by droperidol 0.15 mg/kg and fentanyl 0.007 mg/kg. Propanidid 5 mg/kg was used prior to halothane anaesthesia. Intubation was facilitated by suxamethonium 1.5 mg/kg. Relaxation was maintained by diallylnortoxiferine. Artificial ventilation was performed according to the Engström-nomogram.

The PRA of the peripheral venous blood was determined preoperatively in recumbent and upright position in 12 patients and on the day of operation in all patients 30 min after premedication, 10 min after induction of anaesthesia, 5 and 60 min after opening of the peritoneum, and 4 hr postoperatively. The last blood sample was taken on the morning after the operation. The determinations of the PRA were performed by means of a radioimmunoassay for angiotensin I according to the method of Haber et al. (1969). The results are indicated as ng angiotensin I/ml of serum/hr.

RESULTS

The mean values of the PRA with the corresponding standard errors of all the 25 patients are shown in Figure 1. The PRA increases significantly (p < 0.025) from 3.29 after pre-medication to 4.75 ng AI/ml/hr 10 min after induction of anaesthesia. Five minutes after opening the peritoneum the PRA was 5.01 and 60 min later it was 5.59 ng AI/ml/hr. These values, however, do not differ significantly from the activity after induction of anaesthesia. Four hours after the operation we measured 4.73 and in the morning of the first postoperative day 5.76 ng AI/ml/hr. These levels, too, do not vary significantly from the activity after induction of anaesthesia.

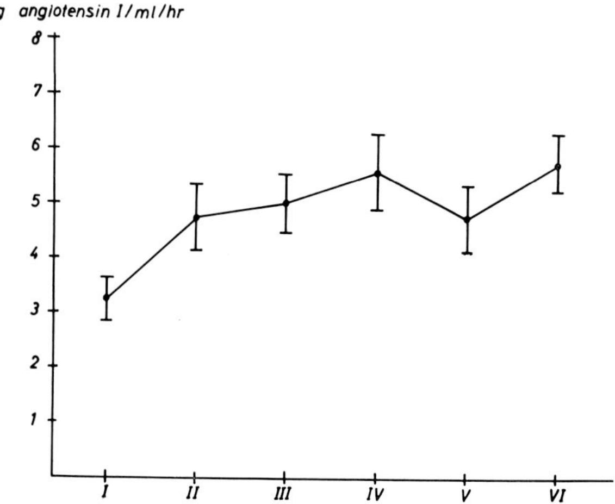

Fig. 1.   *Mean peripheral PRA in 25 patients during the study. I=after premedication; II=after induction of anaesthesia; III=5 min, and IV=60 min after opening the peritoneum; V=4 hr postoperatively; VI=morning after operation. Bracketed lines indicate SE.*

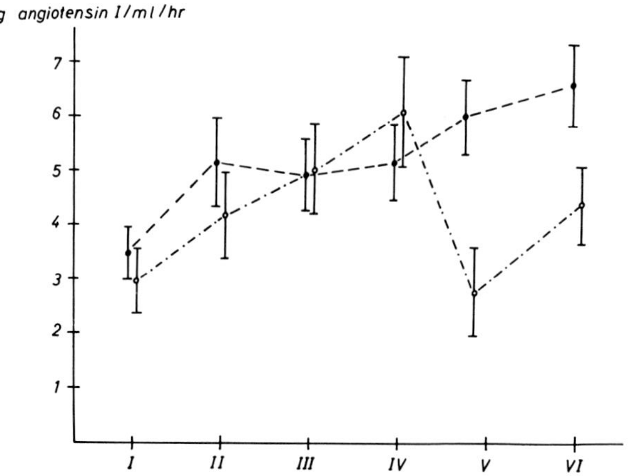

Fig. P.   *Mean peripheral PRA in 14 patients during and following halothane anaesthesia (−.−.−.−) and in 11 patients during and following neurolept anaesthesia (- - - - -). Time of blood samples according to Figure 1.*

The comparison of the 2 anaesthetic methods is plotted in Figure 2. With NLA (n = 14) the PRA rises significantly from 3.51–5.19 ng AI/ml/hr. The further intraoperative activities are 4.98 and 5.19 ng AI/ml/hr and are close to the values after induction of anaesthesia.

With HA (n = 11) a comparable increase from 3.00–4.22 ng AI/ml/hr after induction of anaesthesia occurred. In contrast to the NLA the PRA increased during surgical manipulations to 5.05 ng AI/ml/hr and 6.10 ng/AI/ml/hr. There were however, no significant differences between the corresponding values with NLA and the first activity after induction of HA. Four hours postoperatively the PRA was found to be with NLA 6.09 and with HA 2.83 ng AI/ml/hr. The values of the first postoperative morning were 6.58 for NLA and 4.46 ng AI/ml/hr for HA.

DISCUSSION

There was a significant increase of the PRA after induction of anaesthesia almost equal to the elevation from 3.15 in recumbent to 5.51 ng AI/ml/hr in upright position. During surgical procedures no further elevation could be seen, although with halothane anaesthesia the PRA rose remarkably, but not significantly. These results are different from those of Robertson and Michelakis (1972), who also found an increase of PRA, but not before the midpoint of operation. According to this the increase of the PRA is caused in our investigations by anaesthesia and in that of Robertson by the surgical manipulation. The comparability of the results is limited – Robertson and Michelakis (1972) investigated patients during general and regional anaesthesia in the course of various operations.

The elevation of PRA after induction of anaesthesia could be explained by the measured decrease of systolic blood pressure from a mean value of 130–114 mm Hg – Skinner et al. (1964) demonstrated, that PRA rises due to an acute reduction in blood pressure of 10 mm Hg. This causes a stimulation of the baroreceptors in the vas afferens of the kidney (Tobian, 1966). In our patients there was no reduction of the PRA following the initial increase despite a stabilized blood pressure. This might be explained by special stimulation of the surgical procedures. It is not possible to interpret the different PRA-levels after NLA and HA and further investigations will be necessary.

REFERENCES

Braun-Menendez, E., Fasciolo, J. C., Leloir, L. F., Munoz, J. M. and Taquini, A. C. (1947): *Renal Hypertension.* Charles C. Thomas, Springfield, Ill.
Davis, J. O., Urquhart, J., Higgins, J. T., Rubin, E. C. and Hartroft, P. M. (1964): *Circulat. Res., 14,* 471.
Haber, E., Koerner, T., Page, L. B., Kliman, B. and Purnode, A. (1969): *J. clin. Endocr., 29,* 1349.
Le Quesne, L. P. and Lewis, A. A. G. (1953): *Lancet, 1,* 153.
McKenzie, J. K., Ryan, J. W. and Lee, M. R. (1967): *Nature (Lond.), 215,* 542.
Moore, F. D. and Ball, M. R. (1952): *The Metabolic Response to Surgery.* Charles C. Thomas, Springfield, Ill.
Robertson, D. and Michelakis, A. M. (1972): *J. clin. Endocr., 34,* 831.
Skinner, S. L., McCubbin, J. W. and Page, I. H. (1964): *Circulat. Res., 15,* 64.
Tobian, L. (1966): *Fed. Proc., 26,* 48.

Chapter VIII

Anaesthesia and postoperative care for organ transplantation

Anaesthesia and postoperative care for transplantation. I. Anaesthesia for cardiac transplantation

G. VOURC'H and M. DENTAN

Department of Anaesthesia, Hôpital Foch, Suresnes, France

The problems involved in anaesthesia for cardiac transplantation are not essentially different from those met during any surgical procedure under extracorporeal circulation (ECC). The present study covers 8 cardiac transplantations carried out between January 1973 and March 1974.

MATERIAL AND METHODS

Preoperative assessment (Table 1)

Age varied between 13 and 61 years; the onset of disease before transplantation was between 3 months and 18 years. There is no correlation between the onset of disease and the postoperative course.

Three patients had ischaemic heart disease with left ventricular failure. All had abnormal conduction, and 2 signs of abnormal excitability. Coronary angiography showed severe and widespread coronary obstruction with extensive left ventricular dilatation and akinesia. Two patients had systemic hypertension and moderate renal failure. Five had a non-obstructive cardiomyopathy, with right ventricular failure (2 cases), or global heart failure (3 cases). All had signs of impaired conduction, without abnormal excitability. Preoperative lung function tests showed 4 cases of restrictive lung disease with hypoxia at rest and venous admixture.

Previous cardiac catheterization showed a dramatic reduction in cardiac index, and a raised ventricular end-diastolic pressure. Pulmonary arterial pressure was always high (mean 24–42 mm Hg). All patients had normal liver function, and no gastrointestinal disease.

Anaesthetic technique (Table 2)

Premedication included diazepam (5 cases), or opiates (2 cases). Atropine or scopolamine was administered to all patients, since none had tachycardia.

Induction was achieved by a sleep dose of thiopentone, followed by suxamethonium under electrocardiographic control (ECG). Nasotracheal intubation was carried out; a gastric tube, an oesophageal thermometric probe and a urinary catheter were inserted.

Three venous catheters were considered adequate, one of which was for recording the central venous pressure, preferably through the external jugular vein. The radial artery was cannulated (either percutaneously or by cut-down). The electroencephalogram was monitored throughout.

Table 1. *Preoperative condition*

Case No.	Age	Type of cardiopathy	Onset of disease	Type of cardiac failure	Excitability disturbances	Conduction disturbances	Pulmonary arterial pressure (mm Hg)	Cardiac index l/mm/m^2	Systemic hypertension	Renal insufficiency	Respiratory insufficiency
1	61	Coronary disease	18 years	Left ventricular	+	+ PR↗	?	?	0	0	0
2	48	Coronary disease	16 months	Left ventricular	0	+ LBB	42	0.750	+	+	0
3	43	Coronary disease	17 months	Left ventricular	+	+ LBB	24	2.40	+	+	0
4	26	Cardio-myopathy	18 months	Right ventricular	0	+ PR↗	40	1.22	0	0	Restrictive syndrome
5	13	Cardio-myopathy	5 months	Right ventricular	0	+ RBB	35	1.20	0	0	Restrictive syndrome
6	40	Cardio-myopathy	2 years	Global heart	0	PR↗ +RBB +LBB	?	?	0	0	Restrictive syndrome
7	43	Cardio-myopathy	9 years	Global heart	0	+ RBB	?	0.900	0	0	Restrictive syndrome
8	53	Cardio-myopathy	2.5 years	Global heart	0	PR↗ +LBB	38	1.80	0	0	0

Table 2. *Anaesthetic technique*

Case No.	Age	Weight (kg)	Total duration	Duration ECC	Induction		Maintenance			Complications	Diuretics	Drugs		
					Thio-pentone (mg)	Succinyl-choline (mg)	Curare total dose (mg)	Pheno-peridine total dose (mg)	Others total dose (mg)			NaHCO$_3$	Isopren-aline	Miscellaneous
1	61	78	6 hr	1 hr 30 min	450	80	d-tubo-curarine: 35	12	Diazepam: 20	0		Furosemide +	+	0
2	48	65	5 hr	1 hr 15 min	400	70	Pavulon: 8	7	Droperidol: 20	0		Furosemide +	+	0
3	43	76	4 hr 10 min	1 hr 30 min	500	80	Pavulon: 8 d-tubo-curarine: 20	17	Diazepam: 5	0		Furosemide +	+	0
4	26	58	5 hr 30 min	1 hr 30 min	350	60	Pavulon: 11	10	0	0		0	+	+	0
5	13	41	8 hr	1 hr 45 min	250	50	d-tubo-curarine: 58	11	0		Haemodynamic instability +++	Furosemide +	+	CaCl$_2$
6	40	71	5 hr 30 min	1 hr 15 min	400	80	Pavulon: 10	14	Droperidol: 25	0		0	+	+	0
7	43	71.6	5 hr 15 min	1 hr 15 min	400	90	Pavulon: 8	14	Droperidol: 45	0		Mannitol +	+	0
8	53	47.5	6 hr 30 min	1 hr 30 min	300	50	Pavulon: 12	14	Droperidol: 20	0		0	+	+	CaCl$_2$

Anaesthesia was maintained by various concentrations of nitrous oxide and oxygen, according to the patient's condition. Pancuronium bromide was used in 6 patients, d-tubocurarine in 2 and in a further case who developed marked hypertension. Phenoperidine was used extensively, either alone or in combination with diazepam or droperidol (7 cases).

Heparin was used during the ECG (3 mg/kg) and neutralized by protamine sulfate (1.3 mg/mg of heparin) in slow infusion. Amino-caproic acid was administered at the time of sternotomy (1 mg/10 kg).

Operating time varied between 4.10 and 8 hr with ECC of between 1.15 and 1.45 hr. The period preceding ECC was uneventful. The resumption of spontaneous cardiac activity was easily achieved, assisted always by infusion of minimal doses of isoprenaline; the infusion was continued in the postoperative period. In one case only was cardiac instability encountered (Case No. 5), isoproterenol caused severe tachycardia (180 beats/min) but when it was stopped, marked hypotension occurred. Anaesthesia in this case included d-tubocurarine and phenoperidine, but no droperidol.

Haemorrhage was minimal (mean amount transfused was 1500 ml of ACD blood which was warmed to 37° C).

Postoperative period (Table 3)

The patients remained intubated and were ventilated; they were transferred to the cardiac intensive care unit with ECG-monitoring. A doctor and a nurse stayed at their side for as long as there were any problems; strict surgical asepsis was enforced. The same regime was used as for any open-heart operation.

Ventilation under IPP was used for a variable period (6–72 hr); drainage tubes were kept under suction for 24 hr. Central core temperature was recorded twice daily, and body weight measured daily. ECG, arterial, venous pressure, were monitored, and urine output assessed hourly. Blood gas and electrolyte studies were carried out initially every 6 hr and thereafter daily.

Some points must be stressed: The *ECG* must be carefully analysed for right axis deviation; microvoltage changes with a fall of Barnard index (sum of QRS amplitude in D_1 D_2 D_3) and Shumway index (sum of QRS amplitude in D_1 D_2 D_3 V_1 V_6) must be determined. *Chest X-ray* must be assessed to detect an enlargement of the left ventricle, visualized by 2 silver clips applied during operation. *Blood coagulation* studies are carried out twice daily. *Cardiac output* is measured by isotopes initially twice daily and thereafter daily, while right auricular and pulmonary pressures are recorded at intervals. *Immuno-suppressive therapy* includes azathioprine, corticoids, and purified antiglobulin serum. Oral azathioprine is administered prior to surgery (4–5 mg/kg); the dose is reduced to 0.5–3 mg/kg in the postoperative period, according to the leucocyte count and liver function. Prednisolone is administered i.v. before (5 mg/kg), and after ECC (2 mg/kg) and during the first week, followed by reduced oral doses. Massive doses of both may be required to control rejection. Antiglobulin serum (20 ml), is injected daily first, then every 48 hr. Heparin is infused until the 6th postoperative hr, and antibiotics administered (cefalotin and gentamicin).

RESULTS

Some early, or late complications, have been encountered. There were 2 cases of renal failure receiving corticoids. Other complications are associated with treatment – pneumo-thorax induced by excessive positive pressure ventilation, haemopericardium during heparin therapy (2 cases, requiring surgical drainage). Corticoids may lead to severe hyperglycaemia, psychic disturbance and osteoporosis. Antiglobulin serum was responsible for phlebitis,

Table 3. *Evolution*

Case No.	Pneumo-thorax	Haemo-pericardium	Renal insufficiency	Infection	Rejection	Miscellaneous	Evolution
1	0	0	0	Septicaemia +aspergilloma pulmonary cerebral	8 days-16 days-30 days	Hepatoma	+51 days reject infection
2	0	0	+Furosemide	+Pulmonary	27 days–4 months	Hepatocellular insufficiency 7 months serum hepatitis	Alive 12 months
3	+	0	+Furosemide	+Pulmonary venous	7 days	0	Alive 38 days
4	0	+18th day	+Furosemide	+Pulmonary	7 days–11 months	0	Alive 13 months
5	0	+13th day	0	+Septicaemia	24 days	0	+29 days reject infection
6	0	0	0	+?	?	Low cardiac output, right heart failure	+3 days
7	+	0	0	+Venous	8 days-64 days	0	+69 days rejection
8	0	0	0	+?	6 days	0	+8 days rejection

anaphylactic reaction, but thrombocytopenia did not occur. Azathioprine has induced moderate leukopenia; in one case (Case No. 2) the cause of hepatic insufficiency after 7 months is uncertain.

The 2 major complications are: *Infection*, aggravated by the massive immunosuppressive therapy. It may be localized or generalized, sometimes bacterial, more often viral or fungal. It has been a constant finding in our cases, although of variable severity.

The signs of *rejection* are: (*a*) *electric* – right axis deviation and microvoltage, with a fall of Barnard and Shumway indices; (*b*) *haemodynamic* – fall of cardiac output and index; and (*c*) *biological* – hypercoagulability in spite of adequate doses of heparin.

Other signs, usually late, are disturbances of cardiac excitability, conduction, or ischaemia; hyperthermia; salt and water retention with gain of weight and fall in urine sodium output. Cardiac enlargement, rise of phosphocreatinekinase and lactic-dehydrogenase III also occur.

The onset of rejection varies. In 5 cases (Nos. 1, 3, 4, 7, 8), it was noticed between the 6th and 8th postoperative day, leading to death in one (Case No. 8). It was controlled in 4 cases, but led to further rejection in 3 (Case Nos. 1, 4, 7) with 2 deaths (Case Nos. 1 and 7). Therefore, 3 of 5 patients with early rejection died within 8–69 days. One is still alive, but it is still too early (38 days) to form an opinion. Only one is alive after more than a year.

A late rejection (between 3 or 4 weeks), occurred on 2 occasions (Case Nos. 2 and 5) with a death, and a survival after a year.

In one case, a few hours after the transplantation, a low cardiac output syndrome developed which resulted in death after 72 hr (Case No. 6), due either to the poor quality of the transplanted heart, or to acute right heart failure linked to pre-existing pulmonary hypertension.

SUMMARY

Cardiac transplantation is a very hazardous procedure; it can only be considered when faced with heart failure irresponsive to any other form of treatment (medical, or 'conventional' surgical). Cardiac failure may be due to coronary obstruction or non-obstructive myocarditis. Age over 50 years is considered to be a bad prognostic sign. The duration of the disease is not relevant. On the other hand, gastric ulcer, gout, diabetes, arteritis, organic renal or hepatic disease are contraindications, as well as high pulmonary arterial pressure and pulmonary vascular resistance – a mean of 45 mm Hg appears to be the upper acceptable limit. High constant pulmonary arterial hypertension may account for the early right ventricular failure with low cardiac output observed in some patients.

Anaesthetic problems are in no way different from those involved in open-heart surgery. Premedication must be adequate to alleviate anxiety. Blood pressure fluctuations, and arrhythmia must be controlled as far as possible; we had no problem associated with suxamethonium. Pancuronium has no depressant effect on the circulation but may induce hypertension; it is not clear whether it offers any advantage over d-tubocurarine. The use of central analgesics coupled with diazepam or droperidol has achieved satisfactory conditions. Droperidol may reduce the incidence of arrhythmias induced by isoprenaline.

In the postoperative period constant medical and nursing care must be available, by competent personnel. Infection and rejection are the major complications. In our series, all patients had some infectious complications to a variable degree; all had one or more rejection episodes, the first always before 1 month (it occurred before 2 months in Shumway's series of 29 cases). The date of the first rejection seems to be important – the earlier it is, the poorer the prognosis. A rejection after 7 days is also considered to fall in the same category.

In our series, 5 patients died during the early postoperative period (3 days–3 months) before they had left the hospital. The 3 surviving cases have now 38 days, 12 and 13 months survival.

Anaesthesia and postoperative care for organ transplantation. Lung transplantation: Report of a case

STANLEY A. MASON

Anaesthetic Department, King's College Hospital, London, United Kingdom

The patient was an Iraqui of 40 years who was moribund from cryptogenic fibrosing alveolitis of unknown cause. His disease was progressive and incurable and prior to transplantation he had been dependent on oxygen, even at rest, for 24 hr a day for almost 2 years. He had been well until the age of 15 when he noticed clubbing of his fingers. The clubbing progressed, but he had no other symptoms until he was almost 30 when he developed undue shortness of breath on exertion which had become very severe by the age of 36. Radiology in 1966 showed fine nodulation in both lung fields and laboratory investigations excluded schistosomiasis and other unusual conditions not found in Britain. His overall lung function tests at this time (Table 1) show the typical changes of stiff lungs with a gas transfer deficit.

Table 1. *Results of overall lung function tests*

Test	Patient	Predicted normal
FEV (in litres)	1.84	3.6
VC (in litres)	2.1	4.2
FEV/VC (%)	87	75
Tco (ml/mm Hg/min)	9.0	29.5
Static lung compliance (l/cm H_2O)	0.07	0.3

An exercise test showed a large fall in arterial oxygen tension and a large alveolar-arterial gradient for oxygen. Regional lung function at bronchoscopy indicated a severe progressing fibrosing alveolitis of unknown cause almost obliterating the function of both lower lobes of the lungs, but partly sparing the upper lobes. A lung biopsy was carried out to prove the diagnosis and to exclude alveolar cell carcinoma – histology was typical of a fibrosing alveolitis with pronounced squamous metaplasia of the bronchial mucosa.

PREOPERATIVE COURSE

He was put on prednisone and a weight reducing diet but his lung function and clinical state deteriorated. In 1967 he was given a portable oxygen set. His resting arterial Po_2 was 53 mm Hg which increased to 76 with oxygen. In 1969 he was started on azathioprine

50 mg daily as well as the prednisone. By 1970 his FEV had fallen to 1.4 l and his vital capacity to 1.5 l. His haemoglobin remained raised at 18.2 g/100 ml but his blood volume was 4.7 l. He finally stopped work for almost 2 years and became dependent on oxygen for 24 hr a day. During the few months before transplant he had difficulty in eating or cleaning his teeth. Eventually he was consuming twenty 100 cu. feet cylinders of oxygen per week.

Two weeks prior to transplant he was admitted moribund from a minor chest infection, but recovered with antibiotics; he was so cyanosed and breathless without oxygen that it was impracticable to measure his arterial blood gas tension whilst breathing air. The patient accepted the possibility of lung transplant and waited 9 months for the operation until a suitable donor could be found.

THE DONOR

In March 1971 a boy of 16 years was admitted to hospital having had a cerebrovascular accident – he required ventilating but all investigations including a cerebral angiogram and repeated EEG's showed an inactive brain with no blood supply. When two physicians and a consultant neurologist were both satisfied that cerebral death had occurred, permission was sought from the boy's relatives to use his organs for transplantation. There were three major mismatches when tissue typing was done and the donor's blood group was O positive, whilst the recipient's group was B positive. Although the tissue match was not as good as we would have liked, the excellent state of the donor lung, the hazardous clinical condition of the recipient and the paucity of potential donors encouraged the recommendation of a transplant to the recipient to which he agreed.

THE OPERATION AND ANAESTHETIC

The only premedication given was 10 mg of diazepam administered one hour beforehand to allay anxiety. Because the patient was dependent on 100% oxygen it was decided to rely on powerful intravenous analgesic agents during the operation whilst maintaining automatic ventilation of the lungs with 100% oxygen after complete paralysis with muscle relaxants.

At 21.20 hours, sleep was induced with 80 mg of methohexitone and with the aid of suxamethonium chloride a left Robertshaw double-lumen tube was inserted and its position checked by auscultation. Relaxation was continued with pancuronium bromide and analgesia maintained with incremental doses of intravenous phenoperidine. A total of 19 mg of pancuronium bromide and 10 mg of phenoperidine were used for the 9-hr operation.

The chest was opened through a right posterolateral thoracotomy and cardiopulmonary bypass established using a Temptrol oxygenator. The oxygenated blood was returned to the left femoral artery and flows ranged from 1–3 l/min. The blood gases immediately improved on bypass and a right pneumonectomy was performed. It was a grossly shrunken lung and felt like a hobnail liver. Meanwhile, the donor lung was removed after the ventilator had been stopped and cardiac standstill had occurred. The donor lung was implanted and arterial, venous and bronchial anastomoses carried out. The implanted lung inflated easily and the patient came off bypass without difficulty. The total time on bypass was 114 min and the temperature was kept normal. The warm ischaemic time till blood flow was re-established in the donor lung was 59 min. The blood gas estimations during the course of the operation are shown in Table 2.

At 04.15 he was conscious and responding to speech; however, owing to excessive drainage he was re-anaesthetised and his chest reopened at 04.50. By 06.00 hr the chest was closed again and after removal of the endotracheal tube he was talking and asked to pass urine.

Table 2. *Blood gas estimations during the course of the operation*

Time	Stage of procedure	P_{O_2}	P_{CO_2}	pH	Saturation (%)
26 March 21.20	Induction of anaesthesia	59	83	7.2	83
22.15	Artificial ventilation with pure oxygen	112	78	7.22	97
22.45	Chest opened and lung retracted	39	72	7.23	80
23.46	On bypass	65	49	7.31	93
27 March 01.40	Off bypass new lung ventilated	88	34	7.45	97
03.45	Spontaneous respiration of O_2 with OT tube in place	134	75	7.14	98
08.00	In ward breathing 7 l/min pure oxygen	80	60	7.31	95

His measured blood loss was 6.5 l which was replaced by 8 l of acid-citrate dextrose stored blood. He still continued to drain a lot of blood from his chest drains despite fresh blood and fresh frozen plasma and by the evening it was apparent that blood clot was restricting his new lung. His chest was reopened at 21.45 that night and the clot evacuated. For this operation he was given 50/50 O_2/N_2O to breathe and his saturation remained at 95% with a P_{CO_2} of 50 mm Hg.

POSTOPERATIVE COURSE

The patient's room and adjoining bathroom were both ventilated with filtered air under positive pressure. All staff changed into sterile clothes, scrubbed and wore masks, before entering. All equipment was gas sterilised and all food was made bacteriologically sterile by neutron irradiation. Daily radiographs were taken by inserting the X-ray tube through a polyethylene bag into the room.

From being completely oxygen dependent before transplant he was by the 3rd postoperative day breathing quietly and had a normal colour without oxygen. He was able to walk about the room by the 4th day. By the middle of the 4th week he was taken for a drive to London and subsequently for a short walk in a local park. Six weeks after the operation he walked briskly up steps and about 400 metres without breathlessness, to see a new flat.

His postoperative course was complex and he had many periods of illness, some due to infection, some due to rejection, and the distinction will be discussed later. The first bout of rejection was treated by increasing the prednisone and the azathioprine and the subsequent bouts were treated with anti-lymphocytic globulin. He had a definite bout of infection between the 9th and 14th days when the sputum was frankly purulent and grew *Pseudomonas aeruginosa*. He was treated with gentamycin and cephaloridine the latter being subsequently replaced by tetracycline. Daily postoperative chest radiography showed no definite changes since the time of transplant except for a small area of collapse consolidation between the 9th and 14th days. The original lung remained contracted whilst the new lung was well expanded and showed a good excursion between inspiratory and expiratory films.

On auscultation the breath sounds over the new lung were clear vesicular throughout and it only had persistent rhonchi on two occasions when incipient rejection was suspected. The highest oxygen tension was recorded on the 40th day when he had a saturation of 96%. His FEV on the 43rd day was 1.6 l with a VC of 1.9 l. Technetium-albumin scans taken with a gamma camera on the 15th and 30th posttransplant days both showed that the new lung had all the perfusion except for some to the apex of the old one. A Xenon 133 scan on day 46 showed that the ventilation was distributed in balance with the blood and in the new lung both had a virtually normal distribution from apex to base.

The high doses of prednisone given for immunosuppression caused the patient to develop glycosuria which was controlled by small doses of insulin. There was also a high loss of urinary potassium which despite oral potassium caused a fall in serum potassium.

The patient died on the 53rd postoperative day from two sudden severe haemoptyses. At postmortem a peribronchial abscess had eroded the pulmonary artery.

DISCUSSION

This was a clinically successful lung transplant because (1) preoperative lung tests had shown the nature of his restrictive lung disease so that it could be predicted that the remaining lung would not become over-distended; (2) extreme care was taken to avoid introducing infection; (3) rejection signs were recognised early and treated. Even so infection proved to be the obstacle to success. The anaesthetic problems posed by this patient were easily solved by an anaesthetic team used to cardiopulmonary bypass. The use of one lung anaesthesia is routine for pneumonectomy and presents no problem. Haemorrhage was certainly a problem at the time of operation and in the first 24 hr, but responded to fresh blood and plasma. The operative and anaesthetic problems pale into insignificance compared with the complex problems of infection and rejection subsequent to operation.

Anaesthesia and postoperative care for organ transplantation: Complications of immunosuppressive therapy

AILEEN K. ADAMS

Addenbrooke's Hospital, Hills Road, Cambridge, United Kingdom

Most patients undergoing organ transplantation need immunosuppressive therapy to prevent rejection of the graft. Rejection depends on the genetic disparity of the donor and the recipient. Isografts between identical twins of identical genetype survive indefinitely without treatment. Allografts, grafts between individuals of the same species but of different genotype, provoke a wide variety of rejection response, which is correlated with the degree of antigen disparity shown by donor-recipient tissue typing.

MECHANISM OF ALLOGRAFT REJECTION

Immunologically competent cells in the host are 'made aware' of the histocompatibility antigens possessed by the allograft but not by the recipient. These antigens pass in some form via the lymphatics, the blood stream, or both, to regional lymph nodes. Appropriate cells respond and produce immune lymphocytes and immunoglobulins, which then invade the graft and react with its components to cause its destruction (Herbertson, 1971).

This mechanism may be likened to a reflex comprising an afferent or recognition phase, and an efferent or destructive one.

MODIFICATION OF REJECTION

The mechanism may theoretically be interrupted at several points (Evans and Sells, 1971):
1. Rendering the graft non-antigenic.
2. Preventing the antigenic material from reaching the lymphoid system.
3. Preventing recognition of the antigen.
4. Preventing the central reaction against the antigen.
5. Preventing lymphoid cells from reaching the graft.

Much work has been done on all these methods. Apart from corneal grafts, where the fifth method is successful (these grafts usually survive indefinitely except when they become vascularised), only the fourth approach has proved useful clinically.

PREVENTING THE CENTRAL REACTION AGAINST THE ANTIGEN

Various methods of controlling the immune reaction by suppression of the lymphoreticular system have been used:

1. Ionic radiation – whole body, local, or extracorporeal.
2. Lymphocyte depletion – thymectomy, thoracic duct drainage.
3. Corticosteroids.
4. Antimetabolites – 6-mercaptopurine, azathioprine, methotrexate, cyclophosphamide.
5. Antibiotics – actinomycin C.
6. Antilymphocytic serum (ALs.)

In practice, corticosteroids and azathioprine have been the mainstay for many years, supplemented in rejection crises with actinomycin C and ALs.

SIDE-EFFECTS OF IMMUNOSUPPRESSIVE THERAPY

All these drugs are non-specific in their actions. The side-effects of steroids are well known and their combination with azathioprine depresses the immunological reaction at the same time as exerting toxic effects on the bone marrow, gastrointestinal tract, liver and pancreas, reducing resistance to bacterial, fungal and viral invasion, and eventually producing bone necrosis, arthritic changes, cataracts and occasionally neoplasia (see Table 1).

Table 1.   *Complications of immunosuppressive therapy*

Corticosteroids	Cushing's syndrome
	Diabetes mellitus and pancreatitis
	Gastrointestinal tract ulceration
	Osteoporosis, avascular necrosis and arthralgia
	Cataracts
	Psychoses
Azathioprine	Bone marrow depression
	Alopecia
	Liver dysfunction
	Wasting, and growth retardation in children
Cyclophosphamide	Bone marrow depression
	Oral ulceration
	Nausea and vomiting
	Amenorrhoea and oligozoospermia
Actinomycin C	Bone marrow depression
Antilymphocytic globulin	Local skin reactions
	Serum sickness and anaphylaxis
	Leucopenia and thrombocytopenia
Combinations	Delayed healing and infections
	Neoplasia

In the Cambridge series comprising about 300 renal and over 30 hepatic transplants' the most serious complications have been infection and gastrointestinal haemorrhage.

There are many sources of infection in transplant patients (Evans, 1971). Endogenous sources include the patient's nasopharynx, gastrointestinal tract and lungs, and in renal failure genitourinary tract infections of course are common, whilst vascular shunts inserted for haemodialysis may become infected. Bacterial infections of wounds and of the lungs commonly occur postoperatively and normal commensal organisms may become pathogenic, particularly if antibiotics are used. Patients may harbour latent infections from viruses and fungi, and exogenous infections may be introduced from the atmosphere, from staff and visitors, from dialysers, or from the allograft itself.

Over 10% of our patients have been affected by the herpes zoster varicella virus (Evans,

1973) most mildly, but one developed fulminating varicella from which she died. Candida ulceration of the mouth and oesophagus, and Aspergillus infection in the lungs are both common, whilst cytomegalovirus has been found at postmortem in 42% of our patients who died following renal transplantation (Millard et al., 1973).

Some unusual infections encountered included leprosy and tuberculosis, the former occurred 2 years after transplantation in a patient who had been treated for it 10 years previously, the latter occurred apparently de novo after 6 years, in a patient who had developed inhalation pneumonitis after anaesthesia, progressing to a lung abscess requiring lobectomy. Both were treated successfully without interruption of immunosuppression, but a patient who developed Listeria monocytogenes meningitis died.

In spite of every effort to eliminate infections and to diagnose and treat them early, patients still die from inexorable spreading infections.

Massive gastrointestinal haemorrhage is not infrequent, both from peptic ulcers and from multiple erosions, and in our experience early surgery is indicated, but despite this several patients have died (Evans and Smellie, 1971).

Our experience suggests that, excluding the technical complications of surgery, such as anastomotic breakdown and urinary fistulae etc., almost all the postoperative complications are attributable to the immunosuppressive therapy.

AVOIDANCE OF COMPLICATIONS

The dose of immunosuppressive drugs should be kept to the minimum. Unfortunately, not only is complete histocompatibility testing before transplanting not feasible because of the enormous number of sera required, but there are insufficient organs available for such an ideal to be achieved. In addition, many recipients possess cytotoxic antigens from previous pregnancies or multiple blood transfusions. This underlines the need to avoid blood transfusion even in severely anaemic patients except where lifesaving, and then to use only washed red cells, although even this process does not remove all leucocytes (Joysey, 1971). However, if no major mis-match is shown by tissue typing, many recipients progress well with only moderate doses of drugs and minor side-effects.

All sources of infection must be sought for, and where possible eliminated, before grafting is contemplated. Removal of infected kidneys is essential. During and after operation all reasonable precautions should be carried out, though centres vary in what they consider reasonable, from the extreme of a completely sterile environment, to the compromise, used in Cambridge, of protective isolation (see appendix) with limitation but not exclusion of staff and visitors, until all wounds have healed, when normal activities can be resumed. Prophylactic antibiotics must not be used, but where infections arise they should be treated with narrow spectrum agents, and where renal failure continues, blood levels of antibiotics should be estimated and dosage adjusted accordingly.

The detailed management of immunosuppression is beyond the scope of this paper and in any case is constantly modified. The dangerous triad of rejection, infection and bone marrow depression presents formidable problems for diagnosis and clinical judgement. Rejection episodes require temporarily increased drug doses, but our current philosophy is to regard the transplanted kidney to some extent as disposable – better a rejected and removed allograft in a live patient than the complications, so often fatal, of massive immunosuppressive therapy. Unfortunately, this is not applicable in transplantation of other organs.

Most problems occur in the first 3–4 months. In the long-term some adjustment occurs with a degree of resistance to minor infections such as colds and influenza. Some renal patients require as little as 5 mg prednisone daily, and it is of interest that 2 of 4 surviving hepatic transplant patients are maintained on azathioprine alone without steroids.

Advances in the understanding of immunological responses should result in the development of safe regimes of immunosuppression, and thus remove one of the major causes of morbidity and mortality following organ transplantation.

Appendix

Protective isolation, or reverse barrier nursing, involves confining the patient to his own single room, whilst staff and visitors wear gowns and masks and wash their hands before entering. Linen is freshly laundered and all equipment is kept in the room for the sole use of the patient, or is disposable.

Acknowledgements

I am very grateful to Dr D. B. Evans for his help and advice, and to Professor R. Y. Calne for permission to refer to his patients.

Note added in proof

The regime described has resulted in much less infection, but the sepsis rate is still much higher than in patients not on immunosuppressive therapy. Table 2 shows this improvement. The early series refers to the first 55 patients, the recent series to the last 62 patients in 1974.

Table 2. *Infections following renal transplantation*

	Early series	Recent series
No. of patients	55	62
No. of significant infections	35 (64%)	16 (26%)
Septicaemia	18 (33%)	6 (9.6%)
Pulmonary infections	15 (27%)	6 (9.6%)
Deaths due to infection	16 (28%)	12 (19.2%)

REFERENCES

Evans, D. B. (1971): In: *Clinical Organ Transplantation*, Chapter 7, p. 167. Editor: R. Y. Calne. Blackwell Scientific Publications, Oxford – Edinburgh.

Evans, D. B. (1973): In: *Ciba Foundation Symposium 15* (*new series*), p. 279. Associated Scientific Publishers, Amsterdam – London – New York.

Evans, D. B. and Sells, R. A. (1971): In: *Clinical Organ Transplantation*, Chapter 2, p. 31. Editor: R. Y. Calne. Blackwell Scientific Publications, Oxford – Edinburgh.

Evans, D. B. and Smellie, W. A. B. (1971): In: *Clinical Organ Transplantation*, Chapter 16, p. 248. Editor: R. Y. Calne. Blackwell Scientific Publications, Oxford – Edinburgh.

Herbertson, B. M. (1971): In: *Clinical Organ Transplantation*, Chapter 1, p. 3. Editor: R. Y. Calne. Blackwell Scientific Publications, Oxford – Edinburgh.

Joysey, V. C. (1971): In: *Clinical Organ Transplantation*, Chapter 4, p. 104. Editor: R. Y. Calne. Blackwell Scientific Publications, Oxford – Edinburgh.

Millard, P. R., Herbertson, B. M., Nagington, J. and Evans, D. B. (1973): *Quart. J. Med., 42/167,* 585.

Anaesthesia and postoperative care for organ transplantation: Infection and rejection in lung transplantation

STANLEY A. MASON

Anaesthetic Department, King's College Hospital, London, United Kingdom

Since 1963, 31 lung transplant attempts have been reported most of which resulted in death within one month. The surgical procedure and immediate graft function were generally satisfactory, but the major problems arising in the post-transplant period were associated with ventilation/perfusion imbalance, infection and rejection.

Ventilation/perfusion imbalance occurs in patients with nonrestrictive lung disease such as emphysema. Unequal vascular and terminal airway resistance occurs between the remaining lung and the donor lung and increased vascular resistance in the remaining lung shunts blood to the more compliant donor lung. Inspired air is also trapped in the intact emphysematous lung causing it to overexpand and thus compresses the donor lung with fatal consequences.

The patient in whom we transplanted a lung had fibrosing alveolitis and did not pose a ventilation/perfusion problem. However, we were involved with the other two major complications.

Infection is a major problem after any transplant since the immunosuppressive therapy required to combat tissue rejection also inhibits the natural defence mechanisms against invading organisms. Sepsis is a particular hazard in lung transplantation and can be expected whenever a cadaver lung is used. Following surgery a transplanted lung will be exposed once again to aerial pathogens from the hospital environment. In the case of the lung transplant described elsewhere (*This Volume*, p. 371), special precautions were taken to keep the ambient-air bacterial counts in his room at a level comparable to those recommended for operating theatres. All items of equipment, food and personal belongings were double-wrapped before gas or gamma-ray sterilisation. Outer wrappings were then removed before transfer to the sterile area through an ultraviolet screen.

Cross-infection was minimised by reverse barrier nursing and ECG's and chest X-rays were taken without moving either equipment or technical personnel across into the sterile area. All inhalation agents given during or after surgery were passed through 0.3 μm filters and humidification was avoided. Later during transit to other departments or outdoors a maximum concentration face mask delivering 20 l/min of filtered air was used to ensure protection against aerial contamination.

Rejection is difficult to distinguish from infection after lung transplantation for neither clinical nor radiological signs are distinctive enough to make differentiation possible. In 1971, Munro et al. introduced the rosette inhibition test to assess alterations in peripheral blood lymphocytic activity as an indication of adequate immunosuppression. A result from this test can be reported within 4 hr of venipuncture and can serve as a guide to the amount of drug therapy required to prevent rejection. The test uses anti-lymphocytic globulin (ALG) to inhibit the spontaneous formation of rosettes with sheep red blood cells and a falling titre indicates inadequate immunosuppression. In addition, circulating organ-binding antibodies have been shown to play a role in rejection after transplantation and these can be measured by immunofluorescent techniques.

INFECTION

In the lung transplant described there was clinical evidence of chest infection between the 9th and 14th postoperative days. The patient appeared ill with a raised respiratory rate and required more oxygen. His sputum changed from mucoid to purulent and became excessive: Radiology showed incomplete expansion of the right lung (donor lung). Improvement occurred with antibiotics and infection thereafter was not clinically evident. Findings at necropsy showed little evidence of pulmonary parenchymal infection and polymorphonuclear leucocytes were rarely seen in the alveolar tissue.

REJECTION

As indicated by the rosette inhibition test, changes in the immunological state occurred on four occasions and alterations in clinical features occurred within 24 hr on each of these occasions. The rosette inhibition test first showed inadequate lymphocyte suppression on the 6th day (Fig. 1) but at the same time the patient felt and looked well and showed no clinical or radiological change. An increase in conventional immunotherapy (actinomycin, Imuran and prednisone) improved the rosette inhibition test report. A further episode of inadequate lymphocyte suppression occurred on the 19th day, this time associated with malaise as well as an increased respiratory rate and oxygen requirements. Immuno-suppression was increased this time chiefly by the administration of intravenous ALG. This was followed by both clinical and immunological improvement.

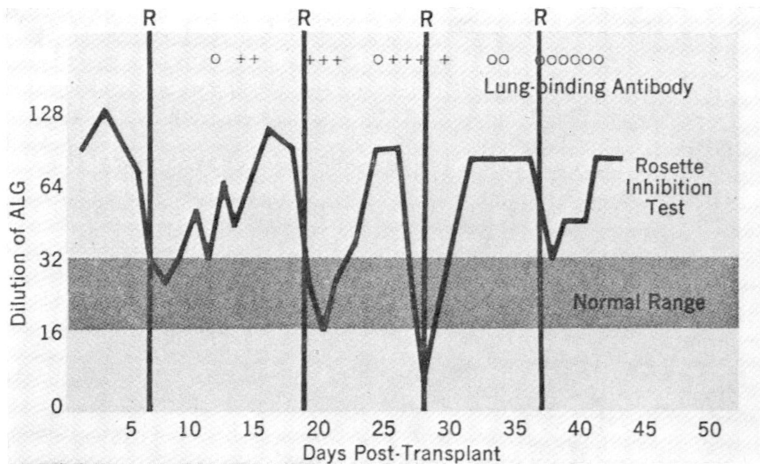

Fig. 1.   *Four episodes of incipient rejection ('R' days 6, 19, 28, and 37) were reflected in the fluctuating ALG titres reported for the lung transplant patient. Although lung-binding antibody (+) typically appeared 48–72 hr before shifts in the ALG titre, none (○) was detected during the last episode.*

Two further similar episodes of inadequate lymphocyte suppression were associated with significant patient deterioration and in both instances a change in the rosette inhibition test preceded signs of clinical deterioration. The episodes responded within a few hours to high dosage intravenous prednisone and there was concurrent improvement in the rosette inhibition test.

The presence of circulating lung-binding antibody was looked for during the last three rejection episodes and in two of the episodes this antibody was found to precede any changes in the rosette inhibition test by as much as 72 hr and to disappear afterwards (see Fig. 1).

PATHOLOGICAL FINDINGS

At necropsy histology of the donor lung showed minimal infiltration with lymphocytes and plasma cells: some pyroninophilic mononuclear leucocytes were scattered as small collections of cells throughout the lung parenchyma. Electronmicroscopy revealed intact alveolar structure with a predominance of tall Type II pneumocytes. Minor nonspecific ultrastructural cytological changes were also evident and the presence of cells in the lymphoplasma series was confirmed. These findings show that rejection was minimal at the time of death and certainly was not the cause of death.

Ulceration of the bronchus on the donor side of the anastomosis penetrating into the pulmonary artery of the right upper lobe was responsible for the massive haemoptysis that occurred. Histologically there was necrosis of both cartilaginous and membranous portions of the donor bronchus.

DISCUSSION

Necrosis of the donor bronchus has been a complication in many lung transplants and is due to the length of donor bronchus used without at the same time attempting to establish an anastomosis of the bronchial artery: the size of this artery makes this impracticable.

Infection has always been a problem in transplant surgery and its presence preoperatively is a serious contraindication to lung transplantation. In the patient described, careful environmental control limited chest infection to 6 days: the rosette inhibition test allowed minimal but effective immunosuppression which no doubt contributed to the minimisation of pulmonary sepsis.

Cellular and humoral mechanisms involved in the rejection response must be monitored and no doubt better methods will be evolved than the ones used in our patient. These tests will not only allow the differentiation of rejection from infection but also allow treatment to be instituted before clinical deterioration takes place.

REFERENCE

Munro, A. et al. (1971): *Brit. med. J., 3,* 271.

Complications of the immunosuppressive drugs in renal transplantation

DAVID TORNOS SOLANO

Unidad de Transplante Renal, Facultad de Medicina, Barcelona, Spain

The transplantation of tissues or organs amongst genetically different individuals of the same species (allotransplantation), stimulates the immune defense systems to reject strange antigens. The immunosuppressives can reduce or inhibit completely mechanisms inducing, in some cases, a prolonged effect. Nevertheless, immune defense systems, apart from those involved in the destruction of the foreign antigens, may be harmful to the patient. The majority of deaths occurring after renal transplantation can be attributed directly or indirectly to the immunosuppressives.

The drugs used in our service are corticoids, azathioprine and cyclophosphamide. The complications observed are: Because of corticoids, aesthetic (cushinoid facies), diabetes, delay in healing, necrosis of the femoral head, osteoporosis of the vertebral column, digestive complications (ulcers, hemorrhage), cataracts, pathogenic and opportunist infections. Because of azathioprine medullary depressions, hepatitis and infections have been observed. Cyclophosphamide has caused alopecias, gonadal lesions and medullary depressions.

Corticoid complications have occurred in patients who have received high dosages, more than 1 mg/kg/day during a period of over a month.

Infections are a common complication in renal transplantation. Several factors predispose to their occurrence. The existence of an infectious focus prior to the transplant, which has been treated inadequately (urinary infections, nasotracheal etc.); secondly, the presence of surgical hematoma etc.; thirdly, leukopenias provoked by the immunosuppressive drugs; fourthly, high dosage of immunosuppressives. In transplants carried out with a cadaver kidney, rejections are more frequent and more intense; this compels an increased dosage of immunosuppressives, resulting, in turn, in more frequent complications.

Of the infections, the most serious and those responsible for a high mortality rate, are those of the respiratory system. These, as with infections in transplanted recipients, can be caused by usually pathogenic agents or by opportunists. The latter make their presence later, and, as stated by Hill (1967), death which occurs as a result of opportunists rarely takes place before the second month after transplantation. Early diagnosis is important including the etiological agent, in order to determine therapy. This is sometimes very difficult, particularly in infections of the lungs, for various reasons. These infections can be mixed and the agent which is cultivated from the sputum is not always responsible for the infection. The clinical onset of lung infections is sometimes very insidious, and it is important constantly to suspect an infection in order to reach a diagnosis. Viral infections, without any signs on physical examination of the chest, can only be diagnosed by means of radiology (see Fig. 1). This is the case of an 8-year-old child who had received a transplant and who had received a high dosage of corticoids because of two crises of rejection. Azathioprine caused considerable leukopenia which forced a suspension of treatment for some days. The child was discharged from hospital and four months later he was admitted once more with a high temperature and coughing. Physical examination of the thorax was negative. Sputum cultures and tracheal aspiration were also negative. Radiology gave the appearance as shown in Figure 1 and this gradually extended during the following days (see Fig. 2).

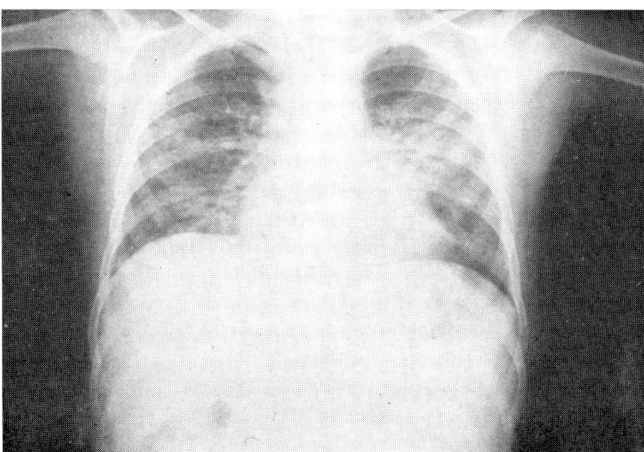

Fig. 1. *Pneumonia image.*

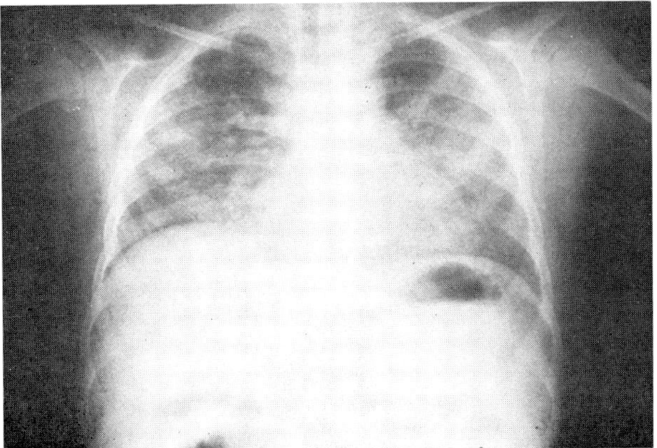

Fig. 2. *The same patient (as in Fig. 1) two days later, the pneumonia image is more extensive and appears on the other side.*

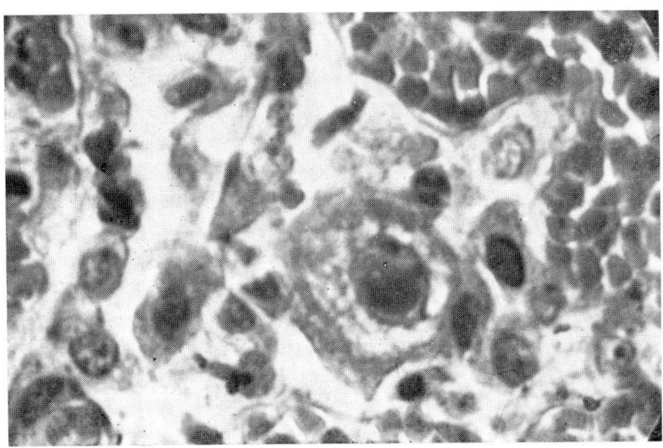

Fig. 3. *Cytomegalic inclusion.*

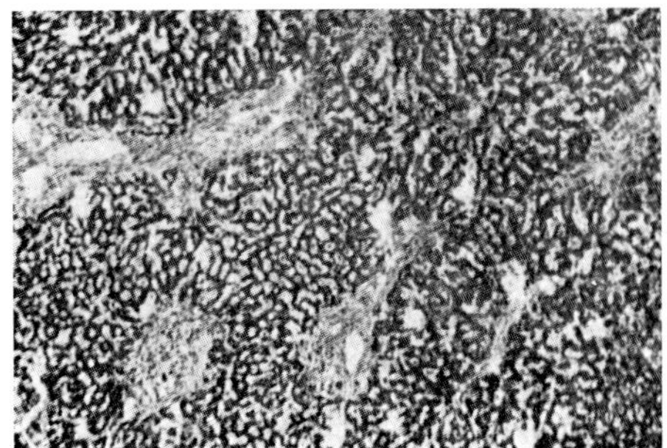

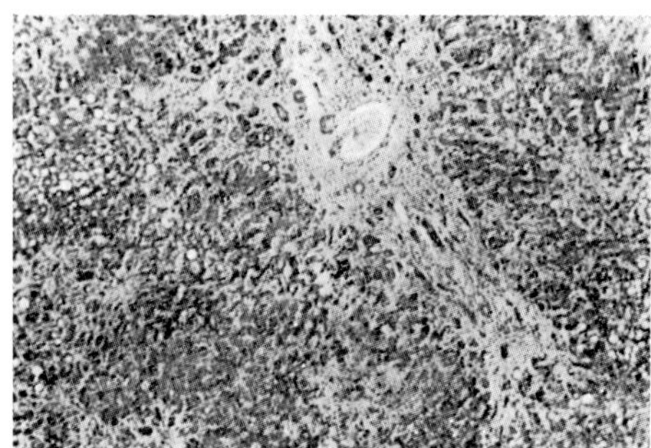

Fig. 4.   *Initial lesions observed two months after treatment with immunosuppressives. Collagenation in the peri-sinuous areas and the presence of a dilatation of the sinusoid can be seen. The portal areas are widened with scarce cellular infiltration.*

Fig. 5.   *Cellular atrophy, large areas of collagenation and portal area with scarce infiltration are seen.*

Auscultation of the thorax continued to be negative notwithstanding extreme dyspnea. The child died from respiratory failure with a pH = 7.19, Po_2 = 32 and a Pco_2 = 30, which proved alveolar capillary blockage. Postmortem histology showed the existence of cytomegalic inclusion bodies (Fig. 3). It is therefore necessary that a total and careful examination of the patient should be carried out, including inspection of wounds, of urine cultures, of drainage, of sputum, of tracheal aspiration, and adequate therapy. If, in the presence of positive radiology, the appropriate therapy, according to culture, does not have any effect, biopsy of the lung should be carried out.

Another of the important problems associated with kidney transplantation is hepatitis. In our service 20% of kidney recipients have presented hepatitis. The presentation of this complication varied between 15 months and 2 years after transplantation. It was manifest clinically by an increase in transaminases, glutamate-oxidases and pyruvates in all patients and by sub-jaundice or jaundice. Fifteen cases of hepatitis were observed during a period of 4 years. During this period, 2 nurses and an assistant presented with jaundice and increased transaminases. An interval between the transplant and the onset of the first symptoms of less than 7 weeks, which is the maximum period of incubation of infectious hepatitis, was observed in 11 of the 15 cases presented: one assistant, one nurse and cases: 1, 3, 4, 5, 7, 9, 10, 11, and 12. Following our experience (Bacardi et al., 1969) hepatic alterations were evidently more severe when azathioprine was increased in 3 patients. The same applied on increasing the dosage of corticoids in 4 patients, 3 of them diabetics and one nondiabetic. Histological examination has been carried out on 15 patients with hepatitis. The lesions discovered show two groups of patients. In the first group there is one diabetic patient who had sub-jaundice with an SGPT increase of up to 300 units/ml. Azathioprine was replaced with cyclophosphamide and after a few days high doses of corticoids were administered for a crisis of rejection; the patient died suddenly a few days later. Necropsy histology showed fatty microscopic degeneration of 40% hepatic cells. The rest of the patients are included in the second group, and the histological lesions show some points in common which are important (Bacardi-Nogueras, 1970). In the initial phase of the process the formation of very fine collagen-substance fibers within the centri-lobular peri-sinuous area as can be seen in Figures 4 and 5. The hepatic travecula therefore progressively atrophy. Portal areas tend to widen, but cellular infiltration is poor. The problem of etiology needs clarification; perhaps it is a question of hepatitis modified by the use of immunosuppressive drugs.

Transplanted recipients may suffer from complications in muscle and joints, particularly the knees and shoulders. Three cases of aseptic necrosis of the femoral head have occurred in this series; two were bilateral and the other was on the right femoral head. All three received cadaver kidneys and high doses of cortisone. The interval between transplantation and symptoms was 6, 4, and 10 months, respectively. In two cases the symptoms began with pain at rest and on movement, but there was no radiological evidence until approximately 8 months later. In the other case, there was X-ray evidence of osteoporosis, 4 months after transplantation, but with no clinical symptoms; symptoms were delayed until a year after transplantation and consisted of a limp of the right leg and 3 months later of the left leg. The appearance 28 months after transplantation is shown in Figure 6. Both femoral

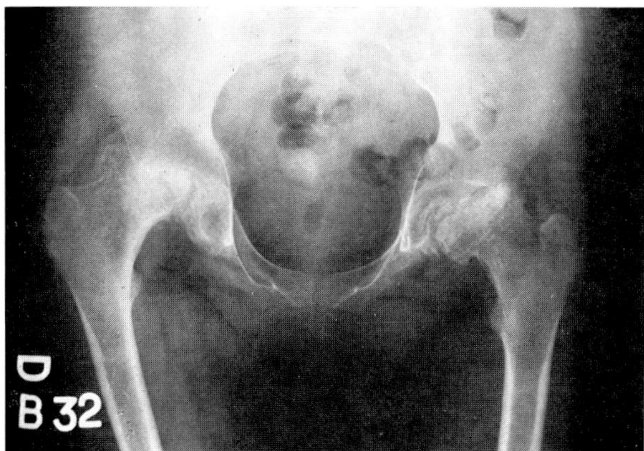

Fig. 6.   *Destruction of both femoral heads.*

heads had been destroyed which forced the patient to walk with the aid of sticks. An arthroplasty of the left hip was performed and 7 years after transplantation a further arthroplasty was carried out on the right side. The pathogenic mechanism has been the subject of many theories. Circulatory disorders with vasculitis, infarcts, and thrombosis occasioned by cortisone, all tend to cause destruction of the bones. Fatty microembolism might be caused by the lipid mobilization which corticoids produce. Local osteoporosis with destruction of the subchrondral osseous lamina by compression could cause deterioration of the articular cartilage. Sinovitis, arthralgias, arthritis (suppurant), myopathies, fractures of the vertebral column, have also been described. Another complication in this series is a case of cataracts in a young man 22 years of age, 4 years after transplantation. Intestinal hemorrhage and one case of colonic perforation have been seen.

Two cases of azoospermia occurred in patients treated with cyclophosphamide, 100 mg weekly, for more than a year.

REFERENCES

Bacardi-Nogueras (1970): *Clin. Med.*, *54*, 11.
Bacardi, R., Caralps, A. et al. (1969): *Clin. Med.*, *53*, 355.
Fisher, D. I. and Bickel, W. H. (1971): *J. Bone Jt Surg.*, *53*, 859.
Heiman, W. B. and Freiberger, R. H. (1960): *New Engl. J. Med.*, *42*, 327.
Hill Jr., R. B. (1967): *Amer. J. Med.*, *42*, 327.

Hill Jr, B. and Rowlands Jr (1964): *New Engl. J. Med.*, *271*, 1027.
Jesserer, H. (1967): *Folia clin. int. (Barcelona)*, *17*, 403.
Lience, E., Caralps, A. and Gil Vernet, J. M. (1971): *Clin. Med.*, *56*, 4.
Richard, L. and Myerowitz, M. D. (1972): *Amer. J. Med.*, *53*, 308.
Rifkund, D. and Thomas, L. (1967): *Amer. J. Med.*, *43*, 28.
Rifkund, D., Thomas, L. and Marchiord, M. D. (1964): *J. Amer. med. Ass.*, *189*, 397.

Liver transplantation: Intraoperative and anesthetic management

J. ANTONIO ALDRETE

University of Louisville School of Medicine, Louisville, Ky., U.S.A.

Of the many thresholds bypassed by medicine in the last decade, organ transplantation is perhaps one of the greatest achievements. Of the various specific organs, it appears that hepatic orthotopic replacement, because of the extent and complexity of the surgical process and the lack of temporary alternative support (such as dialysis or cardiopulmonary bypass), is the most daring.

Patients undergoing liver transplants have had either end-stage liver failure or localized malignant neoplasms. Of the former, alcoholic, posthepatic and biliary (secondary to congenital biliary atresia) cirrhosis have been the most common causes (Starzl, 1971).

Preoperatively, most patients have had an advanced degree of hepatic insufficiency, ascites, hypoxemia, electrolyte imbalances, albuminemia, coagulation disorders, upper gastrointestinal bleeding and occasionally coma.

In the planning of anesthetic management of patients having liver transplantation, several factors must be taken into consideration. First, all commonly used anesthetic agents are at least partially metabolized by the liver, some of them also altering splanchnic blood flow or perhaps they may harm the organ. Second, hemodynamic changes take place since the inferior vena cava and portal vein flows have to be interrupted during the anhepatic period. Third, major derangements in a number of metabolic processes, such as control of blood sugar, acid-base balance, and electrolyte aberrations, all may happen. Last, but not least, in patients with severe hepatic dysfunction, the degradation of most narcotic, barbiturate and tranquilizing compounds is altered. The metabolism of succinylcholine, sympathomimetic amines and most local anesthetics is indirectly dependent on liver enzyme activity.

The seriously compromised physical status of the candidate patients for liver transplantation is aggravated by the semi-emergency character of these operations, which bring about a highly compromised anesthetic risk.

ANESTHETIC AND INTRAOPERATIVE CARE

Induction with titrated doses of thiopental, ketamine or Innovar is carried out and endotracheal intubation performed. Anesthesia is maintained with either light levels of inhalational agents (fluroxene or Ethrane) or neuroleptanalgesic combinations with nitrous oxide/oxygen. Muscle relaxation is achieved by using d-tubocurarine, gallamine, or pancuronium bromide (Aldrete et al., 1969).

Hemodynamic changes

Transoperatively, 'tenting' of the inferior vena cava, or its complete obstruction during the anhepatic phase, impedes venous return to the heart, resulting in a fall of arterial blood pressure. Although portal vein interruption ensues in rapid hemodynamic deterioration and metabolic acidosis in normal individuals, this surgical trespass is better tolerated by cirrhotics because of the collateral vessels from portal hypertension (Picache et al., 1970).

Metabolic alterations

Metabolic acidosis has been a feature in almost every case, resulting from a combination of factors. Clamping of the portal vein and hepatic artery lowers hepatic pH, and the degree of circulating H^+ is usually proportional to the time of hepatic ischemia. This finding has further been confirmed in the laboratory by the observation that lactic acidosis develops after hepatic inflow occlusion in dogs, even when a mesenteric caval shunt was made, thus ruling out splanchnic blood stagnation as a primordial factor (Starzl et al., 1968).

Glucose demand and utilization

Moreover, in the anhepatic state, the conversion of liver glycogen to glucose is impossible since the liver is absent and hepatic integrity is required for the activation of glucose-6-phosphatase, which acts upon the release on demand of free glucose to the blood stream (Harper, 1963). In the postoperative period, muscle weakness, lethargy, and convulsions have been observed in recipient patients when low blood-sugar levels were present.

Serum electrolyte changes

Some changes in serum electrolytes have been noted to follow certain patterns. Hypokalemia has been seen frequently in the post-revascularization period, requiring considerable replacement. The mechanism of this alteration was confirmed in the laboratory (Abouna et al., 1971). Hepatic ischemia causes liberation of intrahepatocytes, potassium ions producing hyperkalemia. However, after blood flow is restored to the hepatic parenchyma, K^+ re-enters the hepatocytes, depleting the plasma pool. Occasionally when large amounts of $NaHCO_3$ were given to offset metabolic acidosis, hypernatremia developed; in these instances one may consider THAM as an alternative (Aldrete, 1969).

Blood transfusions and clotting problems

As mentioned previously, arterial hypotension has occurred rather frequently, produced either by sudden severe blood loss, surgical manipulation, or metabolic alterations. The former has required blood transfusions from 1,000 to over 40,000 ml of blood in few cases. These large volumes of blood loss, the evacuation of ascites and the use of irrigating fluid make estimation of blood replacement difficult. Serial hematocrit determinations and constant attention to estimation of blood loss are needed, along with central venous pressure, urine output and intra-arterial pressure measurements. Large volumes of citrated blood given rapidly can allow for citrate accumulation, even more so in the anhepatic patient with acidosis and underperfusion, resulting in myocardial depression. These effects have been partially offset by the intermittent administration of calcium chloride and $NaHCO_3$ (Aldrete et al., 1969).

During hepatic orthotopic transplantation, depression of coagulating factors of hepatic origin occurs, though it is restored to near normal levels soon after the homograft's function begins to take place. Thrombocytopenia and fibrinolysis have occurred only in a few cases that required large volumes of blood transfused (Groth et al., 1969). Although administration of ε-aminocaproic acid (EACA) and fibrinogen seldom has been indicated, systemic heparinization has been achieved when instances of intravascular coagulation have been diagnosed.

Perhaps the most important factors are adequate preservation of the homograft and prompt restoration of function, bringing the coagulation mechanism back to normal with minimal blood loss.

Other corrective measures

Frequent communication between surgeons and anesthesiologists obviates the development of unilateral complications. Sudden arterial pressure changes should be made known so the surgical team can limit manipulations compromising hepatic circulation to the minimum. Repeated arterial blood gases and pH determinations are mandatory not only to learn the acid-base status, but also the changes in ventilation that may be required, especially when diaphragmatic displacement is impeded by surgical dissection, in underperfused states, or when fluid overload is occurring (Aldrete, 1969).

To prevent hypoglycemia, 50% glucose solutions have been used even before the initiation of the anhepatic period, until its completion; thereafter 5% glucose solution is given continuously throughout the postoperative period. Repeated determinations of blood sugar are made during and after surgery. Postoperatively, due to a large intra-abdominal incision, extensive dissection and the preoperative poor physical condition of the recipient patients, mechanical ventilation is advised until stabilization of vital signs and safe assurance of normal respiratory function (Aldrete et al., 1969).

In conclusion, the anesthetic management of patients undergoing hepatic transplantation requires more than selection of innocuous anesthetic agents and monitoring of vital signs. It demands a full involvement of the anesthetist group into the transplantation team, acquiring knowledge of the various factors involved and actively participating in the decision-making process of therapy, including surgical judgment.

REFERENCES

Abouna, G. M., Aldrete, J. A. and Starzl, T. E. (1971): *Surgery*, 69, 419.
Aldrete, J. A. (1969): In: *Experience in Liver Transplantation*, p. 81. Editor: T. E. Starzl. W. B. Saunders Co., Philadelphia, Pa.
Aldrete, J. A., Levine, D. S. and Gingrich, T. F. (1969): *Anesth. Analg. Curr. Res.*, 48, 802.
Groth, C. G., Pechet, L. and Starzl, T. E. (1969): *Arch. Surg.*, 98, 31.
Harper, H. A. (1963): In: *Review of Physiological Chemistry*, 9th ed., p. 179. Lange Medical Publications, Los Altos, Calif.
Picache, R. S., Kapur, B. M. L. and Starzl, T. E. (1970): *Surgery*, 67/2, 319.
Starzl, T. E. (1971): *Hosp. Pract.*, 6, 47.
Starzl, T. E., Groth, C. G., Bellschneider, L., Moon, J. B., Fulginiti, V. A., Cotton, E. K. and Porter, K. A. (1968): *Surgery*, 63, 549.

Liver support systems

LEO STRUNIN

Anaesthetic Department, King's College Hospital, London, United Kingdom

Normal liver activity embraces the vast majority of metabolic functions and is responsible for homeostasis of carbohydrates, proteins and fat. In liver disease there is impairment or decrease of these functions. Acute liver-cell failure may follow viral hepatitis, the administration of hepatitic or hepatotoxic drugs, hypoxia, hypotension, hepatic artery ligation or hepatic homotransplantation. The effects are multiple and include: ineffective haemostasis, coma, hypoglycaemia, electrolyte abnormalities, hypotension, cardiac irregularities and renal failure. The aetiology of this complex condition is by no means clear and treatment, therefore, is essentially symptomatic (Sherlock, 1969; Williams, 1972), based on the knowledge that the liver has an enormous regenerative capacity if given enough time. The major therapeutic problems are haemorrhage and coma.

About 75 % of all patients suffer bleeding at some time during their illness (Hobbs, 1973). Nasopharyngeal bleeding is particularly hazardous, as inhalation of blood readily occurs in the comatose patient. Bleeding occurs as there is a failure of synthesis of various clotting precursors and an increase in fibrinolysis probably due to intravascular coagulation (Rake et al., 1970).

The pathogenesis of the encephalopathy of fulminant hepatic failure is not clear. It has been suggested that it is due to the absence or short supply of substances needed for normal brain function and usually secreted by the liver into the blood stream (Rueff and Benhamou, 1973). Alternatively, accumulation of neurotoxic substances, such as ammonia, which the liver normally eliminates or detoxifies have been postulated as the cause of hepatic coma. However, no clinical or animal studies have confirmed that any of these suggestions are the actual cause of the encephalopathy seen in acute hepatic failure.

TREATMENT

For acute hepatic failure to be treated effectively encephalopathy has to be reversed, clotting factors restored and the liver must be capable of regeneration. In any given case, however, no initial assessment can be made as to whether recovery is possible. Many forms of treatment have been proposed and success in individual cases has often led to unfounded claims of efficacy.

Corticosteroid drugs, exchange blood transfusion, haemodialysis, extracorporeal liver perfusion and cross circulation have been tried. Review of the literature, however, gives no grounds for the belief that these treatments have made a significant impression on recovery rates (Rueff and Benhamou, 1973; Redeker and Yamahiro, 1973).

Since none of these therapeutic procedures is uniformly successful, attempts are being made to investigate the possibility of making an 'artificial liver' similar to the 'artificial kidney'. Dialysis is capable of removing toxic water-soluble compounds such as ammonia, but will not remove protein-bound compounds. These may, however, be removed by passing the blood over charcoal coated with resins which adsorb protein-bound compounds. This technique is known as haemoperfusion (Wilson et al., 1972) and is simply performed using an arteriovenous shunt, regional heparinisation and a simple blood pump. The initial results of haemoperfusion, combined with fresh frozen plasma infusion and haemodialysis, where necessary, have been very encouraging.

REFERENCES

Hobbs, K. E. F. (1973): *Resuscitation, 2*, 51.
Rake, M. O., Flute, P. T., Pannell, G. and Williams, R. (1970): *Lancet, 1*, 533.
Redeker, A. G. and Yamahiro, H. S. (1973): *Lancet, 1*, 3.
Rueff, B. and Benhamou, J. P. (1973): *Gut, 14*, 805.
Sherlock, S. (1969): *Brit. J. Hosp. Med., 5*, 1257.
Williams, R. (1972): *Brit. med. Bull., 28*, 114.
Wilson, R. A., Webster, K. H., Hofmann, A. F. and Summerskill, W. H. J. (1972): *Gastroenterology, 62*, 1191.

Renal failure: Preoperative problems and their management

LEO STRUNIN

Anaesthetic Department, King's College Hospital, London, United Kingdom

For the purposes of considering patients suitable for renal transplantation only chronic renal failure is appropriate. Many patients, with acute renal failure, may recover normal renal function and need only be sustained by dialysis, often peritoneal, in the meanwhile.

The symptoms and signs of chronic renal failure are essentially similar – regardless of the aetiology. Hypertension, anaemia, electrolyte and acid-base disturbances, the high risk of infection and the dependance of the patient on his veins and arteries for dialysis are the major problems.

DIALYSIS

The advent of dialysis programmes has revolutionised the treatment of chronic renal failure. Indeed, patients may lead a normal life and treat themselves at home.

Two forms of dialysis are available – peritoneal and haemodialysis. The former is most suitable for situations where recovery of renal function is likely, or until facilities for haemodialysis are available. The advantages are that the treatment is cheap, the setting-up is easy and rapid, disequilibrium does not occur, no blood is needed, no shunt is required and there is a minimum of apparatus. The disadvantages are that the process of peritoneal dialysis is slow and therefore not suitable for hypercatabolic states, there is a risk of peritoneal infection and the patient is confined to hospital. In contrast, haemodialysis is rapid and effective. There are, however, a number of disadvantages including the need for expensive, special apparatus, a special hospital site, the risk of disequilibrium, blood may be needed and the patient must have a suitable arteriovenous shunt or fistula.

HYPERTENSION

This is usually controlled by haemodialysis but bilateral nephrectomy may be necessary. Other indications for bilateral nephrectomy are: infection of the urinary tract, large poly-cystic kidneys which may interfere with subsequent transplantation and haematuria. The anaesthetic problems are essentially similar to those for renal transplantation (Jenkins et al., 1973).

ANAEMIA

Most patients compensate for their anaemia by increasing their cardiac output, increasing the 2,3-diphosphoglycerate (DPG) content of their red cells and maintaining a normal blood volume. The decrease in viscosity and shift of the oxygen dissociation curve associated with metabolic acidosis also help.

Blood transfusion is only indicated if anaemia is very severe. There is no long-term effect and the risk of hyperkalaemia, excess iron load, viral B hepatitis and an antibody response which may compromise a future transplant should be borne in mind.

ELECTROLYTE AND ACID-BASE DISTURBANCES

These are usually corrected by haemodialysis. Hyperkalaemia may, however, occur before dialysis can be instituted and plasma levels in excess of 6–7 mEq/l may cause fatal cardiac dysrhythmias. Immediate treatment is by calcium gluconate, sodium bicarbonate and insulin and dextrose intravenously. None of these measures, of course, removes potassium from the body and therefore dialysis should be commenced without delay. Calcium resonium enemas may also be used as intermediate treatment.

OTHER PROBLEMS

Gastrointestinal bleeding may occur due to steroid therapy and increased acid secretion in the stomach.

Serum calcium levels may be low due to acidosis and/or parathyroid gland proliferation. This may lead to pathological fractures and particular care should be taken during surgery. Steroid therapy may also cause avascular necrosis of the bone with further risk of fractures.

SHUNTS AND FISTULAE

For successful haemodialysis an arteriovenous shunt or fistula is required. Unfortunately, these are not simple procedures and refashioning is frequently required. The surgical operating time may be extensive. Both local and general anaesthesia have been used (Savege and Strunin, 1971; Samuel and Powell, 1970). Local procedures have the advantage that sympathetic blockade may assist the surgeon in finding suitable vessels. Recently, Galizia and Lahiri (1974) have described the use of stellate ganglion block with general anaesthesia for this purpose.

REFERENCES

Galizia, E. J. and Lahiri, S. K. (1974): *Anaesthesia*, *29*, 362.
Jenkins, L. C., Maloney, P. J. and Cyr, W. (1973): *Canad. Anaesth. Soc. J.*, *20*, 259.
Samuel, J. R. and Powell, D. (1970): *Anaesthesia*, *25*, 165.
Savege, T. M. and Strunin, L. (1971): *Anaesthesia*, *26*, 498.

Anaesthesia for renal transplantation

G. VOURC'H and P. DUVALDESTIN

Department of Anaesthesia, Hôpital Foch, Suresnes, France

Between 1965 and 1972, 107 renal transplantations have been performed in our hospital. A previous series, including the first successful homotransplantation in man has been reported elsewhere (Kuss et al., 1960; Vourc'h et al., 1961).

In the present study on 103 cases, the major problems encountered before, during and after transplantation, and the technique used are summarized (Table 1).

Table 1. *Surgical procedure carried out in 103 cases of renal transplantations*

	No. of cases
Transplantation + bilateral nephrectomy	47
Transplantation + right nephrectomy	28
Transplantation alone	21
Transplantation + left nephrectomy	3
Transplantation + bilateral nephrectomy and splenectomy	2
Transplantation + left nephrectomy and splenectomy	2
Total	103

BIOLOGICAL PROBLEMS

Advanced renal failure induces severe disorders which may interfere with anaesthesia and surgery and affect:

(a) The cardiovascular system

Hypertension is nearly always present in case of glomerulonephritis and some malformations, less frequently in cases with interstitial nephritis. It is not always controlled by haemodialysis. It may require bilateral nephrectomy and even then blood pressure may take some weeks to reach normal values (Hampers et al., 1967; Safar et al., 1969).

Left ventricular failure secondary to hypertension and increased blood volume is frequent, and anaemia is common. Pulmonary oedema may occur.

Pericardial effusion is usually controlled by haemodialysis but may recur if this is inadequate. Haemopericardium is sometimes observed (Jungers et al., 1972).

(b) Blood and coagulation

Anaemia is the rule, haematocrit being usually around 20%. It is well tolerated owing to an increase of cardiac index (Mostert et al., 1970).

"

Coagulation may be impaired because of platelet dysfunction and a decrease of pro-thrombin consumption (Horowitz et al., 1970).

Heparin required for haemodialysis may still be present at the time of operation due to a rebound phenomenon (Hampers et al., 1966; Kjellstrand and Buselmeier, 1972).

Fresh blood must not be used, and transfusion given with old bank blood, irradiated blood, or packed red cells.

(c) Electrolyte and acid base regulations

These are controlled by peritoneal or haemodialysis. Hyperkalaemia is common, and worsened by acidosis. Treatment is by sodium bicarbonate, and 30% glucose infusions with insulin. Stored blood (21 days) contains 25–30 mEq/l of potassium in the plasma. Hyperkalaemia may be observed in some cases of tubulopathy, and following haemodialysis. Hyper- or hypocalcaemia may be present.

PHARMACOLOGICAL PROBLEMS INDUCED BY RENAL FAILURE

The duration of action of a drug depends upon its diffusion space, its metabolism and its excretion. In case of advanced renal disease, the half-life of some drugs, where the kidneys are the main or only route of elimination, may be considerably prolonged. Bennet et al. (1970) have provided a useful guide for drugs commonly employed.

MUSCLE RELAXANTS

Decamethonium (and all methonium compounds), and gallamine, are excreted solely through the kidneys, and should not be used (Strunin, 1966).

Cohen et al. (1967) and Cohen and Feldman (1970) have shown that although d-tubocura-rine is normally excreted by the kidneys the liver is an alternative route. This has been borne out in clinical practice (Table 2). The dosage, however, must be reduced. In our

Table 2. *Experience in clinical practice*

| Authors | No. of cases of renal transplantation | No. of cases in which d-tubocurarine was used | | Respiratory incidents (No. of cases) |
		Succinyldicholine then d-tubocurarine	Only d-tubocurarine	
Samuel and Powell, 1970	100	93	7	Pulmonary oedema (2) Regurgitation (1) Mixed acidosis (1)
Homi and Smith, 1970	112	–	71	–
Strunin, 1966	36	–	9	Respiratory insufficiency requiring ventilation for 6 days (1)
Soxon	18	–	16	Prolonged curarisation, 26 mg of d-tubo-curarine for 5 hr (1)
Aldrete et al.,	260	102	89	Prolonged curarisation (7)

experience, it has seldom led to prolonged curarisation; in only 16 cases was neostigmine required to reverse it. The doses used were: m = 2.704 ± 0.654 μg of d-tubocurarine/kg/min on 101 patients.

In case of concomitant renal and liver failure, prolonged action may be expected. One patient received d-tubocurarine on 3 occasions: bilateral nephrectomy; renal transplantation, the doses used being 32 and 35 mg respectively, without any sign of residual curarisation (Vourc'h and Conseilier, 1969). Between these two operations he developed hepatitis, and an operation was required to establish an arteriovenous shunt. On that occasion he received 24 mg of d-tubocurarine and showed signs of residual curarisation for 24 hr. Pancuronium bromide appears to share the same fate as d-tubocurarine (Agoston et al., 1973).

Suxamethonium should be a suitable agent since it is metabolised into succinylmonocholine, whose potency is only 1/20th that of succinydicholine, but excreted by the kidneys. One of our former cases showed signs of residual muscle paralysis after succinylcholine infusion (Vourc'h et al., 1961). In the present series it has been used on most patients prior to intubation. Miller et al., (1972), found that it does not increase the blood potassium level in cases with renal failure.

ANAESTHETIC AGENTS

(a) Volatile

Although *cyclopropane* has been used by some (Hampers et al., 1968; Hansen et al., 1972), cases of cardiac arrest have been reported (Levine and Virtue, 1964).

Halothane is widely employed either as sole agent or in combination with other drugs (Aldrete et al., 1971; Gozon, 1970; Hampers et al., 1967; Homi and Smith, 1970; Samuel and Powell, 1970; Strunin, 1966), including muscle relaxants. It has been used in 18 of our cases, but only at the end of the operation, in 0.5–1% concentrations, without complications.

Methoxyflurane has been tried, but its nephrotoxicity is now well-established (Bergstrand et al., 1972; Hollenberg, 1972) and precludes its use.

(b) Intravenous

Barbiturates, other than barbital, are metabolized by the liver. The dose must be reduced (Dundee and Annis, 1955; Freeman et al., 1962; Taylor et al., 1954). Tranquillizers (Reidenberg, 1971) and especially diazepam (Goodman and Gilman, 1970) may be used.

Narcotics are not contraindicated (Bennett et al., 1970), although a case of prolonged action requiring haemodialysis has been reported (Mostert et al., 1971). In our series, morphine, and pethidine have been used in the premedication; and pethidine, phenoperidine and fentanyl as adjuvants. In one case only was respiratory assistance required after 4 mg of phenoperidine in a patient with hepatitis.

The antidiuretic action of morphine, and morphine-like drugs, must be considered. One of our patients (a physician) noticed a reduction in urine output following transplantation after pethidine injections.

(c) Adjuvants

Atropine, commonly used in the premedication, is partly excreted by the kidneys. One of our patients (a physician) mentioned a prolonged action after moderate doses (0.5 mg), following repeated procedures.

ANAESTHETIC TECHNIQUE

Two different situations may occur:

1.   The transplantation is a planned procedure from a living donor. The patient can be prepared by haemodialysis, if required, and the various metabolic and haematologic disorders corrected. Immunotherapy may be started in advance.

2.   It may be done in emergency, from a cadaver kidney, on a patient unknown to both surgeons and anaesthetists, unprepared, sometimes with a full stomach. The assessment of his condition, and the correction of the various metabolic and haematologic disorders, must be carried out in a very short time.

Premedication includes atropine or scopolamine, and a sedative whenever possible. A nasogastric tube is inserted.

Anaesthesia is induced with a small dose of thiopentone, and intubation carried out under suxamethonium; mechanical ventilation is achieved with a mixture of nitrous oxide and oxygen. In our cases, d-tubocurarine was used in all cases but 5 who received pancuronium. Phenoperidine or fentanyl are administered in divided doses. Halothane was used on 18 cases towards the end of the operation.

In 16 cases, neostigmine was required to reverse residual curarisation. 4 patients were left intubated and ventilated for 2 hr, 9 for more than 4 hr; in 8 of them prolonged curarisation is probable; in 1, a patient with hepatitis, central respiratory depression due to phenoperidine (4 mg) occurred.

Venous catheterization must be achieved with utmost care, since:

1.   Shunts or arteriovenous fistula preclude injection in the corresponding limb (blood pressure must *not* be taken on that limb either, lest the shunt or fistula might clog).

2.   The arterial and venous stock must be preserved should haemodialysis be required in the postoperative period.

3.   Strict asepsis must be observed.

The electrocardiogram must be monitored throughout, particularly if metabolic disorders are present.

SURGICAL TECHNIQUE

Two entirely different approaches have been made:

1.   In the early period, the trend was to perform, not only the transplantation, but at the same stage, uni- or bilateral nephrectomy, and possibly splenectomy. It resulted in severe trauma in acutely ill patients, with a considerable risk of postoperative complications, and particularly infection.

2.   A different attitude has recently been adopted. Transplantation alone is carried out, and the wound closed without drainage. The other procedures are achieved independently, either before, or after. This new attitude has considerably reduced the incidence of complications, particularly infection, in patients submitted to immunotherapy.

COMPLICATIONS

No patients were lost during the operation; one, from a previous series died shortly afterwards from hyperkalaemia.

Hypotension was encountered at the time of induction, on 6 cases, (moderate and transient); and during anastomosis, due to haemorrhage, leading to cardiac arrest in one case; this was reverted by external massage and transfusion. Two further cases of hypotension occurred; in one of them the venous catheter was found to be in the pleural space.

4 patients had to be operated again for haemorrhage in the immediate postoperative period.

Postoperative respiratory complications occurred in 3 cases, requiring intubation and tracheal aspiration; this proved fatal in one case.

POSTOPERATIVE COURSE

Most patients are overhydrated before the operation. Two possibilities can be met once the transplantation is achieved: (1) The transplanted kidney does not function. The recipient's haemodynamic condition must be assessed, furosemide and mannitol (if the osmotic load is not already high) administered. (2) The transplanted kidney is functioning. The hourly urine output must be assessed, a negative water and sodium balance being sought.

REFERENCES

Aldrete, J. A., Daniel, W., O'Higgins, J. W., Homalas, J. and Starzl, T. E. (1971): *Anesth. Analg. Curr. Res., 50,* 321.

Agoston, S., Vermeer, G. A., Kersten, V. W. and Maijer, D. K. F. (1973): *Acta anaesth. scand., 17,* 267.

Bennett, W. M., Singer, I. S. and Coggins, C. H. (1970): *J. Amer. med. Ass., 214,* 1468.

Bergstrand, A., Colliste, L. G. and Franksson, C. (1972): *Brit. J. Anaesth., 44,* 569.

Cohen, E. N., Brewer, H. W. and Smith, D. (1967): *Anesthesiology, 28,* 317.

Cohen, E. N. and Feldman, S. A. (1970): In: *Proceedings, Fourth World Congress of Anesthesiologists, London 1968,* p. 410. Editors: T. B. Boulton, R. Bryce-Smith, M. K. Sykes, G. B. Gillet and A. L. Revell. Excerpta Medica, Amsterdam.

Dundee, J. W. and Annis, D. (1955): *Brit. J. Anaesth., 27,* 114.

Freeman, R. B., Sheff, M. G., Maker, J. F. and Schreiner, G. E. (1962): *Ann. intern. Med., 56,* 233.

Goodman, L. S. and Gilman, A. (1970): In: *The Pharmacological Basis of Therapeutics 4th Ed.,* p. 178. Collier-MacMillan, Toronto.

Gozon, F. X. (1970): In: *Proceedings, Fourth World Congress of Anesthesiologists, London 1968,* p. 675. Editors: T. B. Boulton, R. Bryce-Smith, M. K. Sykes, G. B. Gillet and A. L. Revell. Excerpta Medica, Amsterdam.

Hampers, C. L., Bailey, G. L., Hager, E. B., Van Dam, L. D. and Merrill, J. P. (1968): *Amer. J. Surg., 115,* 741.

Hampers, C. L., Blaufox, M. D. and Merrill, J. P. (1966): *New Engl. J. Med., 275,* 776.

Hampers, C. L., Skilman, J. J., Lyons, J. H., Olsen, J. E. and Merrill, J. P. (1967): *Circulation, 35,* 272.

Hansen, D. D., Fernandes, A., Skovsted, P. and Berry, P. (1972): *Brit. J. Anaesth., 44,* 584.

Hollenberg, N. K. (1972): *New Engl. J. Med., 286,* 877.

Homi, J. and Smith, E. R. (1970): In: *Proceedings, Fourth World Congress of Anesthesiologists, London 1968,* p. 679. Editors: T. B. Boulton, R. Bryce-Smith, M. K. Sykes, G. B. Gillet and A. L. Revell. Excerpta Medica, Amsterdam.

Horowitz, H. I., Stein, I. M., Cohen, B. D. and White, J. G. (1970): *Amer. J. Med., 49,* 336.

Jungers, P., Lacombe, M., Neveux, J. Y., Man, N. K., Zingraff, J. and Soucy, P. E. (1972): *Ann. Chir. Thorac. Cardiovasc., 11,* 195.

Kjellstrand, C. M. and Buselmeier, T. J. (1972): *Surgery, 72,* 630.

Kuss, R. et al. (1960): *Presse méd., 20,* 755.

Levine, D. S. and Virtue, R. W. (1964): *Canad. Anaesth. Soc. J., 11,* 425.

Miller, R. D., Way, W. L., Hamilton, W. K. and Layzer, R. B. (1972): *Anesthesiology, 36,* 138.

Mostert, J. W., Evers, J. L., Hobika, G. H., Moore, R. H., Kenny, G. M. and Murphy, G. P. (1970): *Brit. J. Anaesth., 42,* 397.

Mostert, J. W., Evers, J. L., Hobika, G. H., Moore, R. H. and Ambrus, J. L. (1971): *Brit. J. Anaesth., 43,* 1053.

Reidenberg, M. M. (1971): In: *Renal Function and Drug Action,* p. 55. Editors: W. B. Saunders Co., Philadelphia, Pa.

Safar, M., Fendler, J. P., Weil, B., Beuvemery, P., Brisset, J. M., Idatte, J. M., Meyer, P. and Milliez, P. (1969): In: *Actualités Nephrologiques de l'Hôpital Necker*, p. 61. Editors: Editions Médicales Flammarion, Paris.

Samuel, J. R. and Powell, D. (1970): *Anaesthesia, 41*, 165.

Strunin, L. (1966): *Brit. J. Anaesth., 38*, 812.

Taylor, J. D., Richards, R. K., Davin, J. C. and Asher, J. (1954): *Anesth. Analg. Curr. Res., 49*, 323.

Vourc'h, G. and Conseiller, C. (1969): *Thérapie, 24*, 175.

Vourc'h, G., Lecharny, B. and Madre, F. (1971): *Anesth. Analg. Réanim., 28*, 1.

Vourc'h, G., Winckler, C., Germain, A., Miraille, A., Pellati, J. and Cakmur, D. (1961): *Acta Inst. Anesth., 10*, 91.

Aspect of fluid, electrolyte and circulatory problems during anaesthesia for renal transplantation

K. G. DHUNÉR and I. WICKSTRÖM

Department of Anaesthesia I, Sahlgrenska sjukhuset,
University of Gothenburg, Gothenburg, Sweden

In severe renal failure, dialysis and kidney transplantation are commonly used therapeutic methods. Both methods have advantages and disadvantages. The procedure used in a particular case depends upon a number of factors. In Gothenburg, limited facilities for dialysis widens the indications for transplantation, both with regard to age and to the general condition of the patient. As many of our patients receive cadaveric kidneys, the time available for preoperative treatment is short and the patients have to be operated upon even when they are not in the best possible general condition.

Many anaesthetic methods can be used. We have based our technique upon induction with barbiturate, intubation with a single dose succinylcholine and maintained with N_2O and a nondepolarizing muscle relaxant. Sometimes halothane has been added (Table 1). The main problem of anaesthesia in a uraemic patient concerns the effect of renal failure e.g., balance of water, electrolytes, split products of protein and anaemia.

Table 1. *Anaesthetic techniques*

	No. of cases
Barbiturate$+N_2O+O_2+$relaxant	261
Barbiturate$+N_2O+O_2+$halothane	39
Barbiturate$+N_2O+O_2+$halothane$+$relaxant	138
Neurolept II$+N_2O+O_2+$relaxant	4
Total	442

A patient with uraemia may be able to produce water, but cannot excrete electrolytes and products of protein metabolism. Operation can be performed without much preoperative treatment. Other patients may have a marked water retention which will not only result in hypervolaemia but they may also have fluid in the lungs, pleura and pericardium. Such a patient is not a good candidate for operation and should be put on the dialysis programme before transplantation. In Table 2 the number of patients without previous dialyses and the time of the last dialysis before transplantation is shown.

The changes in the water content of the body must be considered. A recently dialyzed patient is hypovolaemic and may be susceptible to falls in blood pressure during the

Table 2. *Dialysis*

		% patients
Not dialyzed		21.5
Regular peritoneal dialysis		2.3
Regular haemodialysis		
Last dialysis before transplantation	1 day	38.0
	2–3 days	25.5
	4 days or more	12.7

transplantation. Fluid therapy must be liberal during the operation. In patients where the tast dialysis before the operation can be timed, as for instance when there are living donors, lhe water content should be reduced only to a normal value. Stability of the blood pressure results. Overhydrated patients have to be watched very carefully. Pulmonary oedema and even cardiac tamponade have been noted. Measurement of CVP is of great importance and of course fluid therapy must be restricted.

Loss of water during the operation must be considered. Transplantation takes a long time and the wound is fairly large. Most interest however, is focussed around the function of the new kidney. Sometimes no urine is produced but sometimes the kidney starts to produce urine within minutes and the production can be more than one litre during the operation.

Uraemic patients are mostly anemic (Table 3). It is discouraging to find how difficult it is to increase the haemoglobin with transfusions to values which are normally required before anaesthesia. However, it is found that uraemic patients have increased peripheral circulation, which is not only caused by haemodilution, but other factors also seem to be involved. The risk of overhydration and immunological reactions which disturb the function of the transplant are the contraindications to blood transfusion. Patients are therefore accepted for anaesthesia with haemoglobin levels above 5 g Hb/100 ml.

Table 3. *Preoperative blood levels*

No. of cases		
Hb	113	($<$ 6 g/100ml)
K^+/s	57	($>$ 5.5 mEq./l)
$TotCO_2$/s	49	($>$ 17 mEq./l)

Total number of cases = 442.

During the operation blood loss may be small, in which case transfusion should be avoided. When the blood loss is greater, packed red cells, albumin and water are given in order to avoid immunological reactions.

Infusion of small molecular dextran is given during the operation for rheologic reasons. The big vessels can be clamped in connection with implanting the vessels from the new kidney. In that way heparin need not be used. Infusion of the hyperosmolar solutions may cause pulmonary oedema. With slow infusion this has been avoided. During the postoperative course early dialysis is used in patients with incipient pulmonary oedema.

Of the electrolytes potassium is of great interest (Table 3). Observation of patients at or above the upper normal value is important since it is known that the potassium level will increase from the time the premedication is given until the operation starts. When the time limit for operation does not allow preoperative haemodialysis an ion exchange resin is given rectally, infusion with glucose and insulin and also peroperative peritoneal dialyses have been used.

The sodium level is low in many patients. This is usually accepted but in some cases added sodium has helped start the diuresis of the transplant.

Metabolic acidosis is not rare and can be corrected preoperatively. However, when acidosis is marked, large doses of bicarbonate may cause a sodium and water load and correction should therefore be done very carefully (Table 3).

As a consequence of the uraemic changes cardiovascular problems will occur during the transplantation.

A newly dialyzed patient with hypovolaemia will be very susceptible to blood pressure falls caused by the anaesthetic technique and by further loss of fluid. These patients need fluid replacement which should be done with extreme care.

Overhydration can result in fluid in lungs, pleura and pericardium and this may result in impairment of oxygen transport, pulmonary oedema and even cardiac tamponade. In this respect it must be pointed out that pulmonary oedema will be held in check by positive pressure ventilation during operation but may cause trouble in the immediate postoperative period. As in every anaesthetized patient, cardiac arrhythmia occurs. In addition, patients with uraemia have other reasons for arrhythmias, for instance, high potassium levels.

Many of the patients are hypertensive and receive one or several, antihypertensive drugs. If possible these drugs should be abandoned one or two days before the operation. This has not been possible in most of our patients nor has it caused trouble.

Occasionally there have been patients who, during the operation, develop a very high blood pressure – diastolic pressure 130 mm Hg or more. Addition of small amounts of halothane has been used to control the blood pressure with good results.

Pancuronium as muscle relaxant in renal transplantations: Comparison with tubocurarine

MLADEN IBLER

Department of Anesthesiology, Glostrup Hospital, Copenhagen, Denmark

Pancuronium is a non-depolarising muscle relaxant which, in comparison with d-tubocurarine, offers the following advantages: lack of ganglion-blocking side-effects, hypotension, moderate stimulation of sympathetic nervous system, insignificant liberation of histamine and modest binding to plasma proteins. Because of its properties pancuronium should be well suited for bad-risk patients undergoing anesthesia, including those submitted to renal transplantation.

Using a newly developed fluorimetric method (Kresten et al., 1973) Agoston et al. (1973) recently proved that following intravenously injected 6 mg dose pancuronium, 11% is excreted unchanged in the bile and 37–44% in the urine. Miller et al. (1973) showed that in anephric patients undergoing renal transplantation the duration of pancuronium blockade is increased only 20–50% following doses ranging from 1.8–5.5 mg. Clinical observations from as far back as 1969 showed that in patients with reduced renal function a cumulative effect may be expected after the third dose (Stojanov, 1969).

This is a retrospective study of the dosage of pancuronium, the relationship between dosage of tubocurarine and pancuronium, the occurrence of postoperative respiratory failure and the side-effects of these drugs in patients undergoing renal transplantation.

MATERIAL AND METHODS

The study group consisted of 38 patients with absent renal function who had 41 cadaveric renal transplantations. The operations were performed as emergencies and the patients were often in poor general condition, with severe anemia, uremia and fluid- and electrolyte disturbances. Anemia and hyperkalemia were partly corrected preoperatively. As premedication pethidine and atropine or only promethazine was given. After gastric aspiration, and preoxygenation, anesthesia was induced with enibomal sodium (Narcodorm ®) 3–5 mg/kg and the patient was intubated after a single dose of suxamethonium. Patients with high serum potassium levels were not given suxamethonium but were intubated after administration of tubocurarine or pancuronium (Table 1). Anesthetic agents employed were halothane, nitrous oxide, fentanyl, dehydrobenzperidol (DHB) or, in one case, ether. After the initial dose of pancuronium 4–6 mg, or tubocurarine 15–20 mg, relaxation was maintained with doses of 1–2 mg pancuronium or 5–10 mg tubocurarine, given when necessary. Most of the supplementary doses of pancuronium were given during the first half of the period of anesthesia, and there were rarely given more than 2 supplementary doses of pancuronium. The ventilation was controlled. The neuromuscular block was reversed with neostigmine

2.5 mg given simultaneously with atropine 1 mg. Evaluation of muscular function after decurarisation was based on the ability of the patient to lift his head and to perform deep inspiration. The duration of anesthesia was counted from the induction till the patient was extubated or transferred from the operating theatre to the respiratory care unit.

Table 2 shows average doses of tubocurarine by different types of anesthesia. Doses of tubocurarine in patients anesthetised with halothane is, as expected, lower than in patients anesthetised with nitrous oxide and fentanyl but the number of patients in the first 2 groups is too small to derive any conclusions. Table 3 gives the doses of pancuronium in patients anesthetised with nitrous oxide and fentanyl, DHB, fentanyl, nitrous oxide and halothane. Here also the dose of pancuronium is somewhat lower in the halothane group than in other groups. Table 4 shows the ratio tubocurarine:pancuronium by different types of general anesthesia; this ratio seems to be in accordance with that stated in the literature for patients with normal renal function, namely between 5 and 10. The frequency of postoperative respiratory failure was the same in both groups (Table 5).

The duration of anesthesia was extremely long in patient No. 1 – almost 7 hr – and blood

Table 1.   *Anesthetic agents employed*

No. of anesthesias	Anesthetic agents	Mean age	Mean Hb (g/l)
12	N$_2$O-fentanyl	35	93
7	DHB-N$_2$O-fentanyl	52	79
20	Halothane-N$_2$O	42	67
1	Halothane-ether	45	101
1	Ether-N$_2$O	36	82

Table 2.   *Tubocurarine dosage in patients without postoperative respiratory failure – mean values*

No. of anesthesias	Anesthetic agent	Creatinine serum (mg/l)	Tubocurarine chloride	
			Total dose (mg)	Dose (mg/kg/hr)
3	N$_2$O fentanyl	105	65	0.240
2	DHB-N$_2$O-fentanyl	88	42.	0.112
11	Halothane	89	38 5	0.163
1	Ether	77	50	0.170

Table 3.   *Pancuronium dosage in patients without postoperative respiratory failure – mean values*

No. of anesthesias	Anesthetic agent	Creatinine serum (mg/l)	Pancuronium	
			Total dose (mg)	Dose (mg/kg/hr)
7	N$_2$O fentanyl	113	8.4	0.030
4	DHB-N$_2$O-fentanyl	102	8.2	0.032
8	Halothane	105	7.2	0.025

Table 4.   *Ratio tubocurarine chloride/pancuronium on mg/kg/hr base*

N$_2$O-fentanyl	8
DHB-N$_2$O-fentanyl	3.5
Halothane	6.5

Table 5. *Tubocurarine and pancuronium dosage in patients with postoperative respiratory failure*

Patient No.	Anesthetic agent and dose	Creatinine serum (mg/l)	Artificial respiration	Tubocurarine	
				Total dose (mg)	Dose (mg/kg/hr)
1.	N₂O-fentanyl 0.25 mg	70	14 hr	45	0.078
2.	Halothane	89	1 hr 20 min	43	0.108
				Pancuronium	
3.	N₂O-fentanyl 0.20 mg	139	2 hr 30 min	13	0.054
4.	N₂O-DHB 7.50 mg				
	Fentanyl 0.20 mg	142	1 hr	7	0.018

loss was 2700 ml. Patient No. 2 lost 2000 ml during operation, and patient No. 3, a young girl who was in better general condition than other patients, evidently received an overdose of pancuronium. It should be noted that the average peroperative loss of blood in patients without postoperative respiratory failure was 860 ml in the tubocurarine group and 900 ml in the pancuronium group.

Systolic hypotension of 10–30 mm Hg was observed in 2 patients after administration of both initial and supplementary doses of tubocurarine, whereas no fall of blood pressure due to administration of the drug was seen in the pancuronium group.

In the material presented a total dose of pancuronium ranging from 7.2–8.4 mg was used. The dose ratio, tubocurarine:pancuronium was found to be between 3.5 and 8, which corresponds to the ratio usually stated for individuals with normal renal function. This fact, as well as the same frequency of postoperative respiratory failure in both the pancuronium and the tubocurarine group, could, from a clinical point of view, suggest that absent renal function influences tubocurarine and pancuronium blockade equally. Except the diminished renal excretion of these drugs, other factors important for the development of postoperative respiratory failures are: a state of increased catabolism with reduction of the muscle mass, excessive bleeding, fluid overload and prolonged time of operation.

According to our clinical experience, use of pancuronium and tubocurarine in patients undergoing renal transplantation, with the exception of the tendency to circulatory instability following tubocurarine, did not reveal any significant difference.

REFERENCES

Agoston, S., Vermeel, G. A., Kresten, U. W. and Meijer, D. K. F. (1973): *Acta anaesth. scand.*, *17/4*, 267.
Kresten, U. W., Meijer, D. K. F. and Agoston, S. (1973): *Clin. chim. Acta, 44/1*, 59.
Miller, R. D., Stevens, W. C. and Way, W. L. (1973): *Anesth. Analg. Curr. Res., 52/4*, 661.
Stojanov, E. (1969): *Arzneimittel-Forsch., 19/10*, 1723.

Spinal anesthesia for renal transplantation: Five years experience at the University of Rochester Medical Center

ROBERT G. MERIN and CLARA L. LINKE

Department of Anesthesiology, University of Rochester School of Medicine,
Rochester, N.Y., U.S.A.

Two of the earliest reports on anesthesia for renal transplantation advised regional anesthesia for the following reasons: superb surgical field; good lower aortic blood flow; no concern about renal excretion of drugs; no interaction of drugs with the biochemical derangements of terminal renal failure; avoidance of tracheal intubation and further interference in already compromised defense mechanisms against infection; and maintenance of airway integrity in the face of a full stomach (VanDam et al., 1962; Wyant, 1967). Although hemodialysis has markedly improved the pathophysiology of renal transplant recipients, most of the considerations that led VanDam and Wyant to choose regional anesthesia for their patients are still pertinent.

Some institutions have used potent inhalation anesthetics (Lofstrom, 1967; Hansen et al., 1972), but the desire by surgeons for the use of electrocautery, and the concern about hepatic and renal dysfunction following halogenated anesthetics has led other groups to rely heavily on nitrous oxide, narcotic analgesics and neuromuscular blocking drugs (Dhuner et al., 1968; Samuel and Powell, 1970; Monks and Lumley, 1972; Latarjet et al., 1973). Although only gallamine is excreted primarily via the kidney (Feldman et al., 1969), there have been several reports of prolonged blockade in these patients after d-tubocurare and pancuronium (Katz et al., 1967; Aldrete et al., 1971; Logan et al., 1974). Indeed one group has adapted a succinylcholine-tetrahydroaminacrine regimen because of such problems (Smith, 1973). Many patients still come to transplantation with hyperkalemia and acidosis (Fujita and Miyazaki, 1973) in spite of maintenance hemodialysis. Arrhythmias with drugs, particularly succinylcholine can be troublesome in this situation (Koide and Waud, 1972). Finally, although perfusion and preservation techniques have prolonged cadaver kidney survival time, many institutions still consider these operations as emergent. Consequently, many patients present with a full stomach. A cuffed endotracheal tube can protect the lungs from gastrointestinal contents, but then the risk of iatrogenic infection and interference with normal tracheobronchial defense mechanisms is introduced. Infection is still the most common complication of renal transplantation (Chisholm, 1972).

After considering the surgical, pharmacologic and pathophysiologic aspects of renal transplantation, we chose regional anesthesia for our patients in 1968. Our transplant team decided at the same time to stage the bilateral nephrectomy-splenectomy which was

* Supported in part by RCDA HL No. 31752 (Dr. Merin) and The New York State Kidney Institute.

routine for our patients at that time, so the surgical field was extraperitoneal and lower abdominal (ideal for lumbar epidural or spinal anesthesia). Our initial experience with continuous lumbar epidural was poor, so we converted to a single high dose spinal anesthetic with tetracaine-epinephrine (Table 1). Of the 55 transplants performed at the University of Rochester Medical Center between August 1968 and December 1973, 45 were anesthetized by means of this technique. After 3 hr of surgery, one of these was supplemented with thiopental-N_2O-halothane. The other 44 were all successfully sedated so that they were responsive to command with small doses of Innovar (total 2–4 ml) or diazepam (total 5–7 mg). Supplemental oxygen (and nitrous oxide after 4 hr of surgery) was given by disposable inhalation therapy masks. Patient acceptance was good enough that subsequent transplant recipients were often reassured by the 'veterans' about the anesthetic technique.

Table 1. *Anesthesia techniques: Planned approach (University of Rochester Medical Center, 1968–1973)*

	Spinal	Continuous epidural	General and continuous spinal	General
No. of cases	45	5	1	4
Donors				
Live 14	11	1	0	2
Cadaver 41	34	4	1	2
Age				
10–15 yrs	3	0	0	3
16–39 yrs	32	4	1	1
40–57 yrs	10	1	0	0
Duration of surgery				
2–4 hr	20	1	0	2
4–6 hr	25	4	1	2
Sedation				
IV only	23	1		
IV + N_2O insufflation	21			
Inhalation	1	4	1	4
Neuromuscular blocking drugs	0	1	0	1
Endotracheal intubation	0	1	1	3
Tetracaine dose (mg)	15.8			
mean range	(10–20)			

Monitoring included continuous electrocardiographic observations in all patients. Successful central venous catheters were passed through a forearm vein in 45/55 patients for pressure monitoring. Arterial blood pressure was measured directly from the arterial limb of the shunt or by auscultation, Doppler or pulse wave detection in patients with fistulae. In view of vessel access problems in this group of patients, we did not cannulate peripheral arteries for monitoring purposes separately.

Elective transplants were transfused with washed frozen red blood cells on the day prior to surgery during their dialysis in order to bring the hematocrit to 25%. Cadaver kidney recipients were treated individually on advice from the nephrologist considering their last prior dialysis. During transplantation, 5% dextrose in water was infused at 0.3–0.5 ml/kg/hr. Blood and fluid losses were replaced as closely as possible with washed frozen red cells and albumin. 44/55 patients needed no more than one unit of red blood cells and only two patients needed more than 3 units (4 and 6 respectively).

Although 26/45 patients given spinal anesthetics were hypotensive at some time during the procedure, (less than 80% of the preoperative blood pressure) blood pressure could usually be easily managed with position, fluids, blood and sometimes vasopressors. Consequently, 8/45 were hypotensive at the time of kidney revascularization and only 2 of these had systolic blood pressures of less than 100 Torr.

There were no permanent neurologic sequelae in our series, although a number of patients had preexisting uremic neuropathy. As VanDam et al. (1962) had reported, there were no post-spinal headaches in our series.

The commonly quoted reasons for avoiding regional anesthesia for renal transplantation include the emotional instability of the patient population, the duration of surgery, abnormal clotting mechanisms, cardiovascular instability and neurologic complications. None of these proved to be a problem in our series. Our experience with spinal anesthesia for renal transplantation has been positive from the standpoint of the patient, surgeon, and anesthetist. We believe that regional anesthesia produces less pharmacologic and physiologic trespass in these high-risk patients.

REFERENCES

Aldrete, J. A., Daniel, W., O'Higgins, J. W., Homatas, J. and Starzl, T. E. (1971): *Anesth. Analg. Curr. Res.*, *50*, 321.

Chisholm, G. D. (1973): *Proc. roy. Soc. Med.*, *66*, 914.

Dhuner, K. G., Lundberg, H. and Peterhoff, V. (1968): *Scand. J. Urol. Nephrol.*, *2*, 31.

Feldman, S. A., Cohen, E. N. and Golling, R. C. (1969): *Anesthesiology*, *30*, 593.

Fujita, T. and Miyazaki, M. (1973): *Tohoku J. exp. Med.*, *110*, 195.

Hansen, D. D., Fernandes, A., Skovsted, P. and Berry, P. (1972): *Brit. J. Anaesth.*, *44*, 584.

Katz, J., Kountz, S. L. and Cohn, R. (1967): *Anesth. Analg. Curr. Res.*, *46*, 609.

Koide, M. and Waude, B. E. (1972): *Anesthesiology*, *36*, 142.

Latarjet, J., Bouletreau, P., Fraysse, G., Gillies, Y. D., Dubernard, J. M., Blitz, M., Bomel, J., Archimbaud, J. P., Orgiazzi, M. F. and Banssillon, V. G. (1973): *Anesth. Analg. Réanim.*, *30*, 337.

Lofstrom, B. (1967): *Scand. J. Urol. Nephrol.*, *1*, 161.

Logan, D. A., Howie, H. B. and Crawford, J. (1974): *Brit. J. Anaesth.*, *46*, 69.

Monks, P. S. and Lumley, J. (1972): *Ann. roy. Coll. Surg. Engl.*, *50*, 334.

Samuel, J. R. and Powell, D. (1970): *Anaesthesia*, *25*, 165.

Smith, B. H. (1973): *Proc. roy. Soc. Med.*, *66*, 918.

Van Dam, L. D., Harrison, J. H., Murray, J. E. and Merrill, J. P. (1962): *Anesthesiology*, *23*, 783.

Wyant, G. M. (1967): *Canad. Anaesth. Soc. J.*, *14*, 255.

Anesthesiological problems in renal transplantation

H.-D. TAUBE and L. STÖCKER

Department of Anesthesiology, University of Essen, Essen, Federal Republic of Germany

Patients elected for renal transplantation usually belong to the high-risk group. Concomitant disorders are frequently: (1) poor general condition; (2) hypertonus; (3) myocardial insufficiency; (4) tendency to pulmonary edema; (5) severe anemia; (6) hypoproteinemia; (7) plasma coagulation disorder especially after hemodialysis; (8) electrolyte imbalance; (9) metabolic acidosis.

Considering the anesthetic management, the inherent risks of each method have to be discussed. Regional anesthesia, preferred in the first years of renal transplantation, almost always causes a marked fall in blood pressure, stabilized only by a considerable amount of fluid infusion. Restlessness or psychic disturbance of the patient requires additional sedation with central depression which becomes similar to general anesthesia.

In our opinion the volatile anesthetics halothane and methoxyflurane are disadvantageous on account of myocardial depression, decreased kidney function and biotransformation to metabolites which are eliminated by the kidneys and have a possible hepatotoxic effect.

In patients with chronic uremia and especially in renal transplantation neuroleptanesthesia (NLA II) is preferred. The well known advantages are the stabilizing effect on the circulation without any depression of cardiac, renal or liver function. For induction, droperidol 0.1 mg/kg and fentanyl 0.005–0.006 mg/kg are injected slowly with simultaneous infusion of 300–500 ml oxygelatine solution. Intubation can be facilitated by suxamethonium 1 mg/kg i.v.; further relaxation is maintained by fractional doses of nordiallyl-toxiferin, initially 0.08 mg/kg.

Important anesthesiological complications are:

1. Hypotension, due to the α-receptor-blocking effect of droperidol, occurs particularly in hypertensive patients.

2. Arrhythmia or asystole after suxamethonium.

3. Prolonged action of suxamethonium, due to the decreased level of pseudocholinesterase in patients following hemodialysis.

4. Inadequate antagonization of nondepolarizing relaxants, or recurarization.

5. Severe and prolonged side-effects of cholinesterase inhibitors.

6. Hemorrhage, due to coagulation disorder.

7. Dysequilibrium after hemodialysis.

In 45 renal transplantations, performed between July 1972 and July 1974, the following complications were noticed. In 4 cases the systolic blood pressure temporarily fell more than 30% during induction, and was stabilized after infusion of 250–500 ml of oxygelatine solution. One case of cardiac arrest, due to suxamethonium during the induction period was treated successfully by transthoracic massage, calcium gluconate and orciprenaline i.v. Four hours earlier the serum potassium had been within normal limits: 5.2 mEq/l. To reduce muscular fasciculation, 1 mg norallyltoxiferin was given i.v. before the suxamethonium (1 mg/kg), which induced bradycardia and asystole. Serum potassium checked at this time was 8.4 mEq/l. 40 g of Resonium A were instilled into the rectum and 100 ml 4% dextrose with 20 units soluble insulin were administered i.v. Two hours later the serum potassium was 6 mEq/l and transplantation was done without further anesthesiological problems.

The use of nondepolarizing relaxants was omitted during the last 2 hr of the operation; however postoperative respiratory insufficiency was noticed in 2 cases. One patient had to be ventilated for 3 hr. The other did not show any muscular weakness after reversal at the end of the operation but 5 hr later developed severe signs of recurarization, which was completely cured by another dose of neostigmine (1 mg).

Cholinesterase inhibitors cause prolonged side-effects in anuric patients. Routine reversal should not be used. In 14 of the 25 cases in the first year neostigmine was given. Two of these patients displayed severe bronchorrhea which required repeated endotracheal suction. Reversal with cholinesterase inhibitors is not now used and elective ventilation is preferred (about 20%).

Coagulation disorders, due to heparin were seen in 2 patients operated on a few hours after hemodialysis. Protamine sulfate was given in one case. The other patient was known to be allergic to the drug and received PPSB, a compound of Factors II, VII, IX and X. No significant bleeding was seen during the transplantation. Two hours later the patient deteriorated rapidly with restlessness, then unconsciousness and generalized convulsions. Autopsy revealed a hemangioma of the cerebellum with subarachnoid bleeding.

Dysequilibrium after hemodialysis is seen sometimes when transplantation follows hemodialysis. An unpredictable shift of electrolytes may cause hypokalemia, which was detected postoperatively in 3 patients who were not polyuric.

Muscle relaxation with pancuronium during renal transplantation

J. A. INGEMAR WICKSTRÖM

Department of Anaesthetics I, Sahlgrens Hospital, Gothenburg, Sweden

Curare and succinylcholine have been frequently used for relaxation during anaesthesia for renal transplantation. The metabolism and excretion of these drugs in patients with renal failure are well known. However, in cases with hyperkalaemia or uraemic neuropathy succinylcholine may cause a dangerous rise of serum potassium. In recently dialysed patients who sometimes are hypovolaemic the ganglion blocking effect of curare may cause blood pressure to fall. Pancuronium is known not to have these effects.

In this series pancuronium has been used in 100 consecutive cases undergoing renal transplantation. The age of the patients varied between 8 and 64 years. About 50% were over 40 years. 74 patients were undergoing regular haemodialysis, 4 regular peritoneal dialysis and 22 had not yet needed dialysis but were uraemic. No extra preoperative dialysis was given. Preoperative blood levels are given in Table 1.

Table 1. *Preoperative blood levels*

	Mean	Range
Hb (g/100 ml)	6.8	4.2–13.0
PCV (%)	21	12–40
Creatinine (mg/100 ml)	10.0	2.6–27.0
Na^+ (mEq/l)	137	122–144
K^+ (mEq/l)	4.4	3.0–6.1
Total CO_2 (mEq/l)	23	10–35

After premedication with meperidine and scopolamine, anaesthesia was induced with hexobarbitone sodium. Endotracheal intubation was made after relaxation with pancuronium. Anaesthesia was maintained with oxygen 30% and nitrous oxide 70%. The patients were slightly hyperventilated with an UR 70 volume controlled ventilator. Incremental doses of pancuronium, 0.5 or 1 mg, were given to maintain a sufficient relaxation. The relaxation was planned so that pancuronium was avoided during the last 45 min of anaesthesia. At the end of the operation the hyperventilation was stopped and atropine and neostigmine were given. Incremental doses of meperidine were given in 63 cases and of fentanyl in 3 cases. Halothane was used in 11 cases. Any slight metabolic acidosis was compensated for only by hyperventilation. In cases with a more pronounced metabolic acidosis sodium bicarbonate was given during anaesthesia. The time between the injection of the intubation dose of pancuronium and the intubation was registered. The degree of relaxation was estimated at intubation, before and 5 min after the injection of neostigmine. Urine production during anaesthesia was recorded.

The average intubation dose of pancuronium was 0.084 mg/kg body weight. By dividing the dose so that one third was given before and two thirds after the barbiturate we have been able to reduce the intubation dose by about 15% without impairing the degree of relaxation at intubation. In this way also the time before the patient is relaxed enough for intubation is reduced. On the average the patients were intubated 2.5 min after the last part of the intubation dose was given. At intubation 38 patients were completely relaxed, 55 were incompletely relaxed but not enough to cause any difficulty and in 7 cases there were minor difficulties owing to the incomplete relaxation. The duration of the first dose of pancuronium was 63 min on average.

The average total dose of pancuronium given was 0.040 mg/kg/hr. There was no significant difference between the total dose given to patients producing less than 20 ml and more than 500 ml urine during the anaesthesia. If those cases with hypotension caused by bleeding or by halothane are excluded, hypotension exceeding 20%, but not 40%, of the preoperative pressure occurred in 10 cases. In an earlier series when curare was used this frequency was 29%. The doses of atropine and neostigmine given at the end of the anaesthesia were 0.015 and 0.034 mg/kg body weight on the average. Before neostigmine was given 4 patients could raise their heads, 52 had spontaneous ventilation, 40 reacted to suction in the endotracheal tube and 4 were completely relaxed. Five minutes after the neostigmine 70 patients could raise their heads and 30 could not but had adequate spontaneous ventilation. Fifteen minutes after the extubation 2 patients had signs of muscular weakness. One of them had received a large total dose of pancuronium. The patients left the recovery ward after a few hours of observation; both had good urine production during anaesthesia. Postoperative blood levels are given in Table 2.

Table 2. *Postoperative blood levels*

	Mean	Range
Na$^+$ (mEq/l)	129	114–144
K$^+$ (mEq/l)	4.5	3.0–6.4
Total CO$_2$ (mEq/l)	20	10–30

If used with care pancuronium is a suitable relaxant for patients with renal failure. The incremental doses should be low and relaxation should be planned so that no dose has to be given late during the anaesthesia. Metabolic acidosis should be corrected while the patient is ventilated. Handled in this way pancuronium causes a low incidence of insufficient postoperative reversal. It also has definite advantages over succinylcholine in not affecting the potassium level and over curare in having minimal influence upon the circulation.

Chapter IX

Anaesthesia and postoperative care in coronary surgery

*Heparin rebound: Studies in patients and volunteers**

N. ELLISON, C. P. BEATTY, D. R. BLAKE,
H. A. WURZEL and H. MACVAUGH III

Departments of Anesthesia, Pathology, and Surgery,
University of Pennsylvania School of Medicine, Philadelphia, Pa., U.S.A.

The term 'heparin rebound' was originally used to describe a state of rebound hyper-coagulability that follows the discontinuation of heparin therapy (Cate et al., 1954). In 1956 Kolff et al. first described heparin rebound as 'a treacherous phenomenon in which heparin is neutralized by protamine sulfate and the clotting time becomes normal in a matter of minutes. However, protamine seems to be eliminated from the blood before heparin is, thus leaving the heparin uncovered as demonstrated by protamine titration.'

Since 1956 there have been many studies, both experimental and clinical, of heparin rebound with varied results. The incidence is reported to vary from those 'who have never seen' the entity and question its existence to others who report a 100% incidence in animals that were studied (Perkins et al., 1959; Thies, 1960). Gollub (1967) had been quite skeptical of the validity of the clinical entity, heparin rebound, and believed it to be a reflection of inadequate technique. When challenged to produce the data which justified his skepticism, he acknowledged that he had none and set out to obtain it. Much to his surprise, he found heparin rebound in 21 of 40 patients as demonstrated by protamine titration after open-heart surgery (Gollub, 1967). Heparin rebound can develop after procedures other than open-heart surgery. Hampers et al. (1966) found it in 11 of 16 patients following hemodialysis and suggested that the phenomenon is 'more common than the literature suggests'.

The time at which heparin rebound occurs after neutralization is equally varied. Heparin in a dose of 3.0 mg/kg has a half-life of approximately 90 min (Olsson and Lagergren, 1963; Estes, 1970). Most cases of heparin rebound have been reported to occur within 8 or 9 hr after heparin neutralization. However, rebound has been reported to develop as much as 18 hr after neutralization of heparin (Hyun et al., 1962).

We designed a study to answer 2 specific questions: (1) How does the incidence of heparin rebound vary with the dose of protamine? (2) When does the phenomenon occur? The study was carried out both in human volunteers followed for 20 hr and in patients who had had cardiac surgery.

STUDIES IN VOLUNTEERS

Heparin, 3.0 mg/kg, was administered intravenously to 6 unanesthetized, fasting, informed volunteers after placement of intra-arterial, peripheral, and central venous lines. Prior to heparinization, blood was sampled for coagulation studies. The Lee-White whole blood

* Reproduced with permission from *Journal of Thoracic and Cardiovascular Surgery* (67, 723–729, 1974), copyrighted by The C.V. Mosby Company, St. Louis, Mo., U.S.A.

coagulation time (WBCT), activated partial thromboplastin time, prothrombin time, and protamine titration were measured as previously described (Ellison et al., 1971). Five minutes after heparin administration, a blood sample was obtained for an in vitro protamine titration to determine the minimum dose of protamine sulfate required to neutralize exactly the heparin activity. In our titration method, 5 test tubes were prepared immediately prior to sampling, with 10, 20, 30, 40, and 50 μg of protamine sulfate added to the 5 tubes. The additives were in solution in μl volumes *, and the tubes were kept at 37°C. Next, 1 ml of the subject's heparinized blood was added to each tube, which was then gently tilted 90° every 30 sec starting 1 min after the addition of blood. The concentration of protamine which produced the shortest coagulation time provided the basis for calculating the protamine dose for reversal. The concentration was multiplied by the estimated blood volume (6.5% of body weight), and this dose of protamine was administered precisely 30 min after the heparin. Adequate neutralization was confirmed by protamine titration as well as by a

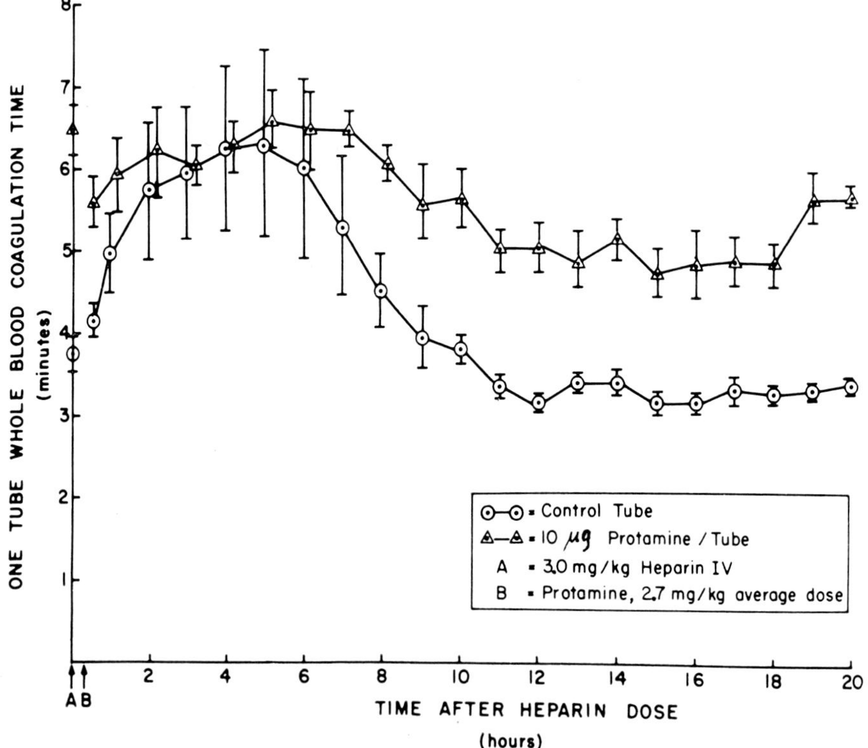

Fig. 1.   *Whole blood coagulation time versus time following heparin neutralization (mean ± standard error of 6 volunteers). Normally the control (or plain) whole blood coagulation time is shorter than the coagulation time after administration of protamine. This is true for the pre-heparinization values and the initial, in vivo, post-neutralization value (points A and B). There was then a progressive decrease in the difference between these 2 values with a minimum difference at the 4th hr. Indeed, no statistical difference could be demonstrated between these values from hours 1 through 7. At all other times these differences were significant at least to the $p < 0.05$ level.*

---

* Use of a microliter syringe (Model 710) with repeating dispenser (Model PB 600–1), available from Hamilton Co., Whittier, Calif., permits accurate delivery of protamine in 10 μg increments.

return of the WBCT to normal. The same coagulation parameters were obtained at 0.5-hr intervals over the next 20 hr. Heparin rebound was defined as clotting in a tube containing 10 μg of protamine/ml of whole blood before clotting in the control tube which contained no added protamine. Mere prolongation of WBCT was not considered to represent heparin rebound.

The average protamine dose required for heparin neutralization was 2.7 mg/kg (range 1.0–3.9), and the average protamine-heparin ratio was 0.90 (range 0.66–1.3). Only 1 volunteer, the individual with the lowest measured protamine-heparin ratio, demonstrated rebound between the 2nd and 7th hr following initial heparinization. Figure 1 plots the average clotting times for the control tubes and the tubes containing protamine against time after the neutralization. It can be appreciated that between the 2nd and 6th hr the average times are much closer, suggesting that subclinical degrees of heparin rebound may have occurred at this time. In every case, the WBCT lenghtened appreciably during this time period.

STUDIES OF HEPARIN REBOUND IN PATIENTS

Two groups of patients were studied after open-heart surgery. The groups were comparable in terms of age, weight, duration of cardiopulmonary bypass, and average heparin dose (Table 1). One group received the minimum dose of protamine required for heparin neutralization, based on a protamine titration. The other group received a larger dose of protamine (359 as compared to 204 mg), approximately equal to the *total* amount of heparin (in mg) administered to the patient and to the pump prime. In all cases, adequate neutralization was confirmed by protamine titration and WBCT.

Figure 2 compares these groups. The protamine-heparin ratio for the low-dose group was 0.56 (range 0.40–0.76) and that for the high-dose group was 1.15 (range 0.81–1.47) when the total amount of heparin administered to the patient and to the pump is considered. These figures are respectively 0.92 (range 0.65–1.25) and 1.80 (range 1.24–1.94) when only the initial heparin dose administered to the patient is considered. In every patient receiving

Table 1. *Comparison of patient characteristics, bypass time, and total heparin and protamine doses*

Dose of protamine	Age (yr)	Height (inches)	Weight (kg)	Bypass time (min)	Dose of heparin (mg)				Dose of protamine (mg)		
					Initial Patient	Initial Pump	Supple-mental	Total	Initial	Supple-mental	Total
Low dose (6 patients)											
Mean	43.3	66.8	67.8	97	204	98	54	356	138	66	204
S.E.	4.5	3.1	9.1	17	28	12	25	47	22	12	30
High dose (6 patients)											
Mean	40.7	65.8	63.7	82	198	76	48	316	334	25	359
S.E.	3.1	2.4	4.8	16	15	12	73	43	52	15	53

There was no significant difference (p > 0.05 by Student's t-test) in the 2 patient groups with respect to age, height, weight, and duration of cardiopulmonary bypass. The low-dose protamine group had a protamine heparin ratio of 0.57 (range 0.40–0.76), and the high-dose group had a protamine-heparin ratio of 1.15 (range 0.81–1.47). Supplemental protamine was necessary for 2 patients in the high-dose group, each of whom received 1,000 ml of bottled, heparinized blood from the pump in the period after bypass.

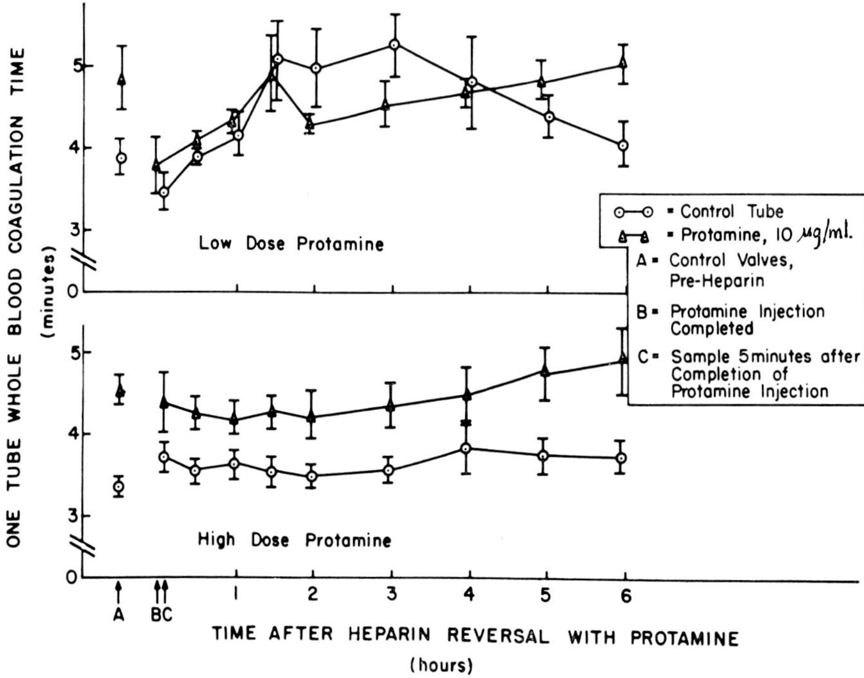

Fig. 2.   *Whole blood coagulation time versus time following heparin neutralization for 2 groups of patients following open-heart surgery. For the low-dose protamine group, the average whole blood coagulation time for the protaminized tube was shorter than that for the control tube between 1.5 and 4 hr, demonstrating that heparin rebound had occurred. At no time was this reversal in the whole blood coagulation time seen in the high-dose protamine group. Results are statistically significant (p < 0.05) in the low-dose protamine group only for the control tubes (point A) and for the measurement at 6 hr; in the high-dose protamine group, all determinations were significant except immediate reversal (point C) and measurements at 1 and 4 hr.*

the minimal dose of protamine, heparin rebound was demonstrated at some time between 1 and 5 hr after neutralization. In 3 cases this rebound was associated with clinical bleeding and necessitated additional protamine. In contrast, none of the 6 patients who received the larger doses of protamine exhibited rebound.

DISCUSSION

Only 1 volunteer demonstrated heparin rebound whereas all 6 patients who received a dose of protamine based on the same technique of protamine titration exhibited rebound. Clearly, these 2 groups were not identical. The patients received much larger amounts of heparin (average 6.3 mg/kg) in divided doses and were heparinized for longer periods of time (pump time 97 min average). In contrast, the volunteers received 3.0 mg/kg heparin, and this was neutralized precisely 30 min after heparinization. It is possible that heparin leaves the circulation over a period of time and returns via the lymphatics and thoracic duct several hours later, which may explain why rebound was seen in patients but not in volunteers (Schreiner, 1958).

The correct amount of protamine to reverse heparin anticoagulation following cardiopulmonary bypass is controversial; various authorities recommend 0–4 times the original dose of heparin (Rothnie and Kinmouth, 1960; Castaneda, 1966; Adkins and Hardy, 1967; Osborne, 1967). Perhaps one of the reasons for this variability in recommended dose is that rarely it is specified whether the recommendations are based on the initial dose only, the initial dose plus supplemental doses, or on the total amount of heparin administered to the patient and to the pump prime. There are other factors which may influence the heparin level at the time of neutralization. These include the decline of levels of heparin in the blood as it relates to the duration of bypass and body temperature (Wright et al., 1964; Pardanani et al., 1970), medication errors (Fantl and Ward, 1960), additional heparin given in the form of heparinized blood (Terhan et al., 1970), or excessive heparin flush for arterial and central venous lines.

The fear of producing anticoagulation in vivo by excessively high doses of protamine has led some to recommend not giving high doses of protamine. In fact, it has been suggested that one possible cause of what appears to be heparin rebound is actually the anticoagulant effect produced by protamine (Anderson et al., 1959). However, we have previously shown that, while protamine possesses a mild in vitro anticoagulant effect, the drug is not a clinically important anticoagulant in moderate overdoses. Thus we do not feel that this is a possible cause of heparin rebound (Ellison et al., 1971). There have been many other suggested causes of heparin rebound. These are listed in Table 2 in the order in which they were suggested.

Table 2.

Date	Suggested cause of rebound
1957	Heparin may be released by red blood cell breakdown (Dodrill et al.)
1958	Heparin may escape from the circulation into the extravascular space and return via the lymphatics and thoracic duct to the circulation many hours later, after protamine has been administered and cleared (Schreiner)
1959	Heparin may be injected into tissues instead of intravenously, forming a depot source for prolonged absorption (Perkins et al.)
1961	A part of the heparin level may be temporarily neutralized by an endogenous antagonist, not otherwise specified. When this antagonist is cleared from the blood, heparin activity is then demonstrated (Perkins et al.)
1962	Protamine may be removed by metabolism or may be combined with other plasma proteins before heparin is removed (Hyah et al.)
1966	Protamine chloride does not produce heparin rebound although protamine sulfate does. This may in part be due to more rapid metabolism of protamine sulfate (Frick and Brogly)
1970	Heparin rebound is seen more commonly with hypothermia (Pardanani et al.). It had previously been shown that heparin levels do not decay as rapidly during hypothermic perfusions (Wright et al., 1964)
1974	For a given heparin level, low levels of platelets result in a more pronounced effect of that heparin level on the coagulation mechanism (Conley et al., 1943). Since thrombocytopenia is a common occurrence following open-heart surgery, it is quite possible that heparin activity may be enhanced

How should the protamine dose following cardiopulmonary bypass be calculated? Ideally, the amount of heparin remaining in the patient may be calculated by subtracting from the total dose that is left in the pump, on the drapes, and in the suction bottles. Since this figure is not readily obtained, Perkins et al. (1959) suggested using a protamine titration to calculate the minimum dose of protamine needed. While this method is accurate and may be useful in cases in which the total heparin dose is not known, we do not believe that it is always necessary as the danger of moderate over-administration of protamine is not great. Furthermore, while the dose calculated by this method will neutralize the heparin activity at that instant, our results in patients suggest that heparin rebound may occur when this minimum dose is administered. The exact amount of heparin given to the patient and to the pump prime is a figure which can be readily obtained and used as the basis for calculating a safe protamine dose. With this figure on hand, a safe dose for oxygenators with small prime volumes may be calculated by means of a protamine-heparin ratio of 1.0, that is, an amount of protamine equal in milligrams to the total dose of heparin. For oxygenators with large prime volumes, an amount of protamine equal to half the total dose of heparin should provide a safe dose (Ellison et al., 1971).

In summary, the dose of protamine required to neutralize exactly the in vitro heparin activity following cardiopulmonary bypass was consistently less than the dose required to prevent heparin rebound. Since moderate excesses of protamine have not been shown to produce clinically important anticoagulant effects and since relatively small amounts of heparin do have clinically important anticoagulant effects, it appears prudent to give enough protamine to prevent heparin rebound as well as to ensure adequate neutralization.

REFERENCES

Adkins, J. R. and Hardy, J. D. (1967): *Arch. Surg.*, *94*, 175.

Anderson, M. N., Mendelow, M. and Alfano, A. (1959): *Surgery*, *46*, 1060.

Castaneda, A. R. (1966): *J. thorac. cardiovasc. Surg.*, *52*, 716.

Cate Jr., W. R., Sadler, R. N., Seitzman, D. M. et al. (1954): *Amer. Surg.*, *20*, 813.

Conley, C. L., Hartman, R. C. and Lalley, J. J. (1948): *Proc. Soc. exp. Biol. (N.Y.)*, *69*, 284.

Dodrill, F. D., Marshall, N., Nyboer, J., Hughes, C. H., Derbyshire, A. and Stearns, A. B. (1957): *J. thorac. cardiovasc. Surg.*, *33*, 60.

Ellison, N., Ominsky, A. J. and Wollman, H. (1971): *Anesthesiology*, *35*, 621.

Estes, J. W. (1970): *J. Amer. med. Ass.*, *212*, 1492.

Fantl, P. and Ward, H. A. (1960): *Thorax*, *15*, 292.

Frick, D. G. and Brogli, H. (1966): *Surgery*, *59*, 721.

Gollub, S. (1967): *Surg. Gynec. Obstet.*, *124*, 337.

Hampers, C. L., Blaufox, M. D. and Merrill, J. P. (1966): *New Engl. J. Med.*, *275*, 776.

Hyun, B. H., Pence, R. E., Davila, J. C. et al. (1962): *Surg. Gynec. Obstet.*, *115*, 191.

Kolff, W. J., Effler, D. B., Groves, L. K. et al. (1956): *Cleveland Clin. Quart.*, *23*, 69.

Olsson, P. and Lagergren, E. K. (1963): *Acta med. scand.*, *173*, 619.

Osborne, J. J. (1967): In: *Cardiac Surgery*, p. 97. Editor: J. C. Norman. Meredith Publ. Co., New York, N.Y.

Pardanani, D. S., Roy, G. and Sen, P. K. (1970): *J. postgrad. Med.*, *16*, 26.

Perkins, H. A., Acra, D. J. and Rolfs, M. R. (1961): *Blood*, *18*, 807.

Perkins, H. S., Osborne, J. J. and Gerbode, F. (1959): *Ann. intern. Med.*, *51*, 650.

Rothnie, N. G. and Kinmouth, J. B. (1960): *Brit. med. J.*, *1*, 73.

Schreiner, R. (1958): *Trans. Amer. Soc. artif. intern. Org.*, *4*, 36.

Terhan, S., Moffitt, E. A., Lundborg, R. O. and Wallace, R. B. (1970): *Surgery*, *67*, 584.

Thies, A. A. (1960): *Thrombos. Diathes. haemorrh. (Stuttg.)*, *4*, 400.

Wright, J. S., Osborne, J. J., Perkins, H. A. et al. (1964): *J. cardiovasc. Surg.*, *5*, 244.

Management of circulatory complications during coronary artery surgery

F. GEORGE ESTAFANOUS

Department of Anesthesiology, The Cleveland Clinic Foundation and
The Cleveland Clinic Educational Foundation, Cleveland, Ohio, U.S.A.

During coronary artery surgery, hypotension and arrhythmias occurring before initiation of cardiopulmonary bypass are more frequent in patients with impaired left ventricular function and patients with accompanying valvular lesions or septal defects. The incidence of hypotension and arrhythmias is increased in patients who manifest the empty heart phenomenon (Wigboldus et al., 1973) with electrolyte disturbances (mainly K) and in those receiving digitalis and antihypertensive and β-adrenergic blocking drugs (Viljoen et al., 1972). Hypotension may occur on opening the sternum and retracting the ribs (Rushmer, 1961; Guyton, 1963). Hypovolemic patients are more vulnerable to hypotension and arrhythmias, especially during manipulation of the heart and cannulation of the great vessels. We make every effort to maintain adequate circulating blood volume guided by the levels of mean arterial, central venous, and left atrial pressures. However, direct observation of heart filling and the response of its different chambers to transfusion can determine the amount of transfusion needed.

We try to maintain the heart rate and rhythm within normal limits, thus decreasing the incidence of hypotension.

When bradycardia, nodal rhythm, and conduction defects occur, atropine sulphate (0.5 mg) is administered, and if it fails to restore the heart rate, isoprenolin infusion (0.4 mg/250 ml) is used. Arrhythmias at this stage are better treated by DC counter shock to avoid myocardial depression.

If hypotension and arrhythmias are recurrent or persistent we prefer rapid initiation of partial cardiopulmonary bypass to avoid repeated use of different drugs (Viljoen et al., 1974). On initiation of artificial bypass, a variable degree of hypotension occurs (Wynands et al., 1970). This can be minimized by maintaining adequate circulating blood volume preferably with whole blood or colloidal solutions. Initially the flow can be increased up to 30% over the predicted values to maintain systemic pressure of 60–100 mm Hg (Tufo et al., 1970).

If hypotension persists a small dose of epinephrine (3–5 ml of 1/50,000 solution) is administered. Usually this restores the pressure and further doses are not needed. Increased peripheral resistance and hypertension during bypass are treated by repeated doses of nitroglycerine solution (0.4 mg/ml). If this fails we use small doses of phentolamine (2 mg).

Early in surgery and during bypass we try to use short-acting drugs and rely on mechanical support of the circulation. This allows better assessment of the cardiovascular status on termination of artificial cardiopulmonary support and consequently we treat hypotension and arrhythmias specifically.

WITHDRAWAL FROM CARDIOPULMONARY BYPASS

On completion of the anastomosis, any abnormalities in pH, blood gases, and serum potassium are corrected and adequate circulating blood volume is ensured.

At this stage gradually diminishing ECG signs of myocardial ischemia are often seen, especially if anoxic cardiac arrest is used. Repeated doses of nitroglycerine (0.25 mg) may be administered intravenously. However, if these signs persist or if there are signs of isolated right or left heart failure, a 22-gauge needle is inserted in the graft to drain any possible air embolism, and satisfactory blood flow in the graft is ensured by an electro-magnetic flow meter. If signs of ischemia still persist, we prefer to keep the patient on partial bypass until any surgical cause of myocardial ischemia is excluded.

After excluding the above factors, if hypotension persists, we correlate the monitoring information available to diagnose the cause of hypotension and we treat it specifically as follows (Estafanous and Viljoen, 1973; Estafanous et al., 1972).

1. Hypovolemia, as manifested by low arterial mean, low central venous and low left atrial pressures and a rising pulse rate, is treated by blood volume expansion. In the presence of left ventricular impairment, changes in left atrial pressure measurements are the most sensitive index of the response of the heart to transfusion.

2. Arrhythmias:

(*a*) If arrhythmias are accompanied by hypokalemia, a bolus of 5–7 mEq KCl is administered intravenously. The serum K level is maintained at about 4–4.5 mEq/l by dilute infusion of KCl 8 mEq/100 ml.

(*b*) Sinus or digitalis-induced bradycardias are treated with intravenous atropine sulfate (0.5–1 mg).

(*c*) Atrial fibrillation is treated by DC counter shock.

(*d*) A rapid ventricular response to a persistent supraventricular arrhythmia is treated by rapid intravenous digitalization.

(*e*) Persistent ventricular arrhythmias are treated with lidocaine 100 mg given slowly intravenously, followed by an infusion, with the rate adjusted to control arrhythmias with minimal myocardial depression.

(*f*) If ventricular tachycardia or fibrillation occur, DC countershock is applied.

(*g*) Arrhythmias refractory to drug treatment are treated by external pacing.

3. Cardiac decompensation, as manifested by falling arterial mean pressure and rising central venous and left atrial pressures:

(*a*) If the pulse rate is between 80 and 100 beats/min, 1 g calcium gluconate is administered, as serum levels of ionized Ca may be depleted during bypass (Moore, 1970).

(*b*) In the presence of a normal or slow pulse rate, particularly when due to conduction defects, a β-receptor stimulant – isoproterenol, 0.4 mg/250 ml – is infused.

(*c*) If the pulse rate is over 100 beats/min, particularly in patients with previous history of heart failure, digitalis is indicated. Lanatoside C (Cedilanid oral), 0.8 mg–1.2 mg, is administered, provided the serum potassium level is above 4 mEq/l. A modified dose is given to patients who have received digitalis previously.

We use peripheral vasoconstrictors as a last resort. A dilute epinephrine infusion (1 mg/250 ml) is preferred because of both its cardiotonic and vasopressor effects. After its use for a short period we observed that in many situations it improves the force of contraction and maintaining adequate blood pressure and it is no longer needed.

REFERENCES

Estafanous, F. G. and Viljoen, J. F. (1973): Paper presented at: 6th International Anaesthesia Postgraduate Course, No. 21.

Estafanous, F. G., Viljoen, J. F. and Loop, F. D. (1972): *Canad. Anaesth. Soc. J., 19*, 160.

Guyton, A. (1963): *Cardiac Output and Its Regulation.* W. B. Saunders Co., Philadelphia, Pa.

Moore, E. W. (1970): *J. clin. Invest.*, *49*, 318.

Rushmer, R. F. (1961): *Cardiovascular Dynamics*, 2nd ed. W. B. Saunders Co., Philadelphia, Pa.

Tufo, H. M., Ostfeld, A. M. and Shekelle, R. (1970): *J. Amer. med. Ass.*, *212*, 1333.

Viljoen, J. F., Estafanous, F. G. and Kellner, G. A. (1972): *J. thorac. cardiovasc. Surg.*, *64*, 826.

Viljoen, J. F., Estafanous, F. G. and Kim, K. (1974): *Brit. J. Anaesth.*, in press.

Wigboldus, A. H., Urzua, J. and Viljoen, J. F. (1973): *J. thorac. cardiovasc. Surg.*, *66*, 807.

Wynands, J. E., Sheridan, C. A., Batra, M. S., Palmer, W. H. and Shanks, J. (1970): *Anesthesiology*, *33*, 260.

A disposable electrode for the continuous in vivo measurement of arterial oxygen tension during heart surgery

PEDRO M. DIAZ, MARTIN I. GOLD, IGNACIO DUARTE and YUNG J. SOHN

Department of Anesthesiology, University of Miami School of Medicine and
Veterans Administration Hospital, Miami, Fla., U.S.A.

The availability of monitoring devices that provide continuous information on the condition of organ systems is very important for the successful completion of surgical procedures in sick patients. Currently available laboratory methods for the measurement of Pa_{O_2} are not completely satisfactory because of (1) delay in obtaining results; (2) errors introduced while the sample is transferred; (3) errors introduced because of differences in temperature between the patient and the electrode; (4) difficulty in observing trends in oxygenation; and (5) inability to detect oxygenation changes which are rapidly reversible. Some of these problems can be obviated, at an increased cost in personnel. A disposable, in vivo electrode for the continuous monitoring of arterial oxygen tension, would eliminate many of the above problems. We have evaluated such a system during heart surgery.

Watanabe et al. (1973) have described a new instrument for the continuous in vivo measurement of blood P_{O_2}. The instrument works on the polarographic principle. The system consists of a 100 μ gold cathode covered with a polymeric hydrophilic gel mounted at the end of a probe, 0.15 inches in outer diameter and designed to pass readily through an 18 inch gauge plastic cannula. The entire length of the probe is coated with hydrophilic gel which is tissue compatible and non-thrombogenic. The gel is tough and is not easily damaged with tissue contact. The probe requires from 10–20 min to reach near equilibrium with full equilibrium being reached in approximately one hour. The anode is placed on the patient's skin, and the body becomes a part of the polarographic oxygen cell. Water and oxygen diffuse through the gel to the gold cathode. Oxygen molecules are reduced, generating current which is proportional to the oxygen partial pressure. The small current produced at the cathode is amplified by a battery operated analyzer with a direct read-out in Torr. The analyzer may be connected to a recorder to obtain a permanent record.*

We have tested the performance of these electrodes in vivo and in vitro and have used them in 32 heart cases, including 19 saphenous vein aorto-coronary bypass operations. We have left the electrode in place during the postoperative period, for as long as 48 hr.

METHODS

In vitro tests

The performance of 4 IBC oxygen electrodes was tested in vitro using an Instrumentation Laboratories Model 237 Tonometer. Three ml of whole blood were placed in the tonometer

---

* The system is manufactured by the International Biophysics Corporation (IBC), Irvine, Calif.

cup. The oxygen electrode and its anode were introduced and secured into the cup with plastic cannulas. The blood in the tonometer was equilibrated with air, for at least 20 min, at 37° C and the electrode calibrated to read (barometric pressure – water vapor at 37° C $\times$ 0.209). The blood in the tonometer was then equilibrated for at least 20 min with various mixtures of humidified oxygen and nitrogen at 37° C.

The gases were mixed by means of an Instrumentation Associates gas mixing pump. The gas mixtures tested had oxygen tension in the range of 38–610 Torr. After equilibration the IBC electrode Po_2 was read, and immediately two samples of the blood were withdrawn and analyzed in two separate Radiometer Digital Acid-Base Analyzers, Model PHM 72. The Radiometer electrodes were calibrated before each sample using humidified air. From the values obtained, the regression coefficients for the IBC electrode and the Radiometer electrode as compared to the tonometer were calculated.

In vivo tests

The performance and usefulness of the indwelling electrode was tested in a series of 32 heart operations. After in vivo equilibration of the electrode for at least 20 min, it was calibrated both internally and from the value obtained from a Radiometer electrode. The patients were then ventilated with various mixtures of nitrous oxide and oxygen. The F_{IO_2} was monitored by means of a fuel cell oxygen analyzer. The patient was allowed to equilibrate at each F_{IO_2} for at least 5 min, at the end of which the indwelling electrode Pa_{O_2} was read at body temperature and the Pa_{O_2} of an arterial blood sample obtained simultaneously was read at 37° C in a Radiometer electrode. 167 comparisons were made and the regression coefficient of the two methods calculated.

The indwelling electrode was left in place during the rest of the operation and in some cases during the postoperative period for up to 48 hr without failing.

RESULTS

The results of the in vitro studies are shown in Figures 1 and 2 and Table 1. In the range

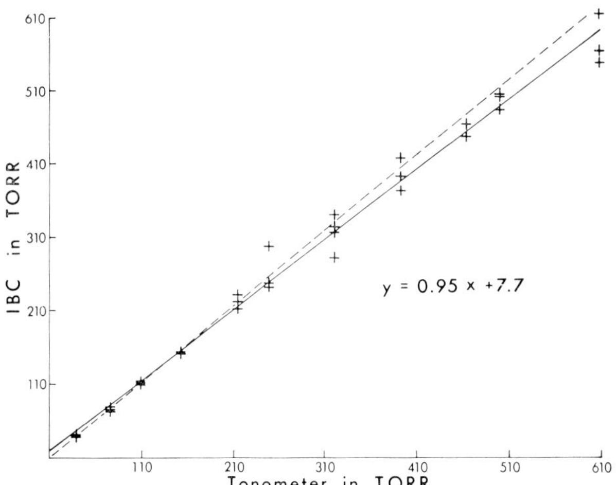

Fig. 1.   *Regression line (solid) of Po_2 of tonometered blood obtained with 4 IBC electrodes, against the theoretical Po_2 in the tonometer. The ideal correlation is represented by the dotted line. Each cross represents one reading with a different electrode.*

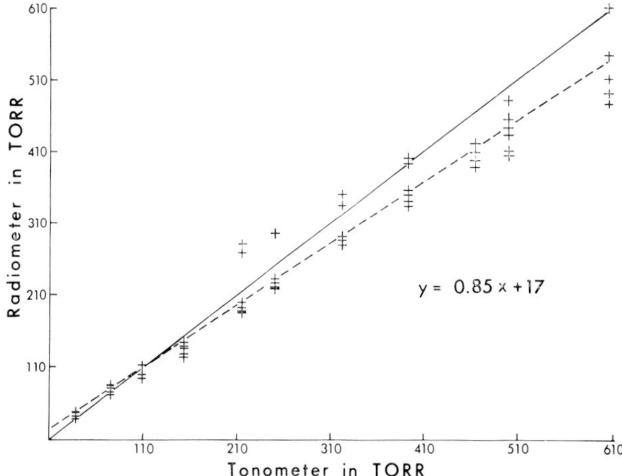

Fig. 2. *Regression line (dotted) of PO_2 of tonometered blood obtained with two Radiometer electrodes, against the theoretical PO_2 in the tonometer. The ideal correlation is represented by the solid line. Each cross represents one reading.*

Table 1. *Comparison of two oxygen electrodes using tonometered blood*

Tonometer	Oxygen tension in Torr					
	38	75	108	153	215	251
IBC electrode	40 ± 1.5	76 ± 2.1	110 ± 2	152 ± 1.4	218 ± 9.6	261 ± 31
(Mean ± S.D.)	n = 4	n = 4	n = 3	n = 4	n = 4	n = 3
Radiometer electrode	42 ± 3.4	79 ± 4.4	96 ± 6.6	135 ± 6.9	214 ± 38	248 ± 36
(Mean ± S.D.)	n = 6	n = 7	n = 6	n = 8	n = 8	n = 6
	323	395	467	503	610	
IBC electrode	314 ± 25	392 ± 23	450 ± 9.8	496 ± 9.9	574 ± 39	
(Mean ± S.D.)	n = 4	n = 3	n = 3	n = 4	n = 3	
Radiometer electrode	301 ± 29	362 ± 29	400 ± 14	442 ± 25	526 ± 53	
(Mean ± S.D.)	n = 7	n = 6	n = 5	n = 8	n = 6	

of 38–503 Torr there is little difference between the values obtained with the IBC electrode and those of the tonometer. At 610 Torr the value from the electrode was 6% lower than the tonometer. The standard deviation of each mean value in the range 38–215 Torr was within 5% of the mean.

The values obtained with the Radiometer electrode were nearly identical to the tonometer in the range of 38–215 Torr with the exception of the value obtained at 152 Torr which was 11% lower than the tonometer. Above 152 Torr the Radiometer electrode reads lower than the tonometer, the mean reading being 14% lower at 610 Torr.

The results of the in vivo comparison of the IBC electrode with the Radiometer electrode are shown in Figure 3. The correlation of the two methods is very good in the range of 60–240 Torr. At values higher than 240 Torr the IBC electrode reads somewhat lower than the Radiometer.

Table 2 shows the high inspired oxygen tensions needed in 11 of our patients to keep an arterial oxygen tension between 90 and 114 Torr in the interval between induction and cardiopulmonary bypass.

Figure 4 is from a tracing obtained in the intensive care unit with a strip chart recorder connected to the IBC analyzer. The patient had been taken to the unit, after resection of an abdominal aortic aneurysm and an aorto-bifemoral graft. The patient had a massive myocardial infarction with hypotension, which resulted in a sharp drop in the Pa_{O_2}. Cardiac arrest occurred and the changes in Pa_{O_2} during an unsuccessful attempt at cardiopulmonary resuscitation are seen in the tracing.

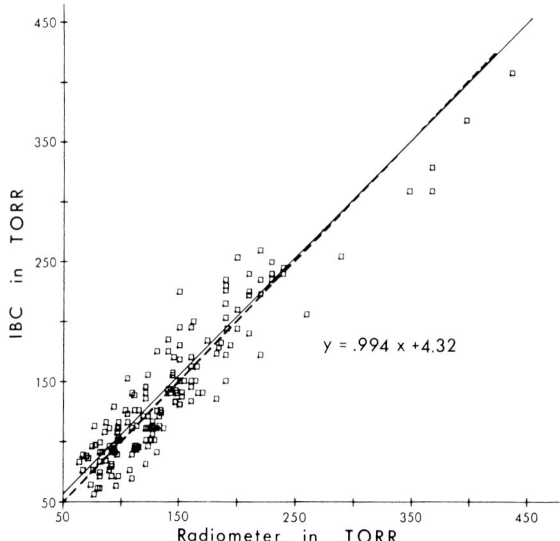

Fig. 3.   *Regression line (solid) of P_{O_2} obtained with IBC electrode in vivo, against values obtained with a Radiometer electrode in vitro. 167 comparisons were made during 32 heart operations. The ideal correlation is represented by the dotted line.*

Table 2.   *High inspired oxygen concentrations needed in 11 heart patients to get a normal Pa_{O_2}*

Procedure	Inspired oxygen tension in Torr	Pa_{O_2} in Torr
ACB	*(a)* 270	95
	(b) 300	96
ACB	270	95
AVR	300	108
ACB	266	95
AVR+MVR	290	110
ACB	304	97
AVR	304	114
ACB	270	96
ACB	290	62
ACB	266	95
AVR	300	90

ACB = aorto-coronary bypass
AVR = aortic valve replacement
MVR = mitral valve replacement

DISCUSSION

The Pa_{O_2} obtained with the IBC electrode correlate better with the tonometer than those of the Radiometer electrode. This is specially true at Pa_{O_2} above 300 Torr. There are several reasons for this. The IBC electrode was calibrated with tonometered blood, while the Radiometer electrode was calibrated with air. No correction for the gas/blood ratio was made. Blood metabolism, most of it in the leucocytes, reduces Po_2 3 mm/min at high Po_2 (Nunn, 1962). There are O_2 losses while transferring the sample from the tonometer to the Radiometer electrode.

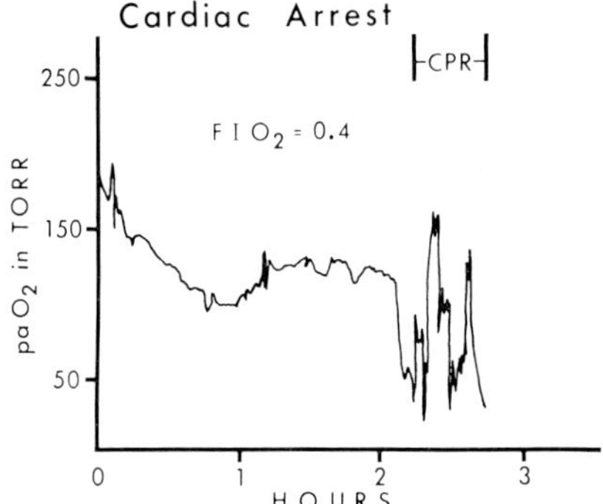

Fig. 4.   *Changes in arterial oxygen tension during a cardiac arrest in a patient monitored with the indwelling oxygen electrode in the intensive care unit. The patient's Pa_{O2} remains stable during a period of 2 hr after arriving at the unit on an F_{IO2} of 0.4. The initial drop in Pa_{O2} is the result of a decrease in the F_{IO2} when the patient came to the unit. Preceding the cardiac arrest, the Pa_{O2} drops from 120–50 Torr in a period of 10 min. At this point, cardiopulmonary resuscitation (CPR) was started unsuccessfully. Notice the increase in the arterial oxygen tension during CPR.*

With both methods there was a downward deviation of the regression line from the ideal, at Po_2 above 200 Torr. It is doubtful that at high Po_2 complete equilibrium of the blood in the tonometer occurs. Errors are introduced because of nonlinearity of oxygen electrodes. This effect becomes evident when the sample Po_2 is far from the calibration Po_2.

From our data it seems that the indwelling electrode has greater accuracy and reproducibility because errors introduced in the transfer of blood samples are avoided.

The in vivo correlation between the indwelling oxygen electrode and the Radiometer electrode is excellent between 60 and 240 Torr. The indwelling electrode Po_2 were lower than the Radiometer electrode at Po_2 higher than 240 Torr. This is probably a temperature effect, since most of these samples were obtained while on cardiopulmonary bypass with the patient at temperatures between 28° C and 30° C. No corrections for temperature were made.

The data from Table 2 illustrate the usefulness of an indwelling oxygen electrode during heart surgery. Eleven of our patients required an F_{IO2} greater than 35% to keep the Pa_{O2} between 90–110 Torr at some stage of the operation, prior to cardiopulmonary bypass. Five of the 11 patients required an increase in the F_{IO2} during this period to avoid hypoxia. With the help of the indwelling electrode it was possible to adjust the F_{IO2} from minute to minute to the patient's individual need. Changes in Pa_{O2} are also used as a gross indication of cardiac function, since decreases in cardiac output are reflected in the Pa_{O2}. This is illustrated by the tracing in Figure 4.

In summary, we have evaluated an indwelling electrode for the continuous monitoring of arterial oxygen tension. The accuracy of the electrode is better than that of standard bench electrodes, probably because errors introduced in the transfer of blood samples are eliminated. The use of the electrode has improved the care of patients coming for heart operations, both during the operative and postoperative periods.

REFERENCES

Nunn, J. F. (1962): *Brit. J. Anaesth.*, *34*, 621.
Watanabe, H., Siegelman, H., Welsh, L. and Spracklen, S. (1973): *Proc. San Diego biomed. Symp.*, *12*, 37.

Routine ventilatory care following coronary artery surgery

F. G. ESTAFANOUS

Department of Cardiothoracic Anesthesia, The Cleveland Clinic Foundation and
The Cleveland Clinic Educational Foundation, Cleveland, Ohio, U.S.A.

After direct myocardial revascularization the blood supply to the myocardium immediately improves. Whether oxygen available to the myocardium is similarly increased will depend largely on the systemic arterial oxygen tension. If the patient is allowed to breathe spontaneously in the immediate postoperative period the following factors may lead to arterial hypoxemia:

1. Circulatory inadequacy will lead to malperfusion, ventilation, perfusion inequalities (Bressler, 1963) and increased shunt effect.

2. Cardiopulmonary bypass, particularly if prolonged, will cause parenchymal hypoxia which will decrease the surfactant. Hemolyzed blood is deposited in the lung tissues. The effect of cardiopulmonary bypass will vary from mild hypoxia to a full-fledged postperfusion lung syndrome (Roberts and Morrow, 1967; Provan et al., 1966).

3. Postoperative pulmonary complications such as atelectasis, hemothorax, and pneumothorax are common.

4. Postoperative pain and the residual effects of muscle relaxants impair respiratory muscle function. The lungs may not be properly expanded, especially if both pleurae were left open at the end of surgery.

5. Central depression of respiration caused by the residual effects of anesthesia, analgesics, and sedatives.

Postoperative spontaneous breathing will require great respiratory muscular effort. This will increase oxygen (O_2) consumption when the supply of O_2 is decreased.

Since the start of myocardial revascularization at the Cleveland Clinic the beneficial effects of prolonged postoperative ventilation have been recognized. This is considered an important cause of decreased incidence of mortality and morbidity. Based on our experience over the past 5 years, we have adopted the following routine ventilatory care for patients who have undergone myocardial revascularization. All patients are ventilated overnight (Viljoen, 1968). In general, a tidal volume of 10–12 ml/kg, at a rate of 10–12 times/min is used and every effort is made to maintain Pa_{O_2} levels of at least 100 mm Hg (Wyands et al., 1970). For this purpose a pressure cycled ventilator, e.g., Bennett P. R. II is used. The machine is compact, does not need electric power, and can be easily operated and serviced. It supplies $F_{I_{O_2}}$ about 0.5, which does not cause oxygen toxicity. If satisfactory blood gas levels are not obtained, or pulmonary congestion or edema occur, a volume cycled ventilator (Emerson) is used. In this case, the pattern of ventilation (tidal volume and respiratory rate) is modified to achieve Pa_{CO_2} of 30–35 mm Hg and a Pa_{O_2} of 100 mm Hg. The minimum possible amount of O_2 is added to achieve this Pa_{O_2}, thus minimizing the possibility of O_2 toxicity, and a suitable dead space is added to maintain the Pa_{CO_2} level.

However, if these measures fail to achieve the above mentioned Pa_{O_2}, or if the $PA_{O_2}-Pa_{O_2}$ difference is > 300 mm Hg, (Moffit et al., 1968) positive end expiratory pressure (PEEP) is applied. However, adequate circulating blood volume must be maintained and small amounts of transfusion may be required to avoid hypotension (Viljoen et al., 1974). In this situation we recommend the use of pancuronium bromide as the muscle relaxant of choice to synchronize the patient with the ventilator, because of its unharmful effects on a hypotensive patient. In general, improvements of Pa_{O_2} levels will allow better myocardial performance (Estafanous and Viljoen, 1974); however, careful and more frequent circulatory monitoring is required.

The incidence of mediastinal and subcutaneous emphysema and tension pneumothorax is increased with the application of PEEP (Kumar et al., 1970), especially if it is prolonged and high levels are used. Lack of synchronization, sudden changes in the preset pressure and volume of the ventilator, and circulatory abnormalities should alert the physician to the possibility of pneumothorax (Estafanous et al., 1974).

In conclusion we have found that the advantages of prolonged postoperative ventilation are (1) adequate arterial oxygenation when severe postoperative hypoxemia is inevitable if the patient is breathing spontaneously; (2) reduction of the work of the respiratory muscles in a situation where adequate spontaneous respiration may be responsible for as much as 50% of the total oxygen consumption (Garzen et al., 1966); (3) the use of large tidal volume helps to re-expand the lungs, especially if the pleura were left open, and decreases the incidence of atelectasis; (4) positive pressure ventilation confers against pulmonary edema especially when the left ventricular function is impaired; (5) fast and efficient resuscitation when circulatory instability is common; (6) minimal anesthetic problems should reopening of the chest for control of bleeding be required; and (7) strong analgesia and sedation are possible, and this decreases the incidence of postoperative myocardial infarction caused by reflex coronary artery spasm (Viljoen and Gindi, 1971).

The use of routine cardiac postoperative pulmonary care almost prevents postoperative morbidity due to pulmonary complications.

REFERENCES

Bressler, R. (1963): *Ann. N.Y. Acad. Sci., 104*, 735.
Estafanous, F. G. and Viljoen, J. F. (1974): *Anesth. Analg. Curr. Res., 53*, 610.
Estafanous, F. G., Viljoen, J. F. and Barsoum, K. N. (1974): *Anesthesiology*, in press.
Garzen, A. A., Seltzer, B. and Karlson, K. E. (1966): *Circulation, 33 (Suppl. I)*, 57.
Kumar, A., Falke, K. J., Giffin, B. et al. (1970): *New Engl. J. Med., 283*, 1430.
Moffit, E. A., Tarhan, S. and Lundborg, R. O. (1968): *Anesthesiology, 29*, 6.
Provan, J. D., Austen, W. G. and Seanell, J. G. (1966): *J. thorac. cardiovasc. Surg., 51*, 626.
Roberts, W. C. and Morrow, A. G. (1967): *J. thorac. cardiovasc. Surg., 54*, 422.
Viljoen, J. F. (1968): *Anesthesia, 23*, 515.
Viljoen, J. F., Estafanous, F. G. and Kim, K. S. (1974): *Brit. J. Anaesth.*, in press.
Viljoen, J. F. and Gindi, M. Y. (1971): *Surg. Clin. N. Amer., 51*, 1081.
Wyands, J. E., Sheridan, C. A., Batra, M. S. et al. (1970): *Anesthesiology, 33*, 274.

Coronary surgery and computerized monitoring-patient care

H. A. FERRARI and FRANCIS ROBICSEK

Department of Anesthesiology, and Department of Cardiovascular Surgery,
Charlotte Memorial Hospital, Charlotte, N.C., U.S.A.

INTRODUCTION

Postoperative care of a patient after coronary surgery may be subdivided into (1) basic nursing, (2) accurate assessment of the cardiovascular state, and (3) prevention and treatment of complications.

Basic nursing is essential in maintaining the patient's physical and mental well-being. Simple measures for his comfort can be neglected if nurses have to spend most of their time in routine and repetitive tasks.

Accurate and continuous assessment of the cardiovascular state of the patient during the immediate postoperative period is essential, if irreversible changes are to be avoided.

Prevention of complications is possible if variations are detected early and corrected immediately. If complications occur, treatment is more effective the sooner it begins.

Since 1967 the Surgical Intensive Care Unit of the University of Alabama Hospital has been employing an IBM 1800 process control computer system in the postoperative care of patients undergoing cardiac surgery. The working hypothesis was that 'much of the analysis and decision making, and certain types of treatment are accomplished best by an orderly set of rules and logic, based upon numerical data' (Sheppard et al., 1972). This system has been used clinically in more than 3,000 patients to do more than just monitor; it has, in fact, been used to perform those interventions that absolutely require human skills. Its usefulness has been clearly demonstrated and reported in several articles (Sheppard et al., 1968, 1972, 1973; Kouchoukos et al., 1971).

Furthermore, in a study by A. D. Little, Inc. of Cambridge, Mass., (Little, 1972), under contract to the National Center for Health Services Research and Development, it was concluded that the information provided by the computerized system is more reliable and accurate and can be retrieved faster than data obtained by conventional manual techniques.

At Charlotte Memorial Hospital we have recently acquired an Advanced Intensive Care System which has been developed taking advantage of the vast experience at the University of Alabama Hospital. It was installed in a 6-bed cardiovascular recovery unit, but initially only 2 beds were connected to the system.

DESCRIPTION OF THE ADVANCED INTENSIVE CARE SYSTEM

The computer-based advanced patient care system performs periodic and demand monitoring, display and out-of-limits alarm of: arterial blood pressure (systolic, diastolic and mean); right atrial or central venous pressure (mean); left atrial pressure or pulmonary artery pressure; rectal temperature; respiration rate; heart rate; urine output; and chest drainage.

"

Additional capabilities of the system include: cardiac output computation (thermal dilution); automatic blood and fluid infusion; acid-base analysis (manual input); electrolytes (manual input); interactive dialogue; history data storage and display; and calibration of inputs.

METHODS

The beds have bedside TV monitors connected to an independent α-numeric-graphic character generator permitting time-shared interaction with the computer from keyboards at the bedside. The TV monitors have α-numeric as well as graphic display capability. A printer periodically produces a printed copy of the patient's data for record keeping purposes. A teletype is used for entering and removing a patient from the system.

It should be noted that light emitting diode isolators are interposed between the patient monitoring system (PMS) and the computer to minimize current leakage.

Urine flow measurement is accomplished by supporting a disposable plastic bag for urine collection on a platform attached to a Statham load cell. The load cell bag and associated electronics are housed in a protective frame equipped with restraining clamps to anchor the plastic tubing. Violation of urine output limits (less than 6 ml in one hour or less than 15 ml/hr, 2 hr in a row) will result in a display on the screen: 'Consider Diuretics'.

Measurement of *chest drainage* is accomplished by use of suction of — 15 cm H_2O to route fluid into a disposable plastic bottle. The bottle sits within the same frame as the urine and a similar load cell system.

A 2-channel recorder permits recording of any of the signals originating from the patient monitoring system.

A special sensor and control system provides the following:

1. Two infusion pumps; one for blood, the other for i.v. fluids. These are occlusive roller type pumps metering 1.0 ml and 0.05 ml per revolution of the control shaft respectively.

2. Pump control and error detection logic. This circuitry responds to computer commands for infusion and detects the existence of bubbles in the outflow line, lack of fluid, cable disconnect and pump lock-up, for both blood and i.v. fluid.

3. Stand-alone logic and controls permitting selection of infusion control at the bedside without the computer. The capability exists to infuse blood and i.v. fluid from thumbwheel settings over the range of 0 ml/hr to 1190 ml/hr for blood, in increments of 10 ml/hr and 0 ml/hr to 99 ml/hr for i.v. fluid, in increments of 1 ml/hr. Resettable counters indicate, at any time, the total volume infused.

4. A transducer stand with elevation control and strain gauge transducers for intravascular pressures.

5. Duplication of all critical circuits controlling pump operation to increase reliability.

All parameters are monitored on a 2-min basis (6 samples each, one second apart). The *status display* is automatically updated every 2 min. In addition, the display can be updated upon demand.

Two independent *alarm systems* are used (standard bedside monitoring equipment alarms and computer alarms) for complete flexibility of alarming on all parameters including computer derived variables. Also, preprogrammed alarm messages are displayed at the bedside monitor as the criterion for the messages are met, e.g., 'replace blood bag', 'arterial pressure damped', 'rectal temperature low', etc. The clinical measurement of *cardiac output* is based upon a thermal dilution technique. *Stroke volume* is calculated by dividing the output in milliliters per minute by the present heart rate. All results are stored and can be retrieved for review at the bedside.

Automatic blood infusion

The rules and logic for the administration of blood employ the *left atrial pressure* and the *blood infused to chest drainage ratio* in a closed loop feedback mode. The limits are set for every patient and when indicated, 1–20 ml of blood (depending on the age and size of the patient) are automatically infused every 2 min until the situation is corrected.

If the amount of blood automatically infused should lag seriously behind that required, the staff can give aliquots of blood rapidly, using the motor driven pump via the computer.

Fluid infusion

This program computes the amount of fluid (D_5W) to be infused by a specified time, dependent on body surface area and then controls the hourly rate of infusion to achieve the desired total. If the infusion is stopped for any reason, a new rate will be computed to correct the deviation.

Acid-base analysis

Determinations of arterial P_{O_2}, P_{CO_2}, pH, oxygen saturation, and hemoglobin are made at desired intervals and the numerical values for these variables are entered manually into the computer. An acid-base balance program is then called to assist in the management of the patient's pulmonary and metabolic sub-systems. This program derives from the blood gas measurements, standard bicarbonate, buffer base, and base excess. The base excess is calculated from the equation of Sigaard-Anderson.

If there is a base deficit, and if the base deficit exceeds 3 mEq/l, therapeutic intervention is indicated. Extracellular base deficit equals 1/4 of the base deficit in mEq/l multiplied by the patient's weight in kilograms. Half of the extracellular base deficit is recommended as the quantity of sodium bicarbonate to be administered initially. The recommendation is displayed at the respective patient's console.

Electrolytes

Manual input of serum sodium, potassium and chloride for storage as history data and for display.

Interactive dialogue

The bedside keyboard in conjunction with a series of interactive display routines, permits dialogue between the user and the system. The clinical staff can direct the computer in the following functions: (1) retrieval of data for review of trends; (2) revision of measurement status; (3) entry and retrieval of blood gas measurements; (4) setting of pressure limits for automatic blood infusion; (5) entry of desired rate for automatic control of infusion; (6) initiation of automatic infusion of intravenous maintenance fluid and blood; and (7) demand for instantaneous measurements prior to expiration of the normal 2-min period.

History data storage and display

At 5-min intervals each patient's measurements (both primary and derived) are stored in the computer. The accumulated data are automatically printed out every four hours. In addition, upon demand, a bedside display of the data may be obtained in either a tabular or graphic format.

The *tabular display* contains the measurements made on a selected patient during a prior period dependent on the time increment selected. The following choices are available from the keyboard:

Time increment	*Past period*
Every 5 min	40 min, plus current
Every 30 min	4 hr, plus current
Every 1 hr	8 hr, plus current
Every 2 hr	16 hr, plus current
Every 3 hr	24 hr, plus current

The *graphic feature* allows plotting of two curves simultaneously; (e.g., heart rate and systolic arterial pressure vs time). The ordinate is scaled to the individual parameter values such that maximum resolution is obtained over the range of values displayed. A choice of time scales of 4 hr and 24 hr is available in increments of 5 min and 30 min respectively.

Calibration of inputs

This program permits calibration of the pressure transducers, the chest drainage and the urine flow system by the computer. The program is interactive, requesting the operator to input values to the transducers and computing and displaying the scale factors and offsets resulting. If these are reasonable, they are stored in the computer and used to convert actual transducer generated voltages during monitoring, to parameter values.

In patients where additional respiratory mechanics data is desired to that obtainable from the Respiration/Apnea module of the patient monitoring system (respiration rate), the option is offered whereby a pneumotach is integrated into the system to measure average tidal volume and minute volume. The pneumotach flow signal is sampled for each breath for 30 sec. The total expired volume excluding breaths under 30 ml is multiplied by 2 to get minute volume, and divided by the number of breaths per 30 sec to get average tidal volume. These calculated values are updated every 30 sec.

The option is offered whereby a capnograph is integrated into the system to measure end expiratory fractional CO_2. This is obtained by sampling the CO_2 concentration curve and determining the maximum point within each 30-sec period.

COMMENTS

Computer based monitoring in the United States has been in the research and evaluation phase for several years, but only recently has moved into the realm of clinical care.

The Advanced Intensive Care System offers:

1. Consistency in data collection.

2. Increase in comprehensiveness of monitoring by: (*a*) acquisition and simultaneous display of several primary physiologic variables; (*b*) computation and display of derived physiologic data.

3. Detection and display of premonitory events, allowing earlier therapeutic intervention.

4. Automatic closed loop blood and fluid infusion.

5. Review of accumulated data.

The care of the patient after coronary surgery has improved with the use of a computer based patient care system. The vast experience at the University of Alabama has shown that, on the average, patients remain connected to the automated system 24 hours or less, making possible an earlier discharge from the Cardiovascular Recovery Unit. The logic and rules for treatment are determined by physicians on the basis of research and experience; the System applies them automatically as instructed.

This system does not replace human beings. By eliminating time-consuming measurements and recordings, nurses and physicians are allowed to provide more intelligent and interesting patient care.

'The seriously ill patient has many labile physiological abnormalities which need to be monitored simultaneously and frequently in order to guide his treatment intelligently. It is our belief that this is best supplied by an on-line computerized system. One has to have and use many instruments to fly a complicated airplane through a storm at night' (Gerbode, 1973).

REFERENCES

Gerbode, F. (1973): *J. thorac. cardiovasc. Surg.*, *66/2*, 167.
Kouchoukos, N. T., Sheppard, L. C. and Kirklin, J. W. (1971): *Cardiovasc. Clin.*, *3/3*, 110.
Little, A. (1972): *Review of Patient Monitoring System, University of Alabama Medical Center*. Arthur D. Little, Inc., Cambridge, Mass. In press.
Sheppard, L. C., Kouchoukos, N. T., Acton, J. C., Fincher, J. M. and Kirklin, J. W. (1972): *J. Ass. Advanc. med. Instrumentat.*, *6/1*, 74.
Sheppard, L. C., Kouchoukos, N. T. and Kirklin, J. W. (1973): *Computer*, *7*, 29.
Sheppard, L. C., Kouchoukos, N. T., Kurtts, M. A. and Kirklin, J. W. (1968): *Ann. Surg.*, *168/4*, 596.

Management of systemic hypertension following myocardial revascularization

F. G. ESTAFANOUS

Department of Anesthesiology, The Cleveland Clinic Foundation and
The Cleveland Clinic Educational Foundation, Cleveland, Ohio, U.S.A.

Systemic hypertension is observed in about 33% of patients undergoing myocardial re-vascularization. It was as frequent following internal mammary implants when no cardio-pulmonary bypass was used, as after aorto-coronary grafts which are performed during anoxic cardiac arrest. The increase in arterial pressure occurs during the first few hours following surgery, particularly in the first four. It occurs in patients already awake and in those still unconscious. The hypertensive episode is not related to pain, ventilatory difficulty, or obvious anxiety; these factors were excluded in a study done in the Cleveland Clinic in 1973 (Estafanous et al., 1973). Our findings concluded that the frequency of hypertension is not related to any specific anesthetic agents. It occurs in patients receiving methoxyflurane anesthesia (Estafanous et al., 1972), neuroleptic agents, as well as in patients anesthetized with morphine (James et al., 1972). Hypertension is not related to hypervolemia, as it occurs in patients with low central venous and left atrial pressures, and these pressures do not rise during the hypertensive episodes. More important is that restriction of infused fluids or blood does not lower the systemic arterial pressure, and further lower the central venous pressure. Our clinical experience emphasizes that patients in whom these episodes develop always need more transfusions following treatment. The hypertensive episodes occur in patients with adequate urinary output with or without evidence of renal dysfunction. Vasopressor drugs were not used in the management of any of the patients we studied, so residual pharmacological effect cannot be incriminated.

Rare causes such as thyrotoxic crises or latent pheochromocytoma can be excluded because of the absence of any other clinical signs and the high incidence of these episodes and their lack of recurrence in the absence of specific medications. The cause of this post-operative hypertension has not yet been determined and one can only speculate regarding its genesis. However, the early rise in arterial pressure following internal mammary implants would throw some doubts regarding the role of improved cardiac performance in such cases, since these implants are followed by a transient period of diminished ventricular performance (McNamara and Urschel, 1969). Our initial studies of the hemodynamic changes in these patients show a trend to decreased cardiac output during the hypertensive episodes. The transient course of this postoperative hypertension, its early development in the absence of obvious fluid overload, its response to a neural depressant agent, and the absence of recurrence in most cases after the initial pressure control, all might suggest a neurogenic mechanism. They are reminiscent of the transient hypertensive episodes that occur at the onset of some episodes of myocardial infarction (Horowitz and Sjoerdsma, 1964; Friedberg, 1966). The increased incidence of hypertensive episodes after myocardial revascularization procedures for coronary artery disease make it tempting to relate them to the coronary reflexes described by Brown (1965) and Peterson and Brown (1971).

Hypertension, especially after major cardiac surgery, can present a serious problem. It increases the work of the myocardium and can predispose to heart failure. It can be complicated by renal failure and cerebrovascular hemorrhage.

During the hypertensive episode, occasional premature ventricular contractions are observed and there is increased oozing from the site of the incision and in the drains. Early in our experience, two serious postoperative complications attributed to hypertension occurred and these initiated our study. The first case was a patient who had ventricular aneurysmectomy and in whom a hypertensive episode was associated with hemorrhage from a previously intact ventricular suture line. In the second patient the hypertensive episode was associated with a sudden severe hemorrhage from the aorta at the insertion line of the saphenous vein graft.

At the moment, the lack of notable complications in our series is credited to the routine early and systemic efforts at reducing blood pressure. Our current practice is to maintain the arterial pressure as close as possible to the preoperative level in normotensive patients, and around the normotensive levels (140/90 mm Hg) in preoperatively hypertensive patients (Viljoen et al., 1974).

Due to the transient nature of these hypertensive episodes, we do not advocate the use of long-acting hypotensive agents in the critical immediate postoperative period.

Pantopon is given both intravenously (10 mg) and intramuscularly at the first indication of hypertension in a conscious patient. It does not significantly affect arterial pressure except in a few obviously uncomfortable patients. Earlier we tried phentolamine hydrochloride (Regitine 5 mg intravenously) and intravenous nitroglycerine (0.4 mg/ml) but their effects on the blood pressure last only 3–5 min. We found that the most effective drug is promazine hydrochloride (Sparine) in reduced doses. The hypotensive effect is due to inhibition of centrally mediated pressor reflexes and α-adrenergic blocking properties. It has a direct vasodilating effect on the blood vessels and it may cause an increase in coronary blood flow (Jarvik, 1970). To avoid sudden hypotension, a dilute solution (5 mg/ml) is injected very slowly intravenously while the arterial mean and central venous pressures are continuously monitored. The dose required varies from one patient to another, but in general, small doses (5–15 mg) are effective when central venous pressure is rather low (5–10 cm H_2O). Normal values in our unit range from 7–12 cm H_2O because of the application of intermittent positive pressure ventilation (Mushin et al., 1969). The larger doses (25–50 mg i.v.) are needed in a few patients who have slightly increased central venous pressure (15–20 cm H_2O). However, in rare instances in which the patients do not respond to promazine hydrochloride, sodium nitroprusside (5 mg/100 ml) drip is used to maintain blood pressure at the level required. Blood or fluid must be immediately available for transfusion if hypotension occurs.

REFERENCES

Brown, A. M. (1965): *J. Phys. (Lond.)*, *177*, 203.
Estafanous, F. G., Tarazi, R. C., Viljoen, J. F. et al. (1973): *Amer. Heart J.*, *85*, 732.
Estafanous, F. G., Viljoen, J. F. and Loop, F. D. (1972): *Canad. Anaesth. Soc. J.*, *19*, 160.
Friedberg, C. K. (1966): *Diseases of the Heart*, p. 605. W. B. Saunders Co., Philadelphia, Pa.
Horwitz, D. and Sjoerdsma, A. (1964): *Proc. Council High Blood Pressure Res.*, *13*, 39.
James, F. A., Rems and Benbau, B. P. (1972): *Anesth. Analg. Curr. Res.*, *51*, 901.
Jarvik, M. E. (1970): In: *The Pharmacological Basis of Therapeutics*, 4th ed., 12/162. Editors: L. S. Goodman and A. Gilman. The Macmillan Press Ltd., New York – Melbourne – London.
McNamara, J. J. and Urschel Jr., H. C. (1969): *Circulation*, *36*, 40 (*Suppl. I*), 67.
Mushin, W. W., Rendell-Baker, L., Thompson, P. W. et al. (1969): *Automatic Ventilation of the Lungs*, 2nd ed., 11. F. A. Davis Co., Philadelphia, Pa.
Peterson, D. F. and Brown, A. M. (1971): *Circulat. Res.*, *28*, 605.
Viljoen, J. F., Estafanous, F. G. and Kim, K. (1974): *Brit. J. Anesth.*, in press.

Lobar pulmonary gas exchange and hemodynamics following open heart surgery*

DEMETRIOS G. LAPPAS, MORTIMER J. BUCKLEY
and MYRON B. LAVER

The Cardiac Anesthesia Group and Anesthesia Laboratories, Harvard Medical School, and
Cardiovascular Laboratory, Department of Surgery,
Massachusetts General Hospital, Boston, Mass., U.S.A.

Large gradients between alveolar and arterial P_{O_2} may appear in patients following open heart surgery. These gradients have been attributed to congestive heart failure and secondary to pulmonary sepsis. Several studies have demonstrated the presence of marked ventilation-perfusion abnormalities secondary to chronic left ventricular dysfunction.

To define the magnitude of the regional abnormality in oxygenation we have studied gas exchange in 9 patients during mechanical ventilation following mitral valve replacement. Catheters were inserted into the right upper and lower pulmonary vein during surgery through left atriotomy and under direct vision. A pulmonary artery catheter (Swan-Ganz balloon-tipped catheter) was inserted through an internal jugular vein. The following measurements were made the morning after operation during mechanical ventilation in semi-supine, right and left lateral positions: pulmonary arterial, left atrial, central venous, arterial blood pressures, cardiac outputs (dye dilution), arterial, mixed venous, upper and lower pulmonary vein P_{O_2}, P_{CO_2}, pH and O_2 contents, esophageal and airway pressures. Derived measurements included: regional (right upper and lower lobe) and total $\dot{Q}_S/\dot{Q}_T$, transmural right and left atrial as well as pulmonary transmural pressures; systemic pulmonary vascular resistance indices and cardiac index. The patients were studied during ventilation ($V_T = 15$ ml/kg body wt) supine, the catheterized lobes dependent and non-dependent with zero-end expiratory pressure (MV with ZEEP) and supine with 8 cm H_2O end-expiratory pressure (MV with PEEP). The results are presented in Table 1.

CONCLUSION

Addition of PEEP to the pattern of mechanical ventilation had no significant effect on cardiac index, pulmonary vascular resistance index or $\dot{Q}_S/\dot{Q}_T$ (Table 1). Calculated right and left atrial as well as pulmonary artery diastole transmural pressures did not change significantly upon addition of PEEP. There was a significantly higher $\dot{Q}_S/\dot{Q}_T$ in the right lower lobe as compared with the anatomically non-dependent (upper) lobe; in fact, $\dot{Q}_S/\dot{Q}_T$ for the lower lobe $(\dot{Q}_S/\dot{Q}_T)_{LL}$ was nearly double the value obtained for the upper lobe $(\dot{Q}_S/\dot{Q}_T)_{UL}$. In patients with a high pulmonary vascular resistance change to the latter position (MV with ZEEP) resulted in a decrease of $(\dot{Q}_S/\dot{Q}_T)_{UL}$ and $(\dot{Q}_S/\dot{Q}_T)_{LL}$ although

* Supported in part by U.S.P.H.S. Grant GM 15904-07.

Table 1. *Results of gas exchange studies in 9 patients*

	Supine MV with ZEEP	Catheterized lung		Supine MV with PEEP
		Dependent	Non-dependent	
Cardiac index	2.49	2.42	2.31	2.42
(L/min/M^2)	$\pm$ 0.52	$\pm$ 0.59	$\pm$ 0.62	$\pm$ 0.66
$\dot{Q}_S/\dot{Q}_T \times 100$	12.9	13.2	13.9	14.0
(total)	$\pm$ 5.9	$\pm$ 4.6	$\pm$ 6.0	$\pm$ 5.47
$\dot{Q}_S/\dot{Q}_T \times 100$	14.9	18.8	15.15	21.6
(right lower lobe)	$\pm$ 11.4	$\pm$ 23.0	$\pm$ 8.1 (n$=$8)	$\pm$ 20.5
$\dot{Q}_S/\dot{Q}_T \times 100$	7.2	8.3	8.6	8.2
(right upper lobe)	$\pm$ 3.9	$\pm$ 1.4	$\pm$ 2.8	$\pm$ 3.7
Pulmonary vascular	5.1	4.9	5.1	5.5
resistance index (units)	$\pm$ 5.1	$\pm$ 4.5	$\pm$ 4.6	$\pm$ 4.3
Right atrial pressure (Torr) Absolute *	12.0 $\pm$ 2.2	—	—	12.6 $\pm$ 3.6
Right atrial pressure (Torr) Transmural	14.2 $\pm$ 2.5	—	—	13.3 $\pm$ 2.9
Left atrial pressure (Torr) Absolute *	14.1 $\pm$ 5.0	—	—	13.6 $\pm$ 6.2
Left atrial pressure (Torr) Transmural	16.3 $\pm$ 5.1	—	—	14.4 $\pm$ 6.2
Pulmonary diastolic pressure (Torr) Absolute *	19.0 $\pm$ 9.8	—	—	17.9 $\pm$ 7.1
Pulmonary diastolic pressure (Torr) Transmural	21.2 $\pm$ 9.7	—	—	18.6 $\pm$ 7.1

* Relative to atmosphere.

the ratio between the two was similar, as in the supine position. The marked regional variations in $\dot{Q}_S/\dot{Q}_T$ suggest that alterations in oxygenation following open heart surgery are closely related to the problems of congestive heart failure or pulmonary venous hypertension rather than extracorporeal perfusion. Brief (30 min) mechanical ventilation with added PEEP had no effect on this pattern of oxygenation.

Hemodynamic response to intravenous calcium chloride immediately following insertion of coronary artery bypass grafts

D. G. LAPPAS, L. DROP, E. D. MUNDTH and M. B. LAVER

Anesthesia Laboratories, Harvard Medical School, Massachusetts General Hospital, and Cardiovascular Laboratory, Department of Surgery, Massachusetts General Hospital, Boston, Mass., U.S.A.

It has been generally assumed that the intravenous infusion of $CaCl_2$ administered to correct inadequate hemodynamic function, results in an increased arterial blood pressure secondary to its positive inotropic action. Previous studies at our laboratories have shown that the hemodynamic response to an increase in plasma ionized calcium varies according to the integrity of autonomic tone. Fifteen minutes following a 5-min infusion of 1 or 2 g of $CaCl_2$, we have noted a marked rise in mean arterial blood pressure secondary to a significant rise in systemic vascular resistance (SVR) but no change in cardiac output. On the other hand, patients who had received deliberate hypotensive anesthesia with halothane and pentolinium tartrate responded with a significant increase in stroke and cardiac indices with no change in SVR.

We have now extended these studies to 14 patients immediately following cardiopulmonary bypass for coronary artery bypass grafts. Left ventricular contractility (dP/dt) was measured by intracavitary manometry and cardiac output by the dye-dilution technique. A rise in ionized calcium level of 0.68 mmol/l was associated with a small increase in dP/dt, an insignificant rise in systemic vascular resistance and mean arterial pressure and no change in cardiac output.

Table 1. *Changes following intravenous $CaCl_2$ administration* *

	Postoperative patients	Patients under deliberate hypotensive anesthesia	Patients with coronary artery bypass grafts
Dose and duration of $CaCl_2$	1 g/5 min	1 g/30 sec	5 mg/kg bolus
Time after infusion (min)	15	3–5	10
n	9	7	14
ΔCa^{++} (mmol/l)	$0.15 \pm 0.11^+$	$0.40 \pm 0.20^+$	$0.22 \pm 0.03^+$
ΔMAP (Torr)	$13.4 \pm 11.6^+$	$14.5 \pm 5.0^+$	4.64 ± 7.6
ΔSVR (dynes/sec/cm^{-5})	173 ± 173†	-15 ± 174	61.2 ± 201.9
ΔSV (ml/beat)	0.2 ± 5.3	9.8 ± 9.5†	2.35 ± 7.01
ΔCO (l/min)	0.13 ± 0.43	0.71 ± 0.75†	0.35 ± 0.55
ΔdP/dt			290.1 ± 344.1†

* Mean $\pm$ S.D.; † $p < .05$; $^+$ $p < .01$.

In view of the known effects of increased contractility on myocardial oxygen consumption and the modest hemodynamic effect found with a 25% increase in ionized calcium levels, there appears little benefit associated with the intravenous administration of $CaCl_2$. Studies are now in progress to evaluate the hemodynamic response to intravenous $CaCl_2$ following rapid infusion of citrated blood in patients following insertion of coronary artery bypass grafts. The effect of chronic administration of propranolol on this response is also being evaluated.

Neuroleptanalgesia with droperidol-fentanyl for coronary surgery

H. A. FERRARI

Department of Anesthesiology, Charlotte Memorial Hospital, Charlotte, N.C., U.S.A.

The noticeable stability of the cardiovascular system in patients receiving droperidol-fentanyl has been observed repeatedly by many investigators. This property should make it the anesthetic of choice in coronary surgery.

In an attempt to corroborate or correct the clinical impression we (Ferrari et al., 1974) measured the cardiac output and related parameters in healthy volunteers not subject to the stress of surgery.

The 15 subjects (age range: 19–28 years) were divided into 3 groups of 5 each in order to evaluate the actions of (1) droperidol (Inapsine), (2) fentanyl (Sublimaze), and (3) droperidol-fentanyl combined in a 50 : 1 ratio (Innovar). They were breathing room air under resting conditions.

The arterial pressure and the electrocardiogram (Lead II) were monitored continuously. Test drugs consisted of 15 mg droperidol, 0.3 mg of fentanyl, or a combination of 15 mg of droperidol plus 0.3 mg of fentanyl, in divided doses, given over a period of 26 min. Just before each cardiac output determination, arterial systolic, diastolic, and electrically integrated mean pressures were recorded. The 6 serial measurements of cardiac output in each subject were performed with the radionuclide-precordial counting technic (Gorten and Gunnells, 1961). Immediately after the cardiac output determination, arterial blood samples were drawn for measurement of pH, Po_2 and Pco_2. The total peripheral resistance (TPR) was calculated. The statistically significant observations were: a slight elevation in cardiac output and stroke volume with both drugs, slight decrease in arterial pressure and TPR when droperidol alone or in combination was given, and decreases in Pao_2 and pH with increases in $Paco_2$ when fentanyl alone or in combination was used. In almost all subjects, variables determined 27 min after last drug administration had returned to baseline levels. No cardiac arrhythmias were observed at any time. A depressant action on the myocardium was not detected with our methods; when changes in cardiac output and stroke volume were significant, mean values were always higher than baseline values.

In clinical practice we use between 7.5–12.5 mg of droperidol and 0.15–0.30 mg of fentanyl for induction of adults. The patient breathes oxygen 100% in the beginning and oxygen-nitrous oxide in a 1 : 1 ratio later on.

The most patent nostril is sprayed with 2 ml of 10% cocaine for topical analgesia and vasoconstriction. An injection of 4% Xylocaine (4 ml) through the cricothyroid membrane completes the topical analgesia, before nasotracheal intubation (Murphy tube, soft cuff) is accomplished with the patient still breathing spontaneously.

After intubation the gas mixture is changed to oxygen 30–40% and nitrous oxide 70–60% and adjusted according to blood gases determinations. The patient very rarely remembers the awake intubation.

A fentanyl drip (fentanyl 0.5 mg in 250 ml of D_5W) is started to maintain analgesia. A muscle relaxant of the non-depolarizing type is used.

During the bypass we keep injecting fentanyl in 0.05 mg increments; our only indication for droperidol is an increase in the perfusion pressure.

At the end of the procedure the patient tolerates the nasotracheal tube very well, is taken to a special recovery unit and placed on a volume ventilator until at least the next morning.

We have experienced basically two problems with this technique: (1) arterial hypotension during induction, usually counteracted by the administration of 5% Albumin and lactated Ringer's solution; and (2) awareness on the part of the patient of noises, conversations, etc., especially during long bypass procedures. The patient never feels pain, but the experience is rather distressing.

Neuroleptanalgesia with droperidol-fentanyl offers many advantages and a few disadvantages. At this point we feel that the advantages justify its use, but are still looking for the ideal anesthetic for coronary surgery.

REFERENCES

Ferrari, H. A., Gorten, R. J., Talton, I. H., Canent, R. and Goodrich, J. K. (1974): *Sth. med. J. (Bgham, Ala.)*, *67/1*, 49.
Gorten, R. J. and Gunnells, J. C. (1961): *J. appl. Physiol.*, *16*, 266.

Anesthesia and postoperative care for coronary artery surgery

J. BECERRA and R. GUDÍN

Department of Anesthesia, Fundación Jiménez Díaz, Madrid, Spain

MATERIAL

Thirty patients underwent surgical treatment for correction of coronary insufficiency by means of aorto-coronary grafts using saphenous veins. Viljoen's technique has been used with slight modifications.

PREOPERATIVE

Circulatory and respiratory functions should be investigated and enquiries made about any drug therapy particularly digitalis, β-blocking, diuretic, monoaminooxidase inhibitors and steroids. Digitalis and β-blockers should be withdrawn 1–3 days prior to surgery. Serum electrolytes, especially potassium, should be carefully assessed. A complete study of the patient's coagulation system should be carried out.

PREMEDICATION

Preoperative sedation is most important. To achieve this, 5–10 mg diazepam (Valium) is given orally the previous night. One hour before the operation, morphine (1 mg/5 kg, up to 10 mg) and promethazine (Phenergan) (1 mg/2 kg, up to 25 mg). No vagolytic agents are used in order to avoid tachycardia and dry mouth.

ANESTHESIA

Since cardiac patients do not tolerate circulatory depression, anesthesia should be light and oxygenation maintained.

Induction

The patient comes to the operating room with a sublingual tablet of pentaerythritol tetranitrate and nitroglycerine. An electrocardiograph is connected and a vein in the right elbow and the radial artery of the left arm are cannulated percutaneously. The latter is used for direct arterial pressures recordings (Mingograf-Elema).

Induction is with thiopentone (Pentothal) (5%) given very slowly until there is evidence of drowsiness, but not exceeding 300 mg. The patient is encouraged to inhale oxygen through a mask, by means of a Magill system to which a Ruben valve has been attached. If hypoventilation occurs respiration is controlled manually.

Pancuronium bromide (Pavulon), 4–6 mg is given at first for intubation and subsequent relaxation.

Maintenance

After intubation, the patient is connected to an automatic ventilator (Engström-300). The Engström nomogram is used to estimate the ventilatory minute volume and measurement of arterial blood gases (Po_2, Pco_2) confirms more accurately that the imposed ventilation is adequate.

The anesthetic mixture is 50% N_2O and O_2. Fractional doses of morphine (2 mg) to a total of 32 mg are given. Morphine lowers peripheral resistance and achieves better tissue perfusion; it may also facilitate cardiac performance without decrease in cardiac output. Muscular relaxation is obtained by repeated doses of pancuronium (2 mg).

MONITORING

Central venous pressure is monitored electronically by a catheter in the external jugular vein, reaching the superior vena cava (Mingograf-Elema). Nasopharyngeal temperature is also recorded. Repeated arterial O_2 and CO_2 tensions, acid-base balance and serum concentration of electrolytes are made. A nasopharyngeal tube and a urinary catheter complete the monitoring.

EXTRACORPOREAL CIRCULATION

The technique employed is the usual one. For treatment of the blood we have a Bentley-Temptrol Unit, assembled in a Sarns' console pump. The heart is electrically fibrillated. It should be pointed out that there is no need to keep the aorta clamped during the whole time of the graft since the proximal anastomosis can be performed while the heart is beating.

POSTOPERATIVE CARE

Respiratory care

The patient is moved to the Intensive Care Unit whilst still intubated and receives controlled ventilation by intermittent positive pressure for at least 12 hr. Extubation is usual the next morning after a clinical and analytic evaluation of the patient (Po_2, Pco_2, chest X-ray, etc.). Oxygen is then inhaled by the patient through a face mask (Ventimask 40%). Intercurrent periods of forced ventilation (Bennett sessions, lasting 10 min every hr) have proved benificial.

Cardiocirculatory care

The early detection and identification of arrhythmias is also important and a pacemaker is useful for their correction; the electrodes are implanted during the operation. In cases of potassium depletion, K should be administered (40 mEq/500 ml 5% glucose) alone or in association with hypertonic glucose or insulin. Ectopic rhythms can be treated with

i.v. lidocaine (1–2 mg/kg). This drug depresses the irritability of the ventricular muscle
and has less effect on contractility and arterial pressure.

Treatment of renal failure

Acute renal failure is due, in most cases, to a prolonged reduction of cardiac output.
If the central venous pressure is low, mannitol should be administered i.v. (250 ml 10%
solution, over 30 min). Mannitol should not be employed if the CVP is high. In those
cases, or when mannitol is not effective, furosemide (20–40 mg by i.v. route) may be used.

Anesthesia management for coronary bypass grafting: A report on 700 cases

JULIO M. GARCIA

St. Lukes Hospital Center, New York, N.Y., U.S.A.

Starting with the preoperative visit, meperidine (Demerol) 1 mg/kg and promethazine hydrochloride (Phenergan) 0.3 mg/kg are given intramuscularly 45 min before induction of anesthesia. Atropine sulfate is given intravenously before or during the induction of anesthesia only if necessary. Before the induction of anesthesia, under local infiltration with 1% lidocaine solution, percutaneous catheters are introduced into the femoral artery and superior vena cava for monitoring of arterial and central venous pressures. Two veins respectively, in the left and right forearms are cannulated percutaneously with No. 14 gauge teflon catheters. The EKG leads are connected and the patient is now ready for anesthesia.

A 2% solution of Na thiopentone is administered to induce anesthesia and succinylcholine is given to facilitate endotracheal intubation. Balanced anesthesia is used, and maintenance of relaxation is accomplished with the use of a long-acting non-depolarizing muscle relaxant. Analgesia is obtained with the use of an intravenous fentanyl and droperidol combination (Innovar). 60% nitrous oxide with oxygen is used. A volume controlled ventilator (Venti-meter ventilator, Air Shields Inc.) is adjusted to maintain arterial blood gases within the normal physiologic range. Blood gases, electrolytes, hematocrit, oxygen content and arterio-venous oxygen (AV) differences are measured at 15-min intervals on Instrumentation Laboratory, Inc., pH blood gas analyser 313 and Flame Photometer 343. When the heart is fibrillating on total cardiopulmonary bypass, the lungs are held expanded with 100% oxygen at 5–7 cm H_2O positive pressure.

Hypotension occurring before, during or following the induction of anesthesia is treated by the administration of an adequate blood volume replacement, and the judicious use of α- or β-vasopressor drips * depending on the circumstances. Hypertension is corrected by the use of α-blockers, ganglioplegics or nitroglycerine.

The cardiopulmonary bypass management includes a disposable blood oxygenator with a priming volume of 1800 ml. Temptrol disposable blood oxygenator (model Q 100, Bentley Laboratories) is used. No blood is used to prime the oxygenator. Homologous blood is added only if the hematocrit of the perfusate falls below 20%. Serum potassium levels are monitored and replaced accordingly into the oxygenator when the perfusate levels fall below 4.0 mEq/l.

---

* Concentration of vasopressor solutions used in drips: (1) epinephrine 4 μg/ml; (2) isoproterenol 2 μg/ml; and (3) norepinephrine 8 μg/ml.

Anaesthesia and postoperative care for surgery in coronary artery disease

O. PRAKASH, E. BOS, J. NAUTA, A. W. DUNCAN, W. HEKMAN
and P. G. HUGENHOLTZ

Thorax Centre, Erasmus University, Rotterdam, The Netherlands

Having observed considerable differences in the intraoperative and postoperative behaviour of patients undergoing surgery for coronary artery disease compared with other surgical manoeuvres, we decided to analyse more closely these variations. Comparisons will be made between patients receiving aortocoronary vein bypass grafts, those having resection of ventricular aneurysms and a group of patients undergoing prosthetic mitral valve replacement.

METHOD

Patients and surgery

A series of 94 patients undergoing surgery for coronary artery disease was compared with 30 patients having replacement of the mitral valve. An analysis of the surgery performed for coronary artery disease is presented in Table 1. Saphenous vein was used for the bypass grafts. Prosthetic valves were used in mitral valve replacement.

Table 1. *Analysis of 94 patients having surgery for coronary artery disease*

Surgery	No. of patients
2 or more coronary bypass grafts	69
Single coronary graft	10
Resection of ventricular aneurysm	15*

* 7 of these patients also had coronary bypass grafts.

Anaesthesia

At the time of the preoperative visit, night sedation was ordered to allay anxiety. All patients were premedicated with Papaveretum, haloperidol and atropine given intramuscularly one hour prior to transfer to the operating room. Prior to induction, ECG monitoring was commenced and intra-arterial and central venous catheters were introduced percutaneously under local anaesthesia. Anaesthesia was induced with fentanyl, pancuronium and a small dose of thiopentone. Maintenance of anaesthesia was with nitrous oxide (60%), fentanyl and pancuronium.

No other inhalational agent was employed. Inhaled gases were humidified to water vapour saturation at 30° C. Intermittent positive pressure ventilation was guided by breath-to-breath analysis of expired carbon dioxide using an infrared analyser. During surgery arterial, right and left atrial pressures, electrocardiogram with arrhythmia detection, mixed venous oxygen saturation, respiratory rate, expired minute volume, total compliance and inspiratory airway resistance were continually monitored by computer. Isoprenaline was used as a positive inotropic agent when indicated. Blood replacement was regulated according to blood loss measurement, preoperative and postoperative blood volume estimation using ^{131}I-labelled albumin and the recorded intravascular pressures. Blood loss measurement was by swab weighing and the volume of blood in suction bottles and drainage flasks.

All administered blood is filtered with the Swank Transfusion which is effective against adhesive aggregates as small as the 10 μm range.

Postoperative care

Monitoring of the above parameters was extended into the postoperative period. Intermittent positive pressure ventilation with 30% humidified oxygen in air was given to all patients. Only when essential was minimal sedation with methadone or diazepam given to provide analgesia or facilitate ventilatory support.

RESULTS

Mortality

Three hospital deaths occurred in the 94 patients undergoing surgery for coronary artery disease and there was one death among the 30 patients who had their mitral valve replaced.

Myocardial infarction

Three patients developed cardiogenic shock due to myocardial infarction. Cardiogenic shock was defined for the purposes of this study as a systolic artery pressure less than 90 mm Hg, a left atrial pressure exceeding 18 mm Hg, associated with evidence of inadequate peripheral perfusion, e.g. urine output less than 20 ml/hr. Intra-aortic balloon pumping was employed in these patients and was successful in 2 cases.

Blood loss

The patients were considered in 3 groups and blood loss measured in the postperfusion period and during the first postoperative day. The results are presented in Table 2. By necessity, the method of blood loss measurement provides an underestimate of total loss.

Table 2.   *Blood loss measurements in 3 groups of patients*

	Blood loss in post-perfusion period (ml)	Blood loss during first postoperative day (ml)
Bypass graft	2,870 ± 1,020	1,650 ± 790
Aneurysm resection	5,404 ± 1,530	2,680 ± 220
Mitral valve replacement	1,093 ± 278	363 ± 333

During both periods, differences were observed between the groups. Blood loss associated with aneurysm resection exceeded that for bypass grafts which was also greater than in mitral valve replacement. These differences are statistically highly significant.

Hypotension

For the purposes of this study, hypotension was defined as a systolic pressure below 95 mm Hg or a diastolic pressure below 60 mm Hg. Hypotension during the postoperative period unrelated to hypovolaemia and presumably due to myocardial insufficiency was observed in 15% of patients with bypass grafts, in 50% of aneurysm resection patients and in 10% of the mitral valve replacements. Mixed venous oxygen saturation was monitored continually with a fiberoptic catheter placed in the pulmonary artery in most patients. All aneurysm resection patients had a mixed venous oxygen saturation below 50% during the first postoperative day. This finding, not seen in the other surgical groups, correlated directly with reduced cardiac output.

Arrhythmias

Ventricular arrhythmias were observed quite commonly in our patients. They can be considered in 2 groups: those unrelated to ventilatory problems and those related to ventilatory problems. Table 3 gives the distribution of arrhythmias due to myocardial irritability amongst the various groups. Table 4 illustrates the causes of ventricular arrhythmias related to ventilatory problems and their incidence. These problems were not peculiar to any particular surgical group and all were reversed by correcting the cause. When tried, they proved refractory to antiarrhythmic agents.

Table 3. *Ventricular arrhythmias due to myocardial irritability*

	No. of patients
Bypass grafts	11
Aneurysm resection	15
Mitral valve replacement	9

Table 4. *Ventricular arrhythmias associated with ventilatory problems*

	No. of patients
Hypercarbia	
due to malfunction of infrared analyser	5
due to respiratory obstruction	3
Hypocarbia due to hyperventilation	8
Enriched oxygen mixture not reaching the patient	1

Duration of ventilation

Intermittent positive pressure ventilation was continued for a range of 6–20 hr (mean 14 hr) following bypass grafts and mitral valve replacement. In aneurysm patients it was maintained for a range of 3–6 days (mean 4 days). No significant respiratory complications were observed in our series.

Urine output and potassium requirements

During perfusion and in the postperfusion period urine output and consequent potassium loss were markedly greater in coronary artery disease patients compared with mitral valve replacement patients. The range of urine output for coronary bypass grafts was 2–4 l compared with 600–1000 ml for mitral valve patients. This high urine output was not continued postoperatively and the mean urine production for coronary bypass grafts was 410 ml in the first 16 hr. Postoperative urine production in mitral valve patients was within normal limits. Potassium supplements were given according to urine output and serum potassium levels. Coronary bypass grafts required 6–10 g of potassium during perfusion and the first postoperative day while mitral valve patients received only 2–4 g.

Temperature

A rise in body temperature, often prolonged, was observed in all groups of patients similar to the findings of other workers. Treatment with surface cooling and rectal dimethylamino-phenyldimethylpyrazolone (Pyramidon®) was frequently employed with mixed success.

DISCUSSION

The observed operative and early postoperative mortality of 3.2% of patients undergoing surgery for coronary artery disease compares very favourably with other series (Cooley et al., 1973; Najmi et al., 1974). The incidence of myocardial infarction following coronary bypass grafts is not known. However, 3 of our patients developed cardiogenic shock due to infarction. Under these circumstances, diastolic augmentation with an intra-aortic balloon pump was employed and 2 of the patients survived. In our experience, excessive blood loss can be anticipated in patients having resection of ventricular aneurysms and to a lesser extent in coronary bypass grafts. This finding is not consistent with all other centres (Stanley et al., 1974). Impaired myocardial function as evidenced by hypotension and reduced mixed venous oxygen saturation was more frequently seen in the aneurysm patients. An isoprenaline infusion was used to counteract this tendency.

Ventricular arrhythmias were common and we would suggest from our series that in all cases a ventilatory cause should first be excluded before the introduction of anti-arrhythmic agents. This relationship of hypercarbia, hypocarbia and hypoxaemia to the occurrence of significant arrhythmias has been described by other workers (Osborn et al., 1971). When the origin of arrhythmias was myocardial irritability the usual antiarrhythmic drugs were employed.

Hypercarbia was sometimes the result of falsely low recordings obtained from the capnograph due to poor calibration and failure to absorb water from the circuit. The latter problem was resolved by insertion of a water absorber. Hypocarbia occurred with hyperventilation due to rapid patient triggering. The single case of hypoxaemia was due to failure to connect oxygen to the ventilator to enrich the air that the patients received. The duration of postoperative intermittent positive pressure ventilation for most patients was short. Aneurysm patients, however, required a longer period of ventilatory support. The postoperative persistence of a low cardiac output state in this group was followed by dyspnoea if ventilation was discontinued too early.

We favour light anaesthesia and minimal postoperative sedation for our patients. Cardiovascular depression is reduced to a minimum and the patient is alert and co-operative in the postoperative period. The absence of significant respiratory complications in our series can at least in part be attributed to this policy. We consider another important factor to be the use of an efficient blood filter to prevent microembolism. Gas analysis and computer-assisted monitoring of ventilation undoubtedly aid in the management of our patients.

SUMMARY

1. Excessive blood loss may occur during and after surgery for coronary artery disease and in particular with resection of ventricular aneurysms.

2. An underlying ventilatory cause for arrhythmias should be excluded.

3. Light anaesthesia and postoperative sedation minimizes cardiovascular depression and shortens the period of ventilatory assistance.

4. Gas analysis and computer-assisted monitoring of ventilation are valuable aids to patient management.

ACKNOWLEDGEMENTS

We are grateful to the nursing staff for their careful recording of observations and to Miss Marianne Wester for typing this manuscript.

REFERENCES

Cooley, D. A. et al. (1973): *Ann. thorac. Surg.*, *16/4*, 380.
Najmi, M. et al. (1974): *Amer. J. Cardiol.*, *33/1*, 42.
Osborn, J. J. et al. (1971): *Surgery*, *69/1*, 24.
Stanley, T. H. et al. (1974): *Ann. thorac. Surg.*, *17/4*, 368.

The anaesthetic problems of direct revascularisation in chronic and acute heart ischaemia

KRZYSZTOF STENGERT, JAN MOLL, ALICJA IWASZKIEWICZ-ZASLONKOWA, PIOTR KINTOPF and MICHAL OGINSKI

Department of Anaesthesiology; II Surgical Clinic; and Scientific and Medical Research Centre, Medical Academy, Lodz, Poland

Direct myocardial revascularisation, which has become more and more frequent in recent years, is the new technique for treating acute and chronic heart ischaemia (Effler et al., 1970; Moll et al., 1972; Pifarre et al., 1971; Scanton et al., 1971; Spencer, 1972b).

Venous aortocoronary bypass or anastomosis of the aorta with coronary sinus provides an additional arterial blood supply and improved blood flow to the heart muscle (Effler et al., 1970; Spencer, 1972a).

In cases of acute coronary insufficiency or impending infarction, direct revascularisation usually prevents ultimate infarction (Edelman et al., 1971; Spencer, 1972a).

The final decision about the method of operation is taken individually and is based on the clinical examination of the patient and selective coronary radiography.

Since 1969, 53 direct myocardial revascularisations have been performed at the II Surgical Clinic of the Medical Academy. The age of patients ranged between 29 and 66 years. Indications and type of operation are shown in Table 1. In 10 cases bypass was performed during total body perfusion. In the remaining 43 cases the operation was performed without cardiac arrest. During these operations, the apparatus for cardiopulmonary bypass was always ready for immediate use. If arterial pressure fell below 70 mm Hg or if dysrhythmias developed during trial clamping of the coronary artery, bypass was instituted. Thirty patients suffered from chronic coronary insufficiency; 21 of them had previous infarcts – between 3 months to several years earlier.

Table 1. *Number of operations performed*

Clinical diagnosis	No. of patients	Post-infarctional stage	Kind of operation				ECG
			Bypass				
			Aorto-coronary left	Aorto-coronary dexter	Bilateral aorto-coronary	Aorto-sinusal	
Impending infarct	12	6	5	3	3	1	2
Recent infarct	11	6	3	3	2	3	4
Coronary disease – advanced stenocardia	30	21	13	9	5	3	4
Total	53	33	21	15	10	7	10

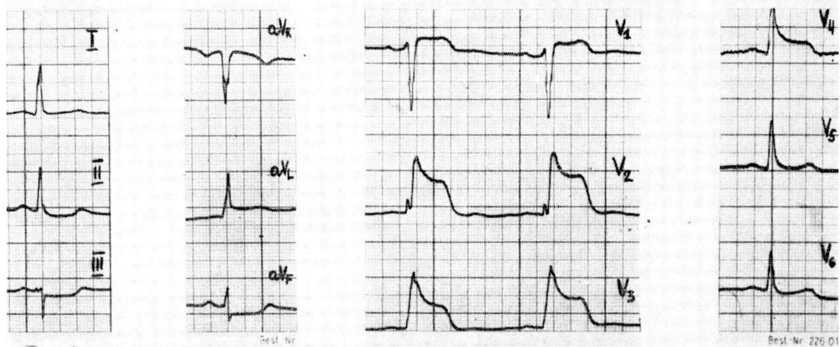

Fig. 1. *ECG at the time of peak coronary pain in a patient with an impending infarct. Lowering of ST section in Leads II, III and aVF and considerable elevation of ST section in Leads V_2, V_3 and V_4.*

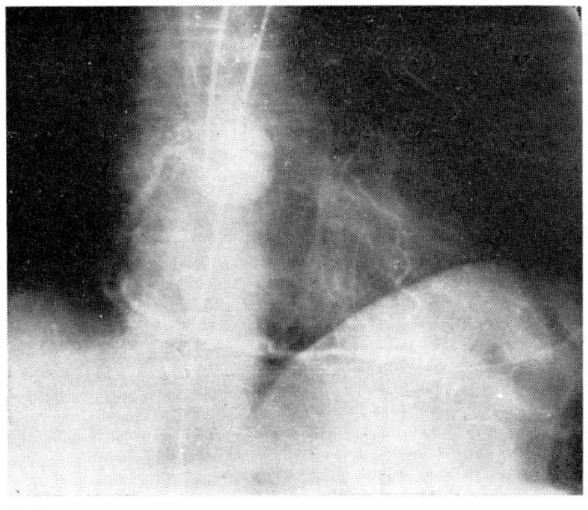

(a)

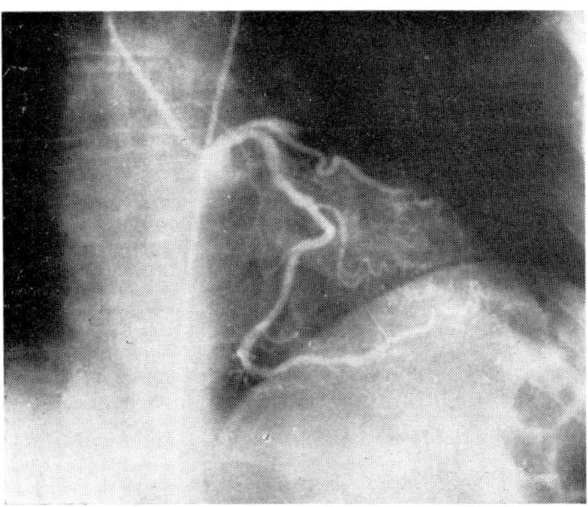

(b)

Fig. 2. *(a) Disseminated arteriosclerotic changes in the right coronary artery; (b) a considerable narrowing of anterior interventricular branch near its main trunk. Disseminated arteriosclerotic changes in the circumflex branch.*

The remaining patients qualified for immediate operation because of an impending infarct. An early decision to perform revascularisation before the complete formation of an infarct prevents further development of shock.

The operations, particularly those performed on patients in severe shock present serious problems for anaesthesia during the preparation for the operation, anaesthesia and post-operative care.

An acute pain is usually combatted with large doses of narcotics and glyceryl trinitrite. Excessive adrenergic stimulation from deadly fear for one's life additionally aggravates the condition. In these circumstances a rapid decrease of cardiac output in the presence of restricted coronary blood flow may lead to the dangerous complications including ventricular fibrillation. This condition is of special clinical importance since it is accompanied by respiratory insufficiency which aggravates hypoxia and results in acid-base disturbances.

The conclusion is that the most important task of the intensive preoperative treatment, besides suppression of pain, is to ensure that cardiac output is adequate for cellular demands and to ensure elimination of carbon dioxide. Among commonly used analgesic drugs,

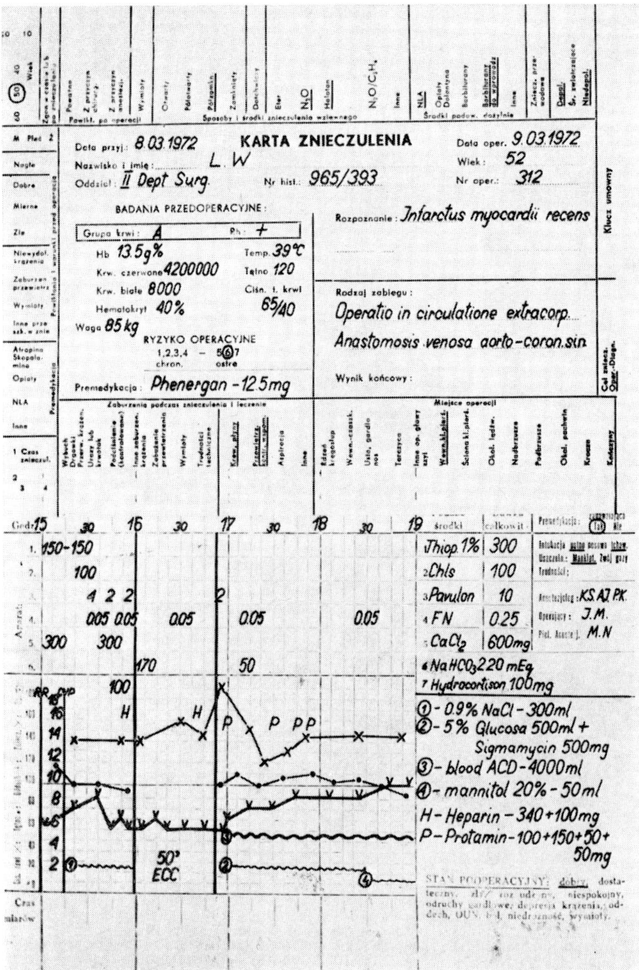

Fig. 3.   *Anaesthesia record.*

which in these conditions include morphine, pethidine and fentanyl, pentazocine (Fortral) seems to be an excellent analgesic since respiration is hardly depressed and there is no effect on the circulation. Good effects are also registered when using a combination of pentazocine with dehydrobenzperidol, provided DHBP is not given to patients with arterial pressure below 70 mm Hg.

The least disturbance of ventilation, irrespective of the start of operation, is an indication to start assisted or controlled respiration immediately.

Low cardiac output was in selected cases treated with β-adrenergic drugs (Isuprel) which when administered in small doses improves circulation and ensures sufficient arterial pressure and tissue perfusion, which can be checked by measurements using ^{133}Xe.

When shock is fully developed and cannot be controlled in this manner immediate extracorporeal circulation is indicated to maintain the blood flow through vital organs. In such situations assisted circulation by means of intra-aortic balloon pumping (IABP) is indicated. When haemodynamic improvement has occurred coronary radiography and myocardial vascularization may be performed (Mundth et al., 1972; Nicholson, 1972; Sanders et al., 1972). Another decisive factor is the elimination of acid-base disturbances and electrolyte-imbalance (particularly potassium). During and after operation it is essential to ensure coronary perfusion. Any fall of arterial pressure or bradycardia immediately after anastomosis, involves poor blood flow with the risk of coagulation in the bypass graft and dangerous ischaemia.

During postoperative treatment, clinical symptoms disappeared in most patients and ECG signs of myocardial ischaemia were reduced.

This is well-illustrated by one patient who was a 52-year-old man, professionally active, admitted to the Intensive Care Unit with sudden symptoms of acute myocardial ischaemia which were confirmed by ECG (Fig. 1).

Acute and increasing coronary pain did not disappear after narcotic drugs and glyceryl trinitrite. Coronary radiography at that time showed an impaired patency of the coronary

Table 2. *Blood-gas analysis during and after the operation*

	Before perfusion	After perfusion	Day 1	Day 2
pH	7.41	7.38	7.48	7.46
P_{CO_2} (mm Hg)	37	34	30	33.5
BE (mEq/l)	—1	—4	—0.2	0
BB (mEq/l)	44.8	45.8	46.2	44
SB (mEq/l)	23.5	21	23.8	24
AB (mEq/l)	23	20	22	23.5
Total CO_2 (mEq/l)	24.1	21	22.9	24.5
P_{O_2} (mm Hg)	149	180	70	90
S_{O_2} (%)	–	–	95	97.2

Table 3. *Blood tests during and after the operation*

	After perfusion	6 hr postoperation	Day 1	Day 3
Na^+ (mEq/l)	143.5	125.3	142.5	143.0
K^+ (mEq/l)	4.50	2.82	4.29	3.98
Cl^- (mEq/l)	99.8	91.4	94.0	97.5
Hb (g%)	–	12.8	–	11
Erytr. (mm³)	–	3850000	–	3350000
Ht (%)	–	37.7	–	33.0

arteries (Fig. 2*a*, *b*). The patient was in cardiogenic shock, the arterial pressure was below 70 mm Hg, pulse rate 120–140/min. Low molecular weight dextran, morphine 5 mg with promethazine 12.5 mg were given. Anaesthesia was induced with 1% thiopental, succinyl-choline, $N_2O + O_2$ and halothane (0.3 up to 0.7 vol%). Muscular relaxation was with 8 mg pancuronium and analgesia was complemented by fentanyl. During cardiopulmonary bypass halothane 0.3 vol% with O_2 was given direct to the oxygenator. The patient's condition was monitored by arterial pressure, central venous pressure, ECG, body temperature and urine output. The record of the anaesthetic procedure is shown in Figure 3. In the postoperative period assisted or controlled respiration was continued during 6–24 hr after the operation and pentazocine was used for analgesia.

The disturbance in acid-base and electrolyte equilibrium was treated in the typical manner and Tables 2 and 3 show the changes in the arterial blood-gas electrolytes in the above patient. Figure 4 shows a subsequent ECG examination.

Out of 53 patients who were operated on 12 died. The causes of their deaths are given in Table 4. In the immediate postoperative period 5 patients died with low cardiac output syndrome. One death, 8 hr after the operation, was caused by a recent clot in the anastomosis. All deaths but one occurred in those patients who had immediate operations for myocardial ischaemia. The condition of these patients was so serious that it was not possible to overcome shock before the operation. Three patients had numerous cardiac arrests during their admission due to ventricular fibrillation which was efficiently reverted by DC defibrillation. In the third week after the operation a further 6 patients died (Table 4). The remaining patients left hospital in a generally satisfactory condition and some resumed work.

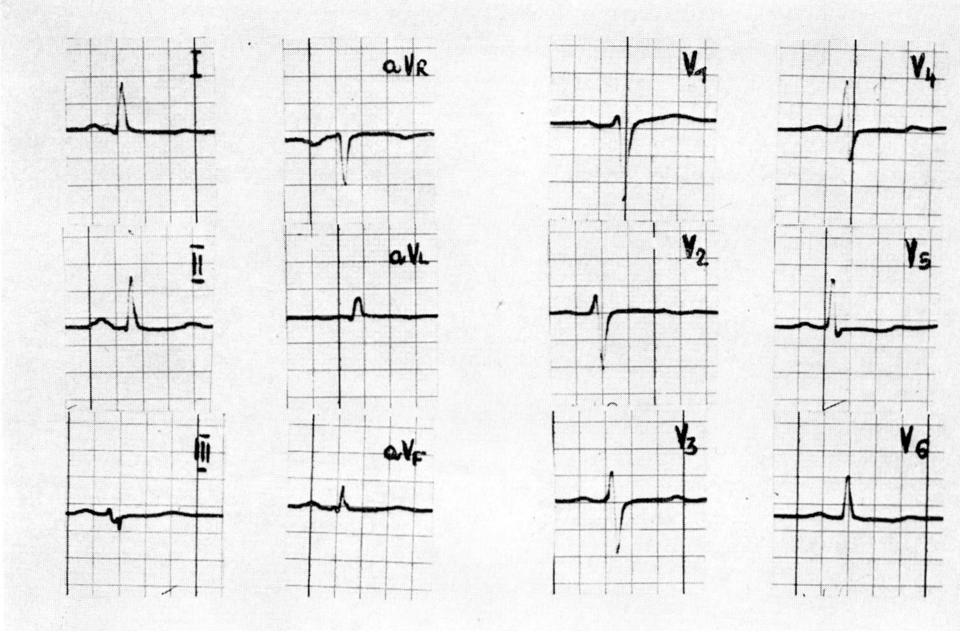

Fig. 4.   *ECG on 25th day after the operation – left aortocoronary bypass. A slight lowering of ST section in Leads II, III and aVF. In cardiac leads, ECG curve near normal level. Slight changes in the ST section probably due to postoperative pallium lesions.*

Table 4. *Cause of death*

| | Diagnosis | | | | | |
| | Early (2 hr–3 days) | | | Late (14–19 days) | | |
	Impending infarct	Recent infarct	Coronary disease	Impending infarct	Recent infarct	Coronary disease
Thrombosis in the region of anastomosis	1	–	–	–	–	–
Low cardiac output	–	4	1	–	–	–
Myocardial infarct	–	–	–	–	1	–
Bilateral bronchopneumonia	–	–	–	1	–	2
Renal insufficiency uraemia	–	–	–	–	–	1
Ileus shock	–	–	–	–	1	–
Total	1	4	1	1	2	3

CONCLUSION

Early decision and the operation of direct myocardial revascularisation in patients with acute myocardial ischaemia generally prevents the development of shock and an infarct. It is essential that the disturbances of acid-base and potassium equilibrium should be corrected at the same time, independent of treatment with analgesic and cardiotonic drugs.

Preoperative and postoperative artificial ventilation considerably facilitates postoperative treatment by ensuring optimum oxygenation of arterial blood and elimination of CO_2.

Assisted circulation is indicated when the circulatory insufficiency prior to operation cannot be controlled by pharmacological treatment.

REFERENCES

Edelman, M., Chętkowska, E., Iljin, W., Moll, J. and Żuchowska, J. (1971): *Kardiol. pol.*, *44*, 387.
Effler, D. B., Favaloro, R. G. and Gorves, L. K. (1970): *J. thorac. Cardiovasc. Surg.*, *59*, 147.
Moll, J., Musia, W., Dziatkowiak, A., Iljin, W., Krzemińska-Pakua, M. and Tracz, W. (1972): *Kardiol. pol.*, *15*, 307.
Mundth, E. D., Buckley, M. J., Dagget, W. M., Sanders, C. A. and Austen, W. G. (1972): *Circulation*, *45*, 1279.
Nicholson, M. J. (1972): *Anest. Analg. Curr. Res.*, *51*, 125.
Pifarre, R., Spinazzola, A., Nemickas, R., Scanlon, P. and Tobin, J. (1971): *Arch. Surg.*, *103*, 525.
Sanders, C. A., Buckley, M. J., Leinbach, R. C., Mundth, E. D. and Austen, W. G. (1972): *Circulation*, *45*, 1292.
Scanton, R., Nemickas, R. and Tobin Jr., J. (1971): *J. Amer. med. Ass.*, *218*, 207.
Spencer, F. C. (1972a): *Progr. cardiovasc. Dis.*, *14*, 399.
Spencer, F. C. (1972b): *Circulation*, *45*, 1314.

Chapter X

The role of the anaesthesiologist in the treatment of multiple injures

Priorities in the immediate management of major injuries

PETER J. F. BASKETT

United Bristol Hospitals and Frenchay Hospital, Bristol, United Kingdom

The natural reaction of most doctors, when confronted by a patient with multiple major injuries at the roadside or on the factory floor, is a feeling of inadequacy in the face of the enormous problems. Only training and practice can overcome this reaction and replace it with the calmness and confidence of knowing what to do urgently and being able to do it.

The first action must be a rapid assessment of the situation and establishment of an order of priority of treatment.

We must ask ourselves 3 questions: (1) What can I do to preserve this patient's life? (2) What can I do to reduce the complications arising from these injuries? (3) What can I do to relieve this patient's pain?

Let us examine these questions in a little more detail.

WHAT CAN I DO TO PRESERVE THIS PATIENT'S LIFE?

Thanks largely to the teaching and skills of anaesthetists, it is now clear that the first priority in the management of any patient with major injuries is to assess and, if necessary treat, the respiratory and cardiovascular function. This may appear to us to be stating the obvious, but there are numerous instances in apparently excellent centres, where vital priorities have been overlooked in the face of other, perhaps dramatic, but nevertheless non-urgent, injuries. One can cite the example of the victim of a car crash with a nasty looking compound fracture of a limb who succumbs in the X-ray Department with a tension pneumothorax which has been missed because his leg injury was more obvious. In preserving life, the first actions must be: (*a*) to ensure a clear and safe airway; (*b*) to assess and support, if necessary, ventilation and oxygenation; (*c*) to diagnose and treat, if necessary, a pneumothorax; and (*d*) to arrest haemorrhage and replace blood loss.

The airway

To anaesthetists, the skill of maintaining a clear and safe airway is our stock in trade and does not usually present us with any major problems. We are experts with a laryngoscope and endotracheal tube but we must remember that our colleagues in the Accident Centre may not be, and that, in a great deal of cases, correct positioning in the semi-prone or lateral position with support of the jaw will be quite adequate. A simple Guedel airway may help but is often difficult to manage in the semi-conscious, restless individual who rejects it and then promptly obstructs his airway again. In these patients, the nasopharyngeal airway is invaluable and, in the author's opinion, is all too infrequently used.

Probably the most difficult airway problem of all is the ruptured trachea or bronchus. This condition can usually be diagnosed by the presence of mediastinal and subcutaneous emphysema. Management is usually extremely difficult – if possible, intermittent positive ventilation should be avoided because it usually tends to make the problems worse. As a last resort, endobronchial intubation may have to be used while surgical repair is carried out. Any intrathoracic tension must be relieved by underwater seal drainage and skin relieving incisions may have to be made as well.

Ventilation and oxygenation

The assessment and support of adequate ventilation is again something that is a basic part of the anaesthetist's skill and should not present a problem to us. In the patients with major injuries, at least 40% oxygen should be given to help compensate for shunting in damaged lung tissue or other circulatory inadequacies at least until blood gas analysis can be carried out.

Pneumothorax

Sucking wounds of the chest must be closed immediately by a firm, airtight pad and bandage. A simple pneumothorax may require to be drained through a Heimlich valve arrangement, or an underwater seal, but is not a matter of extreme urgency. A tension pneumothorax, however, is, and if a proper thoracic drainage catheter is not immediately available, the tension can be temporarily relieved by the insertion of a wide bore intravenous cannula into the pleural cavity. Remember that in a helicopter, the patient often lies on the floor and so a Heimlich valve arrangement is required instead of an underwater seal bottle. This can be simply made out of a length of flaccid rubber sheath (Paul's tubing) tied securely to form an extension of the thoracic catheter.

Haemorrhage and transfusion

Arrest of haemorrhage at a peripheral site is best managed by simple pressure over the bleeding points rather than by application of a tourniquet. Severe haemorrhage into the body cavities is a different matter and requires urgent surgical intervention. Blood loss should be replaced as soon as possible by Hartmann's solution, dextran with a molecular weight of about 70,000 and whole blood as they become available. The problems of setting up an intravenous infusion in the almost exsanguinated patient are all too familiar to us, but if the patient is placed in the head down position, the external or internal jugular or subclavian veins can usually be cannulated successfully.

Failure to respond to blood transfusion at surgery usually indicates severe uncontrolled haemorrhage in an unexplored area but, if this can be ruled out, then massive doses of steroids may be tried to enhance the failing circulation.

WHAT CAN I DO TO REDUCE THE COMPLICATIONS OF THE INJURIES?

The best way to avoid complications of the injuries is to remember what these complications may be and to be diagnostically alert, not only for the obvious injury, but also for the overt. Always remember the possibility of the spinal or head injury. Any patient with a neck or back injury should be treated as if he has an unstable spinal injury and splinted in a spinal board and cervical collar for transport. In this context, it is worth remembering at the scene of a road accident, that it is often better to remove the victim from his vehicle sitting in the car seat, rather than to try to get him out of the seat which will usually mean flexing or extending the spine.

In a patient with a head injury, observation of the level of consciousness, limb movements and eye signs will indicate if there is increasing cerebral compression requiring urgent burr holes or craniotomy.

Limb injuries should be dressed with a simple gauze dressing, haemorrhage controlled and suspected fractures splinted. It is important to avoid converting a simple fracture into a compound one.

Overt damage in the chest must not be forgotten, even though all appears to be well. The ruptured aorta often takes several days to manifest itself, as may a tear in the diaphragm. In the abdomen, rupture of the gastrointestinal tract, bladder, spleen, kidney, liver or pancreas are all potentially lethal conditions which respond well to early diagnosis and treatment.

WHAT CAN I DO TO RELIEVE PAIN?

Analgesia is too often inadequate or even totally omitted in patients with severe multiple injuries. Yet we know that relief of pain brings with it not only humane benefits, but also improvement in the circulation as a result of the reduction in circulatory catecholamines. In providing analgesia in this situation, where both respiration and the circulation are in jeopardy, a number of factors must be taken into consideration, including the effectiveness of the analgesic, its depressant side effects and its route of administration, uptake and duration of action. In the early management of major injuries, we have found that Entonox, a 50% mixture of nitrous oxide and oxygen contained in a single cylinder, has served the purpose best. Nitrous oxide is one of our best proven analgesics with minimal depressant side effects. Its inhalational route of administration ensures a rapid uptake and equally rapid excretion. Using a demand apparatus, the gas mixture can be self-administered by the patient, supervised by paramedical personnel. Alternatively, the gas can be delivered from a continuous flow device to a disposable type oxygen face mask or used in conjunction with a Laerdal Resusci bag or mechanical ventilator.

Entonox can be used in conjunction with small doses of the opiates given intravenously and, together, the combination will give relief of even severe pain. There does not seem to be a lot to choose between the members of the opiate group in this context, given in equianalgesic doses. Pentazocine, however, has claim to some advantage in being free from the rigid controls that other opiates are subject to, and may be just a little less depressant than some other members of the family.

It is worth remembering that anxiety is a major factor in the patient with multiple injuries and pure sedation with a relatively non-depressant agent like diazepam, may enable the dosage of opiates to be drastically reduced, or even omitted, leaving Entonox alone to provide the analgesia.

These resuscitation techniques for patients with major multiple injuries have been developed in hospitals, largely by anaesthetists, and, in the majority of centres, have become an extremely efficient routine. Patients who reach hospital alive and without irreversible damage to a vital organ can usually be well cared for.

A significant improvement in the morbidity and mortality figures is now likely to depend on the application of these resuscitative skills and techniques at the accident site and during transportation.

The title of this symposium is 'The role of anaesthesiologists in the treatment of multiple injuries'. I would put it to you that our role is not only to practise in hospital the skills and techniques and therapy that we hear about at this symposium. We must also take an active part in resuscitation rescue schemes at the accident site in mobile resuscitation units, where we can practise our skills at the earliest possible moment and, therefore, to the best advantage of our patients. We can then see what the problems are of conducting resuscitation in the far from ideal conditions of the roadside, factory floor or inside an ambulance, and amend our techniques to suit these situations. Finally, it is also our place to provide training in resuscitation and care of the severely injured to general practitioners, the ambulance and emergency services and the members of the general public.

The role of the trained nurse in the anaesthesiological treatment of the patient with multiple injuries

B. FL. HAXHOLDT

Department of Anaesthesiology, Glostrup Hospital, Glostrup, Denmark

Patients with multiple injuries, mainly caused by traffic casualties and more rarely by factory accidents, often show symptoms of serious damage to several organs. Such patients are most conveniently treated in an Intensive Care Unit (ICU). In Denmark the anaesthetic departments usually run these units, and are responsible for the management, the coordination of specialist services and the education of the attending staff.

Major hospitals, however, have specialized Intensive Care Units for coronary, nephrological, neonatal or neurosurgical cases. The anaesthetic department must extend its services also to these units, for instance in ventilator treatment of patients with respiratory insufficiency.

The main task of anaesthetists in the treatment of patients with multiple injuries is to support vital functions; the most typical contribution is ventilator treatment. As an illustration, the situation in Glostrup Hospital is described briefly. This is a 1000 bed hospital with more than 40,000 patient admissions annually, covering a population of about 350,000. This hospital is situated 10 km from the center of Copenhagen in an area with many, but new, factories, and with main roads carrying the highest traffic intensity in Denmark.

Table 1 gives an analysis of the ICU patients who received ventilator treatment during the past two years. The largest group of ventilator treated ICU patients suffered from medical and paediatric diseases and the total annual number is close to 400. The second largest group, considerably lower, is of those with multiple injuries, the percentage being approximately 15.

Table 1. *Ventilator treated ICU patients*

Year	Surgical and gynaecological	Medical and paediatric	Neurological	Multiple injuries	Total	Multiple injuries (%)
1972	33	266	17	52	368	14.1
1973	48	268	8	65	389	16.1

Table 2 shows the death rates of ventilator treated ICU patients and reveals an overall mortality of about 40%; the highest rate of mortality, around 60%, is among those with multiple injuries.

In Table 3 the patients with multiple injuries are divided into a mainly intracranially damaged group and into a thoraco-abdominally damaged group often with various fractures. It demonstrates the well-known experience that serious intracranial injury is highly lethal,

Table 2. *Ventilator treated ICU patients (death rates)*

Year	Surgical and gynaecological	Medical and paediatric	Neurological	Multiple injuries	Total
1972					
% deaths	30.3	38.7	41.1	55.8	40.5
No. of patients treated	33	266	17	52	368
1973					
% deaths	27.1	39.2	25.0	61.5	41.1
No. of patients treated	48	268	8	65	389

Table 3. *Ventilator treated ICU patients with multiple injuries*

Year	Total	Mainly intracranial	Mainly thoraco-abdomino-extremical
1972			
No. of patients	52	35	17
Deaths	29	25	4
Death rate	55.8	71.4	23.5
1973			
No. of patients	65	50	15
Deaths	40	39	1
Death rate	61.5	78.0	6.7

as here, with a mortality of 70%. When only slight cerebral damage has occurred, even severe thoraco-abdominal insults and fractures can often be treated with great success, and modest sequels remain. In this group only 24% and 7% died.

The patients with brain damage are usually treated in the Neurosurgical Intensive Care Unit. The other categories of the patients with multiple injuries are treated in the Anaesthetic Intensive Care Unit and Table 4 shows the available staff of doctors, nurses and auxiliary nurses and others, partly in daywork and partly on night duty in our small respiratory

Table 4. *Staff*

Daywork	*On-duty*
3 Consultants	1 Consultant
5 Senior doctors	1 Senior doctor ⎫ Staying 24 hr
2 Special course doctors	1 Junior doctor ⎭ in hospital
6 Junior doctors	1 Staff nurse
1 Ward sister	1 Nurse
2 Staff nurses	1 Auxiliary nurse
14 Nurses	
6 Auxiliary nurses	
2 Orderlies	
1 Engineer	
2 Laboratory technicians	

unit. This staff also treats about 10,000 recovery cases per year, and the doctors supervise 17,000 anaesthetics annually around the clock.

In the definition of the intensive care therapy it is often stated that it implies 24-hr service from the doctor at the bedside. This, however, is utopian in most situations, because during the duty period comprising 2/3 of the 24 hours, the two anaesthetist doctors have to conduct all emergency anaesthetics and resuscitation as well. Consequently, the moment-to-moment therapy has to be given by our specially trained nurses, working for 8-hr periods, and they have gradually taken over many functions formerly considered to be exclusively physicians' work.

Evidently, such nurses must be capable of not only immediately instituting resuscitation on their own, but also of setting-up the ventilators, administering intravenous fluids, including blood, analgesics and sedatives, according to their own evaluation of the changing needs of the patient and naturally following the departmental therapeutic principles. She must master the observation and evaluation of an increasing number of sophisticated parameters and laboratory findings.

Figure 1 gives an idea of the comprehensive and complicated electronic TV-monitoring

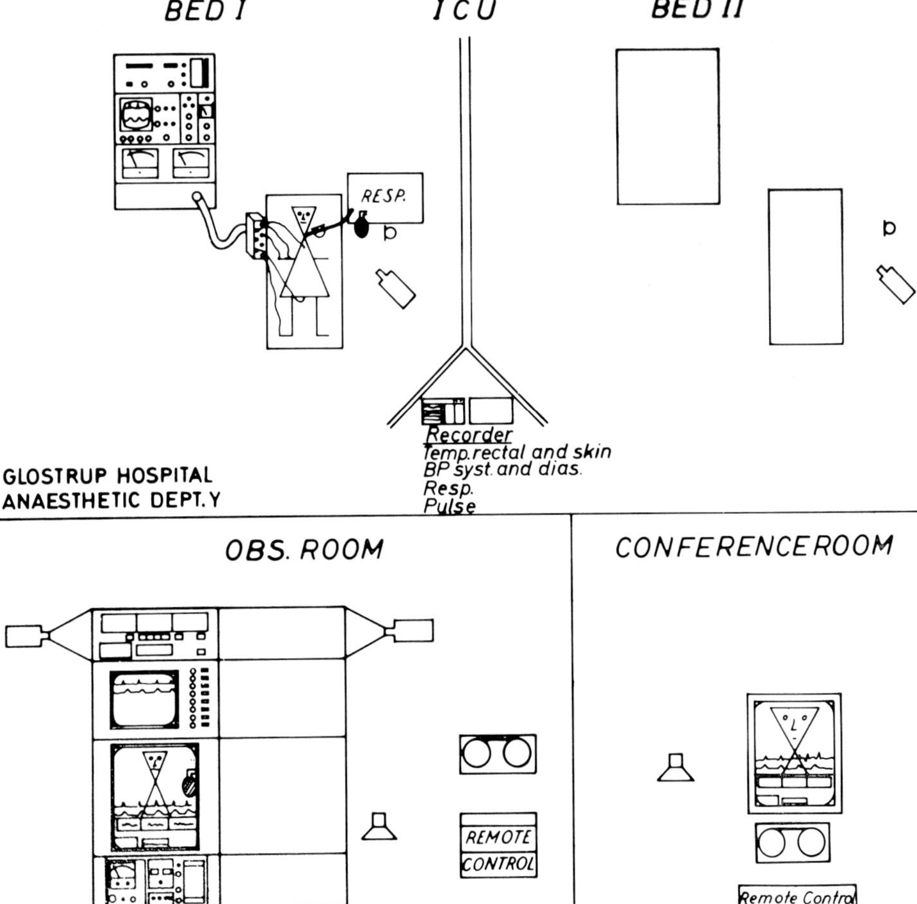

Fig. 1. *Schematic set-up of electronic- and TV-monitoring.*

the nurses must use in the proper way. Two of the bedside monitors have automatic recording and TV cameras. Remote displays of the secondary working areas of the nurses and doctors – recovery room and conference room – enable one person to cover several functions except in the most acute phases. Videotape recorders are connected to the system.

Desirable qualifications for such nurses are previous training in surgical wards, medical wards and theatre work. Further, neurosurgical, nephrological and cardiological experience is a great advantage, as is anaesthetic practice. Of course it is not possible to find these qualifications in a single nurse, so they also have a great task in mutual training.

In Denmark the education of the anaesthesiological ICU nurse is not standardized as yet. In Glostrup the training comprises weekly theoretical lessons, as well as several hours' daily bedside instruction, all given by doctor anaesthetists. Instruction in the use of the electronic- and TV-monitoring is given by our engineers. The nurse acquires skills in performing artificial ventilation, suction and intubation during a rotation to anaesthetics. Audiovisual self-instruction is included in our teaching methods. The importance of the nurses' daily participation in the doctors' conference must be stressed, since this also means teaching of following the considerations and decisions regarding therapy.

Finally, it ought to be pointed out that already in the initial therapy of the multiple injured patients, the specially trained nurse, here the anaesthetic nurse, plays an important role, as she often is more capable than the young doctor-anaesthetist. Not rarely, anaesthetic assistance is needed at the actual site of the casualty, where the nurse with the doctor and the rescue people can give the initial treatment, being in contact with the department by aid of a specially developed walkie-talkie system. Further the nurse is most valuable during the ambulance-transportation, in the casualty-theatre and during the often longlasting, complicated anaesthetic, preceding intensive therapy.

The specially trained nurse is playing an important role in the treatment of the patient with multiple injuries, and we believe it worthwhile to give her extensive and continuous training to obtain the optimum of a successful therapy. The upgrading of the nurses' teaching and of their functions is not the cause, but probably a cause of the encouraging survival rates of multiple injured patients.

The treatment of patients with multiple injuries associated with damage to the spinal cord

C. V. MORPURGO

Istituto Ortopedico Gaetano Pini, Milan, Italy

Anaesthetists are best suited of all specialists to manage patients in the acute stage with spinal cord injury and associated multiple injuries.

The number of these patients is continuously growing in parallel with the increase in road accidents, but even more so as a result of the progress made in the fields of First Aid, transport and treatment of these victims (Cheshire, 1971; Guttmann, 1967). Until a few decades ago these patients were considered incurable and not worthy of attention.

From our point of view, the care of such patients can schematically be divided into 3 stages: the 1st stage begins at the moment of trauma or of the interruption of the functions of the spinal cord and lasts for 7–8 hr; the 2nd stage, from the 1st to between the 3rd and 6th days, comprises the phase of regression of spinal shock, (occasionally this exceeds 20 days); the last stage ends in most instances within 20 days after the accident when the patient can leave the intensive care unit for a ward.

The first hours after the occurrence of spinal cord injury are the most important and crucial for the survival of damaged nervous tissue. During this period, neglect or wrong treatment can cause a reversible lesion to become irreversible: it is known that ischaemia or hypoxia can provoke the release of noradrenaline in the damaged spinal tissues and a subsequent necrosis of nervous cells (Osterholm et al., 1971; Sinha et al., 1971). Therefore, even if the spinal cord is unharmed, incorrect transport or unjustified loss of time can result in irreversible tetra- or paraplegia. Hence the rule is that spinal resuscitation must continue rather than diagnostic investigation or treatment of other injuries.

The anaesthetist has to start respiratory and circulatory resuscitation immediately to improve the general condition of the patient and to avoid or reduce post-traumatic damage to the spinal cord. Otherwise an injury at level C_3–C_5 or any post-traumatic complication at this segment of the spinal cord may result in death from respiratory insufficiency because all respiratory muscles, including the diaphragm, are paralysed. It is wise to keep the body temperature within safe limits (a high fever predisposes to bed sores, difficulties in respiration, acidosis etc.). It is important to control the loss of fluid and electrolytes with infusions, and to correct the tendency to post-traumatic shock. Anaesthesia may also be required for the reduction of a fracture or dislocation of the spine or to treat concomitant injuries.

Any delay may result in the irreversibility of many lesions which were not so serious at first; on the other hand, the decision to perform a laminectomy for exploratory purposes often does no more than to add surgical trauma to the initial accidental injury (Bedbrook, 1966). Therefore, the more sensible decision is to attempt to restore the normal shape of the vertebral canal in the simplest and least traumatic way in order to prevent any difficulties of circulation due to compression or kinking of the vessels (Ducker and Perot, 1971).

Moreover, in these early hours of treatment, it seems justifiable to try to introduce directly into the damaged tissue of the spinal cord drugs to impede the release of noradrenaline, or to counteract its action (Foldes et al., 1957), to prevent the formation of necrotic areas in the grey matter. The use of these substances by normal routes of administration is rendered impossible by their toxicity (e.g. α-methyltyrosine) or by their inability to cross the blood-brain barrier (e.g. d-tubocurarine). Only by direct injection of d-tubocurarine into the subdural space, which was first suggested in 1961 (Morpurgo and Spinelli, 1963), is it possible to keep the dosage effective without dangerous side-effects.

The second stage is characterised by signs of systemic shock and signs of spinal shock: it is a period of great instability of vital functions. The anaesthetist is usually called upon to resolve difficult situations:

Respiratory management

A patient with a high spinal lesion at C_5 and no other associated injury loses two-thirds of his vital capacity (Maglio et al., 1966). Thus, if there is fever, damage to the respiratory tract, the rib cage or pulmonary tissue, respiratory assistance or control via an endotracheal tube or a tracheostomy is essential. There is also a need for careful, sterile suction of secretions, drainage of pneumo- and haemothorax and efficient ventilation of the alveoli because the patient cannot cough actively. The situation must be monitored by pH and blood gas analysis. Care must be taken to prevent pulmonary collapse due to aspiration of vomitus and pulmonary oedema caused by fluid-overloading.

Disorders of circulation

The loss of regulation of vagal tone in the paralysed part of the body makes the control of arterial pressure difficult; in the presence of concomitant damage to the heart or the vessels, the situation deteriorates and readily leads to severe hypotension or cardiac arrest. The blood volume must be accurately maintained. The level of the central venous pressure, which is normally a good guide to the quantity of infused fluids required, can be misleading here, because of the absence of peripheral vascular tone and the impairment of spontaneous ventilation which affects the venous return to the heart.

Body temperature

There is very seldom a need for warming because of deep hypothermia. A rectal temperature of 34–35°C can be safely maintained in order to reduce the oxygen requirement. More often there is dangerous hyperthermia which must be overcome, if necessary, by the techniques for controlled hypothermia. At first we used to give antipyretics, but after the introduction of injections of curare via the subdural space this problem was solved.

Water and electrolyte balance

There is a tendency to water retention which may be enhanced if spinal shock is confused with traumatic shock and the patient is overloaded with fluids in an attempt to correct hypotension. Potassium depletion occurs in the damaged and denervated muscles and the ion is lost in fluids aspirated from the gastrointestinal tract. Other disturbances likely to occur are sodium retention, acidosis and magnesium depletion. All these conditions must be corrected in an adult of average weight by giving up to 300 mEq in 24 hr of potassium and 5 mEq of magnesium, by replacing the fluid loss with a calculated amount and by restricting the use of saline solutions.

Metabolism

The basal metabolic requirement of 1800–2000 kcal/day can rise to 3000–4000 kcal/day in the case of associated infections and hyperpyrexia (Cheshire and Coats, 1966). Insufficient intake of calories leads to rapid depletion of glycogen stores (approximately 350 g) and to increased destruction of body protein. Total intravenous nutrition can be accomplished nowadays with the administration of 1500 ml dextrose (50–60%) and 1500 ml (8.5%) solution of amino acids per day via a catheter inserted in a large vein. Insulin added to the solution or administered subcutaneously in a dosage of one international unit for 5–10 g of sugar has a real value in promoting the access of potassium to the cells and the utilisation of carbohydrates with a reduction in the catabolism of proteins and amino acids. Acidosis can be corrected with bicarbonate.

Gastrointestinal tract

Distension of the abdomen through an excess of gases gives rise to further impairment of the mechanical efficiency of the diaphragm. Paralysis of the intestine promotes the absorption of endotoxins. Acute gastric dilatation, when not corrected, can rapidly cause death. A stomach tube with controlled suction, a rectal tube, oxygen therapy, drugs such as Prostigmine, Mestinon, pantothenic acid, enemas etc. are useful. The subdural administration of curare, by promoting the return of the autonomic reflexes has always been beneficial in this respect. A normal potassium level is essential for the activity of the smooth muscles of the intestinal tract. The administration of nutrients, fluids or drugs by the oral route must be postponed until after the onset of clear signs of intestinal activity. When parenteral nutrition must continue for several days the need for trace elements can be met with transfusion of blood or plasma; it is our hope that the industry will make available a solution of trace substances for this purpose, thus avoiding transfusions with their attendant risk of hepatitis.

Urinary tract

Every complication can be found in these patients with multiple injuries, varying from simple urinary retention to anuria following damage to the renal arteries or systemic shock, or to rupture of the bladder or urinary tract. There is always a tendency to an impairment of renal function, in which case potassium retention and high blood urea occur. Often the assistance of a Renal Unit is required. Subdural curare can prevent urinary retention by promoting automatic emptying of the bladder and thus shortening the period of intermittent catheterisation.

Skin

These patients are very susceptible to bed sores. From the beginning it is necessary to put the patients in the correct position and move them frequently, to give sufficient amino acids, proteins and blood by infusion and to avoid hyperpyrexia.

Superimposed infections

These patients easily contract infections, particularly of the respiratory system, the urinary tract and the bed sores. They need antibiotics from the start and special precautions should be taken to ensure asepsis in every procedure.

Miscellaneous

In giving therapy for pain one must always consider the reduced vital capacity and any eventual damage to the respiratory centre. Five% ethyl alcohol added to the intravenous solutions is a good analgesic which has no respiratory depressant action. It is also a source of calories (5.6 kcal/ml) which is readily metabolised. Muscle relaxation may be necessary for the reduction of fractures and dislocation, but succinylcholine can produce cardiac arrest. Diazepam is efficient in reducing spasticity.

Traumatic shock

The usual therapeutic aids for the treatment of shock must be applied liberally and without delay. Ganglion blockers may, in these cases, upset an already delicately balanced circulatory equilibrium. This is particularly so when the thoracolumbar part of the sympathetic system is affected by the injury. In this case cautious use of noradrenaline or of sympathetic amines may be advised. There is always a need for large amounts of blood, plasma and fluids.

Spinal shock

In the treatment of this condition it is useful to recognise the different mechanisms which can provoke it (Van Harreveld and Stamm, 1954); simple concussion of the spinal cord, hypoxia, oedema, external compression, haematomyelia, laceration and transection of the cord. In the last case spinal shock can be due to the prevailing activity of the inhibitory circuits in the spinal cord (Guttmann, 1973), which are no longer counteracted by the facilitatory influences of the brain. In these patients, drugs which can block the hyperactivity of the inhibitory circuits are effective, as is any measure which diminishes the causes of an abnormally high inhibition (e.g. overdistension of the bladder or of the intestine, fever, pain, cutaneous sores etc.). So it is important to correct all the different pathological conditions provoked by the injury as soon as possible in order to shorten the duration and intensity of spinal shock. On the other hand, any therapeutic intervention, even as simple as the reduction of a fracture or dislocation, always becomes more difficult if delayed. Above all, the risk of circulatory complications and infections, to which these patients are particularly prone, is increased. The subdural injection of d-tubocurarine (0.4 mg) is usually repeated on about the 4th and the 8th days.

The third stage lasts about 20 days at most and represents the time before transference from an intensive care unit to a rehabilitation ward. The patient gradually becomes more stable. Catabolism persists and thus there remains a need for infusions of blood, plasma and amino acids. If, in the preceding stages the treatment has been complete and correct, the anaesthetist has only to deal with the problems arising in the attempt to give stability to the vertebral column. (Often when the cervical spine is damaged, insurmountable difficulties are met during oral or nasal endotracheal intubation; the risk of cardiac arrest caused by succinylcholine increases from the 3rd to the 7th week after the accident.) In other cases, plastic surgery on bed sores or other lesions, which went unnoticed or were left untended in the more dramatic stages of the first days, now takes place. Any pre-existing pathological condition must be carefully watched, because reflex responses caudal to the spinal lesion can be partially or totally abolished and the patient cannot attract attention to subjective symptoms of complications.

In a large accident and orthopaedic hospital of 600 beds, an average of one patient with vertebral fracture is admitted each day. Of these, about 4% have associated injuries, while more than 1% have neurological signs of spinal cord damage. Experience has shown in all these cases that prompt correct treatment is an essential condition for the limitation of permanent damage. The more serious cases call for the ability, the attention and the organisation of a team assembled for the specific purpose of tending these cases and provided with the special equipment they need. In this team the anaesthetist has a definite and predominant role.

Our best results have been obtained in patients admitted a few hours after the accident.

In one case of a fall inside a lift shaft which occurred within the hospital a very successful recovery was made from paraplegia and the associated fractures of the vertebral column, the hip and the feet with minimal disability.

Some cases with spasticity as an end-result may be due to chronic hypoxia of the spinal cord which might have been avoided or corrected with prompt and efficient respiratory and circulatory assistance.

The experience gained with more serious patients enables the anaesthetist to recognise, in many cases with fracture of the vertebral column without subsequent spinal cord damage, the presence of autonomic disturbances which are best treated promptly to avoid complications (impairment of respiratory, intestinal and renal functions etc.)

REFERENCES

Bedbrook, G. M. (1966): *Paraplegia, 4/1*, 43.

Cheshire, D. J. E. (1971): In: *Proceedings, XVIII Veterans' Administration Spinal Cord Injury Conference*, p. 87. Editor: Erich G. Krueger. Washington D.C.

Cheshire, D. J. E. and Coats, D. A. (1966): *Paraplegia, 4/1*, 1.

Ducker, T. B. and Perot, P. L. (1971): In: *Proceedings, XVIII Veterans' Administration Spinal Cord Injury Conference*, p. 29. Editor: Erich G. Krueger. Washington D.C.

Foldes, F. F., Baart, N., Shanor, S. P. and Erdos, E. G. (1957): *Anesthesiology, 18/1*, 163.

Guttmann, L. (1967): *Paraplegia, 5/3*, 115.

Guttmann, L. (1973): *Spinal Cord Injuries – Comprehensive Management and Research, 1st ed.*, Chapter 20. Blackwell Scientific Publications, Oxford, Edinburgh.

Maglio, A., Venerando, A., Dal Monte, A. and Lamberti-Bocconi, F. (1966): *Paraplegia, 4/2*, 116.

Morpurgo, C. V. and Spinelli, D. (1963): *Surv. Anesth., 7/3*, 222.

Osterholm, J. L., Mathews, G. J., Irvin, J. D. and Angelakos, E. T. (1971): In: *Proceedings, XVIII Veterans' Administration Spinal Cord Injury Conference*, p. 17. Editor: Erich G. Krueger. Washington D.C.

Sinha, R. P., Ducker, T. B. and Perot, P. L. (1971): In: *Proceedings, XVIII Veterans' Administration Spinal Cord Injury Conference*, p. 25. Editor: Erich G. Krueger. Washington D.C.

Van Harreveld, A. and Stamm, J. S. (1954): *Amer. J. Physiol., 178*, 117.

Pulmonary sequelae of polytransfusion and their treatment

KARL STEINBEREITHNER

Experimental Division, Department of Anaesthesiology,
University of Vienna, Vienna, Austria

Increasing insight into the nature of the so-called 'progressive pulmonary insufficiency' (Moore et al., 1969) has led to changing concepts of the pathomorphosis of the 'shock syndrome' stressing the important role of the lung as a target organ. In accord with a great number of researchers it is assumed that this is a multifactorial process which, largely independent of aetiological components, induces a well-defined, *uniform reaction syndrome* in the lung (Steinbereithner et al., 1973). According to Mittermayer et al. (1973) an important reason for the fact that such lesions have been observed so frequently over the last few years is a change in the character of the shock syndrome in the broadest sense. As more and more experience is gained in the fields of early volume substitution and in the prevention and treatment of renal failure, the lung is playing an increasingly important role as a 'shock organ' and as a factor which limits resuscitation efforts. Until 7 or 8 years ago this stage was not reached except occasionally.

As far as *pathophysiology* is concerned, the 'hallmarks' were defined precisely by Pontoppidan et al. (1972) so that they may be quoted literally: 'The abnormal pattern of gas distribution, with closure of alveoli or airways, or both; and, secondly, an increase in pulmonary extravascular water, with interstitial oedema caused either by pulmonary vascular congestion or by loss of integrity of capillary endothelium with exudation of plasma into the interstitium. Both conditions . . . result in a reduction in functional residual capacity, a decrease in pulmonary compliance and mismatching of ventilation and blood flow.'

On the basis of the above multifactorial thesis, an analysis (Table 1) of 75 ventilator patients in our ICU who died shows that there are a great number of 'additive' findings which clearly suggest the presence of a *pathogenetic summation effect*.

Table 1. *Role of 'additive' factors in lung pathology (correlation of clinical and postmortem findings)*

	No.	%
Cases investigated	75	–
'Ventilator lung' (VL)	53	70.8
Additional findings in 53 VL-cases:		
Lung trauma	11	20.7
Polytransfusion	10	18.8
Intrapulmonary fat	12	22.7
Lung emboli	6	11.3
Sepsis	13	24.5
Lung abscesses	12	22.7
Acute abdominal processes	12	22.7
Renal failure	14	26.7

ROLE OF POLYTRANSFUSION IN 'ADULT RESPIRATORY DISTRESS'

Although in the literature of the last 10 years (Moore et al., 1969; Miller, 1973) massive transfusion has repeatedly been incriminated for causing pulmonary reaction syndrome, Collins still claimed in 1969 that this is not a serious clinical problem. However, careful clinical and morphological analysis of ventilator patients from various ICU's (Mittermayer et al., 1971, 1973; Steinbereithner et al., 1973) suggested that polytransfusions, or poly-infusions, were involved in a high percentage of the fatal pulmonary cases (Table 1).

Four observations made in 1972 led us to investigate this problem in greater detail. In 3 cases, transfusion of 9 or more blood units was followed, with a variable latent period, by manifestations of acute respiratory insufficiency with corresponding blood gas values (pronounced hypoxaemia, increased $AaDo_2$, hypocapnia). The blood volume was about normal or slightly below; the central venous pressure did not show any major deviation. The thrombocyte counts were subnormal or distinctly reduced. X-ray either showed signs of interstitial and alveolar fluid accumulation (resembling the so-called 'fluid lung') or increased density of a diffuse, 'mottled' appearance similar to the pattern of fat embolism. In all cases ventilator treatment and administration of heparin led to an improvement of the clinical condition, which was also reflected by the results of blood gas analyses.

The course of another case is so unusual that it is worth describing in greater detail. A 13-year-old girl had received a relatively rapid transfusion of 4 blood units in a country hospital because of excessive anaemia (RBC, 1.7 million; Hct 28). This resulted in pulmonary oedema and temporary circulatory failure, with respiratory insufficiency which persisted after resuscitation. During artificial ventilation Po_2 values first ranged from 30–80 Torr and then continued to fall in spite of increased inspired oxygen. X-ray showed diffuse interstitial and alveolar fluid accumulation. After some temporary improvement on the 7th day, acute renal failure occurred; the patient died on the 13th day (terminal hypoxia with Po_2 values of 26/30 Torr in spite of PEEP). The postmortem findings were: 'ventilator lung', necrosis of the renal cortex. A blood group incompatibility could be excluded.

All the cases described above seem to have one thing in common – a direct connection between acute pulmonary symptoms and the administration of large volumes of blood and the absence of other predisposing factors which might be involved in inducing the lesions in the lung.

An analysis of all patients who received at least 7 blood units within 48 hr was carried out in order to discover if polytransfusion alone was as important as the first observation suggested. 'Pure' (uncomplicated) cases of haemorrhage were compared with patients who had other diseases which predisposed them to the development of 'shock lung'.

Seventy-five per cent of patients with intercurrent diseases (Table 2) exhibited distinct pulmonary changes (which were confirmed by findings obtained in patients who died),

Table 2. *Analysis of polytransfusion cases (1972/73)*

	No. of cases	Units blood (mean)	Thrombopenia ($< 100,000$)	Lung 'positive'	No. of deaths	(Lung positive)
Patients with 'additive' factors (trauma, sepsis, renal impairment etc.)	8	13	6	6	3	(3)
Gastrointestinal haemorrhage	13	21	8	5	6*	(2)

* 4 deaths within 48 hr (intractable bleeding).

whereas the corresponding percentage among cases of haemorrhage was only about 40%. This apparently clear difference is not statistically significant ($p > 0.15$). In spite of the small number of cases this seems a definite indication that polytransfusion plays an important role in causing damage to the lung.

Of course, these patients are not representative because the milder cases are not usually admitted to an ICU. Tammisto (1972) observed however, that pulmonary complications occurred in 23% of 75 patients with gastrointestinal haemorrhage who were not treated in an ICU.

PATHOGENETIC FACTORS OF 'TRANSFUSION LUNG' (see Table 3)

Lesions of the capillary wall presumably result from hypoperfusion (ischaemia) of the lung (Moore et al., 1969; Pontoppidan et al., 1972; Gump et al., 1970), *release of vasoactive substances* (Moore et al., 1969; Bergentz, 1970), and vegetative neural effects on the pulmonary vessels (Kinney, 1970; Ulmer, 1970). This assumption is supported by the fact that in all cases observed the 'fluid lung' pattern was a clear feature.

Table 3. *Pathogenetic factors of s.c. 'transfusion lung'*

Predisposing factors (shock, sepsis)
Capillary impairment
  ischaemia (hypoperfusion)
  vasoactive substances
  pulmonary vasoconstriction
Microembolization
DIC
Acute fluid overload
Blood denaturation
Graft vs. host reaction

Closely associated with this is the problem of *acute fluid overload* (Moore et al., 1969; Bachofen-Porchet and Bachofen, 1973), which some authors think is of prime importance.

Microembolization of the lung which results from aggregated blood components (Mosely and Doty, 1970, and others) can probably be controlled nowadays by adequate preventive measures. This factor is by no means as important as is often pretended. Veith et al. (1968) showed that bypassing the pulmonary filter by using intra-arterial retransfusion resulted in the same pulmonary changes as following intravenous transfusion.

The importance of *intravascular clotting* (DIC) (Bergentz, 1970) is extremely difficult to assess. Although a reduction in thrombocyte count is frequent in our patients, even in cases of uncomplicated haemorrhage, this may only be a dilution phenomenon (Miller, 1973). The complete syndrome of disseminated intravascular coagulation occurred once in this series. The fact that postmortem findings have been negative is not absolute counter-evidence, since Sandritter (1973) has been able to prove that adequate volume substitution may cause '*wash-out' of the microthrombi*.

The so-called 'homologous blood syndrome' is fortunately extremely rare. In the case described above it is possible that an acute immunological reaction caused the severe, acute pulmonary oedema and the secondary renal impairment (similar possibilities are suggested by Ward et al. (1968) and by Byrne and Dixon (1971)).

THERAPEUTIC ASPECTS

The following prophylactic and therapeutic recommendations may be made:

Economy in administering blood. This also applies to fresh blood, which is rich in immunocompetent cells. Clinical and experimental data show that extreme degrees of haemodilution can be tolerated so that it is no longer justifiable to replace blood with blood.

Moderate volume substitution. Pontoppidan et al. (1972) recommended that circulatory repletion in high-risk patients should be guided by the *urine volume*, whilst subnormal blood and venous pressure values were accepted, especially since rapid volume substitution may provoke the pulmonary syndrome.

Filtration of blood to avoid microembolism (Swank and Edwards, 1968, and others). This requirement seems fully justified in view of the fact that many disposable microfilters are available on the market.

Precise *supervision* by X-ray and blood gas analyses, as well as *early*, possibly prophylactic *use of a ventilator*. (Since more attention has been given to these cases, no serious complications have occurred.)

Continual *heparinization* with small doses (150–200 units, not more than 500 units/hr). Since only *early treatment* seems to be promising (Miller, 1973; Steinbereithner et al., 1972), and small doses do not cause haemorrhage, the surgical doubts and scruples should be overcome. In addition, heparin has a viscosity-reducing effect because lipoprotein lipase is activated (Ehrly, 1968) which reduces thrombocyte adhesiveness (Stremmel, 1973).

Drug-induced *reduction of the pulmonary vascular resistance* by sympatholytic drugs (Vogel et al., 1971). It should be noted that the increase in the pulmonary arterial pressure may otherwise be as much as 300% (Ulmer, 1970).

Prophylaxis by acetylsalicylic acid. Thorough experimental studies have shown that this substance not only checks the aggregation of platelets but influences the thrombocyte metabolism, preventing a 'release reaction'. With parenteral preparations now becoming available prophylactic use should be considered in all surgical operations involving large blood loss.

Careful *buffering*, because according to Collins (1969) severe acidosis is also injurious to the lung. Our own experience has shown that some care should be exercised, as an overdose may lead to pronounced transfusion alkalosis (Eisterer et al., 1968). Additional *corticoid* treatment may be given which must be supported by forced diuresis and aldosterone antagonists.

Moss and Saletta (1974) have recently suggested a way in which an overall solution to the problem may be found in the near future by stating: 'The era of whole-blood transfusions is probably coming to an end. Resuscitation may ideally be carried out with crossmatched red cells combined with asanguineous fluids.'

CONCLUSIONS

Among the numerous factors possibly causing 'acute respiratory distress syndrome in the adult' polytransfusion may play an important role. On analysis of cases treated in our ICU lung lesions could be demonstrated in about 40% of patients suffering from severe haemorrhage only. Since in animal experiments even autotransfusion led to functional pulmonary changes, polytransfusion not only acts as an 'additive factor' in lung impairment but may also *cause* pulmonary lesions of a minor degree. If this occurs at the same time as other factors injurious to the lung (e.g. shock, trauma, etc.) are operative, then severe pulmonary reaction might ensue. It is important to be constantly aware of this potential danger and to start appropriate therapeutic measures in time, possibly thus avoiding the full development of the lung's reaction.

REFERENCES

Bachofen-Porchet, M. and Bachofen, H. (1973): *Schweiz. med. Wschr.*, *103*, 1.

Bergentz, S. E. (1970): In: *Schock-Stoffwechselveränderungen und Therapie*, p. 419. Editors: Zimmermann and Staib. F. K. Schattauer Verlag, Stuttgart – New York.

Byrne, J. P. and Dixon, J. A. (1971): *Arch. Surg.*, *102*, 91.

Collins, J. A. (1969): *J. surg. Res.*, *9*, 685.

Ehrly, A. M. (1968): In: *Hemorrheology*, p. 773. Editor: Copley. Pergamon Press, London – Oxford – New York – Toronto.

Eisterer, H., Mayrhofer, O. and Steinbereithner, K. (1968): In: *Abstracts, 3rd Congress of the European Society for Experimental Surgery, Munich, 1968*, p. 7.

Gump, F. E., Mashima, Y. and Kinney, J. M. (1970): *Amer. J. Surg.*, *119*, 515.

Kinney, J. M. (1970): In: *Schock-Stoffwechselveränderungen und Therapie*, p. 89. Editors: Zimmerman and Staib. F. K. Schattauer Verlag, Stuttgart – New York.

Miller, R. D. (1973): *Anesthesiology*, *39*, 82.

Mittermayer, C., Pfrieme, B., Vogel, W. and Zimmermann, W. E. (1971): *Langenbecks Arch. klin. Chir.*, *329*, 664.

Mittermayer, C., Thomas, C., Rengholt, R., Schäfer, H., Vogel, W., Martinez, G. and Sandritter, W. (1973): *Klin. Wschr.*, *51*, 37.

Moore, F. D., Lyons, J. H., Pierce, E. C., Morgan, A. P., Drinker, P. A., MacArthur, J. D. and Dammin, G. J. (1969): *Post-traumatic Pulmonary Insufficiency*, Chapter 6. W. B. Saunders Co., Philadelphia, Pa.

Mosely, R. W. and Doty, D. B. (1970): *Amer. Surg.*, *171*, 329.

Moss, G. S. and Saletta, J. D. (1974): *New Engl. J. Med.*, *290*, 724.

Pontoppidan, H., Geffin, B. and Lowenstein, E. (1972): *New Engl. J. Med.*, *287*, 690.

Sandritter, W. (1973): *Klin. Wschr.*, *51*, 1.

Steinbereithner, K., Krenn, J. and Lechner, G. (1972): *Anästh. Informat.*, *13*, 321.

Steinbereithner, K., Krenn, J., Schertler, R., Vecsei, V. and Bauer, E. (1973): In: *Lungenveränderungen bei Langzeitbeatmung*, p. 52. Editors: Wiemers and Scholler. Georg Thieme Verlag, Stuttgart – Leipzig.

Stremmel, W. (1973): *Münch. med. Wschr.*, *115*, 416.

Swank, R. L. and Edwards, M. (1968): *Microvasc. Res.*, *1*, 15.

Tammisto, T. (1972): In: *Abstracts, Internat. Fortb. Kurs. Klin. Anästh., Homburg-Saar, 1972*, Ref. 4.

Ulmer, W. T. (1970): In: *Schock-Stoffwechselveränderungen und Therapie*, p. 93. Editors: Zimmermann and Staib. Schattauer Verlag, Stuttgart – New York.

Veith, F. J., Hagstrom, J. W. C., Panossian, A., Nehlsen, S. L. and Wilson, J. W. (1968): *Surgery*, *64*, 95.

Vogel, M., Mittermayer, C., Burchardi, H., Birzle, H. and Wiemers, K. (1971): *Arch. klin. Chir.*, *329*, 491.

Ward, H. N., Lipscomb, T. S. and Cowley, L. P. (1968): *Arch. int. Med.*, *122*, 362.

The role of the anaesthetist in the care of the patient with crushed chest

J. VAN DE WALLE and H. DELOOZ

Department of Anaesthesia and Intensive Care, and Department of Emergency Medicine,
Academisch Ziekenhuis St. Rafaël, Louvain, Belgium

When confronted with a patient suffering from severe chest injury, the task of the anaesthetist may be 3-fold: therapeutic, organizational and paedagogic.

His therapeutic role consists in resuscitation of the patient, evaluating his vital functions and supporting, or eventually supplementing, these functions should they fail. The vital functions that are principally involved in thoracic injury are the ventilation and the oxygenation of cells. These functions are accomplished by 2 physiological systems: respiration and circulation. A specific thoracic injury, or the general disturbance caused by the shock of the accident may, at various levels, damage respiration and circulation.

AIRWAY

As far as the airway is concerned obstruction may be caused by the tongue falling back if unconsciousness results from cerebral injury or cerebral hypoxia. Airway obstruction can also be caused by foreign bodies such as blood, vomitus or a dental prothesis, and further by direct injury of the larynx, the trachea or the bronchi.

As a free airway is essential for ventilation, it should be maintained patent at all times. Different methods can be used for this purpose:

1. Hyperextension of the head with elevation of the skin and forward displacement of the mandible is standard practice.

2. Use of an oropharyngeal or nasopharyngeal airway, bearing in mind the possibility of gagging and vomiting when consciousness is recovered. Forward lifting of the jaw and an oropharyngeal airway, although quite effective, can only be used for a brief period and is a short-term measure.

3. When the foregoing measures fail, or when respiratory support is likely to be necessary for more than several hours, it is best to proceed with endotrachael intubation. This is the most efficient and safe method for ensuring a patent airway.

4. When endotracheal intubation is difficult or impossible as in a severe laryngeal injury, or when a much longer period of respiratory support must be considered, for example more than 5 days, tracheostomy should be performed. This procedure is also mandatory in the presence of mediastinal emphysema.

VENTILATION

Ventilation of the lungs may be greatly impaired because of depression of the respiratory centre as a result of cerebral trauma, or through diminished breathing caused by pain or caused by paradoxical breathing and 'flail' chest. A less frequent cause of an increase of the dead-space is the diminished perfusion of the lung as a result of vascular trauma, lung injury or lung compression. Dead-space resulting from extensive atelectasis can be another factor contributing to alveolar hypoventilation but it is often hypovolaemia with diminished pulmonary perfusion, which is responsible for the increase in dead-space.

Respiratory depression and hypoventilation caused by 'flail' chest are best treated by controlled artificial ventilation. Assisted respiration, where the inspiratory phase is triggered by the patient's own inspiratory effort, is senseless in these circumstances since assisted ventilation calls for an intact respiratory centre and cannot provide the necessary thoracic splinting in the presence of an unstable chest-wall. Extensive atelectasis is another indication for artificial ventilation, but here one can choose between assisted or controlled ventilation. Hypovolaemia should be corrected as quickly as possible.

The presence of a pneumothorax should be excluded by X-ray examination before starting intermittent positive pressure ventilation. If a pneumo- or haemothorax is present, or when there is severe emphysema, pleural drainage should be instituted before resorting to positive pressure ventilation since a tension pneumothorax, which may be rapidly fatal, can easily occur.

OXYGENATION

Hypoxaemia of the arterial blood is caused by an increase of the physiological shunt. In the presence of thoracic injury, this is especially a consequence of atelectasis resulting from instability of the chest-wall, or as a consequence of pain, compression of the lung by a haemo- or pneumothorax or through direct lung-injury. Later, complicating factors such as shock, cerebral trauma or fractures of the lower limb may lead to progressive lung consolidation.

Arterial hypoxaemia must first be treated by the oxygen therapy. If 60% oxygen does not produce an arterial Po_2 of at least 70 mm Hg, artificial ventilation should be imposed, with all the precautions mentioned above.

OXYGEN TRANSPORT

Oxygen transport is especially dependent upon the haemoglobin concentration and cardiac output. Cardiac output is threatened by hypovolaemia but also by hypoxia and acidosis. Furthermore, direct cardiac injury may lead to cardiac tamponade. Usually, normal cardiac function will return provided that the haemoglobin concentration and the blood volume are normal and that acidosis and ventilation have been corrected. If this does not occur other complicating cardiac factors such as cardiac tamponade must be considered. If tamponade is present, thoracotomy and drainage should be performed after adequate tissue perfusion has been established.

DISCUSSION

In severe chest injury, all these resuscitative measures must generally be continued for several days and it seems unthinkable that the anaesthetist should alone be responsible for their performance. Therefore, the question should be considered as to whether it is good policy for the anaesthetist to leave the operating theatre to perform these tasks, particularly in the presence of a world-wide shortage of anaesthetists. This is certainly a controversial point, but it is our opinion that on account of this situation, it is the task of the anaesthetist to train and to teach others to accomplish these functions and to help organising the necessary infrastructure capable of nursing these patients adequately.

This infrastructure should comprise all the necessary facilities so that patient care may commence at the place of the accident and continue during transportation to the hospital. The facilities of a well-organised emergency department and of an intensive therapy unit are also required.

If the anaesthetist is not capable or willing to perform these supplementary tasks of organisation and teaching, he will still be confronted with these patients but he will be without these facilities. Nevertheless, as the specialist most proficient in resuscitation, the anaesthetist still has the clinical responsibility of the care for the patient with crushed chest.

The anaesthetists in our hospital have tried to organize this 3-fold task.

In the first place, the co-author of this report is responsible for an ambulance system supplying the necessary medical care at the place of the accident. An account of this 'advanced emergency care delivery system' is given elsewhere. The same co-author, together with the anaesthetic, surgical and medical staff, is responsible for the emergency department where all the equipment and personnel, necessary for urgent resuscitative measures, are available on a 24-hr basis. Our anaesthesia department is also in charge of the intensive therapy unit which was started at our hospital in 1965.

During the last 8 years, 34 patients (28 males and 6 females) with severe chest injury were nursed in this unit. Table 1 shows that the incidence in each age group is about equal, except for those under 10 and those above 70 years. There is no relation between the duration of artificial ventilation and age. Twenty-seven patients were artificially ventilated for, on an average, 12 days, with a minimum of 2 and a maximum of 41 days. Curarisation was necessary in 15 out of 27 patients at one time or another during artificial ventilation. Adequate sedation with morphine-like drugs was sufficient for the others. Thirty-one out of the 34 patients had other important injuries: multiple fractures, cerebral contusion or important abdominal injuries.

Table 1. *Chest injuries (1966–1973) – ICU, University Hospital St. Rafaël, Louvain*

Age distribution (yr)	No. of patients	No. of deaths
0–10	2	1
11–20	6	–
21–30	5	2
31–40	5	–
41–50	5	1
51–60	4	–
61–70	4	1
71 and over	3	1
Total	34	

The overall mortality was 6 out of 34 patients (17.6%). The mortality in the group which had artificial ventilation was 5 out of 27 (18.6%). One patient died from progressive pulmonary consolidation. The other deaths were, in part, due to associated neurological or circulatory complications.

CONCLUSION

The good results obtained and the experience gained at our hospital in caring for patients with severe chest injury confirm our opinion that the anaesthetist is, generally speaking, the person 'par excellence' to take up that 3-fold therapeutic, organisational and paedagogic task. His good example, his proficiency and the necessary propaganda, together with the help of the board of directors of the hospital, should make it possible to have the necessary facilities and personnel to fulfil them.

The effect of dextran 40 on capillary flow, transcapillary exchange and tissue acidosis of skeletal muscle in an experimental shock model in the dog*

LENNART K. APPELGREN, DAVID H. LEWIS and ALF K. MEDEGÅRD

Departments of Anaesthesia I and III and Surgery I,
University of Göteborg, Göteborg, Sweden

In the dog the procedure of laparotomy and exteriorisation of the intestines under slight stasis for 2–3 hr will produce a shock state with haemoconcentration, slight fall of arterial blood pressure, tachycardia, tachypnea and the peripheral signs of shock. During the progress of this experimental shock state – with its obvious relation to clinical conditions with splanchnic stasis – tissue acidosis builds up which is only partly revealed in the circulating blood. Indirect evidence for such a 'hidden' acidosis in this shock model is as follows:

1. The tissue acidosis was revealed in arterial blood after replacement of the intestines and closure of the abdomen and intravenous infusion of crystalloid or colloid solutions (Bergentz et al., 1969). Among the infusates used dextran 40 was found to be the most effective means of displaying the tissue acidosis.

2. There is a disturbed transcapillary exchange of water-soluble substances in this shock model, the dynamics of which have been studied by a local tissue clearance technique (Appelgren and Lewis, 1972). In the shock state there was a reduction of the tissue clearance of one of the isotopes used, $^{131}I^-$, suggesting a reduction of the available capillary surface area for exchange and an increased concentration gradient between the tissue and the regional venous blood of muscle tissue metabolites with a transcapillary diffusion similar to that of iodine. After treatment, including infusion of dextran 40, this disturbed transcapillary exchange was returned to control values suggesting in turn a normalization of the concentration gradient following a washout of the 'hidden' acidosis.

Thus there is reason to expect different hydrogen ion gradients between tissue and blood in the control state, in shock and after treatment with dextran 40. It is the aim of the present investigation to present preliminary results with this shock model on the direct measurement of pH in arterial, in regional venous blood from the hindlegs and in muscle tissue and to relate these measurements to the transcapillary exchange and capillary blood flow as measured by the local tissue clearance technique.

---

* The original investigations reported in this communication were supported by grants from the Swedish Medical Research Council (Grant No. B 74-40-X-660-10). The support from AB Pharmacia, Uppsala, Sweden, is also gratefully acknowledged.

MATERIAL AND METHODS

Mongrel dogs were anaesthetized with sodium thiopentone and ventilated mechanically with a constant volume/minute. Catheterization and recording procedures including radio-active measurements and calculations were as described in detail before (Appelgren and Lewis, 1972).

Tissue-blood exchange occurs by transcapillary diffusion from tissue to capillary blood and by perfusion by blood away from the tissue. Perfusion and diffusion can be estimated separately (Appelgren, 1972) by the tissue clearances of one perfusion-limited substance, ^{133}Xe (where the transcapillary diffusion is fast and the tissue clearance equal to capillary flow) and one diffusion-limited substance, ^{131}I$^-$ (where the transcapillary diffusion is the transport-limiting step, slower than perfusion and determined by the available capillary surface area for exchange). The simultaneous determination of tissue clearances of ^{133}Xe and ^{131}I$^-$ was made by measuring the residual gamma activities by an external detector in a small depot in skeletal muscle at different times. From the slopes of semilogarithmic plots of activities against time the fractional disappearance rates were calculated and multiplied by the distribution coefficients tissue/blood times 100 to give tissue clearances in ml/min/100 g tissue.

pH in blood was measured by the micro glass electrode of the Astrup gas tonometer (BMS 3 Blood Micro System, Radiometer, Copenhagen), on the exposed muscle fascial surface by a glass electrode of 2 mm o.d. and within the muscle tissue by a spherical glass electrode of 2 mm o.d. Both the tissue electrodes were according to Glinz (1970) (W. Möller Glasbläserei, Zürich). Electrometer Model 245 (Instrumentation Laboratories Inc., Lexington, Mass.). The glass electrodes were calibrated repeatedly against standard buffer solutions. The regional venous blood was taken through a small indwelling catheter from a deep femoral vein.

Recordings were made during a *control period*, after 2–3 hr of a *shock period* (induced by laporotomy, splenectomy and exteriorisation of the intestines) and after 1 and 2 hr of a *post-shock period* (starting with the return of the intestines, closure of the abdomen and infusion of dextran 40 in 10% solution (Rheomacrodex®, AB Pharmacia, Uppsala, Sweden) 1.5 g/kg within 15 min, followed by 0.5 g/kg/hr.

RESULTS AND COMMENTS

Figure 1 summarizes results of clearance measurements in control and shock and – in a conceptual form – their relation to the arterial, venous and tissue concentrations of the isotopes, the distribution of flow through the muscle microcirculation and the available area for transcapillary exchange. Mean pH values are also indicated (5 measurements in each period in 6 dogs). Note the definition of tissue clearance as the blood with its isotope content leaving the tissue per minute and 100 g tissue being virtually reduced in volume to the isotope concentration which is in equilibrium with the tissue (Fig. 1, middle panel). The upper limit of clearance at any given flow is therefore the flow, as is the case for ^{133}Xe. A lower clearance at any given flow indicates a lower concentration in the venous blood. This represents a less efficient transcapillary exchange and a larger tissue-venous blood gradient (see concentration diagram in middle left panel of Fig. 1).

There were practically no hydrogen ion gradients between blood and tissue in the control period. In the shock period there was a gradient with a hydrogen concentration 2–3 times higher in the tissues than in regional venous blood. Furthermore, as shown before (Appelgren and Lewis, 1972) there was a reduction of iodine clearance by 50–60% compared to control even with no reduction of xenon clearance. This would mean an increase of the tissue-blood gradient from 50% to 75–80% of the tissue concentration (cf. Fig. 1). According to Figure 1

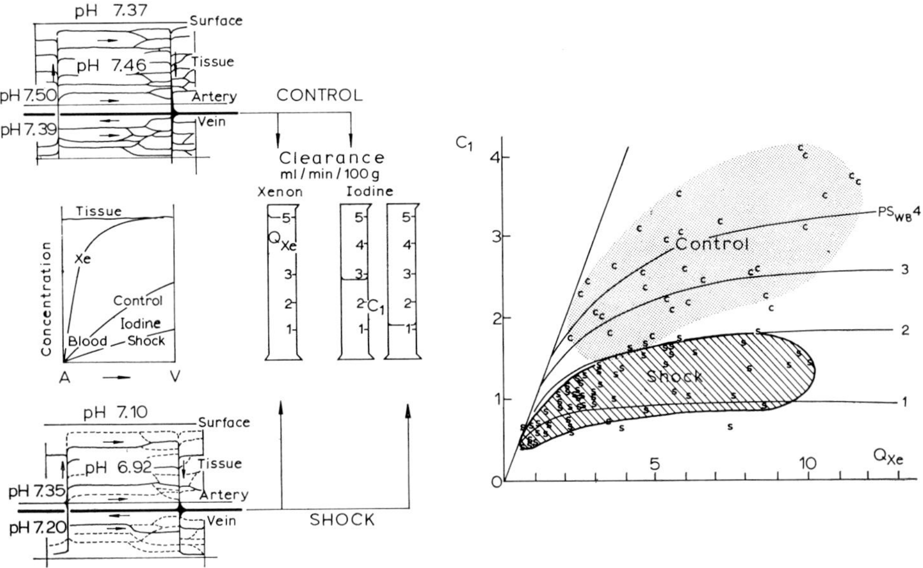

Fig. 1.   *Right panel: Relation between iodide clearance C_I and xenon clearance Q_{Xe} (ml/min/100 g) in skeletal muscle during control and shock. The areas indicated control and shock enclose experimental values in the two periods. The straight line is the line of identity between C_I and Q_{Xe}. For a discussion of the curved lines and PS_{WB}, see Appelgren and Lewis (1972). Left panel: A schematic picture of the capillary bed in skeletal muscle in control (upper panel) and shock (lower panel) and of the concentrations of the isotopes in tissue and in blood along the capillary from the arterial to the venous end (middle panel). (Note equilibrium for xenon at the venous end). pH-values (means of 6 dogs) for arterial and venous blood, on the muscle surface and in muscle tissue are given. Middle panel: Shows clearances conceptually as the volumes of blood of equilibrium concentration between tissue and blood, which have the same amount of substance as the venous outflow per minute per 100 g of tissue. Note that xenon clearance is equal to flow. The comparison of iodide clearances in control and shock is arbitrarily made at Q_{Xe} 5 ml/min/100 g.*

a lower blood flow should increase the passage time through the tissue allowing more time for equilibration between blood and tissue leading to a smaller concentration gradient. Thus it seems reasonable to assume that the increased pH-gradient between tissue and venous blood in shock is not solely dependent upon a very low flow in skeletal muscle but upon a disturbed transcapillary exchange as well.

In the post-shock period there was a normalization with a return of clearance data to the same area in the clearance diagram as in the control period (Appelgren and Lewis, 1972). The pH values in blood and tissue approached each other again, a time dependent process as illustrated by the figures from a typical experiment given in Table 1. With a slow saline

Table 1.   *pH values in blood and tissue at control and at post-shock period*

	pH: control	pH: shock (2 hr)	pH: post-shock period	
			(1 hr)	(2 hr)
Artery	7.28	7.31	7.37	7.37
Regional vein	7.23	7.21	7.31	7,33
Muscle tissue	7.23	6.88	7.12	7.30

infusion instead of dextran 40 there was no restitution within 1 hr and only a slight restitution towards normal within 2 hr.

Thus the tracer kinetic measurements and the pH measurements were at least semi-quantitatively consistent. However, tissue pH is in a complex way dependent not only on tissue-blood exchange of metabolites with acid-base properties but on the state of the buffer systems of blood and tissue and of the aerobic and anaerobic metabolic rates in the tissue. There is at present no exact way to transfer the tracer data of tissue-blood exchange to quantitative data of metabolic exchange and tissue concentrations of metabolites (Appelgren, 1972).

In conclusion, the present data have been produced in a simple and fairly standardized experimental shock model whose clinical counterpart – with an intestinal stasis of the extent and duration used here – should give no treatment problems. Our data clearly illustrate how quickly a disturbed tissue-blood exchange and a parallel tissue acidosis occur and how this can be properly normalized by haemodilution, which was produced by dextran 40 in the present investigation.

REFERENCES

Appelgren, K. L. (1972): *Acta physiol. scand., Suppl.*, 378.
Appelgren, K. L. and Lewis, D. H. (1972): *Europ. surg. Res. 4/3*, 46.
Bergentz, S.-E., Carlsten, A., Gelin, L.-E. and Krebs, J. (1969): *Ann. Surg., 169/2*, 227.
Glinz, W. (1970): *Langenbecks Arch. klin. Chir., 326/2*, 306.

The anaesthetist as an emergency physician: His tasks in the treatment of multiple injuries at the scene of the accident and during transportation

B. GORGASS, F. W. AHNEFELD, W. DICK and R. DÖLP

Department of Anaesthesiology, University of Ulm, Ulm, Federal Republic of Germany

THE TASKS OF THE EMERGENCY MEDICAL SERVICE

Reasons for the organization of emergency medical services

It is a classical postulate that life-threatened patients should be treated as much as possible at the scene by a physician who is familiar with the problems of emergency medicine.

Exact investigation of resuscitation methods, progress by specialization in medicine, and latest scientific findings about the pathophysiology of clinical death meanwhile require special equipment and organization of the medical service in order to keep the patient alive and to prevent severe injuries.

In the Federal Republic of Germany an increasing number of emergency medical services are being organized. Adequately qualified physicians, often anaesthetists, are sent with well-trained emergency medical technicians in specially equipped vehicles or helicopters to the person requiring help.

Principles of treatment

The medical team, the means of transportation and their medical equipments aim for rapid care of the emergency patient. An emergency patient is one whose vital functions and protective mechanisms, which guarantee an independent survival, are impaired by environmental influences or unexpected diseases.

Formerly the local treatment of injuries was often dominant, but now the first-aid measures are primarily designed to maintain, to secure, and to recover vital function. Classical first-aid, dressing and immobilization of fractures are of secondary importance.

THE MULTIPLE INJURY PATIENT

20% of all emergency patients are multiple injuries

The sequence of priorities is important, but some essential principles of trauma must be considered.

In Ulm more than 4,500 engagements have been carried out in about 3 years. About 20% of all engagements were concerned with the treatment of patients after traffic accidents, industrial accidents, and everyday accidents.

Particular medical problems of multiple injuries

The combination of general and local effects of trauma may result in irreversible damage if treatment is delayed or inappropriate. Blood loss of more than 3 l is frequent and if combined with hypoxia leads to renal and pulmonary damage and favours the development of fat embolism.

Pulmonary hypoxia or centrally-induced hypoventilation aggravate cerebral damage.

MEDICAL TREATMENT OF THE MULTIPLE INJURY PATIENT

Elementary diagnostics

Primarily the emergency physician starts with the elementary assessment of vital functions, breathing and cardiovascular system, in order to prevent or remove acute danger to life by quick and appropriate action.

Immediate therapy

(1) Selection of the most injured patients still with a chance of survival. (2) Clearing and maintaining the airway by an oro- or nasopharyngeal tube. (3) Endotracheal intubation in the case of bleeding in the pharynx or vomiting in patients with increasing unconsciousness, or because of the need for artificial ventilation, or aspiration. (4) Ventilation with a self-filling bag at the scene, and possibly with an anaesthesia apparatus in the MICU or helicopter. (5) Infusion of volume replacement solutions through a peripheral or central vein. (6) Cardiopulmonary resuscitation. (7) Occlusion of bleeding of big vessels by pressure bandage, clamping and tourniquet.

Detailed assessment

(1) Removal of clothes. (2) Clinical examination of the head: signs of head injury? (3) Palpation, compression, and auscultation of the thorax: marks of contusion? signs of rib fractures? pneumo/haemothorax? tracheal suction in case of a tentative diagnosis of a bronchial injury. (4) Palpation of the abdomen: marks of contusion? signs of an intraabdominal bleeding or other injuries? (5) Compression of the pelvic girdle, insertion of a catheter into the bladder in case of pelvic fractures or contusion marks in the kidney region. (6) Recording of the wounds and deformations of the limbs. Reposition in case of (*a*) an extreme disposition of the distal fragment, (*b*) lack of circulation distal to the fracture, (*c*) a risk of skin perforation. (7) Immobilisation by a vacuum mattress or a pneumatic splint. Extension by an extension splint only if considerable trauma during transportation can be expected, e.g. rescue in the mountains or under conditions of a disaster. (8) Simultaneous and continuous monitoring of the circulation and respiration at the scene and during transportation which should be performed as carefully as possible and only exceptionally by using the emergency signals under alert conditions. (9) Introduction of anaesthesia as a kind of shock treatment and to gain time after consultation with the clinic on the intercom. (10) Application of analgetics if the diagnostic procedures are completed.

Additional measures

The success of an emergency engagement often depends on additional measures which will be performed at the scene or during transportation.

(1) Especially in rural regions without a technical emergency service, which could be

alerted, the rescue of casualties sometimes presents technical problems. Therefore the emergency physician together with the emergency medical technicians has to initiate those technical rescue measures by simple means. (2) With respect to the conditions of the injuries the emergency physician will have to select the appropriate clinic, which is staffed and medically equipped for the definitive treatment of the patient. (3) Preliminary information to the clinic on the intercom or by telephone if an immediate operation or quick inter-disciplinary action will be necessary. (4) Blood for crossmatching and transport for it during transfer to the hospital. (5) Sufficient information to the colleagues in the clinic on a patient-transfer-record, about the event, the initial findings, the therapeutic techniques, and their effect.

CONCLUSION

The chances of survival for multiple injury patients are significantly improved by exact medical care and monitoring, at the scene, during transport, and by cooperation between the emergency service and the clinic. In addition practice as an emergency physician offers excellent possibilities for training and proficiency of anaesthetists.

Chapter XI

Problems in long-term respiratory treatment

How to avoid cross infections

RUDOLF FREY

Institute for Anesthesiology, University of Mainz, Mainz, Federal Republic of Germany

The first measure in order to avoid cross infection has to be taken by the *architect of the hospital* – he has to see to it that the ward for intensive therapy be provided with a sterile area where each patient is attended to in a separate Intensive Care Room. For visitors he must provide an outside gallery, say around the Intensive Care Room, so that the family of the patient has the possibility to get into contact with him through a window or, perhaps, by means of a telephone or microphone. In the case of patients wanting to have their private atmosphere maintained, it is possible to arrange a glass screen which is transparent only from the inside, while being opaque from outside.

The best example of separated sterile area and visitors' zone may be seen at the University Hospital of the Catholic University in Rome; there, Professor Corrado Manni has, with the assistance of some excellent architects, established a special reception room with adjacent Intensive Therapy Ward and Poison Control Center (fully computerized). In Germany such an Intensive Therapy Ward is about to be constructed with a gallery for visitors in the Protestant Hospital of Hattingen/Ruhr (the understanding for family sentiments seems to be especially developed in confessional hospitals).

The second important point in this connection is the question of *personnel* – each patient must have one nurse at his disposal, i.e. 3–4 nurses, taking into consideration a 6–8-hr shift service; e.g., for 10 intensive therapy beds with artificial ventilation units etc. 40 nurses are needed. The dress of physicians and nurses must be sterile (mouth protection cloth, protection for shoes, hair, etc.). Visitors are seldom allowed to enter the Intensive Therapy Ward (e.g. in case of a patient dying), but then they, too, have to wear sterile clothing.

Climatization – recirculation of air is not allowed. The air admitted must always be fresh, filtered, and sterilized; thus, the room is always kept in a state of slight overpressure, so that it is impossible for germs to enter from outside (e.g. by current of air). The fresh air should be aspirated from the roof, not from the floor, and in no case from a place near the animal test department as, unfortunately, it has been sometimes done with the result of several cases of tetanus. The fresh air must pass a filter which has to be changed often; if this is not done, the filter turns out to be a germ culture medium.

The *respirators* for artificial ventilation must be reliable and safe; here, too, the germ filters must be changed frequently. That part of the apparatus which is in contact with the patient (especially with the inspired and expired air) has repeatedly to be sterilized separately, the remaining parts must be disinfected. There is an important problem waiting for solution by designers and engineers – the future does not belong to the 'giant systems' which are meant to die out very soon, but to the easily manageable systems with small computerized parts, which can be handled without difficulty by physicians and nurses (not only by technicians) and – at least the parts in contact with the patient – be easily sterilized.

For air-moistening devices and supersonic vaporizers one should use only sterilized water; they, too, must be equipped with filters which have to be changed every second day;

at the very latest after one week or before being required for another patient.

One-way material should be used wherever and whenever possible – endotracheal tubes, suction catheters, needles, intravenous catheters etc. are to be used once only and then be thrown away.

Traumatization of the patients' tracheal mucosa must be avoided; today there are special suction catheters for the tracheobronchial tree. Ordinary urological catheters are much less suited for this purpose (in particular for repeated use or long-term ventilation). The special atraumatic tracheal suction catheters are to be preferred. (Manufacturers, among others, Rüsch, Rommelshause, or Sherwood/U.S.A.)

The application of *antibiotics* should be limited to *therapeutic indication* only – routine prophylaxis by means of antibiotics might easily result in a 'survival of germs with best resistance', which would mean a straightforward breeding of 'hospitalism'.

Nutritional problems associated with long-term respiratory care

KARL STEINBEREITHNER

Experimental Division, Department of Anaesthesiology,
University of Vienna, Vienna, Austria

In spite of growing insight into the importance of adequate nutrition in ICU patients, this problem has hardly ever been discussed in connection with prolonged ventilator treatment. This fact seems rather surprising as most of these patients are not able to eat because of their lesion or other reasons (unconsciousness, etc.). Recourse to artificial alimentation, therefore, becomes essential.

On the other hand, most patients requiring long-term respiratory support suffer from hypercatabolism of various degree – as can be deduced from Table 1, which gives some examples. Even when feeding via the normal routes becomes feasible, these increased metabolic demands cannot be met without additional administration of nutrients.

Table 1. *Additional calorie needs (% of normal) in ICU patients*

Elective operation (depending on severity)	15– 40
Fractures of long bones	25
Sepsis-peritonitis	20– 50
Burns	40–150
Cerebral trauma	60–130

(From: Brückner, 1969; Cuthbertson, 1970; Davies and Liljedahl, 1970; Kinney et al., 1970; Haider et al., 1975).

As, at least from the clinical point of view, no substantial difference exists between the composition of nutrient mixtures for enteral or parenteral use, this paper deals solely with components of parenteral nutrition. Personal experiences, gained in an ICU since 1963, are used in order to refrain from interfering too much in ardent discussions presently under way as to dosage, utilization, relative value and/or optimal relations of the various alimentary components. The disadvantage of this 'subjective' approach is counterbalanced, we hope, by a certain reality.

COMPONENTS OF PARENTERAL ALIMENTATION

Primary stress must be upon quantitative and qualitative substitution of the principal nutrients – proteins, carbohydrates, and fats, including the calorie requirements. This does not preclude the importance of many other 'essential' components (electrolytes, trace elements, vitamins, etc.), but these cannot be discussed in greater detail.

Proteins

Proteins, or more correctly, *amino acid solutions* are used since other possible protein substitutes (blood, plasma or albumin) are of restricted value in providing protein-building substances in severe protein catabolism. The majority of authors now agree that it is extremely difficult to cope with the increased protein breakdown in the severely diseased or traumatized patient. Positive nitrogen balances are scarcely obtainable especially in the so-called 'flow phase'. The cause of this catabolic reaction is poorly understood but there is little doubt that the resulting protein deficiency has particularly serious consequences for the ICU (ventilator) patient, which include disturbance of antibody formation, deficient blood regeneration, deficient cell formation, delay in wound healing, deficient synthesis of hormones and enzymes, a tendency to oedema, coagulation disorders, as well as muscular atrophy and decubitus. To counterbalance these severe losses, at least partly, large doses of amino acids have to be administered, the recommended amounts being about 2 g/kg/day (Dudrick et al., 1972*a*, *b*; Wretlind, 1972; Steinbereithner, 1972). Other calorific substances, especially carbohydrates, should be given liberally together with amino acids in order to facilitate their deposition in the muscles and to avoid gluconeogenetic deamination and utilization via another metabolic pathway (Munro, 1972; and others).

The decision regarding which one of the numerous preparations offered by the industry should be chosen, seems of minor importance at present. Critical comparative evaluation of modern crystalline mixtures (low in glycine) yields almost identical retention ratios; this is true also for balanced hydrolysates (e.g. Aminosol) reinvestigated recently (Tweedle et al., 1973; Abrahamson et al., 1972).

Taking into consideration the special situation of the ventilator patient, high protein and adequate calorie intake with concomitant low losses of muscular protein might be *the* critical factor during the *weaning period*. As Teres et al. (1973) have pointed out recently, the nutritional status is of extreme importance in the success of weaning manoeuvres in 'borderline' cases (irrespective of whether oxygen consumption increases on spontaneous ventilation or not; Berry and Pontoppidan, 1968).

Disregarding the rare cases of acute intolerance, metabolic acidosis frequently occurs, especially in children. This is mainly due to an elevated chloride content of some solutions (Heird et al., 1972; Dudrick et al., 1972*a*, *b*); careful daily balance and/or prophylactic buffering are indispensable especially in ventilator cases in order to prevent unfavourable lung effects. Although no absolute contraindications are accepted nowadays, some caution must be recommended in severe liver impairment and/or renal insufficiency (danger of extrarenal azotaemia; Dudrick et al., 1970). If renal impairment is superimposed on respiratory insufficiency, preparations of essential amino acids should be used exclusively; these can influence favourably the course and duration of acute anuric episodes (Abel et al., 1973).

Carbohydrates

Glucose is still the sugar used mainly, being *the* essential nutrient for various organs (e.g. brain), since it reduces endogenous glucose production (Kinney et al., 1970) from other sources and decreases the elevated glucagon output in catabolic states (Felig, 1972). The dangers of *hyperosmolar coma* and severe *hyperglycaemia* (Dudrick et al., 1970) may be avoided by 'titrating' with insulin (Hinton et al., 1971) which also encourages the utilization of amino acids and fat. The mechanism by which glucose and insulin ameliorate protein catabolism after severe shock and trauma (impaired glucose utilization and insulin resistance) is still poorly understood (Kinney et al., 1970; Gump et al., 1973).

Laevulose (*fructose*) which is partly metabolized independent of insulin, replenishes liver glycogen and may promote assimilation of infused amino acids better than glucose. Since it might provoke severe lactacidosis in higher doses, concentrated solutions should be used with caution (Coats, 1972; and others).

The value of various sugar-alcohols (pentitols) or *sugar-exchanging substances* (sorbitol, xylitol, etc.) is still highly disputed, because of deleterious side-effects of long-term administration (Coats, 1972; Thomas et al., 1972). Experience with balanced fructose-glucose-xylitol (LGX) mixtures is still inadequate. Although the carbohydrate problem has still some aspects which need elucidation, these substances play a very important role as a source of calories.

The recommended proportions (according to the literature) of a 'balanced' parenteral nutrition regime comprise (Table 2) 50% carbohydrates. Some authors (e.g. Beisbarth et al., 1973) prefer a somewhat different pattern, with 65% carbohydrates at the expense of fat; other groups (Coats, 1972), try to increase the calorie supply by adding larger amounts of *alcohol*; reports of further experience are awaited.

Table 2. *Recommended proportions of components in parenteral nutrition (% of total calories)*

Amino acids	20
Fat emulsions	30
Carbohydrates	50

A new aspect of great importance concerning high carbohydrate feeding has been observed by Hansen et al. (1972). These authors demonstrated that administration of about 13–17 MJ (3,000–4,000 kcal), 93% carbohydrates, to volunteers with chronic altitude hypoxia led to a significant increase in arterial oxygen tension (and saturation). These data are in agreement with results found by other groups as well as ourselves (Table 3). These investigations were made during spontaneous respiration; the same effect may be seen during artificial ventilation. The fact that raising the RQ to near 1.0 by carbohydrates does increase alveolar oxygen tension, provided $P_{A_{CO_2}}$ is kept constant, can readily be derived from the alveolar air equation. As AaD_{O_2} does not change substantially this carbohydrate effect would yield a proportionally large rise in $P_{A_{O_2}}$ especially under hypoxic conditions.

Table 3. *P_{O_2} response to carbohydrate ingestion*

Authors (condition)	P_{O_2} increase (Torr)
Hansen et al., 1972 (Carbohydrate diet, altitude hypoxia)	6.6 ± 3.7
Steinbereithner and Wagner, 1967 (Fructose infusion, cerebral trauma, hypoxia)	7.2 ± 5.9
Saltzman and Salzano, 1971 (Carbohydrate diet, sea level)	9.3 ± 2.6
Eckman et al., 1945 (Carbohydrate-rich diet, altitude hypoxia)	4.3

Fat emulsions

Considering the increased calorie requirements in severely disabled ICU patients it seems practically impossible to cope with these without administering fat which provides about 9 kcal/g parenterally. When discussing the inherent problems of this nutrient, one always has to take into account the great biological differences between various emulsions (e.g. tolerance, toxicity, elimination rate, uptake by RES, effects on coagulation, etc., Wretlind, 1972); results obtained with different preparations, therefore, cannot be compared.

In burns (Liljedahl, 1972) and after surgery and trauma (Fegetter et al., 1974) fat has been shown to be the main source of energy. Liberal amounts of fat, together with amino acids and carbohydrates, are therefore given as early as possible to our most severe cases. It may be added, that our own group (Haider et al., in press) found ROs around 0.7–0.8 in cerebral trauma, which again suggests that fat is being utilized primarily. Beisbarth et al. (1973) are opposed to this view for various reasons (e.g. unsatisfactory influence on N-losses, poor utilization after trauma, etc.). Carlson (1970) demonstrated a decrease of endogenous FFA mobilization in severe stress by giving fat. This is another indication of fat being a very 'effective energy substrate' (Gump et al., 1973).

Sundström et al. (1973) found reduction in pulmonary diffusing capacity (D_{LCO}, mean decrease 15%) after infusion of intralipid which subsided to normal after 45 min. The authors stress this finding to be of no clinical significance in healthy subjects, but quote a number of papers where (with cotton-seed emulsions!) similar, but more severe effects including hypoxaemia were reported. Steinbereithner and Wagner (1967) did not observe a decrease in arterial P_{O_2} following administration of intralipid in high doses (up to 1.8 g/kg/hr) to chronically hypoxic patients (Table 4) (see also Somerkamp and Giesübel, 1968), and therefore consider this effect to be negligible.

Table 4. *Influence of rapid infusion of parenteral nutrients on arterial P_{O_2}*

Diagnosis	Parenteral nutrient solution (sequence)	Before	After	30	120
		infusion		min later	
Cerebral contusion	Fat	88	88	93	84
	Fructose	85	87	90	80
Cerebral contusion	Fructose	49	49	–	56
	Fat	49	–	59	62
Cerebral contusion	Fat	78	77	84	–
	Fructose	83	93	–	–
Cerebral contusion	Fat	70	69	69	74
	Fructose	Patient expired			
Cerebral contusion	Fructose	53	67	58	58
	Fat	68	69	68	73
Epidural haematoma	Fructose	68	78	83	88
	Fat	73	68	58	58

On the other hand, certain precautions should not be omitted – in spite of the still rather hypothetical role of the lung in fat resorption (Gigon et al., 1966), fat should be withheld in protracted shock and/or fat embolism (even if only suspected), since in these cases, according to own experience, stability of emulsions in the circulation as well as clearing function might be considerably impaired.

CLINICAL PROBLEMS

As to *technique*, it should again be stressed that the nutritional components must always be given *simultaneously*. Any successive administration means wastage and unsatisfactory utilization. Numerous investigations, on the other hand, have proven that a *balanced* intravenous nutrition regime can keep patients in good nutritional state for a relatively long period. This, of course, presupposes that artificial alimentation is started promptly since, in a state of starvation, regeneration and anabolic repair are difficult to achieve.

On the other hand, certain *hazards* of this nutritional regime cannot be denied; for example, infection, hypophosphataemia, massive solute diuresis, and deficiency in vitamins and trace minerals, especially Mg and Zn (Moore and Brennan, 1972). Whereas these hazards may be avoided by careful balance and substitution and close observation, the one real danger is *fluid overload*. Severe catabolism requires sometimes extreme calorie supply ('hyperalimentation' in its true sense); even after careful monitoring of intake and output, overhydration, partly due to metabolic (oxidative) water production, might ensue. The importance of a most careful fluid balance, especially in ventilator cases, supported by diuretics, if required, cannot be overstressed.

Finally, a new therapeutic concept should be mentioned briefly: Cuthbertson's group (Tilstone and Cuthbertson, 1970) as well as Liljedahl (1972) and others, have demonstrated that by raising the environmental temperature above the 'thermoneutral zone' (30–32° C), hypermetabolism, nitrogen and weight loss are, to a great extent, prevented after trauma or in burns. This procedure is now a routine in most modern burn units and might also prove to be valuable in other catabolic states. In this case, not only would therapeutic attitudes have to change but also reconstruction of most of our ICUs would be necessary.

CONCLUSION

In long-term respiratory care, nutritional aspects have frequently been considered to be of minor relevance. Since most of our patients suffer from severe hypercatabolism of various origins, the importance of adequate parenteral (and enteral) alimentation regime as soon as possible should no longer be neglected. Some inherent hazards of this therapy might be of special concern in ventilator cases, particularly fluid overload. These drawbacks, however, are more than outweighed by provision of an improved metabolic status at the commencement of rehabilitation and convalescence.

REFERENCES

Abel, R. M., Beck, C. H., Abott, W. M., Ryan, J. A., Barnett, G. O. and Fischer, J. E. (1973): *New Engl. J. Med., 288*, 695.

Abrahamsson, L., Hakelius, L., Hambraeus, L., Öhlin, S. E. and Hjorth, G. (1972): *Acta chir. scand., 138*, 645.

Beisbarth, H., Krämer, K. and Schultis, K. (1973): *Z. Ernährungsw., 12*, 121.

Berry, P. R. and Pontoppidan, H. (1968): *Anesthesiology, 29*, 177.

Brückner, J. B. (1969): *Zbl. Chir., 94*, 46.

Carlson, L. A. (1970): In: *Energy Metabolism in Trauma*, p. 155. Editors: R. Porter and J. Knight. J. and A. Churchill Ltd., London.

Coats, D. A. (1972): In: *Parenteral Nutrition*, p. 152. Editor: A. W. Wilkinson. Churchill-Livingstone, Edinburgh – London.

Cutbertson, D. P. (1972): In: *Parenteral Nutrition*, p. 4. Editor: A. W. Wilkinson. Churchill-Livingstone, Edinburgh – London.

Davies, J. W. L. and Liljedahl, S. O. (1970): In: *Energy Metabolism in Trauma*, p. 59. Editors: R. Porter and J. Knight. J. and A. Churchill Ltd., London.

Dudrick, S. J., MacFadyen, B. V., Van Buren, C. T., Ruberg, R. L. and Maynard, A. T. (1972a): *Ann. Surg., 176*, 259.

Dudrick, S. J., Steiger, E. and Long, J. M. (1970): *Surgery, 68*, 180.

Dudrick, S. J., Steiger, E., Long, J. M., Roberg, R. L., Allen, T. R., Vars, H. M. and Rhoads, J. E.

502   *K. Steinbereithner*

(1972*b*): In: *Parenteral Nutrition*, p. 222. Editor: A. W. Wilkinson. Churchill-Livingstone, Edinburgh – London.

Eckman, M., Barach, B., Fox, C. A., Rumsey Jr., C. C. and Barach, A. L. (1945): *Aviation Med., 16*, 328.

Fegetter, J. G. W., Tweedle, D. E. F. and Wright, P. D. (1974): *Europ. surg. Res., 6 (Suppl. 1)*, 74.

Felig, P. (1972): *New Engl. J. Med., 287*, 982.

Gigon, J. P., Enderlin, F. and Scheidegger, S. (1966): *Schweiz. med. Wschr., 96*, 71.

Gump, F. E., Long, C. L., Wong, M. and Kinney, J. M. (1973): *Surg. Gynec. Obstet., 136*, 611.

Haider, W. et al. (1975): In press.

Hansen, J. E., Hartley, L. H. and Hogan, R. P. (1972): *J. appl. Physiol., 33*, 441.

Heird, W. C., Dell, R. B., Driscoll, J. M., Grebin, B. and Winters, R. W. (1972): *New Engl. J. Med., 287*, 943.

Hinton, P., Allison, S. P., Littlejohn, S. and Lloyd, J. (1971): *Lancet, 1*, 767.

Kinney, J. L., Long, C. L. and Duke, J. H. (1970): In: *Energy Metabolism and Trauma*, p. 103. Editors: R. Porter and J. Knight. J. and A. Churchill Ltd., London.

Liljedahl, S. O. (1972): In: *Parenteral Nutrition*, p. 208. Editor: A. W. Wilkinson. Churchill-Livingstone, Edinburgh – London.

Moore, F. D. and Brennan, M. F. (1972): *New Engl. J. Med., 287*, 862.

Munro, H. N. (1972): In: *Parenteral Nutrition*, p. 34. Editor: A. W. Wilkinson. Churchill-Livingstone, Edinburgh – London.

Saltzman, J. A. and Salzano, J. V. (1971): *J. appl. Physiol., 30*, 228.

Sommerkamp, H. and Giesübel, W. (1968): *Fortschr. Med., 86*, 251.

Steinbereithner, K. (1972): *Méd. et Hyg. (Genève), 30*, 1675.

Steinbereithner, K. and Wagner, O. (1967): *Agressology, 8*, 389.

Sundström, G., Zauner, C. W. and Arborelius, M. (1973): *J. appl. Physiol., 34*, 816.

Teres, D., Roizen, M. F. and Bushnell, L. S. (1973): *Anesthesiology, 39*, 656.

Thomas, D. W., Edwards, J. B., Gilligan, J. E., Lawrence, J. R. and Edwards, R. G. (1972): *Med. J. Aust., 1*, 1238.

Tilstone, W. J. and Cuthbertson, D. P. (1970): In: *Energy Metabolism in Trauma*, p. 43. Editors: R. Porter and J. Knight. J. and A. Churchill Ltd., London.

Tweedle, D. E. F., Spivey, J. and Johnston, I. D. A. (1973): *Metabolism, 22*, 173.

Wretlind, A. (1972): In: *Parenterale Ernährung*, p. 9. Editors: G. Hartman and H. Berger. Hans Huber Verlag, Bern – Stuttgart.

Long-term ventilation and cerebral circulation

EMERIC GORDON

Department of Neuroanaesthesia, Karolinska Hospital, Stockholm, Sweden

REGULATION OF CEREBRAL BLOOD FLOW DURING NORMAL AND PATHOLOGICAL CONDITIONS

The vital influence of ventilation on intracranial conditions was recognized early by neurosurgeons (White et al., 1942). Knowledge about the delicate mechanisms which regulate cerebral metabolism, circulation and intracranial pressure in which ventilation plays a decisive role is, on the other hand, more recent. The experimental and clinical studies about this subject were presented in several international symposia during the past decade (Ingvar et al., 1968; Luyendijk, 1968; Brock et al., 1969; Brock and Dietz, 1972; Fieschi, 1972), and for more detailed information the reader is referred to these publications. Normal cerebral circulation has well-developed *autoregulation*, which means that the resistance in the cerebral vasculature is regulated so that the flow remains unchanged with changing perfusion pressure (which is defined generally as the difference between mean arterial pressure and the intracranial pressure). This autoregulation fails when the perfusion pressure is less than 30–40 mm Hg, and results in a decrease of cerebral blood flow. The mechanisms reponsible for autoregulation are not yet fully clarified, but it is evident that the arterial carbon dioxide tension (Pa_{CO_2}) and the pH of cerebral extracellular fluid and cerebrospinal fluid (CSF) has a powerful effect on the cerebrovascular resistance (CVR), and as such has a decisive role in the regulation of cerebral blood flow (CBF). An increased Pa_{CO_2} and a low pH thus result in cerebral vasodilatation and a significantly increased CBF, and vice versa, a fall of Pa_{CO_2} and an increased pH leads to cerebral vasoconstriction and lowered blood flow.

Hypoxia and/or hypercarbia strongly affect the normal autoregulation described above (Harper, 1965). These pathological circumstances jeopardize cerebral metabolism and lead very rapidly to intracerebral lactacidosis which results in a more or less pronounced vasoparalysis. CBF will then be pressure-passive, i.e. cerebral oxygenation will be fully dependent upon the arterial blood pressure. The vasoparalysis results also in focal hyperaemia (luxury perfusion, Lassen, 1966) which persists for a long time after the normalisation of the cerebral metabolism (Häggendal et al., 1970).

The changes described above can develop globally in the whole brain, as after a cardiac standstill, but most often they are seen focally or multi-focally, as after head injury, brain tumour or subarachnoid haemorrhage. These focal lesions result in a strongly heterogeneous blood flow. Ventilatory disturbances with hypercarbia accentuate these changes and favour the development of cerebral oedema with increasing intracranial pressure. Oedema is further enhanced by an increased capillary permeability which aggravates the tissue acidosis. These complex mechanisms result in an extension of the lesion to areas of the brain, which were not primarily affected. A vicious cycle is generated, which, if no adequate treatment is instituted, leads finally to a rise in intracranial pressure up to systemic pressure levels until total cerebral circulatory standstill and brain death ensue.

The inhomogeneity of the cerebral blood flow is also the reason for paradoxical flow reactions, the intracerebral steal syndrome (Symon, 1968, 1969). The general feature of the steal syndrome is that measures which normally enhance the CBF (increased arterial pressure or carbon-dioxide tension), will increase flow only in the undamaged regions, while in the damaged areas, where a more or less complete vasoparalysis has already taken place with resultant non-reaction to pressure changes, the circulation is further compromised since blood flow is diverted to normally reacting and healthy areas of the brain. An additional and devastating effect of this paradoxical reaction is the focal increase of tissue pressure by the higher flow in the undamaged areas which again jeopardizes flow in damaged regions by compressing its capillaries.

The control of ventilation undoubtedly has a beneficial effect on these pathological, and many times, life-threatening situations (Gordon, 1971; Rossanda et al., 1966, 1972). Controlled hyperventilation counteracts tissue acidosis both by elevating CSF pH, and by the 'countersteal' phenomenon which implies that vasoconstriction in normally reacting brain tissue reduces intracranial pressure. This pressure reduction enables at least some of the compressed capillaries to reopen and the reestablishment of a better perfusion in the previously ischaemic areas.

CLINICAL APPLICATIONS OF CONTROLLED VENTILATION

This effect of controlled hyperventilation is the basis of this treatment of patients with severe head injuries. This subject has been discussed in detail elsewhere *(This Volume*, p. 784), and therefore will not be considered here.

During recent years, however, the indications of long-term controlled ventilation have been largely extended to other neurosurgical patients. Clinical evidence is now steadily accumulating which shows that patients after elective neurosurgery benefit greatly from ventilator treatment in the postoperative period, especially if the operation was long and technically difficult. Tables 1 and 2 show the number of patients treated postoperatively in our clinic with controlled ventilation classified according to diagnosis.

Table 1. *Number of patients treated with controlled ventilation during 1970–1973*

	1970	1971	1972	1973	Total
Subarachnoid bleedings	12	13	19	19	63
Brain tumours	10	19	10	21	60
Brain injuries	16	24	25	27	92
Intracranial bleedings	11	13	10	30	64
Others	7	7	7	4	25
Total	56	76	71	101	304

Table 2. *Diagnosis and period of treatment of patients with controlled ventilation during 1970–1973*

Diagnosis	No. of patients	Mean time and range (days)	
Subarachnoid bleedings	63	7	(1–21)
Brain tumours	60	6	(1–47)
Brain injuries	92	13	(1–86)
Intracranial bleedings	64	7	(1–36)
Others	25	8	(2–35)
Total	304		

Postoperative ventilator treatment is largely facilitated by the neuroleptanaesthesia now currently used during operations in our clinic. The effect of these drugs is simply not reversed at the end of the operation, but rather increased by small incremental doses of 1 mg of phenoperidine when necessary. The great advantage of this drug is that while the patient is absolutely comfortable and not disturbed by the endotracheal tube or the respirator, he or she is still conscious and the assessment of the neurological status is not hampered. Communication with the patient during ventilator treatment is easy, but despite this it is surprising that after the termination of this treatment, the patient is frequently amnesic for this period.

The length of postoperative ventilator treatment varies depending on the clinical state of the patient. Controlled ventilation can often be abandoned on the first postoperative day and therefore tracheostomy is seldom necessary. Should the patient's condition require more prolonged ventilator treatment either because of unconsciousness or persistent respiratory or airway troubles, this treatment is continued through a tracheostomy.

Our results of long-term ventilator treatment are good but, because of the relatively small number of cases, statistical evidence of an improved postoperative course is not yet available. However, from the experience of the individual cases there is no doubt that the postoperative ventilator treatment has influenced the clinical outcome favourably.

The disadvantages of long-term ventilator treatment in neurosurgical patients are practically negligible and the indications for this treatment are broad. The only limiting factor is, alas, the need for increased personnel and resources in the intensive care unit. On the other hand, when it is clear and proved to be significant by statistical analysis, that a great number of patients can be saved, and severe postoperative complications avoided or reduced by the routine use of long-term postoperative respiratory care, no major elective surgery should be undertaken, without the safeguard of adequate postoperative resources.

REFERENCES

Brock, M. and Dietz, H. (Eds.) (1972): *Intracranial Pressure.* Springer-Verlag, Berlin – Göttingen – Heidelberg – New York.

Brock, M., Fieschi, C., Ingvar, D. H., Lassen, N. A. and Schürmann, K. (Eds.) (1969): *Cerebral Blood Flow.* Springer-Verlag, Berlin – Göttingen – Heidelberg – New York.

Fieschi, C. (Ed.) (1972): *Cerebral Blood Flow and Intracranial Pressure.* S. Karger, Basel – New York – Berlin.

Gordon, E. (1971): *Acta anaesth. scand., 15,* 193.

Häggendal, E., Löfgren, J., Nilsson, N. J. and Zwetnow, N. N. (1970): *Acta physiol. scand., 79,* 272.

Harper, A. M. (1965): *Brit. J. Anaesth., 37,* 225.

Ingvar, D. H., Lassen, N. A., Siesjö, B. K. and Skinhøj, E. (Eds.) (1968): *Scand. J. clin. Lab. Invest., Suppl. 102.*

Lassen, N. A. (1966): *Lancet, 2,* 113.

Luyendijk, W. (Ed.) (1968): *Cerebral Circulation. Progress in Brain Research.* Elsevier Publ. Co., Amsterdam – London – New York.

Rossanda, M., Boselli, L., Castelli, A., Corona, C., Ermino, F., Mardini, M., Porta, M. and Villa, C. (1972): *Europ. Neurol., 8,* 169.

Rossanda, M., Di Giugno, G., Corona, S., Bettinazzi, N. and Mangione, G. (1966): *Acta anaesth. scand., 23/3,* 766.

Symon, L. (1968): *Scand. J. clin. Lab. Invest., 102/13: A.*

Symon, L. (1969): In: *Cerebral Circulation. Vol. 7,* Chapter 3, pp. 597–615. Editor: D. G. McDowall. International Anesthesiology Clinics.

White, J. C., Verlot, M., Selverstone, B. and Beecher, H. K. (1942): *Arch. Surg., 44,* 1.

New methods of control and treatment of flail chest

V. CHULIA CAMPOS, J. ORTUNO BORJA and V. LOPEZ MERINO

Departments of Anesthesiology and Medicine, University Hospital,
Faculty of Medicine, Valencia, Spain

All trauma to the thorax provokes injuries which involve the costal wall and the subjacent pulmonary parenchyma. It is known that the extent of the injury is determined by the age, and the degree of opening or closure of the glottis at the time of the accident. It is possible for a youth with an elastic thorax to have widespread injuries of the pulmonary parenchyma without any costal injuries. In the adult, both in frontal and lateral injury, a costal fracture appears at the point of maximum impact, and an area of fracture in continuity with the thoracic wall which loses its anatomic connections with the result that normal physiology is altered.

Paradoxical movements of the chest wall occur during spontaneous respiration in lateral and anterolateral thoracic injuries. This is claimed to result in a pendulum movement of air (Milic-Emili and Henderson, 1966), and therefore to important disturbances in distribution of gases (Cara et al., 1963).

Air passes from one part of the lung to the other during expiration without exchange with fresh gas. This ventilatory inefficiency may also result in secretions passing from one lung to the other. X-ray screening can be used to demonstrate this effect. This is a mechanical problem and it must be reversed in order to avoid ventilatory failure and its complications. For this reason we have directed our study to its solution.

Borelli in 1674, in his treatise 'Motu Animalium', described the mechanism which permits insufflation of air as a result of the contraction of the respiratory muscles. In 1953 Cara clarified the physical aspects of the mechanics of ventilation. This study sought a simple means of control and measurement of the flail chest in relation to the distribution of inspired gas.

Classifications of flail chest are usually clinical; this discussion is in 4 parts: (a) mechanical; (b) radiological; (c) hemodynamic; and (d) biological.

MECHANICAL

If 2 pneumatic waistcoats are put around the chest of a healthy subject separately for each hemithorax, it is possible to record the pressure changes by means of pressure transducers. An approximate estimate of the parallel variations in intrapulmonary volume can be made.

In the normal subject the curves from each side have the same shape (Fig. 1), but in the injured chest with rib flattening the curves are completely different. The curves obtained also show shifts in time with differences in expansion of each hemithorax, which are related to the degree of mobility of the flail chest and the respiratory frequency. If one respiratory cycle of 360° is considered, the angle of the shift can easily be calculated. Figure 2 shows how the internal pneumatic stabilization leads in many cases to a total correction of the angle of shift; nevertheless, in other cases, this angle is not totally corrected. This means that a certain degree of paradoxical movement remains.

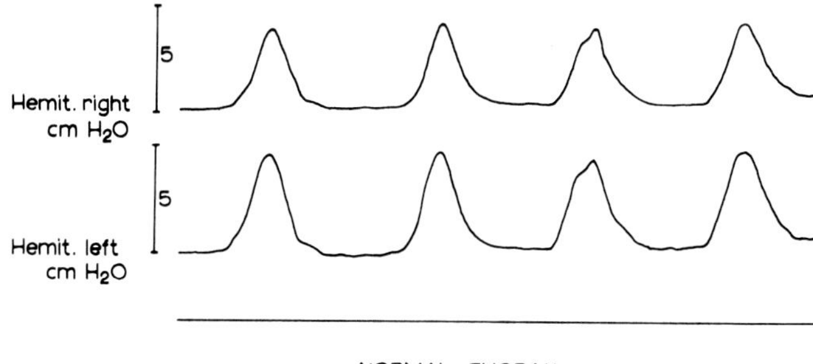

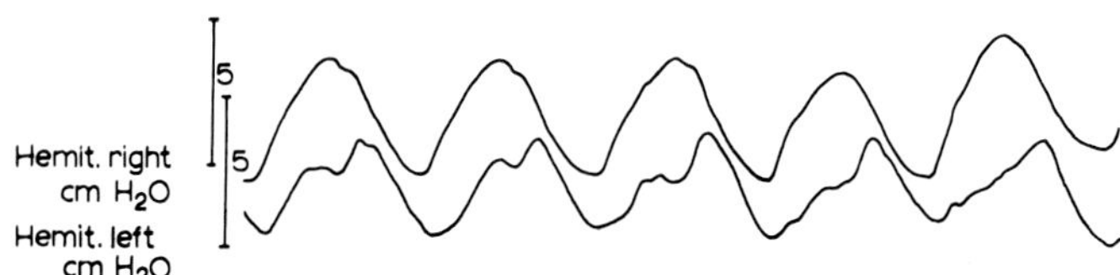

Fig. 1. *Plethysmographic records from each hemithorax using pneumatic waistcoats.*

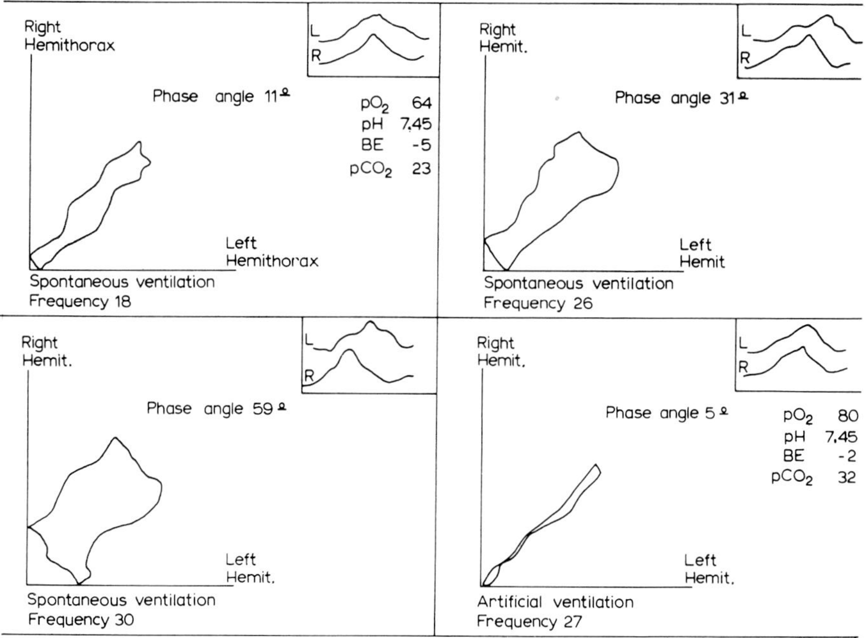

Fig. 2. *Record of plethysmographic curves of a patient with a flail chest. In the top right corner are registered right and left hemithorax curves. The increase in the phase angle during spontaneous ventilation is related with increased frequency, and its total correction with artificial ventilation.*

RADIOLOGICAL

Radiological study enables the degree of approximation or separation of the costal fragments to be assessed in relation to the treatment. At the beginning the internal pneumatic stabilization, due to the increase in functional residual capacity, separation of the fractured ribs is encouraged which delays repair (Fig. 3).

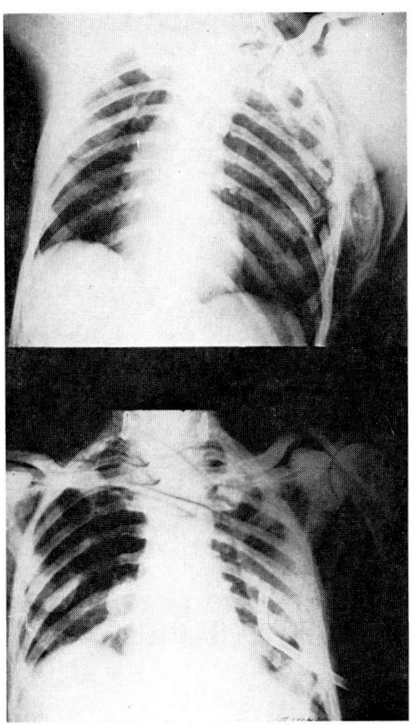

Fig. 3.   *Radiological aspects of a patient with homolateral flail chest. In the top figure the separation of the ribs produced by artificial ventilation with positive end-expiratory pressure (PEEP) can be seen. In the lower figure this has been corrected with elastic bandages.*

HEMODYNAMIC

The effects of artificial ventilation on the systemic and pulmonary circulation have been studied in patients with thoracic injuries.

BIOLOGICAL

Repeated acid base measurement (Po_2, Pco_2, and base excess), can be used to assess ventilatory efficiency, and is a measure of the efficiency of this treatment.

Since the time constants of each side of the thorax (compliance x-resistance) are not always identical, internal pneumatic stabilization does not always eliminate uneven distribution.

This phenomenon has already been observed (Milic-Emili and Henderson, 1966) in different parts of the normal lung, and it is likely to be more obvious in a patient with a flail chest. From the radiological study the costal separation which homolateral hyper-inflation provokes is obvious and this is exaggerated when delayed expiration is used (PEEP).

Some workers have suggested separate inflation of the 2 lungs with 2 ventilators using a modified Carlens tube. This method is inconvenient because the tube must remain in situ for a minimum of 15 or 20 days and it is difficult to obtain even distribution in both lungs.

Elastic bandages have been applied to the injured side during artificial ventilation which allows effective counter pressure to be applied when the vertebral column and the sternum

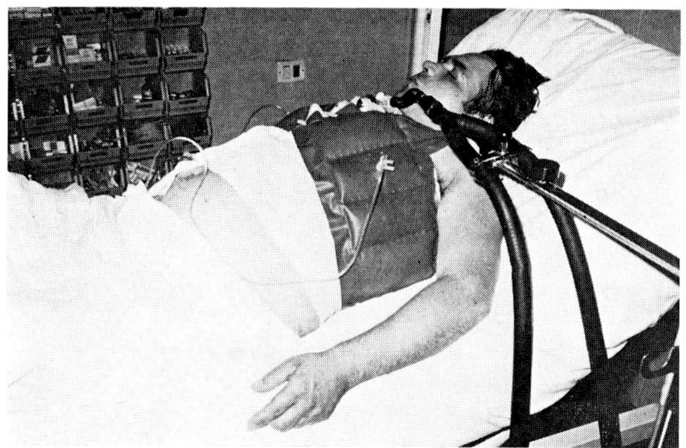

Fig. 4.   *A patient with a flail chest showing the pneumatic waistcoats (dark) and the   astic bandages (white).*

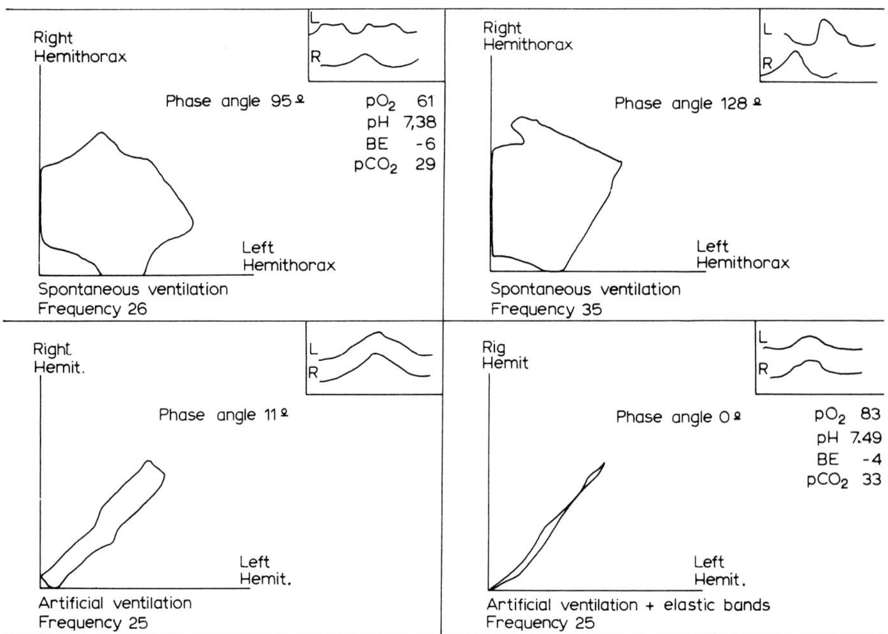

Fig. 5.   *Changes in the plethysmographic curves of one patient with a flail chest. In the top right of each chart are the recorded pressure changes over the right and left hemithorax. The phase angle is determined from an xy plot of these in spontaneous ventilation and in artificial ventilation with elastic bandages. The phase angle is reduced during artificial ventilation with elastic bandages.*

are used as fixed points. The loss of elasticity of the thoracic wall is thus compensated (Fig. 4). The time constants of both hemithoraces are the same and homolateral hyper-inflation is avoided. The efficiency of this treatment is assessed by the same criteria of evaluation of flail chest (angle of shift 0°, union of costal fragments radiologically, and the absence of hemodynamic changes and acid-base measurements) (Fig. 5).

Figure 3 shows the good approximation of the ribs obtained with this method.

Finally, from the orthopedic point of view, the elastic bandages combined with the internal stabilization present enables mobilization of the costovertebral joints by passive physiotherapy. The functional results are improved because the thoracic cage heals more normally.

REFERENCES

Cara, M. (1953): *Le Poumon*, *5*, 371.

Cara, M., Echecter, E. and Poisvert, M. (1963): In: *Proceedings, XIII Congres d'Anesthésiologie* Masson et Cie, Paris.

Maloney, J. V. (1961): *J. thorac. cardiovasc. Surg.*, *41*, 291.

Milic-Emili, J. and Henderson, A. M. (1966): *J. appl. Physiol.*, *21*, 749.

The use of an inspiratory resistance to compensate for variations in patient pulmonary resistance

G. W. BURTON

Department of Anaesthetics, Bristol Royal Infirmary, Bristol, United Kingdom

During intermittent positive pressure ventilation of a patient, the inspiratory flow pattern is dependent partly upon the pressures generated by a mechanical ventilator or by the hand of the anaesthetist, and partly upon the resistances and compliances within the patient and ventilator system.

Changes in air flow and airway pressures are to some extent analogous to those seen in an electrical circuit. Thus, in a respiratory model, the air flow rate is directly proportional to the pressure difference and is inversely related to the total airway resistance (cf. Ohm's Law). Also, as found in an electrical circuit, if we place two airway resistances in series, the overall resistance is equal to the sum of the two taken separately. However, as may be seen from Figure 1, airway resistances differ from electrical resistances in that their magnitude is usually dependent upon the air flow rate; increased values are seen at the higher flow rates and are caused by increasing turbulence within the air stream.

In an electrical circuit, the charging or discharging of a condenser follows an exponential function, governed by the time constant, which is the product of resistance and capacitance. In a lung the rate of filling or emptying is similarly governed by its time constant, in this case the product of resistance and compliance. Figures 2 and 3 show the changes in air flow rate and alveolar pressure, within an artificial lung, associated with the sudden release of an intrapulmonary pressure of 50 cm H_2O. It may be seen from Figure 2 that an increase in airway resistance, when accompanied by a rise in the time constant, produced a slowing of the rate of emptying of the lung. However, when the compliance was also varied, so that a uniform time constant was maintained, the emptying of the artificial lung followed the same pattern (Fig. 3).

During artificial ventilation, the same physical principles apply. The inflation of a lung is dependent upon both the applied pressure and the time constant.

If we look at the performance of a conventional volume pre-set, time-cycled ventilator, we find that changes in patient resistance markedly affect both the inspiratory and expiratory flow rates. Figure 4 shows recordings of the air flow rates and pressures measured within an artificial lung (alveolar pressure) and within the airways and the ventilator. The compliance remained constant at 50 ml/cm H_2O and the airway resistance was varied from 5–50 cm H_2O/l/sec. It may be seen that raising the patient resistance markedly affected the inspiratory flow rate, despite the associated rise in airway pressure.

The expiratory patterns are similar to those seen in Figure 2, a raised airway resistance leading to a lowering of the expiratory flow rate. If the pressure within the lung does not return to atmospheric before the beginning of the next inspiratory phase we have, in effect, a raised functional residual capacity.

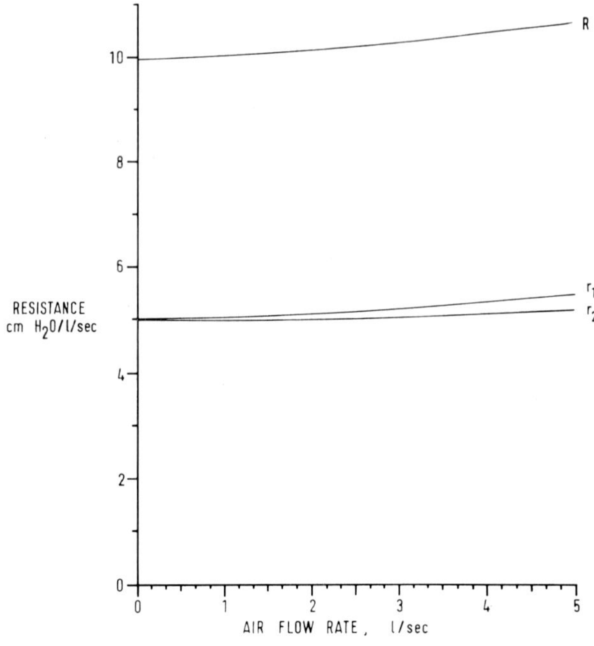

Fig. 1.   *Note that with increasing flow velocity there is a rise in resistance associated with increasing turbulence. (r_1 = resistance of stainless steel woven wire gauze of 59 mm diam., r_2 = resistance of stainless steel woven wire gauze of 84.5 mm diam., R = resistance of r_1 and r_2 in series).*

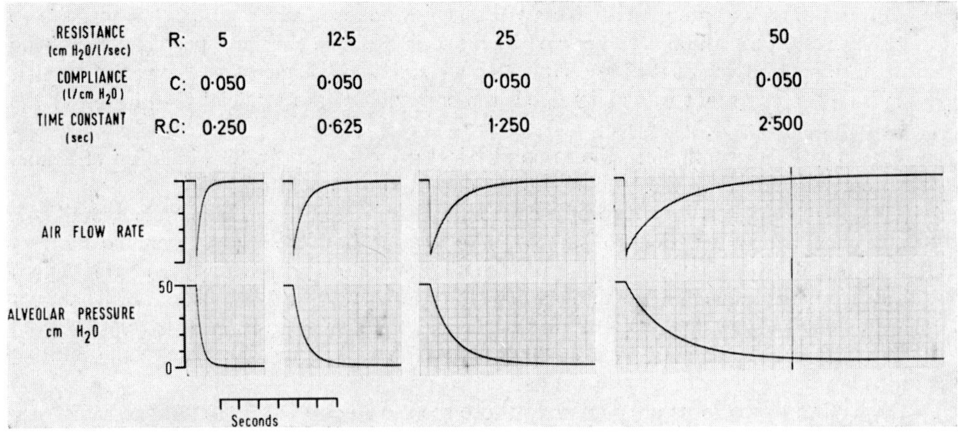

Fig. 2.   *An artificial lung was inflated to a pressure of 50 cm H_2O and the recordings show the effects of sudden release of this pressure. The alveolar pressure indicates the pressure measured within the lung. The resistance component and time constant were varied and the compliance maintained at a constant level.*

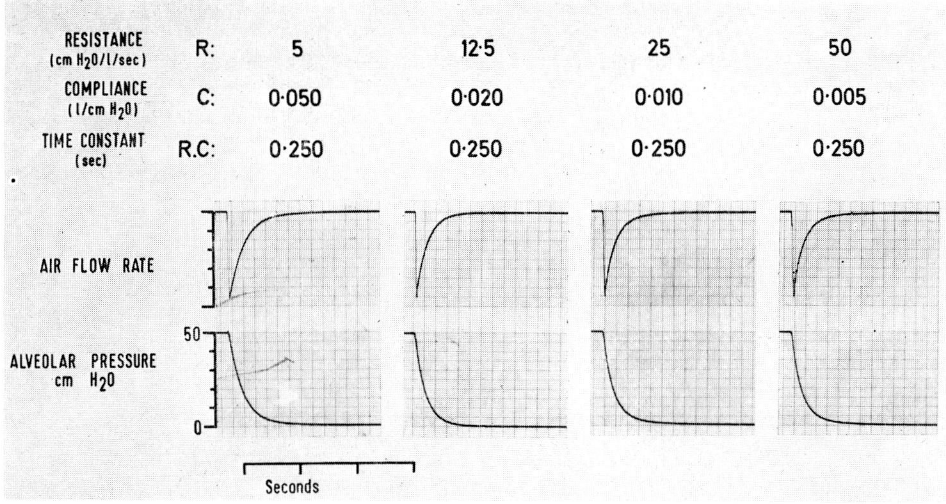

Fig. 3.   *Recordings as in Figure 2, except that the compliance was varied in order to maintain a uniform time constant.*

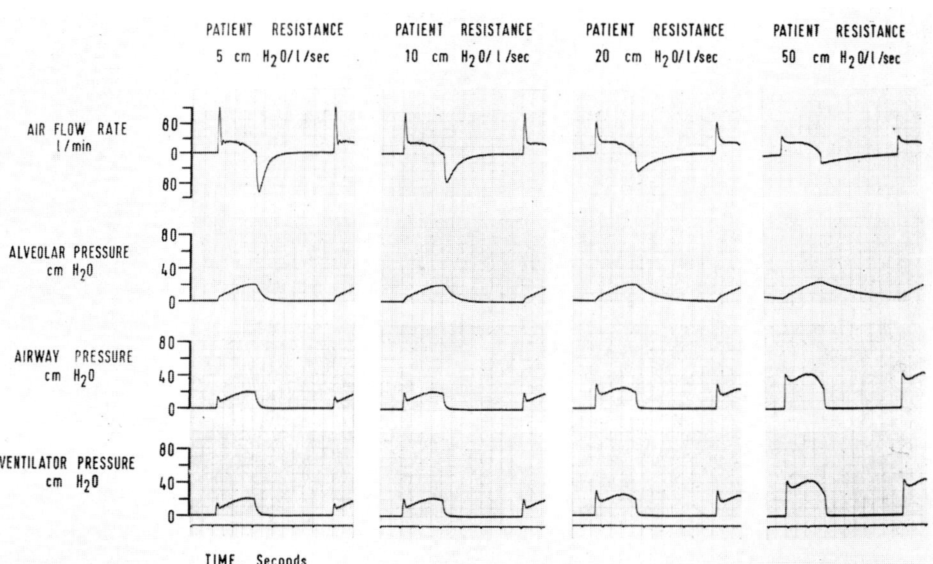

Fig. 4.   *Effects of changes in patient resistance – Cape Mark II ventilator. (Tidal volume = 1000 ml; frequency = 10/min; compliance = 50 ml/cm H₂O). Air flow rate: upward deflection = inspiration; downward deflection = expiration. Alveolar pressure: pressure measured within the artificial lung. Airway pressure: pressure measured in airway immediately before the lung. Ventilator pressure: pressure measured at inspiratory port of ventilator.*

However, during inspiration it is possible to preserve the flow pattern provided that changes in the time constant of the system are avoided. Although it may not be possible to control the patient's resistance or compliance, we can put a variable resistance, or flow control, in the inspiratory line in series with the patient resistance (Fig. 5). By setting this variable resistance at the appropriate level, we are then able to regulate the overall time constant. Provided that the ventilator is capable of generating adequate pressure, it is possible to compensate for very large variations in patient resistance or compliance and to control the inspiratory flow to the lung.

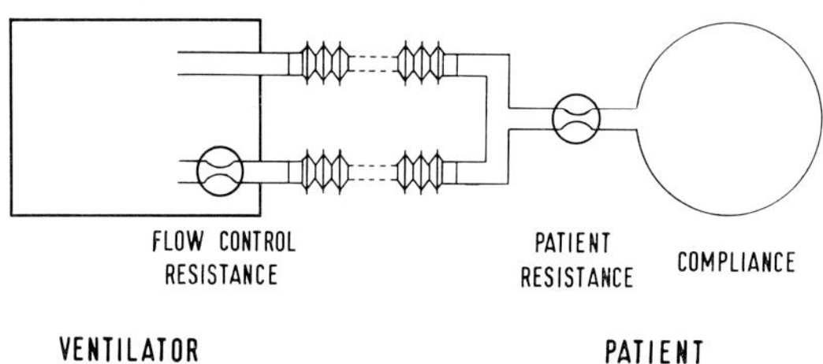

Fig. 5.   *Schematic diagram showing use of a flow control resistance in the inspiratory line. Time constant = (patient resistance + apparatus resistance) × compliance.*

Figure 6 shows recordings made using a ventilator system which incorporates a variable resistance, or flow control, in the inspiratory line within the ventilator. It may be seen that the inspiratory flow pattern remained essentially unchanged despite a 10-fold increase in patient resistance.

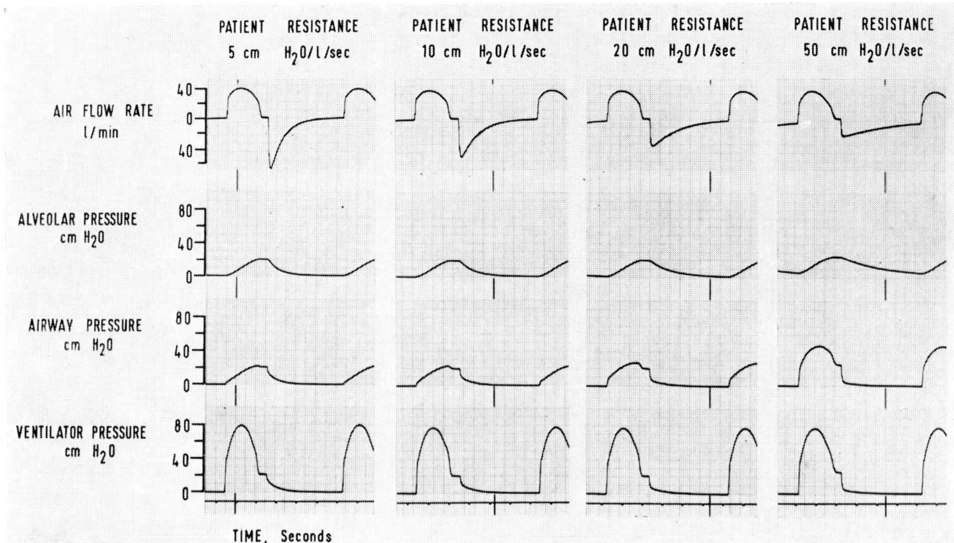

Fig. 6.   *Effects of changes in patient resistance – Cape Bristol ventilator. (Tidal volume = 1000 ml; frequency = 10/min; compliance = 50 ml/cm H2O). Air flow rate: upward deflection = inspiration; downward deflection = expiration. Alveolar pressure: pressure measured within the artificial lung. Airway pressure: pressure measured in airway immediately before the flow control resistance.*

If we look at the distribution of pressure gradients we find that when the patient resistance was 5 cm $H_2O/l/sec$, the alveolar and the airway pressures were very similar, there being only a small pressure gradient across the patient resistance. The lower two traces show large differences in pressure, caused by the relatively large pressure gradient across the flow control resistance. When the patient resistance was raised the resistance of the flow control was decreased, thereby reducing the pressure gradient across it and thus compensating for the raised gradient across the patient resistance.

Use of this flow control resistance not only enables compensation for the variations in airway resistance found in different patients and differing types of tubing or connections in the circuit, but it can also be used to compensate for temporary changes in patient resistance or compliance. One of the problems found during artificial ventilation is the person who fights the ventilator. This calls for immediate action – he may require aspiration of secretions or further sedation, etc. We have found that as a temporary measure, the increase in patient resistance can be overcome by decreasing the resistance of the flow control, thereby maintaining adequate ventilation over the time during which sedative drugs are taking effect. One may then be able to avoid the hasty use of excessive dosages of depressant drugs or the unnecessary paralysis of a patient.

SUMMARY

1. In a ventilator-patient system, changes in pressure and air flow are analogous to those seen in an electrical circuit.

2. The inflation and deflation of a lung are governed not only by the ventilator pressure but also by the time constant of the system – that is the product of total airway resistance and compliance.

3. The inclusion of a variable resistance, or flow control, within the inspiratory line, allows control of the time constant. This therefore enables an inspiratory flow pattern to be maintained over a wide range of variations in patient resistance and compliance.

Clinical experience with a new modular Engström Care System Ventilator

OLOF NORLANDER, MARTIN H-SON HOLMDAHL, GEORG MATELL,
SVEN OLOFSSON and KARL-JOHAN WESTERHOLM

Department of Anaesthesiology, Karolinska Sjukhuset, Stockholm;
Department of Anaesthesiology, University Hospital, Uppsala;
Department of Medical Intensive Care, Södersjukhuset, Stockholm; and
Jungner Instrument Co., Div. LKB Medical, Stockholm, Sweden

Almost 25 years ago the Engström principle for the treatment of respiratory insufficiency was introduced into clinical use (Engström, 1963). Since that time this method has gained universal acceptance and without exaggeration hundreds of thousands of patients have benefitted from this method.

What is the Engström method? Volume-controlled ventilation with an increasing, accelerating inspiratory gas flow with an automatic pressure adaptation to the impedance of the lungs. The patient system is indirectly separated from the driving system which has sufficient power to overcome even the most difficult pathological changes in the lungs. The flow pressure adaptation creates an inspiratory plateau phase which assures the best possible gas distribution. Several modifications of the original ventilator have been made in accordance with medical improvements generally and especially with regard to sterility. The autoclavable respirator 300 was a pioneer in this field. Although these ventilators are extremely useful, there is a need for further simplification of techniques, especially regarding handling by personnel, safety aspects and size of apparatus.

This new Engström Care System Ventilator has solved these problems. It should be regarded as a care system as it satisfies many needs associated with ventilatory control during anaesthesia and intensive care. This new modular ventilator is based on modern technology using pneumatic and electronic components. The ventilator consists of 4 modules each one with a different function. Each module can easily be detached and replaced for service if necessary. The 4 different modules are:

A ventilator part, which uses compressed air as driving force. The characteristics of the ventilator are similar to the original Engström accelerating flow but has in addition possibilities for infinite variation of I/E ratio and frequency from 10–60. It also permits a high inspiratory force for patients with low compliance and high resistance. It may be used in a trigger mode. The ventilator part is equipped with a series of alarm functions in order to facilitate the clinical handling of the patients.

The gas mixtures to the ventilator are fed through a completely new gas mixer, which allows mixing of air and oxygen and oxygen and nitrous oxide with one single control function for mixing percentage and gas flow.

The mixer has an improved accuracy over current flow meters. The technical design of this gas mixer is described elsewhere.

The 3rd and 4th modules of the ventilator consist of a new type of gas meter, which measures volumes independent of the composition and humidity of gases. The displaced expired volumes are measured according to a new concept and the signals derived from the gas meter are electronically processed in the 4th module which displays tidal volume and minute volumes. The accuracy of the volume meter is high and the meter can be used for tidal volumes of 20 ml up to more than one litre. Built into the ventilator is an ultrasonic humidifier with a dosage control which ensures humidification up to 100% according to the clinical situation. All modules which are in contact with the patient's airway can be heat-sterilized. The ventilator is small and compact and can be easily used both in operating rooms and in intensive care wards.

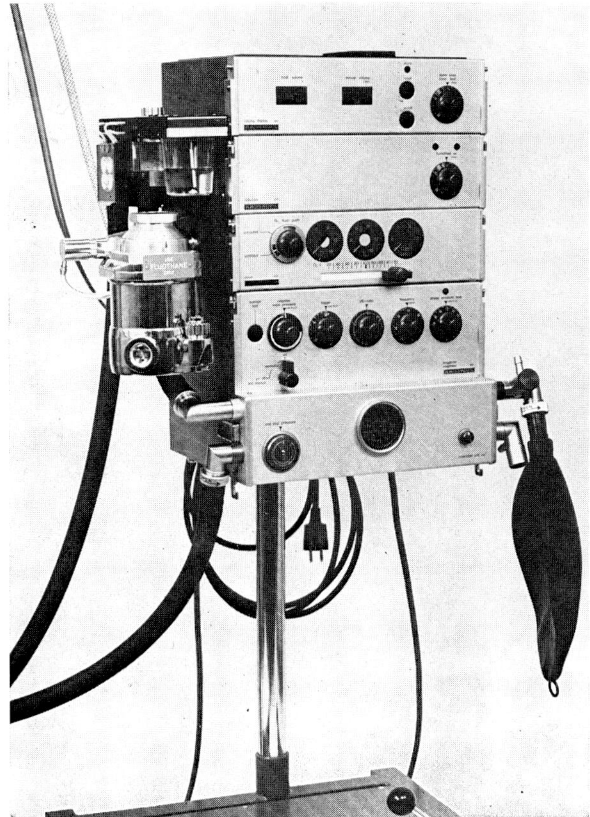

Fig. 1. *The Engström Care System ECS 2000. The modules from top to bottom are: volume display, nebulizer, mixer, and ventilator with patient unit.*

This ventilator has been used for a long trial period in 3 different hospitals – Karolinska Hospital, Stockholm, University Hospital, Uppsala and Southern Hospital, Stockholm. The ventilator has been used in connection with anaesthesia for open-heart surgery for small children and adults, in intensive care for all types of ventilatory failure including asthma, poisoning, chest trauma etc. It has also been used postoperatively in cardiovascular and thoracic surgery. A series of measurements have been compared with the commonly used Engström respirator 300. Studies on the efficiency of ventilation, the effect of various I/E ratios and the expiratory frequencies etc., have been made and the results indicate a clinical performance of the highest quality. It has been used in patients for up to 16 weeks, for poisoning, status asthmaticus, chronic bronchoconstrictive lung disease, ischaemic heart disease (infarction patients), meningitis etc. The synchronization problems sometimes associated with conventional respiratory treatment seem to be minimized due to the specific flow characteristics of the system.

REFERENCE

Engström, C.-G. (1963): *Acta anaesth. scand., Suppl. 13.*

Long-term ventilation with PEEP and the alteration of lung and haemodynamic functions

H. REINEKE, P. LOTZ, R. DÖLP and W. DICK

Department of Anaesthesiology, Centre of Interdisciplinary Medical Units,
University of Ulm, Ulm, Federal Republic of Germany

Clinical experience shows that intermittent positive pressure ventilation can impair lung function (Benzer, 1969; Regele, 1967). The question of aetiology is still open; the ventilation itself, dose of oxygen (Morgan, 1968), the original disease or secondary infection are possible (Kühn and Pichotka, 1948). As a final therapeutic measure an end-expiratory pressure may be used when lung function remains impaired (Gregory et al., 1971).

It is the aim of this report to examine the hypothesis that there is a causal relationship between changes in lung function and intermittent positive pressure ventilation and that an end-expiratory pressure reduces the alterations in lung function qualitatively.

Ten healthy pigs were ventilated for 48 hr with intermittent positive pressure or with a raised end-expiratory pressure. The compliance decreased slightly but not significantly in Group B (Fig. 1).

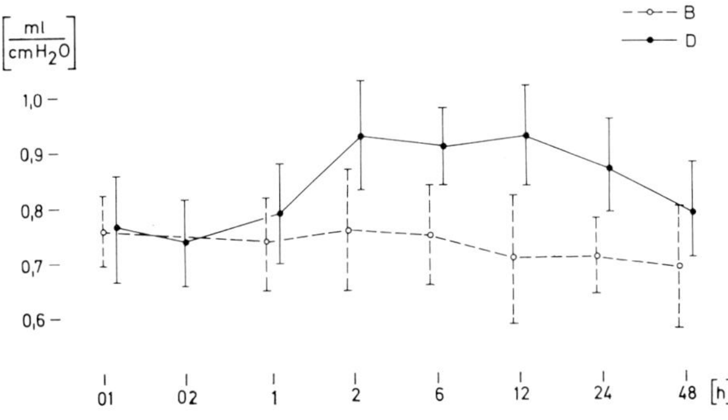

Fig. 1. *Compliance alteration during the 48 hr of continuous ventilation. The point 01 represents the start of the test in Groups B and D. 02 is the first test value directly after the increase of the end-expiratory pressure in Group D.*

In Group D at first the compliance improved significantly above the initial value but it decreased at the end of the period. The final values differ significantly ($p = 5\%$).

At first the proportion V_D/V_T (dead space/tidal volume) remained constant in both groups between the 12th and 48th hr, but later it increased but not significantly (Fig. 2). The Aa_{DO_2} (alveolar-arterial DO_2) as an expression of disturbed ventilation/perfusion matching increased in Group B. The values at the beginning and at the end of the test

"

were similar in Group D. The changes in venous admixture ($Q_S/Q_T\%$) are identical in both groups and increase at the end of the test in both groups (Fig. 3). The cardiac output decreases continuously in Group B until the 24th hr without further significant change (Fig. 4). At first the positively increased end-expiratory pressure reduces the cardiac output. The cardiac output recovers owing to the compensatory mechanisms of the organism so that the final values of the 2 groups do not differ. The pulmonary resistance changes inversely to the changes in cardiac output (Fig. 5).

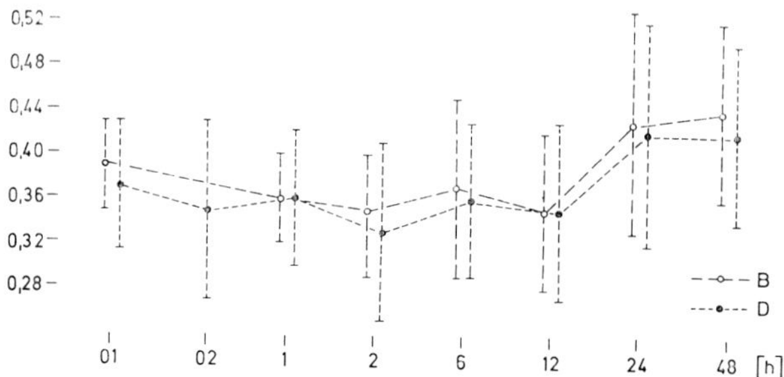

Fig. 2.   *V_D/V_T (dead space/tidal volume) during 48 hr.*

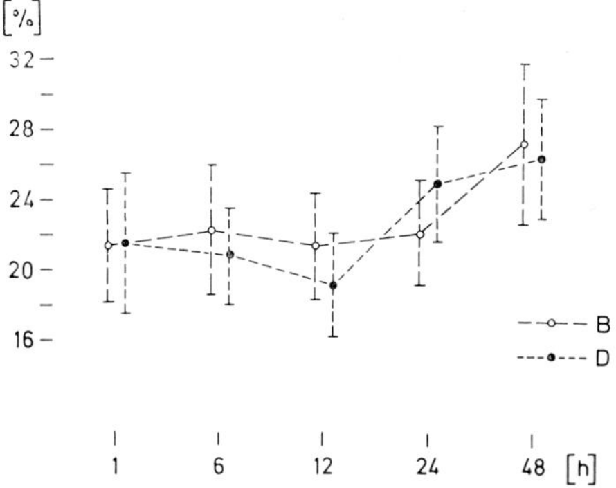

Fig. 3.   *Alterations of Q_S/Q_T (shunt blood volume) in the lungs during 48 hr.*

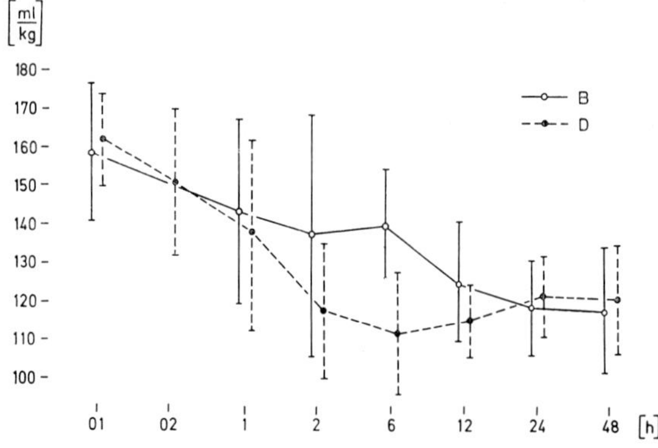

Fig. 4.   *Alterations of cardiac output (ml/min/kg) during the 48 hr of continuous ventilation.*

In contrast to the cardiac output the final values of pulmonary resistance differ significantly at the 5% level. The value of the arterial resistance increases in both groups independent of the technique of ventilation. The increase is continuous and does not differ even qualitatively in both groups.

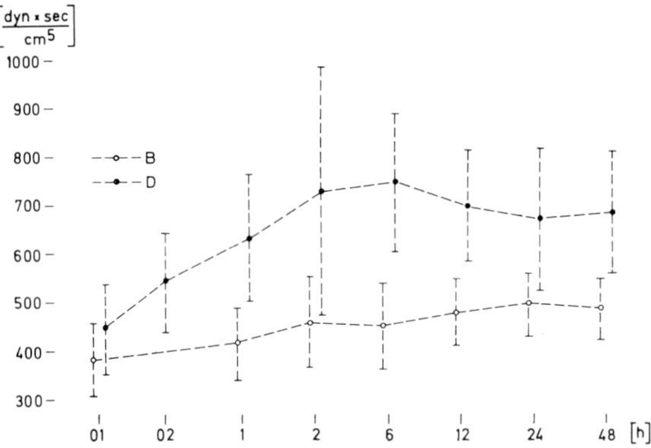

Fig. 5.   *Pulmonary resistance during the 48 hr of continuous ventilation.*

In both series there are found interstitial and alveolar oedema limited to certain alveolar regions. In Group D these are considerably scarcer than in Group B. This is also correlated with the lung weight/kg bodyweight. Isolated hyaline membranes appear as a consequence of mechanical compression of the alveolar oedema by excessive pressure. The tendency to form oedema may be due to reduced formation of lymph or rather to a relative overproduction during artificial ventilation.

The alterations following raised end-expiratory pressure are quantitatively less developed. The tendency toward oedema production is reduced. The cardiac output is affected initially but it adjusts itself. The results imply that ventilation with increased end-expiratory pressure is applicable not only as final treatment but also as an initial method of treatment provided that there is normovolaemia and good cardiac function.

REFERENCES

Benzer, H. (1969): In: *Anaesthesiologie und Wiederbelebung*, p. 38. Springer-Verlag, Berlin – Heidelberg – New York.

Gregory, G. A., Kitterman, J. A., Phibbs, R. H., Tooley, W. H. and Hamilton, W. K. (1971): *New Engl. J. Med.*, *284*, 1333.

Kühn, H. A. and Pichotka, J. (1948): *Naunyn-Schmiedeberg's Arch. exp. Path. Pharmak.*, *205*, 667.

Morgan, A. D. (1968): *Anesthesiology*, *29*, 570.

Regele, H. (1967): *Beitr. path. Anat.*, *136*, 165.

The influence of long-term ventilation on lung morphology

H. REINEKE, K. H. BOCK, P. MILEWSKI and F. W. AHNEFELD

Department of Anaesthesiology, Centre of Interdisciplinary Medical Units,
University of Ulm, Ulm, Federal Republic of Germany

In order to determine if the alterations in the lung which are described as typical of long-term ventilation (Nash et al., 1971; Northway et al., 1967; Regele, 1967) are due to the use of a high concentration of oxygen or to the use of a ventilator, 4 groups 40 pigs were ventilated artificially by different techniques.

Group A: oxygen ($FI_{O_2} = 1$), PPV

Group B: ambient air ($FI_{O_2} = 0.25$–0.3), PPV

Group C: oxygen ($FI_{O_2} = 1$), PEEP (7.5 cm H_2O)

Group D: ambient air ($FI_{O_2} = 0.25$–0.3), PEEP (7.5 cm H_2O)

After 48 hr ventilation the lungs were examined macroscopically and microscopically.

Firstly the lungs of animals in Groups A and C are much pinker than those of Groups B and D. Qualitatively the tendency towards atelectasis is most marked in Group A. The differences of lung weight/kg body weight are related to the technique of ventilation and to the inspired oxygen concentration (Table 1). The consistency of the lung tissue of all lungs is more compact than that of non-ventilated animals. Oedema liquid can be always squeezed out of the lung sections of Group A animals. Macroscopically animals of all other groups seem to be less susceptible to oedema.

Table 1. *Average lung weight, 5% confidence intervals, and statistical comparison*

Group	Mean value	5% confidential interval	Significance (t)	(p in %)
A	20.35	3.33	AB 3.73	1
B	14.59	1.02	AC 3.13	5
C	14.77	2.27	BD 2.41	5
D	12 72	1.43		

The histological results verify the impressions of macroscopic study. To a qualitatively different extent the lungs of all animals show water both in the interstices and also inside alveoli.

Corresponding to the maximum lung weight/kg body weight in Group A the most distinct predisposition to oedema is confirmed histologically in this group. The interstices and the septa are broadened, and the alveoli are filled with liquid and protein (Fig. 1). In many alveoli the protein is compressed mechanically by the intraalveolar excess pressure, and it lines the alveolar septum as hyaline membranes (Fig. 2). The lymphatic vessels appear clearly dilated.

The histological differences between Groups A and B are of a quantitative and qualitative kind. Qualitatively the oedema is evidently less but it affects the interstices and the vessels as in Group A. The qualitative difference is that the liquid does not appear everywhere but it is limited to certain alveolar regions in the extravascular area. Cell infiltrations are not seen in isolated areas. The intraalveolar oedema is condensed to compact formations. Since there is a relation between the weight of lungs and the extent of oedema, it might be concluded that the increase of lung weight is mainly dependent upon the extravasation of liquid into the cellular tissue. Atelectasis occurs less in Group B than in Group A.

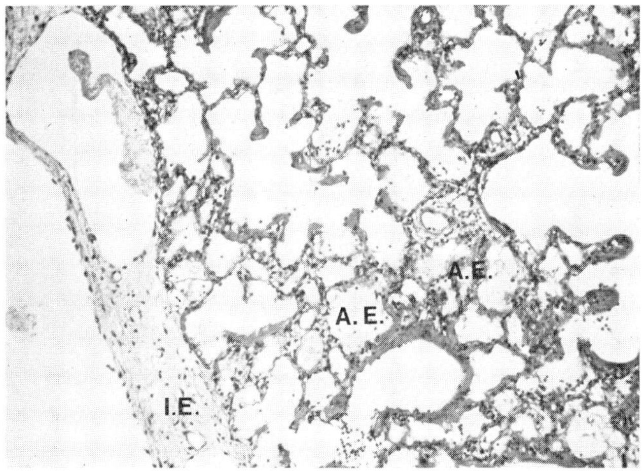

Fig. 1.   *Histological section through the left basal lobe. IE= interstitial oedema; AE= alveolar oedema.*

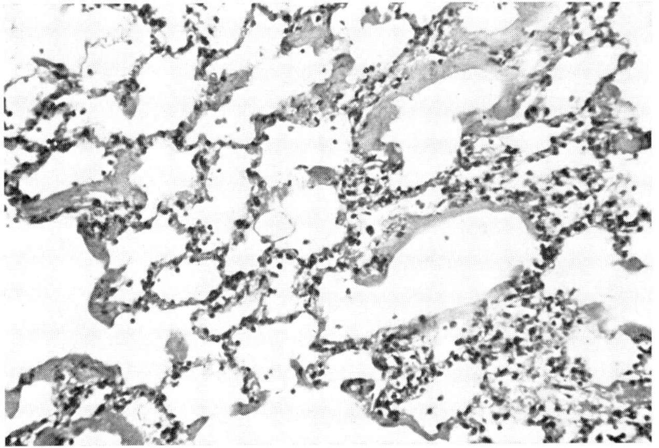

Fig. 2.   *Histological section through vesicles of the lungs whose septum is lined with hyaline membranes.*

For Groups C and D the same description is valid as for Groups A and B, but the pathological alterations are quantitatively less developed. In Group C, as in Group A, an almost general disposition to oedema is noticeable, but only isolated alveolar regions are affected in Group D. Corresponding to the decrease of oedema there are fewer hyaline membranes and none were found in Group D. There is a relation between average lung weight and histological section and that the increase in weight corresponds exclusively to the degree of formation of oedema in Groups C and D.

In summary both the dose of oxygen and the use of a ventilator affect lung morphology. Ventilation by positive end-expiratory pressure reduces the effects. The general formation of oedema in the 2 groups treated with oxygen indicates thoracic vascular damage. The oedema restricted to certain alveolar regions in Groups B and D can be interpreted as an imbalance between the production of lymphatic fluid and its elimination. The influence of increased end-expiratory pressure on the disposition to oedema is not only the consequence of the reduced cardiac output but it also results from the increased mean intra-thoracic pressure by which liquid is pressed effectively out of the cellular tissue.

REFERENCES

Nash, G., Bowen, S. A. and Langlimais, P. C. (1971): *Arch. Path.*, *21*, 234.
Northway, W. H., Rosan, R. C. and Porter, D. Y. (1967): *New Engl. J. Med.*, *276*, 357.
Regele, H. (1967): *Beitr. path. Anat.*, *136*, 165.

*Extracorporeal membrane oxygenation in the treatment of acute respiratory failure**

HARM-PETER DIETRICH **, MAURICE LAMY ***, ROBERT J. FALLAT,
ROBERT EBERHART, J. DONALD HILL and FRANK GERBODE

Department of Cardiovascular Surgery, The Institutes of Medical Sciences, and
Bothin Heart Research Laboratory, Pacific Medical Center, San Francisco, Calif., U.S.A.

There is an increasing awareness of death from acute respiratory failure (ARF) – estimated at about 50,000 per year for the United States. Recent experience indicates that the lungs may heal and patients can recover if prolonged extracorporeal membrane oxygenation (ECMO) can be used to maintain oxygenation during the critical stages of the disease.

Twenty-five patients suffering from generalized hypoxemia due to acute respiratory insufficiency were treated with extracorporeal membrane oxygenation for periods from 12 hr to 19 days after maximum respiratory support with conventional management had failed. Maximum respiratory support means volume controlled continuous positive pressure breathing (CPPB) with inspired oxygen of 100% ($F_{IO_2} = 1.0$) and the use of optimal levels of positive end-expiratory pressure (PEEP) up to 15 cm of water, maximum diuresis, and other appropriate medical regimen (antibiotics, steroids, heparin). Our present minimal criteria and the contraindications for the use of ECMO are outlined in Table 1.

Table 1.

A. Minimal criteria for initiation of ECMO

1. (*a*) Rapidly deteriorating course with: $Pa_{O_2} < 50$ Torr with $F_{IO_2} = 1.0$ for > 2 hr plus maximum respiratory support
   (or)
   (*b*) Deterioration after 48 hr of optimal ventilatory management (PEEP, diuretics, etc.) with $Pa_{O_2} < 50$ Torr on $F_{IO_2} > 0.6$ for > 12 hr
2. Possibility of reversibility of the pulmonary pathology
3. Hypoxemic myocardial or CNS depression

B. Contraindications for ECMO

1. Active bleeding
2. Documented irreversible brain damage
3. Progressively degenerative systemic disease (e.g. cancer, COPD, CNS, severe left heart failure)
4. Over 3 weeks duration

* Aided in part by USPHS grants HE 13150–04 and PHS International Research Fellowship 1 F05 TWO 2/00–01.
** Fellow of the Deutsche Forschungsgemeinschaft, Bonn-Bad Godesberg, Federal Republic of Germany.
*** Chargé de Recherche au F.N.R.S., Belgium.

Using the Bramson membrane oxygenator, 3 cannulation techniques have been employed.

Veno-venous (V-V) bypass was used in the first 6 patients. (Blood obtained from the inferior vena cava was pumped through the oxygenator and returned to the superior vena cava via the internal jugular vein.) Since pulmonary flow is not decreased, pulmonary artery pressure (PAP) remains high and the increase in arterial oxygen tension (Pa_{O_2}) is limited by the actual bypass flow obtained. In an attempt to reduce the PAP and to improve peripheral oxygenation, veno-arterial (V-A) perfusion was used in the next 14 patients. (Blood obtained from the right atrium via the femoral vein was oxygenated and returned retrograde into the femoral artery, so that the entire cannulation could be done via one groin.) Mixing of oxygenator and left ventricular outflow occurs in some higher region of the aorta. Although the benefit of this scheme is the reduction of cardiac and pulmonary blood flow and pressures, the coronary artery and aortic arch blood is still dependent on the biological lung for oxygenation and the Pa_{O_2} is in the lower limits of acceptability. In order to find a compromise between high pulmonary circuit pressure and sometimes inadequate oxygen supply to the lung, heart and brain, a combination of V-V and V-A perfusion was used in the last 5 patients as shown in Figure 1. This combined technique is actually a V-A perfusion with a second arterial cannula placed in the right ventricle via the internal jugular vein, using the tricuspid valve to prevent recirculation. This method allows high bypass flows, yet decreased PAP, maximal control and improvement of oxygenation in both the pulmonary and peripheral circulations, and some protection against particulate matter for brain and heart (Eberhart et al., 1974).

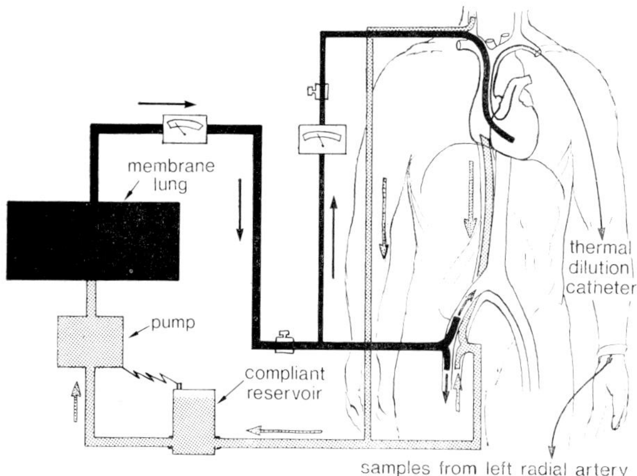

Fig. 1.   *Combined veno-venous/veno-arterial (V-V/V-A) bypass: Blood obtained from the right atrium via femoral vein is oxygenated and returned retrograde to the aorta via femoral artery and to the right ventricle via internal jugular vein.*

Our procedure for following the pulmonary gas exchange in these patients was as follows (Dietrich et al., 1974): Radial artery and pulmonary artery blood gases were determined daily or more often at 4 levels of PEEP (0, 5, 10 and 15 cm of water) and up to 6 levels of F_{IO_2} (usually 0.4, 0.6, 0.8, and 1.0), if clinically possible. For each level of PEEP, separate graphs were drawn depicting Pa_{O_2} on the vertical and F_{IO_2} on the horizontal axis (Fig. 2). Isopleths of shunt-fraction (Q_S/Q_T) were calculated using a mean value for hemoglobin, pH, P_{CO_2}, temperature, and A-V difference; a RQ of 0.8 was assumed. Cardiac output was measured with each determination (Swan-Ganz thermodilution catheter). When a patient was on ECMO, the tests were performed daily in the same fashion while the bypass flow was reduced to 0.75 l/min, thus approximating the prebypass conditions. Figure 2 shows a typical graph of Pa_{O_2} vs F_{IO_2} under PEEP of 15 cm water of a patient (W.R.) for a sequence of days before (day — 1) and during ECMO (days 0, + 4, and + 5). The obtained data demonstrate changes in lung function and characterize the pathophysiological defect: (*a*) 'Severe fixed shunt' (Q_S/Q_T) is shown by day — 1 as Q_S/Q_T changes very little with decreasing F_{IO_2}. This fixed shunt-fraction was found to be very high (50–80%) in all of the patients before they were treated by ECMO. (*b*) Severe ventilation-perfusion abnormality (V/Q) is indicated when Q_S/Q_T decreases with increasing PEEP and increasing F_{IO_2}. In our example, Q_S/Q_T on day + 4 was in the range of 30% on F_{IO_2} of 0.5, but only about 15% on F_{IO_2} of 1.0. This reversibility of Q_S/Q_T with PEEP or increasing F_{IO_2} is a good prognostic factor.

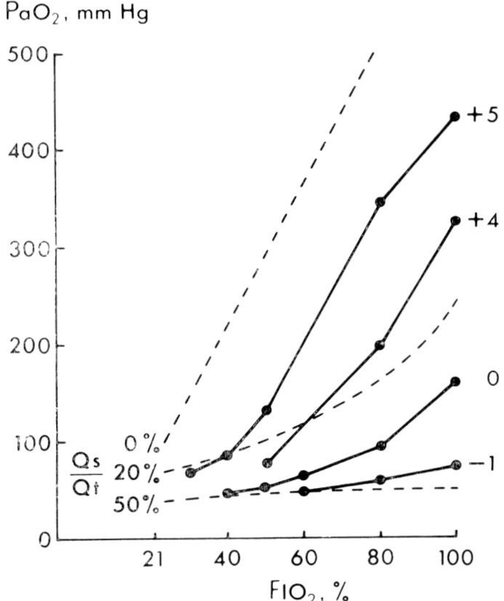

Fig. 2. *Pa$_{O_2}$ vs F$_{IO_2}$ diagram at PEEP of 15 cm water of a patient (W.R.) with severe fixed shunt before ECMO (day —1) and V/Q abnormalities dominating during the further course of improvement on ECMO (days 0 through +5). The patient was ultimately a long-term survivor. The dashed lines represent calculated Q$_S$/Q$_T$ isopleths.*

A summary about the etiological factors of the terminal pulmonary dysfunction and the ultimate clinical outcome of the 25 patients is given in Table 2. Thirteen patients (52%) could be removed from ECMO with improved and acceptable pulmonary gas exchange (Pa_{O_2} > 80–90 Torr) under conventional ventilation at acceptable settings, i.e. F_{IO_2} < 0.6 and PEEP < 10 cm of water. Four of these 13 patients were eventually long-term survivors. The most common cause of death during and after ECMO was progressive lung failure (11 of 21 patients). This progression in the pulmonary pathology, despite sufficient oxygenation and reduction of F_{IO_2} and respiratory pressures to less dangerous levels, indicates the need for more definite criteria of reversibility of the different forms of ARF. Bleeding is the largest risk in the use of ECMO and the second most common cause of death both during and after bypass (5 of 21 patients). The decrease in the level of platelets is the most prominent hematologic effect of bypass. Disseminated intravascular coagulation (DIC)

Table 2. *Etiological factors and eventual prognosis*

Etiological diagnosis	No. of patients	Death on bypass	Taken off bypass	Long-term survivors
Pneumonia	12	8	4	–
Shock-lung, trauma	5	1	4	3
Fat embolism	4	–	4	1
Lung contusion	1	–	1	–
Post-open-heart surgery	1	1	–	–
Respiratory burn	1	1	–	–
Amniotic fluid embolism (septicemia-DIC)	1	1	–	–
Total	25	12	13	4

played a prominent role in the death of 3 patients, in combination with progressive lung failure, and was present to a clinically significant degree in 8 patients. However, since one of the long-term survivors showed reversed DIC and 4 other DIC patients could be removed from ECMO satisfactorily, DIC should not be considered a contraindication or poor prognostic sign unless its underlying cause is uncontrollable. The most critical problem is still selecting patients who have potential reversible pulmonary disease and who have not progressed into the state of irreversible pulmonary fibrosis (Hill et al., 1974).

From our experience we conclude:

1.   Combined V-V/V-A bypass is the most efficient form of ECMO.

2.   Patients with ARF caused by trauma, fat embolism or other effects of non-thoracic trauma, who come to bypass treatment early in their disease, are the most likely to benefit from ECMO – 8 of 9 such patients could be taken off bypass with pulmonary improvement and 4 were long-term survivors.

3.   Infectious cases, who usually come to ECMO later in their course, have a less fortunate prognosis – only 4 of 12 patients with severe pneumonia improved enough to be removed from ECMO, and there were no survivors. Acute viral pneumonia seems to benefit better from ECMO than late destructive bacterial or aspiration pneumonia.

4.   Progressive severe fibrosis of the lungs, bronchopleural fistula and a fixed shunt indicate a very poor prognosis.

REFERENCES

Dietrich, H.-P., Lamy, M. and Fallat, R. J. et al. (1974): *Clin. Res.*, *22*, 199A.
Eberhart, R. C., Lamy, M. and Dietrich, H.-P. et al. (1974): *Trans. Amer. Soc. artific. intern. Organs.*
Hill, J. D., Ratliff, J. and Fallat, R. J. et al. (1974): *J. thorac. cardiovasc. Surg.*

Chapter XII

Functional and biochemical alterations in hyperventilation and hypoventilation

Is it legitimate to interrupt resuscitation?

A. AGUADO MATORRAS

'La Paz' Intensive Care Unit, Public Health Department, Social Security Service, Madrid, Spain

The constant vigilance and attention implied in modern procedures enable many organic functions essential to survival to be maintained, and many medical and surgical treatments to be carried out which, on many occasions, will definitely save the patient's life.

Unfortunately there are other occasions when death is partial, leaving the patient in occupational, social, physical and even psycho-intellectual impairment in 'coma dépassé'.

STATE OF TOTAL INCAPACITY

The doctor who has resuscitated a patient may be faced with 2 situations of total incapacity, quite separate from one another, which will transform a human being into what we have termed a 'hospitalized invalid': (1) total physical incapacity with total or partial retention of consciousness; and (2) total and prolonged loss of consciousness or 'coma dépassé'.

In the first case it is obvious that any resuscitation, by which is understood 'replacement of the vital functions' (respiration, digestion and assimilation, renal excretion) must, on principle, be continued.

Elementary human, civil and medical rights assist the patient in this case. Suppression of them would constitute euthanasia, which is not authorized by the legal and medical codes of most countries; it would be in the nature of purely Spartan selection at the close of life.

KNOWN NON-RECOVERABILITY AND ABSTENTIONIST ACTION

In some situations, however, there may be important shades of difference which can imply decisive variations of legal and medical judgment.

In some hospitals throughout the world it has been decided *not to initiate* treatment for patients with serious and definite organic lesions, including senile involution, when such patients are in a serious state, either because the permanent illness has become more acute, or because there appears a new disease which is important enough to justify the need for resuscitation.

When this attitude leaked out to the public, beginning in England in 1967, it generated some lively polemics in the world press, alerted moralists and judges and opened up new channels in which might run offences listed under 'refusal of assistance'.

Without doubt such medical decisions are endorsed by considerable past and prospective experience and are supported statistically by 'biological terms'. Nevertheless, the judges in this country (and, it would appear, also in others) abstain from taking these aspects into consideration, and interpret the facts with mathematical exactitude in order to defend the rights of the citizens. Taking for example Spanish legislation, we see that Article 570 of the Penal Code says in relation to the *refusal of assistance* that 'refusal of assistance to another person requiring it constitutes a *default of minor seriousness*'. Article 586 of the same Code says: 'Anyone who refuses to offer help when requested to do so by another with a view to avoiding a more serious wrong, provided there is no damage to himself, will be punished by a fine of 250–5000 pesetas and a private reprimand'. Nevertheless, the *refusal of assistance* has not always been considered an infringement of these Articles 570 and 586, but of Article 565 of our Penal Code referring to *'reckless imprudence'*: 'Anyone who through reckless imprudence performs any deed which, should malice be present, would constitute an offence, will be punished by minor imprisonment. Anyone who by infringing the regulations shall commit an offence due to simple imprudence or negligence will be punished by major arrest'.

Certainly the attitude of the doctor in relation to Article 586 and the 'refusal of assistance' may be justified in that it involves 'accumulating economic detriment' not to the person himself but to the *community*, in respect of which the doctor has an obligation not to squander his resources but to use them adequately and intelligently. Nevertheless, Article 565 above clearly places a limit on the adoption of restrictive means of treatment by the threat of grave penalties. Would a preconceived and systematized attitude constitute 'malice' in the opinion of the judiciary, or merely poor interpretation of professional and legal obligations on the one hand, and administrative and internal regulations on the other?

It is evident that the purpose of legislators and judges is to defend the law in absolute terms, and this, as I understand it, on principle invalidates biological statistics, in which it is practically impossible to consider all the variants of each case, refined to the maximum extent. On the other hand it must be admitted that the rigidity of the arrangements and the consequent threat of punishment do provide a warning for those involved and limit, almost always effectively, interpretative abuse of the laws or clear transgression of them.

Though we may agree that the great majority of medical men are honest, maintaining a professional ethic modelled on their own code and on their national laws, transgression of both these is not infrequent, as is the lack of an adequate level of knowledge.

THE RELATIVE NATURE OF MEDICAL KNOWLEDGE

Individual actions

It is certain that the nature of the circumstance constitutes an important and sometimes decisive fact as regards the individual conscience and the legal assessment of each individual situation; but it is no less certain that, in terms of the development of the means available to present civilized society, the decisions to be taken by the doctor in his own field of action are open to question, so long as there remains a lack of more authoritative advice and more effective means of diagnosis and treatment.

The possibility that abstention from actively treating a condition might be acceptable leads us to another consideration, which is also valid in absolute terms – whether on a regional, provincial or local basis – who is it, the individual doctor or the group of doctors, who should decide the question of 'non-intervention', i.e., 'non-resuscitation'? How will a standard of this kind work out in practice? Good sense and individual or team experience find an outlet in practice, and justice rarely intervenes, at least in cases involving house calls in the city or the rural areas.

Action in hospital

Nevertheless, there is a continually growing demand that doctors should take this kind of action within a hospital environment. As we understand it, families differ in their attitudes because of 3 fundamental factors, one of them positive and the other 2 negative:

(1) People continue to put greater faith (often to excess and without any basis) in the

possibilities offered by present-day medicine; and therefore its demands increase, with no allowances made for failure, mistakes, limitations or even helplessness when faced by an illness.

(2) The progressive dehumanization of life in large cities in which, very often, the home is left empty for the greater part of the day because both parents are out at work, conditions a demand (to some extent unjustified) by the family upon society that the latter should take charge of the patient and thus avoid upsetting the daily routine, besides relieving it of the physical and economic burdens imposed by attention to the patient's needs.

(3) Medical decisions are taken on the basis of data obtained from the patient when his family is not present (this being necessary because of hospital organization), which arouses unfounded suspicions in some patients and increases the conditioning referred to under (2) above.

INTERRUPTION OF RESUSCITATION

There are 2 shades of difference involved in interrupting resuscitation: (1) suppressing the procedures whereby the vital functions are substituted; and (2) suppressing all forms of treatment except those concerned with the replacement of vital functions, and thus inhibition in the presence of complications which, while they might respond to treatment, will not resolve the principal illness.

SUPPRESSING THE REPLACEMENT OF THE VITAL FUNCTIONS

This form of action, as we have said, clashes with the standards of modern human rights. Nevertheless, we also know that some primitive societies (nomad Eskimos and some Asian tribes) simply abandon their sick, wounded and senile members who are unable to perform their activities adequately, and that this soon leads to their death. Our society, civilization and religion does not condemn these customs, but neither will it tolerate them within itself, precisely because of the difference between the cultures, ways of life and economic potential, but this does not prevent our society from allowing and planning forms of activity, either between nations or between ethnic groups or social classes within the same nation, driving large sections of the population to poverty, unhealthy conditions or keeping them in this state, thus depriving them, because of lack of hygiene or of food, of the same human and political rights which, apparently, should be enjoyed by all the members of that society.

On the other hand it is demanded of medicine that it should preserve lives that are in a precarious condition, however little may have been done to prevent the illness – or the war.

I do not claim to have discovered that the inconsequence and variability of consciences is a generalized and morally unjustifiable fact, in terms of pure logic. Probably no specific or comparative consideration can avoid the suppression of replacement of the vital functions being legally classifiable as an act, at the very least, of euthanasia.

Our Penal Code considers only one aspect of euthanasia, that in which putting an end to life is done at the request of the person himself (suicide); it does not consider such a decision taken in conjunction with the family and medical advisers of a patient who is irrecoverable. The legal position could be even more serious *.

---

* As far as we are aware, no specific provision is made for the second possibility in the Code and no sentences have been passed in cases of this kind by the Spanish judiciary. Nevertheless, Article 565 and the second part of Article 409 constitute an implicit warning.

At first sight, reference may be made to Article 409 of the Penal Code: 'Any person who assists or incites another to commit suicide will be punished by a major prison sentence **. If he lends himself to the point of perpetrating the death himself, he will be punished by minor life imprisonment ***'.

MINIMUM TREATMENT

From the point of view of medical deontology and Christian morality (and more doubtfully, from the legal aspect), not intervening with unusual remedies in cases of the second group might be justified, so long as adequate knowledge is available and the work is guided strictly by conscience. In fact, the latter must prevail as regards assessment of the other variable, because what are 'unusual remedies'?

The evolution of medicine, of its organization and of the use of its hospitals, is constantly being perfected, and such an assessment is also therefore undergoing constant variations which cannot be quantified absolutely at any moment. Many of the unusual remedies employed years ago are now a matter of everyday routine.

EVALUATION OF THE EXTENT OF FUNCTIONAL REPLACEMENT

In these cases it would be preferable to determine the unusualness of a remedy in terms of the extent of replacement that the remedy offers to the functioning of the body, and in practice this evaluation might give an almost constant average.

On the other hand, one factor that needs to be considered concerns the use of remedies whose availability is limited – as in the case of human blood and its derivatives. At times the reserves may be considerable even if there is a scarcity in general terms. The fairness of its use is open to discussion if we take into account that stocks may be redistributed in order to prevent their being damaged, or may be used for the extraction of sub-products and/or fractions. The difference between products of vegetable, animal or synthetic origin is substantial, seeing that the production of these would only be limited by the economic possibilities of society.

Nevertheless, whether one is concerned with chronic previous pathological conditions, senile involution or the nature of the present lesions, biliary, pancreatic or intestinal fistulae, extensive pulmonary resection with the lung partly affected or in a state of insufficiency, advanced emphysema, irrecoverable quadriplegia, total resection of the intestine, etc., serious problems arise which are certainly not only of a medical nature properly so-called (these could have been determined or at least discussed beforehand), but are of a socio-economic kind – such as the availability of beds in Intensive Care Units and in hospitals in general, and the economic means of maintaining them.

We realize that it is not a question of pushing patients aside without treatment on the grounds that they cannot recover, but of maintaining treatment at the level of our present means and knowledge.

We might recall that the cost of a stay in our Intensive Care Unit was 4.679,— pesetas in 1972 and 5.578,— pesetas in 1973. These figures may be broken down as shown in Table 1.

Analysis of this picture shows:

(1) A percentage reduction in family costs and a reduction of 1.022% or 813.39 ptas. per capita in the income for 1972.

** 6 years and one day to 12 years.
*** 12 years and one day to 20 years.

Table 1. *Breakdown of costs of stay in Intensive Care Unit during 1972 and 1973*

	1972	1973
Medical staff	2,891,095	3,806,964
Auxiliary staff	8,326,752	10,377,052
General services	175,088	227,614
Repayment and maintenance, apparatus	1,647,984	1,812,782
Repayment, installations	302,521	302,525
Food	313,268	369,656
Medicaments	5,097,349	5,422,711
Total	18,754,057	22,319,304

No. of stays (per year)	4,008
Average stay (days)	11
Hospital average	7.2

	No. of cases
Thoracic surgery	90
Neurosurgery	99
General surgery	209
Urology	49
Opthalmology	15
Traumatology	128
E.N.T.	20
Internal medicine	194
Intensive care	29
Total	833

The ratio between the average stay in the Intensive Care Unit and the total stay in the hospital was:
4,679/2,246 = 2.083 (1972)
5,568/2,729 = 2.0403 (1973)
(average of 3 months taken at random in each year)

Additional investment in installations

	1972	1962	Ratio (1963)
Expenses on public health assistance per holder	7,783,03	1,115,37	6.977
Gross national income/family expenses	71,971	72,993	0.985
Family expenses per capita	57,281	18,003	3.181
Expenses on public health and social security per capita	6,847,30	664,93	10.297
Gross national product per capita	79,589	24,664	3.226

(2) An enormous increase (6.977 times) in the cost of Social Security assistance, even though it must be taken into account that a considerable part of the cost is due to the construction and use of new hospitals (18,000 beds in 10 years).

(3) In any case, the total figures for Public Health and Social Security increased 10.297-times in the 10 years mentioned, and this is certainly not due only to the increased Gross

National Product per capita (3.226-times), but also to the increased average expectancy of life and the increased social security payments, etc. – nevertheless, the increase seems very significant.

Spanish society therefore (and I presume this also applies to other countries), is facing progressively increasing medical costs as well as increased costs related to the Intensive Care Units (the increase is slighter, due to the cost of new installations).

CONTRACTUAL RIGHT TO MEDICAL SERVICES

So, can Spanish society (or that of any other country) deny indiscriminately the right that the patient has acquired?

We will consider, not the present situation, but one in the past – the obligation of an individual to join the Social Security system. At such times no limit was set to public health services, any more than is done now. The individual, therefore, contributed for a great part of his life to the progress of medicine and to the maintenance of institutions of which he asked little or nothing, since he remained in good health both in youth and as an adult. He thus acquired a contractual right to medical attendance when he needed it – and logically this is more likely during the last years of his life.

Can this right honestly be disregarded by adducing economic shortages, lack of space or insufficient medical auxiliary staff? In pure logic, certainly not; and as regards the legal aspect this would probably run counter to Principle 10 of the Labour Code, would contravene the general rules of the Social Security system and would ignore the acquired rights already mentioned. But the prolongation of average survival time seems to be a continuous factor: it has not yet reached its ceiling and as far as we can foresee it will not do so for some years to come – but on the other hand, requests for utilization of the health services may also show an increase with age, producing a general increase in total costs and (bearing in mind that the illnesses will become progressively more serious) of the costs of the Intensive Care Units.

This problem clearly goes beyond the doctor's decision. He can do no more than warn the Administration of facts of which he is aware but has not analyzed in depth, and can report to his own Association which will consider the situation. He may also expect to know what will be asked of him in the future, so that he can then decide how to act.

There is no point in evading this problem, nor the fact that anyone (whether in authority or an ordinary citizen) may think that 'the case arising . . .' he may need to resolve it individually.

SELECTION OF CASES FOR ADMITTANCE TO HOSPITAL

Certain attempts at hospital planning in various countries, including our own, have recorded a logical but hazardous tendency; only acute cases, and those to be prepared for immediate surgical operation, are admitted to hospital. But what does the great majority of hospitalized acute cases consist of? How will the burden imposed by the movement of these acute cases be felt? Will not our units be blocked by insoluble cases, becoming every day more numerous in proportion as medicine progresses? Have the aims that have apparently been pursued now been reached or, on the contrary, are we not feeling the effects of the presence of many patients suffering from moderately serious illness, who previously used to be admitted, but who now take longer to cure or who develop sequelae that formerly could have been avoided?

We certainly must face 2 facts – the rights acquired (and paid for) by individuals, and the opportunities for genuine treatment during a prolonged incurable illness.

The solutions would certainly be different from those suggested in an enquiry directed to informed and responsible persons and to jurists, in the abstract; they might decide that the ordinary citizen had simply been swindled if his savings (his contributions) were not ready to be handed over when they were needed (because of illness) without meanness or restriction.

'COMA DEPASSE'

These considerations of the patient's 'right' are entirely relevant to a case known to be incurable, but less so from the medical point of view with regard to 'coma dépassé'.

The criteria of clinical death (cerebral death), established by Schwab and Young in 1968 (absence of sensitivity to pain; absence of osteo-tendinous and autonomic reflexes; absence of respiration; EEG flat (taken for 10 min each hr); carotid angiogram (no intra-cerebral filling) for 8–24 hr at normal temperature and in the absence of any drugs that depress the CNS) are accepted by doctors in most countries. On the other hand, forensic medicine sticks to the old definitions of total death (i.e., cerebral, cardiac, cellular). Is our present experience perhaps insufficient, and has any case meeting these postulates ever survived?

It seems logical, therefore, that jurists, pathologists and clinicians should accept a single criterion of death, even though the simultaneous presence of both sides will be needed in every case, and that whoever lacks sufficient information should be obliged to obtain it from recognized centres or persons.

We do not propose here to enter into a specific discussion of the legitimacy of organ transplants, although this would logically follow, without giving an actual assessment of the individual's prospects of survival as a human, rational and thinking being. The legal and medico-legal fundamentals upon which are based the complete or partial maintenance of life are, if you like, a pedestal not to be stepped upon by the ordinary doctor, but neither do they constitute the armoured redoubt of an immovable doctrine.

I consider that the repeated negative response of the legal authorities to applications for the interruption of resuscitation or for the extraction of organs in case of cerebral death corresponds more to indiscriminate hypersensitivity and to an excess of zeal in the abstract defence of human rights than to any real assessment of the situation. Certainly, survival on the vegetative plane may have been considerable and prolonged, but have we in fact seen, not indeed total or acceptable recovery, but any inkling of the conscious integration of sensation, the workings of elementary intellectual processes, etc.?

It may be argued that, in this sense, there is not very much that present-day medicine can achieve, and that processes of this kind may be in existence in such situations which cannot be demonstrated by our most sophisticated methods. We certainly have to admit the existence of introspective mental processes that occur at times unknown to others, whether they be scientists or not. From the philosophical point of view, and in particular with regard to religious doctrine, acceptance of such a possibility would set up an un-scaleable obstacle.

However, I would dare to venture this suggestion: are we not dealing here simply with a manifestation of legalistic perfectionism, with an atavistic and not well justified fear, or with uncompromising defence of the acquired right?

Without doubt we are obliged to relate our actions to the times in which we live, for otherwise what retrospective judgment might be passed on us for bleeding the tuberculous, comatose or febrile patients, as our predecessors did in the Middle Ages? Still more, what kind of purist opinion do we hold of those who marked the patients who had leprosy, yellow fever or the plague?

In the first of these instances, action was consequent upon the knowledge current at the time; in the second, the aim was to protect the rest of society. What fundamental differences, not merely differences in shades of meaning, can be established in the present cases, in which present-day knowledge assesses the non-viability of cerebral function and can advise or authorize the interruption of resuscitation? If man consists of himself and his circumstances, why do we require of the doctor, and still more of Society, that treatment should be prolonged when it is useless as far as our knowledge goes, and can only lead to a kind of collective suicide as a result of the squandering of our resources on patients who cannot recover?

I should like finally to draw a parallel with medicine in times of war or natural catastrophe, where a single doctor or a team of doctors, generally ill-supplied with material, 'chooses' the cases that can be treated and decides to abandon the more seriously afflicted, because on the one hand they have less chance of surviving and on the other they would take up too much time at the expense of those less seriously hurt, who presumably can be saved.

Still, we must be realistic, and consider whether our Society would be ready to renounce: (*a*) a percentage (how much, and of whom?) of the possibilities of treating those who can recover; and (*b*) some increase of well being (with zero or negative increase) maintained at the level required at any time by public health expense?

Have public affairs administrators, the representatives of productivity sector, jurists and clinicians really meditated sufficiently on this problem? Have not some of them adopted an ostrich-like attitude? Who is competent to resolve this problem – the philosopher, the theologian, the moralist, the legislator, the administrator, the physician, or all of them together?

Certainly my realism may seem excessive, and to many of you crude, sceptical and materialistic; but this is not a question of expressing a precipitate judgment 'for the public good', justifying an archaic or unreal conservatism or a defensive or prudish puritanism; this is something to be thought out alone (in my case too), and perhaps on another occasion it may be possible to express an impartial, honest opinion, not influenced by any process of conditioning.

ACKNOWLEDGEMENT

We express our thanks to Dr Mario de la Mata M.D. (Head of the Central Inspectorate of the Social Security Service), to Dr José Ma. Serrano (Head of the Conjoint Economic Service of the I.N.E.) for the information supplied, and to Dr Luis Nuño for his collaboration in obtaining the economic data.

REFERENCES

Instituto de Estudios Fiscales (1969): *Contabilidad Nacional de España 1954–1964*. Ministerio de Hacienca, Madrid.

Instituto Nacional de Estadística (1973): *Contabilidad Nacional de España 1964–1971 y avance para 1972*. Instituto Nacional de Estadística, Madrid.

Schwab, R. S. and Young, R. R. (1968): In: *Proceedings, Symposium on Recovery Period after Resuscitation, Moscow, 1968*, p. 251. U.R.S.S. Medical Science Academy.

Vicarious elimination of excess CO_2 in chronic hypercapnia treated with mechanical ventilation

M. DE FRUTOS HERRANZ

Intensive Care Unit, Ciudad Sanitaria de la Seguridad Social 'La Paz', Madrid, Spain

Episodes of respiratory insufficiency mark the lives of patients suffering from advanced chronic pneumopathy. These incidents can sometimes be controlled with cardiotonics, bronchodilators, mucolytics, antibiotics, corticosteroids, oxygen therapy and respiratory physiotherapy, but some cases require the use of mechanical ventilators with intubation or tracheostomy and all the inconveniences which accompany them. For example, there are the difficulties in humidifying and warming the inspired air, the increased flow of secretions, risk of bronchial cross-infection, mechanical lesions in the trachea and glottis (hemorrhage, malacia, stenosis), and the need for increased vigilance and work on the part of the ward personnel.

Since the consequences of respiratory decompensation are basically hypoxia, hypercapnia and acidosis, attempts are made to improve these findings whilst avoiding the more aggressive techniques as much as possible.

The most effective action in countering hypercapnia is to improve alveolar ventilation which promotes the respiratory elimination of CO_2, but, the renal elimination of CO_2 can also be increased. The renal function of the patient suffering from chronic bronchopneumopathy may well be adequate, but they are always to some extent overloaded. If treatment is carried out with diuretics, urinary losses of Na^+ and K^+ are combined with the losses of Cl^-, making the synthesis of $NaHCO_3$ difficult and causing a tendency towards acidosis.

When ventilatory assistance is insufficient in the reduction of acidosis and hypercapnia, under certain conditions conservative treatment of the respiratory insufficiency can be undertaken to avoid the need for intubation or tracheostomy. The treatment is based on the promotion of renal elimination of bicarbonate, by inhibition of carbonic anhydrase (CA) to obtain resynthesis of bicarbonate at the expense of the excess CO_2, and buffering with THAM the metabolic acidosis.

MATERIALS AND METHODS

During the period 1971–1973, 248 patients were treated in the Intensive Care Unit of the 'La Paz' Ciudad Sanitaria in Madrid for acute or chronic decompensated bronchopneumopathies, of whom 19 received the treatment described below. A first series of patients has already been reported in the literature (Aguado and Frutos, 1971). The patients studied included 13 men and 6 women aged 37–76 years (mean of 59 years). The causes of respiratory insufficiency are described in Table 1. Six patients received continued respiratory assistance through a tracheostomy. 13 underwent intermittent ventilotherapy with the Bird Mark-8 ventilator with a mask and a ventimask between the sessions. The numbers of test treatments

Table 1. *Causes of respiratory insufficiency*

Exacerbated chronic bronchopneumopathy	14
Bronchopneumonia	3
Pickwickian syndrome	1
Chronic bronchopneumopathy and atelectatic	1

Table 2. *Number of test treatments carried out for each patient*

Patients	Test treatments per patient	Total number of test treatments
9	1	9
7	2	14
1	3	3
1	4	4
1	5	5
19		35

carried out for each patient are shown in Table 2. The scheme of the test treatments was as follows: (1) 250 mg acetazolamide i.v.; (2) 250–350 ml of 0.3 M THAM over 60–90 min i.v.; (3) diet with salt; (4) other treatment included i.v. theophylline, mucolytics, digitalis or antibiotics in the case of infection; (5) ventilatory assistance as described previously.

Estimations of acid-base balance were obtained before the administration of acetazolamide and after 2, 6 and 24 hr, with urinary pH determinations at the same times. Urinary and plasma ionograms were obtained before the administration and after 24 hr. Total urine output was determined daily before and after the test treatment.

The indications for treatment were respiratory acidosis, elevation of P_{CO_2}, a good reserve of base, no plasma Na^+ deficit, and absence of the clinical state of coma. The treatment was not used when there was an additional metabolic acidosis or severe hypoxemia.

RESULTS

The changes in the mean values of the parameters, together with their chronological development, are shown in the tables and figures. The results are comparable with those obtained previously (Aguado and Frutos, 1971) on similar patients (Table 3).

Table 3. *Results*

		Before	After		
			2 hr	6 hr	24 hr
Blood	pH	7.312	7.362	7.355	7.336
	P_{CO_2} (mm Hg)	71.4	66.7	61	52.8
	Base excess (mEq/l)	5.4	6.9	5	1.5
	Na (mEq/l)	141			136
	Cl (mEq/l)	89			94
Urine	pH	5.5	7.8	6.5	6
	Na (mEq/l)	79			116
	Cl (mEq/l)	50			46
	Diuresis (ml)	1,360			2,680

Figure 1 shows that the pH started at a low value, increased to a maximum after the THAM perfusion, and then decreased without reaching the initial level. However, in 3 patients the final pH value was lower than the initial value. The mean P_{CO_2} value showed progressive decrease but in 2 patients this value did not decrease. After a temporary increase following THAM, the base excess level decreased considerably in all patients due to the urinary loss of alkali. As a result, the urinary pH underwent a significant rise, although values very close to the original were found after 24 hr.

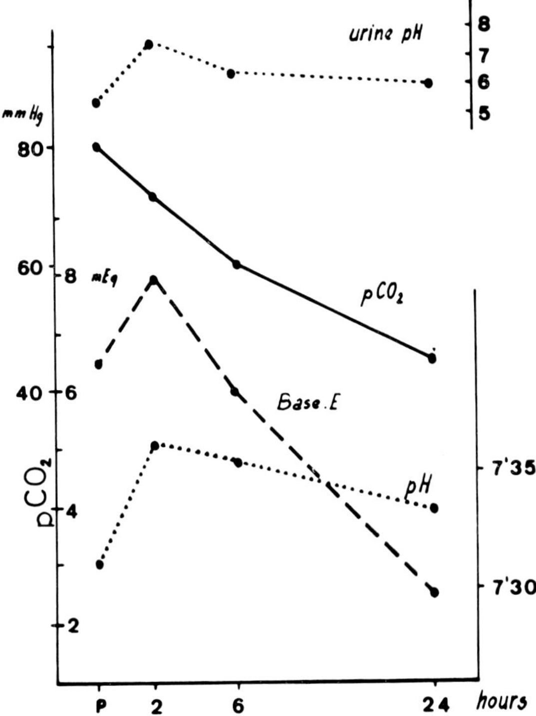

Fig. 1.   *Changes in the mean values of acid-base assays.*

There was a decrease in plasma Na^+ due to the greater urinary elimination, but the blood Cl^- level rose and there was hardly any change in the urinary level (Fig. 2). Urine output increased from the mean 1,360 ml on the day before treatment to 2,680 ml in the following 24 hr.

The state of consciousness and cooperation improved in all patients, which facilitated intermittent respiratory assistance with the mask and respirator in those patients who did not undergo tracheostomy. Apart from the 6 tracheostomized patients who received continuous mechanical ventilation before the start of this treatment, only one of the other 13 patients required subsequent intubation and tracheostomy; the others showed clinical and analytical improvements after one or several treatments with acetazolamide and THAM.

DISCUSSION

The reaction $CO_2 + H_2O \rightleftharpoons H_2CO_3$ is a slow process in vitro, requiring 100 sec to reach

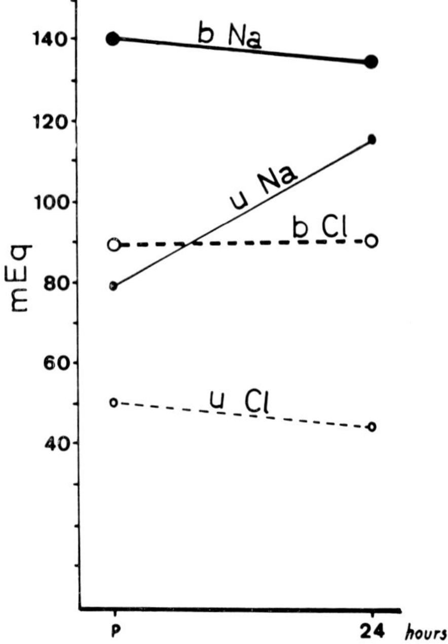

Fig. 2.   *Changes in the mean values of Na and Cl in the plasma and urine.*

equilibrium. However, in vivo it is accelerated by carbonic anhydrase, which is mainly localized inside the erythrocytes and in the renal tubular cells (Tomashefski et al., 1954).

Some sulfonamides inhibit carbonic anhydrase (CA) and their administration causes temporary metabolic acidosis due to the urinary loss of cations. The effects of an intravenous injection of acetazolamide are shown in Table 4. Oral administration causes minimal changes, the most important being urinary alkalinization. Intravenous acetazolamide causes changes similar to those caused by the inhalation of CO_2. In the latter case there is an increase in the tissue P_{CO_2} value due to the exogenous supply, whilst in the former case this increase is due to interference in the process of transportation of the gas from the

Table 4.   *Effects of intravenous acetazolamide*

Increased	Pulmonary ventilation
	$P_{A_{O_2}}$
	Pa_{O_2}
	Cardiac output
	Urinary pH
	Urinary losses of Na^+ and K^+
	Urinary losses of HCO_3^- (loss proportional to CO_2)
Decreased	Blood pH
	$P_{A_{CO_2}}$
	Urinary NH_4^+
Unchanged	Elimination of CO_2 (may vary)
	Content of CO_2 in the plasma
	Oxygen consumption

From: Carter and Clark, 1958; Mithoefer, 1959; Ruiz and Estada, 1968.

tissues to the lung. Normally, CO_2 elimination is a function of alveolar ventilation, the pulmonary blood flow, and the transport mechanisms which depend on CA. When one of these factors is suppressed, normal CO_2 elimination through the lungs can only be maintained by the increase of the other factors. When CA activity is inhibited, both the ventilation and the pulmonary blood flow show an initial increase for a short time in order to maintain the CO_2 elimination.

In the mammalian kidney, CA in the proximal tubule aids the reabsorption of bicarbonate by promoting the supply of H^+ to the tubular lumen. CA catalyzes the dehydration of the intraluminal H_2CO_3 formed by the reaction between intraluminal bicarbonate and the secreted H^+. Inhibition of CA decreases the reabsorption of bicarbonate by decreasing the supply of H^+ and by increasing the pH gradient against which the H^+ must be separated. The reabsorption of Na^+ and Cl^- in the proximal tubule is also diminished (Kunau, 1972).

THAM has been used clinically in the treatment of severe respiratory acidosis. Objective signs of its effects are the increase in pH, the increase in total CO_2 and the increase in CO_2 binding capacity (Darby and Anderson, 1966; Sadoul et al., 1966) as well as the decreases in oxygen saturation and in alveolar ventilation (Sadoul et al., 1966). The depression of ventilation is the one side-effect which must be taken into account in the treatment of patients with chronic bronchopathies.

THAM also behaves as an osmotic diuretic, promoting the elimination of Na^+ and Cl^- and, to a lesser extent, of K^+ and HCO_3^- (Nahas, 1962). The excretion of Na^+ and Cl^- is greater than can be accounted for by their decrease in the plasma, indicating that there is a significant movement of these electrolytes from the tissues into the extracellular spaces. The level of plasma K^+ remains constant despite its extensive elimination, indicating that there is an appreciable loss of K^+ from the cells (Nahas, 1962).

The combined use of acetazolamide and THAM has as its objective the elimination of the excess CO_2 which is present in the crises of respiratory insufficiency, acting in the following ways:

(*a*)   The elimination of bicarbonate by acetazolamide.

(*b*)   The administration of THAM to buffer the acidosis caused by the urinary loss of bicarbonate, and then promoting the formation of HCO^- from H_2CO_3.

$$CO_2 + H_2O \rightleftharpoons H_2CO_3 \qquad \text{(I)}$$
$$(CH_2OH)_3\text{--}CNH_2 + H_2CO_3 \rightleftharpoons (CH_2OH)_3\text{--}CNH_3 + HCO_3^- \qquad \text{(II)}$$

Even with CA inhibited, reaction I is still slow.

In the blood, the values of pH, P_{CO_2} and excess of base in our patients underwent parallel changes. The initial increase in base excess coincided with the formation of HCO_3^- at the expense of THAM and H_2CO_3 according to reaction II, with the consequent elevation of the pH value. The persistence of alkali losses in the urine led to reductions in the pH and base excess during subsequent treatments.

The elimination of bicarbonate and of THAM led to an increase in urinary pH. At the same time there was increased diuresis and increased loss of Na^+, although no significant variations in Cl^- elimination were observed.

During these test treatments we did not encounter the harmful effects described for THAM treatments (e.g. hypoglycemia, respiratory depression, severe K^+ depletion, perivenous burns) since the doses used were neither high nor rapidly infused; supplementary K^+ was given in other infusions, and the THAM injection was through a catheter in a large trunk vein (generally the subclavian).

CONCLUSIONS

1.   The combined treatment with THAM and acetazolamide can be effective in the

correction of acid-base alterations found in respiratory decompensation in cases of chronic bronchoneumopathy, and in the elimination of excess CO_2 by the kidney. The state of consciousness is improved and cooperation during physiotherapy and ventilotherapy is facilitated.

2.   The improvements obtained with this treatment may be temporary if the underlying cause remains and repetition of the treatment may be required.

3.   Lack of response to treatment occurs when previous depletion of Na^+ or Cl^-, or alterations in renal function exist (Aguado and Frutos, 1971).

REFERENCES

Aguado, A. and De Frutos, M. (1971): *Maroc méd.*, *547*, 365.
Carter, E. T. and Clark, R. T. (1958): *J. appl. Physiol.*, *13*, 42.
Darby, T. D. and Anderson, S. J. (1966): *Ann. Anesth. franç.*, *7*, 585.
Kunau, R. T. (1972): *J. clin. Invest.*, *51*, 294.
Mithoefer, J. C. (1959): *J. appl. Physiol.*, *14*, 109.
Nahas, G. G. (1962): *Pharmacol. Rev.*, *14*, 447.
Rector, F. C., Carter, N. W. and Seldin, D. W. (1965): *J. clin. Invest.*, *44*, 279.
Ruiz, S. and Estada, J. A. (1968): *Arch. Bronconeumología*, *5*, 559.
Sadoul, P., Pham, Q. T., Aug, M. C. and Gay, R. (1966): *Ann. Anesth. franç.*, *7*, 585.
Tomashefski, J. F., Chinn, H. I. and Clark, R. T. (1954): *Amer. J. Physiol.*, *177*, 451.

Carbon dioxide regulation and maintenance of the physical stability of the lung during controlled ventilation

A. ARIAS ALVAREZ

Fundación Jimenez Díaz, Madrid, Spain

A rebreathing technique using the Engström volumetric ventilator, models 200 and/or 300, in order to maintain carbon dioxide (CO_2 homeostasis) has been in use for 8 years. Regulation of the minute ventilation ($\dot{V}$) with a graduated dose valve in a closed circuit system is possible. When the soda lime is excluded from the semi-closed system, it is possible to use a fairly accurate degree of rebreathing.

Both during anaesthesia with mechanical ventilation and in long-term support of the lung with controlled ventilation, it is sometimes difficult to keep the arterial carbon dioxide pressure (Pa_{CO_2}) at normal levels with physical stability of the lung. Several techniques are available, such as the addition of dead space or the addition of CO_2 to the fresh gas mixture. Upon removing the carbon dioxide absorber from the semi-closed circuit, the P_{CO_2} in the inspired gas mixture (PI_{CO_2}) will be determined by the proportion of fresh gas ($\dot{V}f$) added to that rebreathed and in relation to the minute ventilation ($\dot{V}_E$), the CO_2 production ($\dot{V}_{ECO_2}$) and the expired partial pressure of CO_2 ($P\bar{E}_{CO_2}$). The relation is shown by the following equation:

$$PI_{CO_2} \times \dot{V}_{ECO_2} = P\bar{E}_{CO_2}(\dot{V}_E - \dot{V}f)$$

This equation applies when the fresh gas inflow rate ($\dot{V}f$) does not exceed half of the minute ventilation ($\dot{V}_E$) (Suwa). When larger tidal volumes (V_T) and consequently bigger $\dot{V}_E$ are used, Pa_{CO_2} may be estimated using the following equation:

$$Pa_{CO_2} = K \, \frac{\dot{V}_{CO_2}}{\dot{V}f} \,.$$

A constant, K (0.863), is used for conversion from fractional concentrations to partial pressure.

The principal aim in using this partial rebreathing technique is to maintain the Pa_{CO_2} within normal ranges or in proportion with the blood or cerebrospinal fluid (CSF) bicarbonate, as in metabolic alkalosis. This partial rebreathing technique allows lung ventilation with larger minute volumes than those of the standard nomograms or in relation to body weight, whilst maintaining the CO_2 homeostasis. With normal lungs, both the carbon dioxide production and the physiological dead space are predictable: consequently, the ventilation requirement may be predicted with considerable accuracy. In lung disease, $\dot{V}_{CO_2}$ and V_D are not normal or predictable. The lung ventilation with large V_T supports the physical dynamics in conditions when these forces are out of balance.

METHOD

Initially the rebreathed volume is established in relation to the fall of Pa_{CO_2}. When the Pa_{CO_2} is about critical, say around 23 Torr, rebreathing of about one third of the $\dot{V}E$ necessary under normal conditions is required. The minute volume of rebreathing is established with the graduated dose valve. This proportion of reinspired gases ($\dot{V}R$) to ($\dot{V}f$) allows a slow and gradual build-up of Pa_{CO_2} to the required level in order to achieve the balance of the Henderson-Hasselbalch equation. At the beginning, there is a delay in the Pa_{CO_2} rise until the rebreathing bag is primed with a Pco_2 higher than the Pa_{CO_2}.

During rebreathing, the mixed venous blood equilibrates with Pa_{CO_2}, giving off or taking up CO_2, depending upon the initial concentration of CO_2 in the bag. Different proportions of $\dot{V}R$ up to complete rebreathing are possible. The time required to achieve the equilibrium of the Henderson-Hasselbalch equation depends on CO_2 production ($\dot{V}E_{CO_2}$), previous loss of CO_2, the capacity of the body stores, and the removal of CO_2 from the tissues in relation to blood perfusion.

The time required to regain a proper level of Pa_{CO_2} is not easy to determine. In some particular pathological situations, the $\dot{V}co_2$ is very low. Since at ordinary metabolic rates, the rise in Pa_{CO_2} varies from 3–6 Torr/min in apnea, with one third rebreathing at a low metabolic rate, the rise per minute would be very small, perhaps in the order of half a Torr per minute. According to our experience, the mean time required to elevate the Pa_{CO_2}, from low levels (20–23 mm Hg) to normal levels, varies from 30–40 min and may sometimes be prolonged to one hour. Continuous or intermittent capnography and/or blood gases estimations every 15 or at least every 30 min are necessary until the desired level is achieved. The infrared method for breath-by-breath analysis cannot be used to estimate Pco_2 with accuracy in patients having large V_D/V_T. The difference between Pa_{CO_2} and PA_{CO_2} estimated by end-tidal sampling, may be very large. Shunting combined with a large alveolar dead space may give a normal $P\bar{E}_{CO_2}$ while the Pa_{CO_2} is actually rising.

In some cases, once the Pa_{CO_2} is restored to the desired level, the cardiac index improves. As a result, tissue perfusion and metabolism increase and the $\dot{V}co_2$ therefore increases. After some time with normal Pa_{CO_2}, if the state of the patient has improved, the partial rebreathing may be reduced and a proper $\dot{V}A$ established to avoid a new larger fall of Pa_{CO_2}. At this moment, if the $\dot{V}A$ necessary to maintain the Pa_{CO_2} within normal levels appears to be lower than that required in relation to sex, height, weight, and body surface, from a nomogram or round figures in relation with body weight, partial rebreathing is reimposed. Ventilation requirements may change frequently, therefore Pa_{CO_2} must be measured several times daily.

Partial rebreathing is particularly useful in conditions in which the $\dot{V}co_2$ diminishes, such as in hypothermia, reduced metabolic rate, prolonged ventilatory control, profound pharmacological sedation, inactivity, low cardiac output, etc. Lung compliance usually decreases in controlled ventilation and is further reduced if small tidal volumes are used. Reduction of the functional residual capacity (FRC) causes a decrease of compliance, increase in V_D/V_T proportion and an increase in the alveolar-arterial oxygen difference $PAaDo_2$ due to venous admixture.

To ventilate patients with large V_T may imply haemodynamic interference especially during the inspiratory phase. The increase in intratracheal inflation pressure may, in part, be transmitted through the alveolus and consequently to the capillary and precapillary vessels. The high intra-alveolar pressure exerts a mechanical effect on the pulmonary capillaries, which are compressed, damming back the blood that circulates through the capillaries. This compression leads to a rise in pulmonary artery and a decrease in pulmonary venous pressure if there is not compensation. However, full haemodynamic compensation for a high end-inspiratory pressure is usually achieved.

INDICATIONS FOR PARTIAL REBREATHING TECHNIQUE

1. In primary respiratory alkalosis when the Pa_{CO_2} is near or under the critical level (about 23 Torr). Spontaneous hyperventilation is hard work and consequently oxygen consumption increases. More water is lost through the lungs and secretions become dry. Controlled ventilation may be necessary in spontaneous hyperventilation, in spite of normal arterial Pa_{O_2}.

2. In respiratory alkalosis due to excessive mechanical ventilation.

3. In obstructive airway disease or with reduced functional parenchyma due to different conditions, such as bronchopneumonia or congested lung (post-transfusional, post-extra-corporeal circulation, post-ventilatory control with pulmonary interstitial oedema probably due to sodium retention, thoracic trauma, crush injury, cardiac failure, etc.), when large ventilatory volumes with high inspired oxygen concentrations to alleviate existing hypoxia and the imbalanced physical dynamics are used.

Because CO_2 diffuses rapidly through the alveolar-capillary membrane and because its dissociation curve is almost linear, hyperventilation partly compensates in one alveolus for underventilation in another alveolus. This does not happen with oxygen due to the shape of the dissociation curve. Partial rebreathing probably recruits a larger number of gas interchanging spaces and expands the semi-collapsed alveoli. Positive end-expiratory pressure (PEEP) has a similar effect possibly by causing an increase in the FRC.

Even during the ordinary mechanically controlled ventilation of normal lungs, the distribution of gases is uneven. In some pathological situations of the lung, partial rebreathing with high tidal volumes can be useful. In these cases, the compliance can be maintained or improved, the atelectasis and micro-atelectasis avoided or corrected, and the proportion of V_D/V_T decreased, while the oxygenation may be improved without resorting to the use of a high inspired oxygen fraction (Fi_{O_2}), intermittent sighing or continuous PEEP.

In situations where there is a deficiency of alveolar surfactant which opposes the superficial forces at the air-liquid interface which tend to cause alveolar collapse, it sometimes may be necessary to ventilate the lungs with larger than normal volumes or to increase the mean intrapulmonary pressure by other means, either by increasing the frequency of ventilation or by applying positive end-expiratory pressure.

SUMMARY

The following situations have, in our experience, benefited from this technique:

1. In denitrogenation, with oxygen, for cases of cerebral air embolism, or in the removal of nitrogen from body cavities (pneumothorax) or hollow viscera (ileus) and avoiding a fall of Pa_{CO_2}.

2. In carbon monoxide poisoning which requires rapid replacement of this gas with oxygen, avoiding the fall of Pa_{CO_2} which thus maintains the cerebral circulation, and encourages the oxygen dissociation curve to shift to the right.

3. To reduce steadily the Pa_{CO_2} in chronic respiratory failure to the required level, and match with the existing bicarbonate in blood or CSF, which thus avoids sudden hypotension, the metabolic implications, electrolyte disturbances, and the alkalosis following respiratory acidosis which may induce mental disturbances and tetany.

Effects of continuous positive airway pressure on lung water balance

G. BÖ*, G. NICOLAYSEN and A. HAUGE

Institute of Physiology, University of Oslo, Oslo, Norway

It is a generally held opinion that continuous positive airway pressure (CPAP) counteracts the development of lung edema. In a recent review (Fishman, 1972) it is stated that this effect is due more to a reduction in venous return than to any direct effect on lung capillaries. Other investigators have failed to reveal any effect at all of CPAP on the lung water content (Alexander et al., 1973). One group even found an increase in lung water content during CPAP (Demling and Edmunds, 1973).

In the present work CPAP has been used at constant pulmonary arterial pressure and/or flow. Rises in alveolar pressure (P_A) and rises in transpulmonary pressure (P_{TP}) must be distinguished. A perfused and continuously weighed rabbit lung preparation (Lunde and Waaler, 1969) has been used. By raising left atrial pressure to a high and constant level,

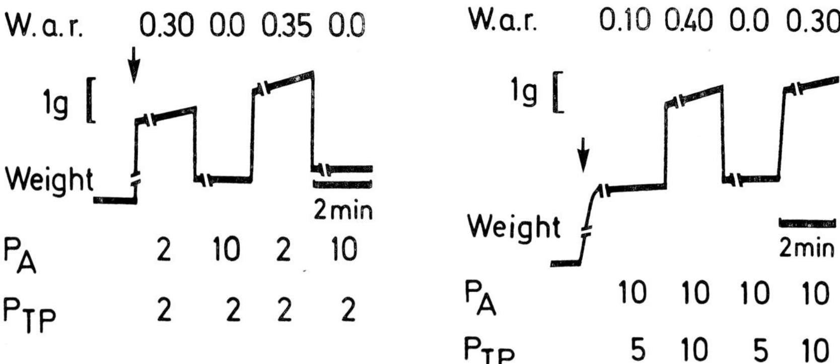

Fig. 1.   *Diagrammatic presentation of effects on rabbit lung weight of changes in alveolar pressure, P_A, at constant transpulmonary pressure, P_{TP}. At zero time (arrow) pulmonary arteria. and left atrial pressure was elevated to 16 and 14 mm Hg respectively. Flow 84 ml/min. The rapid weight changes are interpreted as changes in blood volume. The slow, but steady, changes in weight represents the water accumulation rate, WAR. The figures for WAR are in g/2 min. A selective rise in P_A from 2–10 cm H_2O reduced the WAR by 0.3 g/2 min.*

Fig. 2.   *Diagrammatic presentation of effects on lung weight of changes in P_{TP} at constant P_A. Same experimental setup, abbreviations and units as in Figure 1. Pulmonary arterial pressure 16 mm Hg, left atrial pressure 11 mm Hg and flow 266 ml/min. A selective rise in P_{TP} by 5 cm H_2O increased the WAR by 0.3 g/2 min.*

* Present address: Department of Anaesthesiology, Rikshospitalet, Oslo, Norway.

548

a situation of slow and continuous accumulation of water in the lungs, as judged from the recording of weight, was created. P_A and P_{TP} were varied either separately or in combination, between a high and a low level and the effects on the water accumulation rate (WAR) were observed. In one series of experiments the arteriovenous pressure difference was 2 mm Hg or less, in another it was about 8 mm Hg.

A rise in P_A at constant P_{TP} reduced the WAR in both series of experiments. A rise in P_{TP} at constant P_A caused an increase in WAR in both series of experiments, possibly because of an increase in capillary surface area. A simultaneous and equal rise in both P_A and P_{TP} reduced WAR also in both series.

It is concluded that CPAP may reduce the water accumulation rate in the lungs; the most likely mechanism is an increase in the interstitial hydrostatic pressure around the capillaries.

REFERENCES

Alexander, L. G., Devries, W. C. and Anderson, R. W. (1973): *Surg. Forum, 24*, 231.
Demling, R. H. and Edmunds, L. H. (1973): *Surg. Forum, 24*, 226.
Fishman, A. P. (1972): *Circulation, 46*, 390.
Lunde, P. K. M. and Waaler, B. A. (1969): *J. Physiol. (Lond.), 205*, 1.

The effect of hyperinflation of the lungs on the pulmonary circulation

P. J. R. JEBSON and J. M. HAMPSON

University Department of Anaesthetics, Hallamshire Hospital, and
Sheffield United Hospitals and Northern General Hospital, Sheffield, United Kingdom

The lungs may be subjected to hyperinflation during anaesthesia in such situations as intentional expansion of alveoli or use of excessive tidal volume. This rapid increase of inspiratory pressure is also referred to as the Valsalva manoeuvre (Valsalva, 1707).

This manoeuvre evokes a response from the control systems of the systemic circulation that may be used as a stress test. In part the response depends on the integrity of the autonomic system.

The different nature of the lung vasculature (i.e. a low pressure capacitance/resistance circulation vulnerable to pressure changes) makes the mechanical aspect of high inflation pressures more important and more immediate in effect (Lee et al., 1954). The present study set out to investigate the immediate response of the arterial side of the pulmonary circulation.

METHODS

Eight patients (32–58 years) who were to undergo cardiac catheterisation under general anaesthesia were chosen for the investigation. All were free from heart or lung disease with involvement of the pulmonary circulation.

After routine premedication an anaesthetic technique of N_2O/O_2/relaxant/opiate was used with mechanical ventilation (IPPR).

Following intubation, a frequency and tidal volume from a ventilation nomogram were employed for each individual, normocarbia throughout the investigation being confirmed by arterial blood gas analyses.

Airway pressure (PAW) was monitored by connection of a suitable transducer to the endotracheal tube mount. ECG and heart rate (HR) were obtained from skin electrodes. Percutaneous introduction and advancement of vascular catheters via the femoral vessels enabled the measurement of the systolic, diastolic and mean pressures of the aorta (SAP), pulmonary artery (PAP) and wedge positions (PWP) (Elema-Scholander system).

Cardiac output (pulmonary blood flow) (PBF) estimations were determined by the dye dilution technique, (Indocyanine green) using automatic rapid dye-injection into the pulmonary artery with simultaneous sampling from the aortic arch. The variables were displayed on an oscilloscope and recorded on paper (Mingograf).

Control values on IPPR for the above were obtained from the patient at the peak of inspiration (PAW 7–9 Torr).

The patient was then subjected to hyperinflation of the lungs (PAW 30 Torr) for 7–8 sec. The changes in variables were followed and a blood flow measurement performed by dye injection on release of inflation.

The patient was then replaced on the ventilator and the circulation allowed to stabilise.

RESULTS

From PĀP, PW̄P and PBF the resistance of the pulmonary vascular bed was derived. This resistance may be better termed pre-capillary resistance (PCR) rather than pulmonary vascular resistance (PVR) since calculation of PVR from pulmonary arterial and wedge or left atrial pressures is misleading where inflating pressure exceeds left atrial pressure (De Bono and Caro, 1963).

The control and hyperinflation results obtained were (for brevity only mean pulmonary vascular parameters are shown):

1. PĀP doubled from control to peak inflation
   Mean ($\pm$ SD) of control PĀPs = 14.6 $\pm$ 3.8 Torr
   Mean ($\pm$ SD) of hyperinflation PĀPs = 27.6 $\pm$ 4.9 Torr
       (p $>$ 0.0005)

2. PW̄P: Mean of control PWPs ($\pm$ SD) = 9.75 $\pm$ 2.4 Torr
        Mean of hyperinflation PWPs ($\pm$ SD) = 19.5 $\pm$ 3.07 Torr
        (p $>$ 0.0005)

3. PBF: Mean of control PBFs ($\pm$ SD) = 5.064 $\pm$ 0.74 l/min
        Mean of hyperinflation PBF ($\pm$ SD) = 4.28 $\pm$ 0.285 l/min
        (p $>$ 0.0125)

4. PCR: Mean of control PCR ($\pm$ SD) = 77.7 $\pm$ 40.6 dynes/sec/cm^5
        Mean of hyperinflation PCR ($\pm$ SD) = 153.3 $\pm$ 79.1 dynes/sec/cm^5
        (p $<$ 0.0125)

It was found that the values for control PĀP, PW̄P and PCR were lower than might be expected but compatible with the range found under anaesthesia with IPPR. Though with the Valsalva to each patient, PBF fell and PVR increased, the wide range of individual values is not easily appreciated in the means given. SAP followed the classical response to the Valsalva manoeuvre of initial increase, fall and classical second increase (overshoot). Pulmonary pressures mimicked this progression with more marked changes and slower recovery. HR did not significantly alter in these stages.

DISCUSSION

The vascular responses to this manoeuvre in anaesthetised man are well documented, though the studies have concentrated on pressure changes on the systemic circulation (Price et al., 1951; Lee et al., 1954; Scott et al., 1969; Wayne et al., 1971). The immediate and dramatic fall response of the pulmonary arterial gradient with decrease of flow have not been previously stressed.

In similar Valsalva studies carried out by us whilst monitoring right and left atrial pressure, both values rose, though RAP changed by a higher proportion than LAP. It has been widely held that the initial and predominant effect of hyperinflation is upon the venous return to the right heart rather than as an obstruction to pulmonary arterial flow. Though transmissions of the inflation pressure to the great veins play a part in decreasing venous return, the findings of Scott and colleagues, (Scott et al., 1969) that RAP rise is unaffected by an open chest, throws doubt upon this as the predominant factor in lowering cardiac output. Our results also support observations that high pressure inflation is of more importance to the pulmonary vascular bed than the great veins of the right heart (Brecher, 1956; Lee et al., 1954).

That pressure and flow later recover is reassuring but the observed sudden fall in cardiac output has implications for seriously ill patients, particularly when associated with hypovolaemia and/or ischaemic heart disease. This latter danger has already been reported (Benchimol et al., 1972) and is now confirmed by the findings of our investigation.

REFERENCES

Benchimol, A., Fu Wang, T., Desser, K. B. and Gartlan, J. L. (1972): *Ann. intern. Med.*, *77*, 357.
Brecher, G. A. (1956): *Venous Return*. Grune and Stratton, Inc., New York – London.
De Bono, E. F. and Caro, C. G. (1963): *Amer. J. Physiol.*, *205*, 1178.
Lee, G. J., Matthews, M. B. and Sharpey-Schafer, E. P. (1954): *Brit. Heart J.*, *16*, 311.
Price, H. L., King, B. D. and Elder, J. D. (1951): *J. clin. Invest.*, *30*, 1243.
Scott, D. B., Slawson, K. B. and Taylor, S. H. (1969): *Cardiovasc. Res.*, *3*, 331.
Valsalva, A. M. (1707): *De Aure Humana Tractatus*. G. v. d. Water, Utrecht.
Wayne, T. F., Smith, N. Ty., Eger II, E. I., Stoetling, R. K. and Whitcher, C. E. (1971): *Anesthesiology*, *34*, 262.

Effects of controlled hyperventilation on brain energy and acid-base parameters*

LORENTZ NILSSON

Brain Research Laboratory and Department of Anaesthesia, University Hospital, Lund, Sweden

The well-known fact that hypocapnia leads to a reduction in cerebral blood flow and in addition causes a shift of the oxygen dissociation curve to the left has raised the question whether or not the oxygen supply to the brain can be reduced to such a degree that energy production falls short of the energy demand of the tissue. The purpose of this animal study was to define the effect of induced hypocapnia on the brain tissue concentrations of energetic substrates and to relate alterations of oxidative metabolism to accompanying extra- and intracellular acid-base changes (Nilsson and Busto, 1973). Some of the main results will be discussed.

The brain tissue concentrations of lactate, pyruvate and organic phosphates (phospho-creatine, ATP, ADP and AMP) as well as extra- and intracellular pH values were determined in groups of rats (n = 6–11) hyperventilated to Pa_{CO_2} levels of 20–25 and 10–15 mm Hg for periods of 10 min to 3 hr. The former P_{CO_2} range was chosen since a Pa_{CO_2} of 20 mm Hg is commonly regarded as a safe lower limit while the latter represented excessive hypocapnia. The rats were anaesthetized with nitrous oxide ($N_2O/O_2 = 2/1$). Blood pressure, body temperature, arterial blood gases and pH were monitored in order to exclude variations in parameters other than the arterial P_{CO_2}. At the end of each experiment CSF was sampled and the brain was frozen in situ by pouring liquid nitrogen into a plastic funnel inserted into a skin incision over the cranial vault.

RESULTS AND DISCUSSION

Onset of hyperventilation rapidly decreased the arterial P_{CO_2}'s to the pre-determined values (Fig. 1). Likewise the pH changes were early maximal and did not change significantly when the hyperventilation was prolonged. This was in contrast to the CSF pH (Fig. 2) which was elevated to an initial peak but which then decreased although it never reached the normocapnic value. The lower part of the same figure shows the accompanying pH changes in the intracellular fluid of the tissue. Lowering of the Pa_{CO_2} to 20–25 mm Hg did not give rise to a significant alkalosis but at all points of observation the mean values for the groups were higher than the normocapnic one. More pronounced hyperventilation gave rise to, not a significant alkalosis, but to an acidosis in the early phase of this degree of hypocapnia. However, the homeostatic mechanisms operating were obviously efficient. Thus, after 3 hr, intracellular pH was no longer significantly different from the normocapnic

---

* This study was carried out in collaboration with Mr Raul Busto, senior technician at the Department of Neurology, University of Miami School of Medicine, Miami, Fla., U.S.A.

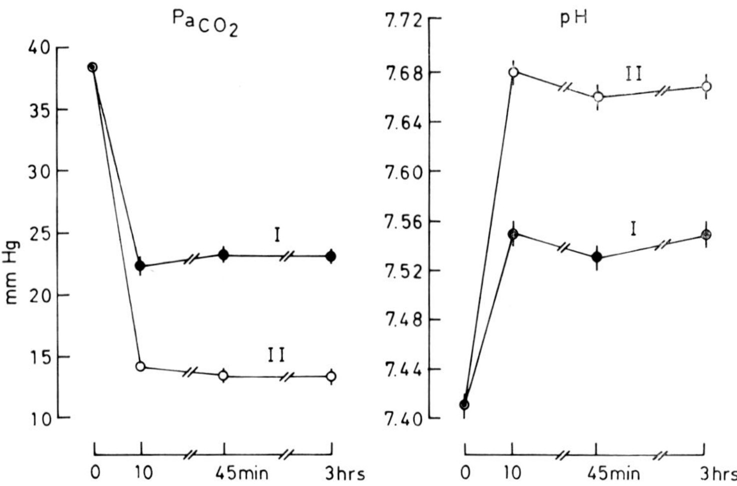

Fig. 1.   *Arterial* P_{CO_2} *and pH measurements in groups of rats hyperventilated to* Pa_{CO_2} *levels of 20–25 or 10–15 mm Hg for periods of 10 min to 3 hr. Each point represents the mean* $\pm$ *SEM of 6–11 values.*

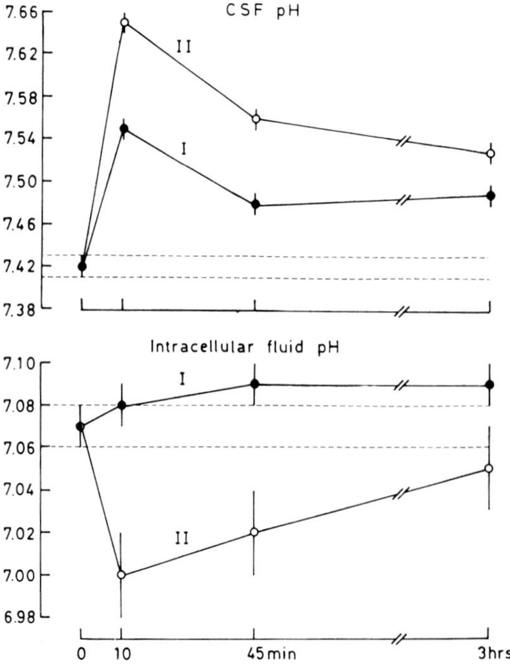

Fig. 2.   *Cisternal cerebrospinal fluid and intracellular fluid pH changes with time in the 2 series of hypocapnic rats. Normocapnic values (broken lines) are represented as* $\pm$ *SEM.*

value. It may be postulated that the very high extracellular (CSF) pH produced in excessive hypocapnia causes a vasoconstriction of such a degree that hypoxia and intracellular lactic acidosis ensue (Fig. 3). The lactic acid (measured as lactate) produced inside the cells immediately starts to diffuse to the extracellular fluid and there it has an acidifying effect

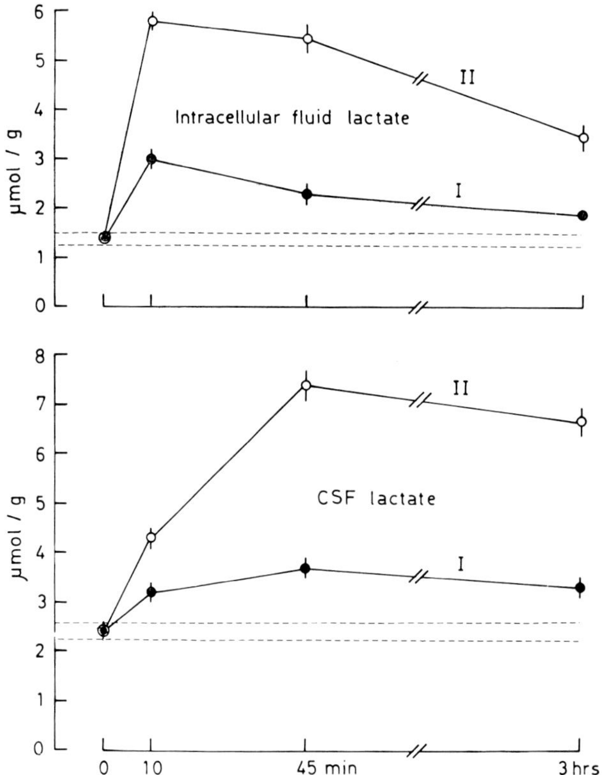

Fig. 3. *Changes in intracellular fluid lactate and cerebrospinal fluid lactate with time in the 2 series of rats made hypocapnic. Normocapnic values (broken lines) are represented as ± SEM.*

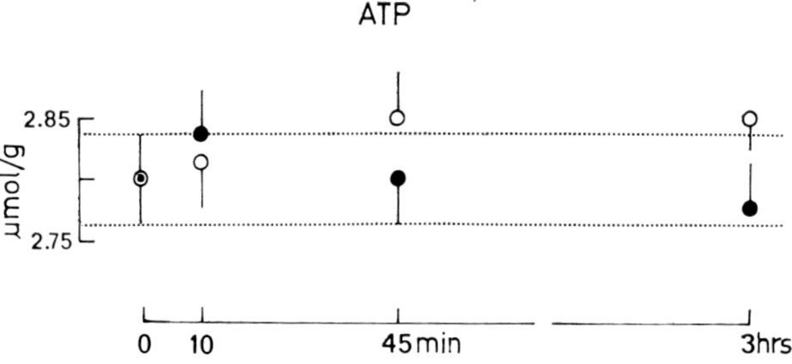

Fig. 4. *Brain tissue concentrations of ATP in the groups of hyperventilated rats. Those ventilated to* Pa_{CO_2} *20–25 mm Hg are indicated with filled symbols. Normocapnic values (broken lines) are represented as ± SEM.*

counteracting the alkalosis and thereby improving blood flow. Due to the diffusion lag the maximum effect is somewhat delayed.

It is concluded that the accumulation of lactic acid as well as of other metabolic acids (cf. Carlsson et al., 1974) explains the normal value for intracellular pH at the P_{CO_2} level 20–25 mm Hg. Further, the results obtained indicate that there is an anaerobic production of lactic acid in the brain at a P_{CO_2} below 15 mm Hg but since the tissue concentrations of ATP (Fig. 4) even at this hypocapnic level did not show significant changes it is necessary to conclude that the tissue hypoxia was of very moderate degree.

REFERENCES

Carlsson, C., Nilsson, L. and Siesjö, B. K. (1974): *Acta anaesth. scand.*, *18*, 104.
Nilsson, L. and Busto, R. (1973): *Acta anaesth. scand.*, *17*, 243.

Chapter XIII

Training and staffing in anaesthesiology

Aims of undergraduate and postgraduate education in anesthesiology

JACK MOYERS

Department of Anesthesia, University Hospital of Iowa College of Medicine,
Iowa City, Iowa, U.S.A.

Undergraduate teaching in anesthesiology is based on the notion that all physicians ought to have some of the technical skills, diagnostic and therapeutic concepts, and clinical judgment that are a part of the daily life of specialists in anesthesiology. The anesthesia scene is an efficient place for medical students to learn these things and anesthesiologists are logical teachers. It is commonplace for us to deal with many important, clinical problems that face other physicians much less frequently, and that derive from other causes.

The demands placed on practicing physicians in one country may differ greatly from those facing doctors in another part of the world. Some of you live in developing nations and must be very self sufficient; others practice in sophisticated medical centers where specialists abound. Consequently, you must specifically relate your objectives of undergraduate teaching in anesthesiology to those skills and capabilities you believe to be required of every physician in your country. This is a most important consideration. In our own part of the world it is not obligatory that all medical graduates be skilled in the administration of anesthesia; so we have learned to emphasize to medical students only those features of what we do that ought to be a part of their life also. Here are some examples of goals we have established for medical students in our University.

1. The student should be able to describe the signs of cardio-respiratory arrest, and discuss their physiological bases. He must be able to outline, step by step, the basic elements of CPR (cardiopulmonary resuscitation) and be able to discuss the rational basis for each maneuver. Finally, he must be able to diagnose arrhythmias commonly associated with cardiac arrest and its therapy, and rationally select appropriate drugs or procedures to correct each arrhythmia.

2. The student must be able to apply basic knowledge and skills in the care and evaluation of comatose patients. He must be capable of using and interpreting monitoring techniques to determine blood pressure, pulse, EKG, CVP, and the patient's response to depressant drugs. We expect the student to demonstrate (on an anesthesized patient) the ability to establish an airway; obtain and maintain a mask fit; and ventilate a patient using the mask and bag, and using mouth to mouth technique. He must be able to intubate the trachea of an adult and of a small child. We require a degree of proficiency such that an 'uncomplicated' patient can be successfully managed, realizing that the 'uncomplicated' patient is as rare as the 'average' man. However, each skill must be demonstrated on a patient whom the teacher feels is not uncommonly problematic for the exercise to be performed.

3. We expect the student to be able to differentiate among possible responses to local anesthetics and to epinephrine mixed with local anesthetics, and to distinguish those which are life threatening from those which are not. An appropriate course of action must be presented. Additionally, the student must be able to outline a rational approach for

performing minor emergency and elective procedures (normally done with local anesthesia) on a patient who says he is 'allergic to Novocaine'. A proper answer will require a knowledge of chemical families, cross sensitivities and side effects of commonly used local anesthetics and their substitutes.

4. Students must learn to apply basic medical knowledge to preanesthetic evaluation and preparation. They must know what findings influence the course of anesthesia, and be able to evaluate risk and physical status in sufficient manner to determine optimal physical condition for surgery and anesthesia. The student should be able to talk appropriately with an adult and with a child about some of the common considerations in anesthesia and he must be able to write rational preanesthetic orders for each.

These are just a few examples. The student can learn from the anesthesiologist equally important lessons having to do with types of hypotension and appropriate therapy, inadvertent intraarterial injection of drugs, postoperative complications (hypothermia, oliguria, delirium, etc.) and respiratory inadequacy in all its manifestations.

In accomplishing these goals of undergraduate education in anesthesiology, it is important for the teacher to remember that he is instructing a young physician, not a future specialist in anesthesia. It is equally important that the student be presented with a full understanding of the basic principles involved in those things he has learned. Otherwise, he will be poorly equipped to transfer his information and skills from the operating room or recovery room scene to his own medical environment in future years. The medical student's recent basic science studies help to make this task easier.

There are many obstacles to required undergraduate experience in anesthesiology for all medical students. However, we remain convinced that our daily work offers to the medical student a number of very important educational experiences that he will not find commonly available from other sources. It is often not easy to convince the Dean or the Curriculum Committee to assign all medical students to the Department of Anesthesia for a modest period of time. Nevertheless, I believe the rewards to the young physician to be well worth the time and effort. Moreover, for recruiting purposes, the favorable by-product of your teaching will be the student's awareness of the scope of anesthesiology and the variety of both basic and clinical research that anesthesiologists perform.

Postgraduate training in anesthesiology is aimed at the development of broadly experienced physicians who will be competent practitioners of the speciality. In this context, the American Board of Anesthesiology currently defines anesthesiology as: 'a practice of medicine dealing with (1) the management of procedures for rendering a patient insensible to pain during surgical, obstetrical and certain medical procedures; (2) the support of life functions under the stress of anesthetic and surgical manipulations; (3) the clinical management of the patient unconscious from whatever cause; (4) the management of problems in pain relief; (5) the management of problems in cardiac and respiratory resuscitation; (6) the clinical management of various fluid, electrolyte and metabolic disturbances.'

A postgraduate training program in anesthesiology should furnish to the would be specialist a number of very important talents and capabilities. First, and some would say foremost, is technical ability. The trainee must acquire technical skill in the administration of anesthesia, by all commonly accepted techniques and employing all commonly accepted agents, even though he expects to restrict his use of some of them at a later date. Technical facility in anesthesia administration is not difficult to acquire; but it does depend upon the teacher's emphasis, the clinical material available, and the extent to which the trainee attaches pride to his effort. It is a very easy thing for any experienced anesthesiologist to remember a host of complications (some minor and inconsequential, but many very serious or even fatal) that resulted not from the anesthesiologist's inadequacy in pharmacology, physiology, or anatomy, but his inability to perform, in safe fashion, the technical skills associated with the administration of anesthesia, supportive intravenous therapy, or ordinary monitoring.

A second aim of postgraduate training in anesthesiology is the trainee's acquisition of mature medical judgment that will allow him to solve the medical problems associated with the care of the patient entrusted to him. This requires that he be not only a specialist in anesthesiology but that he also be a good general physician. He must develop understanding of the interrelationships of disease, surgical metabolic abnormalities, and those factors in a given disease that influence the expected response of the patient to the anesthetic agents we commonly employ. We must continue to emphasize the importance of tailormaking our anesthesia management to specific patients with specific diseases for specific surgical procedures.

Good scholarship is a third goal of postgraduate education in anesthesiology. The teaching staff must somehow establish in its trainees the talent, training and study habits necessary for obtaining, evaluating, and applying new knowledge. The trainee must learn how to learn, and he must be given the tools with which he can rationally adapt, reject or discard both old and new drugs, techniques and concepts.

Here is an excerpt from the brochure we have designed to acquaint prospective trainees with our postgraduate residency program:

'We hope to develop broadly experienced specialists. Teachers trained in various programs present different ideas and methods; supervision is graded and, depending on the resident's progress, varies from strict 'elbow to elbow' monitoring to intelligent neglect. Teaching conferences offer a modest amount of 'spoon feeding' and a wide base of background concepts, facts and experiences from which rational approaches to anesthesia problems and clinical challenges may be derived.

Outside the operating room a resident may expect to find himself acting as resuscitator, specialist in acute medicine, or consultant on a problem involving chronic pain, respiratory insufficiency, poisoning or circulatory dysfunction. In all guises, the resident is taught to approach problems in a scholarly and rational manner and to avoid the futility that attends stereotyped anesthesiology.

To accomplish these ends, the resident staff is served, but not victimized, by a small number of schedules which identify his night and weekend responsibilities, his weekly rotation to the various operating rooms, and the various teaching conferences. These administrative gestures, hopefully, will blend an abundance of clinical teaching opportunities, a minimum of blind obedience, and a staff eager to teach into a postgraduate educational experience that will make the resident a good physician, a responsible anesthesiologist and an eternal student.'

We are not always as successful as we would like to be, and the hard work that goes into our teaching efforts is often unrewarding. I am certain, however, that we would be even less successful and our work even less enjoyable, if we had not thoughtfully established, and if we did not continue to evaluate, our educational aims and the reasons for them.

Undergraduate training in anaesthesia, resuscitation and acute medicine

MARTIN ZINDLER

Department of Anaesthesiology, University of Düsseldorf, Düsseldorf, Federal Republic of Germany

What is the place of anaesthesia in undergraduate education in view of the exploding medical knowledge which is necessary for the treatment of patients, doubling about every 7–10 years, the crowded curriculum approaching the bursting point, considering the fact that only 3%, maximally 5%, of the physicians will actually administer anaesthesia? However, this applies also to the student spending many hours with surgical specialties without ever performing an operation as a physician. As the future physician has to be informed of the possibilities and risks of operative procedures, he has to know about the problems of anaesthesia because he will be associated with patients undergoing anaesthesia in all specialties. It is desirable although not strictly necessary that the student is taught to give anaesthesia.

The important contribution of anaesthesiology to undergraduate teaching is resuscitation and acute medicine, the management of acute life-threatening emergencies. The anaesthesiologist is the expert in keeping the airway open, in artificial ventilation, in treatment of shock.

Considering its importance for every physician, the teaching of resuscitation has so far been neglected. If we do not correct this deficiency in undergraduate training, we shall see the physician standing aside while better instructed life-guards or firemen perform life-saving resuscitation.

In Germany the anaesthesiologists were successful in introducing these ideas in a recent reform of the medical curriculum. In each of these divisions of the medical studies the student is exposed to teaching by anaesthesiologists (see Table 1). Beginning in the winter term 73/74 we had the first experiences with these new regulations with clinical students. In all universities the anaesthesia departments organize these new courses integrating internists, surgeons and neurologists.

According to the catalogue of goals and material which will be required for the first part of the medical examination after the first clinical year the lectures as shown in Table 2 are given. The teaching is patient-orientated bringing groups of 4–5 students into

Table 1. *Reformed medical curriculum in Germany*

	Medicine	6 years	12 terms
Preclinical	First aid course	2nd year	3rd term
Clinical	First medical aid and acute emergencies	3rd year	1st–2nd clinical terms
	Elective anaesthesia and intensive therapy	4th–5th years	3rd–6th clinical terms
Internat	Elective clerkship anaesthesia (4 months) possibly compulsory (1 month)	6th year	7th–8th clinical terms

Table 2.   *Lectures on acute emergencies*

1.	Respiratory insufficiency and arrest	Anaesthesiologist
2.	Respiratory paralysis	Internist
	central (brain trauma, intoxication, infection)	
	peripheral, myasthenia, polyneuritis	
	status asthmaticus	
3.	Cardiac arrest, diagnosis and therapy	Anaesthesiologist
4.	Atrioventricular block, pacemaker,	Anaesthesiologist
	electrical accident, ventricular fibrillation	
5.	Myocardial infarction	Cardiologist
6.	Shock	Anaesthesiologist
	traumatic, hypovolaemic	
	anaphylactic	
7.	Metabolic diseases	Internist
	diabetic coma	
	hypoglycaemic coma	
	hepatic coma	
	coma in electrolyte disorders	
	thyreotoxic crisis	
8.	Cerebral cause	Neurologist
	cerebrovascular accident	
	intracranial pressure	
	cerebral ischaemia	
	acute intracranial inflammation	
	status epilepticus	
9.	Intoxication	Internist
	sedatives	
	alcohol	
	carbon monoxide	
10.	First aid in surgery, fractures, immobilization	Surgeon
	arterial bleeding	
	burns	
11.	Pulmonary oedema	Anaesthesiologist
	near-drowning	
	Accidental hypothermia	
	Heat stroke, insulation	

the anaesthesia, operating and recovery rooms and intensive therapy units. Besides training on manikins in artificial ventilation, cardiac compression and endotracheal intubation, students have the possibility to learn ventilating patients with a mask, start intravenous infusion, etc., and see the activities of the anaesthesiologist in operating rooms and intensive units (Table 3).

The students are greatly interested in the Medical Ambulance Service (Notarztwagen), but in Germany they can go with these ambulance cars only in two universities. In the others, the problems of the special insurance of the students could not be solved.

Particularly informative are experiments in cats or dogs demonstrating the effect of asphyxia until cardiac arrest and resuscitation, treatment of ventricular fibrillation with electroshock and the possibility for every student to intubate a cat.

But good teaching requires time and good teachers. How can a department which has not enough staff and residents for the service to patients in anaesthesia and the demands to the expansion into intensive therapy and emergency aid manage to instruct more than 100 students in small groups, besides all the other activities like training residents, instruction of nurses, in research and other fields? The prime responsibility of a medical school department is to discover, test and deliver the best possible health care. But this includes the education of students and physicians.

Table 3.   *Practical exercises and demonstrations*

Manikin
1. Manikin for cardiorespiratory resuscitation
   Airway
   Mouth-to-nose ventilation
   Ventilation by mask
   Cardiac compression
2. (*a*) Endotracheal intubation, adult and newborn
   (*b*) Venipuncture, needle, canula, butterfly: infusion and transfusion under pressure
3. Diagnosis and therapy of
   Ventricular fibrillation
   Ventricular tachycardia
   Atrial fibrillation and flutter
   Atrioventricular block
   Placement of EEG electrodes

Department of experimental anaesthesia
Endotracheal intubation (cat in ketamine anaesthesia)
Effect of anoxia, hypercarbia until cardiac arrest
Resuscitation, role of drugs
Treatment of ventricular fibrillation

Anaesthesia and operating rooms of surgical specialities
Measurement of blood pressure including Doppler Symptoms of shock
Venipuncture (after local anaesthesia)
Ventilation with mask, controlled and assisted
Oral, nasopharyngeal airway
Endotracheal intubation
Gastric tube, urethral catheter

Recovery rooms
Care of unconscious patients
Airway obstruction
Symptoms of respiratory insufficiency

Intensive-care units
Monitoring ECG, arterial pressure
                central venous pressure
Artificial ventilation
Tracheobronchial toilet
Inhalation therapy
Patient demonstrations:
  Low output syndrome   Myocardial infarction
  Septic shock   Intoxications
  Pleural drainage   Brain trauma
  Management of comatose patients

Emergency admission
Demonstrations without and with patients:
  First surgical aid in the hospital
  Splinting of fractures, pneumatic splints
  Arterial bleeding, tourniquet
  Pneumothorax
  First aid in burns, wounds, open chest

Medical emergency ambulance (Notarztwagen)
Demonstration and use of equipment
First aid and treatment of shock outside the hospital
Stable lateral position of unconscious patients

For the future of our specialty – being the fastest growing specialty in all countries – it is most important and essential to attract more talented students to a career in anaesthesiology. Formerly, most students were not informed about anaesthesia, considering it a technical job of rendering patients unconscious. Anaesthesia had an unfavourable image: that it could be done by nurses and was a secondary service to surgery. Therefore we should make every possible effort to inform the student about the full range of anaesthesiology as part of the work of a physician.

The manpower crisis in anaesthesia with the constantly increasing clinical load and the difficulty in recruiting enough physicians (residents) can only be solved when academic teachers and university departments take on the additional burden to expand and improve their teaching activities. The other possibility, better training and use of nurse anaesthetists, will be discussed later.

Since a major impetus for the decision to become a physician is the satisfaction of helping patients, the teaching in anaesthesiology should be related as much as possible to the process of caring for patients rather than to scientific or technical aspects. Not the achievement of technical skills, but the education of the future physician – to learn, to understand and to grow – is the primary objective.

What other actions can be taken to increase our influence and attract students to choose anaesthesiology as a career? I want to make two suggestions which seem to be applicable in all European countries:

1. Increased *integration of anaesthesiologists in teaching basic sciences*, primarily in pharmacology and also in physiology, covering applied respiratory physiology and possibly in anatomy correlating peripheral neuroanatomy with regional anaesthesia. Anaesthesiology has a unique position between basic sciences and clinical care; it bridges and relates the scientific knowledge to the human art of taking care of sick people. Since the positive decision for a specialty is often made very early, particularly of an active student, it appears favourable that he comes into contact with anaesthesiology as early as possible.

2. The *clerkship* being the best and most effective possibility of teaching should be *increased in number and quality*. The advantage is that this is not confined to university hospitals. In the United States, a preceptorship programme has been instituted since 1968 with excellent results. I propose that every national association of anaesthesiology should institute a similar programme. Certain requirements of good teaching have to be met by the department and the association giving some money per month for each student – if this is not possible, it could be done also by pharmaceutical firms. I hope that this will be discussed further by our American colleagues. I could not imagine a better use of available funds. In conclusion, I wish to stress again that the future of our specialty will be determined by the ability to attract good students to it by our engagement, efforts and success in teaching our students. Let me close by quoting my teacher, Robert Dripps, from *Volume 1/1966* of the series *Clinical Anesthesia*, devoted to Medical Education and Anesthesia, which I recommend warmly to all of you: 'Anesthesiologists who teach the specialty must recognize that they do as much to represent it to students in the way they practice it as physicians and staff members, as in the way they instruct it as teachers. The importance of their having the time and the broad professional interest expected of those who teach and practice in medicine cannot be overestimated.

The great physician-teacher is probably the most effective instrument for attracting people of talent to any medical work.'

REFERENCES

Bruhn, J. G. and Burnap, T. K. (1972): *Anaesthesiology, 37/1*, 79.
Dripps, R. D. (1966): In: *Medical Education and Anesthesia, Vol. 1*, p. 1. Editor: J. M. White. Blackwell Scientific Publications, Oxford-Edinburgh.

Postgraduate training of doctors in anaesthesiology - Sweden

MARTIN H. HOLMDAHL

Department of Anaesthesiology, University Hospital, Uppsala, Sweden

At the present time Sweden has approximately one doctor per 600 people. However, medical school intake has been increased to enable 12 physicians to graduate per 100,000 population yearly; this will allow a doctor-population ratio of 1 to 450 by 1980; a figure which is similar to that of the U.S.S.R. and Israel.

A special government committee has estimated that the number of doctors with specialist competence will be 16,100 in 1985, i.e., a specialist population ratio of 1 to 500. Of this number of specialists 4.4%, or 710, should be anaesthesiologists, i.e., the existing number will be tripled. To attain and maintain this number, the annual output of specialists in anaesthesiology must be around 50. Therefore, from 1977 there is a need for 274 positions for residents, as compared to the 174 existing resident positions in 1972.

These figures demonstrate the tremendous growth of our specialty, and the need for a thorough discussion of the postgraduate training in order, not only to increase the quantity, but also the quality. The existing postgraduate curriculum in Sweden is outlined as a background for this discussion.

Following a 5.5 year medical school curriculum, all doctors must have 2 years of general postgraduate training before obtaining registration. This is similar to house jobs in England or internship in U.S.A. Two months of this period must be spent in an anaesthetic department with intensive-care facilities. Such an obligatory period of training for *all* doctors came with the recognition that every doctor must know how to deal effectively with emergencies and be competent in resuscitation procedures.

After these 7.5 pre-registration years, the period of specialization begins. The present requirement for competence as a specialist in anaesthesiology consists of 4 years of service in specialized departments. As with all other specialties, these years of training are divided into 2 periods. The main period is 3 years and consists of basic clinical training in anaesthesiology. The second period (subsidiary training) is at present one year, and consists of training in other related specialties. For anaesthesiology, such training consists of half a year of service in a surgical clinic and a similar period in a medical clinic. Also, in order to make it possible to include half a year of service in special medical clinics, such as cardiology or clinical physiology, the Swedish Society of Anaesthesiologists has recently requested that the specialization period should be increased to 4.5 years.

Basic training in anaesthesiology must be taken in a hospital with intensive-care facilities, and the hospital must be approved for postgraduate training.

With reference to the role of the anaesthesiologist in intensive therapy the importance of a subsidiary training in medicine, clinical physiology and surgery is clear. Therefore, this part of the training period should be increased rather than decreased. The regulations also include 6 theoretical courses, each of one week's duration, which aim at reviewing the main topics of the specialty and encouraging postgraduate students to read textbooks as well as current literature. These courses deal at present with such subjects as physics applied to anaesthesia, pharmacology of anaesthetic drugs, regional anaesthesia, anaesthesia for special surgery, respiratory physiology and the use of ventilator therapy, and fluid and electrolyte balance. The participants of these courses, which are given on a national basis, go on study leave with full pay. Each course ends with a written examination.

Individual research activity by the student is not required. On the other hand, those wishing to devote their time to research (at present around 10% in anaesthesiology) are accepted for an additional 4-year education leading to a scientific degree, which includes formal courses with examinations and a written thesis. This thesis must contain original work and must be defended in public by a viva voce examination. If the clinical and research training periods are combined, the total period will be shortened to around 7 years.

It may also be of interest to point out that half a year of anaesthesiology is included in the subsidiary training for a specialist in all branches of surgery. We, the anaesthesiologists, interpret this as a sign of recognition of the manifold potential in our specialty.

Finally, medicine is a life-long study and in order to facilitate this, refresher courses for specialists must be given, and taken, at regular intervals.

Product control: Examination or evaluation?

M. K. SYKES

Department of Anaesthetics, Royal Postgraduate Medical School,
DuCane Road, London, United Kingdom

A specialist anaesthetist should have a sound knowledge of those aspects of physiology, pharmacology and anatomy relevant to his practice. He should be capable of assessing the patient's general medical state and should be able to supervise the treatment of medical conditions which may affect the conduct of anaesthesia or surgery. He should be able to make the appropriate clinical measurements when these are required for the assessment of the patient's condition and he should be highly skilled in all the technical procedures associated with the administration of an anaesthetic.

The assessment of a candidate with these potential qualifications obviously presents problems. Methods of assessment vary from the apprenticeship system, with no formal testing, to the theoretical examination. The main advantages and disadvantages of each system may be summarised as follows.

EVALUATION

Ideally the trainee should gain experience in all aspects of anaesthesia under the guidance of a group of experienced teachers who have previously agreed a syllabus and appropriate standard for specialist registration. These teachers should continuously assess the trainee's progress in both the practical and theoretical aspects of the subject and should grant specialist status when the training programme has been satisfactorily completed.

Unfortunately there are many difficulties in the practical implementation of such a scheme. The main problem is that of achievement of uniform standards and the maintenance of those standards from year to year. It is well-known that training programmes are critically dependent on the teaching staff and that, even in the best departments, individuals vary markedly in their teaching ability and in the standard they expect from trainees. The difficulties are compounded if the teacher in a particular subject also assesses the candidate in that subject. Even top rank teachers may transmit a biased viewpoint to the trainee and may then expect that viewpoint to be reproduced when the candidate's knowledge is later tested.

Whilst intellectual bias is certainly a problem, personal bias creates even more difficulties. Few teachers who have had a protracted personal involvement with a trainee can honestly claim that their subsequent assessment is unbiased. Even if the teacher is able to banish personal likes and dislikes from his mind when making the assessment there is a common desire amongst teachers that trainees should successfully complete their training. Few teachers find it possible to be dispassionate in this matter and certification is not infrequently granted to trainees who do not reach a desirable standard.

A further problem concerns the methods used for assessment. Observation of the trainee's response to clinical situations, and of his technical ability obviously provides the main source of information. However, theoretical knowledge cannot be tested satisfactorily by question and answer sessions in the operating room and extra tests must be applied to ensure that the candidate is consolidating his theoretical knowledge. These tests can take the form of regular viva voce confrontations, multiple choice or other written papers.

However, all methods throw a heavy extra load on the teaching staff and require careful preparation and marking. Finally even if the teaching staff is prepared to accept the extra work there is still the problem of ensuring that service commitments do not interfere with the testing programme.

To summarise, continuous evaluation of the trainee probably provides the best method of assessing the trainee's practical ability. However, the evaluation is limited by the period during which the candidate can be observed; it is not free from bias and extra tests of theoretical knowledge must be applied. The greatest problem with the use of evaluation is in equating standards of training throughout a large geographical area.

EXAMINATION

The one big advantage of assessment by examination is that all the candidates at one examination are subject to similar questions posed by a single group of assessors who are chosen for their ability in this field. The candidate's background and personality are not known to the examiners and subjective influences should therefore be minimal. However, it is well known that there are disadvantages.

The most important is the highly artificial nature of any examination, both in form and content. Most examinations are compressed into a short space of time and are held in unfamiliar surroundings. This is unnerving to the candidate who may react adversely under such circumstances. Furthermore temporary illness may invalidate the results. Another objection is that the content of the examination must necessarily be more theoretical than practical. Although some aspects of the subject (e.g. the clinical examination of the patient or the use of some items of apparatus) can be tested under conditions which are not too dissimilar from those existing in clinical practice, much of the examination must necessarily be based on theoretical situations posed by the examiners. The candidate's practical ability therefore remains largely untested and there is a tendency for those with a good theoretical knowledge to pass, whilst many otherwise competent technicians fail.

The third disadvantage is that problems of communication between candidate and examiner are increased. The standard essay-type answer demands a reasonable knowledge of the language which may penalise the overseas candidate. The multiple choice question paper overcomes some of the problems of language but introduces others, for a precise understanding of the question is vital to a correct answer. Furthermore the range of knowledge which can be tested by this method is somewhat limited. The viva voce format is thought by many to be the best answer to the language problem, but many examiners are incoherent and inaudible (as are many candidates) and misunderstandings on both sides are not infrequent.

The fourth disadvantage of the examination system is that candidates tend to concentrate their reading into the sphere of likely examination questions. As a result their general reading suffers and their natural curiosity is often stifled. Involvement in research may also be delayed by the thought of a major confrontation with the examiners. These strictures apply particularly when a specific period is devoted to the assimilation of the basic sciences for practice and theory then appear to be totally divorced. The examination can therefore produce an artificial division between the basic sciences and the practice of anaesthesia. This is ultimately of great detriment to the subsequent intellectual development of the anaesthetist.

What then is the ideal? The answer probably lies in testing the candidate in as many different ways as possible on as many different occasions as possible. Certainly reports from teachers on the candidate's practical ability, clinical judgement and general attitude should be taken into account. The teachers should also be asked to detail the candidate's clinical experience in all the main branches of anaesthesia. However, these statements can only provide part of the information required. They must therefore be augmented with more searching tests of the candidate's knowledge and ability to deal with a particular clinical situation. Multiple choice question papers or essay-type questions could be set by a central examination board and the papers completed at a number of regional centres, although marking would have to be coordinated by a board of examiners. Clinical examinations in medicine could also be held regionally but external examiners would need to be present to ensure reproducibility of standards. Viva voce examinations could also be held regionally but again an external examiner would be required.

Examinations at regional level create many administrative problems and since England is a small country, the tendency has been to centralise the clinical and viva voce parts of the examination, the papers having been sat in London and one other regional centre about 10 days before the oral examinations. In anaesthesia our candidates sit a primary examination in physiology, pharmacology, and physics, clinical chemistry and the principles of clinical measurement. Assessment is by multiple choice question paper, an essay paper and viva voce examination.

In the final examination each candidate sits two written papers on anaesthesia, medicine and surgery, he has a clinical examination in medicine and two viva voce examinations on anaesthesia. Before being awarded the diploma the trainee has to provide evidence that he has completed the prescribed period of training in a hospital which is inspected and recognised by the Board of Faculty but there is at present no direct input from his teachers to the Board of Examiners. It is believed that the examination system provides a stable standard which is applicable to the whole country and which is flexible enough to be adapted to changing patterns of practice. It is felt in the U.K. that this major advantage outweighs the possible advantages of an evaluation system and that although the format of the examination may change, we are unlikely to go back to the system of evaluation which is still favoured in many other countries.

Postgraduate training of nurses in anaesthesia and intensive care

MARTIN H. HOLMDAHL

Department of Anaesthesiology, University Hospital, Uppsala, Sweden

As a basis for discussion the scheme now used in Sweden for training anaesthetic and intensive-care nurses will be presented in detail (new regulations proposed are included).

To enter a nursing school, the trainee must be 18 years old and have completed the 11th academic year of school. These pre-nursing requisites are important when considering the comparable standards to be reached by graduates of similar nursing training programmes in different countries.

Our basic nursing education system has been condensed recently from 3.7 years to five 21-week terms, or 2.5 years as shown in Figure 1. During that time, the nurses have relatively brief exposure to anaesthesia and intensive care. After graduation they have the opportunity to work as assistant nurses in one of the areas requiring specialized training – anaesthesia, intensive care or instrumentation. If, at the end of this time, they wish to

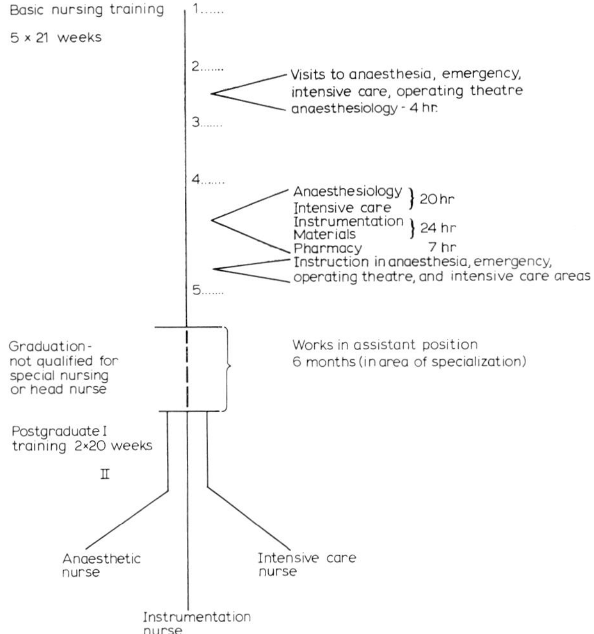

Fig. 1.   *Nurses training programme – general plan.*

572   *M. H. Holmdahl*

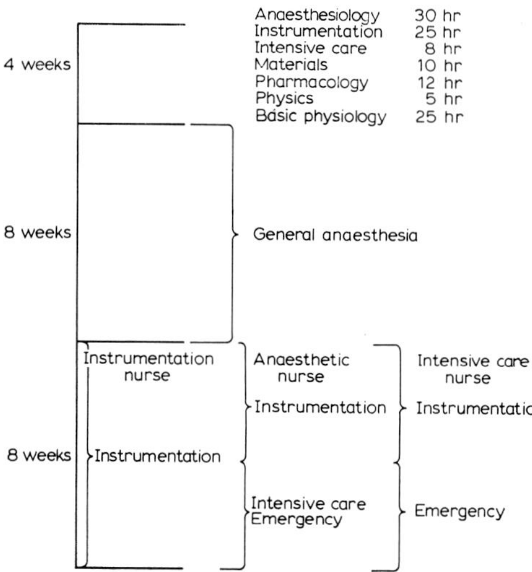

Fig. 2.   *Postgraduate training I – the first 20 weeks.*

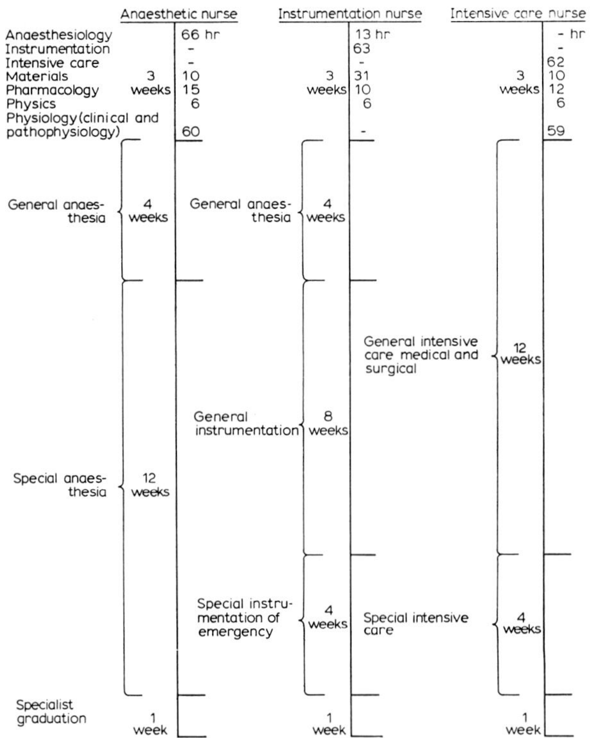

Fig. 3.   *Postgraduate training II – the second 20 weeks.*

study one of these special branches of nursing, they can enter a 40-week postgraduate course (Figs. 2 and 3). Requirements for admission to this postgraduate training are: (1) state registration as a professional nurse, and (2) 6 months' employment as a registered (staff) nurse, except for applicants from the public health nursing programme, who must have a minimum of 2 years' experience. The theoretical lectures given are denoted in the Figures. On satisfactory completion of the course they get a diploma in anaesthesia, intensive care or instrumentation nursing, depending on which course of study was entered. The first 12 weeks of study are identical for all 3 types of special nurse training, but thereafter there is increasing specialization for the various courses of study. Such a system has the following advantages: (1) Fewer teachers are needed because there is less unnecessary repetition of lectures. (2) Nurses graduating from these courses have more appreciation and understanding of the work done by the others, and after graduation they can be usefully employed in any of these 3 areas in an emergency.

In Sweden there are currently 345 nurses in special postgraduate training programmes; of these, approximately 90 will go into anaesthesia. Thus, we anticipate 90 new graduate anaesthetic nurses to enter anaesthesia per year, as compared to 50 new anaesthesiologists. Considering the drop-out rate among nurses, this may ultimately give a doctor-nurse ratio of 1 : 1, as compared to our present ratio of 1 : 2. The estimated number of anaesthetic staff, and the ratio of doctors to nurses will allow for 2 pairs of skilled hands, at least for 'take-off and landing', in all operations, and throughout the more difficult ones on a 24-hr basis.

Anaesthesia and intensive-care nurses: Their background and training

MARTIN ZINDLER

Department of Anaesthesiology, University of Düsseldorf,
Düsseldorf, Federal Republic of Germany

BACKGROUND

One of the major problems of special courses for training nurses in anaesthesia and intensive care is the great difference in knowledge, experience and ability to follow and absorb the teaching.

This can be managed in the *practical instruction* since in the daily practice new nurses work together with more experienced ones. Under the close guidance of the group nurse (4–5 patients) she learns constantly and can always ask.

But the physician who gives *theoretical lectures* does not know the background of the individual nurse coming from different nursing schools and what she remembers of her earlier teaching. The teacher usually overestimates the level of knowledge because, as a rule, only the more advanced nurses ask questions and participate in discussions.

In acute emergencies, every nurse without exception must have enough knowledge to evaluate, decide and act rapidly and correctly. In order to control the effect of teaching on each nurse, it is strongly recommended that frequent tests are employed. This will also increase interest, her own efforts to memorize and hence, the results should improve.

TEACHING PROGRAMME

The recently revised Guide Lines of the German Society of Anaesthesiology and Resuscitation for the special training of nurses in anaesthesia and intensive care are considered. A prerequisite for the course is the normal training and state examination for nurses, which in Germany lasts 3 years.

The requirements of the 2-year course are: theoretical lectures – 240 hr; practical instruction – 640 hr; and clinical work – 74 weeks (of which at least 37 weeks must be in intensive care).

Theoretical lectures and written tests

In Table 1, the suggested topics and hours of the lecture programme are listed. About 50% should be related to general intensive care and resuscitation and 50% to special disciplines (anaesthesia, paediatric intensive care, coronary care, etc.) The lectures are given by physicians.

In these lectures, anatomy, physiology, pathophysiology, biochemistry, pharmacology, physics as well as clinical aspects of anaesthesia, resuscitation and intensive care are discussed in relation to diagnosis, observation and treatment of respective disorders. During the course 10 written tests are given on the topics shown in Table 2.

Table 1. *Theoretical lectures in the 2-year course*

Subject	Total period (hr)
Respiratory function	80
Cardiocirculatory function	40
Kidney and liver function	10
Water and electrolytes	20
Energy and thermal balance	10
Central and peripheral nervous system	40
Endocrine system	10
Blood coagulation	5
Bacteriology and hygiene related to anaesthesia and intensive care	5
Psychology and organization in intensive care	10

Table 2. *Written tests*

Respiratory function
Circulatory function
Renal function, water, electrolyte and acid-base balance
Energy and thermic balance
Central and peripheral nervous system, endocrine system
Artificial ventilation and inhalation therapy
Patient care
Monitoring
General anaesthesia
Regional anaesthesia

Practical instruction and tests

Practical instruction and demonstrations are given by physicians and instruction nurses. During the course for the practical instructions 30 oral tests have to be passed (Table 3). Theoretical lectures and practical instructions are related as much as possible to each other.

Committee for the training programme

This consists of physicians of the various disciplines and the head nurses of the respective units. The committee plans and co-ordinates the training programme and nominates the board of examiners.

EXAMINATION

The 2-year course ends with an examination, divided in 3 parts, written, practical and oral in both general intensive care and a special discipline. At the oral final examinations, an official representative of the government is present.

CONCLUSIONS

The advance in medicine, especially in intensive care, demands knowledge and experience which cannot be gained in the regular basic training in nursing schools.

Table 3.   *Practical tests*

Care during induction and recovery of anaesthesia	Tracheobronchial toilet
Intravenous anaesthesia including preparation	General care of patients in intensive therapy
Inhalation anaesthesia including preparation	Care during artificial ventilation
Regional anaesthesia including preparation	Caloric balance
Injections, infusion, intubation	Preparation and assistance in venous and arterial cut-down
Blood transfusion	Preparation and assistance in tracheostomy
Apparatus and systems for anaesthesia	Diagnosis and emergency measures in acute pulmonary complications
Observation of respiratory function	Disinfection and sterilization
Observation of circulatory function	Documentation and records in anaesthesia
Cardiac resuscitation	Documentation and records in intensive therapy
Life-saving first-aid measures	Introduction and care of catheters and gastric tubes
Cardiopulmonary resuscitation in the hospital	Organization of anaesthesia
Time and volume-cycled ventilators	Organization of intensive therapy
Pressure-cycled ventilators	Handling of material for laboratory tests
Inhalation therapy	Alimentation of patients in intensive therapy

Many activities formerly performed only by physicians have now to be done by nurses who have been trained by special courses. This applies particularly to nurse anaesthetists. However, it should be stressed that anaesthesia can be administered by nurses only under the close supervision and responsibility of a physician.

Quality and success of our intensive therapy depend to a great extent on the quality of our training programme, its careful planning and the engagement of the teachers. The anaesthesiologists must take the additional burden of organizing and improving constantly the training of nurses in anaesthesia and intensive care.

As an additional reward, a good training programme will attract a positive selection of nurses who are willing to learn and to take over responsibility in the demanding and stressful task of caring for our critically ill patients with life-threatening conditions.

REFERENCE

Deutsche Gesellschaft für Anaesthesie und Wiederbelebung (1973): *Anästh. Informat.*, *1*, 28.

Training of emergency medical technicians

J. FREEMAN

Service Universitaire d'Anesthésiologie, Hôpital Cantonal, Lausanne, Switzerland

The use of paramedical technicians to perform first-aid and life-saving measures on their own initiative is accepted in many parts of the world, because it is now established that many regular ambulance personnel recognize both cardiac and respiratory arrest and can perform resuscitation techniques well; well-trained emergency medical technicians can do all that is essential to save and maintain life.

A system of emergency medical care for a region or community should provide for all those types of emergencies which might be reasonably envisaged. The components of such a system comprise first-aid and basic emergency care on the spot, stabilization of the condition of the critically ill and injured followed by transportation with continuing life-support to the nearest appropriate hospital emergency department with surgical and intensive care services. The early application of supportive therapy may contribute significantly to the survival of the acutely ill patient or the accident victim with multiple injuries, but it is rare for adequately-equipped doctors to arrive promptly at the scene, and a doctor is unlikely to arrive first except perhaps in the countryside. Thus the use of emergency technicians can increase the capacity and quality of an emergency medical service. Nevertheless, the training of technicians must be carefully related to the doctor's role in the system and must accord with local needs, i.e. it must be related to the types of illness, accident and catastrophic situations which might occur in the region served, be it urban, suburban or rural.

The use made of emergency technicians varies widely, and the type and degree of their training will depend on the role assigned to them. They may be volunteers or part-time employees serving as a stand-by reserve capable of providing first-aid and basic life-support, including the emergency resuscitation measures in treating cardiopulmonary arrest, or they may be full-time professionals capable of providing advanced life-support for a wide range of conditions; such work includes the definitive treatment of cardiopulmonary arrest, artificial ventilation, intravenous infusion and other intensive care techniques. Emergency technicians may also be specialized, such as those working in trauma teams who are trained in the first-aid, resuscitation and maintenance of the injured (Boyd et al., 1973) or those participating in mobile coronary care who are trained in the principles and techniques of handling cardiac emergencies with or without the remote guidance of a physician (Lambrew et al., 1973; White et al., 1973). Nevertheless, all emergency technicians must be able to act on their own initiative to be effective, and while the duration of training of those to provide first-aid and basic life-support can be comparatively brief, it may take up to 2 years of in-service training to convert an inexperienced ambulance man from a mere stretcher-bearer and driver to an emergency technician capable of providing advanced life-support.

OBJECTIVES OF TRAINING

The main objective of a training programme for emergency technicians is to train personnel to resuscitate and stabilize the condition of critically ill or injured patients and to maintain their condition during transportation to an appropriate hospital emergency centre by acting on their own initiative with or without verbal contact with a doctor. The specific objectives of the emergency system, which are the measurable goals and standards to be established as part of the achievement of their main objective, will be many and varied in accordance with the particular needs and resources of the service and will require careful definition during planning. Having defined the specific objectives of the system, it will be possible to state the objectives of education and training, relating these carefully to the technician's role, the clinical problems, the working and emergency situations anticipated, and also the level of education and pre-existing knowledge and experience of the trainees, which can range from the illiterate (Benson et al., 1972) to experienced ambulance personnel or police (Jaccard and Parisod, 1966). The capability to provide basic emergency care and life-support is usually the objective for volunteer and part-time personnel, while the ideal objective for full-time technicians is the capability to provide advanced emergency care and life-support.

THE TRAINING PROGRAMME

The task of planning a programme is not difficult if the main and specific objectives of training have been well-defined, in which case it is unlikely that an important aspect will be overlooked. Courses may range from 40–600 hr of instruction and in-service training. Both the advice and supervision of doctors with special experience of emergency work is essential for the best results, and the organizers will need the assistance of anaesthetists, cardiologists and trauma surgeons as well as access to the anaesthesia services, emergency and critical care areas of hospitals within the emergency service system, which ideally should be university or teaching centres. The relative amounts of theory, practical work and supervised in-service training must be orientated towards the main objective.

A comprehensive programme would include training in basic and advanced life-support and emergency care in accord with the definitions and recommendations of the International Symposium held in Mainz in 1973 (Frey et al., 1974), including in addition the material necessary to integrate the technicians in the emergency service system.

To train a basic emergency technician the syllabus will comprise the principles and practice of the following:

1. *First-aid*

The management of wounds, application of dressings, enclosure of burns, support and immobilization of fractures, control of visible haemorrhage, clearance and maintenance of the airway, expired air artificial ventilation, and protection of patients from environmental extremes of heat, wet and cold.

2. *Basic life-support*

The emergency resuscitation procedures to maintain life in the absence of pulse and/or breathing, techniques of artificial ventilation without the use of tubes and external cardiac compression.

3. *Basic emergency care*

Use of suction, insertion of pharyngeal airways, administration of oxygen, extrication of casualties, light rescue work, use of traction splints, recognition and immobilization of spinal injuries.

The advanced emergency technician will require in addition to the basic programme, training in the principles and practice of:

1. *Advanced life-support*

The manoeuvres used to prevent cardiac arrest by recognition and correction of life-threatening dysrhythmias, re-establishment of spontaneous circulation by external defibrillation and drugs and the management of shock, which include the setting-up and supervision of intravenous infusions, handling and administration of drugs, inhalational and parenteral analgesia and tracheal intubation.

2. *Advanced emergency care*

This, in addition to basic emergency care and advanced life-support, includes intensive care at the scene and during transfer of patients, observation and care of ill, injured, intubated, artificially ventilated and unconscious patients, bladder catheterization and taking of blood samples.

Both categories of emergency technician will require training in some or all of the following topics: the collection and recording of data essential to the admitting hospital doctor and observations necessary for the evaluation of the emergency medical system; the use, checking and maintenance of the material, equipment and installations of the resuscitation service; the management of simple equipment failure; the use of 2-way radio intercommunication with other components of the emergency service system; the problems of patient care during transport by ambulance, helicopter, stretcher, sledge, chair or boat; the handling and care of crowds, psychotic or suicidal patients; the care of women in active labour and the newborn; the local and regional catastrophe plans, with an understanding of the concept of the plans and the system of command; triage of mass casualties and the assessment of the degree of urgency for care at the first stage of treatment; the measures to be taken to avoid exposure-exhaustion and to avoid electrical hazards, noxious gases and other accidents in damaged or burning buildings and vehicles.

TEACHING METHODS

A preliminary brief course for instructors on the principles and techniques of lectures, demonstrations, practice drills and in particular small group instruction (W.H.O., 1972) before the beginning of the programme will help to establish and maintain the standard of teaching. Theoretical presentations should be didactic, simple and schematic, and teachers should make generous use of audiovisual methods to reproduce reality. Anatomical and physiological presentations should be orientated towards the pathophysiological conditions likely to be encountered. Colour slides of accidents, catastrophes, and the seriously injured, ill and the dead are always impressive and such presentations contribute to the psychological preparation of trainees.

Self-learning techniques are useful to reinforce lectures and demonstrations and to make up for any lack of teachers. Closed-loop films are particularly valuable for the teaching of practical procedures. It is important to prepare text and summaries orientated towards the educational level and training objectives of the trainee technicians.

Practical work should include the use of manikins and simulated situations, not only in the classroom but also in the field. Only frequent repetition will ensure that the capabilities of the technicians will persist in conditions of extreme urgency, improvisation, bad weather and catastrophe. Exposure to emergency work is necessary to stimulate interest and to enhance motivation: trainees should begin to participate in emergency work after preliminary instruction by accompanying trained staff to emergencies, by working under supervision in the hospital critical care areas of the emergency service system in which they are to work, and by participating in catastrophe exercises.

EVALUATION OF PROGRAMME AND PERSONNEL

The evaluation of the trainees and the teaching programme by regular tests and discussion sessions should start from the initiation of the course. Only by such means can gaps in knowledge and lack of understanding be rectified during training and appropriate improvements made in the programme. Acquisition of practical skills can be assessed conveniently with the aid of record cards giving details of attendance at instruction sessions, the quality of return demonstrations and the result of in-service tests. A system of continuing assessment of trainees by their teachers and instructors is valuable both in ensuring a fair result at a certifying examination and in assigning technicians to particular posts or duties.

The prospect of an examination provides an additional incentive to learning. Examinations usually include short-answer question papers, simple multiple choice questionnaires, viva voce examination with pictures and slides, and practical tests on procedures and equipment.

REFRESHER COURSES

Certified emergency medical technicians need refresher courses to maintain their knowledge up to date. However, it is the decay of manipulative skills which presents the greatest problem in maintaining the capabilities of volunteers, part-time personnel and those merely used as an on-call reserve. The deterioration of skills can be minimized by regular sessions of work in a busy admission centre, and probably 10–20 hr per month should be spent in emergency service work. Participation in practice sessions, drills and catastrophe exercises will help to maintain proficiency, personal contacts and a good *esprit de corps*. Annual one-day refresher courses and reassessment of competence at regular intervals of about 2–3 years should ensure the maintenance of a first class emergency technician service.

REFERENCES

Benson, D. M., Esposito, G., Dirsch, J., Whitney, R. and Safar, P. (1972): *J. Trauma, 12*, 408.
Boyd, D. R., Mains, K. D., Romano, T. L. and Nyhus, L. M. (1973): *J. Trauma, 13*, 295.
Frey, R., Ahnefeld, F. W., Nagel, E. L., Poulsen, H. and Safar, P. (1974): *Recommendations of the International Symposium on Mobile Intensive Care Units and Advanced Emergency Care Delivery Systems, Mainz, 1973*. Springer, Berlin.
Jaccard, G. and Parisod, R. (1966): *Méd. et Hyg. (Genève), 24*, 1090.
Lambrew, C. T., Schuchman, W. L. and Cannon, T. H. (1973): *Chest, 63*, 477.
White, N. M., Parker, W. S., Binning, R. A., Kimber, E. R., Ead, H. W. and Chamberlain, D. A. (1973): *Brit. med. J., 3*, 618.
W.H.O. (1972): *Technical Report Series, 489*. World Health Organization, Geneva.

The organization of under- and postgraduate medical education in anaesthesiology

JERZY GARSTKA and WITOLD JURCZYK

Department of Anaesthesiology, Medical Academy, Poznań, Poland

The programme of under- and postgraduate education in first-aid, principles of anaesthesia and intensive therapy in Poland is performed by the Departments of Anaesthesiology at the Medical Academy. The programme of undergraduate medical education is designed for medical students in their 3rd, 4th and 6th courses, for the students of the 3rd and 4th course of dentistry and the 4th course of pharmacy.

The programme for the students in their 3rd year of education comprises 14 hr of lectures on first-aid organization and cardiopulmonary resuscitation (drowning, electric-shock, carbon monoxide poisoning, chemical poisoning, stroke, head and chest injuries, convulsions and cardiac arrest) and 16 hr of practical experience for each student in one of the three ambulances, or mobile care units, under the supervision of the anaesthetists on duty.

For the students in the 4th year, 16 hr of lectures deal with the principles of anaesthesia, local analgesia and intensive therapy. During 5 days of training (4 hr/day) in the operating theatres, the students are taught the technique of intubation, intravenous infusion and the background of anaesthesia.

In the last, the 6th year of education of the medical students, the 15-hr programme deals with clinical anaesthesiology and intensive therapy in different specialties, i.e. surgery, paediatrics, internal medicine, obstetrics and gynaecology. The practical experience is gained in the operating theatres and intensive care units over 10 days (3 hr/day).

The programme for dental students comprises lectures and seminars on first-aid, cardio-pulmonary resuscitation and the principles of anaesthesia and analgesia in dentistry. For the 3rd year students 25 didactic hr and for the 4th year, 35 hr are designated.

A similar programme (30 hr) provides the lectures and practical experience in cardio-pulmonary resuscitation for the 4th year pharmacy students.

Postgraduate education in anaesthesiology in Poland is organised and supervised by the Medical Centre for Postgraduate Education in Warsaw. There are 10 divisions of post-graduate education in anaesthesiology placed in different areas of the country. The education takes place in the Anaesthesiology Department of the Medical Academy and District Hospitals. Each of these divisions organises one 3-month basic course in anaesthesia practice, reanimation and intensive therapy per year, and 2–4 one-month upgrading courses, in different fields of anaesthesia and intensive therapy. The uniform programme is prepared by the Medical Centre of Education.

The programme of education for the basic course comprises 85 hr of theory of clinical anaesthesia and 360 hr of training in the operating theatres and intensive care units and 10 hr of seminar. The teaching programme for the upgrading course consists of 24 hr of lectures, demonstrations and 120 hr of training either in anaesthesia or in intensive therapy. These courses deal with anaesthesia in one of the surgical disciplines. The information courses (refresher courses) in anaesthesia and intensive therapy are held once a year for 3 days in 5 academic centres. These courses comprise lectures and seminars in the recent advances in anaesthesia and intensive therapy and they are intended for consultants and anaesthetists in charge of county and district hospitals.

The number of participants in each of the basic or upgrading courses cannot exceed 12 persons and for the information courses the limit is 20 anaesthetists. The trainees are selected from among many candidates by the district consultants and accepted by the centre. The teaching staff are professors, associate professors and assistant professors and also guest lecturers in related fields from all over the country and abroad.

The trainees are divided into groups of 2–4 persons and undergo training under the supervision of consultant anaesthetists. The most important part of this educational scheme are the hospital days and seminars which are held once a week. Each trainee is obliged to take 3–4 duties per month, either at the hospital or in the mobile care unit. At the end of the courses there is an examination.

All the expenses connected with the organization of courses, tuition, accommodation and living are covered by the Medical Centre of Postgraduate Education. The education and specialization in anaesthesiology in academic and district hospitals take place under permanent supervision of the consultant in anaesthesiology, while candidates from county hospitals are trained at the hospitals periodically once a week.

This situation in anaesthesiology in our country is far from optimal, but results from the great lack of anaesthetists. It is planned that in the near future there will be no other way of specializing in anaesthesia apart from centres representing the highest level of knowledge, skill and facilities in anaesthesia.

Organization of residents teaching programs in anesthesiology

SIMON HALEVY

Department of Anaesthesiology, Columbia University College of Physicians and Surgeons,
New York, N.Y., U.S.A.

The lack of uniformity between existing teaching programs and the paucity of published informations concerning these programs are major difficulties in discussing teaching programs for the residents in anesthesiology. It is, therefore, difficult to describe teaching programs which would be used as an example for an ideal or desirable program. Furthermore, one should not waste efforts to try to develop such ideal programs especially because, as Yamamura observed, 'there are many ways to educate doctors. We should not try to sell the whole world on one system of medical education, and this holds for anesthesiology' (Yamamura, 1967). In addition, it has been acknowledged long ago that one of the most valuable facets of the medical teaching institutions and systems in the U.S.A. is traditional freedom to experiment, to revise curricula and shift goals, with few restraints other than the judgement of those concerned (Austen and Kinney, 1973).

The *first step* in organizing a teaching program in anesthesiology should be to define the framework of its aims and activities, in other words, to devise primary requirements. The present program is a form of graduate medical teaching course, i.e., a system aimed at preparing a physician for a specialty or an advanced academic degree. Subsequently, three major *possibilities* are emphasized: (*a*) a clinical training program, (*b*) an educational program, and (*c*) the common basic 2-year program. The first type of program is primarily designed to create technicians and will therefore require minimum amount of basic science teaching. In contrast, an educational program in addition to providing clinical training, is also designed to develop the habit of independent thinking and scholarship based upon a more comprehensive background. This program would also offer research facilities for interested individuals. The common basic 2-year educational program was created to occupy an intermediate position between the two above mentioned directions. This type of program derives from a necessity but also illustrates the already mentioned basic principle of freedom to experiment. Before a decision is taken in selecting one of the above programs one should be aware, among other things, of some of the consequences. These programs have the tendency to create first and second class citizens, i.e. (1) 'aristocrats,' going into sophisticated research aiming toward academic rewards but also based upon a rigorous scholarly effort, and (2) pure practitioners usually satisfied with their financial rewards.

The decision to select a program is conditioned by the factors which constitute the *second step* of action. The basic idea behind this step is to mold the program holding in mind two major factors: (*a*) the population structure of the residents attending the program at any specific time, and (*b*) the resources available. In the last category are included: (1) the institution offering the program, i.e., its physical resources – facilities, university affiliation, the hospital, etc.; (2) the teachers available in that institution and the students/ teachers ratio within the program; and (3) the financial resources, e.g., teaching grants etc. With respect to the physical resources available, one major problem stands out: the organization of teaching programs in *non university*-affiliated hospitals. To answer this problem, a careful analysis of all factors involved, primarily the residents' and teachers' population and selection of the program, educational or clinical training, is absolutely essential. In any case, teacher facilities should be carefully analyzed both quantitatively (student/teacher ratio) and qualitatively, i.e., who is teaching, qualifications, areas of research, etc. In addition, it is necessary to evaluate other factors: finances, laboratories, number of patients and variety of surgical procedures, library, space, etc. It would be superfluous for instance, to introduce a 10 hr course on statistics applied to research in a non university-affiliated hospital without research facilities. On the contrary, the residents joining such programs would appreciate courses in basic sciences which could prepare them for higher certification or specialty boards. Among these are: applied respiratory physiology, use of ventilators, blood gases monitoring, principles of ECG monitoring, influence of anesthetic agents upon the OR personnel as part of the hospital environment, pharmacology of newer anesthetic agents, anesthesia for various special cases – pediatrics, OB, neurosurgery, etc.

The study of the techniques and organization of basic or clinical *research* is extremely important when research programs are available to residents in anesthesiology. If this exists, statistical analysis is essential, as is the study of a variety of special laboratory techniques related to anesthesiology, such as gas chromatography, cardiac output determination, pulmonary function tests, oxygen consumption, cerebral blood flow determinations, microcirculation, etc. (Anesthesiology Training Committee, 1967). Residents with interest and, especially, with the background and the knowledge necessary should be encouraged to join these programs and attend specialized lectures. Certain limitations however, should be considered. Of these, financial resources are among the most serious since these programs are particularly costly.

There are, however, several special common points which are of use for any teaching program for residents in anesthesiology. Some of these are well-known and well documented and do not require further comments here, e.g., pain clinic or, at least, a minimum of nerve block courses, the treatment of non-surgical chronic pain, inhalation therapy, etc. There are also other important problems which have come into the picture more recently and result from the volume of scientific and clinical information available which has enormously increased over the past 20 years and which demanded that conscientious physicians should be lifetime students (Dryer, 1962; Fink, 1967). To solve this problem within the frame of the anesthesia residency program, a generous allowance of time free to study, i.e., free of clinical responsibilities, should be provided for all residents. This will accomplish two major general objectives: (*a*) continuing education, and (*b*) preparation for examination and certification. It has been shown that the free time to study is more efficiently used when two major tools are at play in teaching programs: (*a*) the organized reading, and especially comments, of leading journals and articles e.g., journal-clubs, and (*b*) the use of modern educational facilities such as audiovisual teaching aids – films, tapes, etc. Free time should be also used to attend major postgraduate courses or refresher courses. Some of the better organized in the U.S.A. are: the annual ASA meeting, the New York State PGA, the Montefiore Medical Center symposium, etc.

A final problem, very rarely discussed, should be considered in any modern teaching program. To bring back *humanism* in our specialty and our professional life is an obligation, and this should start at the resident level (Bonica, 1967). Even though residents do not often perceive the total content of the program and its final aims, they are apt to be responsive to changes within their generation, their social and professional group. Humanism in medicine has a very profound meaning and deserves independent analysis and consideration. Space only permits a brief reference to it here. There has never been a better exposure of this dramatic problem than that which Ignacio Chávez made 16 years ago:

'There is no worse form of spiritual mutilation in a physician than the lack of humanistic culture. He who lacks it may be a great technician in his craft, may be a learned man in his science, but in all else he cannot be but a barbarian, wholly ignorant of that which gives human understanding and sets the values of the moral world. And that is unforgivable . . .

In compliance with the duty imposed by culture, man must immerse himself in the world in which he lives, feeling himself not a stranger, nor even a pure spectator of the social reality that surrounds him . . .

As by a catalytic effect, humanism projected into science invites man to flee from selfish isolation and impels him to work nobly in *collaboration*, at the same time as it offers him a formula to counteract, in large part, the harmful tendencies that rise from specialization – those of the scientist who isolates himself from other men, the specialty that separates itself from other specialties, the medicine which separates itself from other sciences, and the science which divorces itself from culture . . .' (Chávez, 1959).

REFERENCES

Anesthesiology Training Committee (1967): *Status of Research in Anesthesiology*. U.S. National Institute of General Medical Sciences, National Institutes of Health, Bethesda, Md.

Austen, W. G. and Kinney, T. D. (1973): In: *The Future of Medical Education*, Chapter 5, p. 71. Editor: J. Graves. Duke University Press, Durham.

Bonica, J. J. (1967): In: *Education in Anesthesiology*, p. 131. Editor: J. P. Bunker. Columbia University Press, New York – London.

Chávez, I. (1959): *Circulation, 20/4*, 481.

Dryer, B. V. (1962): *J. Amer. med. Ass., 180/8*, 676.

Fink, B. R. (1967): In: *Education in Anesthesiology*, p. 13. Editor: J. P. Bunker. Columbia University Press, New York – London.

Yamamura, H. (1967): In: *Education in Anesthesiology*, p. 107. Editor: J. P. Bunker. Columbia University Press, New York – London.

The significance, organization and practice of studies in anaesthesiology for medical students

H. KREUSCHER

Institut für Anästhesiologie, Städtische Kliniken Osnabrück,
Osnabrück, Federal Republic of Germany

The science of anaesthesiology has hitherto been considered as a specialized subject and on this reasoning it has rarely been included in the undergraduate curriculum. Reforms were considered necessary in the syllabus by the authorities of several countries including the F.R.G. in order to do justice to the educational requirements of a doctor.

The facts which need to be assimilated have increased by approximately 40% within the last 20 years without the original method of teaching being greatly altered. The learning capacity of the student is nearly exhausted and if the mind is overtaxed serious gaps in knowledge may develop. It has reached the stage that teacher and student face a great mountain of knowledge which has to be assimilated. It is not surprising that criticism of, if not a definite refusal to, the growing amount of facts exists.

If the problem of anaesthesiology as a 'learning' subject for students is considered it is necessary at first to be clear about some basic matters.

THE AIM OF MEDICAL STUDY

Years ago the idea of a medical education was that the student should have basic knowledge in all fields and should apply it for the benefit of the population. This idea however needs rethinking because the present specialism within medicine makes new demands upon the future specialist and general practitioner. Therefore it is now necessary that medical training should be a basic education applicable also to specialized subjects. It has to contain structurally the basic matters and encompass effortlessly and without prejudice the important details without gaps. University study can only be a 'basic' education which has to be supplemented by further education or postgraduate studies. The whole purpose of medical study should be that the 'basic doctor' has a chance, in each case, for further medical studies in specialized subjects.

THE PURPOSE OF LEARNING

There is, in the author's opinion, no question that the different sections need to be defined. Some subjects may need to be transferred from one department to another in order that a defined purpose of learning may be achieved. A syllabus for teachers and for students is required.

Departmental interests must be subdued and disciplined within certain boundaries and presentations must be coordinated and adapted according to the needs of the whole and the ultimate purpose.

THE EXAMINATION

In an examination, the understanding and knowledge a student possesses has to be established. The examining-board who have the final responsibility, can visualize the student's capability.

To the question, should 'the basic doctor' have knowledge of anaesthesiology and resuscitation, the answer must be yes, when one considers that with all surgical operations some form of anaesthesia is used. The role of anaesthesia is an important, if not often the determining, risk factor which has to be considered. The students learn surgery not merely to become surgeons but also to give advice to their patients when they themselves turn to other fields of medicine. The conclusion must be to include the study of anaesthesiology. This should also include teaching about basic anaesthetic methods in relation to the operation and the individual risk factors.

The student should be made familiar with the possibilities of and procedure for the treatment of chronic pain with regional nerve block. The phenomenon of pain is an aid to diagnosis and is a therapeutic problem of first importance in modern medicine. This is another gap which must be filled in the education of a doctor. There are only a few specialists who are familiar with the diagnosis and treatment of 'pain-sickness' since the neurological and neurophysiological basis of pain is not thoroughly understood in the present system.

Of special importance is theoretical and practical instruction in resuscitation, that is rehabilitation and preservation of the elementary functions of life. This includes not only the essential resuscitation but also basic intensive care.

Anaesthesiology, more than any other branch, has been appointed this task and with special experience, vital function and clinical research in intensive care, should now make it secure in its claim for teaching students.

The accomplishment of this teaching programme means additional work, which, in view of staff shortages in university departments of anaesthesiology, is a depressing but definite factor.

It must be remembered that the only solution to this situation is to cause the doctor of the future to become acquainted with an attractive subject which not only has real scope for the future, but also has the fascinating combination of applied science and varied clinical work. It is the duty of the authorities and the professors to present or propose to students and their instructors a syllabus which can be added to the education of the 'basic doctor'.

In countries where there is only a written examination there have to be a few particular and consistent questions that have to be presented to the various examination boards. In the F.R.G. there is already such a system. These questions are used as a basis for the verification of the subject in the final examinations.

(For the arrangement of student lessons in anaesthesiology and resuscitation see *Appendix*.)

The effectiveness of teaching can, of course only be recognized by student performance. The student has to prove his ability and not only his knowledge. There can be no doubt, that the traditional form of teaching with solely lessons cannot meet the new demands. Tutoring in small groups, with a reasonable combination of theory and practice, should be carried out by assistant doctors, advanced students and not only by the teachers at Universities. We should notice the objective importance as part of the basic medical education and draw the conclusion to take a greater part in the progress of education for we have this obligation to ourselves, to our colleagues in the future and, of course, principally to our patients.

Appendix

STUDENT LESSONS IN ANAESTHESIOLOGY AND RESUSCITATION

Theoretical section

The following subjects could be presented in the course of 1 year, if 1 or 2 lectures are given per week.

Fundamentals
1. Special effects and side-effects of pharmacological agents used in anaesthesia.
2. Anaesthesia systems and anaesthesia apparatus.
3. Methods of maintaining airway during anaesthesia.
4. Respiration and ventilation.
5. Cardiovascular effects of anaesthesia and operation.
6. Specific anaesthesia techniques.
7. Monitoring of vital functions during anaesthesia and operation.
8. Studies and maintenance of general anaesthesia.

At the end of the section 'Fundamentals' a written test examination should be conducted. Passing the examination should be a prerequisite for further participation in the practical section which, from now on, should run parallel to the theoretical lectures.

Clinical anaesthesia
1. Preoperative measures and premedication.
2. Anaesthesia techniques depending on the kind of surgical procedure.
3. Anaesthesia techniques in extreme age-groups.
4. Anaesthesia techniques for high-risk patients.

Shock
1. Aetiology and pathophysiology.
2. Diagnosis of shock.
3. Therapy of shock.

Reanimation

General postoperative management

Treatment of anaesthetic accidents
1. During general anaesthesia.
2. During regional anaesthesia.

Intensive care
1. Definitions, indications and organization.
2. Methods of maintaning vital functions.
3. Tracheobronchial care in tracheostomized patients and inhalation therapy.

Practical section

The students take part in the operating programme. This should be done in small groups – up to 3 students – who will be taken care of by a senior anaesthetist. They should be instructed in the following:

Recovery room (one week, 4 hr/day)
1. Monitoring the vital functions during the recovery period.
2. Maintenance of the airway with and without aids.
3. Techniques of injection and infusion.

Anaesthesia induction room (one week, 4 hr/day)
1. Manipulation of an anaesthesia apparatus including the control of its functions.
2. Techniques of ventilation and anaesthesia apparatus via an endotracheal catheter or face mask.
3. Technique of endotracheal intubation.
4. Technique of induction and maintenance of anaesthesia.
5. Assessment of the study of anaesthesia and management of anaesthesia.
6. Control of vital functions during operation.

Intensive care unit (one week, 8 hr/day)
1. Principles of intensive care including positioning of the patient, infusion-techniques with the aid of vena cava-catheters, techniques of continuous ventilation using ventilators, care of tracheostomy.
2. Principles of fluid and electrolyte balance.
3. Value of laboratory data.

During final medical examination, the student should pass a written test (multiple choice questions) on the subjects of anaesthesia and reanimation. The subjects may be divided – 18% basic science concerning anaesthetics, 30% clinical anaesthesia, 30% reanimation, 22% intensive care.

Training of specialists in anesthesiology and intensive care at the Bucharest Faculty for Postgraduate Training of Physicians and Pharmacists

GEORGE LITARCZEK and ION CRISTEA

Department of Anesthesiology and Intensive Care, Fundeni Hospital, Bucharest, Rumania

The specialty of 'anesthesiology and resuscitation' was recognized in Rumania in 1957. The teaching of anesthesiology was started a few years earlier, in 1951, only 3 years after the foundation of the Faculty for Postgraduate Training of Physicians and Pharmacists. It consisted of a 2-month course intended to initiate surgeons in modern anesthesia. Some of these surgeons later devoted themselves to the new specialty. After the recognition of anesthesiology as an independent specialty in 1957 a new specialization course was started which lasted 3–6 and, since 1959, 10–12 months. The first courses were held by different specialists such as surgeons, pharmacologists, physiologists, hematologists, etc. Later the newly qualified, mostly self-trained, anesthesiologists joined in, and in 1962, took over the whole task of the specialization courses as well as the refresher courses, obviously in collaboration with other specialists in connected fields. This type of course, lasting from 10 months to 1 year, was an integral part of the 3-year training period for registrars, which was, and is, the compulsory training time for anesthesiologists. During this time, beside the lectures, the registrar had to fulfil another 2 years of practical activity in a surgical center under the direct supervision of qualified anesthesiologists (senior registrar or consultant).

After finishing this period, the registrar had to pass an examination to become senior registrar (specialist). The examination, which is held only in Bucharest under the supervision of the Ministry of Health, is composed of a written test, a practical (anesthesiology) test and a clinical (reanimation-intensive care) test.

The organizational concept of the one-year course during specialization time was to direct the activity of the students into 2 main fields.

The theoretical aspects – for which a programme was set up comprising all the relevant knowledge necessary to an anesthesiologist and reanimatologist for his activity in the operating theatre as well as in the postoperative wards or intensive care units. Sessions concerning blood transfusion, anatomy, minor surgery, pharmacology, statistics and social sciences were also included, and specialists in each of these fields were called upon to give the lectures. The activity in this sector will be extended starting with this year to all 3 years of residency, that is, it will include also the remaining 2 years, which up to now were not under the supervision of the faculty for postgraduate training. During this period beside the practical activity as anesthesiologists, the students will have to finish practical terms and corresponding theoretical lectures in internal medicine (2 months), surgery (3 months), cardiology (1 month), neurology (1 month), pulmonary and cardiovascular investigations (1 month). For all these specialties a corresponding program has been set up. This ncludes the fundamental problems of the surgical intervention, the pathophysiology and treatment of pulmonary, circulatory, excretory, metabolic (fluid and electrolyte balance, acid-base and nutrition) and nervous system from the viewpoint of anesthesiology and intensive care.

The basic course is given in 3 lectures (2 hr/week) over 12 months, usually during the afternoon. The program of this course is divided in 2 parts: anesthesiology and intensive care. The first part is two parallel series of lectures on the pharmacological basis and the technical basis of anesthesiology. The pharmacology is itself divided into 4 parts comprising the 4 main pharmacological aspects of anesthesiology: analgesia, sleep and sedation, relaxation and adverse reactions, including shock. Every anesthesiological technique is described as a pharmacological mosaic into which analgesia enters as a compulsory element. The other 3 elements are related to the operation and the patient. The second part concerns all technical aspects. An important place is given to the techniques of local and regional analgesia used for surgery and therapy.

The section concerning reanimation and intensive care offers lectures about the organization of intensive care units and the main problem of treatment of patients. It emphasizes the technical and theoretical problems concerned with artificial ventilation, extrarenal dialysis, cardiac resuscitation, treatment of acute arrhythmias, problems raised by i.v. therapy, treatment of comatose or poisoned patients etc.

At the end of the course an examination comprising a written (multiple choice) and a practical test is held. Five years experience with this method of continuous teaching and control, compared with the uncontrolled methods showed this to be superior. The homogeneity of the groups trained in this manner is evident when they are compared with former students.

The practical activity of registrars is in the operating theatres and the postoperative and intensive care units of anesthesia and intensive care departments. From the total of 36 months of training the resident has 26 months of practicals in the specialty, which since 1971 is called anesthesiology and intensive care. The rest is occupied in the related specialties.

The programme was set up in direct relation to the tasks which the future specialist will have to face in his work. As in all district hospitals and in hospitals with more than 400 beds anesthesia and intensive care departments are organized, the future specialist will have to solve problems raised in the operating theatres and in postoperative wards and intensive care units.

The efficiency of our courses was good enough to provide sufficient knowledge to more than 500 students.

New techniques in the teaching of anesthesiology

MARK B. RAVIN

Department of Anesthesiology, University of Florida College of Medicine, Gainesville, Fla., U.S.A.

Because of the rapid expansion in the size of medical school classes, it is becoming increasingly difficult to give all students 'hands on' experience. Consequently we have developed and evaluated two animal teaching models to introduce the student to: (1) the techniques of endotracheal intubation (Calderwood and Ravin, 1972), (2) the fundamental pharmacologic principles of uptake and distribution of drugs (Ravin and Tham, 1974), (3) the observation of the signs of clinical anesthesia (Ravin and Tham, 1974), and (4) the principles of cardiopulmonary resuscitation (Ravin and Tham, 1974). In addition, we have adapted the video techniques of athletic coaches and surgeons, including instant replay, to identify errors and improve the motor skills of our anesthesia housestaff (Ravin, 1974).

THE CAT AS A TEACHING MODEL FOR ENDOTRACHEAL INTUBATION

Cats weighing 2–5 kg are anesthetized with an injection of 100 mg of ketamine into the triceps muscle. Within 3–5 min the cats lose their righting reflex, the antigravity muscles of the front legs frequently become rigid and opisthotonos may develop. The swallowing reflex is not abolished, and may be stimulated by salivation. To demonstrate antisialagogic effects, the cats are divided into 2 groups, one of which is given 0.4 mg of atropine in addition to the ketamine. A No. 1 Macintosh blade and a 3.5 mm red rubber endotracheal tube with stylet are used.

Each student practices intubating the trachea until he develops skill and confidence. Students rapidly adapt to the human, the experience gained in intubating the trachea in cats. In a study on the number of trials required for the student to achieve three successful human intubations, students with cat model experience were found to have learned approximately twice as fast as the students who were not exposed to the cat intubation experience.

THE GOLDFISH AS AN ANESTHESIA AND RESUSCITATION TEACHING MODEL

We chose goldfish because they are inexpensive to buy and maintain, yield reproducible results, have physiologic traits which make them particularly suitable for demonstrating anesthesia induction, and their somewhat unique use as a teaching model makes the demonstration more memorable.

The fish are placed in an aquarium beaker one at a time and anesthesia from a gas machine is bubbled into the water at a concentration of 9 % cyclopropane or a concentration of 2% halothane in 2 1 O₂/min. The students, previously informed of the various stages of fish anesthesia, observe and record the progression of anesthetic depths from Stage I through Stage IV. This clinical observation is later correlated with the water anesthetic uptake curves.

Introduction to resuscitation

As soon as the fish has passed into Stage IV (respiratory arrest), it is transferred to another beaker containing aquarium water. If the fish is left untouched, or the water is gently stirred, there is usually no sign of respiratory movement. However, if the fish is gently compressed between the thumb and forefinger so that water is forced through the gills, the fish usually recovers.

Evaluation

This demonstration does not supplant our drug uptake and distribution lecture or the cardiopulmonary resuscitation discussion, demonstration and practice. By using pre- and post-testing it appears that, compared to conventional lecture techniques, the use of the fish model enhances motivation for learning and retention of knowledge.

TEACHING ANESTHESIA MOTOR SKILLS BY REVIEW OF VIDEOTAPED PERFORMANCES

A single manned video camera (Sony AVC-3200) is placed at the foot and to the side of the operating table. The residents are videotaped on half-inch reel to reel tape while they perform an anesthetic induction through endotracheal intubation sequence. Later that day, they review their performance with an attending anesthesiologist. The motor skill sequence is critiqued in terms of technique, inappropriate motion, progression of induction, monitoring, safety and sterility.

The review of videotape performance has several advantages. The student is able to visualize his performance without the handicap of performing simultaneously in a stressful situation. Therefore, objective analysis free from anxiety is possible. The student appears eager to correct his errors, which reinforces the educational value. Motor skill sequences can be compared and counted objectively. Finally, the method appears to be simple, inexpensive and enthusiastically accepted.

REFERENCES

Calderwood, H. W. and Ravin, M. B. (1972): *Anesth. Analg. Curr. Res.*, *51/2*, 258.
Ravin, M. B. (1974): *Anesth. Analg. Curr. Res.*, in press.
Ravin, M. B. and Tham, M. K. (1974): *Anesthesiology*, in press.

Chapter XIV

Electronics in anaesthesiology and resuscitation

Trend prediction and patient monitoring

JOHN A. BUSHMAN and A. GAMBLE

Research Department of Anaesthetics,
Royal College of Surgeons of England, London, United Kingdom

Two main problems are associated with patient monitoring during anaesthesia. The first is concerned with deciding which variables should be measured and the second with how to treat the data once it has been gathered.

With regard to which of the available variables should be measured it is clear that for a monitoring system to have the maximum possible use it must utilise non-invasive techniques. Obviously there is a use for invasive techniques in certain situations where their use may be mandatory. The fact remains however, that invasive techniques are not acceptable to the vast majority of patients who would benefit from some monitoring procedure. If a method is to be widely used it must also be acceptable to the clinician in that it is easy for him to extract the relevant information from the patient. In an operating list consisting of a number of short cases where the anaesthetist may be working without skilled help it is essential that the monitoring method used should be very easy for the anaesthetist to apply, otherwise he will either delay the list by using it or abandon the method.

With regard to the non-invasive methods for monitoring which are available, it is important to extract the maximum amount of information possible from the signals by combining some channels of information to give an additional piece of information. The work described in this paper was done with a Philips patient monitoring system which together with other variables is able to measure the ECG, the pulse and the respiratory waveforms. These variables alone also give information about the pulse amplitude, pulse deficit, cardiac arrhythmias, heart rate and respiration rate. Integral with the cabinet carrying the patient monitoring modules is a 3-channel pen recorder so that we are able to record any of the outputs from the modules.

By combining the pulse deficit module with the blood pressure module, which is normally used invasively, it is possible to measure the blood pressure non-invasively. This is achieved by inflating a cuff round the arm while the pulse amplitude is measured from a finger of that arm. The pulse amplitude is previously adjusted to give a 50% full-scale deflection and then the cuff is inflated. As soon as a pulse deficit is detected then the cuff pressure is measured and recorded as the systolic blood pressure. The cuff is then deflated. The advantage of this system is that the amplitude of the pulse can be adjusted to some arbitrary level, in this case 50% of a full-scale deflection, before the cuff is inflated so that the system is always measuring the same decrease in amplitude whether the blood pressure is high or low at the time of measurement.

In addition, we have shown that it is not strictly necessary using the Philips apparatus to use 5 electrodes to gain this record, the ECG or the impedance pneumogram. The same information can in fact be gained from the placement of only 2 electrodes on the body, one of which can be the diathermy lead and the other can be the anaesthetic mask together with the finger pulse detector.

Having obtained the data non-invasively, by methods that are acceptable to both the

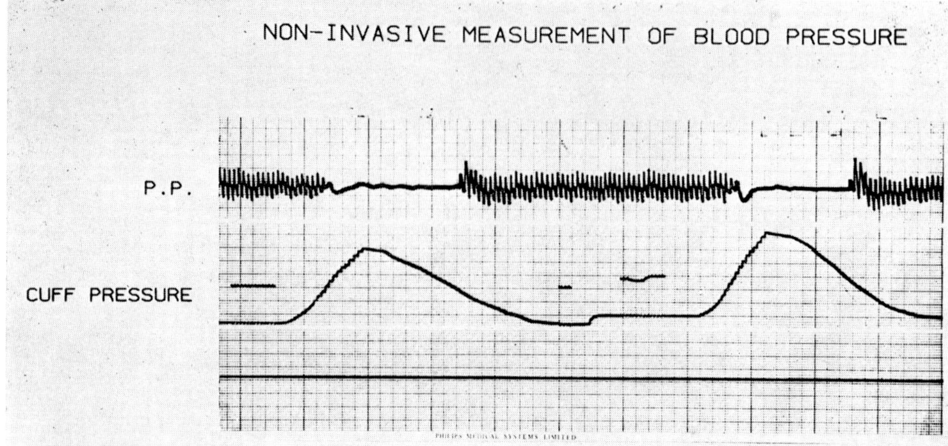

Fig. 1.   *Diagram of cuff pressure and peripheral pulse. This diagram shows the pulse amplitude from a photoelectric transducer on the finger and the pressure in a cuff round the arm on the same side. The top tracing is the pulse amplitude which becomes obliterated at the moment when the pressure in the cuff equals the systolic blood pressure. The lower trace shows the pressure in the cuff together with a calibration pulse, indicating the way the base line and the amplitude can be positioned by controls on the module.*

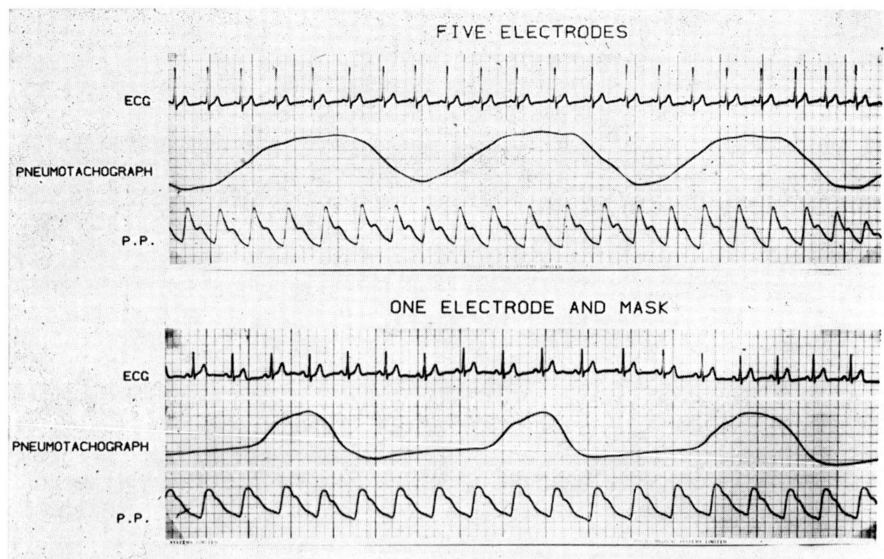

Fig. 2.   *The above diagram shows the ECG and impedance pneumotachograph from a conventional 5-lead system and from one lead attached to the patient and a second lead attached to the mask. Clearly such an ECG is entirely acceptable for measuring the pulse rate, detecting arrhythmias and for noting changes in the waveform.*

patient, in terms of discomfort and the clinician in terms of convenience of application, it is necessary to process it in some way.

In order to do this it is first necessary to establish how often the data requires to be sampled. Since all the high frequency analysis is performed by the analogue equipment, that is the pulse amplitude, pulse deficit and arrhythmias, it is not necessary to perform any fast sampling. It would be wasteful to sample the signals from the analogue modules at a rate which was either faster than required on clinical grounds or at a rate which was faster than dictated by the time constant of the module concerned. If the sampling rate was made much slower than this then information would be lost to the system, which would be acceptable as long as it did not affect clinical decisions on the care of the patient. With these factors in mind it was decided that the channels available from the analogue monitoring system should be logged every 15 sec. The sampling rate is 1 Hz and this data is then averaged every 15 sec. The data logging system runs on a PDP 12 computer. The computer program written in Fortran can manage to log at least 36 inputs in any combination required from one input from each of 36 patients to 6 inputs from 6 patients. The program could be made to run on any computer having 16 K of store, a disk and a plotter.

If the program were rewritten in assembly language or the assembled Fortran program was optimised, the system would be able to manage 6 inputs from at least 12 patients. Any one of the logged channels can be displayed on the visual display unit and within an 8-hr period all the logged data can be plotted on a digital plotter.

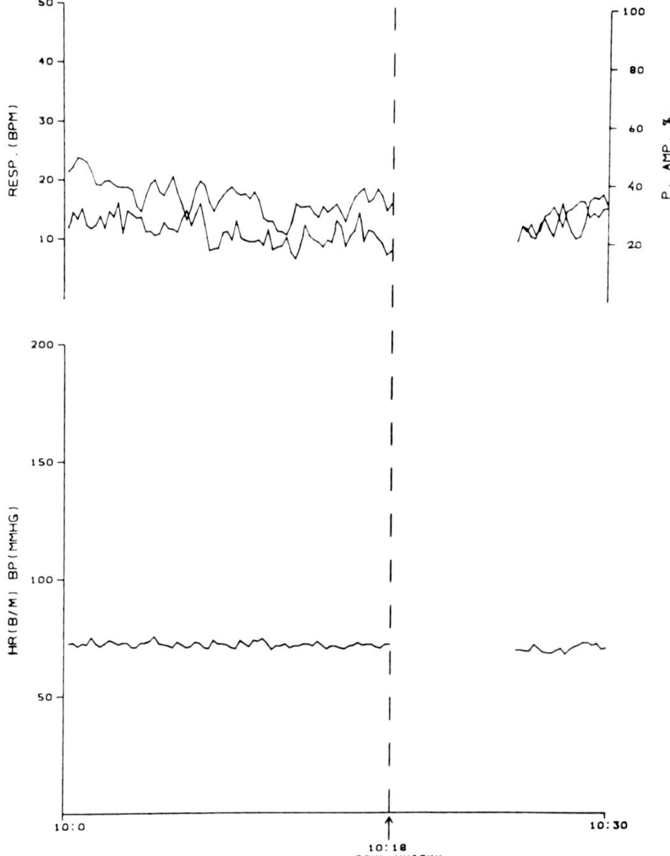

Fig. 3. *This shows the facility for making comments on the final record. This whole system could be custom made to fit any particular chart size or comment format. The variables are normally plotted in different colours. The above record was taken from a volunteer having 50 ml whisky as a stress.*

The plots can be made available in virtually any form. Two forms at present available on the system are an 8-hr plot and a 0.5-hr plot of any section of the 8-hr plot giving a 16 to 1 expansion of the time scale. Prior to the actual plotting but incorporated in the plotting package is the facility to enter comments which appear at the relevant times on the abscissa of the plot.

A number of different approaches are being made to the problem of trend detection. Unless sensitive methods are used to establish the development of a trend it will not be observed until it is so well established that any clinical advantage which might have been gained is lost as the measured variables will eventually be obviously outside normal limits. However, if the method is too sensitive it will alarm on trends which are destined to return to normal having never constituted any threat to the stability of the patient.

A number of separate methods have been evaluated. These include Trigg's tracking signal (Trigg, 1964), Patient Condition Factor (Hope et al., 1973), the cusum method, a cusum and area under the error curve method, a method using continuous integration of the signal and then examining the change in the slope of the integral and lastly an empirical method based on a number of discrete decisions made by the program.

These methods fall into one of two categories. In the first are those methods which can be thought of as analogue approaches, though they may in fact be performed by a digital computer technique. These methods perform a series of mathematical operations on the data and produce a running statistic on the probability of the development of a trend which if continued would be detrimental to the patient. In the second category are those methods where a number of tests are performed on each piece of data logged. Depending on the result of these algorithms the processing may be changed to a different set of algorithms considered to be more pertinent to the present data in the light of the history of that data.

Each of the above approaches works well in certain circumstances but not in all circumstances and at this time it is likely that a method which utilises certain aspects of both of the above categories is likely to prove the best.

Because the physiological variables normally measured from patients are controlled by homeostatic mechanisms which attempt to keep the measured variables close to normal, it is not until the system has been so severely stressed that homeostatic control fails, that any large change will be seen in the measured variable.

Though some of the methods described show some promise there are still many problems to be overcome in the detection of trends in servo-controlled system which may be suffering a long-term stress due to disease but which is otherwise at rest. The most promising line of investigation at this time is the examination of trends following a short-term stress. In this case both the amplitude of the response to the stress and the time for the measured variables to return to normal is indicative of the stability of the system.

REFERENCES

Hope, C. E., Lewis, C. D., Perry, I. R. and Gamble, A. (1973): *Brit. J. Anaesth.*, 45, 440.
Trigg, D. W. (1964): *Operational Res. Quart.*, 15, 271.

Simple monitoring systems

M. A. NALDA

Department of Anesthesiology, University of Salamanca Faculty of Medicine, Salamanca, Spain

The constant development of anesthesiology and resuscitation and thus the increase both of surgical possibilities and of the treatment of patients in critical situations, require some patient monitoring systems which make the operating room or the recovery room look like a space ship full of complex machines which in turn require technical capabilities in the fields of physics, electronics and mathematics.

Modern medicine requires dynamic supervision of a series of parameters that our predecessors did not need, since they practiced static medicine. The only way to achieve this dynamism is to base it upon continuous monitoring of patients. The monitoring era is at a peak, and a difference has developed between the economic ability of hospitals to be monitored as a whole or in part. It is important to realize that the most perfect monitoring installation is only useful to follow-up different parts of a patient, since the care of the patient as a whole can only be done directly by the physician who is caring for the patient and who considers him as a total unit.

When a patient is monitored, a series of biological phenomena can be visualized at the same time as they are occurring so that preventing them or treating them becomes easier. From the study of the records obtained over long periods of time, useful information is available and details which would otherwise go unnoticed are recorded.

All this assumes a guarantee for the patient being monitored, and a relatively quick recovery of the initial investment incurred in the purchase of the material since, as a result of better care, many superfluous treatments are avoided and resuscitation suspended or not started in patients who are not salvageable using current methods which are undoubtedly very costly. It is important that specialists should not feel impotent, because they are in economically weak centers and cannot obtain adequate monitoring apparatus which they regard as ideal. In many places there is a great selection of very costly gadgets, which are not used adequately, and thus their real utility is well below its potential.

Monitoring has been super-inflated and an enormous quantity of parameters can be recorded but they are not always as necessary or as useful as they may seem at first sight. In our opinion there are some essential observations which may be made with relatively simple methods and with machinery from which reliable information can be obtained even though the apparatus is not ostentatious.

Display screens with digital output of recorded values have increased recently but this form of display is not very practical, especially during prolonged monitoring. Digitally expressed values, with continual changes in the figures may be dangerous – the figures are easy to observe, but, given rapid changes, it is very difficult to memorize and retain all the variations that occur and also it is quite possible that these changes may occur without notice. The danger is much greater if more than one patient is monitored simultaneously, since there will be a pile-up of different colored data in our minds, which cannot be evaluated and are practically impossible to transcribe onto paper.

Analog monitors, on the contrary, with or without an oscilloscope, provide either a simultaneous or a paper record. For multiple or prolonged monitoring, this is the only valid system. It is always more practical, comfortable and useful to study curves written on calibrated paper, than to consult hundreds or thousands of numbers, whose transcription may be laden with errors because of tiredness or sheer monotony. There is also available slow recording, 2–3 cm/hr, or intermittent recording which avoids the expense of kilometers of paper, but is also difficult to handle and analyse after collection.

The following parameters have been claimed to be indispensable criteria: (1) vital signs: systolic arterial pressure, diastolic arterial pressure, mean arterial pressure, first derivative of arterial pressure, left arterial pressure, heart rate, pulse, temperature; (2) respiratory measurements: minute volume, tidal volume, respiratory rate, compliance, nonelastic airway resistance, work of respiration; (3) alveolar gas analysis: oxygen uptake, respiratory quotient, end-expiratory CO_2 partial pressure, alveolar oxygen tension, inspired oxygen concentration; (4) blood gas analysis: arterial oxygen tension, venous oxygen tension, pH, arterial CO_2 tension, venous CO_2 tension, standard bicarbonate, base excess; (5) serum electrolytes: K, Na, Cl; (6) cardiac output determinations: Fick method, dye dilution method, cardiopulmonary blood volume.

However, these are not necessary for adequate treatment of a patient; the really indispensable parameters must be the following.

Cardiopulmonary function

ECG must be continuously displayed with a cardioscope, and with a recorder. In the operating room it may suffice to use a cardioscope, but in the recovery room, graphic recording is necessary. Pressures, systolic and diastolic arterial, or in their absence, the mean arterial pressure, to which one has got to get accustomed. In certain cases it is interesting to know and record pulmonary arterial pressure. CVP must be monitored in all patients. Plethysmography is very useful in shocked patients since the peripheral circulatory situation can be assessed. The pulse wave, however, is difficult to record continously. Venous return, though not a common parameter, is one that can be very useful in recovery.

Ventilatory function

Frequency and rhythm are 2 fundamental parameters in patients with spontaneous respiration. Minute and tidal volume must be measured rigorously; alveolar ventilation must be followed. When mechanical ventilation is used, the inflation pressure and waveform of the ventilator should be recorded in order to obtain the maximum information from the machine.

Respiratory function

The respiratory parameters indicate the results of ventilation and is the only measurement which is really useful in determining the adequacy of ventilation and gaseous exchange. Nevertheless, it is difficult to measure these parameters in a continuous manner and as a result, generally speaking, usually they are poorly controlled. Inspired O_2 and expired CO_2 concentrations are the values of interest.

Even though it is actually possible to monitor in a continuous manner the values of blood gases, this type of recording still offers some problems yet not resolved by the bioengineers. So the laboratory still continues to be indispensable for the correct determination of these periodic checks.

Nervous function

The continuous monitoring of the EEG is indispensable in certain types of operations but it must not be omitted in some patients in recovery since from the study and analysis of the recordings obtained therapeutic information of great importance may be gathered. Eight electrodes are necessary.

Metabolism

Patients in recovery need a series of measurements; some of them, like temperature, may be monitored in a very satisfactory way. Others, like diuresis or weight, still pose problems for electronic recording.

The oxygen consumption and cardinal parameters of ventilation must be likewise monitored for a long time.

The meaning of simultaneous monitoring of respiratory minute volume and end-tidal CO₂

H. OEHMIG

Krankenhauswissenschaftliches Institut 'Dr. N. P. Petri',
Frechen-Marsdorf, Federal Republic of Germany

Ventilation is stimulated by a raised arterial carbon dioxide tension; the higher the P_{CO_2} the more vigorous is spontaneous ventilation in both rate and tidal volume.

This mechanism works automatically as a servo-system. In artificial respiration a patient is ventilated manually or by means of a ventilator. If a Wright respirometer or a Draeger volumeter is used the volume of each breath can be determined. But even these simple instruments are very rarely in use or not even available in the operation room. Figure 1 shows normal respiratory minute volume of between 6 and 8 l/min and a 'normal' end-tidal CO_2 concentration of about 5.5 vol%, which is about 40 mm Hg.

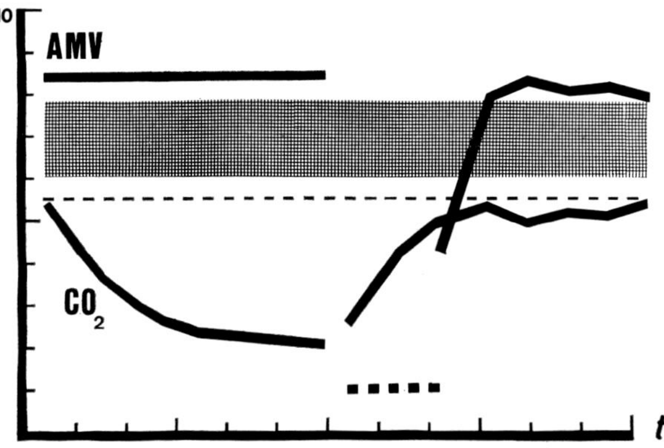

Fig. 1.　*Respiratory minute volume (AMV) and end-tidal CO₂ concentration during overventilation and recovery.*

If a patient is ventilated with more than his 'normal' volume per minute, the end-tidal P_{CO_2} will fall within the next 15–20 min to very low levels. A patient with such a low P_{CO_2} may not breathe spontaneously. If there is ventilation the P_{CO_2} rises over the following 5–10 min and the patient starts breathing spontaneously. This delay may cause hypoxia due to apnoea. No patient should be left apnoeic for more than 1–2 min.

When the patient finally starts breathing, the increasing P_{CO_2} causes the respiratory minute volume to increase until the volume is adequate to maintain a P_{CO_2} of 40 mm Hg.

Figure 2 shows another situation. Here is a patient who was overventilated for a period of time and now has low P_{CO_2}. At the end of the operation the patient is ventilated with a low respiratory minute volume to allow the carbon dioxide to rise. At the very moment

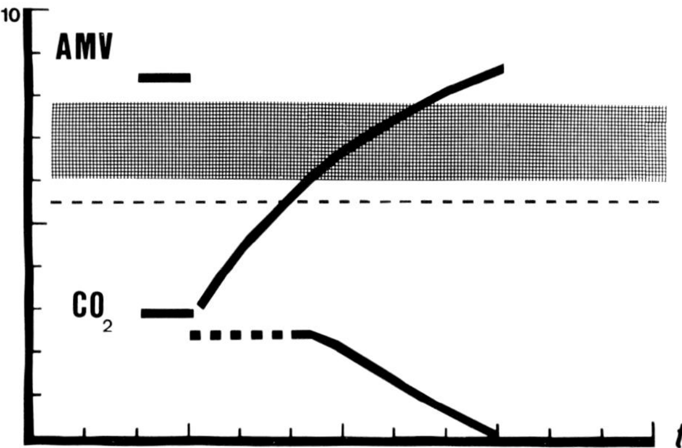

Fig. 2.   *Respiratory minute volume (AMV) and end-tidal CO_2 concentration after overventilation and recovery under the influence of a respiratory-depressant drug.*

the end-tidal CO_2 comes close to its normal level, spontaneous respiration starts. But this patient has respiratory depression, caused by a hangover from an overdosage of barbiturate, of an opiate, or a muscle relaxant. As a result, respiration never reaches its normal value and the respiratory muscles become fatigued and the minute volume decreases and the end-tidal CO_2 increases. Finally respiratory arrest occurs.

The differential diagnosis of apnoea at the end of an operation is facilitated by the use of a CO_2-analyser such as a Capnograph (Fig. 3) connected to the endotracheal tube.

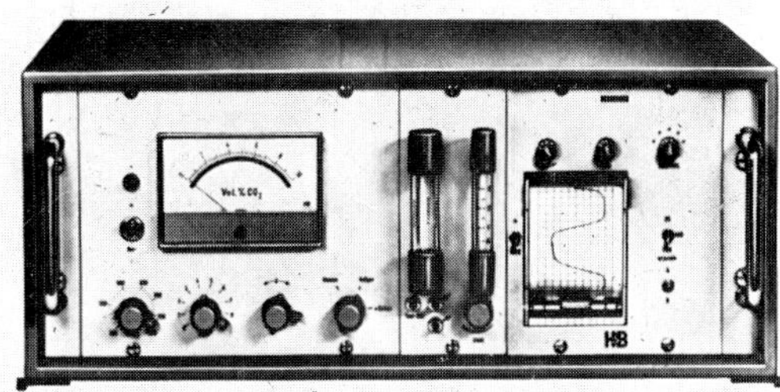

Fig. 3.   *Capnograph and recorder.*

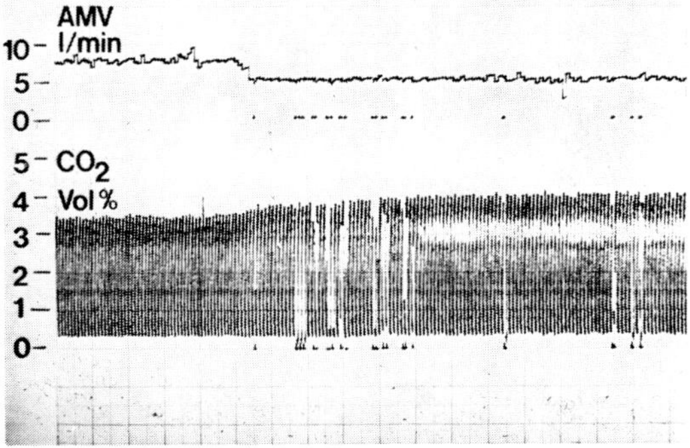

Fig. 4.   *Respiratory minute volume and end-tidal CO_2 recording.*

Capnography, continuously during anaesthesia with spontaneous or controlled respiration, informs the anaesthetist about the presence of under- or overventilation.

A recording of the end-tidal CO_2 concentration and the respiratory minute volume is shown in Figure 4. For long-term monitoring both curves are necessary.

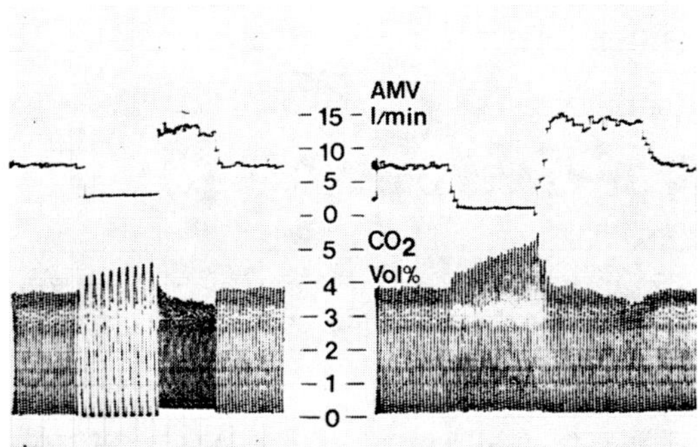

Fig. 5.   *Left: alterations of end-tidal CO_2, depending on respiratory minute volume by changing respiratory rate. Right: result of changing tidal volume.*

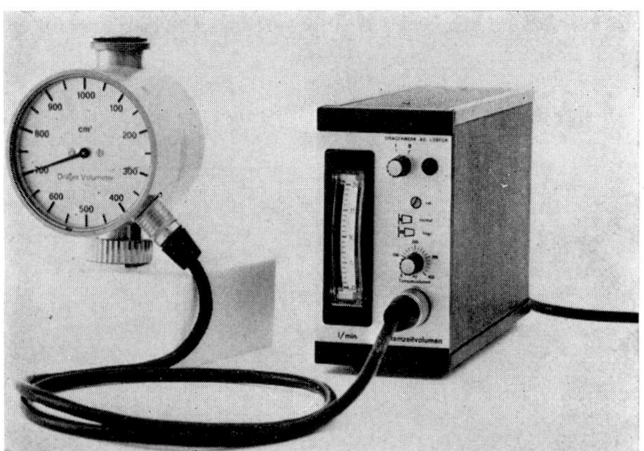

Fig. 6.   *Volumeter with computer which measures respiratory minute volume breath by breath.*

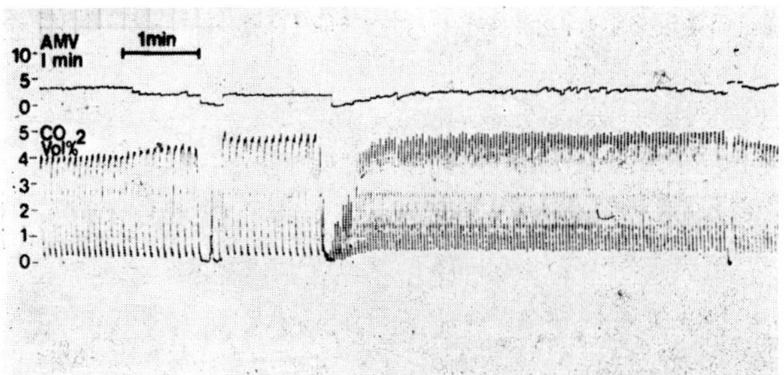

Fig. 7.   *Recording of respiratory minute volume (upper trace) and end-tidal CO_2 at the end of an operation – increasing CO_2 by reducing minute volume of controlled respiration. Spontaneous respiration starts immediately after cessation of automatic ventilation.*

In Figure 5 the upper trace shows the minute volume; the lower curve at its upper edge, the end-tidal CO_2 value. As can be seen, the minute volume has been altered by changing the frequency (left part of this Figure). The CO_2 curve follows immediately and appropriately. On the right the *tidal* volume was changed. The result is practically identical. Thus, provided that the minute volume is adequate the CO_2 remains within normal limits.

These curves were obtained by means of a Draeger volumeter with an electronic pick-up (Fig. 6). On the right is a small computer which computes *breath by breath* tidal volumes in relation to time. Minute volume is displayed on a meter and recording is possible.

A further example of the clinical value of this device which is now commercially available is given in Figure 7. At the end of an operation a patient was ventilated with a minute volume such that the CO_2 values stayed around 4 vol%. In order to stimulate spontaneous respiration, the patient was ventilated with a reduced minute volume, so that the CO_2 went up to 5 vol%. The patient was able to breathe spontaneously and regulated his CO_2 concentration to its normal level around 5 vol%. This example shows clearly that at the end of an operation the patient is able to breathe spontaneously provided that there is no hangover from depressant drugs. Maintenance of natural end-tidal CO_2 only can be achieved when proper measurements are made. It is claimed that anaesthesia is safer as a result of continuous monitoring of end-tidal CO_2 and ventilation.

dV or dot dV: A critique of flow-volume slope analysis*

STEPHEN N. STEEN[1], ROBERT CRANE[2], BERNARD STEIN[3]
and SAMUEL GASSTER[4]

[1] Department of Anesthesiology, UCLA School of Medicine,
Harbor General Hospital Campus, Torrance, Calif.,
[2] Department of Surgery, Montefiore Hospital,
Albert Einstein College of Medicine, New York, N.Y.,
[3] Biomedical Electronics Laboratory, Anaheim, Calif., and
[4] Massachusetts Institute of Technology, Cambridge, Mass., U.S.A.

INTRODUCTION

The Conference Report from the Workshop on Screening Programs for Early Diagnosis of Airway Obstruction concludes that 'a mass screening program for early detection of chronic bronchitis and emphysema should not be undertaken at this time' (Macklem et al., 1974). This recommendation is based on their findings that there are insufficient predictive correlates between the changes in the pulmonary parameters of airway obstruction and the course of the disease. The ratio of the forced expiratory volume in one second to the forced expiratory vital capacity ($FEV_{1.0}/FVC$), from British experience, suggests that it is somewhat better than questionnaires for diagnostic screening. Closing volume and closing capacity measurements are believed to be more sensitive to obstruction in small airways than measurements of $FEV_{1.0}$. Flows that occur at specific volumes in the course of a forced expiratory maneuver have not proven reliable as predictors. A number of investigators (Dayman, 1961; Mead et al., 1967; Paerdaens and Van der Woestijne, 1971; Murray et al., 1972) have explored the slope of the expiratory flow-volume curve. This is a rate constant whose inverse is the more familiar time constant relating resistance and compliance of the lung. This derived parameter is a measurement of the elastic recoil and has been determined from the geometry of the cross-plot (Hyatt et al., 1961). Instantaneous calculation of the slope ($d\dot{V}/dV$) of the maximum expiratory flow-volume (ME$\dot{V}$V) curve may be performed by either analog (Whipp et al., 1973) or digital (Steen et al., 1974) computers.

METHODOLOGY

From the calculus, $d\dot{V}/dV$ may be shown to be $d(\log_e \dot{V})/dt$ (Steen et al., 1972) which demonstrates that $d\dot{V}/dV$, the slope function, is completely determinable from the time course of the flow ($\dot{V}$ versus t). Flow through a pneumotachograph (Fig. 1) causes a pressure

*   This investigation was supported in part by General Research Support Grant 5 S01 RR05551–12 from the National Institutes of Health.

drop (proportional, over a limited range, to the flow through the device). A differential pressure strain gage transducer may be used to sense the pressure drop and provide, with the appropriate electronics for excitation and amplification, an electrical signal proportional to the flow. The existence of a flow signal permits the generation of signals analogous to volume (V), the natural logarithm of flow ($\log_e \dot{V}$) and the time-rate of change of the natural logarithm of flow [$d(\log_e \dot{V})/dt$] by time-integration, logarithmic conversion and time-differentiation, respectively.

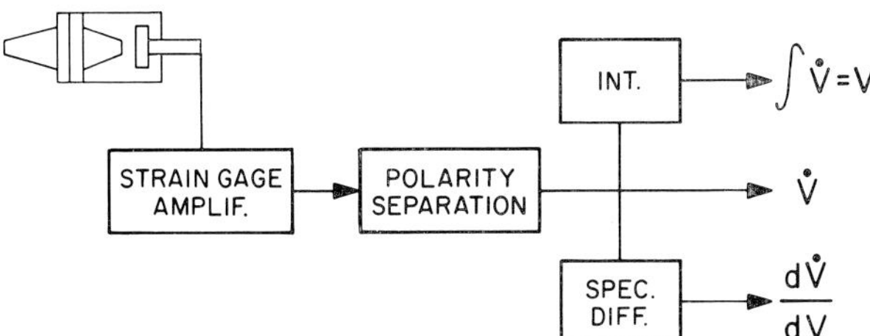

Fig. 1. *System block diagram: Pneumotachograph-pressure transducer (top left) receives excitation from and is amplified by strain gage amplifier. Polarity separation is used to exclude inspiratory signals. Int. refers to time-integration. Spec. Diff. is a special differentiator acting as a $d(\log_e \dot{V})/dt$ operator.*

Ultra-stable electronic integrators have been developed for on-line ventilatory volume computations (Steen and Crane, 1968) and the accuracy of the output volume is limited only by the baseline stability of the input flow signal. Logarithmic amplifiers are available that provide a true logarithmic output for a 4-decade range of input voltage. From Figure 2, it is evident that a 1000-fold more gain is required for the 0.001–0.01 volt decade than that required for the 1–10 volt decade. The high gain at low input signals accentuates system noise which is an inherent limitation of this electronic approach. Electrical differentiators functionally approximate ideal (mathematical) differentiation and may be either passive (R-C networks) or active (electronic), differing only in their gains and frequency responses.

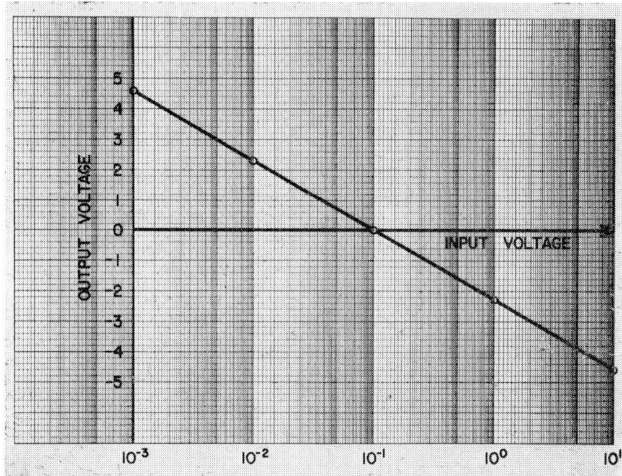

Fig. 2. *Transfer function: Four-decade logarithmic converter. $2.3 \log_{10}\dot{V} = \log_e \dot{V}$.*

The output, for a constant amplitude input, increases linearly with frequency (ω in radians per second), since the derivative of $\sin \omega t$ is $\omega \cos \omega t$. Thus, system noise, usually of high frequency content, is further amplified, with additional deterioration of the signal/noise ratio.

Analog computation of $d\dot{V}/dV$, based on the aforementioned sequence of operations, may be readily displayed directly in scalar form (time course) or may be cross-plotted versus developed volume. The latter mode of presentation, whilst potentially the most useful, is limited by existing display devices. The cathode ray oscilloscope, with an electron beam having minimal inertia, is able to reproduce signals and noise with maximal fidelity and frequency response (Fig. 3). The flat-bed, electromechanically operated X-Y recorder, is characterized by a writing arm with significant inertia which results in poor response to the high frequencies contained in forced expirations (Fig. 4).

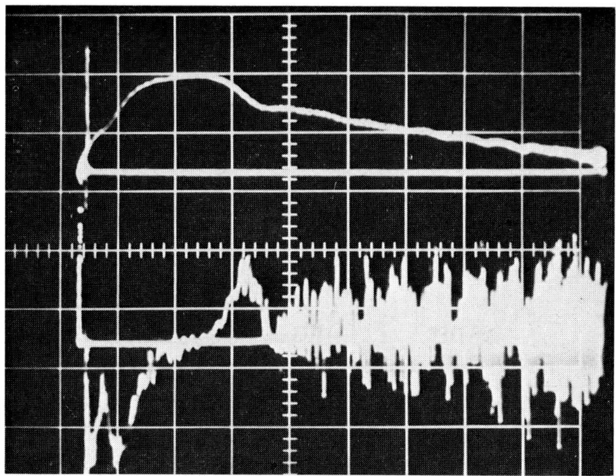

Fig. 3. *Oscilloscopic display of forced expiratory maneuver: Upper tracing is MEV̇V curve lower tracing is dV̇/dV versus V.*

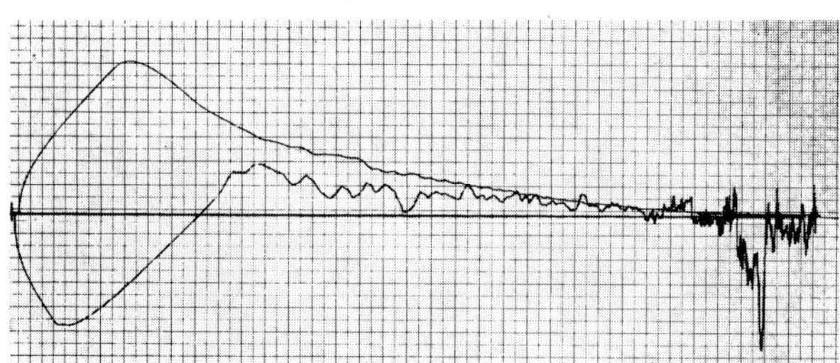

Fig. 4. *Electromechanical recording of forced expiratory maneuver: Unipolar tracing is MEV̇V curve, biphasic tracing is dV̇/dV versus V.*

Utilization of a general purpose mini-computer to perform the same sequence of operations in the binary world requires digitization of the analog flow signal (A/D conversion resulting in a series of discrete points, each of which is represented by its own bit pattern). The sampled flow data would be numerically integrated to produce another set of bit patterns in order to represent the developed volume (V) in digital format. Logarithmic conversion, using 'read only memory' (ROM), would be applied to these same flow bit patterns to provide a further set of bit patterns corresponding to the natural logarithm of the flow (log$_e$ $\dot{V}$). Numerical differentiation of the digitized log$_e$ $\dot{V}$ signal would yield a digitized version of d$\dot{V}$/dV as the end result. A typical example of computer-derived data appears in Figure 5 in which both $\dot{V}$ and d$\dot{V}$/dV are plotted versus time (t) rather than V for the same forced expiratory maneuver. That portion encompassing peak flow, where d$\dot{V}$/dV changes polarity, is presented on an expanded scale in Figure 6.

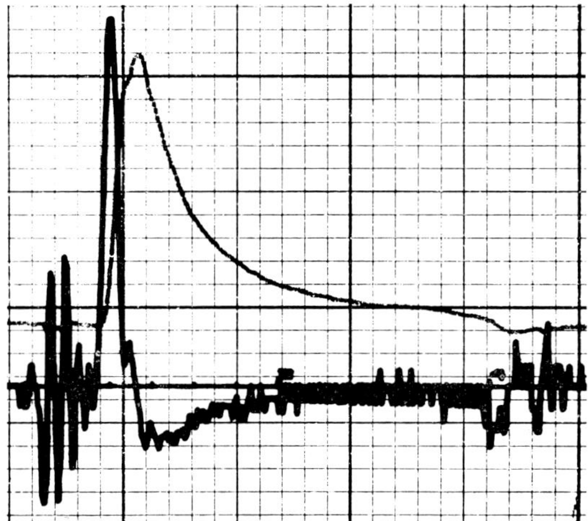

Fig. 5. *Digital computer output of forced expiratory maneuver: Unipolar tracing is MEV̇t curve, biphasic tracing is d$\dot{V}$/dV versus t.*

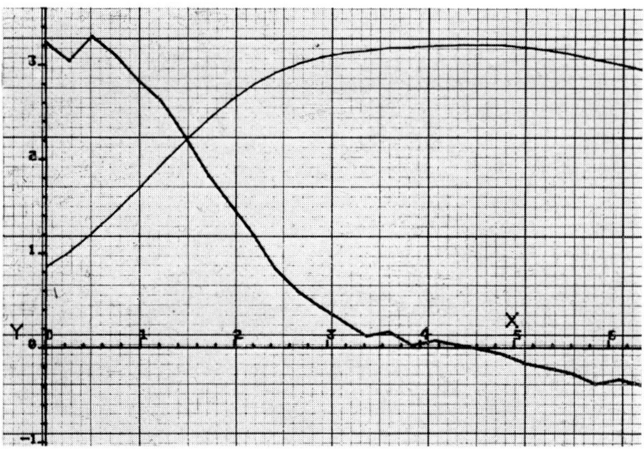

Fig. 6. *Digital computer output of forced expiratory maneuver: Detail of Figure 5 in the region encompassing $\dot{V}_{max}$.*

DISCUSSION

During a forced expiratory maneuver the slope d$\dot{V}$/dV of the terminal segment of the MEV̇V curve is often relatively constant in normals. An indicator of correct computation is the co-existence of the first zero crossing of the slope (d$\dot{V}$/dV) occurring at the same time (which implies the same volume) as does peak flow ($\dot{V}_{max}$) (Figs. 3, 5 and 6). With this criterion, values of $d\dot{V}/dV$ may be accepted at any time or volume (e.g. at 50% of the FVC). Signal/noise deterioration inherent in the analog technic results in excessive noise (Fig. 3, lower tracing) which precludes accurate readability. Attempts to minimize noise by electronic filtering have limited the signal band width resulting in a horizontal shift of the zero crossing relative to $\dot{V}_{max}$. This shift is analogous to that occurring when an X-Y recorder (Fig. 4) was used, in which the band width of the displayed signals is limited by inertial factors (mechanical filtering). Such shifts cast doubt as to whether the displayed relationship between $d\dot{V}/dV$ versus time or developed volume is correct. The signal-to-noise ratio of the initial flow signal is not degraded when operated on by a digital computer. As a result, $d\dot{V}/dV$ is relatively noise-free, and there is no shift in zero crossing (Fig. 5).

CONCLUSIONS

The slope function, $d\dot{V}/dV$, with acceptable noise and with an accuracy confirmed by the zero crossing criterion has been obtained by digital computation – the technic of choice. The rapid rate of development of microprocessors and their incorporation in special purpose digital computers should result in low cost pulmonary function measurement systems. Accordingly, the availability of an instrument to compute $d\dot{V}/dV$ would enable rapid accumulation of reliable data from mass screening programs that might prove useful in the early recognition of pulmonary disease.

REFERENCES

Dayman, H. (1961): *Amer. Rev. resp. Dis.*, *83*, 842.

Hyatt, R. E., Schilder, D. P. and Fry, D. L. (1961): *J. appl. Physiol.*, *13*, 331.

Macklem, P. T. et al. (1974): *Amer. Rev. resp. Dis.*, *109*, 567.

Mead, J., Turner, J. M., Macklem, D. T. and Little, J. B. (1967): *J. appl. Physiol.*, *22*, 95.

Murray, J. F., Greenspan, R. H., Gold, W. M. and Cohen, A. B. (1972): *Calif. Med.*, *116*, 37.

Paerdens, J. and Van der Woestijne, K. P. (1971): *Proc. roy. Soc. Med.*, *64*, 1240.

Steen, S. N. and Crane, R. (1968): *Anesth. Analg. Curr. Res.*, *47*, 276.

Steen, S. N., Crane, R. and Whipp, B. J. (1972): In: *Proceedings, 25th Annual Conference on Engineering in Medicine and Biology*, *Vol. 14*, p. 249. The Alliance for Engineering in Medicine and Biology, Arlington, Va.

Steen, S. N., Stein, B. and Gasster, S. (1974): In: *Abstracts, IV European Congress of Anaesthesiology, Madrid, 1974*, p. 74. Editors: A. Arias, R. Llaurado, M. A. Nalda and J. N. Lunn. Excerpta Medica, Amsterdam.

Whipp, B. J., Crane, R. and Steen, S. N. (1973): In: *Digest, X International Conference on Medical and Biological Engineering, Dresden 1973*, *Vol. 1*, p. 142. Editors: R. Albert, W. Vogt and W. Helbig. The Conference Committee of the X International Conference on Medical and Biological Engineering, Dresden.

*Non-invasive patient monitoring: Expectations and reality**

J. WEINMAN

Rogoff Laboratory for Biomedical Engineering,
Hebrew University Hadassah Medical School, Jerusalem, Israel

The title of this lecture suggests a critical evaluation of the techniques for non-invasive patient monitoring. As such an evaluation was recently published (Weinman, 1971), the intention here is to analyse the difficulties and perspectives of non-invasive patient monitoring in a more general way.

Recently, two reviews on patient monitoring have appeared, one by Gardner (1972) and the other by Fowler (1972) – both are unsatisfactory. Although the authors are concerned with a clinical environment, many of the methods described are not really applicable under clinical conditions and others were tested only in a few cases.

The paper published by Maloney in 1968 entitled *'The trouble with patient monitoring'*, describes well also the present situation. The root of the 'trouble' is not however, as claimed by Wolf (1971), the lack of 'an appropriate technological climate in the hospital' which can be altered only by a 'radical change in . . . the training'; the trouble stems rather from the exaggerated claims made by bioengineers and manufacturers regarding the performance of equipment for non-invasive patient monitoring. As a result, large sums have been spent on elaborate installations which often remain idle or are little used.

The disillusionment thus caused should in no way detract from the importance of patient monitoring. Because most physiological variables are under the influence of several control loops and regulatory processes of the biosystem are interlocked in a complicated way, physiological events have to be monitored over long periods of time in order to obtain an insight into the behaviour of the variables investigated. It is, therefore, important to understand why long-term non-invasive patient monitoring is in trouble.

The expression 'non-invasive patient monitoring' combines two concepts: the first refers to non-invasive acquisition of diagnostic data and is as old as medicine itself, while the concept of monitoring was introduced into medicine only recently, primarily under the impact of engineering. The two activities are independent of each other: it is possible to acquire diagnostic data *non-invasively without monitoring* and it is also possible to *monitor* physiological variables using an *invasive* technique. A discussion of non-invasive patient monitoring has therefore to concern itself *first* with techniques for non-invasive data acquisition and then with problems which arise when these techniques are combined with long-term monitoring.

RE-DEFINING THE TERM 'NON-INVASIVE'

The term 'non-invasive' describes methods for the observation or measurement of physiological variables without penetrating the physical boundaries of the biosystem. In the past,

---

* Supported in part by grants from the Rogoff Foundation and from Mrs. L. Teruzzi.

when information reached the physician only through his subjective senses (i.e. vision, touch or hearing), diagnostic techniques were truly non-invasive. This remained so when transducers, placed peripherally to the biosystem, became available; they provided permanent, objective records of the variables observed and extended non-invasive techniques to physiological events not directly accessible to the human senses, such as the electrical activity of the heart or the brain.

At present, however, newly developed diagnostic techniques – such as ultrasound, isotope scanning, photo and impedance plethysmography or X-ray diagnosis – have deprived the term 'non-invasive' of its unambiguous meaning. These techniques are, by design, invasive, despite the fact that the transducers are situated outside the biosystem. Each method employs a carrier consisting of mechanical, nuclear, radiant or electrical energy, capable of penetrating the boundaries of the biosystem. Information is acquired by letting events occurring inside these boundaries modulate the carrier. That invasion is indeed taking place is demonstrated by the damage caused to the biosystem by too large an amplitude of the carrier or too long an exposure to it.

Despite what has been said above, there is little doubt that the risky heart catheterization and the relatively harmless ultrasound, represent different approaches to diagnostic data acquisition, even if both techniques are de facto invasive. It is apparently not the 'non-invasiveness' which makes one of the approaches more acceptable to the clinician than the other but some other more important property of the technique. This is well understood by the industrial engineer whose task is in some respects similar to that of the clinician. The engineer must be able to test complicated machinery without interfering with its normal performance and to search for faults inside a product without damaging it by the test procedure. Techniques which fulfil these conditions are appropriately termed 'non-destructive techniques' (NDT). Non-destructive techniques use ultrasound, visible and infrared light, electric and magnetic fields, X-rays and other approaches which may be either invasive or non-invasive, but must be non-destructive in the sense defined above.

The task of the clinician is similar to that of the engineer; he has to investigate the performance of the human biosystem without interfering with its normal controls, and to search within the body for a malfunctioning organ without inflicting injury. For this purpose the clinician uses similar tools, namely light, ultrasound and X-rays. It is, however, more difficult to meet the condition 'not to interfere with the normal performance' when a human subject and not a machine is 'tested'. Factors such as fear, discomfort, pain and anticipation have to be avoided because they may easily change the functional baselines and falsify the results. Taking this into account, non-destructive diagnostic technique could be defined as follows: a diagnostic procedure which does not disturb the normal physiological conditions which existed before the test was started and does not cause damage or endanger the biosystem unduly. Providing the above conditions are met, it is, however, unimportant whether the diagnostic procedure is invasive or non-invasive. For example, the implantation of a tiny diode in order to stimulate a nerve by RF waves has been described as 'minimally invasive' (Schuder and Gold, 1974). The procedure is, however, without doubt fully invasive, but can be termed 'non-destructive' if it can be shown that the 'normal physiological conditions' were not disturbed and the injury inflicted negligible.

For the purpose of this paper, the expressions 'non-destructive' and 'non-invasive' will be used synonymously, because the latter appears in the title and the former is not yet widely used in the clinical literature.

THE NON-INVASIVE TRANSDUCER

The non-invasive acquisition of qualitative or quantitative physiological data requires the use of non-invasive transducers, and the challenge to develop these transducers has been taken up by many workers. During the last decade, numerous papers on the subject have appeared in both clinical and bioengineering journals, but from a clinical point of view the results are often disappointing. An example illustrating this point is the number of transducers available for the non-invasive recording of arterial volume pulses. The volume pulse (VP) is a variable carrying significant cardiovascular information; palpation of the radial pulse was until not long ago a routine diagnostic procedure. Terms such as 'pulsus celer', 'tardus' and 'mollis' (Houssay, 1955) were coined by clinicians in order to be able to communicate subjective tactile information to their colleagues. Palpation has, to a great extent, been abandoned because it is rightly felt that describing the pulse is a poor substitute for the permanent record now made possible by the modern non-invasive VP transducers (of the capacitive, piezoelectric or photoplethysmographic kind – to name only some of the existing types). Indeed, many workers have shown how the shape of non-invasively recorded VP reflects various cardiovascular disease states, others have described how VP recordings can be used to measure the peripheral pulse wave velocity (a variable related to the elasticity of the arterial wall) and still others have explained how systolic time intervals (related to cardiac contractility) can be measured if, in addition to the ECG and phonocardiography, the carotid VP is recorded. Van der Hoeven et al. (1973) recently reported non-invasive measurements based on carotid VP recordings; the latter were obtained with a newly developed piezoelectric transducer (Van der Hoeven and Beneken, 1970). Their results are indeed promising: VP recorded non-invasively and blood pressure pulses recorded simultaneously with a catheter show almost identical shapes, and systolic time intervals measured invasively and non-invasively are almost identical. With such results, one would *expect* a conclusion recommending the use of the transducer in clinical practice. Instead, at the end of the paper (Van der Hoeven et al., 1973) one reads with astonishment that: 'In order to establish the clinical value of the technique, measurements should be made in a similar manner in a number of (additional) patients. Preliminary results obtained seem *to imply* that this technique *promises* to be a useful aid in clinical diagnosis.'

Why only a 'promise' if the results are so convincing? Based on my own experience with the photoplethysmographic transducer I dare to suggest that the authors are probably aware of the poor reproducibility of recordings obtained from the same patient at different sessions (Weinman, 1971). A diagnostic method is of little use if the clinician cannot be sure whether a different result (here a different VP shape) is due to the patient or to the variability of the technique (here a different transducer versus artery position). This is a drawback common to many and probably to all types of non-destructive pulse wave transducers. Brecht and Boucke (1953) who devised the capacitive transducer reported this drawback; Weinman (1971) and Weinman et al. (1973, 1974) observed it in many recordings with the reflection photoplethysmograph. Hardy and Eadie (1972), referring to the ultrasound probe stated unequivocally: 'Little can be concluded from the shape of the tracing obtained' because 'by varying the angle of the probe . . . to the vessel axis, by changing the pressure . . . to the skin . . . it is possible to obtain a variety of . . . tracings . . . so variable that little can be concluded from the shape.'

These critical remarks, which in a different form may also apply to some other non-destructive transducers, should in no way detract from the merit of workers whose ingenuity has made possible non-invasive devices and methods. However, most of these workers prove only that a specific non-invasive diagnostic technique has 'a great potential value', is on the 'brink of becoming a clinical tool,' or 'shows promise and is under further investigation,' and so on in a vein familiar to readers of clinical and bioengineering journals in which non-invasive devices are described. However, one has the impression that the ultimate purpose of many workers is to prove that a specific non-destructive method is *in principle* possible and to publish their findings in the hope that other investigators will undertake the task of converting the promising results into a clinical tool. This attitude is not difficult to understand. The road from a feasibility study to a final clinical tool is a thankless one. There is seldom financial reward in it and the project is often too technical and not 'basic' enough to be of interest to a student collaborator for an academic thesis. In addition the undertaking is usually difficult because of the complicated relationship between the primary physiological variable, accessible only invasively (for instance, the blood volume) and the secondary variable related to it, which can be measured non-invasively, such as electrical impedance or the optical opacity.

Because of these difficulties, the task of turning a promising non-invasive method into a clinical tool cannot be successfully undertaken by a clinician working in a busy clinic with a heavy patient load. Specially organised research centres with a scientifically trained staff, technical facilities and a low enough patient load to allow research without impairing patient care are needed for this purpose. Projects aimed at converting a promising non-invasive technique into a clinical tool demand, in order to succeed, effort, persistence and a research strategy often resembling miniature Manhattan or Moon Projects. Non-destructive techniques used by industry are evaluated and perfected in technical universities by engineer-scientists, or in special centres for Non-Destructive Technique Research, such as the one at the Atomic Energy Research Establishment (AERE) at Harwell. Without a similar attitude and without establishing small units and larger centres for evaluating and perfecting non-invasive diagnostic techniques, attached to medical schools, hospitals and technical universities, many of these techniques will remain interesting articles in scientific journals, ending with conclusions similar to those of Fenton and Vas (1973) that: 'Although interpretation of these measurements is difficult owing to the indirect nature of the transducer, the ease of application and simplicity of the transducer give it *significant* potential value in the field of atraumatic cardiac diagnosis.' The reaction of the clinician who wants to use the 'potential value' of the non-destructive method may well find expression in the remarks of Rodbard (1972) on the apex cardiogram: 'There is a vast literature about the apex cardiogram, but the method itself has severe limitations in reproducibility and interpretation of the qualitative data. We were never able to obtain consistent recordings on the same person under the same circumstances.'

NON-INVASIVE MONITORING

We are at present conditioned to associate monitoring with automatic data acquisition and automatic real-time interpretation of the collected data. In principle, however, monitoring should not be automatic. Monitoring implies continuously or periodically measuring the values of or observing the patterns of physiological variables in order to evaluate the performance of the biosystem and intervene when a crisis threatens; it implies record keeping to draw conclusions about trends but it does not imply automation in data collection and in data interpretation.

In its simplest form monitoring can be performed by a nurse sitting at the bedside and recording, at fixed time intervals, pulse and breathing rate, temperature, blood pressure and other physical events accessible to measurements either directly by human senses or with the help of simple instruments. The nurse can also monitor events which cannot be expressed in numbers but which can be observed, such as breathing pattern, skin colour, behaviour of the patient, his verbal communications and other observable but not easily measurable physiological variables – an activity which can conveniently be termed 'pattern recognition'.

At a higher technical level, monitoring becomes 'transducer-assisted monitoring': here some of the physiological variables can be measured by transducers and indicated continuously on electrical pointer instruments; entries can be made whenever a pointer reading is judged to be significant. *None* of the transducers, however, can replace the 'pattern recognition activity' of the human observer.

The next higher level of monitoring can be termed 'recorder-assisted monitoring'. The advent of pen-recorders has made possible not only the continuous monitoring of measurable variables but it also added a new dimension to monitoring, namely, *pattern recognition of signals* appearing on the recording chart. The pattern of an ECG with its extrasystoles and arrhythmias, the pattern of an EEG with its spikes, the pattern of pulse rate variations and many other signal patterns can be monitored and their diagnostic significance appreciated. Recorder-assisted monitoring also enhanced the usefulness of many non-invasive transducers. The poor reproducibility of a pulse wave transducer, for instance, becomes unimportant when only the change in shape of the waveform, due to the use of a vasoactive drug, is of interest.

The effectiveness of recorder-assisted non-invasive patient monitoring can be constantly increased by developing new transducers. This process, however, increases the intellectual load placed on the human observer who has to interpret and correlate a large amount of data, often in a limited period of time. A pilot in a cockpit with its complicated instrument board proves that an operator can be trained to cope intelligently with a vast amount of information. Further progress in recorder-assisted patient monitoring would eventually demand a similar level of skill from human observers. It is doubtful whether the medical profession could train them in sufficient number or afford their cost. The timely advent of computer-assisted monitoring has helped to avoid this dilemma. As yet only pilot projects are in existence; there seems however, to be little doubt that in the next few years computer-assisted monitoring will become commonplace. To facilitate this process future workers should be made aware both of the possibilities and the limitations of the new techniques. They should be taught to view the computer as a logbook in which all the transducer-collected data (values or patterns of the monitored variables) are automatically entered and stored, to be recalled at will for inspection and analysis. They should realise that the computer can be looked at as a huge textbook, whose pages can be turned quickly and re-ordered in any convenient way and to which new, updated pages can constantly be added. Such a textbook will put a vast amount of information at the disposal of the clinical staff. On the other hand, it should be made clear that the term 'computer-assisted monitoring' has to be understood literally; the computer can assist but not replace the human observer in drawing conclusions and making decisions. These limitations are due to the poor pattern recognition capabilities of the computer. Because of this, the computer is unable to monitor with sufficient confidence, pathological patterns in the ECG or EEG. In addition, even such variables as cardiac or respiratory rate or repetitive blood pressure determination with a pressure cuff cannot be computer-monitored although seemingly no pattern recognition is required. These measurements are often contaminated by noise due to patient movement. The human observer can easily recognise the noise pattern and disregard it, while the computer, without this capability, will sound an unnecessary alarm. Ten years ago, it was this difficulty which prompted Pask (1965) to express the view that the best monitoring device would not be a computer but a dab of adhesive glue placed between the finger of a nurse and the radial artery of the patient – the nurse performing the pattern recognition and sounding the alarm. Today, the solution is in principle similar, but more efficient: it is again the nurse, but now with her eyes glued to the screen of a scope where physiological variables of more than one patient are displayed, who performs the pattern recognition, alarms the physician and initiates the recording of the emergency. When computer-assisted monitoring will become a reality, this latter function, but not the nurse, will become redundant because the whole sequence of events which led to the crisis will be retrievable from the computer memory.

However, in the meantime, the medical community should be forewarned not to purchase computer-assisted monitoring equipment before making sure that it is already fully operative and not still in a developmental stage. Hospitals, concerned primarily with patient care, should *under no circumstances* be allowed to serve as manufacturers' pilot plants. This function should be performed by scientifically oriented clinical research centres. Performance validation of computer-assisted monitoring projects by such centres will be of value not only to the user but also to the manufacturer because this is the only effective way to speed up marked acceptance of new and, especially, expensive equipment.

The ultimate technical level of monitoring is computer-automated patient monitoring. I would not dare to exclude the possibility that it will become a reality some time in the future. This, however, will not happen before man understands how pattern recognition is accomplished by the human brain. The still crude and unsatisfactory, but nevertheless interesting, attempts to perform automatic ECG and EEG analysis indicate that medical research centres are actively participating in these efforts.

REFERENCES

Brecht, K. and Boucke, K. (1953): *Pflügers Arch. ges. Physiol.*, *257/6*, 490.

Bushman, J. A. (1972): *Brit. J. Hosp. Med., Suppl.*, 42.

Fenton, T. R. and Vas, R. (1973): *Med. biol. Engng*, *11/5*, 552.

Fowler, N. O. (1972): *Advanc. intern. Med.*, *18*, 283.

Gardner, R. M. (1972): *Ann. Rev. biophys. Bioeng.*, *1*, 211.

Hardy, D. G. and Eadie, G. A. (1972): *Brit. J. clin. Pract.*, *26/1*, 3.

Houssay, B. A. (1955): In: *Human Physiology*, *2nd ed.*, Chapter 21, p. 206. McGraw-Hill Book Co., Inc., New York, N.Y.

Maloney, J. V. (1968): *Ann. Surg.*, *168/4*, 605.

Pask, E. A. (1965): *Proc. roy. Soc. Med.*, *58*, 757.

Rodbard, S. (1972): In: *Clinical Usefulness of Sphygmorecording*, p. 1. Editors: S. Z. Binenbaum and H. M. Hochberg. Roche Medical Electronic Division, Cranbury, N.J.

Schuder, J. C. and Gold, J. H. (1974): *IEEE Trans. biomed. Engng*, *BME-21/2*, 152.

Weinman, J. (1971): In: *Proceedings, 9th International Conference for Medical and Biological Engineering, Melbourne*.

Weinman, J., Hayat, A. and Raviv, G. (1973): In: *Digest, 10th International Conference for Medical and Biological Engineering, Dresden*, p. 103.

Weinman, J., Hayat, A. and Raviv, G. (1974): In: *Biomechanics*. Editor: D. N. Ghista. Marcel Dekker, New York, N.Y. In press.

Van der Hoeven, G. M. A. and Beneken, J. E. W. (1970): In: *Progress Report No. 2*, p. 19. Editor: B. van Eijnsbergen. Institute of Medical Physics TNO, Utrecht.

Van der Hoeven, G. M. A., Beneken, J. E. W. and Clerens, P. L. A. (1973): *Neth. J. Med.*, *16*, 70.

Wolf, H. S. (1971): *Postgrad. med. J.*, *47*, 12.

A computer program for blood-gas analysis

J. M. CAVANILLES

Residencia General, Hospitalet de Llobregat, Barcelona, Spain

Although blood gas equations, nomograms and a blood gas slide-rule are available for calculation and derivation of respiratory and acid-base data of clinical interest, this is a tedious and time-consuming procedure. The increasing availability of computer facilities in hospitals offers a means of performing these calculations. Many of the blood gas equations contained in books and medical journals, are not readily usable in computer programs or in other calculating devices. To facilitate this, a number of the standard blood gas equations have been transformed into equations which are suitable for use with these devices.

CORRECTED P_{O_2}, P_{CO_2} AND pH FOR PATIENT'S TEMPERATURE

Severinghaus' formulae (Severinghaus, 1966) are transformed in the following equations.

(1) $\quad P_{O_2}B = P_{O_2}37 \cdot 10^{0.031 \cdot (B-37)}$

(2) $\quad P_{CO_2}B = P_{CO_2}37 \cdot 10^{0.019 \cdot (B-37)}$

(3) $\quad pHB = pH37 - [0.0146 - 0.0065 \cdot (7.4146 - pH37)] \cdot (B-37)$

The subscript '37' means that the parameter was measured at a temperature of $37°C$; the subscript 'B' means patient's temperature.

CALCULATION OF PATIENT'S P 50 AND OXYHEMOGLOBIN DISSOCIATION CURVE

The calculation of these parameters is performed in the following way:

(*a*) Mathematical representation of the standard oxyhemoglobin dissociation curve with the following equation (Aberman et al., 1973):

(4) $\quad S_{O_2} = \sum_{i=0}^{i=7} K_{i+1} \cdot (P_{O_2} - 27.5/P_{O_2} + 27.5)^i$

where

$$K_1 = +51.87074 \quad K_2 = +129.8325 \quad K_3 = +6.828368 \quad K_4 = -223.7881$$
$$K_5 = -27.95300 \quad K_6 = +258.5009 \quad K_7 = +21.84175 \quad K_8 = -119.2322$$

(*b*) Correction of the standard curve in relation to the pH and base excess of the blood sample, and the temperature at which the sample was measured (Severinghaus, 1966); this is performed as follows:

(5) $\quad P_{O_2/1} = P_{O_2/2} \cdot 10^{0.024 \cdot (T_{l_1} - T_{l_2})} + 0.48 \cdot (pH_{l_2} - pH_{l_1}) + 0.0013\ BE$

where subscripts $|_1$ and $|_2$ represent 2 actual values of the temperature and pH.

(*c*) P 50 is calculated (Severinghaus, 1971) as:

(6)   P 50 $= 26.6 \cdot$ measured P_{O_2}/calculated P_{O_2}, where 26.6 is the normal P 50, measured P_{O_2} is the actual value of the partial pressure of oxygen of the blood sample at its pH, BE and measurement temperature, and the calculated P_{O_2} is the partial pressure of oxygen which should have the sample of blood to match the measured oxygen saturation of the sample at its pH, BE and measurement temperature considering the blood has a normal P 50.

(*d*) Every point and the oxyhemoglobin dissociation curve of the patient at standard conditions are obtained changing in the equation the factor 26.6 for the corresponding partial pressure of oxygen for 10% saturation (P 10), 20% saturation (P 20) — 100% saturation (P 100).

(*e*) In order to get the actual oxyhemoglobin dissociation curve for the patient's condition (temperature, pH and BE) the whole curve obtained as explained in paragraph, (*d*) is corrected to the patient's condition with equation (5).

OXYGEN CONTENT (KELMAN AND NUNN, 1968) AND CONSUMPTION

(7) $O_2^{CONT} = 1.34 \cdot \dfrac{S_{O_2}}{100} \cdot Hgb + 0.0031 \cdot P_{O_2}$

the arteriovenous oxygen difference is $O_2 A - V = $ Arterial $O_2^{CONT} - $ Venous O_2^{CONT} and the oxygen consumption, $O_2^{CONT} = O_2 A - V \cdot$ Cardiac Output $\cdot$ 10.

PULMONARY SHUNT

The magnitude of the venous admixture (fraction of the cardiac output which is not oxygenated in its passage through the lungs) is given by the following formula (Bergreen, 1942):

(8) $\dfrac{Qs}{Q_T} = \dfrac{Cc - Ca}{Cc - Cv}$

where $\dfrac{Qs}{Q_T}$ is the pulmonary shunt as a fraction of the cardiac output. Ca and Cv are the oxygen content in arterial and central venous (Cavanilles et al., 1972) or pulmonary artery blood respectively and Cc is oxygen content in the pulmonary capillary optimally oxygenated; Cc is calculated from mean alveolar P_{O_2} in the following way:

(9) $P_{O_2}A = F_{I_{O_2}} \cdot (PBAR - PH_2O) - Pa_{CO_2} \cdot \left(F_{I_{O_2}} + \dfrac{1 - F_{I_{O_2}}}{0.8} \right)$

where $F_{I_{O_2}} = $ inspired fraction of oxygen, PBAR $=$ barometric pressure, $PH_2O = $ patient's water vapor pressure and $Pa_{CO_2} = $ arterial P_{CO_2}. From mean alveolar P_{O_2}, oxygen saturation and subsequently oxygen content of the pulmonary capillary is calculated.

CO_2 CONTENT AND PRODUCTION

The blood total content of CO_2 is calculated with the Kelman's equation (Kelman, 1967):

(10) $CO_2\ TOT = 2.22 \left[d \cdot \dfrac{Hct}{100} + \left(1 - \dfrac{Hct}{100} \right) \right] CO_2\ PL$

where Hct is hematocrit and CO_2PL is plasma CO_2 content; $CO_2PL = SOL \cdot PCO_2 \cdot$
$\cdot (1 + 10^{(pH - pK)})$;

SOL represents the dissolved CO_2 in plasma and equals to $SOL = 0.0307 + 0.0057 \cdot$ body temperature $+ 0.00002 \cdot$ body temperature (Aberman et al., 1973); d represents the intraerythrocyte CO_2 and is calculated as follow: $d = D \cdot CO_2 \, PL$, where

$$D = DOX + (DR - DOX) \cdot \left(1 - \frac{SO_2}{100}\right); DOX = 0.590 + 0.2913 \cdot (7.4 - pH) - 0.0844 \cdot$$

$\cdot (7.4 - pH) \cdot (7.4 - pH)$ and $DR = 0.664 + 0.2275 \cdot (7.4 - pH) - 0.0938 \cdot (7.4 - pH) \cdot$ $\cdot (7.4 - pH)$. The arteriovenous CO_2 difference and the production are calculated in the same fashion as the arteriovenous difference and consumption of oxygen.

REFERENCES

Aberman, A., Cavanilles, J. M., Trotter, J., Erbeck, D., Weil, M. H. and Shubin, H. (1973): *J. appl. Physiol.*, *35*, 570.

Bergreen, S. M. (1942): *Acta physiol. scand.*, *4 (Suppl. II)*, 1.

Cavanilles, J. M., Shubin, H. and Weil, M. H. (1972): *Fed. Proc.*, *31*, 348.

Kelman, G. R. (1967): *Resp. Physiol.*, *3*, 111.

Kelman, G. R. and Nunn, J. F. (1968): *Computer Produced Physiological Tables*. Butterworth, London – Sydney – Washington.

Severinghaus, J. W. (1966): *J. appl. Physiol.*, *21*, 1108.

Severinghaus, J. W. (1971): In: *Respiration and Circulation*. Editors: P. D. Altman and D. S. Ditmer Federation of American Societies for Experimental Biology, Bethesda, Md.

Telemetry systems and their practicability in medicine

J. EICHLER, I. LOBSIEN and ST. POHLERT

Central Anaesthesia Department, Medical University Lübeck,
Lübeck, Federal Republic of Germany

Biotelemetry is the transmission of biological signals to remote recording apparatus or measuring instruments. The transmission can be telegraphic or wireless. Grant called the stethoscope the first medical telemetry apparatus.

Some authors sharply separate a special form of telemetry i.e. the record of biological data on storage systems, e.g. on magnetic tape for prolonged recording. After the end of the recording, playback is possible. The Holter-Avionics-System is one well-known system.

The idea of biotelemetry is not new. Fifty years ago Einthoven practised biotelemetry in Leiden. He transmitted electrocardiograms by wires into his laboratory. Einthoven employed this technique because his newly-developed string-electrometer could only be transported with the greatest difficulty and each transportation had to be justified.

The telemetry, for example, that of an electrocardiogram, can also be carried out by normal trunk-lines with frequency-modulated audiosignal. A resident doctor could transmit an ECG to the nearest hospital with a special department and it would be interpreted there. This is useful in countries with a low density population; instead of sending the patient to the hospital to obtain an ECG, its transmission there is quicker and cheaper. Furthermore, the diagnosis is facilitated because an expert interprets the ECG. Up till now the biotele-

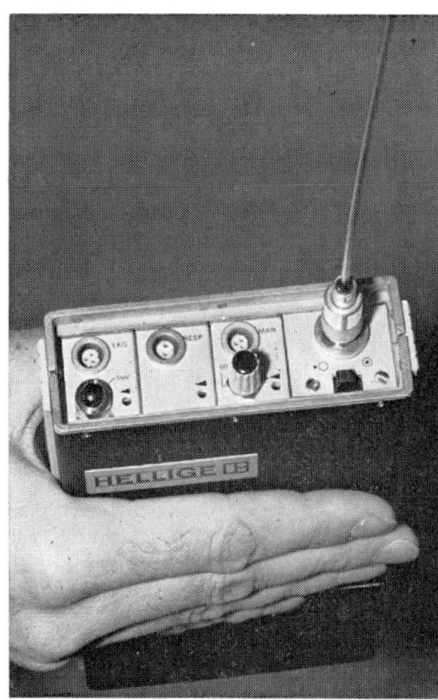

Fig. 1. *Sender of the Hellige telemetry plant (same size for 1- or 3-channel operation).*

metry has essentially meant the transmission of the ECG with particular reference to the heart rate.

For telemetric transmission of biological data the following considerations are of importance: (1) The patient must be in his own environment so that it is possible to reveal stress under natural conditions and not only under laboratory conditions. (2) Tests for fitness for work or sport (ski-jumpers, rowers, pilots) can be carried out by wireless transmission under natural conditions. (3) The telemetric transmission of data is very important, when a patient who requires continuous supervision at an intensive nursing station needs transfer to the operating theatre for X-rays, or for a tracheotomy. This temporary removal does not interrupt continuous supervision.

There is no limit concerning the size or weight for the receiver, which are usually mains-powered, but the nature of the transmitter necessitates compromise.

In Western Germany there are several frequencies for wireless telemetry which are also

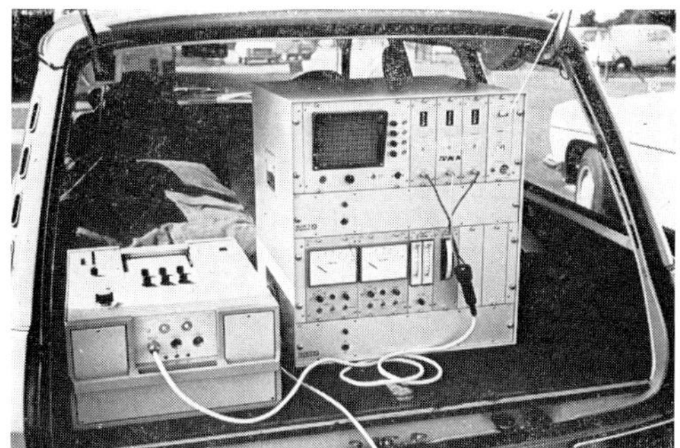

Fig. 2.   *Receiver of the 3-channel telemetry plant (right) with 3-channel writer (left).*

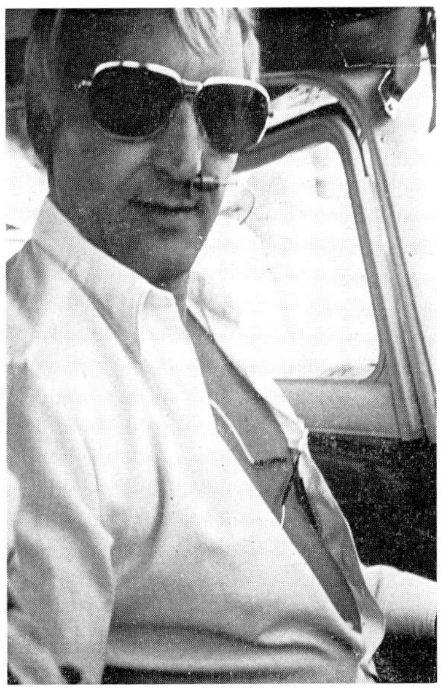

Fig. 3.   *Thermistor for registration of breath frequency and cable for registration of ECG (leading off V_5).*

used by the 3 systems: (1) Siemens (Telecust 36): (frequencies: 36.61–36.79 MHz). (2) Hellige: (frequency approximately 150 MHz; 8 frequencies (Figs. 1 and 2)). (3) Messerschmitt-Bölkow-Blohm: (frequency = 433.4–434.4 MHz).

Transmission of 3–10 values, depending on the apparatus.

The range of the apparatus in built-up areas is about 500 m–10 km by transmission in open unobstructed areas.

ASSESSMENT

In the case of the intensive care unit our telemetry plant is routinely employed for supervision, and the sender is then operating on mains electricity and not by a battery or an accumulator. In our aero-medical service several tests were performed.

In the clinic a utilizable ECG and a faultless pulse frequency derived from it was transmitted up to a distance of 50 m from lying, standing and running patients. An X-ray plant in operation did not interrupt the transmission.

In the case of the running test muscle potentials could not be avoided. Generally V_5 was used in order to avoid these muscle potentials. The respiratory frequency was recorded by a thermistor (Fig. 3).

RESULTS

Recording within the clinic

(*a*) Figure 4 shows the ECG of a 25-year-old patient, who was admitted to the clinic after an accident in a highly drunken state. The patient was restless, excited and in an emotionally unstable state, she cried nearly without pause and rolled to and fro in her bed. During the supervision the heart frequency varied between 100 and 150 beats/min. In spite of the excitement an almost faultless ECG was obtained.

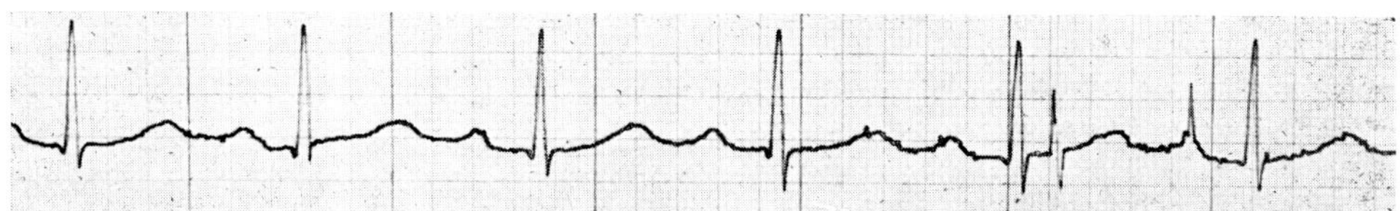

Fig. 4.   *ECG of a 25-year-old drunk patient, after an accident. Disturbing impulses by muscle potentials with high motoric excitement. Pulse-frequency on an average of 100/min (distance of transmission 35 m within the area; paper support 50 mm/sec).*

(*b*) Figures 5a and *b* show the ECG of a volunteer (36-years-old, 96 kg weight). Figure 5a: Stationary at a distance of transmission 50 m with intermediate X-ray-plant. Heart frequency 72/min. Figure 5b: At the double, the pulse increases up to 150/min.

Tests on using aero-medical service

Not only *flying trainees* but also flying trainers are exposed to measurable stress. Figures 6a–c show cardiac and respiratory frequencies of a 51-year-old flying trainer in different phases. The flying trainee flies, the trainer observes and corrects. The muscle potentials on the ECG and the long *pauses in breathing* are signs of the intense concentration during

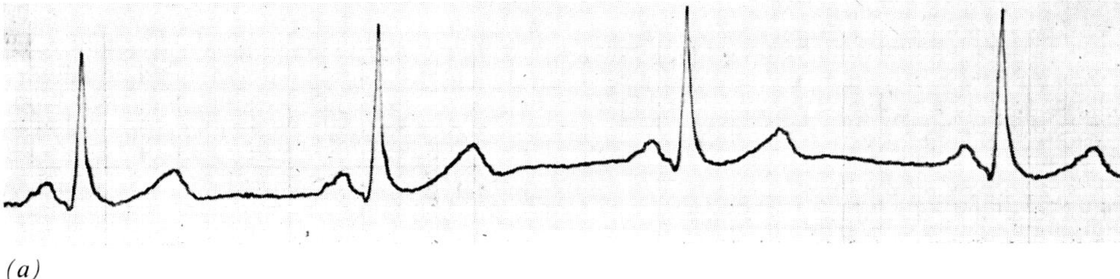

(a)

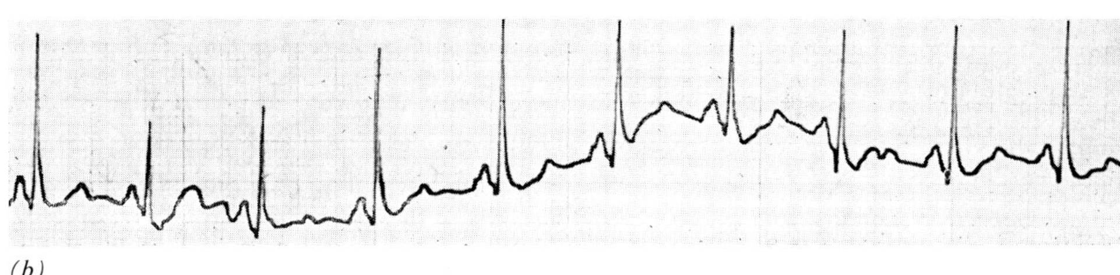

(b)

Fig. 5. *(a) ECG of a 36-year-old test person, 96 kg weight, stationery. Distance of transmission 50 m with intermediate X-ray plant (pulse frequency 72/min; paper support 50 mm/sec). (b) The same person in double. Distance about 40 m. Disturbing muscle potentials and perhaps scouring electrodes (pulse frequency 150/min; paper support 25 mm/sec).*

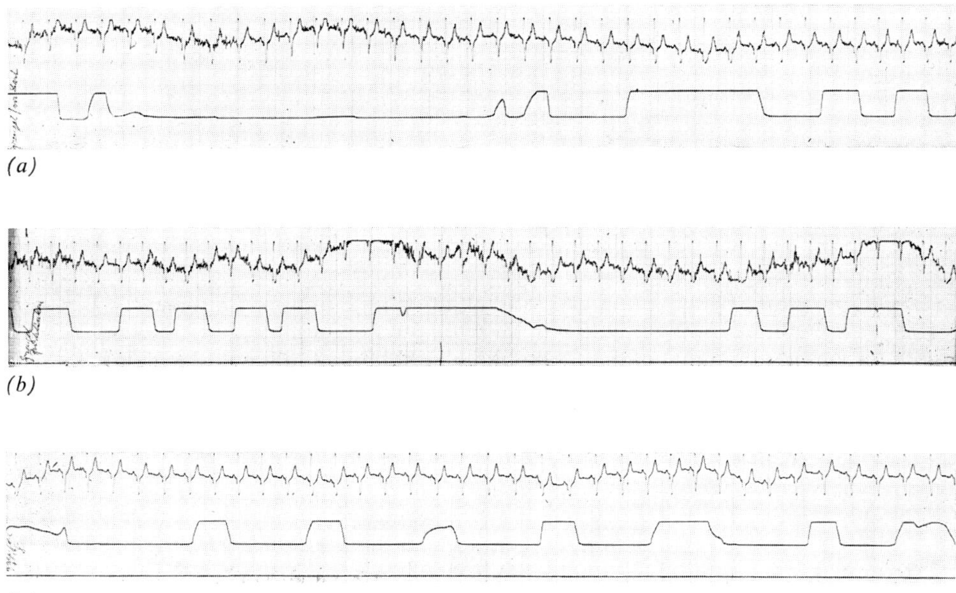

(a)

(b)

(c)

Fig. 6. *(a–c) Test person, Spr., 51-year-old, gliding flight trainer; control of trainee (heart frequency 90/min; paper support 25 mm/sec). Before the start and during releasing overlapping of ECG by muscle potentials and in a + b long breathing pauses as a sign of intense concentration. (a. before the start; b. during releasing; c. free flight).*

the supervision of the flying trainee. Pauses in the breathing of pilots up to 20 sec duration are always seen during concentration, especially during the landing-approach. According to these tests this frequency should be regarded as a more sensitive indicator of concentration than the heart rate.

REFERENCES

Demling, L. and Bachmann, K. (1970): *Biotelemetrie*. Georg Thieme Verlag, Stuttgart.

Eichler, J. (1967): *Z. prakt. Anästh. Wiederbeleb.*, 2, 270.

Eichler, J. and Lobsien, I. (1970): In: *Biotelemetrie*, p. 81. Editors: L. Demling and K. Bachmann. Georg Thieme Verlag, Stuttgart.

Holter, H. J. and Glassclock, W. R. (1961): Quoted by: Ullrich, G. J. (1970).

Ullrich, G. J. (1970): In: *Biotelemetrie*, p. 1. Editors: L. Demling and K. Bachmann. Georg Thieme Verlag, Stuttgart.

Monitoring of cardiac function by impedance cardiography during and after heart surgery

E. HARTUNG, M. NADJMABADI and M. ZINDLER

Department of Anaesthesia, University of Düsseldorf,
Düsseldorf, Federal Republic of Germany

Thoracic plethysmography (impedance cardiography) may now be regarded as a satisfactory method for the determination of the stroke volume (SV), provided its limitations are observed. A personal comparative study with the thermodilution method, consisting of 260 separate measurements, revealed a correlation of $r = 0.63$. However, the main advantage of impedance cardiography lies in the fact that it is not invasive and may be applied continuously for days on end without discomfort to the patient. Siegel et al. have studied the question to what extent impedance cardiography may be applied to inotropic parameters and have found that between the first derivative of thoracic impedance (dZ/dt), the maximal rate of pressure increase in the left ventricle $(dP/dt)_{max}$ LV and the ECG, there exists a direct correlation.

Figure 1 shows the analysis of the recording as recommended by Kubicek et al. From above downwards: the phonocardiogram, ΔZ, (dZ/dt) and the ECG of a healthy adult.

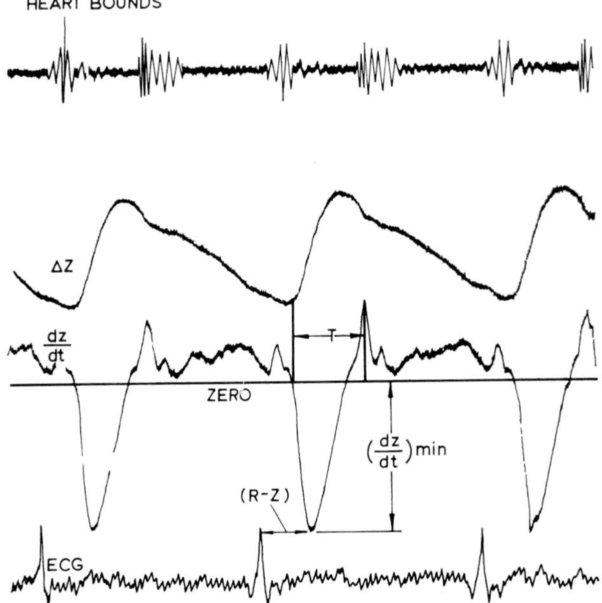

Fig. 1. *Analysis of the recording.*

Note T, the ejection time of the ventricle, but particularly also $(dZ/dt)_{min}$ and the $(R-Z)$ interval which extends from the R-wave of the ECG to the Z-wave of the first lead of thoracic impedance. With a view to simplification, Heather correlated $(dZ/dt)_{min}$ and the $(R-Z)$ interval (Table 1). The resulting index, named the Heather index, might well prove to be of clinical importance, since it offers a possibility of continuously and non-invasively collecting data indicative of changes of the inotropism with reasonable accuracy and with

Table 1.   *Correlation of intervals*

Heather index

$$\frac{(dZ/dt)_{min}}{(R-Z)}$$

the possibility of computer analysis. Especially in bad-risk cases this would be highly useful. Accordingly, in 10 patients subjected to open-heart operations with the aid of the heart-lung machine, the Heather index has been compared with the $(dP/dt)_{max}$ of the left ventricle on the basis of 559 separate determinations (287 of them before, and 272 after surgical correction of the lesion).

MATERIAL AND METHODS

We did not consider it justifiable to introduce a catheter-tip manometer into the left ventricle just to test this method. Consequently, we have made a comparative study in a number of cases in whom open-heart operations with pressure determinations were indicated. In these patients, the left ventricle was punctured directly under visual control by a steel needle (length 6 cm, external diameter 1.25 mm, 18-gauge) and connected with a pressure converter (Statham P 23 Db) by means of a cardiac catheter (Rüsch X-ray No. 10). By means of a differentiating element (PDD-2 Analog computer, Mescher) $(dP/dt)_{max}$ was recorded directly. Adhesive aluminium band electrodes, 6 mm wide, were attached to the chest wall at the usual sites, although in order to protect the sterility and the thoracic incision over only two-thirds of the circumference. These electrodes were connected with the IFM/Minnesota impedance cardiograph model 304A. A separate ECG, made by means of needle electrodes in the usual leads, (dZ/dt), $(dP/dt)_{max}$ LV and the pressure in the ascending aorta c.q. the radial artery were recorded by means of a Schwarzer Physioskript 6-channel recorder and stored on tape (3M). The inherent resonance of the manometer system amounted to 50 Hz, the inertia of the recording system to 270 Hz, so that $(dP/dt)_{max}$ could be measured with adequate accuracy.

Table 2.   *Patients and number of measurements*

Diseases	Before operation	After correction	Total
3 Aortic stenosis	189	35	224
3 Aortic insufficiency	58	166	224
1 Mitral stenosis	15	4	19
1 Coronary artery disease	25	–	25
1 Fallot tetralogy	–	36	36
1 VSD plus aortic insufficiency	–	31	31
Total	287	272	559

Table 2 shows the clinical material and the number of individual measurements. Comparative measurements before and after valve replacement were carried out in 3 patients with aortic insufficiency, in 3 cases of aortic stenosis and in one of mitral stenosis. In one patient with coronary dysfunction measurements were only performed before surgery, and in one with Fallot's tetralogy and one with ventricular septal defect with aortic insufficiency, measurements were only carried out after surgical correction. No good correlation between the Heather index as an inotropic parameter and $(dP/dt)_{max}$ LV could be demonstrated.

In Figure 2 the Heather index is plotted on the ordinate and $(dP/dt)_{max}$ LV on the abscissa. The dots represent values of separate, successive cardiac actions, the shaded squares the values after implantation of the aortic valve. It is interesting to note that dP/dt_{max} changes very little (from 6300–5200 mm Hg/sec) whereas the Heather index is more than doubled after the valvular replacement (from 7–17).

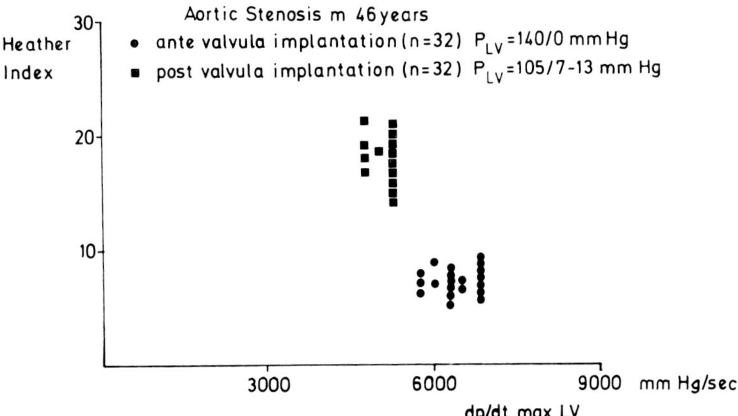

Fig. 2. *Comparison of Heather index and dP/dt_{max} LV.*

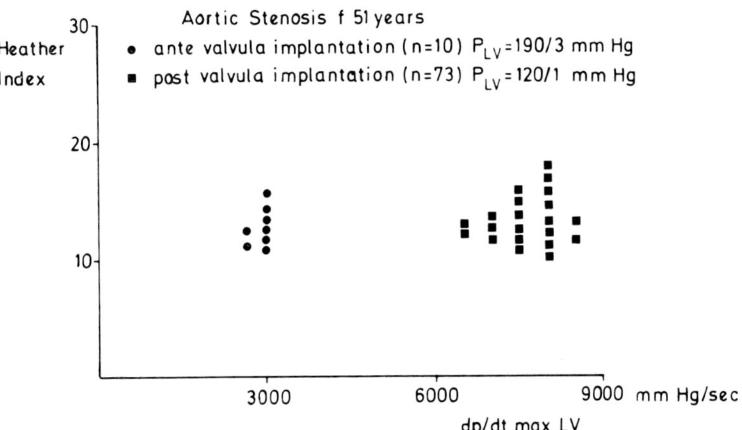

Fig. 3. *Comparison of the Heather index and dP/dt_{max} LV.*

Figure 3 shows the opposite. Once more, the Heather index is plotted on the ordinate, and $(dP/dt)_{max}$ LV on the abscissa. This time, we see that after valve replacement, again shaded squares, $(dP/dt)_{max}$ is more than doubled (from 3100–7600 mm Hg/sec), whereas the Heather index has changed very little (from 15–14).

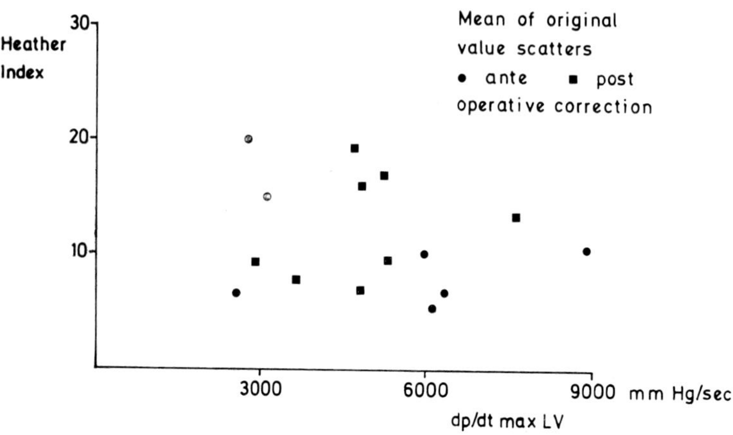

Fig. 4. *Comparison of mean values (10 patients).*

Figure 4 shows the mean values for the individual patients, of $(dP/dt)_{max}$ LV as well as of the Heather index before (the dots) and after surgical correction (the shaded squares), represented by one symbol for each individual case. It is clear that there is no significant correlation between the Heather index and the $(dP/dt)_{max}$ LV. This was also confirmed by computer analysis.

DISCUSSION

This finding contradicts the investigations carried out by Heather and also by Siegel et al. We have been unable to explain the discrepancy. Admittedly, Heather has also studied cardiac patients, but dP/dt was not measured directly, but the ejection phase calculated from the evacuation of the left ventricle as observed angiographically. Changes of inotropism were achieved in some cases by physical effort. Siegel et al. and Moritz et al. have influenced the heart of normal dogs by means of norepinephrine, isoproterenol, pentobarbital and *E. coli* toxin. These workers are unable to establish the part that is played by this difference in circumstances of the investigation, viz., in Heather's study, physical stress on the affected heart, in the case of Siegel et al., pharmacological effects on the healthy heart and in our own study, surgical correction with cardiac ischemia in hearts most of which had sustained preceding damage. Shortening of the impedance electrode by one-third did not affect (dZ/dt); this was checked in all patients.

In conclusion it may be stated that according to our preliminary findings, the Heather index is not suitable for the evaluation of the inotropism in patients to be subjected to open-heart operations.

On-line monitoring of cardiac output, arterial blood pressure and heart rate during and after cardiac surgery with a new computer (COC)

R. PURSCHKE [1], K. H. WESSELING [2], K. FALKE [1] AND S. TARBIAT [1]

[1] Institute of Anaesthesiology, University of Düsseldorf, Düsseldorf, Federal Republic of Germany, and [2] Institute of Medical Physics TNO, Utrecht, The Netherlands

The reliability of calculating stroke volume and cardiac output on a beat-to-beat basis from the arterial pressure pulse contour has been shown in dog experiments (Kouchoukos et al., 1970; Nichols et al., 1972; Purschke et al., 1974a) and under clinical conditions (Purschke et al., 1974b) (Fig. 1).

In this study a new apparatus (Wesseling et al., 1972), computing cardiac output from the aortic pressure wave-form was tested in cardiac surgical patients during and after surgery.

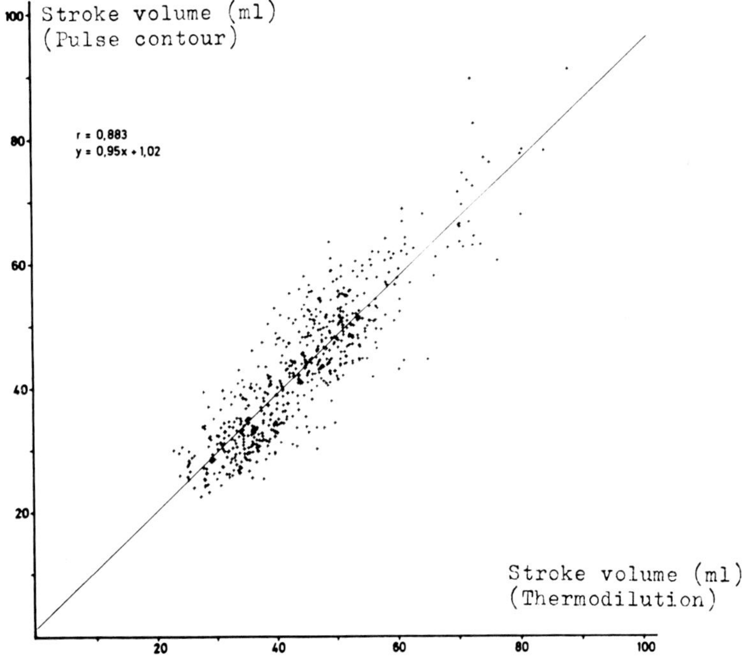

Fig. 1. *Comparison between pulse contour stroke volume and thermal dilution stroke volume (n = 605; pooled data of 13 patients after cardiac surgery).*

METHOD

Reference cardiac output was measured by thermal dilution (TD) using 3-F-thermistor probes in the pulmonary artery (devices cardiac output computer Type 3750).

For comparison, only the pressure pulses during the dilution time were used, in this way truly simultaneous cardiac output estimations could be made.

A total of 494 measurements were made during monitoring periods up to 4 days.

RESULTS

Satisfactory agreement was obtained between the TD and COC pulse contour cardiac outputs, despite large minute-to-minute variations in cardiac output, heart rate and aortic blood pressure in some patients (Fig. 2).

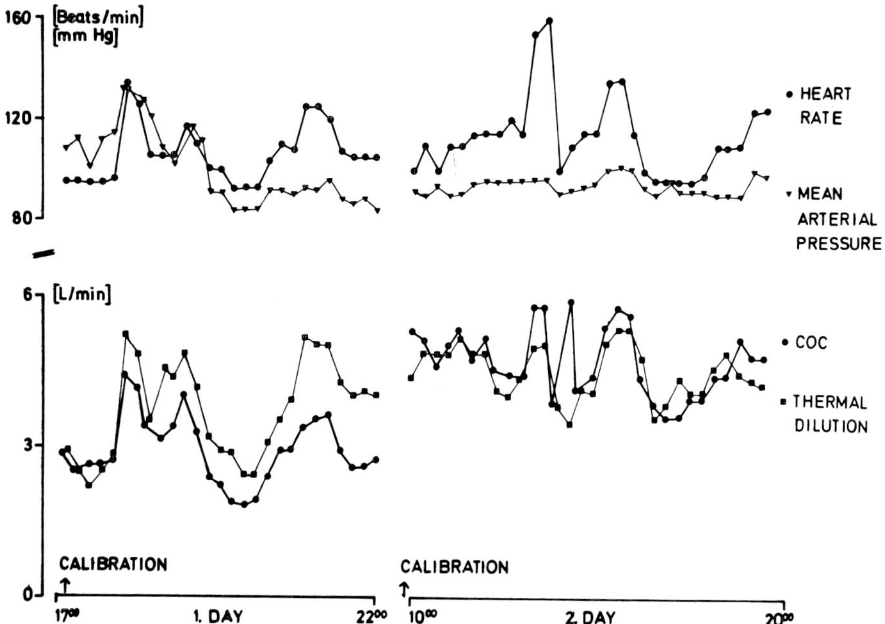

Fig. 2.   *Comparison between thermal dilution cardiac output and cardiac output calculated by the pulse contour computer (COC) (Pat. E.M., aortic valve replacement). Calibration factor was determined each day.*

Simultaneous measurements of cardiac output showed the COC computer to have a smaller scatter than the thermal dilution method when compared 3–8 times in essentially stable conditions: thermal dilution 4.3 ± 0.4 l/min; COC computer 4.2 ± 0.2 l/min.

Due to this small scatter it was possible to observe in one patient a decrease in cardiac output of 15 % within 15 min without any change in heart rate and mean arterial pressure; the patient was developing cardiac tamponade (Fig. 3).

Such a trend, had it been observed with a standard intermittent method, would probably have been ascribed to random fluctuations. On-line monitoring with the COC computer showed it to be a continuous smooth downward trend.

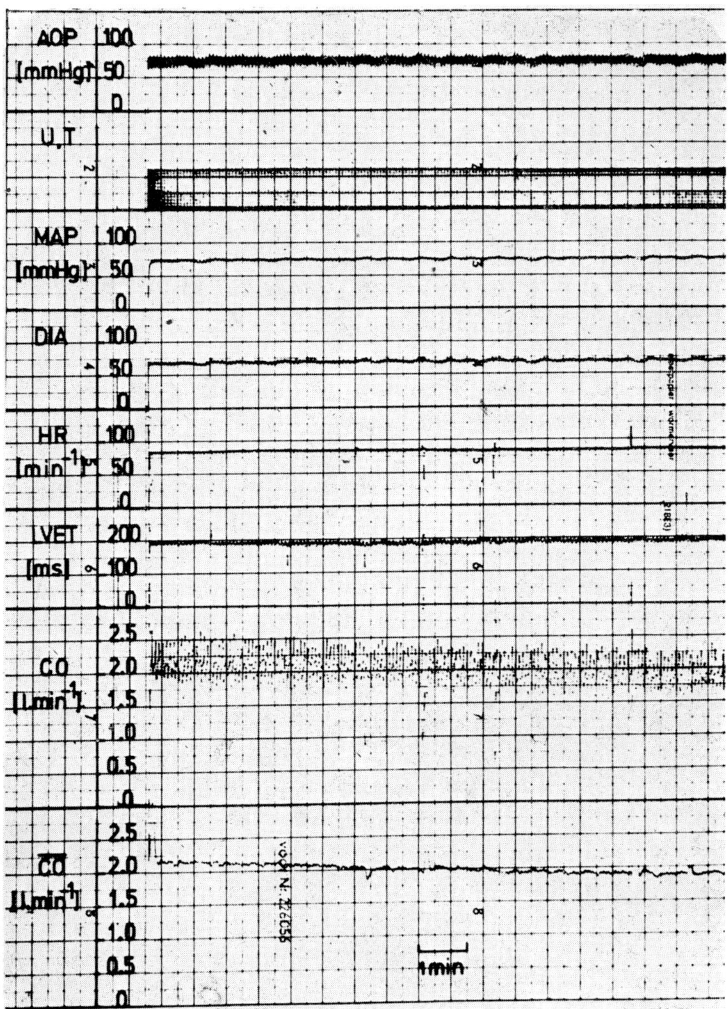

Fig. 3. *On-line recording of aortic blood pressure (AOP), mean arterial pressure (MAP), heart rate (HR), left ventricular ejection time (LVET) and cardiac output (CO) by the COC in a patient developing cardiac tamponade.*

DISCUSSION

On-line monitoring of vital functions is a major problem in the intensive care of critically ill patients. The results of this study show that the computation of the stroke volume from the aortic pressure wave-form offers a relatively simple, clinically useful method for on-line monitoring of cardiac output, heart rate and arterial blood pressure.

The early detection of short-time variations in cardiac output is an important advantage, especially under conditions with severe arrhythmias.

However, difficulties may arise from disturbed pressure curves fed into the computer. The method depends on the accurate detection of the ventricular ejection time and on the integration of the area under the systolic part of the aortic pressure curve (Kouchoukos et al., 1970; Wesseling et al., 1972). If the integration of this area is completed too early or too late, large errors in cardiac output estimations occur. Thus, for reliable cardiac output readings repeated checks of the pressure curve are necessary.

REFERENCES

Kouchoukos, N. T., Sheppard, L. C. and McDonald, D. A. (1970): *Circulat. Res.*, *26*, 611.

Nichols, W. W., Wesseling, K. H., De Wit, B. and Weber, J. A. P. (1972): In: *Abstracts, III International Conference on Medical Physics, Göteborg, 1972*, Abs. 19.6.

Purschke, R., Pütz, E. and Arndt, J. O. (1974a): *Anaesthesist*, *23*, 483.

Purschke, R., Brucke, P. and Schulte, H. D. (1974b): *Anaesthesist*, *23*, 525.

Wesseling, K. H., Nichols, W. W., De Wit, B. and Weber, J. A. P. (1972): In: *Abstracts, III International Conference on Medical Physics, Göteborg, 1972*, Abs. 19.5.

Wesseling, K. H., Smith, N. T., Nichols, W. W., Weber, J. A. P., De Wit, B. and Beneken, J. E. W. (1973): *Paper presented at:* Boerhaave Course on Measurement in Anesthesia, Leiden, 1973.

Chapter XV

Documentation in anaesthesiology

Computerized rationalization, distribution and documentation of medicine consumption

JOHS. O. HAGELSTEN

Department of Anaesthesiology, Kommunehospitalet, Copenhagen, Denmark

In nearly every country in the world the proportion of the National Income, spent on Health Care is steadily increasing. A typical acute hospital in an economically developed country requires a staff/in-patient ratio of about 3 to 1, and personnel costs are a very great part of the total hospital expense. If possible these personnel costs should be cut down by using modern technical equipment, for example, relevant sized computers.

In order to control Health Care costs it is primarily necessary to know what these costs consist of, and it may be especially within this area that computers can provide some important information. Those responsible for the running of a department must be able to document why and for which purposes these enormous costs are spent – and these *are* really enormous. For example, in Sweden, which is particularly advanced in Health Care, during the period from 1963 to 1972 Health Care costs rose by 316% compared to an increase in general price levels of only 45%. During the same period wages and salaries increased by 90%. The proportion of Sweden's Gross National Product absorbed by Health Care is continually increasing. It has been calculated that if the present growth rates are maintained, Health Care costs will exceed the Gross National Product of Sweden in the year 2001. Of course this will not happen but this extreme prognostication illustrates the urgency of bringing costs under control.

Apart from the personnel, another big expense item in a modern hospital is the expense of medical drugs. The number of such drugs is constantly increasing, and it is more and more difficult to choose rationally among all these progressively more active agents.

COMMITTEE FOR SELECTION OF MEDICAL DRUGS

Around 1960 the probably first Committee for Selection of Medical Drugs was appointed in Sweden, and in 1970 the creation of a similar committee was initiated by the Directorate of the Municipal Hospitals of Copenhagen. The task was to rationalize and document the consumption of medical drugs in the hospitals to obtain better economy and to prepare computerized requisition and documentation of medicine consumption. Recommendations have been worked out, these being:

1. to recommend drugs with optimal pharmaco-therapeutic effect;

2. to evaluate which preparations of medical drugs are available in the most expedient forms;

3. to obtain an essential reduction in the number of drugs with practically the same effects; and

4. in the choice between so-called identical drugs to make the pharmaceutical treatment the cheapest possible. The economical advantages are to a wide degree obtained by simpli-

fication of storage and distribution of medicine from the Hospital Pharmacy by recommending a standard assortment of medicine, supplemented according to the special demands of the different departments. The Committee is entitled to expect that the recommendations for the about 300 'standard drugs' are followed in the daily routine, and deviations should be logically motivated, optimally by published controlled clinical and biopharmaceutical trials.

In the work of choosing among 'identical' drugs, it has turned out that the demands to the pharmaceutical firms concerning relevant information also about biopharmaceutical and pharmaco-kinetic properties of the different drugs should be increased in the future.

The problem of too many medical drugs with the same action has been especially big within hospitals, where new doctors are constantly arriving and leaving, and consequently the local assortment of medical drugs is constantly increasing by addition of individual 'favorite drugs'. Practically all departments in the Copenhagen Municipal Hospitals have contributed with special knowledge to the work of the Committee. Of course the Committee has only been able to suggest and not dictate the use of certain drugs, but within certain areas the importance of equalization has been especially stressed and also understood, e.g. the use of digitalis-preparations and anti-coagulants.

Most colleagues have been very positive concerning the suggestions for more rational treatment, especially within areas which are in the periphery of their specific interests.

Until now the Committee has been mainly occupied with the rationalization of the consumption of medical drugs and preparation for computerized requisition and distribution of such drugs, but other tasks for the Committee are obvious, for example pharmaco-kinetic investigations, toxicological investigations, and planning of clinical trials of new drugs etc.

As example of the rationalization can be mentioned that the group 'analgesics' now consists of only 7 drug preparations, and similarly the group 'fluid and electrolyte balance' consists of only 15 recommended preparations. Earlier there were, within this area, a colossal number of drugs, different both quantitatively and qualitatively.

COMPUTERIZED REQUISITION OF MEDICINE

The first wards in the new Hvidovre Hospital, built by the City of Copenhagen, were opened in March 1974, and the work there is partly to be based upon a computer (Univac 9480) with Uniscope terminals and printers (type 800 and DCT 1000), while the cards are processed by Optical Mark Readers (Hewlett Packard 7260 A). The computer is programmed to register basic data of all in-patients, and takes care of arranging tests from the clinical laboratory, X-ray examinations, specified patient-menu items, delivery of goods from the central supply, and finally requisition of medicine from the pharmacy to the wards.

Furthermore more or less 'general information'-type messages may be communicated to all or only some of the display terminals. Every Scandinavian has a specific Personal Identification Number, so the identification problem is easily solved by the general use of this. Furthermore every physician in Hvidovre Hospital will be furnished with a Medicine Requisition Identification Card to be used instead of personal signature. The National Health Service has agreed to this arrangement, so that a doctor's personal signature is not necessary as a general rule within this system, which has been the case until now.

The system of requisition of medicine within Copenhagen City Hospitals was until now performed by so-called 'pharmacy books', which were handwritten, while the new system is based on optical readable cards. Each department of the hospital works out a list of a standard assortment of drugs, mainly based on the recommendations of the Committee for Selection of Medical Drugs, and modified to specific demands. Hereafter each ward receives a number of Standard Requisition Cards (of plastic), corresponding to the contents of the assortment. When one or more drugs are wanted, information from these cards is communicated via the Uniscope display-terminals and the computer to the hospital pharmacy. When a message has been delivered to the terminal, it can be checked on the display-scope whether the contents correspond with the demands, before the data are communicated via the computer to the hospital pharmacy. In the pharmacy the demands are written out by a printer to create a 'packing list'. Routine requisitions can be communicated, if necessary, via the public telephone network, by a terminal consisting also of a reader and maybe a printer.

If a department wants a drug which is not in the specific standard assortment, it has to be ordered on a special requisition card, which has to be filled out manually, as has been the case until now in the   pharmacy books'. It is consequently more difficult to choose a synonymous drug which is *not* in the standard assortment, and this fact has undoubtedly a certain educative effect – teaching people to stick to the recommended drugs.

IMPROVED DOCUMENTATION

The computer is programmed to produce monthly, or more frequently, a detailed documentation of the consumption of, among other things, medical drugs. By this technique a possibility is created for effective steering of the production and stock in the hospital pharmacy, and department- or area-accounts can be produced easily and uniformly at any time.

This computerized documentation has great advantages both concerning safety and economy, and it is also able to document possible misuse of narcotics or other agents at an earliest possible stage.

Why keep anaesthetic records?

D. D. C. HOWAT

St. George's Hospital, London, United Kingdom

Some anaesthetists keep detailed records of all the anaesthetics they give; others tell us that they keep none. Yet I do not believe there is really any doctor who keeps no notes at all about the patients under his care. I propose to deal here with the reasons for records in anaesthesia and to point out some of the problems involved, for we all know that they exist.

The diaries of John Snow, which have only recently been brought to the attention of anaesthetists (Atkinson, 1970), contain notes of all but the first 46 chloroform anaesthetics which he gave during the last 10 years of his life. He recorded that, on the occasion of Queen Victoria's confinement in 1853 'Dr. Locock thought the chloroform prolonged the interval between the pains and retarded the labour somewhat'. This is perhaps the earliest record of the effect of an anaesthetic agent on the course of labour. The first anaesthetic records in the United States were kept by Codman and later by Harvey Cushing at the end of the last century, and a paper was read at the Massachusetts General Hospital in 1903 on the recording of blood pressure during operation (Beecher, 1940). At the 10th Annual Congress of Anaesthetists in New York in 1931, Tovell and Dunn made the following observation:

'The need of an intensive study of alternative anaesthetic agents and methods is imperative. Only large series of cases will suffice if adequate data are to be obtained and conclusions with any degree of accuracy formulated. Tabulation of results suitable for comparison and evaluation is difficult. If some hundreds or thousands of values of a variable have been noted merely in the arbitrary order in which they occurred, the mind cannot grasp the significance of the record' (Tovell and Dunn, 1932).

Twelve years later, Nosworthy described in *'Anaesthesia'* his now well-known punch card which he had been using for over 6 years (Nosworthy, 1943). In the very next article in the same journal, Ayre (of T-piece fame) described a very simple record form. He referred to war-time difficulties and looked forward to the day when 'each hospital has its own department of anaesthesia, staffed by whole-time specialist anaesthetists with technical and other facilities at present conspicuous by their absence' (Ayre, 1943).

In 1954, Mushin described the Cardiff anaesthetic record system which also relies on a complementary punch card system, and stressed the importance of an annual review of the in-patient work in a hospital (Mushin et al., 1954). His reasons for keeping detailed records, were as follows (Mushin, 1953):

1. They give information about the personal activities of anaesthetists.
2. They supply the anaesthetist with interest and information while he is in the operating theatre.
3. They give a regular and comprehensive picture of the work of the hospital.
4. They supply a knowledge of the death-rate in the hospital and of changes in the types of drugs used over a period of time. He pointed out that they are of no value in research unless the record has been designed after the problems to be investigated have been formulated.

In 1965, the British Ministry of Health suggested the standardisation of all anaesthetic and operation records (British Ministry of Health, 1965). The Association of Anaesthetists of Great Britain and Ireland devised a record sheet which, it was felt, might be of use throughout the British Isles for those anaesthetists and hospitals who had not already designed their own. After much discussion, a very simple form was produced. It was not intended to replace those already in use or to be used for research purposes, but was to encourage anaesthetists to record the data which they felt were important before, during and after operation. It was also recommended that the form should be distinctively marked for easy recognition amongst the patient's other notes, although it was suggested that a dark blue colour might not be suitable for our specialty! The standardisation of records has not yet been achieved and the Association of Anaesthetists' record form has never been printed, although some hospitals copied the final draft.

In the last 10 years, the importance of keeping adequate records in the intensive care ward has been recognised; this has coincided with a great increase in the possibilities offered by the computer in recording, sorting and interpreting physiological and pharmacological data (Cliffe, 1967; Osborn et al., 1963). The suggestion has seriously been made that anaesthesia as a specialty may disappear, since technical personnel will be able to perform the necessary mechanical functions, while the control of the patient's physiological state is automated. Anaesthesiologists will then increasingly practice medicine (Forrest and Bellville, 1967). Whatever the future may hold for our specialty, the computer offers a means of release from detailed personal record-keeping, but it is very expensive to instal and maintain. Most of us are still working under such conditions that our recording must be done by hand, both in the operating theatre and in the intensive care ward. As the years pass, we find a mass of papers accumulating, for which we may or may not eventually have some use, but we all know what usually happens. Inevitably the day comes when there is no more room to store them. Let us be quite clear, therefore, why we should keep records at all.

1. We need a current record of the course of the anaesthetic or the state of the patient in the operating theatre or the intensive care ward. A good doctor always keeps a note of the changes in his patient's condition and of the drugs he gives, so that he can modify his treatment without having to rely on memory alone. It is a good discipline for the doctor and therefore indirectly benefits the patient. We all know how difficult it is for an anaesthetist working by himself to keep an adequate record, particularly during a busy list of relatively short cases. Even when this is achieved, the preoperative and particularly the postoperative details concerning the patient are frequently neglected, being confined to a brief note of the premedication given and sometimes the entry 'recovery satisfactory'.

2. A record of the patient's reaction to anaesthesia or to treatment may be invaluable at a later date, if further anaesthetics or therapy are required. One asks the questions: 'Did anything go wrong last time? If so, why? Can I avoid trouble this time?' Yet it is common to find that the same techniques and drugs have different effects on different occasions and the value of the previous record is probably less when a second anaesthetist is involved, except when there has been an unusual technical difficulty or an abnormal reaction to drugs (Morton, 1953).

3. A written record is important in cases involving litigation or during the investigation of a death associated with anaesthesia and operation. Although of no benefit to the patient, this is perhaps the single, most compelling reason for adequate documentation. In my hospital, the anaesthetic record and the patient's written consent to operation are combined in the same sheet.

4. The keeping of records is essential in providing a bank of information for retrospective studies in later years. Certainly it is valuable in the regular revision of anaesthetic practice or acute medical care and in forming the basis of discussion of methods and techniques within a hospital department (Mushin, 1953). Its worth is less obvious when

positive information is sought about, for example, the effects of drugs, although it may have a certain negative value. The various retrospective studies of the possible hepato-toxicity of halothane revealed many gaps in the record systems of the hospitals involved in the investigations. The findings were of great interest, but they were hardly conclusive (Mushin et al., 1964; National Halothane Study, 1966), although they may help to determine the nature and content of a prospective study or to ensure the reporting of important data (Inman and Mushin, 1974).

Each hospital group has developed its own recording system and no two are identical either in the operating theatre or the intensive care ward. The record usually has to be duplicated, so that one copy can be filed in the patient's general notes and another kept in the anaesthetic department. If this is not done, the difficulties of looking back through the notes may be complicated by having to retrieve all the records from a central store and a significant number may be lost.

If we are going to devote time, energy and money to automated systems of documentation, we must be quite clear why we are doing it. Hallén has made a computer programme from data compiled in the Karolinska Hospital in Stockholm, based on the patient's age, weight, condition, previous anaesthetic experience etc., so that the choice of a particular anaesthetic technique can be made automatically (Hallén, 1973). This is an excellent aim, but is applicable only to that particular department. Other workers in other units will have to formulate their own programmes, since variations in technique and ability are so great.

We must remember that information can be wrongly supplied, or not supplied at all, to the system; mechanical and electrical faults can invalidate or paralyse the recording and interpretation of the data. The computer is still our servant and can only act on our information. It has great possibilities, but is our information good enough?

REFERENCES

Atkinson, R. S. (1970): In: *Proceedings, IV World Congress of Anaesthesiologists, Londen, 1968*, p. 197. Editors: T. B. Boulton, R. Bryce-Smith, M. K. Sykes, G. B. Gillet and A. L. Revell. Excerpta Medica, Amsterdam.

Ayre, P. (1943): *Brit. J. Anaesth.*, *18*, 180.

Beecher, H. K. (1940): *Surg. Gynec. Obstet.*, *71*, 689.

British Ministry of Health (1965): In: *Standardisation of Hospital Medical Records*, p. 25. Her Majesty's Stationary Office, London.

Cliffe, P. (1967): *Postgrad. med. J.*, *43*, 195.

Forrest Jr, W. H. and Bellville, J. W. (1967): *Brit. J. Anaesth.*, *39*, 311.

Hallén, B. (1973): *Acta anaesth. scand., Suppl. 52.*

Inman, W. H. W. and Mushin, W. W. (1974): *Brit. med. J.*, *1*, 5.

Morton, H. J. V. (1953): *Proc. roy. Soc. Med.*, *46*, 739.

Mushin, W. W. (1953): *Proc. roy. Soc. Med.*, *46*, 739.

Mushin, W. W., Rendell-Baker, L., Lewis-Faning, E. and Morgan, J. H. (1954): *Brit. J. Anaesth.*, *26*, 298.

Mushin, W. W., Rosen, M., Bowen, D. J. and Campbell, H. (1964): *Brit. med. J.*, *2*, 329.

National Halothane Study (1966): *J. Amer. med. Ass.*, *197*, 775.

Nosworthy, M. (1943): *Brit. J. Anaesth.*, *18*, 160.

Osborn, J. J., Badia, W. and Gerbode, F. (1963): *J. thorac. cardiovasc. Surg.*, *45*, 500.

Tovell, R. M. and Dunn, H. L. (1932): *Anesth. Analg. Curr. Res.*, *11*, 37.

The Hoechst biomedical data base

GEORG-E. UNGER

Hoechst AG., Arzneimittel-Informationszentrum, Frankfurt/Main, Federal Republic of Germany

The permanent increase in scientific publications, the so-called 'information explosion', influences to quite some extent the daily work of the medical profession. The exponential increase is easily demonstrated by a few figures: at present, in the field of biomedical literature, about 14,000–16,000 journals are published per year, with about 700,000–1,000,000 single publications; this means about 2,000–3,000 publications per day. Today about 30,000 diseases are known, annually about 400–600 new ones can be added. Doctors today have about 40,000–60,000 medical drugs at their disposal. This is a 10-fold increase in the last 30 years. Newest calculations state, that every 24 min a publication in chemistry is written, and that every 34–35 min a medical publication appears.

Generally, every scientist doing research needs up to 60% of his working time to produce information. There is practically no scientist who can read more than 5% of the original literature in his field of interest. The information flood leads thus to a considerable increase in information as well as to a lack of it. Accurate knowledge, i.e. finding the correct information, means a considerable time-saving and a considerable saving of cost. 'Not *more*, but the *right* information is needed.'

These few introductory words show the demands which have to be put to an international medical literature information system in order to follow-up all tendencies in modern biomedical as well as chemical-pharmaceutical research. Private enterprise, especially the pharmaceutical industry, has developed for itself various methods of eliminating the shortcomings encased in the 'flood of information'.

The 'Biomedical Drug Data and Information Centre' was established in 1969 by Hoechst AG. The pressure of increase in medical information in all disciplines of medicine and biochemistry became so urgent that the decision to have an automated on-line medical data literature system became imperative.

Data material in differentiated form is today already available on magnetic tape, e.g. Biomedical Abstracts, Chemical Biological Activities, Excerpta Medica, Derwent Ringdoc, Toxicon, International Pharmaceutical Abstracts etc. In September 1972 the first terminal-orientated data base was started. Since then we have more than 20 months experience with terminal-orientated dialogue-researches. In the meantime we have acquired about 2,300,000 documents. In the first phase of the development we used the magnetic tapes of Excerpta Medica. The program complex for this data system had been developed at Hoechst AG using the IBM-program DPS (Document Processing System) which had to be stripped down to its bases and changed completely in order to create a data base with on-line retrieval.

The organisation of data units, which will later be the elements of the search, is the responsible factor for effectiveness of a data-information system. All coded data, which was contained on magnetic tapes, had to be translated into clear text and had to be organized into special columns. For example, the names of the authors, institutions, address, descriptors, classification etc. The DPS is working with inverted data bases, in order to find quickly all the terms wanted in one search.

FORMAT OF DOCUMENTS

The following categories are stored in the system: authors; institution or address; title of publication in English; original title in original language; bibliographical data; language of the original; country of the original; descriptors – (a) primary terms (about 16,000 compulsory, but synonym free terms from the total field of medicine), (b) secondary terms (formal terms such as 'review', experimental animals, ways of application etc.), (c) free terms (explanatory terms), (d) trade marks, (e) name of manufacturer, (f) Coden-code of the periodical, (g) classification code (this is a classification code containing about 4,000 poly-hierarchical groups, into which each publication is classified), (h) abstract, (i) Wiswesser Line Notation for chemical formulae.

FORMULATION OF A QUERY

Due to the fact that the total 'document' including the abstracts are stored, all categories of words within the document can be used for a search. In order to find the proper terms the hierarchical orientated classification, as explained above, can be used. Furthermore the use of the primary and secondary terms allow the query to be specified.

It is a well-known fact that, as soon as indexing and searches are not in one hand – and this is always the case in commercially available data bases – the searcher might encounter difficulties in finding the specific descriptor which the indexer used, even if all the rules and regulations of indexing are observed. Because of this it was decided to store the abstract text as well, so that both could be used in a search. Reading in these abstracts is very often the only way to find hidden data or to specify unclear queries. A searcher has quite a number of possibilities for these words on the terminal; the words can come from all categories of the document. The search procedure is according to Boolean logic. In addition there are word extensions responding simultaneously to indexing terms with different endings (truncation).

Limitations may supply the position of a number of descriptor terms connected by 'and', i.e. the distance between words within the sentence on paragraph. Additional limitation can enable the additional requirement to be made, so that the document found should contain certain data in the categories mentioned above, i.e. certain authors, languages, etc.

Besides the 'and' linkage (in order to narrow the search) certain conditions can be demanded, e.g. that the indexing words connected by 'and' appear not only in the same document, but also within the document in a certain context. Or the word should appear in the same paragraph, or in the same sentence or within one sentence with a predefined distance from a certain word. Another help in the search is the use of synonyms.

Most diseases are described in literature under several different synonyms. The same drug is often listed under many different names. As the tragedy of thalidomide most clearly showed, a drug cannot be rapidly identified unless it has a universally understood and accepted name: i.e., an international non-proprietary name. Equal confusion exists in the medical sciences. Misunderstandings arise not always as a result of any disagreement in principle, but simply as a result of semantics. This situation obviously hampers the effective retrieval of information. It is clear that important observations are lost, simply because they are indexed under different synonyms.

Synonyms account for nearly half of the medical terminology in any language. Some of the terms used are obsolete, many incorrect, and others little used except in specific geographic areas or by particular schools of thought. For instance, *Candida albicans* is discussed in the literature under more than 170 different synonyms. Every clinician has been confronted at one time or another with the large number of synonyms.

Furthermore we can use comparative operants such as 'greater than', 'smaller than', 'within', etc. Besides the 'and' linkage (in order to narrow the search) certain conditions can be demanded, e.g. connected by 'and' appear not only in the same document, but also within the document in a certain context. Or the word could appear in the same paragraph or in the same sentence with one predefined distance from certain words. For example, a search can be made for the words 'rheumatic' and 'fever' and demand that the word 'fever' should appear right after the word 'rheumatic', symbolized by ($+$ 1). Furthermore enlargement of the indexing words can be made by word roots, e.g. the word 'rheumatism' can be searched for by a truncation ($). This would mean that all entries in our dictionary for the word 'rheuma' would be shown on the terminal screen and we would then receive all variations of the truncated word 'rheuma', such as: rheumatic, rheumatica, rheumatism etc. Any of the new words can be introduced into the search in order to find the proper expression.

TERMINAL

The Terminal, which was installed at Hoechst in 1972, is an IBM 2770 with an IBM 2265 visual display unit with console and an IBM 2203 printer. The terminal is via a modem connected on-line with the computer IBM/370–158–VS, situated at a distance of about 3 km. Our data base receives annually about 250,000 documents on 8 IBM 3330–11 discs and can daily be used during working hours. At night additional batch searches can be made.

SEARCH DIALOGUE ON THE TERMINAL

Searches are entered via the console on our terminal and sent to the computer. The program searches relevant inverted data bases, thereby considering the linkages and special conditions of the search; after 10 sec the statistics appear on the visual display screen, i.e. the frequency with which individual indexing terms appear in the stored material and the number of documents in the context research in which they appear. This also applies to logical configurations within the index terms, and is a very useful aid, showing the frequency or rarity of indexing words and the occurrence and frequency of logical linkages between the words. Then the first document is shown at the display screen and can actually then, should it qualify for the search, be printed via the printer.

The user has therefore the possibility of testing on the visual display screen the relevance of each individual document. Should the documents not really qualify for the search he can start a new formulation of the query. In case this also does not satisfy, one can search with the descriptors, classification or the so-called free text terms from the abstracts and restart a new search formulation. The already mentioned 'or'-linkages, are the synonym list and the truncation as already discussed and will give good results.

In order to support the search further, 7 parameters are possible: descriptor list; synonym list; classification scheme; Coden-code list; country code list; language code list; and Wiswesser Line Notation list. These are partly in microfiche.

Principally all documents found can completely be printed out. This equals the normal format of literature documentation as usual. A one-paged document is printed within 15–20 sec. It is furthermore possible to print out only the titles or other categories such as authors, titles, and journal description.

In these cases the shorter titles can be printed one right after another, otherwise each document is one page only. It is natural that the various documents can be selected for printing purposes.

FURTHER DEVELOPMENT

Very good results with this information system led us to the conclusion to have, as from January 1975, 5 more terminals within our company. In addition there will be terminals for our 5 associated companies within Germany, as well as one terminal at our agencies in Paris, Amsterdam and London. Further connections are planned to Austria, Denmark etc.

Preparations for this scheme were made a year ago. Especially for the enlargement of the storage capacities up to 16 discs with the IBM 3330–11 and the IBM 3270/75 terminals and the change from DPS to STAIRS-VS. With this new version 14 terminals can be connected and can simultaneously and independently of each other use the enlarged storages of up to 1,000,000 documents (this is about 3 years).

The question may now arise why Excerpta Medica and not Medlars has been used for such an extensive documentation? Due to the fact that Medlars is already installed in the United States and Europe, a comparison between Medlars and Excerpta Medica revealed that Medlars concentrates more on compactness in the searches and in its answers, and does not offer the same excellent access possibilities as the Excerpta material for a terminal-orientated on-line retrieval system. It has been found that the Excerpta material is far more thoroughly indexed and the polyhierarchical link categories cover the entire medical literature. This fact, and the addition of a very good retrieval program, makes the Excerpta Medica material far more easily accessible. The biomedical information retrieval system, as it is functioning today, is already covering more than 300 ad-hoc searches per month besides SDI's. The fact that quite a number of terminals will be connected with the system by the middle of this year, indicates clearly that the new STAIRS program, along with an enlarged disc storage, has been the correct way to achieve a safe and successful information service.

Anaesthesia record system with a mark page reader

H. LUTZ and P.-O. HILDEBRAND

Institute for Anaesthesiology and Reanimation, Faculty for Clinical Medicine Mannheim,
University of Heidelberg, Mannheim, Federal Republic of Germany

Whereas formerly anaesthesia was only mentioned cursorily, nowadays the process of anaesthesia is usually recorded by means of a formal document. In addition, the notes contain data on the preoperative findings and information on the immediate postoperative course in the recovery room. The data may be regarded as an expression of careful and conscientious patient supervision and should be accessible to evaluation for legal and scientific reasons. The data are not only evidence of acts performed and of correct functioning of individual department or collaborators but they are also an indispensable basis for answers to questions in the field of insurance or law (Lutz, 1970).

In the past few years, the problem of retrieval of this information has been studied intensively. Various methods of data processing have been used (Mushin et al., 1954; Hagelsten and Bennike, 1964; Yeakel, 1964; Giercke and Hutschenreuther, 1965; Brückner et al., 1968; Kleinheisterkamp and Fassl, 1968; Wawersik, 1970; Norlander, 1970; Hallén, 1973).

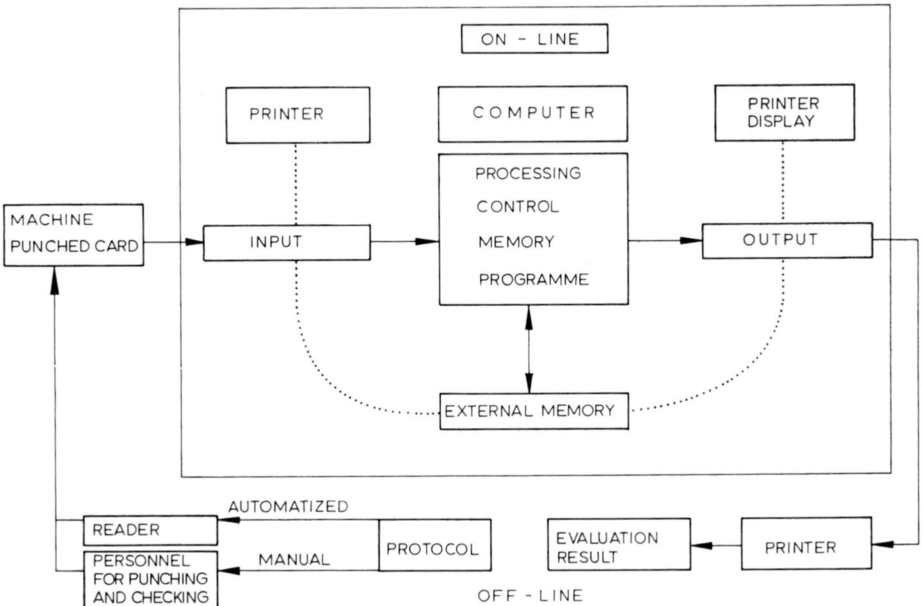

Fig. 1. *Scheme of documentation with mark pages.*

Since 1969 experience has been gained with the technique of off-line processing (Lutz, 1970; Lutz and Hildebrand, 1972) (Fig. 1). In the planning of our system of documentation the following requirements had to be fulfilled: (1) frequency distributions (e.g. the number of anaesthesists in the various disciplines); (2) personnel requirements in the surgical disciplines; (3) involvement of collaborators with the department of anaesthesia; (4) analysis of interrelated problems (e.g. distribution of complications in circumscribed anaesthesia procedures).

For this, it was necessary to substitute for the edge-punched card the machine-punched card. The equipment required was made available by courtesy of industry.

It was assumed that in the near future there would be a shortage of personnel for documentation in anaesthesia departments, so that the anaesthetist must carry out documentation of anaesthesia himself, without spending too much time. The central problem in this respect was the direct conversion of the data collected to data suitable for computer processing. An anaesthesia record was developed which has a 'mark page' in addition to the pages for recording in ordinary writing. This 'mark page' can be evaluated fully automatically by means of a mark reader after the printed mark spaces have been filled out. This eliminates loss of time and personnel for coding and conversion, which is still necessary for punching and checking of machine-punched cards in other systems of documentation.

MARK PAGE

The mark page of DIN A4 format, contains descriptive collective items printed vertically at the margin of the page. The order of printing was chosen in such a manner to correspond as much as possible with the practical procedure. Three main categories can be distinguished: (1) preoperative phase, (2) course of anaesthesia, and (3) recovery room and transport report. The differentiated structure of the mark page permits variable response to numerous problems, according to accurately defined criteria. This increases the validity of the data collected and permits a comparison between different patients and clinics.

The *preoperative section* of the mark page contains data for identification of the patient (date of birth, sex, height, weight). Identification of clinic and anaesthetist is by means of an internal cipher code. Definite classification of the anaesthesias forms the basis of computer determination of performance (Fig. 2).

The site of operation is classified topographically according to 10 main regions in a vertical column. Specification of the organ involved – in as far as this is relevant for anaesthesiology – is on a horizontal line with up to 9 positions. The surgical procedures can be classified in 18 ways. Related concepts such as puncture and incision are taken together as equivalent. An operation catalogue, still to be elaborated, will contribute to standardized definition.

The various intercurrent diseases of a patient can be recorded only by way of overall assessment and are of varied importance for the course of anaesthesia. On the basis of previous experience, cardiac diseases were given a detailed specification. Preoperative findings include parameters such as Hb, haematocrit, urea, creatinine, potassium, Quick test and urinary findings. In addition the blood pressure, ECG findings and possible blood gas analysis are specified. The preoperative category is completed by risk grading and premedication chosen.

The *course of anaesthesia* starts with data on the method. Peripheral and spinal conduction anaesthesia, the local anaesthetic used and the usual anaesthetics for intravenous or inhalation anaesthesia are specified. Specification of dosage is not included, since the value of such information does not justify the space required. Data are included on relaxants used and the nature of the ventilation. The technique of airway maintenance is clearly

Anaesthesia record

| Anaesthesia book number | Name |

Clinic	0	100	200	300	400	Site	500	600	700	800	900
	0	10	20	30	40	of therapy	50	60	70	80	90
	0	1	2	3	4		5	6	7	8	9

| Anaes-thetist | 0 | 10 | 20 | 30 | 40 | | 50 | 60 | 70 | 80 | 90 |
| | 0 | 1 | 2 | 3 | 4 | | 5 | 6 | 7 | 8 | 9 |

Anaesthesia book No.	0T	10T	20T	30T	40T	Patient identi-fication	50T	60T	70T	80T	90T
	0T	1T	2T	3T	4T		5T	6T	7T	8T	9T
	0	100	200	300	400		500	600	700	800	900
	0	10	20	30	40		50	60	70	80	90
	0	1	2	3	4		5	6	7	8	9

Sex

Date of birth	0	10	20	30						
	0	1	2	3	4	Day	5	6	7	8	9
	0	10								
	0	1	2	3	4	Month	5	6	7	8	9
	0	10	20	30	40		50	60	70	80	90
	0	1	2	3	4	Year	5	6	7	8	9

Weight (kg)	0	100				Weighed or estimate					
	0	10	20	30	40		50	60	70	80	90
	0	1	2	3	4		5	6	7	8	9

Height (cm)	0	100	200			Weighed or estimate					
	0	10	20	30	40		50	60	70	80	90
	0	1	2	3	4		5	6	7	8	9

	Nose sinuses	Mouth jaw	Teeth	Cranium	Head	Intrac.	Eyes	Ears	Skin face	Other
	Thyr.	Parath.	Tons. Pharynx	Larynx	Neck	Trach.	Vessels	Cervical spine	Skin and soft tissues	Other
				Lungs						

Fig. 2. *Excerpt from a mark page.*

defined, as is the position of the patient. Special measures such as gastric tube, hypotension or hypothermia can also be recorded if desired.

Because intraoperative patient-monitoring has increased, the section on 'monitoring' has been amplified to 16 positions.

In our opinion, the manifold peroperative complications can only receive an overall classification. If the total number is small, manual evaluation of the original pages on the basis of a list is preferred. The data on peroperative complications are completed by stating whether the condition could be controlled or not. For operations associated with significant blood-loss the latter is specified as a percentage of the nominal volume, either estimated or measured.

The bulk of the available space is occupied by data on infusion and transfusion therapy. Initially a compromise had to be made between the accuracy of data on the nature and dosage of fluid therapy and the space available. Intraoperative additional medical therapy is included insofar as some important groups of drugs are mentioned. It should be noted, however, that the analysis of problems of interaction, for instance, offers a greater chance of success with real-time processing (Norlander, 1972, personal communication).

Since the time of anaesthesia per se gives only an approximate idea of the time spent by the anaesthetist, the time spent between the onset of anaesthesia and transport to the ward or recovery room is now recorded.

Finally, further hospital progress of the patient is specified, with particulars on the condition of the patient when transferred to the intensive care unit if necessary.

The *final part* of the mark page is only filled in when the patient goes through the recovery room. This contains data on particular disturbances in the recovery room, the duration of stay, fluid therapy and department to which the patient is transferred.

DATA COLLECTION

The mark page should be filled out during the anaesthesia or immediately afterwards by the anaesthetist responsible. Experience over a period of several years has shown that this can be done. The time required is short: 3–4 min/page. Before the completed page is filed it is given a current number on the basis of an anaesthesia record book. The protocols are collected daily and checked for completeness. Experience has shown that without such built-in checking the error rate becomes unacceptable and the use of data processing becomes dubious.

DATA PROCESSING

Weekly, the records are transferred to the computer centre and evaluated by the mark reader. Checking of the data for formal and logical errors leads to exclusion of the erroneous records, which must be corrected by the anaesthetist responsible. The most frequent cause of rejection of a record is incompleteness, i.e. absence of one or more marks.

Continuous storage of the data on magnetic tape permits early statistical evaluation of the material. At present print-out of the results is done twice a year. This is done with an overlap in time of some 14 days. On the basis of an error-tracing programme, absent records, duplications and erroneous records are listed and returned to the anaesthesia department for correction. Print-out of the results contains 21 lists, some of them 3-dimensional. The array has been chosen so that important collective items can be inter-related. For instance, identification of the anaesthetist is carried out according to number, time and nature of the anaesthesias, as are the site of operation, risk-grading and condition of the patient on transfer.

Additional lists give data on methods of anaesthesia and peroperative complications, condition of the patient on transfer and particulars in the recovery room. Therefore the total print-out is very comprehensive. Each list can be retrieved separately if desired. Evaluation of certain questions such as determination of anaesthetist performance, requires manual evaluation of the tables.

EXPERIENCE

The mark system has been used as a routine system for anaesthesiological documentation since 1969. Its primary tasks were: (1) determination of simple frequency distributions, and (2) analysis of correlation questions.

Previous experience was limited, so that the mark page had to be changed repeatedly. For instance, the attempt to document the postoperative course for up to 4 weeks after the operation had to be discontinued. Excessively detailed data-collection should also be avoided. For instance, data on the dosage of anaesthetics used did not yield the information expected. The space was subsequently used for other items. For instance, data on blood-loss were included so that the relation to blood substitution and infusion therapy could be determined. Data on the activity of the anaesthetist was found to be a valuable addition. Although at present the frequency of rejection of records is still relatively high, this is due to insufficient checking in the department. On the other hand a comprehensive checking-programme ensures a high accuracy of the data. The method of mark reading described for anaesthesiological documentation can be regarded as a successful experiment since the amount of work required from the individual anaesthetist is small. Collection of the data can be done during the anaesthesia. There is no extra work required for coding. A comprehensive checking programme increases the validity of the data collected. Comprehensive listing of the data permits essential conclusions on the scope and nature of the performance in a department and of the individual anaesthetist.

REFERENCES

Brückner, J. B., Bonhoeffer, K. and Mertens, W. (1968): *Anaesthesist, 17*, 135.
Giercke, H. P. and Hutschenreuther, K. (1965): *Anaesthesist, 14*, 339.
Hagelsten, J. O. and Bennike, K.-Å. (1964): *Ugeskr. Laeg., 126*, 527.
Hallén, B. (1973): *Acta anaesth. scand., Suppl. 52*.
Kleinheisterkamp, U. and Fassl, H. (1968): *Anaesthesist, 17*, 382.
Lutz, H. (1970): *Z. prakt. Anästh. Wiederbeleb., 5*, 35.
Lutz, H. and Hildebrand, P.-O. (1972): *Anaesthesist, 21*, 292.
Mushin, W. W., Rendell-Baker, L., Lewis-Faning, E. and Morgan, J. H. (1954): *Brit. J. Anaesth., 26*, 298.
Norlander, O. (1970): In: *Medical Computing, Progress and Problems*, p. 227. Editor: M. E. Abrams. Chatto and Windus, London.
Wawersik, J. (1970): *Z. prakt. Anästh. Wiederbeleb., 5*, 6.
Yeakel, A. E. (1964): *Anesth. Analg. Curr. Res., 43*, 66.

Differentiation and importance of certain classification characteristics for statistical comparison of anaesthesiological data

J. WAWERSIK, S. ONNASCH and B. VÖLCK

Central Department for Anaesthesia, University of Kiel, Kiel, Federal Republic of Germany

Data processing in anaesthesiology necessarily depends on certain local conditions and circumstances. Therefore it is not possible to develop a system for anaesthesiological documentation for general use or of more than regional scope. Nevertheless an attempt should be made to obtain at least uniformity in the determination of certain basic characteristics, to permit comparison of anaesthesiological data between various teams and clinical institutions.

The fundamental problems of electronic data-processing are effective identity characteristics to link the data to the individual patient and complete an early data collection. These conditions are certainly not easily fulfilled in anaesthesiological practice. Although it has become universal practice to make an anaesthesia record every time anaesthesia is performed, its composition and its completion during the anaesthesia raise difficulties.

IDENTITY CHARACTERISTICS

The difficulties mentioned already apply to the collection of identity characteristics (Fig. 1). In emergencies the patient's name and date of birth may not be known. Secondary checking and, if necessary, completion of the so-called I-number in the anaesthesia protocol in large anaesthesiological departments requires such a large staff that this cannot be done in practice.

According to personal experience 10% anaesthesia records are incomplete in this respect and after correction of errors about 1%. For this reason our personal technique of electronic data-processing so far excludes repeated anaesthesias. Consequently, an essential classification characteristic is necessarily omitted, although it is definitely impossible to answer certain questions.

TIME FACTOR AND DATA REDUCTION

Timely data-collection during anaesthesia may also cause difficulties when intraoperative complications arise and numerous therapeutic measures are necessary for surgical or anaesthesiological reasons. For exact analysis of the course of anaesthesia with time it is therefore indispensable to check such a record after anaesthesia has been terminated. This again requires extra staff and becomes impracticable. Therefore one should consider to what extent time-correlation of the course of anaesthesia can be omitted.

Main entry No	Date		Weekday/Weekend	Clinic	In/out patient	Date of birth	Age	Sex	Name	Weight	Site of operation	Nature of operation	State of development	Onset of anaesthesia	Duration of anaesthesia / technique / Narcotics / Relaxants	CNS / Respiration	Defect / Anhydraemia / Shock-ileus	Hypotension / Respiratory depression / Cardiac arrest	General treatment	Anaesthesist
01900	03	72	50	20	2	250966199	06	0	C21	175	01	3	10	050	3302301020	1000000000	000000	000	04	00
01901	03	72	50	20	2	999966295	06	0	555	175	C1	5	C9	03C	2300301030	1000000000	000000	000	02	00
01902	03	72	10	12	2	020720199	52	0	C79	848	01	3	10	230	1301303120	3000100000	000000	200	11	00
01903	03	72	10	33	2	060733199	39	0	555	1C0	44	2	17	0C8	1203001050	1410000000	000000	000	05	00
01904	03	72	10	33	2	170623199	49	0	559	100	44	2	17	0C8	1202001050	1010000000	000000	000	08	00
01905	03	72	10	30	2	240765199	07	0	C21	227	76	4	13	075	2300301020	3010000000	000000	000	09	21
01906	03	72	10	33	2	281248299	24	0	559	227	76	2	08	035	1302303070	1040000000	000000	000	08	00
01907	03	72	10	33	2	040117159	55	0	559	100	44	2	C9	015	1202001050	1010000000	000000	000	08	00
01908	03	72	10	33	2	040117199	55	0	999	100	44	2	18	010	1202001050	1010000000	000000	000	03	00
01909	03	72	10	33	2	060733199	39	0	599	100	44	2	C9	0C3	1202001050	1410000000	000000	000	03	00
01910	03	72	10	33	0	170623199	49	0	559	1C0	44	2	10	01C	1202001050	1010000000	000000	000	03	00
01911	03	72	20	20	2	041015299	57	0	C63	174	C1	3	17	035	1302301020	1100000000	000000	200	11	00
01912	03	72	20	12	2	280928199	44	0	C75	122	01	4	09	310	1301303220	3010400000	004000	720	11	21
01913	03	72	20	25	2	C60371299	00	9	CC9	911	41	2	10	025	2200300010	4000000000	000000	000	15	00
01914	03	72	20	25	2	260531299	41	0	C63	921	01	2	08	080	1301303030	5000000000	000000	200	15	00
01915	03	72	30	12	2	180338199	34	0	C84	713	C1	3	13	185	1301303120	3000000001	000000	200	11	00
01916	03	72	30	12	2	999969199	03	0	C14	124	79	5	09	220	2300301040	2010000000	101000	000	02	00
01917	03	72	40	25	2	130966299	06	0	C19	841	41	2	C8	015	1202300010	5000000000	000000	000	15	00
01918	03	72	40	25	2	300636299	36	0	559	921	41	2	C4	0C5	1002000010	5000000000	000000	000	15	00
01919	03	72	40	25	2	130570299	02	0	C55	911	41	2	C9	03C	2200300010	4000000000	000000	000	15	00
01920	03	72	30	10	2	210919199	53	0	C89	434	18	5	19	13C	1302503020	2100102500	000000	710	02	11
01921	03	72	40	10	2	120513299	59	0	C62	931	C1	1	08	07C	1302303020	3000400000	000000	200	05	00
01922	03	72	40	25	2	090430199	42	0	C35	842	17	2	08	120	1301303130	1000000000	000000	000	15	22
01923	03	72	30	10	2	190760299	12	0	C30	384	C1	3	C8	3C0	1301503125	7010021000	000000	760	13	14
01924	03	72	40	22	1	130163199	09	0	999	163	01	3	10	0E0	1302301020	1010000000	000000	000	14	00
01925	03	72	40	22	1	240264199	C8	0	999	163	C1	3	C9	075	1302301030	1010000000	000000	000	14	00
01926	03	72	40	23	2	081254299	18	0	555	620	4C	3	12	030	1202301020	1000000000	000000	000	07	22
01927	03	72	40	23	2	070754299	18	0	999	620	4C	1	13	025	1202301050	7000000000	000000	000	07	22
01928	03	72	40	10	2	171104199	68	0	C52	322	01	4	10	220	1302105120	3002000000	000000	340	09	23
01929	03	72	40	10	2	121100299	72	0	559	312	01	4	12	055	1302303120	1000200001	000000	200	16	00
01930	03	72	40	11	2	151252199	20	0	999	931	C1	4	11	1C5	1302303020	3000000000	000000	200	05	20
01931	03	72	40	16	2	230813199	59	0	C71	927	76	4	10	C30	1302301120	3000100000	000001	000	21	03
01932	03	72	40	16	2	190601199	71	0	C44	927	76	4	11	03C	1302501020	7000002000	000000	000	21	00
01933	03	72	40	10	2	291069299	03	0	C10	364	C1	5	C8	25C	2300303025	3000020000	000000	720	02	08
01934	03	72	40	10	2	260692299	80	0	C59	312	C1	4	09	1C5	1303703020	1000600000	000000	200	02	15
01935	03	72	40	10	2	999999299	05	0	559	412	01	5	C8	06C	2200301050	2000000000	000000	000	02	15
01936	03	72	40	11	2	050602199	70	0	999	461	C1	4	09	075	1302303120	5000201000	000000	200	05	20
01937	03	72	40	10	1	130355199	17	0	999	841	41	3	09	035	1202300040	1000000000	010000	000	07	[illegible]
01938	03	72	40	14	1	190568199	04	0	559	611	4C	3	08	010	1202300010	4000000000	000000	000	07	[illegible]

Fig. 1. *Punch card disposition and excerpt from the data. Each line corresponds to the contents of one punch card. Cards with incomplete data on the I-number are marked. (From: Central Department for Anaesthesia, Kiel University, 1972.)*

Nevertheless, overall time-scale for certain events in relation to the course of anaesthesia is definitely desirable. This is especially valuable for the differentiation between the induction, maintenance and recovery.

Certain periods of an anaesthesia show a higher incidence of complications than others. For certain events this is already known in detail, for example the increased risk of vomiting, regurgitation or aspiration during induction and recovery and the frequent occurrence of circulatory depression during induction. This study could be extended.

Correlation with time may have additional information value about causal relationship between preoperative and intraoperative risk factors and intraoperative complications. One should realize, however, that inclusion of the time course of the anaesthesia in the catalogue of risk factors using electronic data analysis necessitates restriction in other respects. This may be illustrated by the example of preoperative risk factors. If a suggestion in the anaesthesiological literature is followed, it is easily possible to have 91 different diagnoses amongst the preoperative findings in the patient (Table 1). Such differentiation would result in tables so large that a survey becomes impossible. This is due to the fact that preoperative risk factors may not only manifest themselves alone but also in any combination. This may be illustrated by an example (Table 2).

If one assumes that extreme age entails an increased risk of anaesthesia it must be accepted that diseases of the respiratory tract in connection with extreme age imply an additional

Table 1.   *Risk factors. (From: Mushin et al. (1952): Brit. J. Anaesth., 24, 298. Anaesthetic record (revised Jan., 1968), The United Cardiff Hospitals.)*

Respiratory system:
Bronchitis – acute
Bronchitis – chronic
Tuberculosis
Upper respiratory infection – acute,
   recent, chronic
Asthma
Pneumoconiosis
Respiratory obstruction
Emphysema
Dyspneoa
Neoplasm of respiratory system
Cyanosis
Tracheostomy
Pleural effusion
Pneumothorax
Lung resection
Others (specify)
Smokers cough – state consumption
   Sputum-add X (box 24 or 27)
Genitourinary system:
Impaired renal function
Others (specify)
Alimentary system:
Oral sepsis
Peptic ulcer
Haematemesis
Jaundice
Impaired liver function
Nausea and vomiting
Recent meal – hr
Others (specify)

Pre-anaesthetic complications
Cardiovascular system:
Peripheral:
   Hypotension (below 100 mm Hg systolic)
   Arteriosclerosis
   Hypertension – diastolic above 90 mm Hg
   Hypertension – diastolic above 120 mm Hg
   Others (specify)
Heart:
   Congenital heart disease
   Thyrotoxic heart disease
   Rheumatic heart disease
   Syphilitic heart disease
   Coronary heart disease
   Congestive heart failure
   Auricular fibrillation
   Arrhythmia (other)
   Heart block
   Angina
   Enlarged heart, clinical, X-ray
   Oedema
   Others (specify)
      add X if ECG evidence
Blood:
   Anaemia – below 12 g
   Anaemia – below 10 g
   Coagulation defect
   Others (specify)
Metabolic:
   Thyrotoxicosis
   Goitre (non-toxic)
   Diabetes – stable
   Diabetes – unstable
   Dehydration
   Loss of weight
   Obesity
   Febrile
   Others (specify)
   Electrolyte imbalance (specify)

Gynaecological:
Menstruating
Pregnant (state duration)
Toxaemia of pregnancy
Others (specify)
Central nervous system:
Marked apprehension
Irrational
Epilepsy
Coma or drowsiness
Other mental complications (specify)
Vascular:
Cerebral haemorrhage, embolism or thrombosis
Other intracranial vascular lesions (specify)
Paralyses:
Paralysis (specify)
Others:
Raised intracranial pressure
Fractures of the skull
Infections – meningitis or abscess
Neoplasm of central nervous system
Others (specify)
Iatrogenic:
Steroids
Hypotensive drugs
Phenothiazines
Monoamine oxidase inhibitor
Others (specify)
Anticoagulants
Other preanaesthetic complications:
Relevant deformities (specify)
Allergic conditions
Neoplasm not elsewhere specified
Foetal distress
Impairment of general health by surgical diagnosis
Glaucoma
Others (specify)

increase of that risk. The presence of 3 risk factors, e.g. extreme age and respiratory disease in connection with cardiovascular disease would further increase the risk of anaesthesia. In the same manner, concurrence of 4 and more factors should be considered. A study on the connection between preoperative risk factors and complications in the course of anaesthesia is therefore only convincing if all possible combinations of the various risk factors are correlated to all possible combinations of complications. The number of such combinations can be calculated (Table 2).

If from n elements i $\leqslant$ n elements are to be selected without regard to their order, then

$$C_{n,i} = \frac{n!}{i!\,(n-i)!}$$

From this it results that 256 different combinations are possible if the preoperative risk factors are divided into 8 classes. If the complications of anaesthesia are divided into 6 classes 64 different combinations ensue. The resultant contingency table therefore consists of 256 lines and 64 columns (Fig. 2). Condensation of all possible preoperative risk factors into only 8 classes and of all possible complications into only 6 is a problem. Practice shows, however, that the distribution of the events in such a contingency table is extremely irregular, despite concentration in a few classes, and is largely concentrated

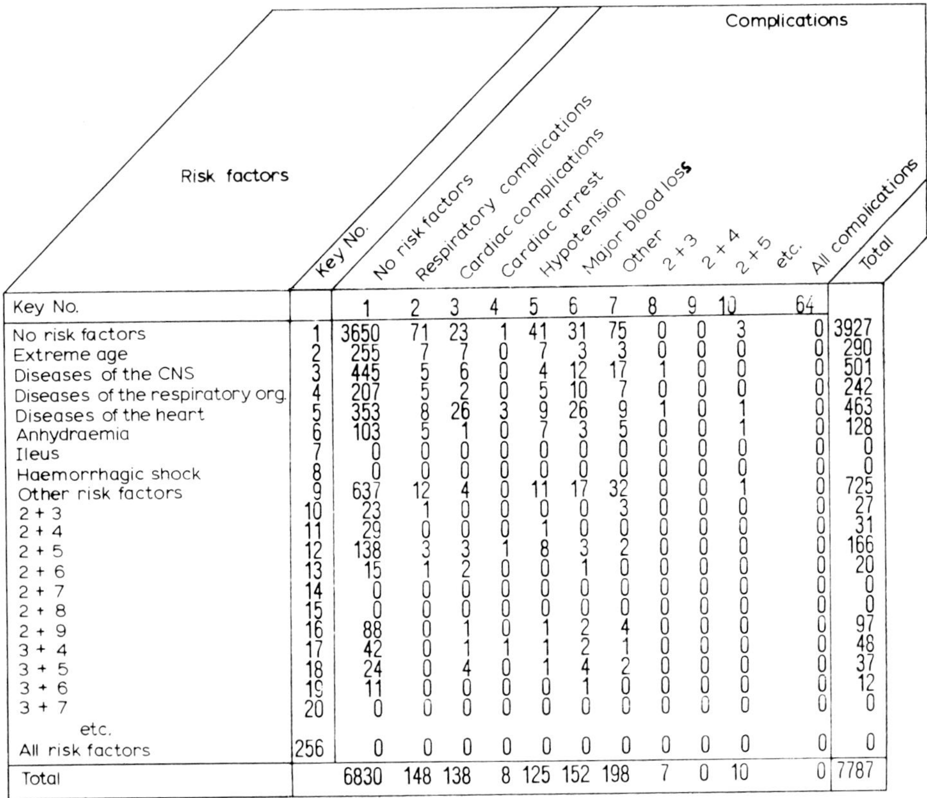

Risk factors \ Complications (Key No.)	No risk factors (1)	Respiratory complications (2)	Cardiac complications (3)	Cardiac arrest (4)	Hypotension (5)	Major blood loss (6)	Other (7)	2+3 (8)	2+4 (9)	2+5 (10)	All complications (64)	Total
No risk factors — 1	3650	71	23	1	41	31	75	0	0	3	0	3927
Extreme age — 2	255	7	7	0	7	3	3	0	0	0	0	290
Diseases of the CNS — 3	445	5	6	0	4	12	17	1	0	0	0	501
Diseases of the respiratory org. — 4	207	5	2	0	5	10	7	0	0	0	0	242
Diseases of the heart — 5	353	8	26	3	9	26	9	1	0	1	0	463
Anhydraemia — 6	103	5	1	0	7	3	5	0	0	1	0	128
Ileus — 7	0	0	0	0	0	0	0	0	0	0	0	0
Haemorrhagic shock — 8	0	0	0	0	0	0	0	0	0	0	0	0
Other risk factors — 9	637	12	4	0	11	17	32	0	0	1	0	725
2 + 3 — 10	23	1	0	0	0	0	3	0	0	0	0	27
2 + 4 — 11	29	0	0	0	1	0	0	0	0	0	0	31
2 + 5 — 12	138	3	3	1	8	3	2	0	0	0	0	166
2 + 6 — 13	15	1	2	0	0	1	0	0	0	0	0	20
2 + 7 — 14	0	0	0	0	0	0	0	0	0	0	0	0
2 + 8 — 15	0	0	0	0	0	0	0	0	0	0	0	0
2 + 9 — 16	88	0	1	0	1	2	4	0	0	0	0	97
3 + 4 — 17	42	0	1	1	1	2	1	0	0	0	0	48
3 + 5 — 18	24	0	4	0	1	4	2	0	0	0	0	37
3 + 6 — 19	11	0	0	0	0	1	0	0	0	0	0	12
3 + 7 — 20	0	0	0	0	0	0	0	0	0	0	0	0
etc.												
All risk factors — 256	0	0	0	0	0	0	0	0	0	0	0	0
Total	6830	148	138	8	125	152	198	7	0	10	0	7787

Fig. 2. *Excerpt from the evaluation table for intraoperative (anaesthesiological) complications on preoperative risk-factors for planned operations. (From: Central Department for Anaesthesia, Kiel University, 1972.)*

Table 2.   *Combination of i, n elements selected from n elements without regard to order. For the number $C_{n,i}$ of the combination the following applies:* $C_{n,i} = \dfrac{n!}{i!\,(n-i!)}$

Groups for risk factors (n=8)		Groups for complications (n=6)	
i	$C_{n,i}$	i	$C_{n,i}$
0	1	0	1
1	8	1	6
2	28	2	15
3	56	3	20
4	70	4	15
5	56	5	6
6	28	6	1
7	8		
8	1		
Total	256		64

in the firstlines and columns (Fig. 2). From this it follows that single or several complications are definitely rare in patients with one or even more risk factors. Therefore, there is a small chance that a suspected causal relationship can be demonstrated statistically. Using this data-analysis differentiation of risk factors and intraoperative complications in more than 6–8 classes is hardly useful. Naturally, within this limitation there is still the problem of deciding which factors are to be specified. In the personal evaluation plan (Fig. 2 and Table 3) time factors are not considered. Instead, preoperative risk factors are divided into the global categories of: (1) diseases of the central nervous system; (2) diseases of the respiratory tract; (3) diseases of the heart.

In addition, the following are specified separately: (4) extreme age; (5) septicaemia, dehydration and/or burns; (6) ileus; (7) haemorrhagic shock; and (8) others.

In contrast, intraoperative complications are divided into 6 categories only: (1) respiratory

Table 3.   *Groups (classification) for risk factors and complications – electronic data processing of anaesthesiological data in the clinics of Kiel University*

Group	Risk factors	Group	Complications
1	Extreme age (1 or 70 yr)	1	Respiratory complications
2	Diseases of the CNS	2	Cardiac complications
3	Diseases of the respiratory tract	3	Cardiac arrest
4	Diseases of the heart	4	Hypotension group
5	Anhydraemia and/or sepsis and/or burns	5	Major blood loss
6	Ileus	6	Other complications:
7	Haemorrhagic shock		difficulties in injection
8	Other risk factors:		difficulties in intubation
	obstruction to larynx, possible alcohol intake		increased blood pressure
	instability of cervical vertebral column		allergy
	allergy		technical complications
	diabetes mellitus		other
	nephropathy and/or uraemia		
	diseases of the liver		
	hypertension		
	other		

complications; (2) cardiac complications; (3) cardiac arrest; (4) hypotension; (5) major blood loss; and (6) other.

This classification is observed primarily for all correlations with preoperative risk factors and/or intraoperative complications.

DATA DIFFERENTIATION

In addition to specific preoperative risk factors there is another criterion from which an inhomogeneous complication risk ensues within anaesthesiological observation series. This involves general organizational conditions under which patients come for surgery. In the first place anaesthesia is carried out for planned surgery. These cases come for surgery after a clear surgical diagnosis has been made and the general condition has been subjected to

Table 4. *Frequency of complications during anaesthesia for planned operations, emergencies and polyclinical surgery in correlation to preoperative risk factors*

| | Complications | Risk factors | | | | | | | | |
| | | (Kiel, 1971/72) | | | (Heidelberg, 1970) | | | (Bruchsal, 1969) | | |
		Yes	No	Total	Yes	No	Total	Yes	No	Total
Planned operations	Yes	876	402	1278	897	443	1340	203	258	461
	No	3952	4622	8574	3750	6442	10192	695	1860	2555
	Total	4828	5024	9852	4647	6885	11532	898	2118	3016
Emergencies	Yes	357	15	372	338	53	391	92	15	107
	No	953	203	1156	954	669	1623	134	264	404
	Total	1310	218	1528	1292	772	2014	226	279	511
Polyclinical surgery	Yes	44	32	76	51	34	85	11	6	17
	No	390	545	935	626	1798	2424	48	361	409
	Total	434	577	1011	677	1832	2509	59	367	426
Total	Yes	1277	449	1726	1286	530	1816	306	276	582
	No	5295	5370	10665	5330	8909	14239	880	2482	3362
	Total	6572	5819	12391	6616	9439	16055	1186	2758	3944

Table 5. *Frequency of intraoperative (anaesthesiological) complications in 3 different observation series*

| Complications | Kiel, 1971/72 | | Heidelberg, 1970 | | Bruchsal, 1969 | |
	n	%	n	%	n	%
Yes	1726	14	1816	11	582	15
No	10665	86	14239	89	3362	85
Total	12391		16055		3944	

Comparison for material	χ^2
I and III	1.68
I and II	43.98
II and III	35.62
For all groups	59.71

comprehensive diagnostic examination. Possible existing risk factors are identified with a very high level of reliability. In emergencies the situation is different. These patients must be immediately operated upon on account of an acute disease or injury. As a rule there is no time for detailed anamnesis or comprehensive preoperative diagnosis with optimum pretreatment of the general condition. Finally the third group consists of patients where a polyclinical operation is carried out. This group is characterized in clinical practice by the fact that preoperatively only an orienting anamnesis and examination of the general condition is carried out. These patients also generally receive anaesthesia without optimum pretreatment of the general condition. Differentiation of anaesthesiological observation series into patients with or without preoperative risk factors on the one hand, and planned operations,

Table 6.   *Frequency of preoperative risk factors in 3 different anaesthesiological observation series*

Risk factors	Kiel, 1971/72		Heidelberg, 1970		Bruchsal, 1969	
	n	%	n	%	n	%
Yes	6572	54	6616	41	1186	30
No	5819	46	9439	59	2758	70
Total	12391		16055		3944	

Table 7.   *Percentage complication frequency for planned operations, emergencies and polyclinical surgery*

Material		Planned operations (%)	Emergencies (%)	Polyclincial surgery (%)
I (Kiel)	With risk	18	27	10
	Without risk	8	7	6
	Total	13	24	8
II (Heidelberg)	With risk	19	26	8
	Without risk	6	7	2
	Total	12	19	3
III (Bruchsal)	With risk	23	41	19
	Without risk	12	5	1
	Total	15	21	4

	Comparison between material	χ^2
Within planned operations	I and II (with risk)	2.09
	I and III (with risk)	9.85
	I and II (total)	10.57
	I and III (total)	9.04
Within emergencies	I and II (with risk)	0.39
	I and III (with risk)	16.87
	I and II (total)	12.50
	I and III (total)	2.47
Within polyclinical surgery	I and II (with risk)	1.25
	I and III (with risk)	3.79
	I and II (total)	28.15
	I and III (total)	6.15

emergencies and polyclinical surgery on the other can lead to alteration of the results on data analysis, as can be demonstrated by the example of 3 different groups of patients (Table 4). These were: (1) an observation series of 12,391 consecutive anaesthesias (clinics of Kiel University); (2) 16,055 consecutive anaesthesias (clinics of Heidelberg University; and (3) 3,944 consecutive anaesthesias (Kommunales Krankenhaus Bruchsal).

The 3 clinical institutions serve a different area and the work is also different.

A survey of the intraoperative complications shows a global complication frequency of 14% in Group I, 11% in Group II, and 15% in Group III (Table 5).

On the basis of statistical analysis the difference of 1% in the frequency of complications in materials I and III is within the range of incidental variations. The difference between materials I and II and between II and III is statistically relevant (Table 5). Therefore in material II (Heidelberg, 1970) the frequency of complications is lower than in the other 2.

After division of the patients with or without preoperative complications the percentage of patients with risk factors is the highest in Group I (Kiel, 1971/1972) (Table 6).

If the information is classified into elective operations, emergencies and polyclinical surgery, the results are fundamentally different (Table 7). The frequency of intraoperative complications is practically identical for Groups I and II, in contrast to the global comparison of the complication frequency, whereas without differentiation an apparent difference had been found (Table 5). In contrast, the complication frequency is distinctly higher in Group III. This finding only applies to planned operations in patients with risk factors and in emergencies with risk factors (Table 7).

It should be emphasized that from such a result no conclusions about the quality of anaesthesia can be drawn, for a complication risk determined by anaesthesia depends on additional factors not included in this study. The findings should serve only to show that comparison of anaesthesiological observation series of different teams may lead to entirely different results, when the information is grouped according to certain criteria. Therefore it is important to attempt maximum reduction of the characteristics included in the documentation of anaesthesiological data, and also to aim at uniformity in the determination of certain basic characteristics.

REFERENCES

Lutz, H. (1970): *Prakt. Anästh. Wiederbel.*, *5*, 45.

Mushin, W. W., Rendell-Baker, L., Lewis-Fanting, E. and Morgan, J. H. (1952): *Brit. J. Anaesth.*, *24*, 298.

Wawersik, J., Köhler, C. and Wagner, G. (1973): *Meth. Inform. Med.*, *12*, 222.

Introduction of new data and codification in the anesthetic recording

M. C. BELDA, V. CHULIA CAMPOS, R. PERIS, F. SANZ and J. AGUILAR

Department of Anesthesia, Faculty of Medicine, University of Valencia, Valencia, Spain

The accomplishment of any cyclic review or research needs the availability of documents and data. Adequate recording is essential because of the increasing importance of anesthesiology in hospital medicine, its progressive development and its close relationship with surgery.

This anesthesiology service has collaborated with the Center of Documentation and Information of the Faculty of Medicine of Valencia and introduced a new recording system for anesthesia. This system, which is being used in all surgical procedures, is still at an experimental stage but aims to satisfy all the requirements of clinical and research use.

METHOD

The anesthetic recording is divided into 2 parts.

(1) The 'classic' anesthetic record, which includes: (*a*) a methodical test to evaluate the general state of the patient in relation to anesthesia; free space for observation and results of investigations (blood pressure, pulse, breathing, routine laboratory data), which must be completed before surgery. (*b*) an anesthetic record in the strict sense (this must be made in the theatre, at the time of the operation, and it encourages thorough observation of the patient); the 'classic' anesthetic record is printed on a thick card, for easy handling in the theatre.

(2) The model, i.e. the booklet of records where data are written, is to be processed by a computer. The data are printed in an autocopy form that can be detached from the booklet, and each copy can be sent for perforation and processing. The model reproduces the information contained in the first part of the record, but detailed and organised according to the needs of processing.

Some data, like sex, weight, height, type, emergency, administrative situation, constant values related to premedication and medication are only present in the first sheet of the model, so that reading is easy. There are 180 items, each one coded, and a space left for observations – with a capacity for 164 characters.

The coded information includes: *identity data:* clinical record number, birth date, admission date, operation date, department; *physical characters:* sex, weight, height, emergency, administrative situation (private, insurance, accident, etc.); *premedication:* agent and dose, related constant biological values; *preanaesthetic findings:* cardiovascular, renal, respiratory, metabolism, allergy, previous medication; *pre- and postoperative diagnosis; operative techniques; type of anesthesia* (technique, ventilation, system); *medication during anesthesia* (agents and total doses); *quantitative data on blood volume* (loss and replacement); *constant biologic values related to anesthesia; complications during surgery and 36 hr postoperative period; time of start and end of surgery; patient's condition on leaving the operating room; death:* time until death; *anesthesiologist code number.*

The coding system involves 3 simultaneous processes: precodification (e.g. preanesthetic findings); direct transcription (every biologic value); codification with special coding help (diagnosis code, operative technique, chemical agents, etc.).

In every case, the name of the agent, diagnosis, etc. is placed besides the code number (to be noted later).

These 3 processes are combined with the following purpose: to enable recording by the anesthesiologist, avoiding the use of code until the information on the sheet is complete; to enable easy reading of the model itself without consulting the code.

The record may now be separated, so that the complete model copy could be processed and the complete recording (the original booklet) remains in the clinical record of the patient.

RESULTS

This method provides a guarantee of complete study and observation of the patient in the anesthetic, clinical and surgical fields. It can be used in most anesthetic procedures.

Processed data is available for any clinical review, statistics or research. Individual anesthetic data for individual patients is available. The activities of a service of anesthesiology, its performance, and the work level of each member is known. Similar information regarding the Department of Surgery is also available. The system can be used for organizational purposes. Pre- and postoperative investigation of the patient is encouraged. The educational value of the record is clear.

REFERENCES

Committee on Clinical Anesthesia Study of the American Society of Anesthesiology, Inc. (1960): *Anesthesiology, 21*, 557.
Galla, S. J., Scwarzbach, R. S. and Buccigrossi, R. (1969): *Anesthesiology 30/5*, 565.
Moore, D. C., Brindenbaugh, L. D., Bagdi, P. A., Brindenbaugh, P. O., Stander, H. and Thomas, G. B. (1968): *Anesthesiology, 29/3*, 595.
Morisot, P. (1973): *Anesth. Analg. Réanim., 30/4*, 793.
Sanchez, P. and Switkin, D. J. (1969): *Anesth. Analg. Curr. Res., 48/6*, 1008.
Yeakel, A. E. (1964): *Anesth. Analg. Curr. Res., 43*, 66.

A process control computer for controlling anaesthesia*

D. DAUB [1], R. VOM HÖVEL [2], G. KALFF [1] and R. REPGES [2]

[1] Abteilung für Anästhesiologie, and [2] Abteilung für Medizinische Statistik und Dokumentation, Rheinisch-Westfälische Technische Hochschule, Aachen, Federal Republic of Germany

The Medical Faculty of the Technische Hochschule of Aachen is planning an extended information system for its new hospital, which will be ready for use in 1976. It is our conviction that, when developing such a system, the more complex parts should be tackled first. Thus, the requirements of the superior aspect can be taken into consideration in subsequent planning of the more limited subsystems.

Anaesthesiology involves the science of the different branches of surgery and cooperation with internal medicine, such as laboratory diagnosis, haematology, roentgenology, neurology, and even psychosomatics is essential. From most medical disciplines the anaesthetist needs information, the importance of which can only be determined during operation. In order to enable him to decide upon his measures immediately in a crucial situation, a documentation system is needed which has a large memory capacity and a short retrieval time. Because the patient is in an unstable state, not only during operation, but also during intensive care, a multitude of data has to be taken into consideration with all its variability and mutual interdependence – a typical task for a computer.

There are already extended documentation systems (Bonhoeffer and Brueckner, 1970; Wawersik, 1970) as well as mere monitoring facilities (Chodoff and Gianaris, 1973; Shrubin et al., 1971; Clark et al., 1971), but most of them do not combine both possibilities.

It is our opinion that, in the field of medicine, real time data processing is not possible without extensive documentation of data as a background. This because of the character of all medical work, which is based not only on calculable functions, but to a great extent on the experience of the respective physician and on empirical research. Proceeding from those fundamental considerations, the Aachen Anaesthesiological Documentation and Monitoring System is conceived in such a way that it should cover all the needs of the department, which is to say that every anaesthesia done by a staff member should be documented, supervised and assisted by the computer service.

The combination of documenting and monitoring functions requires a special hard-ware configuration. Our system uses an AEG 60–50 process control computer with a 32 K 24 bit words core memory linked with an AEG 60–10, 32 K 12 bit words machine for the pre-processing of on-line acquired data. As peripheral storage the 60–10 has a drum (128 K 12 bit words), the 60–50 two exchangeable 9.6 million bytes disks and one magnetic tape unit. Supplementing devices are: a punched-card reader, a punched-tape reader and a tape punch for internal organisation only. A line-printer is the only part of the system which produces hard copy which is of particular use in the field of medicine, the records which are required for the case history. The anaesthesiological staff works only with 16 XDS

---

* Supported by Bundesminister für Forschung und Technologie DVM 022.

colour visual display units, which are to be installed in the different operating-theatres and in the intensive care units of the department.

These displays are the interface between man and machine. Communication is very important since the success of the system depends upon the cooperation of the clinical staff, which is a sine qua non for the introduction of electronic data processing into the hospital. Utmost simplicity in the handling of the system during routine work is the aim, and this is achieved by the use of masks in the communication subsystem.

The cathode ray tube display devices (Xerox BC 100) are used as an inquiry-response system for the dialogue between medical operator and computer. On the one hand, they display alphanumerics and graphics sent by the computer; on the other hand, they receive numerical values and text or pilot information from the operator with the aid of a keyboard composed of primary typewriter keys and some special keys. The terminal incorporates a memory for storing the actual contents of the screen and a protected field facility, which enables the computer to protect specified areas of the screen from being altered by the terminal operator.

On the screen, which has 960 character positions in 24 lines, masks in protected field mode, presented by the computer to the operator, contain free areas, in which requested replies are to be written using the keyboard. Thus the information sent by the computer can be used like a blank form or a voucher. This method does not give rise to dialogue line by line, but fills a screen at a time; this takes account of the fact that the user mostly demands larger sections of data belonging one to another and that values to be stored usually occur in groups.

Input is either a free alphanumeric text or numeric information for qualitative or quantitative answering of questions. When qualitatively describing characteristics out of a given quantity of possible statements, the right ones are selected by one or more figures according to the multiple choice method. Since the problem of a standardized medical metalanguage has not yet been solved conclusively and thus the processing of alphanumeric data may be equivocal, the multiple choice method is used as often as possible.

Whenever the terminal is activated and the contact with the computer is taken up, one of 4 function keys must be depressed first of all. With the help of the so-called survey mask which then appears, one can, for instance, claim information about a patient whose data file has already been opened, or tell the computer that anamnestic and diagnostic data for a new patient is to be entered. In the first case, a push of the same function key causes a mask to appear into which one must feed the patient's identity, the kind of data one wants to know and the authorizing code. In the second example, a mask is generated by which the personal data of a new patient can be entered as well as information related to organs for which pathological diagnoses and anamnestic data have been found. In accordance with this input, masks are then displayed onto which anamneses and diagnoses may be noted. Thus, after one mask is filled a following mask is generated automatically. The kind of mask which appears is generally determined by a logical tree- or network. In this structure, the branching or skipping of masks always happens as a function of the answer given on the preceding mask. Before a new form is shown on the screen, the plausibility of the data which were entered is checked – their correction or confirmation may be demanded – or processors, for example for trend analysis, for the generation or actualization of graphics or for decision-making, may be initiated.

The necessity of leaving a branch temporarily, in order to gain information about the state of a patient in another operating-theatre or about the schedules of the other operating-theatres, has also been taken into consideration. Another function key serves this purpose. When it is depressed, the original contents of the screen are stored and the survey mask is presented. In this way, one may enter a new branch in which one proceeds as usual. In order to leave this branch and return to the former, one has to press this function key again.

The display of a new screen may be initiated not only by the function keys, but also by emergency interruptions caused by the critical values of a vital sign acquired on-line. Alarms of inferior priority are announced by a bell installed on every terminal. If such an alarm occurs, the user can decide whether he wants to receive the message at once or whether he wants to complete his input first.

The soft-ware intended for the medical user has to be implemented within the structure of the basic soft-ware represented by data documenting and retrieval subsystems. This conglomeration of programs will be developed in 3 phases, depending on the extent of their fundamental statistical prerequisites. The first group of programs will relieve the medical personnel from certain routine work, as they will fulfil, for example, the following functions:

1. Documentation of the anaesthesia to be filed in the patient's record (as laid down by law), and standardized summary about anaesthesia and intensive care to be sent to the family doctor.

2. Stock-keeping of all items needed in the department.

3. Listing of all demanded catalogues for the residency program.

4. Composition of service schedule-record of overtime work.

5. Scheduling of available assistants and operating-theatres of the department at a given time.

6. Clearing-systems to relieve paramedical and administrating personnel.

The second group of soft-ware is dedicated to the facilitation and safety of medical work. It will be used during the first stage of the development of the system, because mathematical data-processing is not involved. An outline of some of those programs is:

1. Values which hitherto have been taken from nomograms will be calculated in order to avoid errors in reading. The following are needed for anaesthetic work: Engström nomogram, presenting the parameters of ventilation; the Siggard-Andersen nomogram for Astrup analysis; the Richterrich and the McLean nomograms.

2. Many interrelations between different organic parameters are known, but most of them, though mathematically recorded, are not yet used in everyday work because of the lack of computing capacity. Among them are: the determination of efficacious drug concentration depending on given doses, degradation, solubility, excretion; the evaluation of electrolyte blood concentration as a function of infusions; and all problems of balancing out physiological factors.

Contrary to the above described functions, the last section of the medically oriented soft-ware package requires an extended mathematical analysis of all data and their mutual correlations. For this reason, its realization may only be considered after sufficient experience of data acquisition and statistical evaluation.

1. The decision-aiding subsystem will allow impending critical situations to be diagnosed by registering signs which are deduced from statistical experience together with known physiological interdependences.

2. The same aim will be achieved by calculating the time-trends of vital parameters as a function not only of time, but also of other changing data involved in physiological regulation.

Our endeavours will culminate in the construction of a sophisticated model of anaesthesia and intensive care. This will have to be done by a multidisciplinary approach to the problem; the most important prerequisites are the knowledge of physiology, pharmacology, pathology and anaesthesiology, which will supply us with the framework, and the statistical interactions, which will fill the open structures. The model will be the basis of an anaesthesia simulating program for the training of students, residents and paramedical personnel involved in anaesthesia, and it will help develop the regulation of certain subsystems in anaesthesia and intensive care.

REFERENCES

Bonhoeffer, K. and Brueckner, J. B. (1970): *Z. prakt. Anästh. Wiederbeleb.*, *5/1*, 41.
Chodoff, P. and Gianaris, C. (1973): *Computer biomed. Res.*, *6/4*, 371.
Clark, J. S., Veasy, L. G., Jung, A. L. and Jenkins, J. L. (1971): *Computer biomed. Res.*, *4/3*.
Lutz, H. and Hildebrand, O. (1972): *Anaesthesist, 21/7*, 292.
Shrubin, H., Weil, M. H., Palley, N. and Afifi, A. A. (1971): *Computer biomed. Res.*, *4/5*, 460.
Wawersik, J. (1970): *Z. prakt. Anästh. Wiederbeleb.*, *5/1*, 6.

Documentation of anesthesiological activity in the emergency medical service

B. GORGASS, W. STOTZ, M. SCHORR and F. W. AHNEFELD

Department of Anesthesiology, Center for Interdisciplinary Medicine,
University of Ulm, Ulm, Federal Republic of Germany

In the past, emergency medical services almost exclusively took care of transportation. 'Cooperation' with this clinic consisted only of handing over the patients. Important details about the symptomatology at the scene and about possible changes of findings often could not be obtained or used on account of the absence of qualified accompanying personnel. In an ambulance equipped for intensive medical care, statements of findings could be taken and controlled therapy started. Today, after reorganisation of the EMS in the Federal Republic of Germany, more and more emergency physicians and qualified emergency medical technicians are assigned to mobile intensive care units and rescue helicopters, thus securing instant treatment of emergency patients. An elementary diagnosis is possible at the scene. The immediate life-saving measures are often followed by important changes of symptomatology; these changes should be reported to the clinic, together with information about the emergency circumstances and therapeutic measures. For this purpose a documentation sheet has been developed by the rescue center established at the Federal Defense Forces-Hospital and the Department of Anesthesiology of the University of Ulm.

Under the title 'Information for the receiving hospital' all necessary details are confined to 2 pages. An attempt was made to reduce the written information to a minimum by omitting the so-called 'normal findings' and by preparing a form with the most frequent pathological findings.

This sheet is intended to be used for patients in all fields of emergency medicine, including neonatology, toxicology, traumatology and internal medicine.

KIND OF EMERGENCY

A classification of the kind of emergency, covering over 4,000 emergency missions, gave the following distribution: acute illness 36.7%; traffic accidents 27.4%; secondary transports 15.6%; suicide, crime 7.9%; industrial accidents 3.5%; household accidents 3.2%; and others 5.7%.

Missions itemized under 'others' concern blood- and organ-transports or search missions by helicopter. Information on this matter and information about accident-details are noted on an additional line.

INITIAL FINDINGS

A subdivision in groups of symptoms is as follows:
State of consciousness Somnolent/abnormal reaction; unconscious with protective reflexes;

unconscious without protective reflexes; pupils, dilated and fixed.

Neurological state Anisocoria, left > right, left < right; convulsion; vomiting; restlessness.

Respiration Cyanosis, blocking of the respiratory system; dyspnea; aspiration; asthma, gasping respiration; pulmonary edema, apnea.

Cardiovascular system Preshock, extrasystoles; shock, standstill of the circulation; bradycardia; fibrillation; tachycardia; asystole.

Injuries/fractures Cranium/cerebrum; thorax; pelvis; eyes/face; heart, lower extremity; upper extremity; lung; acid burn; vertebral column; abdomen; burn.

Additional information Two lines are kept free for possibilities which are not identified above.

CHANGES OF FINDINGS

Changes of the findings at the site of the emergency and during transportation, concerning the group of symptoms, written down by hand, are as follows: state of consciousness; neurological state; respiration; and cardiovascular system.

PRELIMINARY DIAGNOSIS

At the end of the first page the preliminary diagnosis is recorded and attested by the emergency physician. On page 2 , resembling an anesthesiological record, the measures conducted and the development are documented. In Ulm the medical measures are distributed as shown in Table 1.

Table 1. *Distribution of medical measures in Ulm*

	No.	%
Maintaining or restoring respiration	837	21.2
Maintaining or restoring heart functions, shock treatment	1,428	36.0
Surgery	520	13.2
Ascertaining death after resuscitation attempt	106	2.7
Ascertaining death, no resuscitation	118	3.0
Others	949	23.9
Total	3,958	100.0

21 % patients required measures for maintaining or restoring respiration. This begins with clearing the airway as the simplest measure and ranges from O_2 therapy to artificial respiration and intubation. Emergency intubations must be performed in case of hemorrhage, in the nasopharyngeal space, aspiration after vomiting or sudden apnea under hypoxemic conditions, without relaxation, and under conditions which, in the clinic, would be classed as an anesthetic incident.

35 % patients required measures for maintaining or restoring the circulation or for shock-treatment, such as pulse, pressure and electrocardiographic control, infusion, external cardiac compression, medicinal and electrotherapy. Quantitatively, shock prevention by intravenous infusion predominates. Depending on the urgency this will be accomplished by EMT under medical supervision for training purposes. On the other hand, puncture of central veins, external cardiac compression, defibrillation and antiarrhythmic treatment

in case of circulatory failure occur in such large numbers that the entire team, by alternating assignments, becomes proficient in these complex activities within a brief period.

The surgical measures conducted in 13% of cases were mostly less dramatic and involved splinting, stopping of bleeding and applying dressings. No special surgical training was required for their performance.

In more than 4,000 missions, neither emergency tracheotomy, nor emergency amputation or even more complicated surgery has been required.

2.7% resuscitations, which partly had to be carried out under extremely adverse conditions, such as cramped space, cold, rain and occasionally in the presence of a large crowd of on-lookers, however, always according to the same principles and using the same equipment as in the hospital, were without success.

The term 'others' comprises alleviation of pain, sedation, anesthesia and lavage of the stomach. Detoxication measures, such as gastric lavage and forced diuresis are usually initiated at the scene before the actual transport.

On the documentation sheet simple symbols are used for: pulse, cardiac massage, blood pressure, defibrillation, artificial respiration, dose of medicaments, in/extubation, start of transport.

At the University-Clinic of Ulm the use of this documentation sheet has proved a success. Its introduction is to recommend its use to similar working emergency medical services in the Federal Republic of Germany and in foreign countries.

On some problems of the computer-oriented documentation of anesthesiological 'complications'

R. KOEPPEN, K. BONHOEFFER, A. KAPP, E. TENHOF and I. HOSSELMANN

Department of Anesthesiology, University of Köln, Köln, Federal Republic of Germany

There can be no doubt that anesthesiological complications including all those special events which deviate from the norm in connection with anesthesia should be recorded and processed so that the (patho-) physiological processes can be properly understood with the result that treatment could be improved.

In connection with the above recording of anesthesiological complications, there has been, up to now, a tendency to confine it to the collection of serious events (aspiration, laryngo-bronchospasm, pulmonary edema, cardiac arrest) and phenomena such as arrhythmia, tachycardia and bradycardia, hypertension and hypotension (Bonhoeffer and Brueckner, 1970; Borchert et al., 1972; Brueckner et al., 1968; Goetz, 1972; Kleinheisterkamp and Fassl, 1968; Lutz, 1972; Moore et al., 1968; Wawersik et al., 1973).

In some anesthesiological records, therapeutic measures can be encoded, but with no strict correspondence between the event and the measure taken (Borchert et al., 1972; Lutz, 1972). However, in none of the hitherto published records suitable for computerized processing is it possible to correlate directly a sign and its cause.

What do data of mere signs really signify? At the best one can, detached from the individual case, link them with age, sex, preanesthesiological risks, technic, manner and location of the operation, etc. Knowledge gained in this manner may sometimes be of interest to the department, however, it is frequently misleading because it may lead to the erroneous conclusion that 'in abdominal surgery halothane provokes arrhythmias more frequently than neuroleptanesthesia'.

In order to obtain useful information about some interesting event it is necessary, in our opinion, to encode all those circumstances relevant to the event in a manner acceptable to a digital computer.

Figure 1 displays the encoding scheme of our anesthesia data record for special events, which consists of 8 identical blocks in which one can encode up to 4 individual observations. By means of the example in the first block, displayed in Figure 2, it becomes apparent that each occurrence of interest can be encoded when broken up into the following characteristics: when did the event occur? – box designated for time (Zeit); how often/long? – box designated for frequency of occurrence (Häufigkeit); in connection with which event already encoded? – box designated for connection (Zusammenhang); which symptom? – boxes designated for symptom of the event (Symptom); which cause? – boxes designated for cause of the event (Ursache); which therapeutic/prophylactic measures have been taken? – boxes designated for therapeutic measures (Therapeutische Massnahmen); with what success? – box designated for success of therapy (Therapieerfolg); at which system pressure? – boxes designated for systolic and diastolic pressure (in mm Hg); at which heart frequency? – boxes designated for frequency.

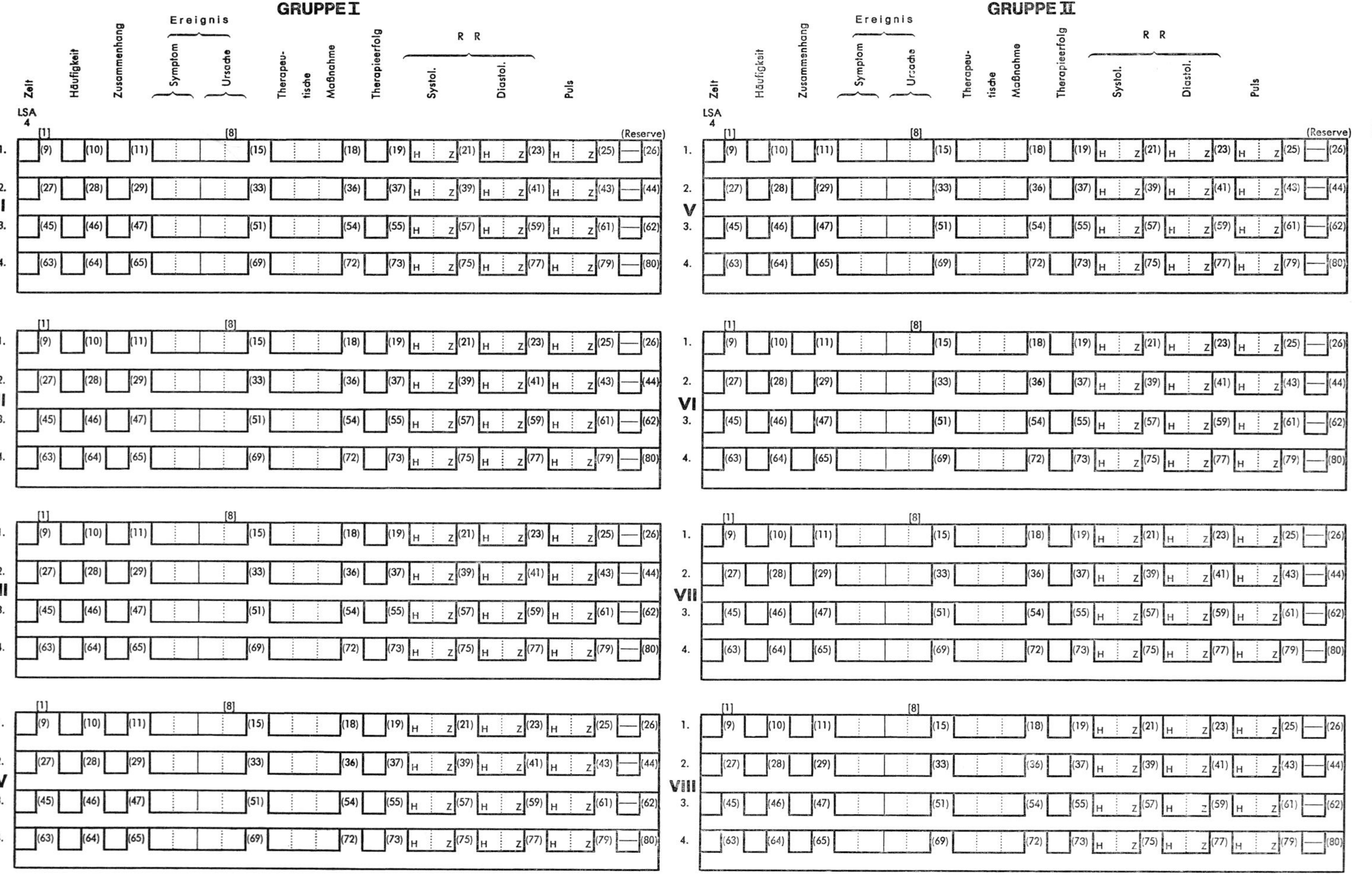

Fig. 1.   An example sheet of the complete scheme for the encoding of special events.

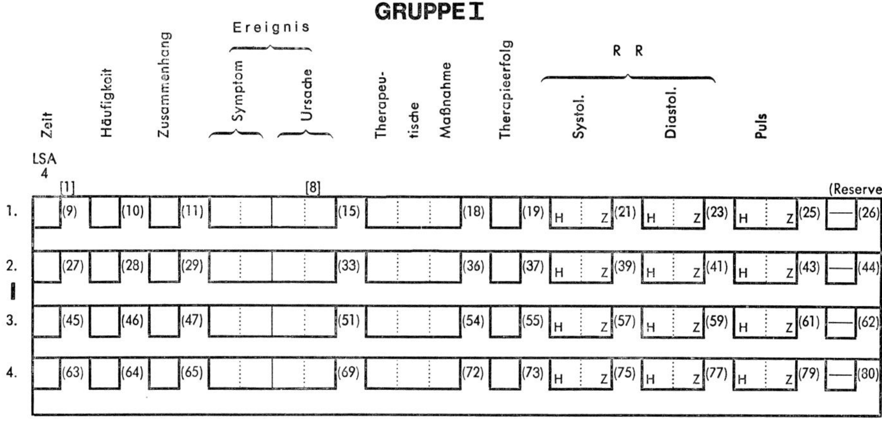

Fig. 2. *The first of the 8 blocks (as on Fig. 1) for the encoding of special events.*

EREIGNIS,dessen
- <u>Symptom</u>:

00.. Kreislaufstillstand		50.. Laryngospasmus	
01.. Kammerflattern		51.. Bronchospasmus	
02.. Kammerflimmern		52.. Stridor	
03.. Asystolie		53.. Lungenoedem	
04.. Exitus		54.. Aspiration, Magen-Darmsaft	
05..		55.. " , n.z.b. Flüssigkeit	
06.. ven. Systemdruck erhöht		56.. " , Fremdkörper	
07.. " " erniedrigt		57.. übermäßige Sekretion	
08.. art. " erhöht		58..	
09.. " " erniedrigt		59..	
10.. abnorme Frequenz		60.. Lähmungen, zentral	
11.. abnormer Rhythmus		61.. " , peripher n.z.b.	
12.. S.-A.- u. a.-v.-Block		62.. Krämpfe	
13.. Schenkelblock		63.. Pupillen lichtstarr, weit	
14.. regelm. supraventr. Rhythmus		64.. Anisokorie	
15.. " ventrik. "		65.. n.z.b. motorische Aktivität	
16.. supraventr. Extrasystolen		66.. n.z.b. psychische Aktivität	
17.. ventr. monotop. ES		67..	
18.. " polytop. ES		68..	
19.. absolute Arhythmie		69..	
20.. Parasystolie		70.. gemessene Urinmenge zu gering	
21.. "Ischämie-EKG"		71.. keine meßbare Urinmenge	
22..		72..	
23..		73..	
24..		74..	
25..		75..	
26..		76..	
27..		77..	
28..		78..	
29..		79..	
30.. f^* erhöht, V_T^* erhöht		80.. Verletzung, n.z.b.	
31.. f^* erhöht, V_T^* erniedrigt		81.. Paravasat	
32.. f^* erniedrigt, V_T^* erhöht		82.. Würgen, Übelkeit	
33.. f^* erniedrigt, V_T^* erniedrigt		83.. Erbrechen (ohne Aspiration)	
34.. Apnoe		84.. Singultus	
35.. Cyanose		85.. Schwitzen	
36.. art. O_2-Untersättigung		86.. Flush	
37.. ven. O_2-Untersättigung		87.. Körpertemp.-Erhöhung	
38.. resp. Acidose		88.. Körpertemp.-Erniedrigung	
39.. resp. A kalose arteriell		89.. n.z.b. Elektrolyt-Erhöhung	
40.. metab. Acidose		90.. n.z.b. Elektrolyt-Erniedrigung	
41.. metab. Alkalose		91..	
42.. SR bei CR		92..	
43.. erhöhter Beatmungsdruck		93..	
44..		94..	
45..		95..	
46..		96..	
47..		97..	
48..		98.. symptomlos	
49..		99.. n.z.b. unerwünschtes Symptom	

f^* = Atemfrequenz
V_T^* = Atemzugvolumen (AZV)

Fig. 3. *Code numbers and their meaning for symptoms (see text for explanation).*

For each of these aspects, there exists, in a special encoding booklet, a list of criteria with associated code numbers, an example of which can be seen in Figure 3.

The symptom code numbers 00 through 21 pertain to the most important information about heart function and blood circulation, those between 30 and 45 and from 50 up to 57 to unwanted events concerning ventilation etc. Code numbers not allotted, like those from 22 and 44 respectively onward can be used for symptoms hitherto not included. Thus, a complete reorganization of the encoding system is avoided when new symptoms are added. Hence, code number 99 (which means: an unwanted symptom which is to be designated somewhere else in the record) will be used less and less; correspondingly, having recourse to the original record will be superfluous. Looking at the list of causes of special occurrences (Figure 4) one can discern 4 main groups: (1) from 00 through 23 individual risks of the patient (which have already been taken into account at another place within the record); (2) from 30 through 59 anesthesiological measures taken; (3) from 80 up to 86 inadequate anesthesiological management; and (4) from 90 through 97 influences stemming from the surgical actions.

The direct correlation of symptom and cause stipulated above is, from a technical point

```
EREIGNIS, dessen
- Ursache:


..00 zum Eingriff führende Erkrankung    ..51 Blut,-ersatz,rel.überdos.
     des Pat. (LSA 1/ 57)                ..52  "   ,-  "   ,normodosiert
..01 präanästh. Risikofaktor, Nr. 1      ..53  "   ,-  "   ,unterdosiert
     (LSA 2/ 11)                         ..54 Lokalanästh.,rel. überdosiert
..02 präanästh. Risikofaktor, Nr. 2      ..55  "             ,normodosiert
     (LSA 2/ 14)                         ..56  "             ,rel.unterdosiert
..03 präanästh. Rf., Nr. 3 (LSA 2/ 17)   ..57 n.z.b. Medikament,rel.überdos.
..04   "        "  , Nr. 4 (LSA 2/ 20)   ..58  "         "      ,normodosiert
..05   "        "  , Nr. 5 (LSA 2/ 23)   ..59  "         "      ,rel.unterdos.
..06   "        "  , Nr. 6 (LSA 2/ 26)   ..60 inkompatibles Medikament,n.z.b.
..07   "        "  , Nr. 7 (LSA 2/ 29)   ..61 inkompatible Narkoseart
..08   "        "  , Nr. 8 (LSA 2/ 32)   ..62 "anästhesiefremdes" Medikament
..09   "        "  , Nr. 9 (LSA 2/ 35)        n.z.b.
..10   "        "  , Nr.10 (LSA 2/ 38)   ..63 Lagerung
..11   "        "  , Nr.11 (LSA 2/ 41)   ..64 Raumtemperatur
..12   "        "  , Nr.12 (LSA 2/ 44)   ..65 Körpertemperatur erhöht
..13   "        "  , Nr.13 (LSA 2/ 47)   ..66 Körpertemperatur erniedrigt
..14   "        "  , Nr.14 (LSA 2/ 50)   ..67
..15   "        "  , Nr.15 (LSA 2/ 53)   ..68
..16   "        "  , Nr.16 (LSA 2/ 56)   ..69
..17   "        "  , Nr.17 (LSA 2/ 59)   ..70 Intubation
..18   "        "  , Nr.18 (LSA 2/ 62)   ..71 intermitt.pos.press.breath.
..19   "        "  , Nr.19 (LSA 2/ 65)   ..72 Wechseldruckbeatmung
..20   "        "  , Nr.20 (LSA 2/ 68)   ..73
..21   "        "  , Nr.21 (LSA 2/ 71)   ..74
..22   "        "  , Nr.22 (LSA 2/ 74)   ..75
..23   "        "  , Nr.23 (LSA 2/ 77)   ..76 n.z.b.Manipulation an Ober-
..24 Laborbefund (LSA 1/ 43 - 48)             flächen
..25 Dauermedikation (LSA 1/ 49 - 54)    ..77
..26 Prämedikation                       ..78 verlegter Tubus (Block)
..27                                     ..79 Extubation
..28                                     ..80 n.z.b. inadäquates management,
..29                                          außer ..81 - ..86
..30 Hypnotikum I, relat. überdosiert    ..81 inadäquat.manag.:medikament.
..31    "          , normodosiert             Basisprogramm (..30 ff.)
..32    "          , relat. unterdosiert ..82 inad.manag.:medik.Adjuvans
..33 Analgetikum, relat. überdosiert     ..83 inad. Technik: Konnektion
..34    "          , normodosiert        ..84 inad. Technik: Apparat
..35    "          , relat. unterdosiert ..85 inad. apparat. Überwachung:
..36 Relax.nicht depol.,rel.überdos.          nicht durchgeführt
..37    "    "      "   ,normodosiert     ..86 inad. apparat. Überwachung:
..38    "    "      "   ,rel.unterdos.         Fehlinterpretation
..39 Relax.depolaris.,rel.überdosiert    ..87
..40    "    "        ,normodosiert       ..88
..41    "    "        ,rel.unterdosiert   ..89
..42 Hypnotikum II, rel. überdosiert     ..90 Op.-Einfluß auf Herz
..43     "           ,normodosiert       ..91 Op.-Einfluß auf Kreislauf
..44     "           ,rel.unterdosiert   ..92 Op.-Einfluß auf Respiration
..45 Volatilum, rel. überdosiert         ..93 Op.-Einfluß auf Endokrinum
..46    "       , normodosiert           ..94 Op.-Einfluß auf ZNS
..47    "       , rel. unterdosiert      ..95 extrakorp.Zirk., partiell I
..48 Kristall.Flüss., rel. überdos.      ..96    "        "    , total
..49    "        "    , normodosiert      ..97    "        "    , partiell II
..50    "        "    , rel. unterdos.    ..98 n.z.b. Ursache
                                         ..99 Ursache nicht erkennbar
```

Fig. 4.   *Code numbers and their meaning for causes (see text for explanation).*

of view, without problems. However, difficulties will occur when the cause of an event is complicated, ambiguous or hidden.

In such cases, a discussion of the events with experienced members of the department should precede the additional coding. If, in spite of comprehensive studies, it is impossible to establish a cause for some symptom, all factors under discussion can be encoded; if this is impossible too, one has to content oneself with entering code number 99 (cause unknown).

A relatively simple encoding example of a complex event is shown in Figure 5. Going from left to right, the meaning of the numbers in the first row is: before the operation; short; no connection with other symptoms already encoded; reduction of the arterial system pressure; caused by a relative overdosage of the barbiturate – kind and dosage to be found at another place of the record; increased by Effortil®; successfully removed; from a pressure level of systolic 80 to diastolic 30 mm Hg; and a pulse rate of 140/min.

The meaning of the numbers in the second row (the same meanings of the numbers omitted) is: additional coincident cause of the reduction of pressure; volume deficiency of the patient; by means of colloidal volume substitution; successfully removed.

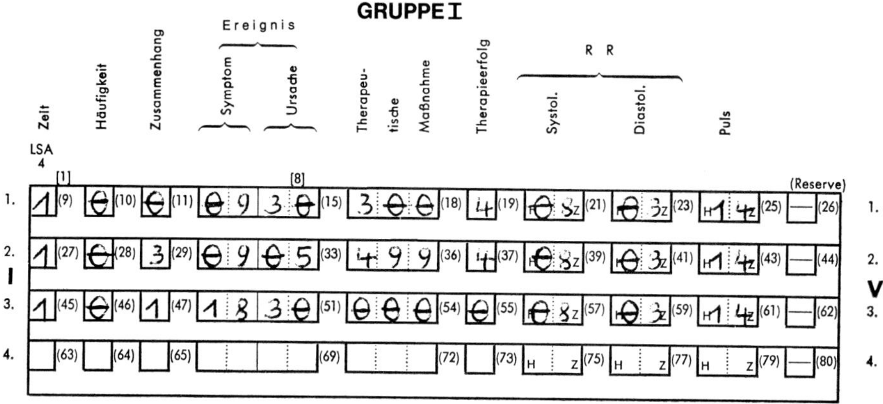

Fig. 5. *An example for encoding a complex event.*

The meaning of the numbers in the third row is: and brought about by the 2 above-mentioned causes coincident occurrence of; polytopic ventricular extrasystoles; for which an antiarrhythmic therapy proved unnecessary; since they disappeared upon the application of the above measures.

This example is meant to elaborate 2 points:

1. Having recourse to the original record will yield no additional information and in view of the volume of the material collected over a longer time, this is to be desired.

2. Such voluminous collections of special events can no longer be processed manually, e.g. by means of marginal-punch cards (Herden and Lawin, 1973; Rehnig, 1967); the use of digital computers is justified.

During the 2.5 years of use of our new anesthesia data record it has become apparent that most of the members of the department are able to encode even special events correctly. Upon removing the remaining technical difficulties with the hardware, first results will follow shortly.

REFERENCES

Bonhoeffer, K. and Brueckner, J. B. (1970): *Z. prakt. Anästh. Wiederbeleb.*, 5, 41.

Borchert, K., Benad, G., Thierbach, F., Kampehl, H.-J., Franke, H. and Bindernagel, U. (1972): *Zbl. Chir.*, 97, 1612.

Brueckner, J. B., Bonhoeffer, K. and Mertens, W. (1968): *Anaesthesist*, 17, 135.

Goetz, E. (1972): *Anaesthesiol. Inform.*, 5, 191.

Herden, H.-N. and Lawin, P. (1973): In: *Anaesthesiefibel, 1st ed.*, p. 199. Georg Thieme-Verlag, Stuttgart.

Kleinheisterkamp, U. and Fassl, H. (1968): *Anaesthesist*, 17, 382.

Lutz, H. (1972): *Anaesthesiol. Inform.*, 5, 183.

Moore, D. C., Bridenbaugh, L. D., Bagdi, P. A. and Bridenbaugh, P. O. (1968): *Anesthesiology*, 29, 595.

Rehnig, H.-J. (1967): *Dtsch. Gesundh.-Wes.*, 22, 2479.

Wawersik, J., Koehler, C. and Wagner, G. (1973): *Meth. Inform. Med.*, 12, 222.

Difficulties in documentation of psychological follow-up of patients' sensations after different anesthetics

HANS-PETER STEGBAUER, WILHELM ERDMANN and RUDOLF FREY

Johannes Gutenberg University, Mainz, Federal Republic of Germany, and
University of Alabama, Birmingham, Ala.,U.S.A

Psychological follow-up of patients' sensations after anesthesia has been given little attention up to now, except with some special substances like ketamine where the drug-induced psychological sensations were obvious.

In reality, uncomfortable sensations after anesthesia are most common. The patient qualifies the anesthesia and anesthesiologist based on these negative side-effects. This documentation of patients' sensations is important for the success of the anesthetist in the patients' mind. Thus, it should be possible to develop guidelines for consideration of the psychological effects, as well as circulatory, respiratory and intoxicatory effects, when a decision is made to determine which of the available anesthetics or methods should be applied (Höhn, 1974; Sonntag, 1974; Steffens, 1974; Tangerding, 1974; Zum Felde, 1974).

934 patients have been interviewed by means of personal conversations and psychological testing regarding their experience with the applied agent or method. The documentation of patients' sensations due to anesthesia has been determined by the following items: (1) Into what phase of the anesthesiological treatment does the patient project the sensation? (2) What was the nature of the sensations? (3) Were they due to the anesthetic or to the manipulations, intubation, etc., which accompanied it? (4) Did the patient have anesthesiological experience before, which could be used as a basis of comparison?

According to this, the documentation plan is, in general, organized as follows: (1) sensations during induction; (2) intraoperative sensations; (3) sensations after operation – awaking, dreams (e.g. horror trips), side-effects due to the anesthetic (headache, vomiting, etc.), side-effects due to manipulation (e.g. throat pain); (4) general consideration of anesthesia and, if possible, comparison between different anesthetics.

In addition to these statements, in Part I of the documentation plan, all data are registered concerning patients, the anesthetic administered, anesthesia performance, and additional treatment with other agents. A first documentation plan was shortened to adjust it to statistical documentation demands (Table 1).

RESULTS

Preliminary results prove the applicability of the new documentation plan: (1) concerning the psychological feelings of the patients; and (2) concerning postoperative symptoms due to anesthesiological manipulation, e.g. intubation.

Table 1.   *Documentation of psychological follow-up studies of patients' sensations due to anesthesia*

Part I

Anesthetic agent:	□□
Patient data: Name _______________________________	
First name _______________________________	
Age	□□
Sex	□
Profession _______________________________	
Height	□□□
Weight	□□□
Premedication	□□
Additional medicaments used	□□
Way of administering anesthesia	□□
Operation to be performed	□□
Position of patient	□
Name of anesthetist	□□
Duration of anesthesia (min)	□□□
Duration of surgical procedure (min)	□□□
Anesthetic risk group	□
Hb (g%)	□□
Hct (Vol%)	□□
Blood loss (ml)	□□□
Complications	□□

Part II

Did you become aware of falling asleep?	□□
Did you have intraoperative sensations?	□
Description:	
Did you awake directly after operation?	□
Did you have dreams?	□
Were the dreams comfortable, uncomfortable, neutral?	□□
Description:	
Did you have other side-effects?	□
What kind of side-effects?	□□
Description:	
When did postoperative pain begin (min)?	□□□
Did you feel afraid of anesthesia?	□
How did you find this anesthesia?	□
Would you be ready to submit once more to the same anesthesia?	□
Did you have anesthesia before?	□
Which kind of anesthesia (if known):	□□□
How did you find this anesthesia in comparison to the former one?	□

The printed fields are for statistical information thus allowing the results to be put into keys: 1 field allows 9 pieces of information; 2 fields allow the registration of 81 different pieces of information.

Psychological sensations and postoperative side-effects due to anesthetic drugs

The percentage of the total amount of psychological side-effects due to anesthesia reaches 30% (Table 2). Postoperative side-effects like vomiting and headaches e.g., are even higher with 45% of the total of the anesthetized patients thus affected. Significant differences in the rate of side-effects exist between ketamine and the other anesthetics involved in the

Table 2. *Psychological sensations and postoperative side-effects due to anesthetic drugs*

Anesthetic procedure		Psychological sensations		Postoperative side-effects	
		Yes	No	Yes	No
Ketamine in total	473	237	236	218	255
Epontol	11	1	10	3	8
Althesin	67	3	64	47	26
Dehydrobenz peridol+fentanyl	106	8	98	35	71
Thiopentone+halothane	203	18	185	88	115
Ketamine+halothane	46	10	36	39	7
Ketamine+Penthrane	32	4	28	2	30
Total	938	281	657	432	512

present study (Table 3). The amount of psychological sensations is significantly higher after ketamine application than it is when using other anesthetic agents. This difference in negative psychological side-effects due to ketamine anesthesia amounts to 5-times as high a rate than with other forms of anesthesia.

Table 3. *Difference in rate of side-effects between ketamine and other anesthetics*

	Psychological sensations (%)	Postoperative side-effects (%)
Ketamine	50.1	46.1
Other anesthetics	9.5	44.7
Total	29.9	45.4

As ketamine proved to be an ideal anesthetic concerning the vital parameters in a series of more than 3,000 ketamine anesthesias performed in our clinic – above all in critical care patients – it seemed to be necessary to try to avoid psychological sensations by combination of ketamine with other agents, like different psychotropic substances. The documentation revealed the results as shown in Table 4.

Table 4. *Psychological sensations after ketamine anesthesia*

	Yes	No	Percentage of sensations
Ketamine (air)	144	53	73
Ketamine+Tacitin	44	149	23
Ketamine+Hal/N_2O	10	36	22
Ketamine+others (N_2O, DHB, γ-hydroxybutyric acid, Valium, Dominal	49	34	59
Total	247	272	47.6

When ketamine was combined with benzoctamine sulfate (Tacitin ®), the percentage of psychological sensations decreased from 73% after ketamine as sole agent, to 23%. This seems to be a very good result compared to those cases where ketamine was only used as induction anesthetic but still with 22% of side-effects. When ketamine is combined with other agents, including psychotropic substances like Valium and Dominal, the amount of side-effects is only reduced to 59%.

Postoperative side-effects due to anesthesiological manipulation

The documentation also includes side-effects due to intubation. A comparative study on side-effects of tubes with low pressure cuffs and those with the commonly used high pressure cuffs revealed a statistically highly significant preference for tubes with low pressure cuffs (Table 5).

Table 5.   *Side-effects due to intubation*

	No side-effects	Side-effects	Total
High pressure cuff tubes	44	156	200
Low pressure cuff tubes	43	29	72
Total	87	185	272

The side-effect group was divided into 3 categories:

(*a*)   Light complaints: no severe cough, little pain, little pressure feeling; symptoms disappeared after 12 hr.

(*b*)   Medium severe complaints: coughing, pain, hoarseness; symptoms continued more than 12 hr.

(*c*)   Severe complaints: general tracheobronchitis and laryngitis, obstructive symptoms, cough with expectoration for a longer period.

A comparison of complaints being recorded after intubation with high pressure cuffs and those being registered after intubation with low pressure cuffs demonstrated a significantly higher rate of the percentage of medium severe and very severe side-effects for the high pressure cuff tubes (Table 6).

Table 6.   *The side-effect group divided into 3 categories*

Side-effects group	a (%)	b (%)	c (%)	Total
High pressure cuff tubes	59.6	32.7	7.7	100% (156)
Low pressure cuff tubes	75.9	20.7	3.4	100% (29)

a = light complaints; b = medium severe complaints; c = severe complaints.

SUMMARY AND CONCLUSIONS

A documentation plan has been developed for statistical documentation of postoperative patients' sensations due to anesthetic agents and manipulations. The documentation plan has been applied for follow-up studies in 934 patients. Psychological sensations during the phase of falling asleep, the intraoperative phase and the postoperative phase due to anesthesia are registered, in addition to postoperative side-effects and complaints due to anesthetic manipulations. Some results reporting the need and the applicability of such a plan have been stated briefly.

Ketamine in general, has an extremely high rate of psychological side-effects, up to 50% (other anesthetic agents, 9.5%), while other postoperative side-effects of ketamine such as vomiting, headache, etc. are the same compared to other agents. When ketamine is used as sole agent, the rate of psychological sensations increases to more than 70%; a combination of ketamine with psychotropic agents, especially benzoctamine sulfate (Tacitin), reduces the rate of psychological sensations to nearly 20% of patients so treated.

A comparison of postoperative side-effects after intubation with the 'high pressure cuff' tubes (78%) used so far and the newly developed and propagated 'low pressure cuff' tubes (40%) reveals a real advantage of low pressure cuff tubes and, in addition, severe side-effects such as general tracheobronchitis become less frequent.

The development of a plan to statistically document side-effects other than vital ones seems to be extremely important. Since patients qualify the anesthesiologist according to their experience with the anesthesia, taking into account all side-effects, the decision as to what kind of anesthesia or method to be applied should be based upon current results of good statistical documentation.

REFERENCES

Höhn, R. (1974): *Die Prä-, Intra- und Post-Narkotische Empfindungslage des Patienten nach Neuroleptanalgesie*. Thesis, University of Mainz.

Sonntag, G. (1974): *Die Prä-, Intra- und Post-Narkotische Empfindungslage des Patienten nach Althesin (CT-1341)*. Thesis, University of Mainz.

Steffens, I. (1974): *Zur Bedeutung der Intubation mit Kontrollierten Niederdruckmanschetten im Anästhesiologischen Routinebetrieb*. Thesis, University of Mainz.

Tangerding, B. (1974): *Die Prä-, Intra- und Post-Narkotische Empfindungslage des Patienten nach Halothannarkose*. Thesis, University of Mainz.

Zum Felde, H.-P. (1974): *Träume und Halluzinationen während und nach Ketaminenarkosen und deren Unterdrückung durch Benzoctamin*. Thesis, University of Mainz.

Need for a practical anaesthetic record

ENRIQUE VAZ HERNANDEZ

Ebro 8, Seville, Spain

From the first it has been taught that there is a need to record the different aspects of anaesthetic work, and there are many advantages to this system. However, there is one question which has prompted this presentation: Why is this practice so rare?

In the author's opinion the bad practice may be manifest by incomplete or approximate anaesthetic records or by absent records. The cause of this is the disproportionate complexity of the records in relation to the scant value of the results which are obtained.

There is no justification for a preanaesthetic questionnaire filled with questions about aspects which cannot be considered when the anaesthetic method is chosen owing to lack of possible variation. Neither is it logical to plot an anaesthetic graph with many physiological parameters which can only occasionally be used in practice. Some records include incidents and postanaesthetic complications which are not recorded later, even in the event of their happening.

Inaccessibility of records for subsequent study is another source of discouragement. Systems of data processing are rare in our country, at least as far as anaesthesiology is concerned and this results in loss of much information which could otherwise be studied. In consequence of this, and based upon the experience with the use of more than 8 different types of anaesthetic records (some personally designed for other hospitals) the fundamental principles of a practical record will be outlined.

The essential process is that data must be recorded if an anaesthetic record is to be useful. This must be obtained accurately, clearly, and systematically. In centres where the teaching of anaesthesia is performed, the records should be printed so that the existence of definite circumstances is indicated with no more than a convenient mark. This encourages beginners in the specialty to remember the questions and necessary investigations, and simplifies the preanaesthetic assessment for all surgical patients, for everybody.

The record is folio in size and consists of a single sheet. The front is divided into 4 unequal parts which contain respectively: *1st part* – the heading of the Hospital Centre; personal details of the patient; location of the patient in hospital; diagnosis which led to operation; operation proposed, and whether it is urgent, planned or as an out-patient; surgeons and anaesthetists; date and time of operation; medical history to which the record corresponds.

In the second part the history of anaesthetic interest is collected. The most important details are printed in red, which are the only ones used in emergencies. *2nd part* – age; sex; previous respiratory ailments of interest (nasal obstruction, common colds, coughs, expectoration, bronchitis, asthma, others); previous circulatory ailments of interest (dyspnoea, oedema, thoracic pain, dizziness, alteration in the arterial blood pressure, varicose veins or phlebitis); previous digestive ailments of interest (jaundice, vomiting, diarrhoea, time of last food intake); previous urinary ailments of interest (irritations, infections, oliguria); previous genital ailments (date of next menstruation, abnormal pregnancies and births); previous nervous system ailments (loss of consciousness, convulsions); previous metabolic ailments (diabetes, obesity, malnutrition); previous infections (fevers, rheumatism, polio); previous haematological ailments (anaemia, haemorrhages, transfusions); previous allergic ailments (medicinal, others); habits (smoking, alcoholism, physical exercise); previous treatments (corticoids, antidiabetics, insulin, hypotensive drugs, cardiotonics, antidepressives, salicylates, antibiotics, barbiturates, etc.); result of previous anaesthesias (good, bad, with incidents, with complications).

In the third part, the physical examination and clinical tests are reported. *3rd part –* weight; height; constitutional type; colour and appearance of skin; state of the superficial venous network; state of the ocular reflexes; state of the rhinopharynx (teeth, prosthesis, etc.); cervical, dorsal and lumbar columns; respiratory rhythm, rate and depth; duration of breath-holding; respiratory auscultation; spirometry; thorax X-ray; number, rhythm and intensity of the peripheral pulse; maximum and minimum BP; cardiac auscultation; ECG; examination of limbs looking for varicose veins and phlebitis.

The fourth part of this side is dedicated to analytic exploration. *4th part –* in blood (haemoglobin, number of red blood cells, blood glucose, proteins, blood urea, electrolytes, acid-base status, blood group, coagulation study); in urine (density, albumin, sediment, sugar, cetona, pigments, bilious salts and urobilin); a space on this side is used to indicate the risk on a scale from 1–4; below is indicated the pre-medication, with a code number which can correspond to a series of premedicant drugs.

The other side of the page is divided into 3 parts. The following are specified in the upper part:

(*a*) Type of anaesthesia: general, spinal, regional, local.

(*b*) Induction, followed by a blank space where the drugs of a codified list are specified.

(*c*) Intubation: No, Yes (oral, nasal, transtracheal), calibre of tube, existence or not of obstruction and record of intubation difficulty.

(*d*) Respiration: spontaneous, assisted, artificial (manual or mechanical).

(*e*) Respiratory system: open, semi-open, semi-closed, closed (circle, to and fro, with absorption of CO_2, without absorption of CO_2).

(*f*) Position of patient: supine, prone, lateral, genupectoral, gynaecological, sitting, Trendelenburg, antitrendelenburg.

(*g*) Maintenance of the anaesthesia with a blank space where the drugs of a codified list are specified.

The middle zone or 2nd part of this side is dedicated to anaesthetic graphs. In its upper part some lines are reserved to note down data and medication during anaesthesia, these being numbered according to a codified list to facilitate the subsequent collection of data and its analysis.

Underneath this is the graph upon which are plotted the pulse, maximum and minimum blood pressure, number of breaths, temperature, central venous pressure, etc.

In the lower part data is about ventilatory pressures, quantity of oxygen, gaseous and volatile anaesthetics; serums, blood, plasma expanders etc.

In the last and lowest part of the page a space is reserved for the 'immediate postoperative information'.

(*h*) Final state of patient: conscious, unconscious, with reflexes, with guedel airway, intubated or tracheotomized.

(*i*) Immediate complication: perivenous injection, intraarterial injection, mucous lesions, dental lesions, severe lack of oxygen, cough, secretions, cyanosis, laryngeal spasm, broncho-spasm, sweating, hiccough, vomiting, bronchial flooding, tachycardia, bradycardia, arrhythmia, hypotension, hypertension, transfusion reaction, prolonged unconsciousness, others.

(*j*) Data about the state of patient at the time of leaving the recovery room, or to intensive care; time, pulse rate, BP, consciousness, pain, diuresis.

(*k*) Lastly: later complications – prolonged hoarseness, lesion of vocal cords, atelectasis, pneumonia, postural nervous paralysis, hepatic lesion, renal failure, vomiting, other.

It is believed that with this type of record, and with the possibility of analysis, valuable data can be obtained, for the progress of our specialty, not only in the field of investigation but also by providing adequate information for future anaesthetists.

Even though there is necessity for great effort in analyzing this information without a computer system, it is believed that it is worthwhile in order to accustom anaesthetists in training to systematically collect data.

This anaesthetic record could also be the basis for a computerized recording system, when the circumstances permit.

Chapter XVI

Acupuncture

Introduction

H. BENZER

Ludwig Boltzmann Institute of Acupuncture, Vienna, Austria

Acupuncture-analgesia is acupuncture's youngest child. In contrast, acupuncture therapy has a long history; it has been practiced in China since the Stone Age. The oldest acupuncture needles, found in China, are about 7,000 years old.

Acupuncture is only a part of traditional Chinese medicine. Aside from massage, physiotherapy, inhalation therapy, and plant therapy, it still plays a leading role among diagnostic and therapeutic methods.

Acupuncture remained unknown to the Western world for a long time. It was probably introduced in Europe in 1671 by a Jesuit missionary; in 1929 classical Chinese texts were translated by Soulié de Morant. Since that time, schools exist in France where acupuncture therapy is systematically practiced with success. Austria too has a notable tradition. The name Johannes Bischko is closely linked to this tradition. His tireless work resulted in the establishment of a scientific institute for acupuncture (the Ludwig Boltzmann Institute of Acupuncture, Vienna).

The first operation under acupuncture-analgesia was performed in China in 1958. In the years following, 50–60% of all operations were performed with acupuncture-analgesia. In China today, the rate is probably 15–20% of all operations. However, such percentages should be looked at carefully, since they depend on incomplete information in the Chinese literature, or are estimated on the basis of reports of various delegations that visited China. Bonica assumes that in the whole of China, less than 10% of all operations are performed at present with acupuncture-analgesia

Reports about acupuncture-analgesia became known to the Western world in 1971 for the first time. In Vienna acupuncture-analgesia was seen in a Chinese television film. The reaction of the Viennese School of Anesthesiology was one of scepticism.

Nevertheless, already at the beginning of 1972, a tonsillectomy was performed under acupuncture-analgesia for the first time in the Western world under the guidance of Dr Johannes Bischko in Vienna. At this time, a group at the Vienna Institute of Anesthesiology, together with the Ludwig Boltzmann Institute of Acupuncture (Director: Dr J. Bischko) began to analyse critically acupuncture-analgesia clinically and experimentally. The problem was examined in an unbiased manner. Euphoria based on Chinese results and scepticism on the basis of negative observations in China, were eschewed. Personal clinical and experimental experience was sought.

This symposium presents the present status of research in acupuncture-analgesia, as far as it applies to the Western world, in the most objective manner possible.

Despite success in China, and successful acupuncture-analgesia in the Western world, acupuncture-analgesia seems to have little practical significance at the present time. Similarly, there is little scientifically-based knowledge about the mechanism of this form of analgesia.

Acupuncture analgesia in the People's Republic of China

O. MAYRHOFER

Department of Anaesthesiology, University of Vienna, Vienna, Austria

Between the end of April and early May, 1973, a delegation of three anaesthesiologists and one bioengineer visited the People's Republic of China, upon invitation of the Ministry of Health in Peking. The object of this visit was to study the practice of acupuncture analgesia, to report on our own experiences in this field and to exchange views on the practical and theoretical aspects of acupuncture analgesia with our Chinese colleagues. One week each was spent in Peking and in Shanghai. In both cities we visited three hospitals and observed a total of 25 procedures under acupuncture analgesia.

GENERAL REMARKS

In all the hospitals visited, there were no other guests at the time and there was complete freedom to move from one operating theatre to another and observe everything.

Each patient was seen from the very beginning, that is from the moment he was brought awake into the operating theatre. The acupuncture technique, the electrical stimulation, the operation and the transport back to the ward were all witnessed. Through interpreters and with the help of English-speaking Chinese colleagues, contact was maintained with patients throughout the procedures. During all the operations, filming, photography and videorecordings were allowed. Moreover, at our request, permission for collecting telemetric data was obtained.

In two specially organised meetings, all the theoretical and practical problems of acupuncture analgesia were discussed with Chinese anaesthetists, acupuncture specialists, gynaecologists, and paediatricians. The Chinese physicians repeatedly stressed the problems of incomplete analgesia and the frequently unsatisfactory insufficient muscular relaxation.

Patients for acupuncture analgesia are selected according to their individual viewpoint. Only those who are cooperative and do not oppose the method are chosen. Some types of procedures are unsuitable for acupuncture, for instance major tumour surgery, operations on the extremities, exploratory laparotomies – in fact operations, the extent and duration of which cannot be predicted.

THE OPERATIONS

Tables 1 and 2 show the operations observed in the three hospitals. For the lobectomy only one needle was used. This needle was placed on the dorsum of the forearm of the same side between the middle and distal third, through the interosseous membrane and manipulated, with poking and twisting movements, throughout the entire operation. In

Table 1. *Operations in Peking, April 30–May 4, 1973 (Total No.=12)*

Type of operation	Age	Sex	Profession	Acupuncture points		Premedication	Intraoperative additive analgesia
				Extremities-Body	Ear		
Cervical disc	44	m	–	+	+	–	0.5 ml 1% procaine
Inguinal hernia	36	m	–	+	—	–	–
Appendectomy	30	m	Worker	+	—	–	2 ml 1% procaine
Tooth extraction	40	m	–	+	—	–	–
Tooth extraction	40	m	–	+	—	–	–
Tooth extraction	5	f	School child	+	—	–	–
Caesarean section	27	f	Teacher	+	—	–	
Ovarian cyst	27	f	Worker	+	—	–	50 mg meperidine
Lobectomy	32	m	Engineer	+	—	0.3 mg scopolamine / 10.0 mg morphine	50 mg meperidine
Stomach resection (B-II)	48	m	Worker	+	+	0.3 mg scopolamine	50 mg meperidine
Thyroidectomy	55	m	Worker	—	+	0.2 mg scopolamine	50 mg meperidine
Hysterectomy	40	f	Worker	+	—	100 mg Nembutal / 0.2 mg scopolamine	50 mg meperidine

Table 2. *Operations in Shanghai, May 7–10, 1973 (Total No.= 14)*

Type of operation	Age	Sex	Profession	Acupuncture points		Premedication	Intraoperative additive analgesia
				Extremities-Body	Ear		
Detachment of retina	33	m	Worker	+	+	100 mg Luminal	–
Prostatectomy	68	m	Sailor	+	–	100 mg Luminal	–
Stomach resection (B-I)	41	m	Worker	+	–	–	50 mg meperidine
Thyroidectomy	31	f	–	+	–	–	–
Thyroidectomy	36	f	–	+	–	–	–
Thyroidectomy	37	f	–	+	–	–	–
Tumour of testicle	66	m	–	+	–	–	–
Laminectomy	47	m	Farmworker	—	+	–	–
Tumour of hypophysis	36	f	–	+	–	100 mg Luminal / 50 mg meperidine	–
Craniopharyngioma	24	m	Singer	+	–	100 mg Luminal / 50 mg meperidine	–
Ventricular septum defect	14	m	School boy	+	+	100 mg Luminal / 50 mg meperidine	0.1 mg fentanyl / 4 ml 0.5% lidocaine
Nasal septum	26	m	Worker	+	+	–	–
Stomach resection (B-II)	44	m	Worker	+	+	–	5 ml 1% procaine
Tumour cerebellum	58	m	–	—	+	–	–

all other operations, electrostimulation was applied to the acupuncture needles with a weak low-voltage current from batteries at a frequency of 2–3/sec.

SPECIAL OBSERVATIONS

Minute-to-minute cooperation between surgeon, patient and acupuncturist appeared to be excellent. The patient was informed about what was going on but was also distracted from discomfort by being given sips of tea or slices of apple. The general condition of most patients throughout the procedures seemed to be good. No patient complained about pain sensation; there was never any groaning or grumbling. Postoperatively all patients appeared to be in good shape. All surgeons worked quickly, smoothly, and gently.

In some instances, the patient was not completely free from pain. The operation was then stopped for a few minutes while the anaesthetist talked to the patient and gave him some meperidine i.v. The most unsatisfactory procedure was the prostatectomy. This old man was obviously in great pain when the adenoma was mobilized. He was sweating and squeezing the acupuncturist's hand.

20–25% of all operations performed in China are now done under acupuncture, usually with electrical stimulation of the needles, and on the average about 10% are failures. The best results can be achieved on the head and neck region, whereas intra-abdominal procedures appear to be the least satisfactory.

In the Shanghai Institute of Physiology, a group of neurophysiologists are trying to determine objectively the effects of electroacupuncture in animal experiments. Their results seem to suggest an explanation which can be related to Melzack and Wall's theory of the gate-control of pain.

CONCLUSION

All in all, the impression gained was that there is a distinct physiological effect detectable following acupuncture with electrical stimulation. The pain threshold is raised in most instances, but complete analgesia is almost never achieved. The remaining gap to complete analgesia for satisfactory operative conditions must be bridged by persuasion and/or drugs. The Chinese patient may be more understanding and cooperative but, as has been proved in Vienna over the past three years, the European patient can also be operated upon successfully under acupuncture analgesia.

Telemetric ECG data (*biorhythms*) from operations under acupuncture analgesia in the People's Republic of China

H. THOMA

Bio-technical Laboratory, II Surgical University Clinic, University of Vienna, Vienna, Austria

Modern medical techniques allow measurement of biological variables outside of the laboratory. By this means, phenomena can be objectively represented, which could not otherwise be demonstrated. The most important condition is that the apparatus should be fully portable and easy to manipulate. This apparatus is unfortunately not commercially available. While on a visit to China, a home-made apparatus was used to record and store the ECG during surgery performed under acupuncture analgesia. The apparatus, consisting of a miniature transmitter, receiver, and tape recorder, is powered by batteries and was transported as hand-luggage by plane. (Development and construction of this apparatus and of the reproducing-set was done in the Biotechnisches Laboratorium der II. Chirurgischen Universitätsklinik Wien.)

MEASUREMENT, MATERIAL, EVALUATION

Before surgery started, a choice was made from the list of operations during which the ECG was to be recorded. In each case 2 miniature transmitters were attached to the patient by adhesive electrodes, before any needling. The transmitters were attached by adhesive tape, if possible in front of the chest, at right angles to each other. Once applied, it was impossible to correct the position of the transmitters during preparation for, or during the course of, the operation, as they were covered by sterile drapes. The 2-channel transmission has several advantages. Because the take-off is at right angles, the larger ECG amplitude can be recorded; recording is still possible, even if the electrodes of one transmitter drop off. High frequency disturbances on one frequency can be eliminated by switching to the other frequency. The transmitters are protected against high voltage interference, but no ECG recording is possible during electrocautery. The time sequence was kept by exact recording of events and time markings on the tape, and by synchronization of marks on the tape. The recordings were taken on the following operations under acupuncture analgesia: hypophyseal tumour, appendectomy, caesarian section, cyst of the ovary, lobectomy, detachment of the retina, VSD. Naturally in VSD we encountered the greatest difficulties. The electrodes of one transmitter came loose during the skin preparation, the second transmitter was in an unfavourable position so that only a small amplitude was recorded. Non-isolated electrical apparatus in eye surgery showed up as disturbances in the evaluation, but could be eliminated later. The recordings in Peking were interfered with, on one channel, by a local radio transmitter on UKW frequency (94.4 MHz).

In the evaluation in the laboratory the variations of the sound were demodulated and at the end of the analog tape recorder the ECG is available for further evaluation (Fig. 1). This evaluation was done on a fully automatic analyzer of our design. From the QRS complex the apparatus analyzes the absolute amplitude of the R, Q, and S wave, and the duration measured from beat to beat. The registration of these parameters seems more suitable since the word 'pulse-rate' is related to the unit time of a minute, and since modern apparatus can accomplish an integration over at least several beats. This apparatus does not measure the biorhythm correctly. Figure 2 shows the approximate course of a heart rate curve, high frequencies correspond to high amplitudes, written in the negative. A saw tooth voltage, triggered by the QRS complex, is continually reduced until the next beat stops its course. The lowest point corresponds to the most recent period in milliseconds. This maximal value is stored in the apparatus until the next beat. The apparatus also analyzes the difference in amplitude of succeeding R waves. This factor, in a quiet subject, corresponds to his respiration. The special advantage of this apparatus is that the respiration can be charted from the ECG (Fig. 1) and the periodicity of this also indicates the rate of respiration.

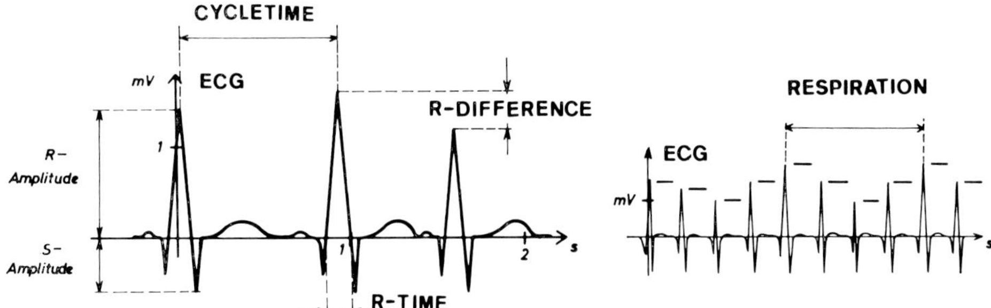

Fig. 1.   *Measured values of the automatic QRS-analyses.*

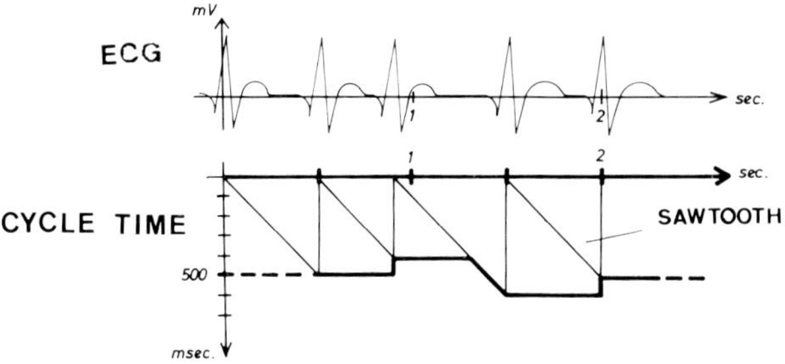

Fig. 2.   *Measuring of the periodic duration without integration.*

RESULTS AND DISCUSSION

Exact measurement of the beat-to-beat interval of the heart allows conclusions in regard to various conditions of a subject (Fig. 2). It is certain, for example, that spontaneous pain causes at least temporary changes in the heart rate. Beyond that the analysis of the field of so-called 'biorhythms' is still undeveloped. A gross classification of these rhythms is possible.

692   *H. Thoma*

Biorhythms occur mainly when the pulse is quiescent; with increasing rate their amplitude declines. A physically and psychologically quiet subject always has a regular rhythm, even if the amplitude of the individual rhythmic wave varies. The anaesthetized subject has no biorhythm, but has an almost exactly regular pulse rate. The excited person, in relation to the intensity of the excitation, shows disturbances of his rhythm, leading possibly to a definite dysrhythmia.

On this basis in general, these patients in China were either restless and excitable, or tired and sleepy. An anaesthetic-like state is excluded, since all patients showed evidence of biorhythms, unless there was a state of excitement. The body-build of these patients varied greatly from a sensitive engineer (lobectomy) to a pyknic worker (detachment of the retina). In most patients, there was no evidence of preoperative sedation with drugs. Although in the pyknic patients, with their stable functions, no such statement can be proved. However, massive reactions to sudden occurrences, such as the entrance of the surgeon or the preparation of the skin, were often recorded. The reliability of our method of recording is confirmed in that the regulatory mechanisms of the body apparently do not recognize any racial differences. These functions are comparable to those of any European patient in an awake state.

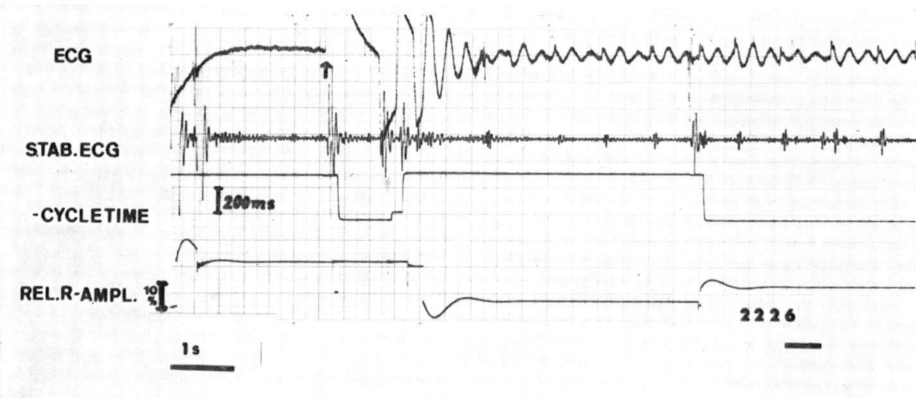

Fig. 3.   *Open heart operation, VSD, defibrillation (see arrow).*

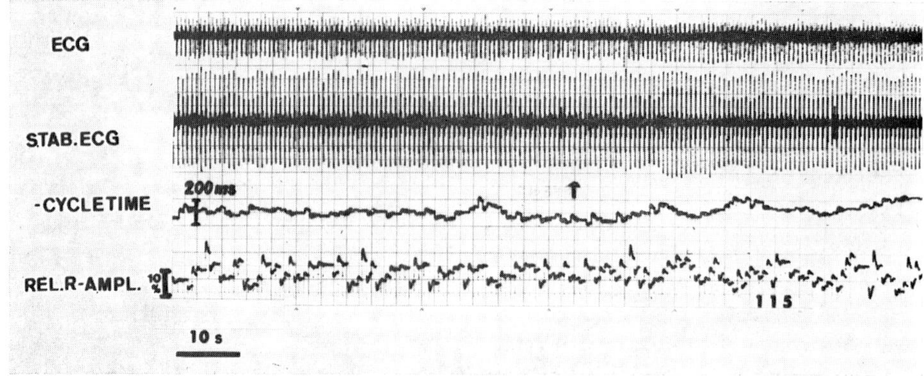

Fig. 4.   *Ovarian cyst, skin incision (see arrow) – no pain! The process of breathing can be seen in the relative R-amplitude.*

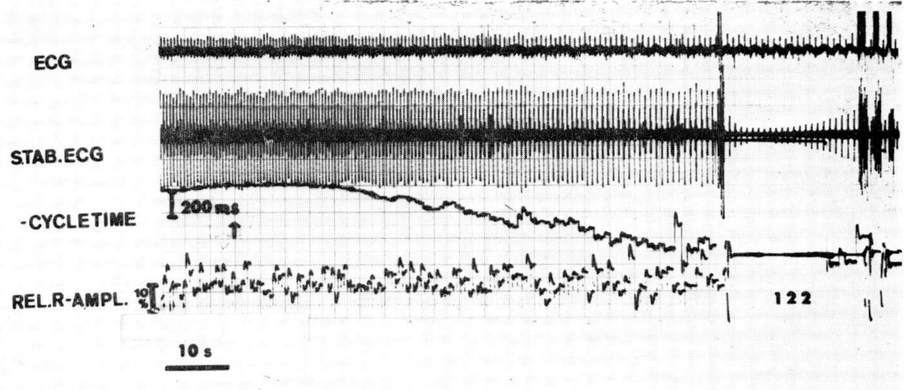

Fig. 5. *Lobectomy, skin incision (see arrow) – fear (pain?) before and during skin incision. Biorhythms 35 sec after incision. Artefacts at the end of the picture.*

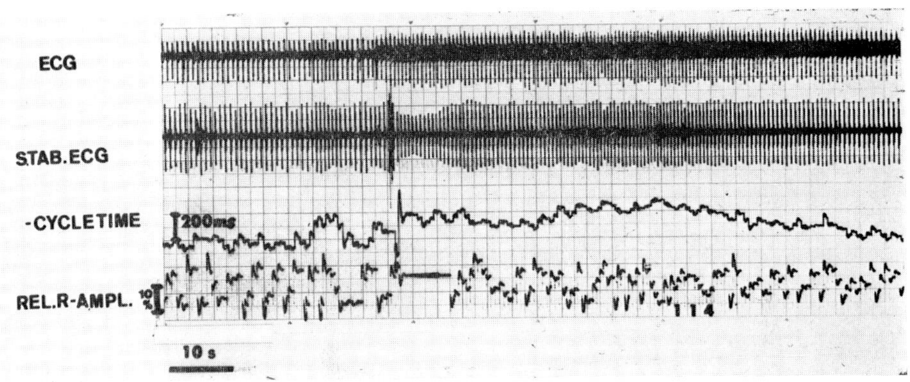

Fig. 6. *Section, massive pulse-rate reaction at the cold washing of the operation field.*

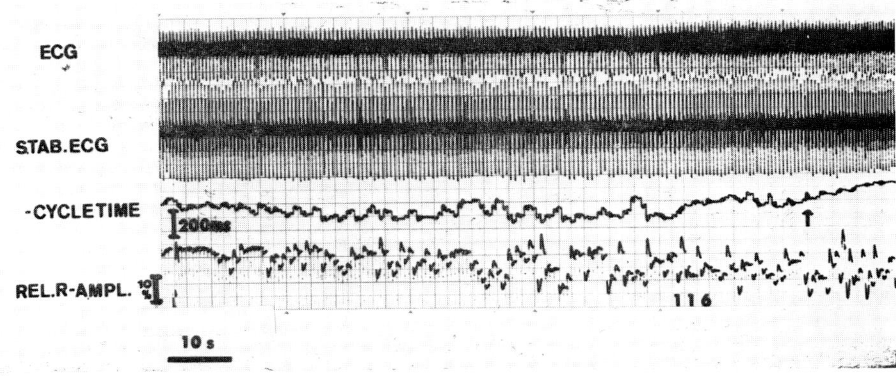

Fig. 7. *Section, rhythms of rest before skin incision (pain?).*

Acupuncture is unable to suppress reflexes. Slowing of the heart occurred when traction was applied to the mesentery or to the eye (appendectomy and detachment of the retina).

The hypothesis that acupuncture has a stabilizing effect on the circulation is also generally untenable; changes in the pulse rate of $\pm\ 100\%$ during the course of an operation tend to contradict this view.

Comment about the sensation of pain in the Chinese patients is naturally very difficult. Pain is a psychic occurrence and therefore it is hard to be objective. In order to try to be objective about pain, 3 methods have been used albeit imperfectly: (1) observation of the patient, in order to recognize signs of pain; (2) leading questions, which is a method often used in psychology; and (3) measurement of psychologic parameters. In the author's opinion, pain does not occur if, on the basis of all these 3 methods, no criteria for pain are to be found.

This goal is set rather high, since there are many causes for apparent signs of pain (e.g. reflex changes of function). In regard to these cases, there were a number of instances in which, on occurrence of operative insults, for example the skin incision, no criterion of pain was observed, nor measured, nor admitted on questioning. On the other hand, there were several instances where a possible pain caused an increase in pulse rate, but direct questioning yielded a negative answer (see Figs. 3–7). Disturbance from electroacupuncture occurs on the ECGs and the frequency of the stimulating impulses is therefore recorded.

FINAL REMARKS

About 150 examples of records, each of about 2 min duration, were prepared. It is necessary to measure physiological functions in order to be objective about psychic phenomena. There is a definite psychic component in acupuncture and the necessity for personal contact with the patient for the optimal results of acupuncture is always stressed in China. After analysis of the heart rate and respiratory rate, the psycho-galvanic skin reaction and the relative centralization need to be measured. In order to achieve this, a miniaturized apparatus is now available and it would be of interest to synchronize recordings of several different parameters.

It is important that medical science, by special measurement, explains acupuncture by objective experiments, rather than by speculative hypotheses. These original observations on patients may be a small step towards the solution of this problem.

Acupuncture analgesia in the western world

H. BENZER and G. PAUSER

Department of Anesthesiology, University of Vienna, Vienna, Austria

A year and a half ago, a team of physicians, together with the Boltzmann Institute for Acupuncture in Vienna, began work on the problem of clinical and experimental acupuncture analgesia at the Vienna Institute of Anesthesiology. This is a critical report which is as objective as possible, and is intended as an interim statement.

A Chinese television film showed how analgesia was achieved through a needle inserted in the lower arm, making a lobectomy possible without intubation or artificial respiration. At that time anesthetists' opinions were divided.

At the Vienna Polyclinic Hospital, in March 1972, under the direction of Johannes Bischko, a tonsillectomy with acupuncture analgesia was successfully performed for the first time. Thereafter, the Vienna school of Anesthesiology decided to involve themselves intensely with this new form of analgesia. After step-by-step experiments, acupuncture was used in the clinic in premedication, against postoperative pain, and for the induction of labor.

The first time acupuncture was used for tonsillectomy, the needles were turned manually throughout the operation in order to achieve analgesia. Aside from skill and awareness, manual turning demands the constant presence of an acupuncturist during the entire operation, and is, in certain circumstances, painful for the patient. An electroacupuncture apparatus was therefore developed. After a series of volunteer experiments the appropriate current was found so that an analgesic effect analogous to that achieved by turning the needles could be achieved. In June 1972, a tonsillectomy with electroacupuncture was performed. A D and C was also done under acupuncture analgesia. In order to test the effectiveness of acupuncture analgesia in the throat region, this form of analgesia was used for the incisions necessary for the pacemaker probe.

During a visit to China in the Spring of 1973, the rather skeptical attitude of Chinese colleagues and, at the same time, the absolute negative response of other western observers concerning acupuncture analgesia were noted with interest. Notwithstanding this, on the basis of newly gained knowledge and personal past experience up until that time, the program of clinical investigation was continued at our Institute.

In order to determine the success or failure of analgesia, a special rating scheme was designed. In this rating scheme, pain is judged subjectively by the patient and objectively by a neutral observer. Further, the patient's respiration, movements, facial expression, perspiration, and circulation are described according to a particular scheme.

Each group is divided into 4 categories, for which points from 1–4 are given (for example, subjective pain rating: 1 point if the patient experiences no pain; 2 points if he experiences bearable pain; 3 points for intense pain; and 4 points for unbearable pain). Thus, there is a total of 7 points for the most successful case, and 28 points for a complete failure, in which case, of course, an anesthetic is then administered. Cases with a total of between 7 and 14 points are regarded as successful.

A total of 119 operations have been performed with acupuncture analgesia up until

Table 1. *Acupuncture analgesia (Department of Anesthesiology, University of Vienna, and Ludwig Boltzmann Institute for Acupuncture, Vienna)*

Procedure	No. of cases	Acupuncture points
Tonsillectomy	48	Large intestine 4, lung 11
D and C	22	Stomach 36, spleen 6
Cesarean section	1	Stomach 36, spleen 6, urinary bladder 27–31, local needles
Laparotomy	2	Stomach 36, 44, spleen 6, local needles
Appendectomy	1	Stomach 37, spleen 7, local needles
Herniorrhaphy	9	Liver 3, spleen 7, local needles
Intrajugular pacemaker	12	Ear-points
Cardiac surgery (sternal fissure)	20	Pericardium 6, lung 7, ear-points
Thyroidectomy	4	1. Ear-points
		2. Large intestine 4, pericardium 6
		3. Punctum nervosum (Chang)
Total	119	

the present time (Table 1). Tonsillectomies were performed on 48 patients. The needles were stimulated electrically. For electrical stimulation, we use a stimulation length of 0.5 msec, a current intensity of 1–10 mA, and a potential of 0.5–20 V, at a frequency of 3–25 Hz. As a rule, points farther away from the operative field are stimulated with a slower frequency, and those close to the operative field with a more rapid one. The details of the various cases are given in Table 1. In 20 cases of open-heart surgery where the thoracotomy was done by sternotomy, a special combined anesthetic was used. The neuroleptic, haloperidol (dehydrobenzperidol) with the 'physical analgetic' acupuncture was combined. As a rule, the patients received the usual drug premedication or a premedication with acupuncture. Immediately before the incision, 25–50 mg pethidine were given to the patients. In only a few cases, additional local anesthesia through a sponge in the operative region was employed. During tonsillectomy, the throat was sprayed with lidocaine to reduce the swallowing reflex.

On the basis of specific observations, it was discovered that the patient's report of the analgesia immediately postoperatively differs remarkably from the opinion expressed a few weeks later. In one case, that after acupuncture analgesia for a cesarean section, the patient reported immediately postoperatively that she had felt no pain at all. Three weeks later, she described the course of the operation to a newspaper reporter as completely painless. However, a few weeks later, this same patient reported to her family doctor that she had felt intense pain during the operation! Thus, it was recently decided to survey all the patients, on whom an operation with acupuncture analgesia had been performed, about their opinion after a longer period of time had elapsed. A questionnaire was sent to these patients, in which they were asked if they would choose acupuncture analgesia again and for what reason. The patients were also asked again about pain during the operation. If so, the patients rate the pain as: (*a*) hardly felt, (*b*) bearable, (*c*) intense, and (*d*) extreme to unbearable. In other questions, the patients were invited to express their opinion about acupuncture analgesia for other patients.

This report involves the results from 52 questionnaires. The overall result of acupuncture is divided into the following categories: *excellent* – if the patient reports that he would undergo another operation with acupuncture analgesia and that he experienced no pain or it was hardly noticeable during the operation; *good* – if the patient would again undergo an operation with acupuncture analgesia and reports having hardly felt pain or had bearable pain; *moderate* – if the patient would again choose acupuncture analgesia, but reports having experienced bearable to severe pain during the operation. Excellent, good, and moderate are summarized as a positive result. The analgesia is regarded as a failure if the patient would not undergo the next operation with acupuncture analgesia, and reports having experienced intense to unbearable pain during the operation. In all the 52 cases, the operation was performed throughout with acupuncture analgesia. The results of this survey on 52 patients are shown in Table 2.

From these preliminary results of an ongoing investigation, one can infer that under certain circumstances, on certain patients, and in certain operations, acupuncture analgesia can be regarded as a possible variant to the methods of anesthesia in the western world.

Table 2. *Criteria to evaluate results of acupuncture anesthesia (preliminary report of a follow-up study in 52 patients)*

	Procedure				
	Tonsillectomy	Herniorrhaphy	Thyroidectomy	Cesarean section	D and C
Excellent: Same type of analgesia desired for any surgery in the future *No pain*	11	4	1	0	1
Good: Same type of analgesia desired for any surgery in the future *Hardly notable to bearable pain*	12	0	1	0	0
Moderate: Same type of analgesia desired for any surgery in the future *Bearable to severe pain*	2	1	2	0	0
Failure: No acupuncture analgesia desired for any surgery in the future *Unbearable pain*	14	2	0	1	0
Total	39	7	4	1	1

MECHANISM OF ACUPUNCTURE

At first, it must be stated that at present there is not enough knowledge and that speculative theories are rife. On the basis of experience, it is suggested that acupuncture analgesia is a form of combined anesthesia (Table 3). Experience has shown that acupuncture alone

Table 3. *Mechanisms of analgesia*

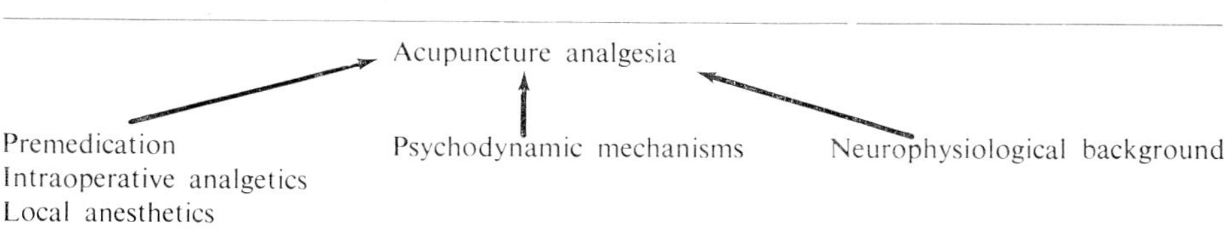

cannot guarantee sufficient freedom from pain during an operation. Thus, it is necessary to give premedication and very small doses of analgetics or local anesthetics during the operation.

Psychodynamic mechanisms may also play an important role. Eighteen out of 26 experts who have been questioned are of the same opinion, 7 deny any psychodynamic effect (Table 4). However, these mechanisms cannot involve hypnosis. Finally, though, it must be noted that the importance of psychodynamic mechanisms does not minimise the value of acupuncture. Any method dealing with a pain problem must involve some suggestion.

Table 4.   *Questionnaire to acupuncture experts*

	Yes	No	No answer
China experiences	8	18	0
Experiences in clinical use	13	13	0
Experiences in treatment of postoperative pain	14	7	5
Experimental experiences	14	10	2
Psychological features	18	5	3
Future of acupuncture in surgery	13	11	2
Future of acupuncture in pain relief	22	1	3
Concerned with problem of acupuncture	22	2	2
Quack?	1	25	0

Type of surgical operations: dentistry, tonsillectomy, tracheostomy, thyroidectomy, appendectomy, cesarean section, mastectomy, herniorrhaphy, D and C, pain relief during labor, gall-bladder removal, removal of nerve tumor. Number of operations varies from 4–321; success rate varies from 0–100%, mostly about 50–75%.

This mechanism could be a significant 'conditioner' for any superimposed neurophysiological phenomenon. Table 5 illustrates a triangle of anesthetist, surgeon and patient whose interaction plays an important role. Mutual contact between the 3 personalities is significant, particularly if the anesthetist has a strong personality. The importance of these factors does not decrease the value of acupuncture analgesia but, on the contrary, increases its value. The necessary explanation given to the patient immediately before

Table 5.   *Role of interaction*

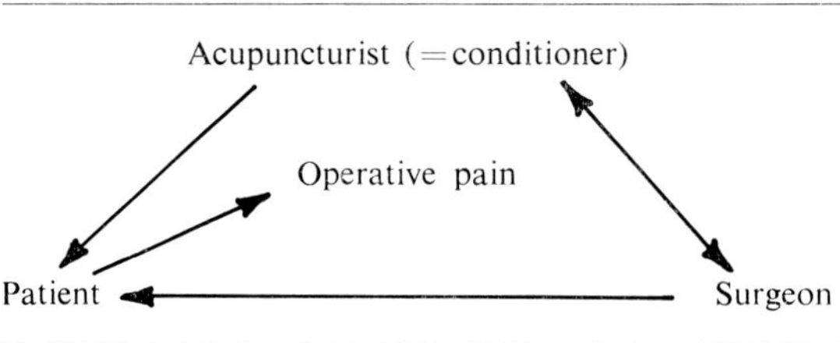

the operation that he will feel the surgeon's manipulation during the operation, but that this will not be felt as pain, is an essential part of this contact. Acupuncture analgesia can be described as inhibiting the pain sensation, though not interfering with the sensitivity to pain. Thus, the operation must be explained to the patient, and the patient himself must stay in contact, though not excessively, with the anesthetist. In our opinion, the introduction of active collaboration establishes a complex condition of trust in the patient, and this helps to convert the hypalgesia achieved through acupuncture to analgesia.

Patients who wish a repeated acupuncture analgesia especially want active contact with the operating team. In particular, it seems that witnessing the operation increases the sense of trust and makes the analgesia successful. The patients continually stressed that the postoperative progress was more favorable as a result of acupuncture. Some actual quotations were as follows: 'Only one who is psychologically suited to the operation can be a proper patient.' 'I think acupuncture analgesia could be a routine method in anesthesia, but unfortunately most patients lack the incentive.' 'It is a useful method for small operations, but one has to have the correct psychological attitude.' An 82-year-old man, undergoing herniorrhaphy with acupuncture analgesia, said: 'I would like this method again because I am suffering from arteriosclerosis, emphysema and troubles with my circulation; I am an opponent of all chemical compounds; I was pleased to be able to experience the operation consciously; I believe in this method!'

Table 6 summarises the preliminary conclusions which are based on individual experiences, and reflect the opinion of a total of 26 competent scientific investigators in Europe and America, by means of a questionnaire.

Table 6. *Future role of acupuncture analgesia in surgical practice in western countries*

(*a*) Basic research on pain mechanism
(*b*) Hardly any practical significance
(*c*) Possible meaning in selected patients for: dental surgery; ENT surgery (tonsillectomy); minor surgery; obstetrics and gynecology (cesarean section); cases of hypersensitivity to drugs.
(*d*) Only available type of anesthesia.

No final statement on the future of acupuncture analgesia is possible at the present time. More precise knowledge about the mechanism is necessary. Those questioned unanimously stressed that acupuncture analgesia is very valuable, that through this method research on pain during operations has been greatly stimulated. At present, acupuncture analgesia has hardly any practical significance. A situation could arise which would make the use of acupuncture analgesia necessary, such as when the patient's general condition excludes general or local anesthesia, or when hypersensitivity to drugs exists. Acupuncture analgesia can be used in the fields of medical dentistry; ear, nose and throat surgery, in tonsillectomies and minor operations; and sometimes in herniotomies and D and C. Acupuncture analgesia might also be particularly important in obstetrics.

Finally, acupuncture analgesia would be useful if, through personnel or mechanical shortages, other methods of anesthesia are not available.

Experimental studies and theoretical considerations about acupuncture effects

M. HAIDER, E. GROLL-KNAPP and C. REICHMANN

Department of Environmental Hygiene, University of Vienna, Vienna, Austria

Besides clinical trials of acupuncture analgesia, systematic and well-controlled experiments are necessary to obtain objective results and to clarify the underlying mechanisms. Such investigations have to be multidimensional. It is necessary to control physiological parameters and psychological aspects. The changes of neurophysiological data for example, neuron-activity, the EEG and the more differentiated process of cerebral activity, for example, evoked potentials and slow potential changes have to be taken into account. Other indices which can be used are pulse rate, electromyogram, electrodermatogram etc. Objective determination of threshold changes may be gained by different psychophysical methods. More general changes of pain sensation and attitudes of the subject may be evaluated by means of different scaling procedures.

In our studies we used these physiological and psychological indices under rigorous experimental conditions. In one study 16 young volunteers (8 male, 8 female) were tested with a special Algesimeter in 3 situations: control, acupuncture and placebo acupuncture. In each situation 2 tests were performed, one before and one after a 20-min acupuncture with electrostimulation, respectively before and after a 20-min placebo acupuncture. In the control situation there were 20-min rests between the 2 tests. Algesimeter tests were performed 20 times on each of 5 points on the subjects' throats. Steel acupuncture needles were inserted into the points circulation 6, sexuality, large intestine 14 and typical ear points. They were electrostimulated with an original Chinese pulse generator. 'Placebo points' were chosen near the above mentioned acupuncture points. Only the acupuncturist but neither the subject nor the investigator knew whether a real or a placebo acupuncture was performed ('double-blind design'). Subjective scaling of pain on a 9 point scale was applied after needling and 5 times during each Algesimeter test. The pulse rate was monitored continuously. The Taylor manifest anxiety scale was administrated before the tests began.

The Algesimeter data showed only very small changes. In the control situation the second test showed some lowering of the pain threshold. This might have been effected by local changes in the tissue or by some learning influences. Acupuncture and placebo acupuncture showed no such lowering of the threshold and there was no significant difference between these two. This may indicate some influence of the needling and of the electrostimulation but cannot be interpreted as a specific effect of acupuncture.

Much clearer differences could be demonstrated by the subjective scaling of pain. In the control situation the pain was stronger in the second test scored than in the first one. This is consistent with the Algesimeter data and shows that the subjects were more sensitive to pain. Acupuncture and placebo acupuncture showed, compared to the control situation, a significant lowering of pain appreciation judgements. This effect was much more pronounced during genuine acupuncture.

Pulse rates were lowered during the second test but only with acupuncture were they significantly lower. In a second study only one acupuncture point, stomach 35, was needled and compared to placebo and control situations. Here the EEG was continuously monitored and evoked potentials for click stimuli were computer-analysed. Slow brain potential changes (expectancy wave) were observed.

For theoretical consideration at least three possible mechanisms to explain acupuncture analgesia have to be discussed.

Firstly, of course, the classification of the effects of acupuncture analgesia as a special class of phenomena not explicable by known physiological or psychological mechanisms. In that case it is necessary to introduce special exploratory concepts like 'energy flow in meridians'.

Secondly neurophysiological and neuropsychological models may be taken into account. Experiments on cell activity, investigations on neurotransmitters and electrophysiological parameters like EEG, evoked potentials and slow potential changes will have to be integrated to find out possible interactions (e.g. 'gating' mechanisms) on different levels of spinal and cerebral functioning. More complicated mechanisms like masking, 'single channel' influences and shifts of attention may be considered.

A third viewpoint may be to explain the observed changes on a purely psychological basis. In that case it may be assumed for example that the effects of acupuncture analgesia are mainly produced by a special and extreme kind of 'social interaction', depending on learning and personality factors as well as on the context of the general social surrounding and the psychosocial commitments derived from traditions.

At present it seems to be most appropriate to assume a hierarchical interaction system in which the above mentioned neurophysiological, neuropsychological and psychosocial mechanisms integrate. The data of experimental investigations show that primary effects on pain thresholds are either absent or small, perhaps only manifest in greater variability of response. Under the influence of secondary factors like attention, learning, personality and social interactions rather stronger and more lasting changes of 'reactions to pain' may develop. Such 'reactions to pain' may include cognitive evaluations as well as autonomic and motor reactions. As an example, for personality trait influences, in our studies the more sensitive and more anxious subjects showed a greater effect of acupuncture. For the psychosocial influences it is obviously important what the acupuncturist and the acupuncture itself 'represents' to the subject. The social interaction will lead some subjects to reinterpret many only secondarily induced changes as primary effects of acupuncture. This influence will reinforce the reduction of pain; the more personal, social, cultural, political and traditional forces are operating in this special kind of 'transference situation' the better.

Measurement of pain threshold (algesimetry) during acupuncture

M. BAUM

Institute of Anaesthesiology, University of Vienna, Vienna, Austria

The determination of pain threshold is one of the most difficult and most disputed problems in the measurement of biological processes. The multiplicity of methods indicates that there is no single satisfactory procedure. The problem of algesimetry is 2-fold: first, the production of a defined, continually increasing, painful stimulus, and second, the choice of a parameter which responds to pain.

A painful stimulus can be electrical, mechanical, thermal or chemical, with subdivisions existing in each group. The evaluation of pain is independent of the method by which the pain is produced. Pain evaluation in the simplest sense can be a subjective statement ('it hurts') or a defensive withdrawal reaction. Alternatively the evaluation can be attempted by objectively charting certain biological parameters (blood pressure, heart rate, respiration frequency, psychogalvanic skin response). In animal experiments these attempts at objectivity are extended to neurophysiological methods especially monitoring the discharge frequency of individual cells.

In attempting to measure objectively the hypoalgesic effects of acupuncture in voluntary subjects certain methods are self-exclusive. The painful stimulus has to be applied to a part of the body for which effective acupuncture points exist, for example the throat, thorax or the teeth. Thus a method of producing pain by ischaemia, by applying a tourniquet, is excluded. The methods chosen for this experiment consist of the application of a controllable pain stimulus by puncture. For this purpose a simple algesimeter was developed. A reservoir contains compressed air under the pressure of 3 atmospheres. By means of a solenoid value the reservoir is connected to a 5 ml glass syringe, via a flow regulator, so that the velocity of the plunger which carries the needle which will apply the painful stimulus, can be controlled. A precision manometer measures the pressure in the syringe; the pressure is a parameter of the force with which the needle is pushed into the skin. The tip of the needle is grinded to a diameter of 0.2 mm under a microscope to avoid piercing the skin but producing a definite feeling of sharp pain. In order to localize exactly the area of the skin which is used, a pattern is pasted on the neck of the subject; the needle can be applied in 5 different locations which can be duplicated with a variation of not more than 0.1 mm. This ensures that the same density of pressor-receptors is always met during the repeated measurements. The whole measuring cycle is controlled by the subject by means of a push-button which initiates the movement of the needle. The pressure of the needle then rises in a linear fashion during the next 5–10 sec until a painful sensation is produced. A second touch on the push-button returns the needle to its original position, while the manometer stores the value of the pressure exerted. After 3–5 sec the subject initiates another needling. In this way each of the 5 points of the pattern is needled 20 times so that 100 measurements result.

Fifteen subjects were tested in a double-blind study, on 3 consecutive days, in a random fashion. The values were compared of the pressure tolerated on starting and the value during acupuncture, the starting value and value during acupuncture at an atypical point (= placebo acupuncture) and the starting value with the value without acupuncture. Statistical evaluation shows that in 72% experiments the result for starting values and the result of values obtained during the experiments were of the same pattern regardless of acupuncture, placebo acupuncture or no acupuncture. Hypalgesia could not be documented even as a statistically nonsignificant tendency. The only difference, and this is not significant, consists in a greater dispersion of values for intensity of pain during acupuncture; in other words there was greater uncertainty amongst the subjects with regard to pain.

Electrical measurement of the stimulus threshold with special reference to the effect of acupuncture

E. STICH

University Dental School, University of Vienna, Vienna, Austria

Measurements of the stimulus threshold on the tooth pulp were made using electrical stimulation of the tooth pulp with the intention of demonstrating the nature and significance of the analgesic effect of acupuncture as objectively as possible. The problem is to determine with acupuncture in the relevant regions of the body whether charges occur and especially if there is an increase in the stimulus threshold for peripheral pain stimulus.

A Chinese electrical acupuncture stimulator was used to produce an acupuncture anaesthesia in the teeth. In all subjects, 2 acupuncture points were chosen, the colon region, D_4, and the infraorbital region. Measurements are taken at high frequencies and the results are continually recorded on paper. The apparatus consists of 3 parts, the pulse generator, a control system and a recorder. The pulse generator produces the stimulating current in the form of constant current pulses with continually increasing current from 0–125 μA. The impulse frequency is 5/sec.

This series of impulses were lead through the tooth pulp of upper second incisor, on which a specially designed electrode was placed. This electrode stays fixed on the tooth during the whole trial. The electrical circuit leads from the generator over the tooth electrode through the pulp and connects through the body to an indifferent hand electrode which is fitted with a push button to interrupt the electrical stimulus. When the electrical current has risen to the stimulus threshold, the subject cuts off the series of impulses by using the push button.

The control apparatus causes an immediate interruption of the impulse series. The intensity of the current of the last impulse corresponds to the stimulus threshold and this is transmitted to the recorder where it is registered on the paper strip in relation to time and amperage. The control apparatus instigates the pulse generator to provide the next series of impulses.

Approximately 500 measurements of the stimulus threshold per hour are obtained and from these, the exact, precise recordings of the size and time of the stimulus threshold. The examples in Figures 1 to 3 illustrate this phenomenon. Figure 1 gives the values of the stimulus threshold during the effect of buccal local anaesthetic on a left, upper, second incisor (1 ml 2% lidocaine solution plus 4 mg % noradrenaline). The following points can be seen on the record:

(1) the preanaesthetic, physiological, stimulus threshold (27pA); (2) the duration of the injection (1 min); (3) the latent period from the beginning of the infiltration (*a*) to the beginning of the increase in stimulus threshold, and (*b*) to the increase of the stimulus threshold above the maximum stimulating current; (4) the rapid increase in stimulus threshold at the onset of the effect of the local anaesthetic; (5) the duration of action; (6) the (in contrast) more gradual decrease in effect; (7) the postanaesthetic stimulus threshold, which is slightly increased in comparison to the preanaesthetic threshold.

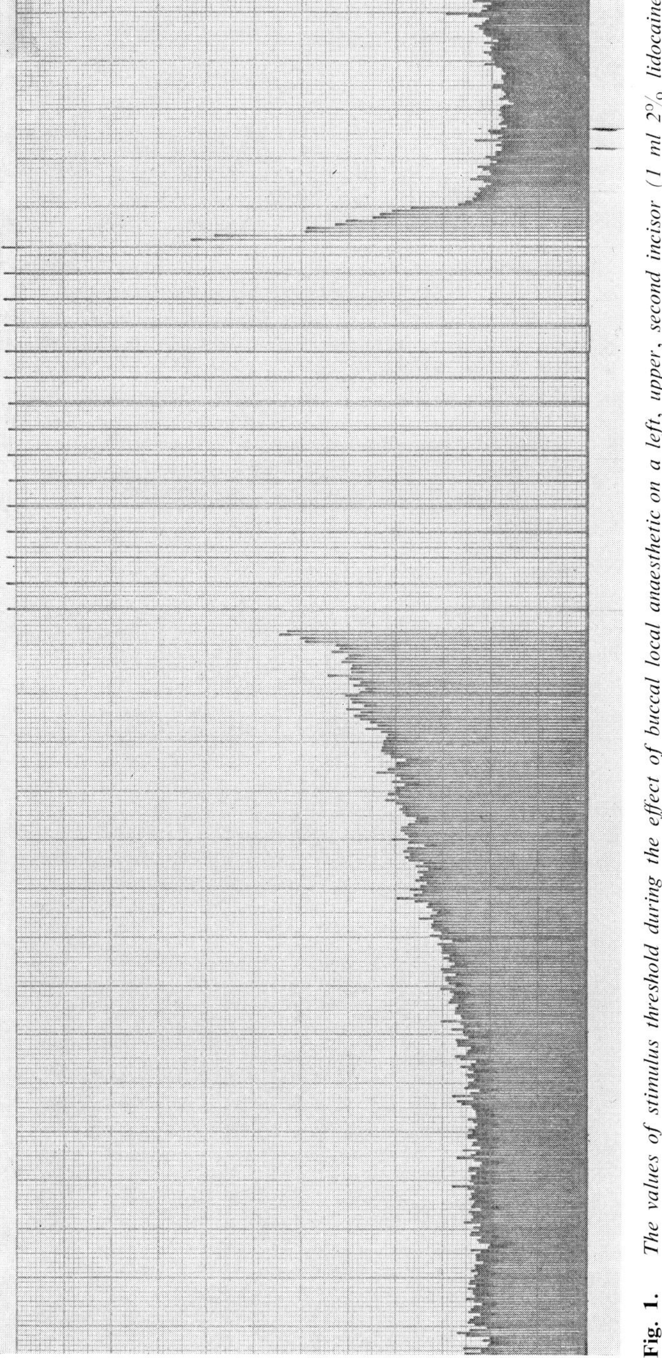

Fig. 1. The values of stimulus threshold during the effect of buccal local anaesthetic on a left, upper, second incisor (1 ml 2% lidocaine solution plus 4 mg% noradrenaline).

Figure 2 shows a record of measurements of stimulus threshold on a subject who had received 10 mg morphine. The stimulus threshold stays the same although psychical changes occurred. Figure 3 shows the results following acupuncture (acupuncture region D_4 and the infraorbital region). No increase in stimulus threshold could be demonstrated.

The advantages of this method compared to other methods of individual measurements are the automation of the control system and the recording apparatus. Because of the frequency of measurements, a reliable average measurement can be calculated. Accidental fluctuations, partly psychic (attention, distraction, etc.) partly vegetative (circulation, breathing) can be evened out, and technical mistakes in measurement, e.g. leakage of current due to moisture on the tooth, can be recognized immediately and corrected.

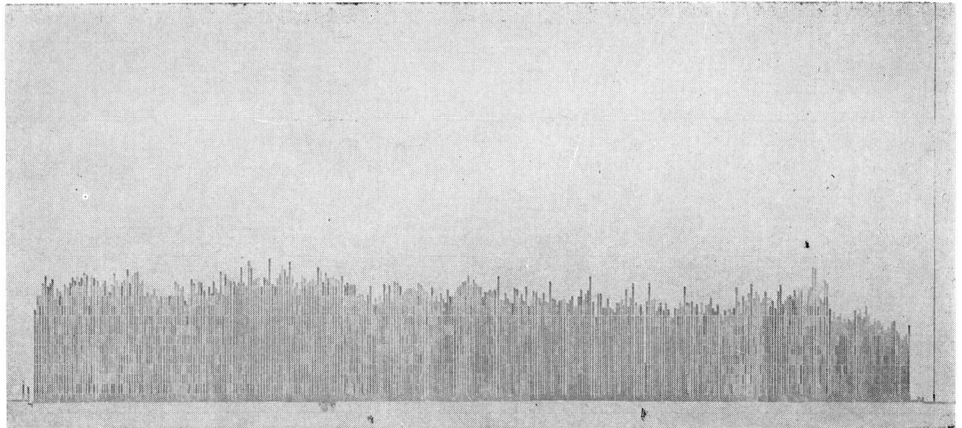

Fig. 2.   *A record of measurements of stimulus threshold on a subject who had received 10 mg morphine.*

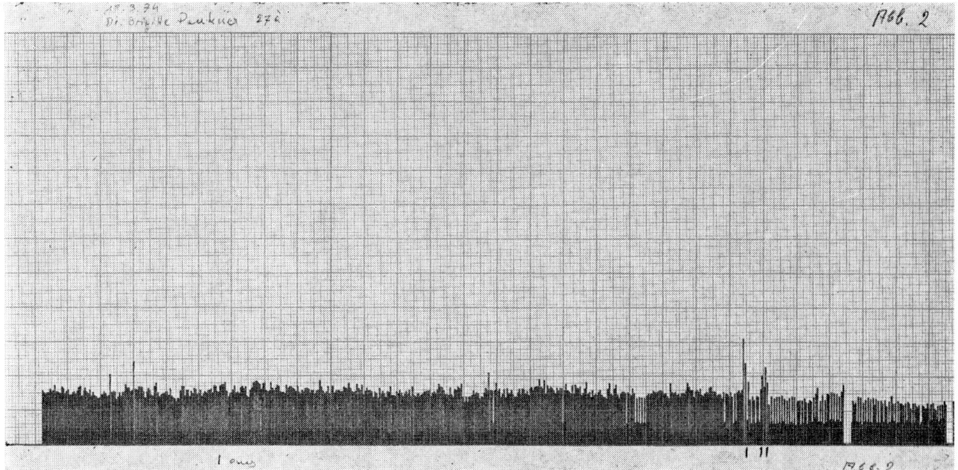

Fig. 3.   *Results following acupuncture (acupuncture region D_4 and the infraorbital region).*

RESULT

In none of the 12 subjects did acupuncture cause increase in the stimulus threshold. The same applies to morphine used as a comparison. Local anaesthetics always demonstrated clearly changes in the stimulus threshold with differences between different drugs and different vasoconstrictors. However, it should be mentioned that one subject, on whom the measurements of stimulus threshold were made, underwent 6 difficult tooth extractions under acupuncture. This was carried out with relative freedom from pain but no increase in the stimulus threshold could be demonstrated either.

Our results disagree with those of a group of Swedish authors (Andersson, Ericson, Holmgren and Lindquist) who demonstrated in their subjects, under similar conditions, a constant, small, increase in the stimulus threshold.

DISCUSSION

The experience 'pain' can be understood as a combination of 2 complicated processes. One includes all physical-chemical and neurophysiological mechanisms from the original pain stimulus through the stimulation of the receptors and the afferent sensory pathways in the 'pain' nerve fibres to the thalamus. This is the afferent system of pain stimulation. The other process includes all psychic and central neurophysiological phenomena, which are active because of the pain stimulus and involve the whole physical and psychical condition of the organism. This causes the evaluation of the pain stimulus and is the central system.

To confirm the above viewpoint, the pain-relieving or pain-removing drugs can be divided into 3 groups according to their points of attack: (*a*) drugs that operate on the peripheral nervous system and temporarily increase or decrease the pain stimulation, e.g. local anaesthetics; (*b*) drugs which operate on the central nervous system and influence the evaluation of pain to such an extent that the pain or the experience of a painful stimulus is temporarily increased or relieved (e.g. morphine); and (*c*) drugs with a combined effect.

The drugs from Group *a* (and *c*) provide a definite increase in the stimulus threshold. The drugs in Group *b* cause no increase. Acupuncture can be included in this group.

Acupuncture does not seem to interfere with the pain stimulus of the above stimulation mechanism, but works directly on the central nervous system. Using this hypothesis, it is possible that the stimulus threshold, that is the threshold for the stimulation which, under certain circumstances, can be converted into pain, can be determined during an acupuncture anaesthesia.

Stimulus threshold and pain threshold are not identical. The physiological stimulus threshold shows, in contrast to the pain threshold, no large, individual, and synchronised variations and it can be exactly determined by most subjects. It is lower than the pain threshold, so that by measurements the value of the stimulus threshold is determined first and the impulse series is cut off before the pain threshold is reached.

In conclusion, the stimulus threshold can be measured, but is not increased by acupuncture. The pain threshold is probably increased but is not easily measurable. Therefore, we can hardly measure the effect of pain or the effect of acupuncture anaesthesia with electrical measurements of the threshold.

Acupuncture anesthesia: The point of view of an American anesthesiologist

FRANCIS F. FOLDES

Departments of Anesthesiology, Montefiore Hospital and Medical Center, and
Albert Einstein College of Medicine, Bronx, N.Y., U.S.A.

I was requested to present the views of American anesthesiologists on acupuncture anesthesia (AA). Since there are differences of opinion between various American anesthesiologists especially with regard to the significance of the various factors for the success of AA and to the applicability of AA in the U.S.A., I cannot comply with this request. Instead of this I shall give you a brief account of the observations made in the course of a recent trip to the People's Republic of China (PRC) on AA research and the clinical use of AA in the PRC. Following this I shall relate to you my own views on the importance of the various complex factors that contribute to the success of AA in the PRC and will hazard some predictions on the applicability of AA in the Western world.

The observations to be related were made between May 1–22, 1974, when as a member of an Acupuncture Anesthesia Study group sponsored by the Committee on Scholarly Communication with the People's Republic of China, I had the privilege to visit the PRC. Our group consisted of 4 anesthesiologists, 5 neural scientists, 1 psychologist, 1 social scientist and a representative of the Committee on Scholarly Communication with the People's Republic of China. A comprehensive report of the group will be published, hopefully, in the near future. We observed 48 surgical procedures performed under AA in 15 hospitals in Peking, Shanghai and Kwangchow. We also had the opportunity to observe and/or discuss the results of experimental studies with AA on laboratory animals and human volunteers, in several Basic Science Departments of Medical Schools and Research Institutes.

Our Chinese hosts were extremely hospitable, showed the greatest concern for our comfort and did everything possible to make our stay in the PRC not only profitable, but also pleasant. I would like to express my sincere gratitude, individually and collectively to our hosts for the many courtesies extended to us.

OBSERVATIONS MADE

Animal experiments

It was demonstrated in the various research centers visited that neural activity evoked by noxious stimuli at various levels of the central nervous system could be partially or wholly inhibited by electrical or mechanical acupuncture stimulation.

In intact rabbits, restrained in a hammock, decreased sensitivity to radiant heat could be achieved by acupuncture stimulation. According to some Chinese investigators, however, decreased sensitivity could only be achieved in about 50% of the rabbits whom they termed 'clever rabbits'. The possibility that the 'still reaction' may have influenced the outcome of these experiments could not be excluded.

Human studies

Studies on human volunteers, not observed but related, to us indicated that pain threshold to experimental pain caused by potassium iontophoresis or pinprick can be raised by acupuncture stimulation. According to some Chinese investigators the increase in pain threshold was uniform all over the body, while others found a greater increase in some, than in other parts of the body. Chinese investigators also disagreed on the significance of the site of stimulation. Some emphasized the importance of the stimulation of classical acupuncture points (e.g., Ho-Ku, Tsu-San-li) for the elevation of the pain threshold while others were of the opinion that these points are only relatively specific. In evaluating the results of these studies it should be considered that the volunteers were aware of the nature of the acupuncture stimulus (Teh-Ch'i') and both they and the investigators were undoubtedly highly motivated to come up with positive results.

Clinical use

The clinical observations made related primarily to the operations. Our team had no opportunity to observe patient selection or preparation, and our information on these important aspects of anesthetic management is based solely on the sometimes conflicting statements made to us in different institutions. Thus, for example, we were told by some that old patients are less suitable and by others that they are more suitable than young adults for AA. Yet others told us that old age does not make any difference, but young children are not suitable subjects for AA. In some Children's Hospitals, however, AA is used, but we had no opportunity to observe AA in children.

We were told that AA is usually employed in good risk patients in whom the diagnosis is well established and no operative complications are expected. The advantages of AA and the disadvantages of general anesthesia are emphasized to the patients in whom the use of AA is contemplated. Those who voluntarily select AA are then usually subjected of acupuncture testing. If they do not tolerate acupuncture stimulation or if the needling does not produce the desired sensation of Teh-Ch'i', they are considered unsuitable for AA. The course of surgery is discussed with those selected and they are forewarned about the sensations to be experienced and are told that they might feel some pain or discomfort during surgery. They may or may not be visited again one or more times by the acupuncturist and/or the surgeon. The importance of patient cooperation with the members of the surgical team for the success of AA is also emphasized at these visits. Patients, especially before intrapleural operations, may also receive respiratory physiotherapy and are taught slow regular, abdominal breathing, Ch'i'-Kung.

Most, but not all patients, receive intramuscularly 100 mg pentobarbital sodium and/or 0.3 mg scopolamine hydrobromide 1–3 hr, and 30–50 mg Dolantin hydrochloride (meperidine) intravenously 10–15 min before skin incision. AA was often supplemented by infiltration of the skin, peritoneum, muscles, intercostal nerves or deep structures, presumably the vagus or autonomic ganglia, with 0.5–1.0% procaine or lidocaine.

All 48 operations witnessed by our group could be finished without having to resort to major supplementation. In 13 out of the 48 patients, however, there were signs of pain and/or discomfort that indicated that the procedure would not have been tolerated by Western patients. It was my impression that the operating conditions provided by AA (e.g., lack of muscular relaxation) would be unacceptable to our surgeons for intraperitoneal surgery.

The patients' physical condition during and immediately after surgery was excellent even when major intrapleural surgery, involving complete collapse of one lung, was performed without respiratory assistance or significant increase of the oxygen concentration of the inhaled gas mixture.

A PERSONAL VIEW OF THE MECHANISM OF ACUPUNCTURE ANESTHESIA

In my opinion AA is primarily a socio-political and psychological technique with a possibly minor contribution from the neurophysiological effect of needling.

The relatively minor role of needling is indicated by the findings that: (*a*) only hypalgesia and not analgesia can be produced by acupuncture stimulation in experimental animals and human volunteers; and (*b*) there is wide variation in the number, location and mode of stimulation of the acupuncture needles utilized in the provision of equally good operating conditions for the same surgical procedure in different institutions. Thus, for example, AA for craniotomy may be produced by placing one needle in the ear, or 2 needles in the ear and 2 needles in the lower extremity, or several needles in the vicinity of the operative field; for thoracotomy with one needle in the arm or 2 needles in the arm or up to 8 needles placed at various points; and for gastrectomy 6–8 needles placed at various sites in the vicinity or away from the site of incision.

The primary effect of acupuncture stimulation is probably due to the distraction of the patient's attention from the surgical stimulus by constant stimulation of one or more points. The needling probably also has a placebo effect and serves to reinforce the positive suggestions regarding the efficacy of AA made during the preoperative visit.

If, as I believe, the needling in itself contributes little to AA, which are those other factors that make possible the undoubtedly successful application of AA in the PRC?

Most, if not all patients before entering the hospital, are favorably influenced toward AA. They are told in the course of lectures, seminars and discussion groups regularly attended by all levels of the population in the PRC that AA is originally Chinese, that it is supported by their wise and universally adored leader, Chairman Mao as a prime example of combining Chinese and Western medicine and that it was suppressed by Liu Shai-chi's counter-revolutionaries. In the hospital this inclination toward AA is further increased by medical workers who are highly motivated to make AA, this great Chinese contribution to medicine, a success.

As described earlier, patients are carefully screened and in those selected, suggestions regarding the advantages of AA are reinforced by needling. The importance of their cooperation with the acupuncturist and the surgeon for the success of AA is also emphasized to them.

The psychologically prepared patients, who expect to experience some pain and discomfort are usually premedicated with sedatives and/or analgesics, but not to the point that they are unable to cooperate and so that they remain receptive to the continuous psychological reinforcement given by the acupuncturist who is in constant contact with the patient during surgery.

Although it is unlikely that there is any difference between normal individuals of different populations in the conduction and perception of noxious stimuli, the effect of pain and the reaction to it may be influenced by social and psychological factors and by the determination not to exhibit any manifestation of pain experienced. Such traits are by no means limited to the Chinese. Martyrs of the early Christian era and American Indians of the not too distant past were repeatedly described to be able to tolerate torture without showing any sign of pain. Even today there are tribes in New Guinea on whose females, adult circumcision is practiced without anesthesia. The Chinese are hardy, determined people, used to exertions in the course of their everyday life that would not be tolerated by most members of Western societies. Furthermore, it was my impression, that the highly motivated Chinese patients were determined not to show any signs of pain they may have experienced. This determination was evident from the great reluctance of even those patients who did exhibit signs of pain during surgery, to admit anything but minimal discomfort, when questioned later.

Competent, fast and gentle surgery and the willingness of the surgeons to adapt their technique to the operating conditions provided by AA also contribute significantly to the undoubtable success of this technique in the PRC.

THE APPLICABILITY OF ACUPUNCTURE ANESTHESIA IN WESTERN SOCIETIES

In my opinion, in the absence of the motivating socio-political factors, the unwillingness of our patient population to tolerate even minimal discomfort and the insistence of surgeons on operating conditions that are not always provided by AA, this technique, that works well in the PRC will not have wide applicability in our Western civilization. It is conceivable that AA will be successful in the hands of a few anesthesiologists with unusual suggestive power for certain surgical procedures in a limited number of patients. In these patients the socio-political factors operating in China will have to be replaced by other equally strong motivating factors.

Because of the extensive publicity received by AA in the news media and the prevailing sociological climate it will be necessary to conduct clinical trials with AA in the U.S.A. and other Western countries. In my opinion, however, these trials will have a negative result and AA will never play a significant role in the care of our surgical patients.

Acupuncture in pain

E. ALVAREZ SIMÓ

Joaquín Maria López 27, 3° D, Madrid 15, Spain

By the criteria of western medicine, acupuncture analgesia remains a mystery. In oriental medicine, it is an accepted phenomenon which however has not yet been fully explained. The fact remains that by using meridians and a series of points around them, it is possible to control various symptoms and to interrupt the transmission of pain.

For the western neurologist, pain results from a noxious stimulus to a nerve ending or receptor neurone, and is experienced in man as a disagreeable sensation in the stimulated areas. The pain phenomenon is also an alerting mechanism for the neuromuscular and vegetative systems. The total experience of pain is very complex involving neurophysiological, biochemical and psychological interactions; particularly important are influences arising from the reticular formation, and of course, psychological factors.

Modern concepts of pain take into account actual pain pathways, the 'simple' perception of painful stimuli at certain levels of the nervous system, the effects of emotion on pain, and the relationship of consciousness to pain.

For the scientific practitioner of acupuncture, be he western or eastern, acupuncture acts through definite neurological mechanisms, although its effects are enriched by the intuition that the good physician usually possesses. The physician's gifts of keen observation and an ability to integrate varying concepts appear in the old Chinese texts, and eastern medicine is of course considered the oldest in the world.

Acupuncture surely illustrates that there is a fundamental relationship between skin and nervous system – a relationship rediscovered in western medicine following embryological studies on ectodermal structures.

The meridians with their internal connections (by which for example we can modify some abnormalities of cortical and subcortical function by stimulation of the foot) may have their conceptional counterpart in the homunculus of modern neurology.

Both western and eastern acupuncturists have confirmed that transverse meridians are related to the corresponding metamera, and that the visceral-cutaneous segments are also intimately related to the longitudinal and transverse meridians of the segmental organization of the cerebrospinal axis.

To return to the western neurophysiological viewpoint, pain and touch stimuli activating peripheral receptors are relayed to the central nervous system by way of two different kinds of nerve fibers. The first kind, known as delta fibers, are myelinated, 3–4 μm in diameter, and conduct rapidly. The second, C fibers, are 0.5–2 μm in diameter, and conduct slowly. When fibers reach the spinal cord, accompanied by afferent fibers from the viscera and blood vessels, they divide into ascending and descending collaterals which spread over 2 or 3 segments to form the dorsolateral tract of Lissauer.

Some C fibers form the ipsilateral posterior pathway ventral to the posterior horn (Foester and Gagel). Connections, both direct and indirect via internuncial neurones (Rolando substance, Lecho II of Rexed) with the principal neurones are complex and give rise to the spinothalamic tract.

The spinothalamic tract originating in the posterior horn passes across the midline ventral to the central canal and travels rostrally in the anterolateral part of the cord on the contralateral side, but dividing into 2 main pathways:

a. The lemniscal system, forming the spinothalamic tract, which is monosynaptic, composed mainly of delta fibers, and is phylogenetically recent. These fibers are myelinated, 6–12 μm in diameter, and carry information (concerning sudden and localized pain) to the neothalamus.

b. The extra-lemniscal system, phylogenetically more ancient, made up of C fibers (immyelinated, predominantly 3–4 μm in diameter) polysynaptic with diffuse connections at different levels and mediating persistent or poorly localized pain stimuli. This system forms a larger tract relaying to the paleospinal thalamus, and seems to be involved with arousal and self-preservation. Perception of pain seems to depend particularly upon this pathway.

With respect to facial pain sensation, the lemniscal pathways pass through the principal sensory nucleus of the trigeminal, and pain and temperature fibers from the trigeminal, the facial, the glossopharyngeal and the vagus proceed into the spinal tract of the trigeminal. These two pathways are respectively projected to Lissauers tract and to the substantia gelatinosa of Rolando, giving rise to two crossed bulbar-thalamic pathways. One is dorsal (neospinothalamic) associated with the lemniscus, and projecting to the ventro-postero-medial thalamic nucleus, and the other ventral (paleospinothalamic) projecting to the reticular formation and the diffuse thalamic system.

Many different brain structures contribute to the perception of pain including the reticular formation, thalamus, rhinencephalon, hypothalamus and the neocortex – each with its specific role in pain perception. The thalamic system appears to have particular importance in determining 'emotional tone', the hypothalamic-rhinencephalic system vegetative and emotional reactions to pain, the autonomic system endocrine changes (via the pituitary) and the neocortex in the consciousness of pain.

Different western theories have attempted to explain the mechanism of pain sensation. The theory of Wall and Melzack (1965) proposes the existence of specialized fibers and the role of a particular organization of painful stimulation. According to this theory, the experience of pain depends on the balance between impulses in small and large fibers, with higher centres limiting the transmission of impulses into extra-lemniscal systems.

Lim (1965) defends another theory. He proposes the existence of pain-producing substances. He distinguishes between immediate pain and delayed pain. The 'first alarm system' relays immediate pain due to the traumatization of cutaneous endings, and the 'second alarm system' relays stimuli arising from tissue substances such as histamine, serotonin, bradykinins, neurokinin (the latter named by Lewis 'P-substance'). These substances are liberated by vasodilatation and increased vascular permeability accompanying ischemia and produce hyperalgesia when the insult is removed.

How do eastern doctors view the mechanism of pain transmission? Through my knowledge of acupuncture and my conversation with traditional and modern acupuncturists, I conclude that there are meridian circuits comparable to western neurophysiological and biochemical circuits. Besides this, acupuncturists believe that there are other less specific ways for the control of this mechanism, rather similar perhaps to modern communication systems in which codes permit the use of a single line for different messages, avoiding duplication of pathways.

With an understanding of the physiology of pain, how could acupuncture produce analgesia? If we consider that pain is a disturbance of the physiological equilibrium, of the Yin-Yang polarity, and bearing in mind that natural actions have equal and opposite reactions, we might propose that if there are physical or chemical elements capable of producing an excessive reaction in one area, there may exist other elements which are capable of opposing these and bringing about a return to equilibrium. It is clear that they exist, since we can restore equilibrium by a simple act such as placing a needle in a specific point, stimulating some physical circuits and regulating the equilibrium of ions by its intervention in the milieu.

Before beginning physiological investigations about pain production, it is necessary to consider the role of psychological factors. We should first exclude hypnosis, a real phenomenon but limited to 10% of patients. Acupuncture, according to Japanese work at Nakayama, can be effective in 90% of patients. Verification is simple; if needles are placed in areas which do not correspond to acupuncture points, the required result will either not be obtained or will be very modest in suggestible individuals. One indisputable argument in favour of acupuncture is its efficacy in animals.

It is not in context to describe the mode of action of anesthetic agents, local and general. Anesthesia is obtained, however, by a greater or lesser intoxication of the nervous system (*'True transgression of the physiological order'* – see H. K. Becker (1961): *Actual situation and perspectives of the anaesthesia. Triangle 1*, pp. 11–15). We must consider instead what acupuncture can do and indicate the levels of pain control and analgesia which it can produce without a 'toxic handicap'.

In acupuncture there are long and short circuits, local and distant points. Modern Chinese acupuncturists such as Dr Chao-Son Teng, think that the pathways involved are lemniscal, and that with acupuncture we act primarily upon the thalamic level. His research at the Taiwan School (which we visited during our recent stay in China), has verified at autopsy that patients with lack of pain sensation in life had lesions of the thalamic intralaminar zone. They drew the conclusion that analgesia acts on this intralaminar zone through inhibitory influences transmitted via the proprio-spinal-reticular-thalamic pathway.

They have observed, in the studies concerning 'needle-pain abolition', 3 phenomena relevant to acupuncture:

1.   In order for acupuncture to be effective it is necessary to feel the needle, to feel the 'CHI'. This is a sensation radiating upwards and downwards. Actuation is not effective.
2.   When the needle is introduced deeply and correctly, these sensations do not amount to pain.
3.   If the needle is placed only in the skin, there is little benefit, but it becomes effective if deeply placed.

With respect to intradermal and small needles, as often used in Japan, it seems that they can be effective if they are introduced for 24 hr or for some days. We do not use them as occasionally, when placed around the orbit for example, they can produce a sympathetic reaction, showing that these receptors are different from those concerned with pain. Large needles soothe not only somatic but also visceral pain.

The Taiwan workers postulate that when the sensation arising from a needle reaches the intralaminar nuclear zone, pain inhibition occurs by 2 mechanisms:
a.   Via the secondary zone of the cortex. Where this is destroyed absence of pain but preservation of other sensations are found.
b.   Another route goes to the primary sensory cortex; a lesion at this level produces a total loss of sensation including pain.

They thus consider that through one or both pathways it is possible to inhibit pain, the 'pain centers' being localized in the complex nucleus of the thalamus, the primary sensory cortex, ventro-lateral or median thalamic areas, and in the secondary sensory cortex via the thalamic posterior nuclei.

Is this inhibition physical or physico-chemical? I have been considering this problem for several years, and reviewing the results obtained on an impressive number of patients who have benefited from acupuncture. The inhibition of pain is 2-fold; besides acupuncture, I complete treatment with medicines based on oligoelements elaborated with a high molecular division permitting them to act as catalysts for altered metabolism, and with these methods I have been able to duplicate the effects achieved with acupuncture.

I also think, and here I agree with well known acupuncturists such as La Fuye, that these micro-traumatizations should act similarly to homeopathy, based on the fact that infinitesimal doses of drugs, some of them very toxic, can alternate the symptoms or diseases which, in greater doses, they can produce.

Some of these facts are evident but it remains hard to explain in terms of physical circuits how it is possible to produce analgesia or to suppress any other symptoms. For example, from ear points one can influence every kind of disorder, independently of the classical meridians. What role do ionic changes, produced by rupture of cell membranes by the needle, play? The physiological laboratory is the current arbiter of scientific truth. In our official research centres I have been unable to find the right person to undertake the full investigation of the physiological basis of acupuncture, and thus I discuss the idea with a view to stimulating interest in this important problem.

REFERENCES

Will be supplied by the author upon request.

The origin of acupuncture dates as far back as thousands of years in China and has long been used for alleviation of pain and therapy of diseases. Acupuncture together with herb medicine had played a most active part in curative means until the introduction of European medicine. The details of its therapeutic procedure were published before Christ in such books as 'Huang Di', 'Nei Ching', 'Lin Shu' and 'Su Wen' which we can read even today.

In recent years, however, it has been reported in China that this time-honored acupuncture is utilized for anesthesia at surgical treatments in a number of cases. Acupuncturing special points of the body lowers the sense of pain in the corresponding special region, thus enabling operation. On the other hand, there is a simple doubt whether or not acupuncture anesthesia actually enables surgical treatment and, in fact, many Western doctors have suspicion on its effects. Here, I would like to introduce our experiences in which we carried out surgical treatment and medical tests in the neurosurgical region by utilizing acupuncture anesthesia.

The subjects were patients in the Department of Otorhinolaryngology, Showa University and in the Department of Neurosurgery, Tokyo Teishin Hospital. With respect to medical tests, PEG and air myelography were conducted for 81 and 10 cases, respectively (Fig. 1).

No.	Initials	Age	Sex	Test	No.	Initials	Age	Sex	Test	No.	Initials	Age	Sex	Test	No.	Initials	Age	Sex	Test
1	O.S.	45	M	Air Myelography	27	S.T.	28	M	PEG	53	N.O.	25	M	PEG	79	I.H.	40	M	PEG
2	M.Y.	58	M	Air Myelography	28	K.S.	30	M	Air Myelography	54	K.Y.	53	M	PEG	80	K.M.	46	M	PEG
3	F.S.	31	M	PEG	29	S.W.	44	M	PEG	55	K.S.	30	M	PEG	81	T.K.	17	M	PEG
4	F.Y.	21	F	PEG	30	K.M.	54	M	PEG	56	T.S.	9	M	PEG	82	H.U.	24	F	Air Myelography
5	N.K.	46	F	PEG	31	H.T.	42	M	PEG	57	S.K.	30	M	PEG	83	Y.K.	30	F	PEG
6	C.S.	58	F	PEG	32	S.S.	32	M	Air Myelography	58	K.A.	25	M	Air Myelography	84	S.K.	15	M	PEG
7	H.K.	32	M	PEG	33	K.N.	30	F	PEG	59	N.H.	30	M	PEG	85	F.K.	32	F	PEG
8	K.K.	28	M	PEG	34	H.T.	42	M	PEG	60	G.O.	53	M	PEG	86	K.C.	68	M	PEG
9	S.M.	23	M	PEG	35	K.Y.	43	M	PEG	61	H.S.	61	F	PEG	87	S.M.	43	M	PEG
10	S.H.	36	M	PEG	36	K.A.	25	M	PEG	62	T.I.	39	M	PEG	88	H.S.	39	M	PEG
11	S.H.	32	F	PEG	37	M.T.	46	M	PEG	63	W.S.	45	M	Air Myelography	89	U.K.	58	M	PEG
12	S.K.	27	M	Air Myelography	38	F.K.	30	F	PEG	64	T.I.	39	M	PEG	90	D.C.	44	F	PEG
13	O.H.	34	M	PEG	39	T.A.	51	M	Air Myelography	65	E.Y.	23	M	PEG	91	O.S.	40	M	PEG
14	K.M.	30	M	PEG	40	H.K.	42	M	PEG	66	K.S.	42	M	PEG					
15	I.K.	24	M	PEG	41	K.I.	44	M	PEG	67	E.Y.	23	M	PEG					
16	T.Y.	32	M	PEG	42	C.H.	42	F	PEG	68	H.U.	9	M	PEG					
17	H.J.	31	M	PEG	43	T.Y.	26	F	PEG	69	S.H.	22	M	PEG					
18	A.T.	22	M	PEG	44	S.N.	50	M	PEG	70	T.D.	72	M	PEG					
19	D.T.	24	M	PEG	45	T.O.	30	M	PEG	71	O.S.	55	F	PEG					
20	T.Y.	33	M	PEG	46	T.N.	57	M	PEG	72	K.K.	23	M	PEG					
21	S.K.	27	M	Air Myelography	47	N.M.	20	M	PEG	73	K.G.	75	M	PEG					
22	F.T.	43	M	PEG	48	W.K.	30	M	PEG	74	T.K.	17	F	PEG					
23	H.K.	36	M	PEG	49	O.S.	46	M	PEG	75	O.M.	45	M	PEG					
24	K.K.	65	F	PEG	50	Y.K.	32	M	PEG	76	S.K.	50	M	PEG					
25	G.Y.	50	M	PEG	51	K.S.	28	F	PEG	77	K.S.	50	M	PEG					
26	M.M.	30	F	PEG	52	T.K.	24	M	PEG	78	M.T.	17	M	PEG					

Fig. 1. *Number of cases tested under acupuncture anesthesia.*

716

Surgical treatment was performed in the following 35 cases, 4 cases of PVG, 3 cases of cranioplasty, 4 cases of chronic subdural hematoma, one case of epicranial formation, 2 cases of pituitary tumor, one case of brain tumor (metastasis of lung cancer to the brain), 6 cases of epicranial laceration, 2 cases of hypogrossofacial anastomosis (skin suture of child's leg), and one case of attachment of male 'Ommaya' tube and so on (Fig. 2). Among the cases of medical tests, favourable effects were found except in 3 cases of PEG and 2 cases of air myelography. As for the cases of surgical treatment, operation could not be conducted at all in one case of pituitary tumor but the effect persisted until the treatment of the tumor in the other case.

1	F.F.	58	F	L—PVG
2	K.S.	45	F	L—Chronic Subdural Hematoma
3	D.H.	48	F	L—Scalp Laceration
4	F.F.	58	F	L—Hypogrossofacial Anastmosis
5	O.S.	46	M	L—Chronic Subdural Hematoma
6	C.S.	58	F	Pituitary Tumor
7	S.S.	45	M	L—Cranioplasty
8	S.T.	18	M	R—Cranioplasty
9	H.K.	33	M	Pituitary tumor
10	S.S.	45	M	L—Scalp wound
11	Y.U.	32	F	R—Hypogrossofacial Anastmosis
12	W.S.	44	M	R—Ventriclopleural Shunt
13	I.S.	31	M	R—Cranioplasty
14	K.M.	67	M	R—Chronic Subdural Hematoma
15	K.T.	35	M	L—Scalp Laceration
16	K.H.	66	M	Brain Tumor(metastasis of lung carcinoma)
17	A.G.	7	M	Skrin closure of L lower extremity
18	S.T.	9	M	bilateral P V G
19	K.S.	35	M	R scalp wound
20	O.S.	52	M	R chronic subdural hematoma
21	S.T.	9	M	OMMAYA tube
22	K.G.	40	M	Laceration of R forehead
23	K.H.	26	M	lipoma of occipital region
24	Y.E.	23	M	L P V G
25	K.S.	35	M	R scalp wound
26	Y.E.	23	M	R P V G
27	N.T.	32	M	tumor of R shoulder
28	H.H.	36	M	Osteoma
29	O.S.	55	F	R—PVG
30	T.K.	17	F	R—PVG
31	S.H.	60	M	R—Cranioplasty
32	T.K.	17	F	OMMAYA tube
33	K.K.	25	M	Scalp Laceration
34	I.M.	31	M	Depressed Fracture
35	Y.K.	30	F	R—PVG

Fig. 2. *Number of cases operated under acupuncture anesthesia.*

SELECTION OF ACUPUNCTURING POINTS

Conspicuous effects were noticed successfully in the other cases except one case each of cranioplasty and epicranial suture.

Acupuncturing points utilized in these surgical treatment are classified into 'main holes' such as 'Ho Ku',* 'Nei Kuang'* and 'Tsu San Li'* and into 'supplementary holes' such as 'I Fong',* 'Fung Tsu',* 'Chu Tsu',* 'Hou Shi',* 'Jia Che',* 'She Kuang'* and 'Pai Jie'.* 'Main holes' indicate points located in the head, neck and the body, and the main holes

---

* These are special names of body parts in Chinese medicine.

given above are also known as 'original holes' or 'mother holes' to which acupuncture can be applied safely without any ill-effects. 'Ho Ku' has been utilized in acupuncture from of old as a point for treatment of sore throat, belly-ache, and brachial paralysis. In the same way, 'Nei Kuang' is known to be effective for coughing and headache and 'Tsu San Li' for belly-ache and brachial paralysis.

The 'supplementary holes' are such points as utilized to improve 'alleviating effect' when distinct anesthetic effect cannot be obtained by the sole acupuncture of the main holes. The acupuncture anesthesia is usually done as follows: when acupuncture is performed into point(s), the presence of needle sensibility, in other words 'response', so called by acupuncturists or named 'Tu Chi' in China, should be confirmed and then the needle(s) is electrified with a Chinese electric anesthesia machine. In our case, both sides of 'Ho Ku', 'Nei Kuang', and both sides of 'Tsu San Li' are electrified for 30–40 min, which lowers sense of pain at the face, head, neck and navel, and makes surgical treatment of those parts possible. The sense of pain drops down to 6–7 in comparison with 10 of the normal one.

Acupuncture anesthesia has by no means a painless effect but more accurately 'an alleviating' effect that enables operation. It appears that there is not always sufficient consistency between regions where sense of pain lowers and the anatomical nerve supply. Further, no definite boundary can be drawn between such regions and those where sense of pain never lowers. The relation between acupuncturing points and region of lowered pain is still wrapped in mystery. One of the characteristics of acupuncture anesthesia lies in that it lowers only sense of pain but has no effect upon senses of pressure, temperature, biblation and shaking. In addition, acupuncture seems to have a delicate effect upon blood pressure, making hypotension higher and hypertension lower. That is the reason why acupuncture has been said from of old to have *a delicate accommodative action on the human body.*

In the strict sense of the word, old acupuncture and today's acupuncture anesthesia are not identical. The old one is 'Chu Chen' which means putting a needle, while today's one is 'Nen Chen' which means twisting a needle, or is electrified acupuncture because little lasting effect can be expected in the former. The stimulating effect of the latter is by far the higher than that of the electrified acupuncture. In surgery as well, less bleeding is usually observed than with an anesthetic. Little effect on blood pressure, pulse, and respiration is noticed and the 'alleviating effect' lasts 2–3 hr following extraction of needle after operation. In fact, in our own cases, an analgesic was scarcely administered. A patient has a clear consciousness and can eat and drink during operation. It appears that better results can be expected under such a condition as a patient can eat and drink and is informed of the progress of his own operation (this is different from mesmerism). It is also required that a patient can see the external world freely.

As mentioned above, postoperative administration of analgetics is hardly needed and the control of respiration that is required after total anesthesia is not necessary. Accordingly, an oxygen tent is not used in ordinary circumstances. In many cases the patients were able to eat and drink after operation and were able to walk to the lavatory. Furthermore, ill-effects such as nausea and vomiting that are usually observed after total anesthesia were not recognized.

APPLICATION EXAMPLES OF ACUPUNCTURE ANESTHESIA

Based on these experiences it may be said that general anesthesia, local anesthesia and acupuncture anesthesia are not antagonistic but complementary. Whereas in operation in the neurosurgical region treating in particular the functions of body, the result of operation under general or topical anesthesia cannot be evaluated until coming round from narcosis due to the motor paralysis and to the impediment of consciousness, in acupuncture anesthesia in which consciousness is kept normal and there occurs no paralysis, the result of operation can be evaluated instantly. Thus, acupuncture anesthesia in neurosurgical treatment is said to be one of the best applications. In our experiences, the anastomosis between hypoglossal nerve and facial nerve can be given as a good example. Electric stimulus was given to a branch of hypoglossal nerve by making the patient put out his tongue during the operation to confirm the excursion of the tongue and to identify that the nerve is not the hypoglossal one itself but its branch, and then the anastomosis with facial nerve was carried out. The following 2 examples are given as the other suitable applications.

The first example is of a 66-year-old male. The administration of Breomycin for treatment of his carcinoma of the penis induced fibrosis in the lung. In addition, WPW syndrome was detected through EKG in this patient and acupuncture anesthesia was applied to remove his chronic subdural hematoma. Second example is of a 60-year-old male who subjected to lobectomy of the right lung due to adenocarcinoma. Acupuncture anesthesia was applied for craniotomy to treat cerebral metastasis in the right hemisphere of the brain and a satisfactory result was obtained.

Total or local anesthesia is also applicable to these cases but considering the progress during and after operation, acupuncture is presumably better. In the unsuccessful case of pituitary tumor, 'Ho Ku', 'Nei Kuang', and 'Tsu San Li' were used as main holes together with 'Pai Jie' and ear needle as supplementary ones. No problem occurred at the incision of skin and no pain was complained of at craniotomy and the incision of meninges.

The lower part of pars temporalis of meninges is the sensorial area of trigeminal nerve where the alleviating effect was confirmed by acupuncturing the abovementioned points. At the same time, the sense of pain at the sella turcica was lowered though not sufficiently. In spite of some alleviating effect in both skull and sella turcica which are commonly under the control of trigeminal nerve, it is very interesting that a certain difference in alleviation between them was observed. It should be noted here that extensive pain of the skin at craniotomy and an echoing sensation in the whole head at the use of neuroairtome during craniotomy are inevitable by acupuncture anesthesia.

We have only a limited number of clinical experiences and have to increase these hereafter. Faults of acupuncture anesthesia lie in that it is not effective in every symptom, that it accompanies some pain at the incision of skin, and that the tonus of the muscle remains during operation of the abdominal parts. In the neurosurgical region, however, the tonus of the muscle does not matter very much and hence acupuncture anesthesia is regarded to be more suitable. We employ acupuncture also to pains of cancer. Although it cannot be concluded definitely owing to the lack of cases tested, it seems to be effective in 'a certain stage' of cancer (see Fig. 3).

As you can see, acupuncture anesthesia has recently moved into a new limelight but its functional mechanism is still clouded with mystery. On the basis of our experiences, however, the best result is obtained when acupuncture is carried out by selecting points according to legends handed down from ancient times.

In order to explain the mechanism of acupuncture anesthesia, some persons insist on the gate control theory but from clinical experiences I am rather negative: (1) Since the muscle contraction occurs at the electrification with a Chinese electric anesthesia machine, is the antidromic stimulation not involved? (2) Does it not control pains at the upper part than the spinal cord, i.e., the upper part including the *reticular formation of the brain-stem?* (3) In particular, is not the *reticular formation* of the brain-stem involved? We have such impressions, judging from the fact that acupuncture anesthesia is more effective in the abdominal part and the pectoral limb than in the pelvic limb and further effective in the head and neck than in the pectoral limb and that it is not very effective in the surgical treatment of the spinal cord.

The reason why the sense of pain at the head, neck, and navel is lowered by acupuncturing

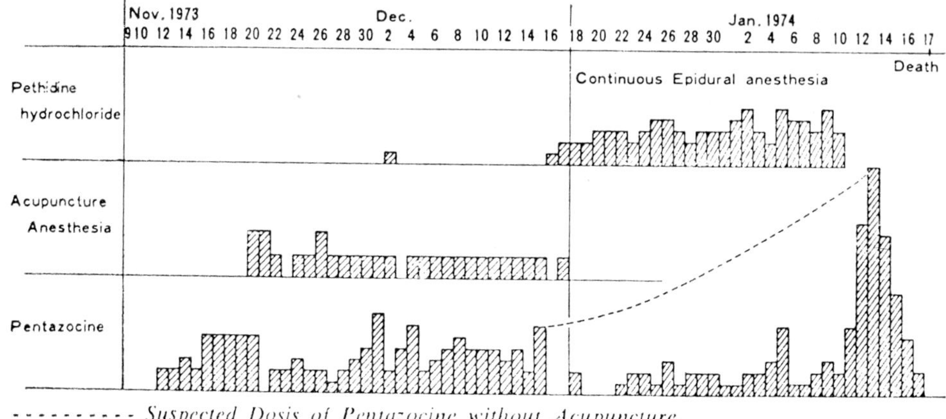

Fig. 3.   *Case of a 40-year-old woman (K.A.), with clinical diagnosis peritonitis carcinomatosa and pathological diagnosis ovarian tumor (?). History: 1971, right mamma carcinoma operated; 1972, abnormal swelling of the lower abdomen; Jan., 1972, admitted to hospital – abnormal increase of ascites; July, 1972, lumbago, metastasis to chest and lymph node; Oct., 1972, discharged; Nov. 9th, 1972, readmitted due to lumbago, abnormal abdominal swelling, general malaise and intractable pain; Nov. 20th, 1972, acupuncture anesthesia began; Dec. 2nd., 1972, very severe abdominal pain, lumbago and general malaise presented, pethidine hydrochloride applied for the first time; Dec. 18th, 1972, continuous epidural anesthesia began (acupuncture no more effective); Jan. 17th, 1974, died. Note: At the beginning and middle stage of intractable cancer pain acupuncture anesthesia is effective but at the end stadium acupuncture is no more effective. Continuous epidural anesthesia and a large amount of pethidine hydrochloride were applied.*

such *acupuncture points* as 'Ho Ku' and 'Nei Kuang' that are located apart from the head and neck is utterly unknown and awaits clarification.

It is difficult to reckon the effect of acupuncture as a simple one, considering that acupuncture has been utilized from of old not only for anesthesia but for treatment of hemiplegia, dysacousis, stiff neck, scapulohumeral periarthritis, vertigo, and nausea in addition to various long-established treatments. The gate control theory may throw light on the effect of acupuncture upon alleviation of pain, but is inexplicable for its effective actions on various diseases mentioned above. On the basis of the multifarious effects of acupuncture, it should be judged that the working point of acupuncture lies in the brain stem, i.e., reticular formation of brain stem rather than in the spinal cord. However, it is fairly difficult to give direct proof that acupuncture acts on the reticular formation of the brain stem, because of its complexity as already stated. In order to prove this, optokinetic nystagmus (OKN) which is called EEG of the brain stem, was employed. As OKN, however, is not applicable to normal subjects, such cases as are suspected to have some lesion in the brain stem, that is, *cases created by the Will of God*, have to be selected. One of the suitable cases is idiopathic congenital nystagmus. Accordingly, one case of jerking type nystagmus and another case of pendular type nystagmus were selected: *Case 1.* jerking type nystagmus, 35-year-old male; *Case 2.* pendular type nystagmus, 10-year-old male.

RESULT

Acupunctured points were: Ho Ku, Nai Kuang and Tsu San Li on both sides. Electrization was performed with a Chinese electronarcosis apparatus. OKP tests were carried out before electrization and 40 min after electrizaton. The optokinetic stimulation was conducted at angular acceleration of 4° up to 160° and subsequently at —4° C up to 0°. The results were recorded at a paper speed of 1 mm/sec and of 5 mm/sec with an electronystagmograph (ENG) manufactured by Sanei Electric Co.

It is clearly seen that the optokinetic nystagmus was facilitated, when OKP tests are compared before and after acupuncture as shown in Figures 4, 5 and 6. Here, I will try only to mention the result of Case 2.

DISCUSSION

It is said that idiopathic congenital nystagmus shows only nystagmus and lacks other neurological symptoms. Congenital nystagmus which could be caused a posteriori, for example, by head injury, is regarded to be attributable to a slight impediment in the brain stem and is very much hereditary. The idiopathic congenital nystagmus is closely related with and influenced by alertness and sleep. The alertness is connected with the level of consciousness and further with the ascending activating system of the brain stem, in particular, reticular formation, which may bring on a change on nystagmus. This means

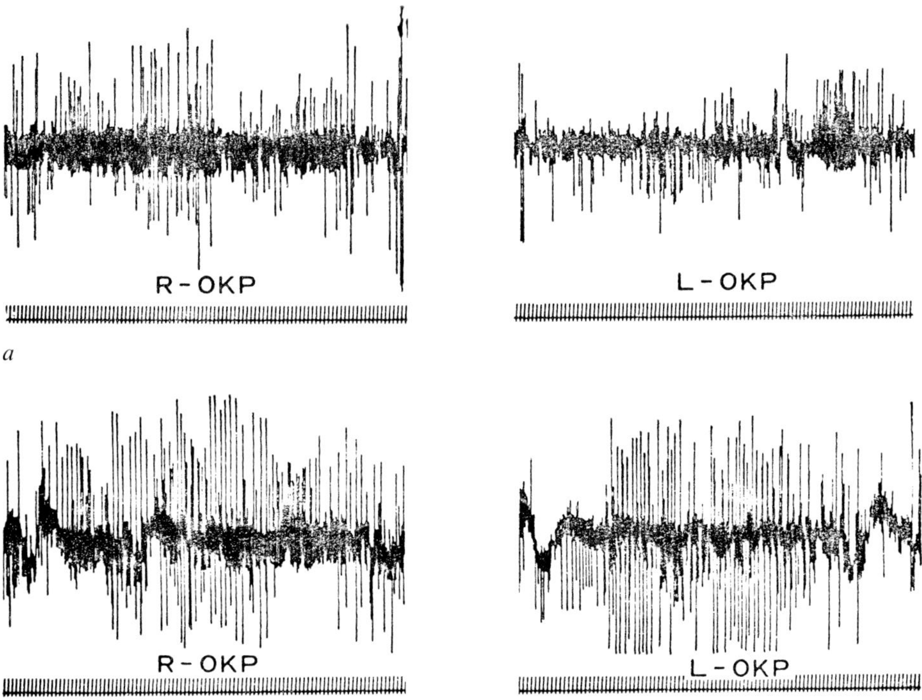

Fig. 4. *(a) Before acupuncture, and (b) after acupuncture. Note: Remarkable facilitation of optokinetic nystagmus after acupuncture (optokinetic pattern shown here).*

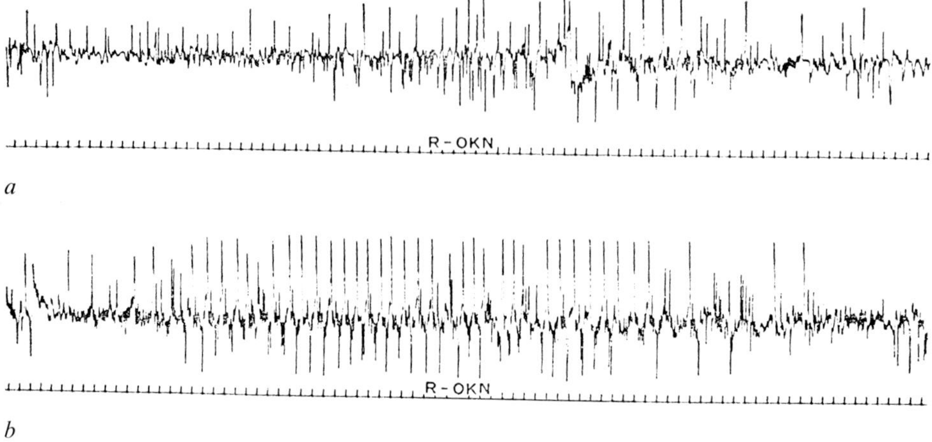

Fig. 5.   *(a) Before acupuncture, and (b) after acupuncture. Note: Remarkable facilitation of optokinetic nystagmus obtained after acupuncture (right OKN).*

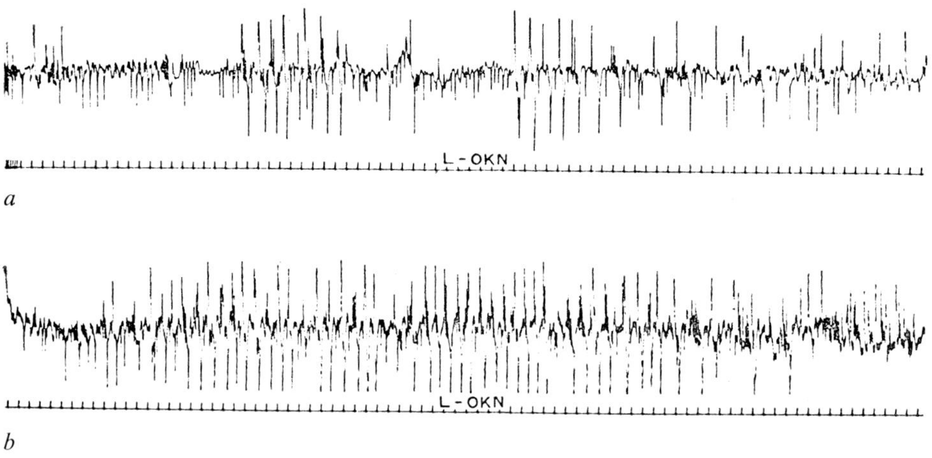

Fig. 6.   *(a) Before acupuncture, and (b) after acupuncture. Note: Remarkable facilitation of optokinetic nystagmus obtained after acupuncture (left OKN).*

the presence of a simultaneous influence upon optokinetic nystagmus. The facilitation of OKN for optokinetic stimulation by acupuncture is presumably caused by its effect on the reticular formation. The optokinetic nystagmus consists of a slow phase that is pursue eye movement and of a quick phase that moves reflectively and rhythmically. The effect of acupuncture upon OKN should be supposed at present not to be an influence upon the quick and slow phases but to be a facilitation to OKN itself.

As the exact lesion is not yet known for idiopathic congenital nystagmus, the origin of this morbid nystagmus remains unsolved. But the effect of reticular formation on OKN can be grasped because the frequency of OKN is apparently increased, for instance, by calculation. Therefore it may be said that acupuncture has an effect on reticular formation,

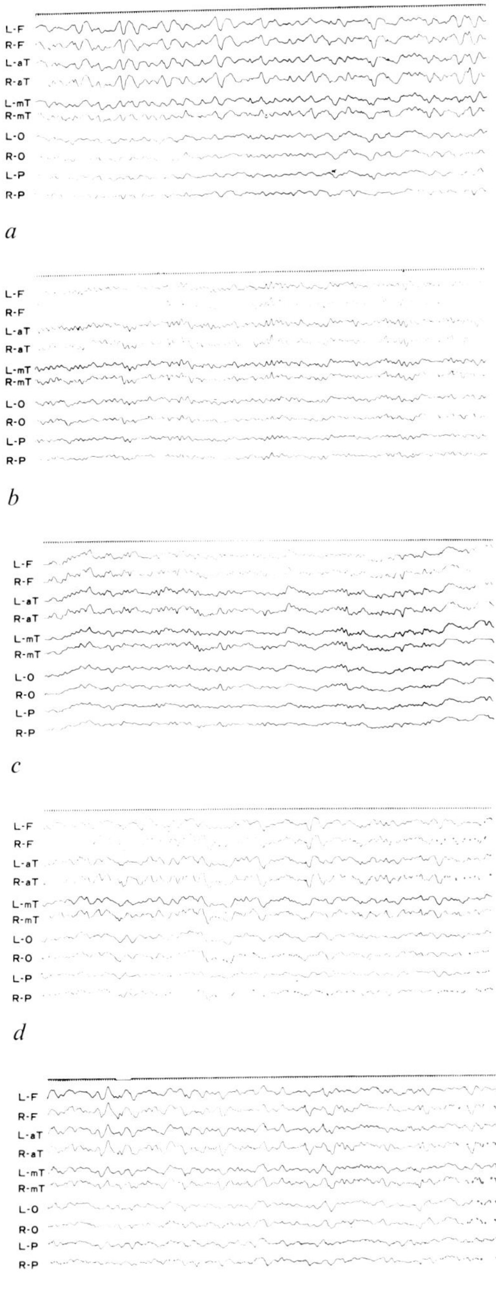

Fig. 7. *(a) Before acupuncture, (b) just after acupuncture (60 min acupuncture stimulation 0), (c) 30 min after acupuncture, (d) 60 min after acupuncture, and (e) 120 min after acupuncture. Note: facilitation of EEG after acupuncture, this effect lasting for 120 min after removal of the needle. This EEG facilitation may be caused by the stimulation of the ascending activating system in the brain stem.*

resulting in facilitation of OKN. But it is difficult to suppose that the effect has an influence upon the ascending activating system because the fact that some of the patients (not all) fall asleep during acupuncture is inexplicable if acupuncture should have an effect on this system and give some influence upon the level of consciousness. On the contrary, it should be supposed that the abovementioned facilitation to idiopathic congenital nystagmus works also on the ascending activating system, inducing some patients to lead euphoric facial expression during operation and the other patients to sleep (by monotonous and rhythmical stimulation).

I will explain acupuncture's effectiveness to reticular formation by citing another case – that of a 55-year-old female. Right acoustic tumor was observed at the cerebellopontine angle during operation. Subtotal removal of the tumor as large as a small hen's egg was done through operation. Postoperative course was not smooth and she died 31 days after operation. Figure 7 (a–e) shows EEG record taken 3 days prior to death, which was attributed to a gradual softening of the brain stem. The cause of death may be due to clipping of the medial or central side and cutting of fine arteries fed from the basilar artery to the brain stem. From the 14th postoperative day, α-activity tended to be activated by acupuncture (needle stimulation) in EEG records. EEG shows that activation was observed even 60 or 120 min after needle stimulation. In other words, Θ-wave becomes α-wave and Δ-wave becomes Θ-wave by acupuncture activation.

Even after removal of the needle, after-effect of acupuncture stimulation was observed in EEG up to 60 or 120 min after stimulation. This conforms well with the clinical experiences that, even after the removal of the needle during acupuncture anesthesia, its effect lasts for 1–3 hr. It is well-known that EEG is facilitated by peripheral high frequency stimulation. Needle stimulation, 2-3-4/cps (low frequency stimulation) is different from the abovementioned high frequency stimulation.

Reticular formation in the brain stem is said to be related to the maintenance of level of consciousness.

Magoun describes that the ascending activating system in the mid-brain stem acts to maintain the level of consciousness. In this case, gradual softening of brain stem results in gradual destruction of the ascending activating system, thus lowering the level of consciousness. At this time (Θ-wave and α-wave were observed in EEG from approximately the 5th day after her death) it is considered that peripheral acupuncture stimulation acts on reticular formation, especially ascending activating system, and ascending activating system activated by acupuncture facilitates brain function (Θ-wave becomes α-wave, Δ-wave becomes Θ-wave as shown in the figure).

How to explain the activation of reticular formation by needle stimulation? It may be considered that neurohumoral function was activated by needle stimulation.

Serotonine and catecholamine contained more in the raphe of brain stem have a close relationship with each other. However, needle stimulation facilitates the release of catecholamine, and its chemical substance is related to activation of reticular formation, which may result in continuation of acupuncture's effectiveness.

The relationship between acupuncturing points and pain-lowered region, and between the positions for needle insertion selected and curative effect of particular diseases awaits elucidation. Hereafter we intend to solve these problems.

ACKNOWLEDGEMENT

This paper is dedicated to courageous La Fu Sing, U Ching Fang, Dr Chang Wei Shui, Monardau, Ou Ching Shii, and many unknown heroes of Taiwan, China, 28th February, 1975.

*Possible pathway of large intestine meridian**

MING K. LIN

Department of Anesthesiology, National Taiwan University Hospital, Taipei, Taiwan

Acupuncture analgesia, using Large Intestine Meridian 4 (LI/) allowed Caldwell Luc operation to be performed without any pain. Is this due either to hypnosis or to the acupuncture? With modern medical knowledge it is difficult to understand this phenomenon. This report is an observation based on Western medical views about the relationship between the sensory innervation of the hand and face in acupuncture practice, namely Large Intestine Meridian.

MATERIAL AND METHODS

This study was carried out with patients either for facial operations or for pain treatment at the National Taiwan University Hospital. The patients were adult, for Caldwell Luc operations, and scheduled for local anesthesia. Each patient was premedicated as usual for local anesthesia. The non-surgical patients suffering from maxillary cancer pain or from trigeminal neuralgia were also subject. A simple explanation was given to them about the insertion of the needles in their skin.

The acupuncture points LI_4 and Pericardium Meridian 6 (P_6) were employed for operations or for the treatment of pain. In some cases Heart Meridian 1 (H_1), stellate ganglion and the fibres from the first thoracic sympathetic ganglion (T_1) were also used. After the needle was inserted at these points, 2 pairs of electrodes of a stimulator generating a pulse at 2–3 V, 3–4 Hz were connected between LI_4 and P_6. If the feeling of numbness was above both elbows, the surgeon was instructed to begin surgery without asking or testing for a painful response. If pain occurred a local anesthetic agent was added; these cases were failures. The cases with tolerable pain or no pain were successes.

Some other experiments on cadavers about the anatomy of Stomach Meridian 36 (S_{36}) and LI_4 with the observatory results were described in the discussion section for related considerations.

RESULTS

There were 59 cases of Caldwell Luc operations (56 by acupuncture and 3 by T_1 block with 2% Xylocaine 3 ml each), 4 cases of maxillary cancer, and 7 trigeminal neuralgias (4 by acupuncture and 3 by T_1 block). In the cases for operation 28 were completely free of pain, 5 had tolerable pain. In the pain clinic, all patients had pain relief.

There were 3 types of complication experienced in this study. None of them, however, was serious. There was one case of pneumothorax. One case of vagal stimulation occurred in a patient for Caldwell Luc operation.

---

* This study was financially supported by the National Council on Science Development of the Republic of China.

About 5 min after bilateral T_1 block, the patient felt very sleepy, with warm cheeks, but pupil sizes were unchanged and there was analgesia of the maxillary gingiva. The blood pressure fell. About 8 min later respiration became diaphragmatic with small tidal volumes. Oxygen was given by mask with assisted respiration for the next 20 min. Thirty-five min after the blocks the tidal volume became adequate. Then the operation was carried out without additional anesthetics; the analgesic effect lasted for 2 days.

There were 3 cases of anterior chest pain.

DISCUSSION

On the basis of our experience acupuncture analgesia definitely exists. The gate control theory (Melzack and Wall, 1965) is believed to be an explanation for this analgesic effect, but many other phenomena including the pathway of meridians are still unknown. There are many reports (Chang, 1973; Chian et al., 1973; Nakatani, personal communication; Dembeck, 1974) that points of acupuncture are directly or indirectly related to the nervous system. However, there is no explanation of the relationship between the hand points, such as LI_4, for operations above the neck for analgesic effect. Kim (1965) advocated that there is a new 'Bonghan system' while Chian et al. (1973) denied fluid theory. S_{36} was found near the anterior tibial nerve, but not the nerve per se, but on the interosseous membrane (Fig. 1). LI_4 was also found near the median nerve and seemed to be on the fascia interossea volaris (Fig. 2).

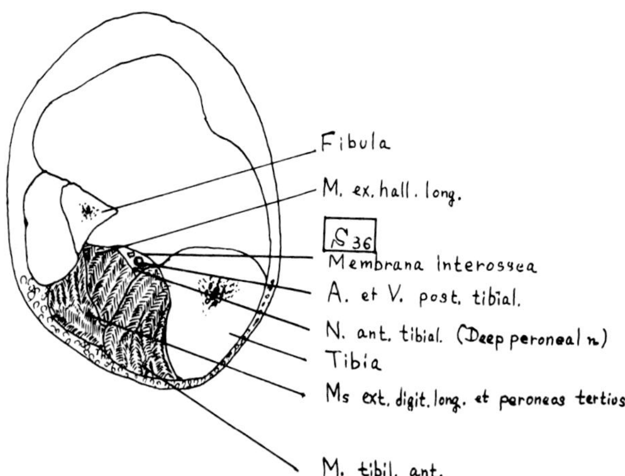

Fig. 1.   *Cross section view of right leg at the level of S_{36}.*

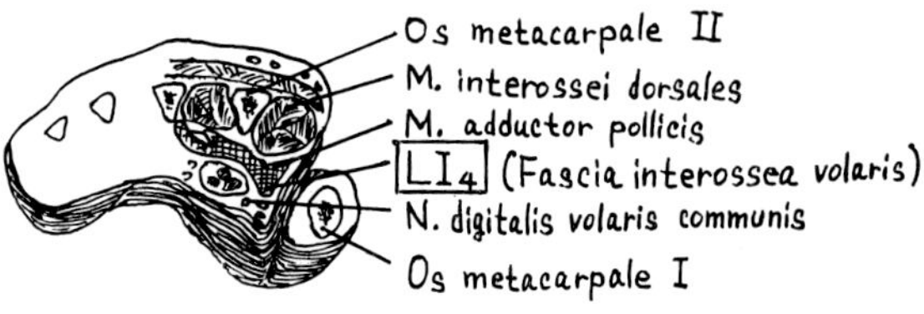

Fig. 2.   *Cross section view of right hand at the level of LI_4.*

A characteristic fainting reaction occurred after needling LI_4 with nausea and vomiting accompanied by cold sweating, bradycardia and hypotension. These symptoms are very similar to those following reflex inhibition of the heart. Thus acupuncture at LI_4 must have some relationship with autonomic nervous system as per the theory of Nakatani (1972). But the fainting reaction did not occur in 6 patients with hyperhydrosis in our series who had bilateral second and third thoracic sympathectomies. On the other hand, utilizing 8 clinical patients who had injury of either radial or ulnar nerve, LI_4 seemed related to the median nerve which receives neurons from fifth cervical nerve to second thoracic nerve. The stellate ganglion may possess acupuncture effectiveness, thus ganglion block was intended for Caldwell Luc's operations in 3 cases, for trigeminal neuralgia in 2 cases and for shoulder pain in one case. The former was not successful and caused more bleeding. The latter gave some pain relief. These results led to consider blocking bilateral T_1 from the dorsal side for the Caldwell Luc operations on 3 occasions and for pain in 3 patients. The result was that the operations could be done with one success and with 2 partial successes, and all trigeminal neuralgias were relieved for 24 hr. The third division of trigeminal nerve terminating at the third cervical level (Kerr, 1963; Imai and Kusama, 1969) in the spinal cord does not seem to be involved. This may indicate that T_1 ganglion plays an important role in the relay of afferent impulse of the sympathetic from the face.

The second question is, if T_1 is concerned with the communication of afferent impulse, then its effective area must be found in the T_1 innervated zone; above the fourth thoracic dermatome (T_4).

Experiments were further carried on in 8 patients either using LI_4 and P_6 with electrical stimulations, or T_1 block with 2% Xylocaine 3 ml for operations and trigeminal neuralgia. A hypoalgesic zone was found above the fourth thoracic dermatome in 4 patients; this was hyperalgesic in 2 and unaffected in 2. Thus analgesic zones below T_5 and T_{12} were also found from celiac and from second lumbar paravertebral sympathetics (L_2) respectively. This may indicate that all dermatomes of the skin are supplied afferent fibres from each plexus, i.e., T_1, celiac, superior and inferior mesenteric ganglions respectively, in addition to sensory innervation. These innervated zones would be different from, and wider than, the regular spinal segment. The present study involved only clinical observations with limited numbers of patients; the study needs to be continued.

REFERENCES

Chang Y. T. (1973): *China Sci. 1*, 28.
Chian, T. Y., Chang, T. T., Chu, S. L. and Young, L F. (1973): *China Sci., 2*, 157.
Dembek, Z.: *A Contribution Towards the Comprehension of Acupuncture and its Physiological Bases.* In press.
Imai, Y. and Kusama, T. (1969): *Brain Res., 13*, 338.
Kerr, F. W. L. (1963): *Brain, 86*, 721.
Kim, H. (1965): *Morphological and Functional Structure of Acupuncture Meridian.* Kakyotsuho.
Kuba, M. (1974): *Acupuncture Analgesia*, Koseido Co., Tokyo.
Melzack, R. and Wall, P. O. (1965): *Science, 150*, 971.

Acupuncture analgesia for the treatment of trigeminal neuralgias: A series of 41 cases

PANG L. MAN [1] and ALLEN CHEN [2]

[1] Northville State Hospital, Northville and
Department of Psychiatry, College of Medicine, Wayne State University, Detroit;
and [2] Department of Anesthesiology, Annapolis Hospital, Wayne, Mich., U.S.A.

'There is only one pain that is easy to bear and that is the pain of others' said a famous surgeon. It is also the pain that we feel or suffer that enables us to survive before detrimental or fatal consequences develop. Pain is a warning signal, a symptom of underlying disease. The physician must try to diagnose the cause of pain and eliminate or reduce it to a subjectively tolerable level; sometimes they fail.

Among the patients who suffer most from chronic intractable pain are those with trigeminal neuralgia who experience unpredictable lightning or jabbing pain. In order to ease this pain they are usually treated with analgesics, narcotics, nerve block and/or surgical interventions. Often, the success rate is very disappointing. Those who fail to respond to all methods of treatment soon realize that they are relegated to trials of various narcotic drugs or are shunned by the physician who realizes he cannot help them further. These unfortunate patients become depressed and dependent upon narcotics to lead any form of normal life.

Acupuncture is a household word not only in the homeland of China but also in scientifically oriented North America. The 2-gate control theory as proposed by Man and Chen (1972*a*) to explain the mechanism of acupuncture analgesia is the synthesis of both Eastern and Western medical technology. Based on this theory, the senior author (P. L. M.) successfully tested it on himself and his family (Man and Chen, 1972*b*). We further applied this knowledge in dental, surgical and clinical practices (Man, 1973; Man and Chen, 1973, 1974). On the basis of this experience, the authors have treated a significant number of patients with trigeminal neuralgia who had not responded to conventional methods of therapy. This communication intends to report the result of this treatment modality.

METHOD

The selected patients had an established diagnosis of trigeminal neuralgia. The clinical symptoms and findings were reviewed by the authors to exclude other illnesses which might simulate this condition. The so-called atypical facial neuralgia is automatically ruled out in the study. Patients who had a psychiatric illness were excluded from the study. Their past and present medical histories show typical clinical symptoms of recurrent episodes of intermittent burning, aching, hyperesthesia to flank sharp pain of one or more branches of the Vth cranial nerve.

Classification of severity of pain

1. *Mild.* Paroxysmal attacks of burning, aching or hyperesthesia to sharp pain at times and the interval is spaced over several days to several weeks. The patient can conduct a normal working life without taking analgesics.
2. *Moderate.* The attack of pain is considerably more often, carbamazepine, diphenyl-hydantoin and narcotics relieve the pain only to a certain point.
3. *Severe.* More frequent paroxysmal attacks of sharp or lightning pain day and night – as many as 40 attacks in 24 hr. The medications in category 2 do not relieve the pain; the patient is depressed and may contemplate suicide at one time or other; he is unable to work or carry out a normal daily life.

Procedure

The following steps were used as a guide to acupuncture treatment: (1) The acupuncture needles are inserted into different branches of the trigeminal nerve depending on the branch involved. The insertion of the needle into the various branches of the Vth cranial nerve is based on the description of Bonica (1953). The most commonly affected branches are the supraorbital, supratrochlear, infraorbital and mental branches. (2) It is important to elicit paresthesia when inserting the acupuncture needles since this indicates that the nerve has been encountered. (3) Maintaining stability of the needle in the supraorbital nerve is rather difficult because of the anatomical structure which is deficient of adequate tissue to hold it in place – therefore a horizontal approach is recommended for the following reasons: (*a*) the needle will encounter both supraorbital and supratrochlear nerves at the same time; (*b*) the needle will be more stable than in the vertical position. (4) Connect the needles with the electronic pulsating machine which delivers bipolar waveform, 40 μsec at mid amplitude, 150 pulses/sec, 280 V at 10 KΩ load. The actual current output is about one milliamp. (5) During this half hour, the patient is instructed on how to increase the electrical current steadily upward at every 5-min interval to the point that the sensation is tolerable without discomfort. (6) The patients are treated once a day for 3–4 days, then 2–3 times a week when the pain is considerably under control. If there is no pain or very little pain, then a regime of once a week, once every two weeks, or once a month is followed. If there is still no pain then the patient is discharged from the clinic.

RESULTS

The outcome of treatment is defined as follows: (1) *Failure.* No change of severity of pain at the end of 8–10 treatments. (2) *Mild improvement.* Experienced to some degree relief of pain, and takes less analgesics. (3) *Moderate improvement.* Severity of pain reduced from severe to moderate as described earlier and takes very small amount of analgesics and the pain is tolerable. (4) *Marked improvement.* No pain or nearly no pain, no need to take analgesics (see Tables 1–3).

Table 1. *History of the patients*

No. of cases	Sex		Average age	Average duration of illness (yr)	Severity of pain			No. of surgical interventions	
	M	F			Mild	Moderate	Severe	Once	More than once
41	16	25	64	8.4	1	11	29	9	3

Table 2. *Branches of the Vth cranial nerve involved*

Side of the face		Branch affected most commonly or in combination						Single branch involved		
Right	Left	1st	1st+2nd	2nd	2nd+3rd	3rd	all	1st	2nd	3rd
26	15	0	8	9	9	6	9	17	35	24

Table 3. *Number of treatments and clinical responses*

Mild improvement	Moderate improvement	Degree of improvement							
		Failure		Mild		Moderate		Marked	
		No.	%	No.	%	No.	%	No.	%
After 3.5 treatments	After 5.6 treatments	4	9.9	1	2.2	9	22	27	66

DISCUSSION

All of our patients had been treated with analgesics, narcotics, procaine and/or alcohol nerve block, denervation of the Vth nerve branches or gasserian ganglion and they all failed to achieve significant relief of pain. Nine or 22% of the cases had received some type of surgery, namely transection or removal of one or more parts of the Vth nerve. Of the 3 surgical cases having failed to respond to acupuncture, 2 had been operated upon twice at the site of gasserian ganglion and one had a neuroma of the 3rd branch of the Vth nerve. Surgical intervention in these cases was a complete failure. These figures are quite alarming in that although one-fourth of the patients will eventually receive some type of surgical treatment, they fail to achieve pain relief. Carbamazepine is non-specific for the reatment of this ailment. Its cost and toxicity are well recognized. Narcotics such as meperidine and codeine are not only ineffectual after being taken for a reasonably long period of time but the patient usually will develop other problems such as narcotic addiction. Surgical treatment may or may not relieve pain permanently and again the patient frequently suffers the consequences of the operation which include disfiguration, paralysis of the face, lacrimation, etc.

With acupuncture analgesia, 88% of the patients have had relief of pain after an average of 5.6 treatments and began to feel better after an average of 3.5 treatments. The result is quite satisfactory but not surprising, based on our experience with other types of pain syndromes. Acupuncture analgesia seems to be an ideal treatment modality for the trigeminal neuralgic patients. Other findings concur with existing statistics of trigeminal neuralgic patients (Hassler and Walker, 1970) i.e.: age approximately 50, female more frequently affected than male. The right side of the face was more frequently affected than the left, 2nd branch of the Vth nerve usually more involved than others.

The basic mechanism of acupuncture analgesia is derived from neurophysiology, neuro-anatomy and pain physiology which form the backbone of the 2-gate control theory. The recent work of Campbell and Taub (1973) also substantiates our hypothesis although for some unknown reason they never mention the word 'acupuncture' analgesia. Inasmuch as we are working towards the same goal of pain relief this is inconsequential. Wen and Cheung (1973) by using the same technique, were successful in the surgery of trigeminal neuralgia. The authors are confident that more and more research will be carried out in acupuncture analgesia which warrants the attention of the medical profession.

In this series, 3 patients are still free from pain over a 1-year period. The long-term acupuncture analgesic effect is being followed-up closely.

REFERENCES

Bonica, J. (1953): *The Management of Pain.* Lean Febiger, Philadelphia, Pa.
Campbell, J. N. and Taub, A. (1973): *Arch. Neurol., 28*, 347.
Hassler, R. and Walker, A. E. (1970): *Trigeminal Neuralgia.* W. B. Saunders Co., Philadelphia, Pa.
Man, P. L. (1973): *Handbook of Acupuncture Analgesia.* New Jersey Fieldplace Press, New Jersey.
Man, P. L. and Chen, C. H. (1972*a*): *Dis. nerv. Syst., 33*, 730.
Man, P. L. and Chen, C. H. (1972*b*): *Curr. ther. Res., 14*, 390.
Man, P. L. and Chen, C. H. (1973): *Dent. Surv., 27.*
Man, P. L. and Chen, C. H. (1974): *Mich. Med., 73*, 15.
Wen, H. L. and Cheung, S. Y. C. (1973): *Amer. J. Acup., 1*, 105.

Treatment of herpes zoster with acupuncture

SVEN ERIK NIELSEN

St. Elisabeth County Hospital, Copenhagen, Denmark

Herpes zoster is a disease of viral origin with a characteristic skin eruption affecting the dermatomes of one or seldom 2 or more peripheral nerves. The disease is usually accompanied by burning and stabbing or neuralgic pain of varying intensity in the affected area. The skin eruption normally dries up within 2–4 weeks but the pain may persist for months or even years – the condition known as postherpetic neuralgia. Many different treatments have been tried to shorten the duration of the acute pain and prevent the development of chronic pain. So far blocking of regional sympathetic ganglia seems to have been the most successful technique. This treatment of herpes zoster pain was introduced to Denmark by Colding in 1964 and has since his report of favourable results (Colding, 1966) been widely used by Danish anaesthesiologists.

Two years ago I noticed that 2 symmetrical acupuncture points in the back of the neck termed 'Feng Chi' or gallbladder 20 were reported 'supposedly vaso-sympathetic' (Mann, 1972). To test this information these 2 points were needled in a female patient attending for her 2nd stellate ganglion block because of severe zoster pain in the left shoulder region. The pain disappeared within 7–10 min and stayed away for 4–6 hr. After 2 more acupunctures she remained pain-free. Encouraged by this result acupuncture was tried on all succeeding zoster cases and by now the method has been used in 60–70 patients.

The present report concerns 25 consecutive patients with painful herpes zoster seen in a pain clinic from March to October 1973. One patient, an 80-year-old male was excluded from the series since he had a sympathetic ganglion block after admission to hospital for psychiatric reasons. Before that he had 2 successful acupunctures. The remaining 24 patients were exclusively treated with acupuncture.

Age and sex distribution and localisation of herpes zoster are shown in Table 1. The technique of the acupuncture is very simple. No matter whether the zoster affected the head, the body or the extremities the needles were inserted in the same 2 points in the back

Table 1. *Age and sex distribution and localisation of herpes zoster in 24 patients treated with acupuncture*

No. of patients	Age (yr)	Sex		Localisation		
		M	F	Cervical	Thoracic	Lumbar
3	0–20	2	1	1	1	1
4	21–40	3	1	1	2	1
5	41–60	2	3	1	3	1
12	> 60	5	7	0	12	0
24		12	12	3	18	3

of the neck (see Fig. 1). The points are located in the concavities which can be palpated in the suboccipital region just lateral to the trapezius muscle at the level of the mastoid processes. The needles, which are Chinese acupuncture needles with a length of 1 inch and a diameter of 0.3 mm, were inserted in the points to a depth of 1–2 cm pointing towards the opposite eye. The needles were stimulated by rotation until the patient reported a feeling of tension or pressure around the needle – what the Chinese call the 'Chi' sensation. The needles were left in place for 20 min. The 'Chi' sensation was again caused by rotation after 10 min and again just before removal of the needles. When the needles had been inserted the patients were asked to report any sensation which they might experience during the next 20 min. They were not told what might happen and the investigator tried not to be suggestive.

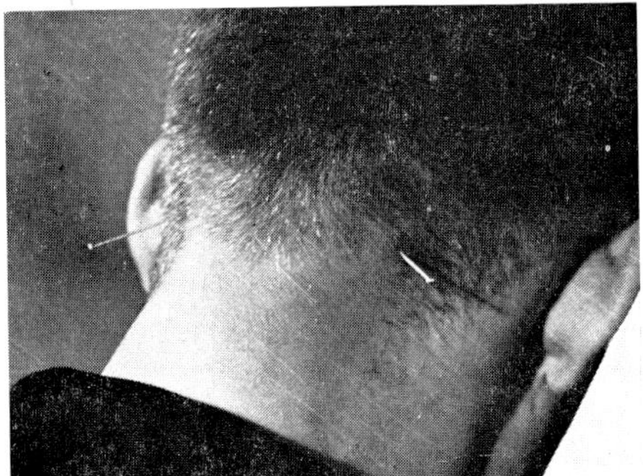

Fig. 1. *Acupuncture points for the treatment of herpes zoster.*

The typical report from a patient in pain was that the pain relief started 6–8 min after the needling and that pain had completely disappeared 5–10 min later. The pain-free period usually lasted for 2–10 hr and the pain was often of reduced intensity when it recurred. The acupuncture was repeated daily or every 2nd day until permanent pain relief was achieved. The 24 patients had a mean pain duration of 5.4 days from the beginning of the treatment. An average of 4.2 acupunctures were needed with only a small difference between the younger and the older age groups.

Table 2 shows that patients who attended for treatment within the first week of the eruption had earlier pain relief and needed fewer acupunctures than those attending later in the disease. The same importance of an early institution of treatment was emphasized by Colding (1969) concerning sympathetic blocks.

Table 2. *Pain duration in 24 patients with herpes zoster treated with acupuncture (AP)*

No. of patients	Duration of eruption before treatment (weeks)	Period after which free of pain (days)	No. of AP
17	< 1	3.7	3.1
5	1–4	6.6	5.2
2	> 4	17.0	10.5

It is often stated that pain is more severe and of longer duration in the geriatric zoster patient. If a treatment is claimed to be beneficial it should therefore be effective in this age group too. In 3 series of largely untreated patients (Rogers and Tindall, 1971; De Moragas and Kierland, 1957; Molin, 1969) one half to two thirds of the patients above the age of

60 had a pain duration of more than 4 weeks (Table 3). By contrast 75% of the 12 elderly patients of the present series were pain-free within 2 weeks, and only one had pain lasting for more than 4 weeks after the skin eruption.

The patient in concern was an 82-year-old female who did not attend for treatment until 6 weeks after the skin eruption. She became pain-free after 11 acupunctures, but one month later she had recurrence of her pain which did not react to further acupunctures. She was the only patient of the present series who developed postherpetic neuralgia.

Table 3. *Duration of herpes zoster pain in patients above the age of 60 in different investigations (figures in %)*

	Rogers and Tindall, 1971 (243 patients)	De Moragas and Kierland, 1957 (430 patients)	Molin, 1969 (90 patients)	Present material (12 patients)
0–4 weeks	53.1	32	50	91.6
>4 weeks	46.9	68	50	8.4*

* One patient who did not attend for treatment until 6 weeks after skin eruption.

The way in which acupuncture works in herpes zoster is obscure but probably the action is effected via the sympathetic nervous system in one way or another. More than half of the patients experienced sensations of heat in the head and often in the hands during the acupuncture. A few could even report a feeling as if a wave of heat was rolling from the head through the body to the extremities. In one elderly female patient who experienced pronounced heat sensations in the head and the hands during several acupunctures thermography was performed – a diffuse increase in skin temperature of her face during 20 min acupuncture was seen, reaching a maximum of 3–3.5°C on the cheeks.

The results from acupuncture treatment of herpes zoster and a few cases of posttraumatic dystrophy treated in the same way are promising and seem comparable to those obtained by sympathetic blocks. The present series is small and should be considered a pilot investigation. A controlled trial is going on. The method is practically without discomfort to the patient and no complications have been observed.

REFERENCES

Colding, A. (1966): *Manedsskr. prakt. Laegegern.,* *44*, 123.

Colding, A. (1969): *Acta anaesth. scand.,* *13*, 133.

Mann, F. (1972): *The Treatment of Disease by Acupuncture,* 2nd ed., p. 62. William Heinemann Medical Books Ltd., London.

Molin, L. (1969): *Acta derm.-venereol. (Stockh.),* *49*, 569.

De Moragas, J. M. and Kierland, R. R. (1957): *Arch. Derm.,* *75*, 193.

Rogers, R. S. and Tindall, J. P. (1971): *J. Amer. Geriat. Soc.,* *19/6*, 495.

Clinical experience with acupuncture anaesthesia

P. J. PÖNTINEN and ANTERO SORASTO

Department of Anaesthesia, Kainuu Central Hospital, Kajaani, and
Kalajoki District Hospital, Kalajoki, Finland

Acupuncture, an ancient Chinese art of healing, although practiced also in Europe for some 200 years, has recently gained widespread interest in Western medical centres. This has mainly been due to acupuncture anaesthesia, which is a new form of acupuncture started in China in 1958. These trials on acupuncture anaesthesia were started 2 years ago. The main purpose was to determine whether acupuncture affects pain and if so, whether surgical anaesthesia is possible. This report presents the experience gained from the first 52 operations performed under acupuncture anaesthesia.

MATERIAL AND METHODS

Patients volunteered for acupuncture anaesthesia for tonsillectomies, dental procedures and thyroidectomies. Their sensitivity to acupuncture was determined before operation. The age of the patients ranged from 15–69 years. Sex distribution was equal. The points for these operations were selected according to the reports from China (König and Wancura, 1973; Shanghai Acupuncture Anaesthesia Coordinating Group, 1973), and Vienna (Benzer et al., 1972). The exact location of points was confirmed with an electric resistance meter (Acumeter, Begmer Electronics) and by the patient's sensations. Manual, mechanical or electric stimulation (Begmer Acu. Begmer Electronics) of needles was used.

RESULTS

The success rate in real operations was very low. In trials for tonsillectomies 15% were successful. In dental surgery the results were more promising and 60% gave excellent or good results. Both thyroidectomies were successful. Details are presented in Tables 1–3.

DISCUSSION

It seems established that acupuncture works in Western people (Benzer et al., 1972; Lanza, 1973; Kubista et al., 1974; Spoerel, 1974). At the beginning of our trials neither the volunteer nor the acupuncturist could know the result of needle stimulation. When the Ho Ku point was stimulated to induce analgesia for tonsillectomies in the first 150 subjects, 76% reacted positively to stimulation. In 80% of these cases the analgesia appeared on the ipsilateral side. In 20% the analgesia was better on the contralateral side. Later on when analgesia for

Table 1. *Tonsillectomies (30 operations)*

Acupuncture points	
Ho Ku (Li 4)	30
Chao Chang (L 11)	22
Nei Ting (S 44)	1
Ear	1
Stimulation	
Manual	24
Mechanical	2
Electrical	4
Effect	
Both sides	23
One side	7

Table 2. *Dental operations (20 patients)*

Main acupuncture points	Local points		Location	Effect
	Upper jaw	Lower jaw		
Li 1, 4	S 2	S 3, 5	Upper jaw	+
(K 27)	Si 18	Cv 24	Lower molars and premolars	+(+)
Ear points			Lower incisives	(+)–

Table 3. *Thyroidectomy*

Age	Sex	Acupuncture points		Type of stimulation	Induction	Maintenance	Effect
		Body	Ear				
57	F	Ho Ku Fu Tu Nei Koan	Shen Men	Electrical 120/min	30 min	4 hr	Excellent *
69	F	Ho Ku Fu Tu Nei Koan	Shen Men Jiao Gan	Electrical 120/min	50 min	1 hr 50 min	Excellent *

* 20 ml 0.5% lidocaine for skin analgesia.

dentistry was attempted it first appeared in the molar area spreading slowly towards midline in most cases. In some cases instead of the teeth the contralateral tonsillar area became analgesic. In most cases the induction time using low frequency electric stimulation was from 40–50 min. These findings seem to confirm that the effect is not due to hypnosis. The success rate in similar operations in China has been reported to be over 90% (Lowe, 1973; Shanghai First People's Hospital, 1973). The same rate was achieved in our later tests on medical students under experimental conditions without the anticipation of an operation. The great difference of success rates is at least partly due to the fact that our patients will not accept the level of anaesthesia of Groups 2 and 3 in Chinese reports (Shanghai Acupuncture Anaesthesia Coordinating Group, 1973).

Controversies of clinical findings with theories of mechanisms of acupuncture

The sensations on limbs under acupuncture cannot be explained by present-day theories·
These sensations are always present when satisfactory analgesia is achieved; when this is
combined with feelings of sleepiness and calmness, the 'deqi state' exists. Humoral mechanisms could explain the general effect of acupuncture (Shanghai Acupuncture Anaesthesia
Coordinating Group, 1973). The theories of peripheral nerve stimulation including the
'gate control theory' by Melzack and Wall (1965) only partly explain the effects of acupuncture. For instance the best acupuncture point for thyroidectomies, Fu Tu, is situated
on the peripheral nerve trunk behind the sternocleidomastoid muscle. In the same way
the best local points for dental analgesia are situated on the trigeminal nerve. However,
excellent analgesia for dentistry and for tonsillectomies was obtained through points situated
on the feet or hands. This cannot be explained easily by segmental thinking. It seems established that the pain threshold is slightly raised whenever areas like feet, hands, face and
ear are stimulated, but the effect is markedly increased when correct acupuncture sites are
used (Man and Baragar, 1973; Research Group of Acupuncture Anaesthesia, Peking, 1973).

Selection of acupuncture points

Selection of points seems to be confusing. The same points are used for many different
operations and at the same time there are many different schemes for each operation. This
is due to the fact that there is the choice between the meridian points, the segmental points
and the points with central calming and pain relieving effects. In addition there are the
local ear points and the centrally acting ear points. In a test situation often the stimulation
of one specific point is enough to induce surgical analgesia. As the tension then increases
more points are needed to deepen the analgesia. The points from different groups have an
additional effect on analgesia. In most cases, when slow frequency electric stimulation is
used, the induction time varies from 40–50 min. In approximately 15% of cases induction
is faster (10–15 min.). These patients are very sensitive to acupuncture and the analgesia
is perfect locally and is combined with a good 'deqi' effect. On the basis of these trials the
patients can be divided into 3 groups: the first including some 15% of people with fast
induction and complete analgesia and a good 'deqi' effect; the second with slow induction
and from complete to reasonably good analgesia with a slight 'deqi' effect; and the third
group with seemingly no response other than slight general pain threshold increase.

In the literature it has been stressed that during acupuncture anaesthesia the vital functions
are stable (König and Wancura, 1973; Shanghai Acupuncture Anaesthesia Coordinating
Group, 1972). Pulse rate, blood pressure and respiratory rate were remarkably stable
during thyroidectomy, but these findings need further confirmation.

Postoperative period

The postoperative period has been almost pain-free in most of the patients and the mucous
membranes have healed quickly. Acupuncture has been used to relieve pain postoperatively
also in cases where operations have been performed under local or general anaesthesia.

CONCLUSION

At present acupuncture anaesthesia is still at the trial stage. The success rate is too low for
routine work. In most cases it is too laborious and time-consuming and not deep enough
for Western patients. On the other hand the stability of vital functions during operations
and very rapid healing postoperatively has been striking. At least it can be said that acupuncture anaesthesia is worthy of further trials.

REFERENCES

Benzer, H., Bischko, J., Kropej, H., Pauser, G., Baum, M. and Toma, H. (1972): *Anaesthesist*, *21/11*, 452.

Kubista, E., Kucera, H., Benzer, H., Pauser, G. and Bischko, J. (1974): *Anaesthesist*, *23/2*, 93.

König, G. and Wancura, I. (1973): *Einführung in die Chinesische Ohrakupunktur*. Haug Verlag, Heidelberg.

Lanza, U. (1973): *Minerva med.*, *64/40*, 2112.

Lowe, W. C. (1973): *Introduction to Acupuncture Anesthesia*. Hans Huber Verlag, Bern-Stuttgart.

Man, S. C. and Baragar, F. D. (1973): *Canad. med. Ass. J.*, *109/6*, 609.

Melzack, R. and Wall, P. D. (1965): *Science*, *150*, 971.

Research Group of Acupuncture Anesthesia, Peking Medical College, Peking (1973): *China Med J.*, *3*, 35.

Shanghai Acupuncture Anaesthesia Coordinating Group (1973): *Acupuncture Anaesthesia. An Anaesthetic Method by Combination of Traditional Chinese and Western Medicine*. Shanghai.

Shanghai First People's Hospital, Shanghai (1973): *China med. J.*, *2*, 17.

Spoerel, W. E. (1974): *Canad. Anaesth. Soc. J.*, *21/2*, 221.

Postoperative treatment of pain by means of electroacupuncture: Preliminary communication

RODOLFO L. RODRÍGUEZ

Belizario Dominguez 2485 Pte., Monterrey, Mexico

One of the earliest references about pain is found in the 4th book of the Nei-Ching which is a classic work of Chinese medicine. A legendary doctor Pien Chiao practiced in the year 190 B.C. with great ability; operations were painless by means of acupuncture. The effect of acupuncture on certain illnesses such as migraine where pain is the principal symptom is well known. Patients who have suffered it for years have been able to obtain relief and this is one of the reasons why acupuncture has had so much attention in recent years.

Last September I had the opportunity of assisting at the First World Symposium on Acupuncture and Chinese Medicine held in San Francisco. It was my first contact with this system of cure as old as one of the oldest cultures, and which in recent decades has been applied in anesthesiology since anesthesia is possible by means of acupuncture.

In order to understand acupuncture, I will try to explain it in simple terms. The Chinese describe the organism as a system of meridians or channels through which flows the vital energy called Chi. Throughout the length of these meridians there are stated to exist points, in which the insertion of needles produce special effects, amongst them, the elimination of pain. Theoretically, in order to cause anesthesia by acupuncture certain points of the meridians which pass through the region or organ must be stimulated.

Likewise, there exist points in the ear and nose whose stimulation is utilized in the general treatment of acupuncture. This treatment can be for a particular organ or for a region of the body. These points are particularly sensitive in the treatment of pain. In obstetrical anesthesia the method could have advantages, because no drugs would be used for anesthesia, thus eliminating the risk of harmful effects on the newborn. Anesthesia by electroacupuncture has been attempted by using the points described by doctor Rocia (Turin) in 2 cesarean operations with very satisfactory results.

A few days later I attended a patient with bilateral fractures of the lower jaw who had eaten a full meal minutes before the accident. This seemed a clear indication for the use of acupuncture anesthesia. The stimulation points used were the same as those used for the extraction of teeth, and were bilateral Li1 and Li4, plus St44 of the meridian that passes through that particular region.

With 2 doses of fentanyl 0.1 mg, and 10 mg of diazepam, the operation of wiring the inferior and superior dentures was completed successfully without the patient feeling pain.

Prolonged postoperative analgesia was marked and drugs were not needed in these cases. The favorable results obtained further stimulated my interest in the field.

Table 1. *Postoperative treatment of pain following general surgery with electroacupuncture*

	No. of cases
Tonsillectomy in children	8
Tonsillectomy in adults	2
Removal of papilloma of the larynx	1
Umbilical hernia and appendectomy	1
Cholecystectomy	1
Cholecystectomy repair of diaphragmatic hernia and appendectomy	1
Exploratory laparotomy	1
Total	15

Table 2. *Postoperative treatment of pain with electroacupuncture*

	No. of cases
Oral surgery	1
Plastic surgery of burns (grafts)	1
Total	2

Table 3. *Postoperative treatment of pain with electroacupuncture in orthopedics*

	No. of cases
Hallux valgus unilateral	1
Hallux valgus bilateral	2
Triple arthrodes s of the foot	1
Fracture reduction of the lower jaw	1
Surgical reduction of fracture in both arms	1
Surgicaι reduction of fracture in one arm	1
Surgical reduction of fracture in both legs	2
Surgical reduction of fracture in both legs and 1 arm	3
Surgical reduction of pseudoarthrosis of the arm	1
Surgical reduction of fracture of the patella	1
Lumbar laminectomy	1
Total hip replacement	1
Meniscectomy	1
Exploration of the radial nerve	1
Total	18

METHOD

The control of postoperative pain was attempted by stimulation with an electrical current of 12 V at 200 Hz, over a period of 4–6 or 8 hr. This current reaches the body at predetermined points through special needles.

Table 4. *Postoperative treatment of pain by electroacupuncture in gynecology and obstetrics*

	No. of cases
Ovarian cyst	2
Bilateral bartolinectomy	1
Colpoperineorrhaphy	2
Vaginal hysterectomy and colpoperineorrhaphy	2
Total abdominal hysterectomy and colpoperineorrhaphy	2
Total abdominal hysterectomy	9
Removal of the cervix, vagina, and pelvic exenteration	1
Cesarean sections	8
Total	27

Table 5. *Postoperative complications in patients treated with electroacupuncture for pain after surgery.*

	No. of cases	%
Nausea and vomiting (more than once)	5	8.33
Paralytic ileus (24–48 hr)	2	3.33
Analgesic during induction	10	16.66
Postoperative pain that needed strong analgesic after treatment (Mecoten, Demerol)	2	3.33
Paralytic ileus (more than 48 hr)	1	1.66
Postoperative pain that needed mild analgesic after treatment (Neomelubrine tablets or Mecoten tablets)	22	36.66
Without analgesics in the postoperative phase	18	30.00
Total no. of cases	60	

DETAILS

Postoperative control of pain with electroacupuncture was attempted in 60 cases, 10 males and 50 females, whose age ranged between 2 and 78 years. At the end of the operation, when there is still some residual analgesia before the patient awakes from a general anesthetic, or before the effect of a regional block has disappeared, the patient is transferred to the recovery room, or to his hospital room, where the acupuncture analgesia is commenced.

Occasionally, it is necessary to administer a sedative, until the acupuncture analgesia begins to take effect, which takes 15 or 20 min of electrostimulation. Meanwhile the patient begins to fall asleep and if questioned, complains of a slight pain, which finally disappears.

The arterial pressure and pulse rate tend to decrease slightly but remain within normal limits.

Respiration is quiet, and of normal amplitude once the required period of stimulation necessary to produce postoperative analgesia has passed, the stimulator and the needles are withdrawn. The patient remains sedated, quiet, and complains of slight pain on movement which disappears immediately when the patient is still.

During the first day after the operation the patient is kept under a strict diet, and a continuous infusion of glucose for hydration is maintained. The intestinal motility recovers early, often on the same night. After a mild hypnotic the patient who is free from pain has a good night's sleep and can get up and start eating the next morning.

COMMENTS

The number of satisfactory results observed, in regard to the absence of pain and the postoperative progress without serious complications, is really impressive. The main postoperative complications were nausea and vomiting and paralytic ileus. All the cases of nausea were in children posttonsillectomy, in whom swallowing of blood was causative – it always disappeared in 24 hr.

Four cases of paralytic ileus occurred and lasted up to 48 hr; for each of these cases there was an adequate surgical explanation and the patients were discharged from hospital within 5 days of surgery.

DISCUSSION

The results obtained in these cases are so different from personal experience over 37 years of professional practice that they may seem incredible.

It has been shown that stimulation of point Gv. 14 produces reactions mediated through the diencephalic organovegetative centers, and shown by an increase of phagocytic activity and by the normalization of fibrinolytic levels in the blood.

Acupuncture is followed by changes in brain biopotentials, recorded on the electroencephalogram.

In respect of its beneficial action on pain, without entering further discussion about the 2-gate theory of Melzack and Wall, it maintains that stimulation of the nonconducting pain fibers $\alpha\beta$ will block the C-conducting pain fibers, at the level of the substantia gelatinosa in the posterior horn. The second gate is most important for the control of pain, because on stimulation of points on the face or on the ears the impulse travels directly through cranial nerves to the thalamus, and painful stimuli are blocked before the cortex is reached.

In the cases presented of the control of pain by electroacupuncture, this theory would explain the exceptional results achieved, by the combined stimulus of auricular and facial points, associated with the stimulation of the peripheral nerves.

Electroacupuncture deserves an intensive clinical trial. With greater knowledge and experience these techniques might become of general everyday use, thus achieving the goal of Primum Non Nocere in the treatment of postoperative pain and providing, in this way, a real and positive benefit to mankind.

Note added in proof

Changes in the technique: the induction of the electroacupuncture stimulation is applied immediately after the surgical procedure is begun.

The points used have been mostly auricular, after techniques described by J. H. Niboyet in the book *L'anesthesie par l'acupuncture, Maisonneuve*, Paris 1973, plus 2 needles at the sides of the incision.

The electrostimulation has been prolonged up to 12 or 24 hr with improved results. A combined, very mild analgesia after surgery, on the other side has been used. 20 ml of fentanyl in 500 ml of 5% glucose, administered with a micro droper, 15 drops/min. The amount used in 24 hr never exceeds 0.4 mg in the first day, which is a homeophatic dose. The initial notation of the discussion holds true, every patient treated is the best proof of the good results obtained.

Chapter XVII

Ethical aspects of resuscitation

Introduction

RAMON DE LA FERIA

Serviço de Anestesia e Reanimação, Centro de Chirurgia Toracica, Lisbon, Portugal

The selection of subjects and the method of conducting this meeting are scientifically based in order to emphasise the basic principles of medical ethics. Man's very presence in society and the implications of a community spirit involve considerations of an individual's right to live and right to die. This problem must be considered in conjunction with the established moral ethics for each society, the extensive medical and technical developments especially with regard to resuscitation, surgery and immunology, the concepts of death and the risk of only partial survival of the human body.

Man must be defined as a whole; he has a personality which may be strong and which may be more or less established in a given society. However, even mentally defective patients or those who have completely alienated themselves from their environment have, as human beings, just as much right to be helped by the society to which they belong and the right to medical care.

The reason for medical treatment is to prolong a patient's life and to mitigate his suffering. In prolonging life however, suffering may be continued and both psychic and physical suffering may be involved. The physician may thus face an impossible choice: he must choose between orthothanasia, i.e. the mitigation of suffering, or dysthanasia, i.e. the prolongation of life by whatever means. Resuscitation techniques have advanced to such an extent that their maintenance results in serious ethical problems. If medicine is practised in relation to the environment of the patient then a solution is possible. However, the conscientious demands of the patient, the relatives, society and even the physician himself, cannot always be met. The extent to which a physician can oppose the request of his patient to be spared further suffering in the face of a short prognosis needs further examination.

Man and the community in which he lives cannot be separated since they are each the consequence of the other. Respect for man must be balanced by the important interests of the community. Neither can be separately considered. If partial anatomical and physiological survival is contemplated for an individual this must be related either to his own request or that of his relatives.

A particular example of this problem is heart transplantation. Immunological difficulties, public criticism and poor results all combine to condemn this therapeutic activity. There are limitations to resuscitation if this is to serve society: these limitations are both clinical, social, ethical and not least, economic.

Psychological and ethical aspects of reanimation

BARAHONA H. FERNANDES

Clinica Psiquiátrica, Hospital Santa Maria, Lisbon, Portugal

It was the wish of the chairman of this Symposium that a Professor in medical psychiatry and psychology should take part in the discussion of the problem of the ethics of reanimation. In addition a medical anthropological point of view has in the past been defended and applied in practice; this may justify any brief intervention on the psychological and ethical aspects of this subject.

The use by the physician of the technics of reanimation must be included in the general perspective of human medicine, for the sick man, provided by professionals with the purpose of saving life.

The aim should be to save not only a life but also a personality. The word 'reanimation' itself includes 'anima' (mind), which suggests that the idea is really to recover a personal existence which is vital, psychological, social and also cultural-spiritual.

The medical act of reanimation with its complicated technics, is only justified in the ethical sense if it means recovering a life which may have a meaning. It will be unjust, immoral and should be forbidden if this is not the intention.

A stratified and hierarchical model of the 'personality in a situation' includes several categories: (1) inorganic; (2) biological; (3) psychological; (4) socio-cultural. In a man in a 'normal' state these form a unity. In a state of coma only the first 2 structural organizations are active. If the reanimation technics are stopped the breathing, circulation, general and cerebral metabolism also cease. This is death; it rests only the first category (inorganic) in disorganization. If reanimation succeeds, spontaneous function of biologic vital functions returns and life goes on.

Will this be sufficient? Who is the man who survives after a state of more or less prolonged alteration or total loss of consciousness with 'life' under these artificial conditions?

Experience in psychopathology shows that the troubles of unconsciousness are in principle, reversible. From the state of coma, the patient can change to states of torpor, mental confusion, amnestic syndrome, etc. until total 'lucidity' occurs. Other psychopathological syndromes may also occur, the so called 'transition syndromes' (Durchgang-syndrome, Wieck) such as conditions of incoherence, depression, exhaustion, paranoid states etc. – these are also reversible. There are, however, other states which are not reversible to the same extent: the conditions of prolonged amnesia (Korsakov syndrome) and especially conditions of deterioration of cognitive and conative functions (psycho-organic syndromes) and several neuropathological states (pyramidal, extrapyramidal deficits, etc.). All these are 'organic' deficits that occur in consequence of ischemic, metabolic, mechanical and other severe lesions of the brain.

The decision to delay or to continue with resuscitation, with the consequent alternative of death or the progressive serious consequences, cannot, of course, be taken by the patient himself. It is quite different from dangerous surgical operations with which the patient may or may not agree. Such a serious decision must then be taken by the doctor or by the resuscitation team, with the consent of the family and those legally responsible.

This is one of the most dramatic decisions with which we are confronted in medicine, not only as technicians, but as men of conscience and responsible for our actions.

Philosophically this may correspond to what is called by Karl Jaspers a 'limit-situation' (Grenzsituationen). These situations express the radical character of man as a being which has not only 'Nature', but gives him in a deep sense the right perspective of the horizons of human behaviour and of the human awareness of his own death, pain, fear and guilt.

It is not possible to analyse thoroughly such a difficult subject. The critical situation of resuscitation cannot be experienced by what Jaspers called 'illumination of existence' and the awareness of frustration and of the limits of Man himself.

The situation of reanimation is a very peculiar one. There is a real possibility of death, pain, or a fight for life. The situation for the patient is an objective crisis – living or not living; becoming or not becoming a Man. What is peculiar is the limit-situation for the doctor himself: he is facing the possibility of another person's death, of a man who is his patient but to whom he is unattached by family ties or friendship but by the doctor-patient relationship. The problem is now not one of theoretical knowledge, technical keenness, but one of ethical responsibility and professional deontology.

It is therefore justified that these ethical aspects are discussed. However, this is only the legal manoeuver to get into a 'code' these norms for behaviour, rules or 'commandments'. In the last analysis it concerns and implies, the medical values and virtues of good or just medical behaviour and also the authenticity, fullness and purity of feelings and attitudes which motivate and stimulate the doctor in his relation with his patient.

It is, of course, basically important to fulfill the legal prescriptions of the code of ethical duty. Considering its relationship with socio-cultural and historical aspects, it may change from one country to another, even according to political and socio-cultural factors. Therefore, because of the diversity of the adopted customs the position may be questioned, as are the ethics of medicine also questioned.

The controversial tendencies of 'anti-culture' and 'anti-medicine' are widely discussed. The 'mutation of values', shown by Nietzsche, does not imply such excessive nihilistic positions. On the contrary, each new conquest of science requires an ethical position. Since Socrates this has been a constant theme of philosophy which is not only theoretical, but is also directly linked to practical life and the personal and social existence of man.

We are here not to 'learn' how we should act or which 'rules' we should follow in this limit-situation of reanimation. This is very important of course, but the human values in question lie beyond the 'codes'. These human values are the deep human feelings and tendencies about the worth of life and existence.

In our problem it is not enough, as it is in religious practice to obey to the revealed commandments against which we should not 'sin'. Nor is an abstract theory, such as the Schopenhauerian representation of moral principles, able to help.

Since Kant, Scheller and Nicolai Hartmann, the Ethic is changing. Utility, altruism, nor the so-called 'eudemonism', even on its modern social form, are no longer sufficient. The generalized search of modern times for well-being, profit, utility, happiness, extended to the greatest number of men, is changing from a mean to an end of life. Thus men become blind to the values of understanding and feeling of the meaningfulness of human existence. Other ethic theories, such as those of C. D. Broad, C. Stevenson and R. M. Hare help the analysis of the problem, but it is not possible to discuss it further.

Concerning the problem of reanimation we would like to point out that the decision whether to prolong or not to prolong a man's life with reanimation technics is only morally legitimate, ethically just and valid, if it aims to fulfill real human needs. As a result of this the patient may effectively change from a vegetative life to an authentic personal life and, as far as is possible, in possession of his full personality.

Instead of objective facts (state of breathing, circulation, metabolism, nervous activity, etc.) this is a consideration of quite a different kind – the *values*.

These are not what exists but what should exist. In the peculiar case of the reanimation situation, fundamental values must be considered, especially those concerning the patient. In the first place is the basic value of life, upon which all the other values depend. The critical situation is that the primordial value of to be or not to be is mooted, that is, to remain or not remain alive. Only on this vital basis can the search continue for a life force, equilibration, health and also other personal values, such as the capacity to react, activity, sensitivity, feelings, wishes, intentions, conscious personal decisions and attitudes of our own and others, and the values themselves.

It is an ethical problem to decide if reanimation should be attempted or not and with what intensity, and by what means etc., which the specialists are here analysing and discussing.

It is not only usefulness that is valuable. The usefulness of the means must be justified by the ethic character of the ends. The main problem is that from the creature in a state of coma can emerge a personality who may have a certain sense in life and find a certain significance in existence after reanimation.

In any decision about reanimation all these values should be considered. The usefulness of each specialized technic, the talent of using them in an efficient way and proper to the situation, and their constant modification with time depending on the changing situation must be also considered. But above all it is the harmonization with reality and the style with which everything is accomplished which is important. The patient is a person with his own humanity. This is a relation of the highest order when it is with another man who only later, or nevermore, may reply to it with affection and understanding. Everything that is done must be with a modest awareness of our potential but with at the same time, an enthusiasm for creativity.

The knowledge of the wise and the courage of acting with faith in our own efforts and dedication must be kept in perspective – at liberty but always aware of the limits of our actions. In a word: act with responsibility.

It is not possible to develop the theme further. The limit-situation of reanimation puts us precisely before the primordial ethical problem of being a medical man. Since Hippocrates these questions have always been considered and discussed. In our times, with the progress and the primacy of technics these problems are aggravated so that one must always be aware of the limits of our actions and of our duties.

In reanimation not only the 'know-how' should be considered but, as physicians, the purpose of our practice must be considered so that both the means and the ends may be ethically valid.

The validity of starting resuscitation

M. A. NALDA

Department of Anesthesiology, Faculty of Medicine, University of Salamanca, Salamanca, Spain

Of all the dramatic situations through which a doctor has to live, perhaps the most difficult is the occasion on which a decision is made to start or maintain a resuscitation. The recuperation or loss of a human life may depend on the application of medical knowledge, techniques and professional standards.

In my opinion, there is no doubt that resuscitation must be started or maintained whenever the possibility exists of saving a life that would otherwise be lost due to the failure of natural response and defense mechanisms.

The first problem is to determine whether an extreme situation will be susceptible to a resuscitative effort.

All who work in this field have experienced the desperate case which is medically and humanely unsalvageable, but which nevertheless in an inexplicable manner, has managed to recover completely. This may cause personal doubt with consequent danger and detriment of performance. It is these exceptional cases which encourage perseverance and therapeutic efforts on many occasions even when the futility of the effort is obvious.

Outside the hospital resuscitation must be improvised, because normally there are no appropriate instruments for the task, but in spite of this a truly useful attempt must be made. Inside the hospital the approach to the problem is fundamentally different, since normally, all the necessary apparatus for resuscitation is available.

The right to die is one of the fundamental human rights which should be respected. It may be that physicians are unable to respect this right.

The problems of resuscitation cannot be divorced from this debate. The Kafkaesque climate existing in some Resuscitating Teams and Intensive Care Units, in which serious psychological problems abound because all available space is filled by noisy monitors, fans, vacuum extractors and other instruments, is really frightening.

Doctors and nurses of these services are themselves terrified at the possibility of being patients in such places. McKegney speaks of an 'Intensive Care Unit syndrome', while Egerton et al. in a more alarmist view, describe an 'ordeal' and Nahum refers to it as the 'dementia of medical progress of these units'.

Social isolation, monotony, passivity, the hopes of the patient and individual tolerance to the psychic and somatic stress are all factors which tend to be ignored. It is unquestionable that much energy, hours of work and finances are wasted in the pretence of maintaining alive some patients who are truly dead.

Dystanasia, a new term in medical deontology, pretends to delay for as long as possible and by all means, the moment of death, and thus causes in many cases, the start of a life of vegetation supported only by artificial means, by techniques and respirators.

The World Health Organization postulates (1968) are not always observed to identify total or irreversible death: absence of reception and response (coma); absence of spontaneous respiration and movements; areflexia; absence of cardiac activity (spontaneous activity); flat EEG; persistence of all these findings for at least 24 hr. As a result the doubts and tribulations of physicians are multiplied, and the moral problems may become overwhelming.

To invoke religious principles would be totally invalid because of the number of religions represented amongst resuscitating specialists but, it may be important for Catholics to notice the words of Paul VI to the Congress of the World Federation of Catholic Physicians: 'the principle of respect for human life enforces us to maintain this as much as is possible, but not to pretend to prolong it by all means until a totally vegetable life exists'. This may be an important moral factor to encourage Catholics to decline to start resuscitation when they consider a patient totally, psychologically or psychically dead – there are many other religions to consider.

Superficial appreciation of these concepts makes those, whose professional standards do not go beyond tradition or a superficial veneer, vacillate, and even though perhaps moved by a 'purely professional' finality absurd attempts are made to recover patients.

It is clear that there is an international preoccupation about the unequivocal diagnosis of death. The doubt does not seem to disappear with years of professional practice, but on the contrary, it seems even greater, and it rises to unexpected levels in the Resuscitation Teams and Intensive Care Units.

In conclusion resuscitative efforts should be started and maintained whenever the possibility exists that a human life can be salvaged. Resuscitation should not be started or should be stopped as soon as it is certain that whatever it is that makes us individual persons, has been lost.

REFERENCES

Cantero, F. (1972): *Rev. esp. Anest., 19/4*, 495.
Egerton, N. and Kay, J. H. (1964): *Brit. J. psychiat. soc. Work, 110*, 433.
Lopez Ibor Jr, J. J. (1973): *Act. luso-esp. Neurol., 1/5*, 661.
McKengey, F. P. (1966): *Conn. Med., 30*, 633.
Nahum, O. (1965): *Conn. Med., 29*, 771.

The problems of medical morality in connection with the donor and the recipient of transplants with particular reference to heart transplants*

A. MILHAUD

Department of Anesthesia-Reanimation, Centre Hospitalier Régional d'Amiens, Amiens, France

It was, perhaps, an error for this subject to be entrusted to the author, who is neither religious, nor a lawyer, nor a moralist but is an anesthesiologist.

Madame de Sévigné (Fig. 1) of the seventeenth century, was not, it seems, at the forefront to progress in her epoch, since she said: 'Just one look at the doctors makes one not wish to offer his body' which is in marked contrast to Rembrandt (Fig. 2).

Transplants are of interest to the anesthesiologist from different points of view; anesthesia, resuscitation of the recipient, the diagnosis of cerebral death, the maintenance of the donor, organization, coordination of the teams, consideration of the relatives and technics of storage are all important matters.

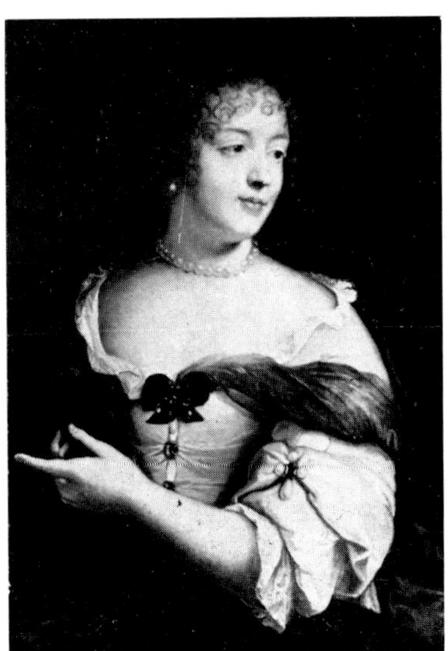

Fig. 1.   *Madame de Sévigné.*

* Supported by grants from Institut de Recherches Picard pour la Medecine d'Urgence (I.R.P.M.U.).

One hundred subjects in the state of cerebral death have been managed in Amiens of which 35 have been maintained for 12–72 hr, and donated their kidneys; 40 of the 70 kidneys have been grafted with immediate success with aid of the French transplant association. Unfortunately, for a year, it has become very difficult to obtain permission from the families although this may be a particular problem for France, and for which there is no simple explanation.

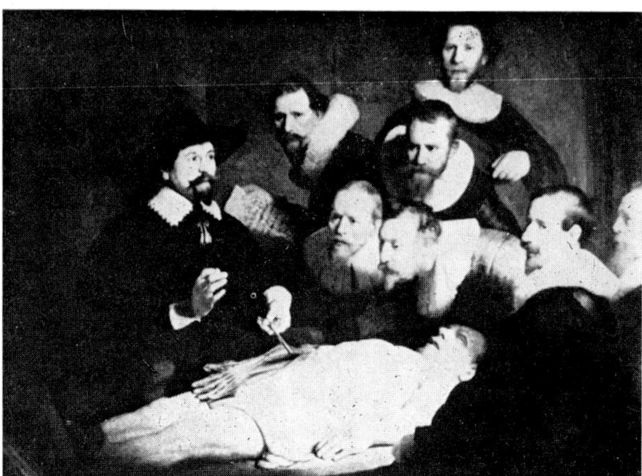

Fig. 2.   *Rembrandt's: The anatomy lesson.*

The lessening in the numbers of donors is itself attributed to certain publicity in the press which has received too much attention; Montaigne could not say more: 'The doctors have the advantage in that their failures are buried, but their successes are walking in the sun'.

In May 1968 in France, the Order of Medicine stated that 'The Council of the Order is afraid of the facts publicly accorded to types of therapeutics, which is actually a nuisance to the progress of science'.

Madame Cara-Beurton said at a seminar in Amiens in April of 1973 (Cara et al., 1974): 'Ethics are the science of morality: they define and analyse human sentiments which orient the individual in his daily life'. (These are the 'vertus morales' of Aristotle: the force, the temperance and the justice.) The moral must help man to live, by a just appreciation of good and evil, and a union of the forces of the soul. It must permit conciliation and safeguard those individuals who have requirements in the communal life. The role of morality is in the conscience, and man is entirely free of good or of evil usage of his will. Thus it is this that establishes through the ages of *rules of morality*, determining the structure of different societies: it is in fact difficult to discuss the rules of morality and their scope, because different solutions are found from one relation to the next. The 'morality' is in perpetual change, in relation to technical progress and also to the political and economic situation. For example, when, in May 1963, we proposed the use of organs from a subject in a state of cerebral death, many doctors were ignorant of the work of Wertheimer, Goulon, Mollaret and others on this subject, and condemned it as immoral.

On the other hand, all have admitted at last that the use of kidneys ex vivo of a parent, is perfectly legitimate.

Prof. Hamburger meditated over the problems of morality posed by the methods of substitution and of transplantation, and declared that 'when it is a question of the generosity of a both sane and responsible father or mother who insists calmly and deliberately to offer one of their own kidneys for transplantation to their child dying of chronic uremia it is not possible to deny the dignity of their desire'. The voluntary donor is becoming more and more rare since the progress in transplants from cadavers makes living transplantation offend medical morality (Fig. 3).

Removal from cadavers or, more precisely from subjects in a state of cerebral death, are considered to be legitimate by almost all physicians and also by the public in the greater part of the world, based on the criteria of cerebral death. Some borrowed quotations of a remarkable book by Doll (1970), counsellor of the appellate court of Paris, will be used as proof of these 2 affirmations:

'The Christian religions admit that the body receives eternal life with the purification of the soul. However, other religions separate the body and the soul and thus a definite character is assigned to both.'

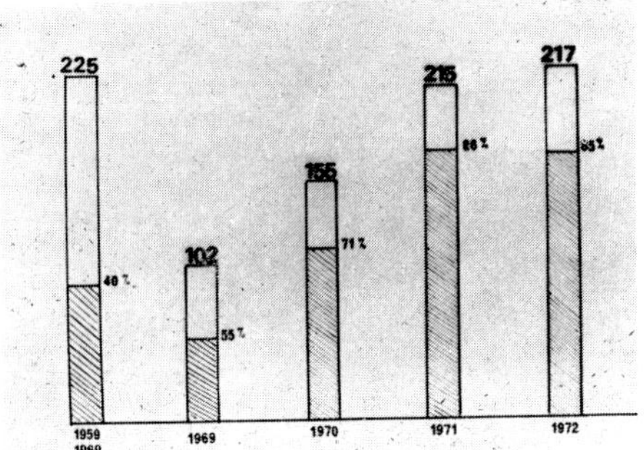

Fig. 3. *Number of renal transplants in France (white area = related donors; shaded area = non-related donors).*

For the Catholic church, the intangibility of 'the cadaver is not a dogma', on the 13th of May 1956 Pope Pius the XII declared formally, at a meeting of his congress about keratoplasty.

'Rabbi Kaplan had expressed the agreement of the Jewish religion, with the announcement of the catholic church; we are not surprised by this decision because of the common root of the both religions.'

A public opinion poll taken by the I.F.O.P. (1968) asked those polled 'would you authorize, after your death, the removal of certain organs for transplantation, to aid the survival of another individual?' 65% of those persons (in France) answered yes (in England 80% and 70% in the U.S.A.).

French decree No. 47-0257 of 20 October 1947 (J.O. 25 October 1947) specifically states: 'However, in the hospital establishments listed by the Minister of the Public Health and of the Population, if the chief of the department considers that a scientific or a therapeutic interest exists, the request for autopsy and the removal of organs, even in the absence of the authorization of the family, should be practiced *without delay*. In this case the death must be witnessed by and confirmed by 2 physicians of the establishment with the duty to employ all the processes known to be valuable to the Minister of the Public Health, to assure the reality of death'.

It is impossible to cite all the legally relevant texts to the removal of organs, since there are many in the greater number of countries which try to facilitate the practice of transplantation.

For example Spanish Ordonnance of 17 February 1955 confirms the provisions of Article 6 of the law of 18 December 1950, 'in case of violent death, the judges of instruction have authorization power, according to the circumstances, to allow the removal of parts of the cadaver for transplantation, when the clinical necessity is evident, and when the replies to the following conditions are satisfactory:

1. When the deceased has during his life, given his permission by an authentic method.
2. When the members of his family, with whom he has lived, give the authorization.
3. When it is impossible to contact or find the family, but that this will not present any opposition to the procedure.'

Then we remember that on the 2nd of February 1968 the soviet Minister of Health, Petrowsky, had for himself given the 'green light' for heart transplants.

Thus, there are only the Moslem countries which maintain opposition to the removal of organs from cadavers for religious reasons. In effect, to be able to attain the paradise of Allah, the believer must reach his rewards with his complete person. Therefore, during his terrestrial life an amputation of a limb or organ is possible but after death his body must repose intact.

On the other hand, if it is necessary for a moslem to receive an organ transplant, his religion would authorize the operation because the organ would aid his survival. Jehovahs witnesses oppose completely organ transplantation in any manner into their bodies, in fact refuse to accept serum or blood transfusions; thus the grafting of organs is not accepted.

In summary, but for a few exceptions, religion does not present a barrier to the performance of organ transplants, since it lengthens individual freedom to complete his terrestrial life, if he is willing.

Therefore, Doll has proposed for France a donor card. It would resemble closely the medallion system used in the U.S.A. having: name, first name, blood group and donor for eyes, for kidneys, as is now used in the greater number of States. In greater Pittsburgh, Pennsylvania, many thousands over the age of 18 years, wear one such medallion around their necks or on their wrists.

In the case of cerebral death, the doctors are given the responsibility to estimate that the death of the brain is synonymous with death. There is practical unanimity about the definitions of cerebral death.

In France (1966), a Ministerial circular was prepared which clarified the problem, and the following are some of the extracts.

This decision would especially be based: 'on the methodical analysis of the circumstances in which accidents are caused; on the entirely artificial character of the continuation of respiration; on the total abolition of all reflexes, complete hypotonus and dilation of the pupils; on the total loss of an electroencephalographic signal (no trace, no possible reactivity) spontaneous or stimulated by all possible artificial means for a sufficient period, in the absence of sedative drugs; the irreversibility of functional death could perhaps serve to establish agreement where one of these signs is absent – such absence should not permit the declaration of death; the certification of death of a patient submitted to prolonged intensive care is confirmed finally following consultation between 2 physicians'.

In the U.S.A., there exists no active legal definition of death. A committee composed of 12 well-esteemed Harvard University Professors of Medicine, in August 1968 decided that a doctor does have the means of saying that the brain is dead.

In April 1973, it was insisted by many of the Amiens Seminar (A.A.F. – Cara et al., 1974) that there are other paraclinical criteria than the electroencephalograph; for example arteriovenous jugulocarotid differences, concentration of enzymes in the cerebrospinal fluid, cerebral scintigraph, electroretinograph, and echoencephalograph, etc. As for these criteria which are clinical, the best clinical sign is probably apnea, which is demonstrated at the time of disconnecting from the ventilator which is done *in pure oxygen, after denitrogenation,* to suppress the extreme hypoxemia and the risk of causing circulatory arrest. This is a simple technic, and is a test which extends over 20 min; the arterial P_{O_2} does not drop below 250 mm Hg.

The moral problems concerning the recipient of a transplant do exist, because apart from renal transplantation the results are such that comparison is possible between the effectiveness of transplantation and that of other therapeutic technics especially chronic hemodialysis.

There are problems which are particularly acute concerning heart transplants. Most industrialized countries have the equipment and the medical/surgical teams who have practiced some form of cardiac transplantation. However, most hesitate to carry out the procedure, because, for once, technical progress is one step behind the progress of moral principles. There are 3 major factors in this delay.

Firstly, it is now possible to be certain that patients suitable for transplant have a prognosis as long as a month and, if they do, whether their physical state might not accept a transplant. Secondly, it is impossible to stop rejection completely. Thirdly, prolonged extracorporeal circulation is not yet sufficiently developed to work for days or weeks.

The Shumway statistics remind us all that of 70 heart transplants, less than 20 survive, and all except one, survived less than 3 years.

Mr. Kornprobst made a very pertinent remark on the subject: 'One can imagine that the father of a family, a man of important affairs, perhaps an author, or an artist might prefer the risks of survival, with the same possibility of danger, and the shelter of a treatment may prolong his life for months, whereas a transplant could cause immediate death.'

CONCLUSION

In the author's opinion it is desirable that heart transplants remain exceptional for mainly technical reasons, and until animal experimentation solves the technical problems. The economic questions merit study (a heart transplantation is much more expensive than esophageal surgery).

Barnado said: 'It is immoral to bury a heart while it can still serve'. In paraphrase it is possible to conclude: 'It is immoral to bury a kidney while it can still serve'.

REFERENCES

Cara, M. and Milhaud, A. et al. (1974): *Ann. Anest. franç.*, *15 (Special Issue)*, 1.

Doll, P. J. (1970): *La Discipline des Greffes des Transplantations et des Autres Actes de Disposition Concernant le Corps Humain*. Masson et Cie, Paris.

Doll, P. J. (1974): *Paper presented at:* XXXIV Congrès International de Langue Française de Médecine Légale et de Médecine Sociale, Liège, 1974.

Milhaud, A. (1964): *Ann. Anest. franç.*, *5*, 639.

Brain death

A. CÉU COUTINHO

Department of Neurosurgery, Hospital Júlio de Matos, Lisbon, Portugal

Limitations of time and space make it impossible even to summarize the various aspects of brain death, namely etiopathology, physiopathology and biochemistry, morphology, diagnosis and prophylaxis. Therefore only some aspects of the problem more related to medical deontology will be discussed.

Concepts, inherent to human thought and indispensable to the process of thinking, are generalizations and abstractions, which do not exist as such in Nature. As abstractions and generalizations they do not correspond exactly to the objects of knowledge, one of the main goals of science being to render that correspondence more and more precise, in an 'infinitely asymptotic progression', as Engels wrote. Life and death, as concepts, are not entities which exist as such in the living or the dead; entities that beings possess or do not possess. These terms correspond to phases of material processes; processes in which life contains death and vice-versa, each one being inconceivable without the other; the concepts of life and death are considered in their dialectic unity, accepting that life is 'special ways of handling energy' (Morrison, 1971) or a peculiar form of movement of matter; not only spatial movement but movement or transformation characterized by the laws of Biology (Oparine, 1961). In this context death is the cessation, the nonexistence or the negation of life, that is the negation of that kind of movement. In addition, concepts have a historical basis, and historical evolution, not only in relation to an individual's history but also to the history of humanity. The concepts of life and death are not exceptions.

When faced with a particular case and the decision of life or death, i.e., when the concepts become operative, a certain number of criteria must be put forward in order to know if biological movement exists or not. This is particularly difficult in such a complex being as the human, that itself has parts which can live even after separation from the whole, and as a consequence of the fact that death is a process and not an event. This difficulty is further enhanced when the diagnosis of death must be made within short periods, such as when organ and/or tissue transplantation is foreseen. These criteria and their development are reviewed.

Halley and Harvey (1968), Beecher et al. (1968), Kantrowitz (1969), Morison (1971), and Kass (1971) discuss death as a *process* or an *event*. This discussion is closely related to our subject and will answer the question of Mollaret and Goulon (1959): 'where to place this fraction of a second, which separates death from life?' In the great majority of cases (if not all) death of man or of one of his organs, the brain inclusive, is a process. Perhaps the sudden carbonization of the whole body by the explosion of an atomic bomb makes a rare exception to this. What is an event is our decision, at a given moment of this process, to consider it irreversible. The event of diagnosing death is, of course, determined by the medical belief of the impossibility of resuscitation or by the prohibition of law to do it, e.g., capital punishment. Two examples will perhaps make it clear. The condemned does not die biologically at the precise moment the guillotine cuts his neck; in this case, after decapitation, the heart continues to beat and the brain to live for some time. In some cases at least, the condemned does not die at the exact moment at which the current of the electric chair stops his brain functioning or his heart beating; in this latter case he could even sometimes be resuscitated, by defibrillating his heart. It is the law which wants, decides his death at that precise moment and forbids his resuscitation.

This decision has been taken at different moments during the process of death in different eras and according to the medical knowledge of those eras. It can be predicted that, in the future, with the accumulation of further knowledge, the diagnosis of death will be made on criteria different from those of the past and of today.

To the classical concept of *clinical death*, based mainly on the respiratory and cardio-circulatory standstill, to the concept of death, based on the total and irreversible failure of the spontaneous respiratory, cardiovascular and CNS (central nervous system) functions, a new one has been added, as a result of the possibility of employing the new techniques of resuscitation and the need for removing organs and/or tissues for transplantation as soon as possible. This new concept – *biological death* (Negovskii quoted by Hockaday et al., 1965), *functional death* (Halley and Harvey, 1968), *partial death* (Leel-Ossy and Torok, 1972), *dissociated brain death* (Kramer quoted by Steinbereithner and Kucher, 1972) – is based on the death of the whole brain alone, in spite of the artificial maintenance of the cardiovascular, respiratory, renal, digestive and other functions, by resuscitation and intensive care techniques, which have enabled 'true isolated heart-lung preparations' (Jouvet, 1959; Wertheimer et al., 1959), or 'the clinical equivalent of the heart-lung prepa-ration of the physiologist' (Mollaret and Goulon, 1959) to be maintained for a long time. In fact, once the irreversible anatomo-functional disintegration of the structures which are the seat of mental life and which command the vegetative, sensorial and motor life of the individual is accomplished, it is now lawful to permit the disintegration of the rest of the body, that is, to permit thereafter the natural evolution of the process of death. If we consider a human organism as alive when it is a composite whole which constitutes an integrated functional unit (Kass, 1971), integration that in man is mainly dependent on the CNS, then we must assume that the disintegration of this functional unit, through brain irreversible disintegration or death, is the equivalent of the death of that organism, although some of its parts continue to live in the same body, in another organism by transplantation, or in cell cultures. The difficulty arises mainly in determining the moment of irreversibility of this disintegration process.

In the mind of scientists, a new concept of death – *social death* or *social brain death* – can arise in the future. It would consist of the irreversible annihilation of relation life, in spite of the maintenance of a rudimentary mental, sensorial and motor life and the normal respiratory, cardiovascular and other vegetative functions – when in fact the individual has lost his personality and liberty and no longer has 'rational' characteristics. Some persist in a state comparable to that of anencephalic monsters. The chronic postcoma syndromes, in which the patients although 'alive', are totally lost in relation to family and social life are examples of such states. It is known that these syndromes are a consequence of partial brain death, of more or less extensive lesions of the cerebral hemisphere cortex and/or white matter and/or some other subcortical structures. The following statement of the Declaration of Sydney (1968) should be remembered '. . . clinical interest lies not in the state of preservation of isolated cells but in the fate of a person'.

A series of new problems would arise for the medical team and for the legislator, if a new concept of death based on these clinical pictures were to be elaborated in the future. For instance, problems of orthotanasia (Beleza, 1973; Dias, 1973) since it is likely that euthanasia will continue to be forbidden.

The following experimental and clinical data permit an understanding of the complexity of brain anatomical organization and pathology and of the difficulty of diagnosing partial and total brain death.

According to Cohen (1973), at least in vitro, cortical slices from the brain of developing and mature rabbits revealed the same sensibility to anoxia. On the other hand, the brains of the fetus and of the newborn seem to tolerate ischemia and anoxia better, on account of lower metabolic rate, poikilothermia and anaerobic source of energy (Himwhich et al., 1941). Kabat (1940), working with dogs of very different ages, concluded that the revival times after brain ischemia diminished gradually from 20 min at the age of 10 days to 6 min in the adult animal; he verified also that the resistance of the brain to ischemia or to anoxia decreases rapidly after birth and then more slowly with advancing age.

With some peculiarities according to the etiology, and the presence of vascular variants and other cerebral conditions prior to the lesion, it is known that there are some areas in the brain more vulnerable than others. In a given individual the more profound and phylogenetically older regions (brain stem and spinal cord) are more resistant than the cerebral hemispheres (Mollaret and Goulon, 1959; Hamlin, 1964). For example, the revival time of the spinal cord after ischemia is approximately 15 min (Gelfan and Tarlov, 1955). In the cerebral cortex itself, ischemic lesions are more frequent in the occipital than in the frontal lobes. The third, fifth and sixth laminae of the cortex are more vulnerable than the second and the fourth (Brierley, 1972).

Grey and white matter have different sensitivities to different noxious stimuli. On the other hand different populations of neurones have different resistance to anoxia; for example, the motoneurone somas of the spinal cord are more sensitive to O_2 lack than the interneurones (Gelfan and Tarlov, 1955); the Purkinje cells of the cerebellum are more vulnerable and the granules more resistant (Brierley, 1972).

Various regions of the brain and of the spinal cord are not equally perfused and there are some areas with terminal or almost terminal capillary circulation which, therefore, are more liable to ischemic or anoxic lesions than others. Variations of the cerebral arterial pattern, so frequent in the Willis' poligone, will also influence the distribution and severity of the lesions. Variations of chemical composition of different brain regions will definitely influence their resistance to various noxae.

Some chronic and seemingly stable brain lesions have, in fact, an evolutive character and manifest themselves clinically only months or years later. This is the case of many post-traumatic and postencephalitic epilepsies and postencephalitic parkinsonism, due to the surreptitious progress of degeneration of nerve fibers or of the extension of an apparently innocent cerebral scar, which invades previously healthy areas (Strich, 1969).

It is understandable, therefore, that all these facts allied to the high complexity of the organization of the brain, make the study of its functions and dysfunctions and the diagnosis of its death a difficult task for the clinician. In fact, the whole brain, not only in the case of local injury, but also in that of general pathological causes, does not die at the same time. and it can occur that some areas are destroyed and others more or less spared or subjected to reversible lesions.

Thus between the healthy brain and the totally dead brain, there are a number of intermediate degrees of partially dead brains with corresponding clinical pictures of impairment of its sensorio-motor, vegetative and psychic functions. Different degrees of deterioration of these functions correspond to the different localization and extension of the lesions. The 'appalic syndrome' of Kretschmer, the 'akinetic mutism' of Cairns, the 'prolonged unconsciousness stupor' of French, the 'white matter degeneration' of Strich, the 'post-comatose' or 'vigile decerebrate stupor', the 'postcomatose psychomotor dissolution', the 'persistent vegetative state' of Jennet and Plum, the 'prolonged comas' of Le Beau, the 'anoetic complex' of Duensing, the 'postcomatose hypertonic stupor' of Fischgold and Mathis, in which the individual has completely or nearly completely lost his relation with the environment, with dementia, and destruction of his personality and liberty, are examples of such lesions that produce true social death. There is the same doubt about these patients as Gomez (1972): 'Does he continue to be a person?' With modern techniques of resuscitation such clinical pictures are becoming more and more frequent. It is still particularly difficult or impossible, in the acute phase of partial lesions, to know in what measure they are reversible or will end in irreversible and more or less disabling brain lesions.

It is clear that in the absence of resuscitation centers, the diagnosis of death is most frequently based on the old criteria of death, because the great majority of people 'die their 'own death', as Torga, a colleague of ours and a great Portugese writer says. The problems of brain death arise most frequently in resuscitation centers and intensive care units mainly when organ and/or tissue transplantation is foreseen. Once resuscitation has been initiated the diagnosis of the patient's death is made by the death of his brain.

Nowadays most medical teams make such a diagnosis by the conjugation of a number of data, whose meaning and importance cannot now be discussed. The value of the complementary means at the disposal of the medical team is still subject to controversy, as well as details of their interpretation and their technical execution. Nevertheless difficulties with respect to the diagnosis of total brain death have been greatly reduced in recent years, although some problems are still awaiting solution, especially with respect to an early diagnosis, in connection with possible organ and/or tissue removal for transplantation.

Since one pathognomonic sign or instrumental datum of total brain death, to provide an early diagnosis, does not yet exist, the team which has to make the decision must employ the means at its disposal, choosing the most reliable and most feasible. These include EEG, SEEG (stereoelectroencephalography), cerebral angiography, radionuclide studies, chemical and cytologic CSF (cerebrospinal fluid) examination, echoencephalography, rheoencephalography, vestibular stimulation, oxygen carotid-jugular gradient, cerebral biopsy, etc.

A few authors think that these are not the means to make a diagnosis of brain death with absolute certainty (Bricolo et al., 1972). Most authors, however, place more confidence on the means at their disposal. For instance Wertheimer et al. (1959) state that, with a certain number of data, it is possible ' . . . to make with certainty the diagnosis of *irreversible* CNS death', and Gros (1972) states that echoencephalography, γ-scintigraphy, cerebral angiography, intracranial-arterial tension equilibrium, per se or in combinations are sufficient to diagnose cessation of the cerebral circulation and hence brain death, even before 24 hr of isoelectric EEG have elapsed or the clinical picture of coma dépassé is established.

The majority of authors base the diagnosis of brain death on the history (the etiology of the process is most important), the clinical picture of coma dépassé and isoelectric EEG. Mohandas and Chou (1971) however, think that if the clinical neurophysiological criteria of brain death are met, the value of an EEG is questionable. These criteria are standardized at the University of Minnesota Health Sciences Center as follows: (1) no spontaneous movement; (2) no spontaneous respiration when tested for a period of 4 min at a time; (3) absence of brain stem reflexes: (*a*) dilated and fixed pupils, (*b*) absent corneal reflexes, (*c*) absent ciliospinal reflexes, (*d*) absent Doll's head phenomena, (*e*) absent gag reflex, (*f*) absent vestibular response to caloric stimulation, (*g*) absent tonic neck reflex; (4) a status in which all of the findings above remain unchanged for at least 12 hr; (5) brain death can be pronounced only if the pathological processes responsible for States 1 through 4 above are deemed irreparable with presently available means.

It would be very interesting to make the diagnosis of brain death merely on clinical grounds, but this point 5 raises a big problem in applying these criteria – which processes are deemed irreparable? Plum (1972) who agrees with the possibility of a purely clinical diagnosis of brain death, answers in a certain measure, this question in '*Processes of Structural or Anoxic Brain Injury*'.

Disagreement also exists between those authors who make the diagnosis of brain death 'in the presence of heart beat and relatively normal blood pressure' (Hockaday et al., 1965), or in cases in which 'the circulation may be intact' (Plum, 1972), and those who make such a diagnosis only with the full clinical picture of coma dépassé, i.e., if cardiovascular collapse supervenes after discontinuing cardiocirculatory support measures.

The above mentioned criteria of the Minnesota University do not even refer to the cardio-vascular situation.

In any case it would be desirable for a diagnosis of brain death to be made by a team of at least 3 members – an internist, a resuscitator and a neurologist or neurosurgeon – a team that should not include anybody pertaining to a team eventually involved in a transplantation of an organ or tissue from the patient. The advice given by Beecher et al. (1968) to turn off the respirator only after declaring the patient dead should be stressed. This is very important from a legal point of view, as otherwise the medical team can be incriminated of homicide or, at least, euthanasia.

Whilst the diagnosis of brain death is merely a medical problem, organ removal for transplantation must be discussed with the patients family.

REFERENCES

Ad Hoc Committee of the Harvard Medical School to Examine the Definition of Brain Death (1968): *J. Amer. med. Ass., 205/6*, 337.

Beecher, H. K. et al. (1968): *J. Amer. med. Ass., 205/6*, 337.

Beleza, J. (1973): In: *As Técnicas Modernas de Reanimação*. Ordem dos Avogados. Porto.

Bricolo, A., Ore, G. D., Pian, R., Benati, A. and Turella, G. (1972): In: *Proceedings, IV European Congress of Neurosurgery*, p. 561. Avicenum, Prague.

Brierley, J. B. (1972): In: *Scientific Foundations of Neurology*, p. 243. William Heinemann Medical Books, Ltd., London.

Cohen, M. M. (1973): *Biochemistry, Ultrastructure and Physiology of Cerebral Anoxia, Hypoxia and Ischemia*, p. 1. Editor: M. M. Cohen. S. Karger, Basel.

Dias, J. F. (1973): In: *As Técnicas Modernas de Reanimação*. Ordem dos Advogados. Porto.

Engels, F.: In: *Dialectique de la Nature*, p. 237. Sociales, Paris.

Gelfan, S. and Tarlov, I. M. (1955): *J. Neurophysiol., 18*, 170.

Gomez, F. C. (1972): *Rev. esp. Anest., 19*, 495.

Gros, C. (1972): *Neuro-chirurgie, 18*, 37.

Halley, M. M. and Harvey, W. F. (1968): *J. Amer. med. Ass., 204/6*, 423.

Hamlin, H. (1964): *J. Amer. med. Ass., 190/2*, 112.

Himwich, H. E., Alexander, F. A. D. and Fazekas, J. F. (1941): *Amer. J. Physiol., 134*, 327.

Hockaday, J. M., Potts, F., Epstein, E., Bonazzi, A. and Schwab, R. S. (1965): *Electroenceph. clin. Neurophysiol., 18*, 575.

Jouvet, M. (1959): *Electroenceph. clin. Neurophysiol., 11*, 805.

Kabat, H. (1940): *Amer. J. Physiol., 130*, 588.

Kantrowitz, A. (1969): In: *The Moment of Death*, p. 66. Editor: A. Winter. Charles C. Thomas, Springfield, Ill.

Kass, L. R. (1971): *Science, 173*, 698.

Leel-Ossy, L. and Torok, P. (1972): In: *Proceedings, IV European Congress of Neurosurgery*, p. 567. Avicenum, Prague.

Mohandas, A. and Chou, S. N. (1971): *J. Neurosurg., 35*, 211.

Mollaret, P. and Goulon, M. (1959): *Rev. neurol., 101*, 3.

Morison, R. S. (1971): *Science, 173*, 694.

Oparine, A. (1961): In: *La Vie et l'Evolution*, p. 5. La Nouvelle Critique, Paris.

Plum, F. (1972): In: *Scientific Foundations of Neurology*, p. 193. William Heinemann Medical Books, Ltd., London.

Steinbereithner, K. and Kucher, R. (1972): In: *Intensiv Station Pflege Therapie*, p. 515. Georg. Thieme Verlag, Stuttgart – Leipzig.

Strich, S. J. (1969): In: *The Late Effect of Head Injury*, p. 501. Charles C. Thomas, Springfield, Ill.

Wertheimer, P., Jouvet, M. and Descotes, J. (1959): *Presse méd., 67*, 87.

Chapter XVIII

Neuroanaesthesia

Control of intracranial pressure

JOHN BARKER

Division of Neuro-anaesthesia, Institute of Neurological Sciences, Glasgow, United Kingdom

Recent advances in techniques of monitoring intracranial pressure have given great impetus to the management of neurosurgical cases. Monitoring has proved of value in diagnosis, therapy and prognosis and, for the anesthesiologist it has been of particular value in the intraoperative management of these cases.

TECHNIQUES OF MONITORING INTRACRANIAL PRESSURE

Lundberg (1960) first demonstrated the value of continuous recording of intracranial pressure (ICP) in the management of patients with space occupying lesions and intracranial hypertension of other origin. He displayed several waveforms including plateau waves and made it clear that single isolated measurements of subarachnoid or intracranial pressure were of little value. Nowadays it is commonplace in many neurosurgical clinics to transduce intracranial pressure and continuously display this. However, there are certain disadvantages to catheterisation of the lateral ventricle which include loss of cerebrospinal fluid, infection and limitation of monitoring time, and recently devices have been invented to record ICP extradurally, subdurally and from brain itself. In all systems sensor and transducer act as detector but in the extraventricular methods there are problems of calibration, correction for drift and fluid penetration of the system. This makes it difficult to measure absolute pressure though recording of changes in pressure are possible. Telemetry is a difficult technique because of problems in getting a suitable energy source and reliable in vivo calibration.

FACTORS INFLUENCING INTRACRANIAL PRESSURE

Ventricular fluid pressure (VFP) monitoring is preferred in some centres because it is possible to have control of CSF drainage and Lundberg (1960) has emphasised the importance of immediate diagnosis and treatment which in some cases may be lifesaving. Miller and Garibi (1972) studied the intracranial volume/pressure response (VPR) during continuous monitoring of VFP in 20 patients by inducing small increases in the volume of fluid in the lateral ventricle. They added 1 ml saline or withdrew 1 ml CSF and found a direct relationship between VFP and VPR. By giving early warning of the stage at which small increases in volume cause large increases in ICP these measurements can help in the prevention of brain tightness or elastance (inverse compliance). Leech and Miller (1974b) have shown that mannitol significantly reduced both VFP and VPR in patients with intracranial hypertension, the reduction of VPR being significantly greater than that of VFP. Similarly the reduction in VPR was more marked than VFP reduction 24 hr after the start of steroid therapy. Their results suggest that both forms of therapy can reduce VFP and make the intracranial contents less susceptible to steep rises in pressure with addition of volume to the cranium. In studies in primates Leech and Miller (1974*b*) also showed that there was less effect on elastance with hyperventilation though ICP is reduced. Furthermore Rowed et al. (1975) suggest that any beneficial effect of hypocapnia on ICP is likely only to be temporary. It seems, therefore, that mannitol has a double action in reducing brain water volume and periventricular elastance, while having little effect on cerebral blood flow. Thus it provides a more satisfactory method than hyperventilation in protecting the brain against the dangers of ICP (Leech and Miller, 1974*b*).

Changes in mean arterial blood pressure can also influence intracranial pressure. The simultaneous recording of ICP and MABP can be very useful in diagnosis because they allow easy estimation of perfusion pressure. Brain compression and increased ICP can cause arterial hypertension, bradycardia and respiratory irregularities but this relationship is very variable (Johnston et al., 1970). A possible source of increased intracranial volume is cerebral oedema. When there is focal oedema, a rise in blood pressure can increase its volume and extent (Klatzo et al., 1967). The concept of a 'breakthrough' of autoregulation by hypertension alone with the possibility of hyperperfusion followed by brain oedema has received publicity recently (Skinhøj and Strandgaard, 1973; Byron, 1973; Rosenblum, 1974). Following studies in primates Leech and Miller (1974*a*) suggest that arterial hypertension in patients with increased ICP is likely to have a deleterious effect by increasing brain elastance.

MONITORING OF ICP DURING ANAESTHESIA

Nowadays it is commonplace to monitor ICP during neurosurgical anaesthesia (Nornes and Magnaes, 1971; Shapiro et al., 1973; Becker et al., 1974); the induction of anaesthesia and the use of volatile agents are known to cause acute rises of ICP, the effect being more marked in patients with space-occupying lesions (Jennett et al., 1969). Certain mechanical factors such as the application of a head clamp or the insertion of a Gigli saw during operation can also cause acute rises in ICP (Shapiro et al., 1973). Endotracheal intubation may cause an arterial pressure response which can initiate a rise in ICP if autoregulation of the cerebral circulation is impaired. Continuous ICP monitoring can give warning of these rises and give guidance for the drainage of CSF or administration of mannitol. It can also be of use in positioning the patient for surgery (Becker et al., 1974). Nornes and Magnaes (1971) measured supratentorial epidural pressure during posterior fossa surgery and advised against rapid and extensive drainage of the ventricles because this may set up a secondary rise in ICP. Rapid and extensive spinal subarachnoid CSF drainage in aneurysm surgery may also result in acute arterial hypertension and cardiac arrhythmias which may be related to brain stem distortion (Aitken, personal communication). Finally the termination of anaesthesia can be associated with rises in ICP and MABP (Leech et al., 1974).

CONTROL OF ICP DURING NEUROSURGICAL ANAESTHESIA

The avoidance of a stormy induction is, of course, mandatory in neurosurgical anaesthesia as is the provision of anaesthesia, sufficiently deep to avoid straining during the operative procedure. Shapiro et al. (1973) have recommended the use of thiopentone by bolus injection of 1.5 mg/kg to prevent rises in ICP, especially those caused by mechanical factors. This is probably achieved by the cerebral metabolic depression produced by the barbiturates. Michenfelder and Theye (1973) suggest that thiopentone diminishes energy requirements of the brain by reducing its function. The protective action of barbiturates in canine acute focal cerebral ischaemia suggests they should be considered for anaesthesia in surgery requiring cerebral vessel occlusion, for example, intracranial aneurysm surgery (Smith et al., 1974). Other agents such as neuroleptanalgesic drugs are also useful supplements to nitrous oxide-oxygen anaesthesia. Volatile agents should be eschewed in patients with space occupying lesions although Adams et al. (1972) recommend their use in low concentrations combined with hypocapnia.

All patients presenting for neurosurgery should be ventilated but excessive hyperventilation is unnecessary and may be harmful. Indeed, Harp and Wollman (1973) feel that with present information patients with cerebrovascular disease or intracranial disease of any sort should be kept normocapnic.

The use of the osmotic dehydrating agent mannitol is to be recommended because of its effect in reducing brain elastance. Spinal drainage or ventricular drainage should only be used cautiously. In observations in patients having aneurysm surgery in this Institute, a drainage rate of spinal subarachnoid CSF of 5 ml/min or less did not produce any hypertensive response or ECG changes.

Attempts should be made to keep the blood pressure (MABP) in the range 70–100 mm Hg though short periods of hypertension to 40–50 mm Hg may be justified, for example in order to make an aneurysm slack and suitable for clipping. If MABP is kept below 40 mm Hg for a long period it may be associated with loss of autoregulation in the post-hypotensive period (Keaney et al., 1972). Any acute rise of blood pressure at this stage may quickly induce cerebral oedema.

It may not always be a wise policy to have the patient wide awake at the end of an operation. If anaesthesia is deep enough this might avoid the adverse effects of extubation and termination of anaesthesia. A slow emergence may be desirable though this may sound heretical to the neurosurgeon.

MANAGEMENT OF HEAD INJURIES

ICP monitoring is a valuable technique in the management of patients with brain damage (Johnston et al., 1970).

There has been a resurgence of interest in the uses of barbiturates and hypothermia in these cases. The long acting drug pentobarbitone used in conjunction with hypothermia and artificial ventilation has been recommended to reduce persistent intracranial hypertension (Shapiro et al., 1974).

Controlled ventilation as a specific therapeutic measure in severe head injuries continues to be recommended because of its effects in reducing ICP, improving brain perfusion, correcting intracerebral acidosis and improving oxygenation. However, there are still some doubts about the value of this method of treatment (Barker, 1975).

REFERENCES

Adams, R. W., Gronert, G. A., Sundt, T. M. and Michenfelder, J. D. (1972): *Anesthesiology, 37*, 510.

Barker, J. (1975): In: *Conservative Management of Head Injuries.* Editor: M. S. Albin. Excerpta Medica, Amsterdam. In press.

Becker, D. P., Young, H. F., Vries, J. K. and Adams, W. E. (1975): In: *Proceedings, 2nd Symposium on Intracranial Pressure, Lund.* Springer Verlag, Berlin – Heidelberg – New York. In press.

Byron, F. B. (1973): *Lancet, 1*, 766.

Harp, J. R. and Wollman, H. (1973): *Brit. J. Anaesth., 45*, 256.

Jennett, W. B., Barker, J., Fitch, W. and McDowall, D. G. (1969): *Lancet, 1*, 61.

Johnston, I. H., Johnston, J. A. and Jennett, B. (1970): *Lancet, 2*, 433.

Keaney, N., Pickerodt, V. W. A., McDowall, D. G., Coroneos, N. J., Turner, J. M. and Shah, J. M. (1972): *Brit. J. Anaesth.*, *44*, 623.

Klatzo, L., Wizniewski, H., Steinwell, D. and Streicher, E. (1967): In: *Brain Oedema*, p. 554. Editors: L. Klatzo and B. F. Seitel. Springer Verlag, Berlin – Göttingen – Heidelberg – New York.

Leech, P., Barker, J. and Fitch, W. (1974): *Brit. J. Anaesth.*, *46*, 315.

Leech, P. and Miller, J. D. (1974*a*): *J. Neurol. Neurosurg. Psychiat.*, *37*, 1099.

Leech, P. and Miller, J. D. (1974*b*): *J. Neurol. Neurosurg. Psychiat.*, *37*, 1105.

Lundberg, N. (1960): *Acta psychiat. scand. (Suppl.)*, *149/36*, 1.

Michenfelder, J. D. and Theye, R. A. (1973): *Anesthesiology*, *39*, 510.

Miller, J. D. and Garibi, J. (1972): In: *Intracranial Pressure*, p. 270. Editors: M. Brock and H. Dietz. Springer Verlag, Berlin – Heidelberg – New York.

Nornes, H. and Magnaes, B. (1971): *J. Neurosurg.*, *35*, 541.

Rosenblum, W. I. (1974): *Lancet*, *1*, 310.

Rowed, D. W., Leech, P., Reilly, P. C. and Miller, J. D. (1975): *Arch Neurol.*, in press.

Shapiro, H. M., Galindo, A., Wyte, S. R. and Harris, A. B. (1973): *Brit. J. Anaesth.*, *45*, 1057.

Shapiro, H. M., Wyte, S. R. and Loeser, J. (1974): *J. Neurosurg.*, *40*, 90.

Skinhøj, E. and Strandgaard, S. (1973): *Lancet*, *1*, 461.

Smith, A. L., Hoff, J. T., Neilson, S. L. and Larson, C. P. (1974): *Stroke*, *5*, 1.

Anaesthesia for paediatric neurosurgery

J. A. PUIG

Departamento de Anestesia-Reanimación, Ciudad Sanitaria 'La Paz',
Facultad de Medicina, Universidad Autónoma, Madrid, Spain

The smoothness with which the average neurosurgical operation proceeds in infancy and childhood today, and the marked reduction in morbidity and mortality incident to such surgery, can in a large part be credited to advances in anaesthesiology and the greatly increased availability of experienced personnel in this field.

The basic principles of neuroanaesthesia for children are the same as for the adult, viz. a good airway, adequate ventilation, a slack brain, minimal bleeding, sufficient neuro-vegetative protection with monitoring of vital functions and light anaesthesia to facilitate the postoperative neurological assessment, etc. Some aspects, however, are especially important, for example, body temperature, replacement of blood loss, fluid-electrolyte and acid-base balance. If these requirements are fulfilled, it is often impressive to see how well even the smallest infants tolerate several hours of major surgery.

METHODS

Preoperatively, respiratory, circulatory, nutrition, fluid-electrolytes, intracranial pressure (ICP) and general state are thoroughly investigated. If there is a doubt about fitness for operation, surgery should be postponed, provided that the risk of delay is negligible. During surgery, careful monitoring of cardiovascular, respiration, temperature, and blood-gasometry values is performed.

Newborns and children between 1 and 6 years of age may need nothing more than atropine for *premedication*; sedative drugs are not used because of the danger of depressing ventilation with a resultant increase in the ICP. On many occasions, vitamin K is administered due to the immaturity of hepatic enzymes.

The ideal method for *induction* is thiopentone plus succinylcholine for endotracheal intubation. In other cases, induction is with nitrous oxide-oxygen and halothane. Intubation is possible and the intravenous line is established later for fluid and drug administration. In both cases, endotracheal tubes must be 'non-kinking', of the correct size, scrupulously clean, accurately placed, and firmly secured to prevent serious accidents.

MAINTENANCE OF ANAESTHESIA

Nitrous oxide-oxygen and neuroleptanalgesia (Palfium-haloperidol or fentanyl-droperidol in small doses) for children over 7 years of age in order to obtain a decrease of ICP. In neonates and infants up to 6 years, anaesthesia is maintained by nitrous oxide-oxygen and halothane. In both groups of cases, mechanical intermittent positive pressure venti-lation (IPPV) with Engström or SF-4 ventilators is used. Paralysis of spontaneous respiration is achieved with d-tubocurarine or pancuronium. This technique reduces the ICP by decreasing the cerebral blood flow (CBF) due to the low arterial P_{CO_2} (25–30 mm Hg). Moreover, mechanical ventilation is quite beneficial because the baby is relieved of respiratory workload, the total amount of anaesthetic agents are reduced and postoperative recovery is rapid.

In posterior fossa surgery, constant observation of monitoring systems is essential. Extrasystoles, dropped beats, bigeminal rhythm and other irregularities serve as warnings. Occasionally, when the patient is breathing spontaneously, a simple Ayre's T-piece or a Digby-Leigh system with a heater-humidifying gas device is used. The ICP is monitored by Lundberg's technique (intraventricular catheter placed 12–24 hr before operation, pressure-transducer and paper-inscription kit). In those cases with a high ICP and where ventricular drainage is not possible, a rapid intravenous infusion of mannitol 20% and furosemide is given with a strict control of electrolytes and diuresis.

EXTUBATION

We oxygenate the child for some minutes before extubation and at the same time oral and pharyngeal secretions are removed.

TEMPERATURE CONTROL

With the advent of air conditioning, intubation and controlled respiration, the danger of hyperthermia has almost disappeared. Accidental hypothermia is a real cause of morbidity and mortality and precautions must be taken to avoid it.

Young children lose heat rapidly by convection and radiation and their shivering is ineffective in the production of heat. The length of operation, cold anaesthetic gases, absent muscle activity, and exposed brain, increase the heat loss.

The baby's body is covered with an electric mat-blanket, heated to a maximum of 39° C and anaesthetic gases are humidified and saturated with water vapour at 37° C. Blood for transfusion is also warmed to the same temperature in a thermostatically controlled heater.

BLOOD LOSS

Haemorrhage may be great. The need for blood replacement and the possibility that this may be necessary with great rapidity should therefore always be anticipated. Compensation for blood loss is poor in children and therefore it is important that intravenous access is assured (catheter).

Warm fresh blood must always be used for transfusion to avoid the dangers due to hyperkalaemia due to storage. If this is not available, stored blood plus calcium gluconate is used to minimize the effect of citrate. Prevention of metabolic acidosis is achieved by adding the correct dose of sodium bicarbonate (mEq). In very long operations, intraoperative haematocrit and haemoglobin determinations may be useful in addition to blood infusion, in order to avoid the danger of excessive replacement.

WATER AND ELECTROLYTE BALANCE

Intravenous catheters should include a 3-way stopcock to permit flushing and injection of drugs. Calculation of fluid requirements must be strictly observed according to body weight and laboratory determinations.

POSTOPERATIVE PERIOD

Dilutional hyponatraemia after operation necessitates restriction of the total amount of liquids given parenterally during the first 2 or 3 days and this fluid should be given as water and sugar (dextrose or fructose 5%). Persistent losses of fluid and electrolytes by vomiting, diarrhoea, cerebrospinal drainage, or bleeding, must be exactly evaluated and treated.

Postoperatively, careful monitoring continues and special attention should be paid to the level of consciousness, changing neurological signs, body temperature, cardiovascular and respiratory rates, radiological and laboratory controls, prophylactic antibiotics, suitable posture and, if necessary, reduction of cerebral swelling (dexamethasone) and antiepileptic treatment.

At all times, close cooperation with neurosurgeons is essential and a good atmosphere of humanity should be encouraged.

Some recent studies of the action of drugs used in neurosurgical anaesthesia

D. GORDON McDOWALL

Department of Anaesthesia, University of Leeds, Leeds, United Kingdom

There are many extensive reviews of the effects of anaesthetic drugs on the cerebral circulation (e.g., Smith and Wollman, 1972; McDowall, 1975). In this paper some of the more recent work on this subject is summarized.

ALTHESIN

It has long been known that thiopentone reduces cerebral blood flow, cerebral metabolic rate and cerebrospinal fluid pressure (Horsley, 1937; Pierce et al., 1962). The effects of the new steroid anaesthetic, Althesin, are similar – as shown in Figure 1 (Pickerodt et al., 1972). In the quoted study it was shown that 50 μl/kg Althesin reduced internal carotid blood flow by 21% and grey matter flow by 40% in lightly-anaesthetized baboons. There was marked depression of electrical activity, with an accompanying 46% reduction in cerebral oxygen uptake. With the reduction in carotid blood flow intracranial pressure fell. The fall in intracranial pressure has been shown by Turner et al. (1973) to occur also in man, and to be greatest in patients with elevated intracranial pressure. For these reasons Althesin is a useful agent in neurosurgery and neuroradiology; the rapid clearance of active drug from the circulation at the termination of anaesthesia giving it an advantage over thiopentone which, in all other respects, is very similar in its action on cerebral circulation and metabolism.

The metabolic theory of cerebral circulatory control would relate the reduction in cerebral blood flow with Althesin to a primary reduction in cerebral metabolic activity mediated, possibly, by the mechanism of brain tissue P_{CO_2} and pH changes. In an attempt to study the time course of these relationships Coroneos et al. (1973) measured the time lag between the first EEG depression and the beginning of the cerebrovascular reaction to

Table 1. *Time relationships (in seconds)*

Beginning of brain arrival of Althesin	5.4 ± 0.2
Peak brain Althesin arrival	7.6 ± 0.3
Start of B.P. reduction	8.2 ± 0.4
Start of EEG slowing	9.1 ± 0.4
Start of carBF decrease	10.9 ± 0.4
Start of carotid vascular resistance increase	11.8 ± 0.3

Means ($\pm$ standard errors) for time course of Althesin effects on the brain and cerebral vasculature in baboons following central venous injection of 50 μl/kg Althesin. (Based on Coroneos et al., 1973.)

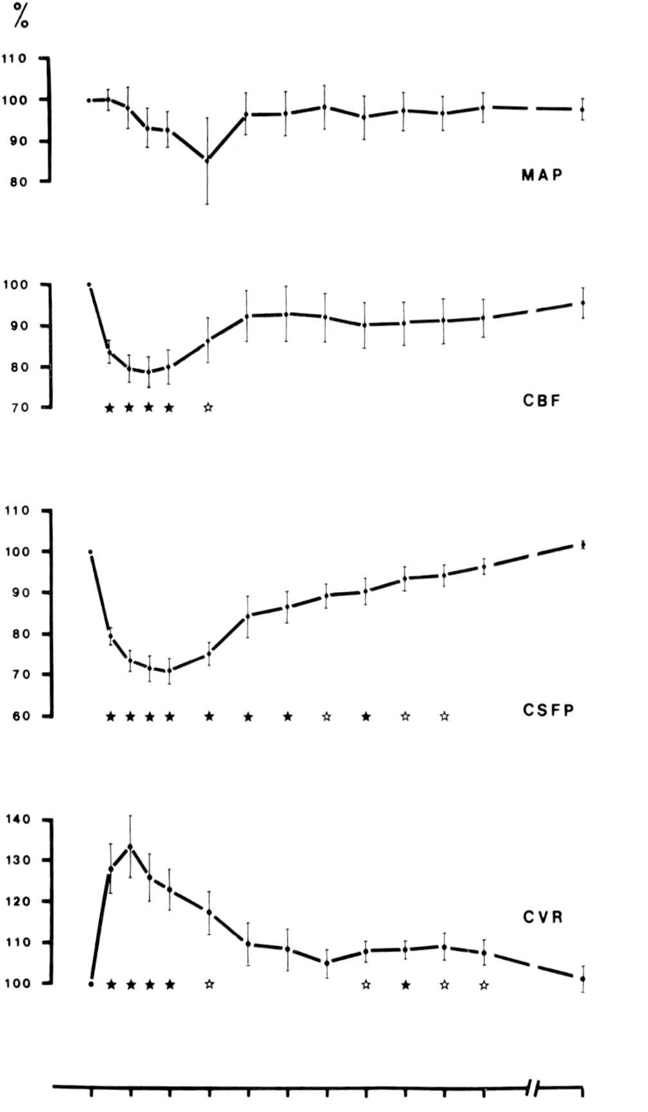

Fig. 1. *Effects of 50 μl/kg Althesin on mean arterial blood pressure, carotid blood flow, cerebrospinal fluid pressure and carotid vascular resistance in normocapnic baboons lightly anaesthetized with nitrous oxide, oxygen and 0.5% halothane. ★ = p < 0.01; ☆ = p < 0.05. (Reproduced from Pickerodt et al., 1972, by courtesy of the Editor, British Journal of Anaesthesia.)*

the metabolic change. The time relationships are given in Table 1, from which it will be seen that the time lag was of the order of 3 sec. Calculations based on the known cerebral metabolic rate and the solubility of CO_2 in brain tissue (Siesjö, 1962) indicate that the maximum change in brain tissue P_{CO_2} which could occur in these 3 sec would be less than 0.5 mm Hg. Further experiments by Keaney et al. (in preparation) have ruled out

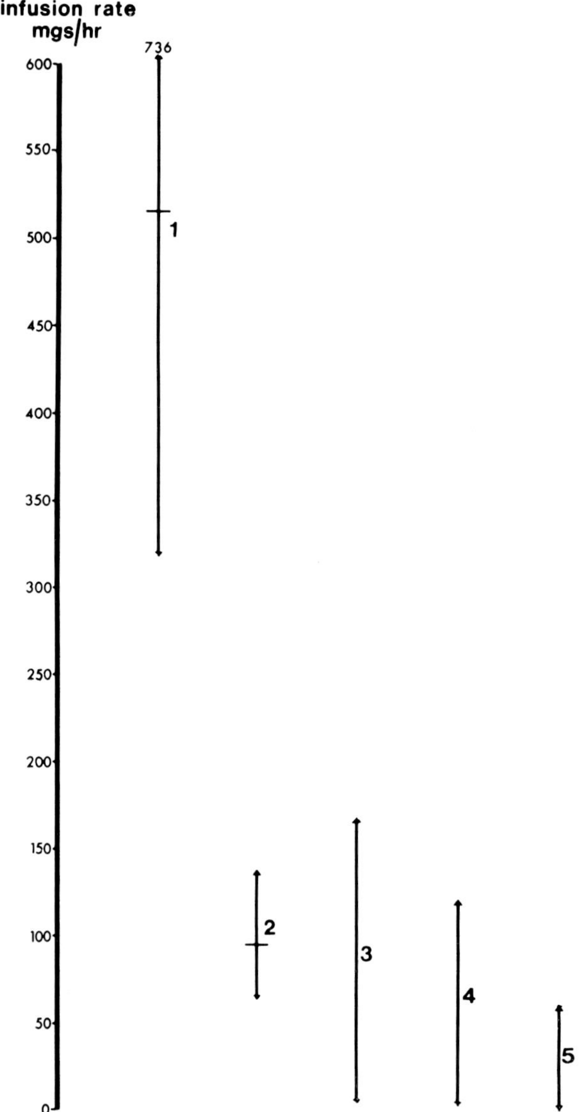

Fig. 2.   *Nitroprusside infusion rates in clinical and animal experimental studies; the bars indicate mean values and the extremities of each line the upper and lower limits. (1) is the dose rate employed in 4 baboons which developed irreversible circulatory failure after correction for body weight difference between baboons and man. (2) gives the same data for 4 baboons which responded normally to sodium nitroprusside. (3), (4) and (5) give the same information for 3 clinical studies of nitroprusside dosage used to produce hypotension for surgery. (3) from Taylor et al., 1970; (4) from Turner et al., in preparation; (5) from Jones and Cole, 1968. (Reproduced from McDowall et al., 1974, by courtesy of the Editor, British Journal of Anaesthesia.)*

a significant neurogenic component to the cerebrovascular response to Althesin-induced metabolic depression.

Effect of induced hypotension CO₂ responsiveness and autoregulation

Autoregulation of cerebral perfusion to changes in blood pressure is not impaired by light anaesthesia (Smith et al., 1970). However, after a period of halothane-induced hypotension to a mean blood pressure of 30–35 mm Hg for 2 hr, it has been shown that autoregulation is impaired for a period thereafter (Keaney et al., 1973*b*). Similar changes occur following hypotension induced by nitroprusside anaesthesia (Keaney et al., 1973*a*). During halothane-induced hypotension to a mean blood pressure of 45 mm Hg, the cerebrovascular response, to Pa_{CO_2} changes is abolished in baboons (Okuda et al., 1974). Hyperventilation during hypotension would therefore appear not to reduce cerebral blood flow further.

Toxicity of sodium nitroprusside

Sodium nitroprusside, when used as a hypotensive agent, dilates the cerebral circulation, as it does other vascular beds; consequently, a sudden rise in blood pressure during sodium nitroprusside infusion can lead to elevation of intracranial pressure (Turner et al., 1974).

Overdosage of sodium nitroprusside can lead to progressive circulatory failure associated with a severe metabolic acidosis in both blood and cerebrospinal fluid. Cerebral oxygen uptake falls to very low levels at toxic dosage, but is not affected by dosage in the clinical range. The toxic dose has been established in baboons, and tentative extrapolation to man on a weight basis has been attempted (McDowall et al., 1974). The results of these calculations are illustrated in Figure 2. The highest dose rate in an experimental animal which recovered normal blood pressure after nitroprusside hypotension would be equivalent in man to 140 mg/hr given over 2 hr, while the lowest dose rate employed in an animal which did not recover normal blood pressure would be equivalent to 320 mg/hr over 2 hr. A recent report in the literature (Merrifield and Blundell, 1974) of toxicity occurring in man would appear to corroborate these experimental findings.

In my view, sodium nitroprusside is a useful agent for hypotension during neurosurgical anaesthesia, but it should be employed with a rigid limitation on the upper dose levels. If resistance to its action is encountered, as it may be (particularly in young patients), then, rather than progressively increase the dosage of nitroprusside, supplementation of its hypotensive action by halothane is very effective, probably because halothane acts mainly on the myocardium (Prys-Roberts et al., 1972), while nitroprusside has a mainly peripheral vascular action.

REFERENCES

Coroneos, N. J., Keaney, N. P., Lane, J. R., McDowall, D. G., Pickerodt, V. W. A. and Turner, J. M. (1973): *J. Physiol. (Lond.), 232,* 30 P.

Horsley, J. S. (1937): *Lancet, 1,* 141.

Jones, G. O. M. and Cole, P. (1968): *Brit. J. Anaesth., 40,* 804.

Keaney, N. P., McDowall, D. G., Turner, J. M., Lane, J. R. and Okuda, Y. (1973*a*): *Brit. J. Anaesth., 45,* 639.

Keaney, N. P., Pickerodt, V. W. A., McDowall, D. G., Coroneos, N. J., Turner, J. M. and Shah, Z. P. (1973*b*): *J. Neurol. Neurosurg. Psychiat., 36/6,* 898.

McDowall, D. G. (1975): In: *The Basis and Practice of Neuroanaesthesia.* Editor: E. Gordon. Excerpta Medica, Amsterdam. In press.

McDowall, D. G., Keaney, N. P., Turner, J. M., Lane, J. R. and Okuda, Y. (1974): *Brit. J. Anaesth., 46,* 327.

Merrifield, A. J. and Blundell, M. D. (1974): *Brit. J. Anaesth.*, *46*, 324.

Okuda, Y., McDowall, D. G., Ali, M. M. and Lane, J. R. (1974): *Brit. J. Anaesth.*, *46*, 316.

Pickerodt, V. W. A., McDowall, D. G., Coroneos, N. J. and Keaney, N. P. (1972): *Brit. J. Anaesth.*, *44*, 751.

Pierce, E. C., Lambertsen, C. J., Deutsch, S., Chase, P. E., Linde, H. W., Dripps, R. D. and Price, H. L. (1962): *J. clin. Invest.*, *41*, 1664.

Prys-Roberts, C., Gersh, B. J., Baker, A. B. and Reuben, S. R. (1972): *Brit. J. Anaesth.*, *44*, 634.

Siesjö, B. K. (1962): *Acta neurol. scand.*, *38*, 98.

Smith, A. L., Neigh, J. L., Hoffman, J. C. and Wollman, H. (1970): *J. appl. Physiol.*, *29*, 665.

Smith, A. L. and Wollman, H. (1972): *Anesthesiology*, *36*, 378.

Taylor, T. H., Styles, M. and Lamming, A. J. (1970): *Brit. J. Anaesth.*, *42*, 859.

Turner, J. M., Coroneos, N. J., Gibson, R. M., Powell, D., Ness, M. A. and McDowall, D. G. (1973): *Brit. J. Anaesth.*, *45*, 168.

Turner, J. M., Powell, D., Gibson, R. M. and McDowall, D. G. (1975): In: *Proceedings, 2nd International Symposium on Intracranial Pressure, Lund, 1974*. Springer Verlag, Berlin. In press.

Anesthesia in the sitting position

MAURICE S. ALBIN, PETER J. JANNETTA, JOSEPH C. MAROON,
ALFRED TUNG and J. EUGENE MILLEN

Departments of Anesthesiology and Neurological Surgery,
University of Pittsburgh School of Medicine, Pittsburgh, Pa., U.S.A.

INTRODUCTION

For neurosurgical procedures on the posterior cranial fossa and high cervical region, the sitting position offers many distinct advantages over other positions since it provides for good surgical access to the site of operation, allows for mechanical gravitational drainage of blood away from the surgical field (thus permitting easier hemostasis) and permits a better view of the facial area in order to monitor evoked responses from cranial nerve stimulation. Conversely, the upright position can have profound cardiopulmonary effects in the anesthetized patient and because of the gravitational gradient between heart and foramen magnum, the danger of air embolization becomes important. The change from the supine to the erect position may be poorly tolerated and this may be especially true in the elderly and/or poor-risk patient.

The purpose of this report is to give some of our experiences relating to the prevention, detection and treatment of air embolism; to show the cardiopulmonary responses to positional changes during anesthesia; to evaluate physiological intraoperative reactions; and to offer suggestions relative to the use of the sitting position.

In this study 200 patients, all undergoing varying neurosurgical procedures in the sitting position, were used as subjects. Our routine of right atrial catheter implantation, ECG, arterial and venous pressure monitoring, end expiratory CO_2 measurements, frequent discontinuous blood gases as well as a standardized type of anesthesia (narcotic, muscle relaxant, 50:50 N_2O-O_2 and controlled ventilation) allowed for the collection and evaluation of many physiological parameters (Table 1). In addition, 110 patients (50 decubitus lateral, 30 supine and 30 prone) having other neurosurgical procedures were monitored with Doppler ultrasound for air emboli (Table 2).

Table 1. *Incidence of air embolism with Doppler detection*

Institution	No. of patients	Air detected	%
Oxford University	23	5	21
Mayo Clinic	69	27	39
University of Pittsburgh	200	52	26
Total	292	84	29

Table 2.   *Air embolism – position*

Position	No. of patients	Detectable air	%
Supine	30	0	0.0
Prone	30	0	0.0
Lateral	50	2 *	4.0
Sitting	200	52	26.0

* Both patients with gradient from right atrium to foramen magnum of 15 and 18 cm respectively.

AIR EMBOLISM [1–10, 12, 13]

All 200 patients were observed for clinical evidence of air embolism as well as having a Doppler ultrasonic air bubble indicator (DUBI) positioned on the precordium over the right atrium. Doppler detection has been hindered because of radio frequency (RF) interference generated by the electrocautery units. In this series we used a Roche Medical Electronics battery powered Fetasonde Doppler unit containing a squelching circuit that deactivates annoying RF cautery noise. The characteristics of this unit have been described in an earlier publication (Maroon and Albin, 1974). As can be seen from Table 2, air was detected in 52 of 200 patients (26%) with symptoms developing in 6 patients (hypotension arrhythmia). Air volumes ranging from 2.0–100 ml were aspirated via the right atrial catheter (Table 3). It is interesting to point out that our calibration sensitivity remains around the 0.25 ml level. Another important factor was the visual verification by the operating neurosurgeon in 25 cases after primary Doppler detection when air could be seen moving through the venous system.

Table 3.   *Air embolism – symptomatology and amount of air aspirated in 52 patients*

Ml	No.	Symptoms	Mortality
2.0–4.0	30	0	0
5.0–9.0	5	0	0
10–19	5	0	0
20–29	3	0	0
30–39	2	0	0
40–49	2	0	0
50–99	4	Hypotension	0
100	1	Arrhythmia, Hypotension	0
Total	52		0

Our findings emphasize the point that the DUBI serves as an early warning detection system to alert the neurosurgical team that a potential hazard is operant. The presence of a right atrial catheter and other monitoring devices mentioned above can only help to minimize and/or abort the development of frank clinical reactions.

CARDIOPULMONARY RESPONSES [1, 3, 4, 8, 9, 11, 14, 15, 16]

Eight patients were studied to evaluate cardiopulmonary responses that take place while moving from the supine to the sitting position under general anesthesia. Their ages ranged from 41–56 years (mean 44.6), and all were ASA Physical Status I except for one patient who was ASA II, indicating their relatively good health. All patients were subjected to posterior fossa cranial nerve explorations and had no evidence of intracranial lesions or increased intracranial pressure.

Premedication was standardized with morphine, diazepam and scopolamine, all given intramuscularly one hour prior to entering the operating room. After induction with thioamylal and intubation under succinylcholine, anesthesia was maintained with morphine, $50 : 50$ N_2O-O_2 and curare. All patients were on controlled ventilation with tidal volumes and airway pressures noted. After the patients were anesthetized, appropriate catheters and instrumentation were introduced. Leg wrapping from toe to groin was carried out prior to anesthesia and a 'G' suit was not used.

The study was divided into five time and position periods (Table 4): No. 1, supine, taking place after anesthesia induction and steady state; No. 2, after moving the patient from supine to 45°; No. 3, from 45° to 90°; No. 4, at 90°, one hour later; and No. 5, in the supine position again after termination of the procedure.

Table 4. *Position – % change*

	No. 1 Supine	No. 2 45°	No. 3 90°	No. 4 90°	No. 5 Supine
Cardiac index	–	—3	—14	—20	+10
O₂ transport	–	—3	—14	—19	+11
SVR	–	+11	+40	+80	+27
Mean arterial pressures	–	0	+9	+38	+27

Cardiac index was calculated from indocyanine green dye dilution cardiac outputs (CO) and body surface area; O_2 transport from cardiac output and O_2 content; and systemic vascular resistance (SVR) from CO and blood pressures.

The results are shown in Table 4 calculated in percentage mean changes from baseline; supine position No. 1.

Physiological changes appear to be negligible when going from supine to 45° position. Stressful responses start occurring immediately after reaching the 90° position and become more marked at the hour interval at 90° in position No. 4. Note the increase in SVR, mean arterial blood pressure and decrease in cardiac index and oxygen transport. Even after assuming the supine position at termination of the procedure, SVR and mean arterial pressures were still elevated.

These findings would indicate the considerable cardiovascular challenge involved in going from supine to the sitting position in the relatively healthy patient; that a 'stable increased' blood pressure may mark an inadequate or marginal perfusion; and that care should be exercised in subjecting the elderly and/or poor-risk patient who does not have active compensatory mechanisms to this position. The critical correlation between these changes and cerebral perfusion dynamics have yet to be done.

REFERENCES

1. Bitte, E. M. and Goebert Jr., H. W. (1966): *Pacif. Med. Surg.*, *74*, 22.
2. Edmonds-Seal, J. and Maroon, J. C. (1969): *Anaesthesia*, *24*, 438.
3. Gardner, W. J. and Dohn, D. F. (1956): *J. Amer. med. Ass.*, *162*, 274.
4. Hewer, A. J. H. and Logue, V. (1962): *Anaesthesia*, *17*, 476.
5. Maroon, J. C., Edmonds-Seal, J. and Campbell, R. L. (1969): *J. Neurosurg.*, *31*, 196.
6. Maroon, J. C., Goodman, J. M., Horner, T. G. and Campbell, R. L. (1968): *Surg. Gynec. Obstet.*, *127*, 1236.
7. Maroon, J. C. and Albin, M. S. (1974): *Anesth. Analg. Curr. Res.*, *53*, 399.
8. Martin, J. T. (1970a): *Anesth. Analg. Curr. Res.*, *49*, 577.
9. Martin, J. T. (1970b): *Anesth. Analg. Curr. Res.*, *49*, 588.
10. Michenfelder, J. D., Martin, J. T., Altenburg, B. M. and Rehder, K. (1969): *J. Amer. med. Ass.*, *208*, 1353.
11. Millar, R. A. (1972): *Brit. J. Anaesth.*, *44*, 495.
12. Munson, E. S. and Merrick, H. C. (1966): *Anesthesiology*, *27*, 783.
13. Shenkin, H. N. and Goldfedder, P. (1969): *J. Amer. med. Ass.*, *210*, 726.
14. Tindall, G. T., Craddock, A. and Greenfield Jr., J. C. (1967): *J. Neurosurg.*, *26*, 383.
15. Ward, R. J., Danziger, F., Bonica, J. J., Allen, G. D. and Tolas, A. G. (1966): *Aerospace Med.*, *37*, 257.
16. Wilson, R. D., Overton, M. C., Waldron, R. L. and Snodgrass, S. R. (1966): *J. Amer. med. Ass.*, *198*, 970.

Hypotension in the operative treatment of intracranial aneurysm

R. R. AITKEN

Department of Anaesthesia, University of Western Ontario, and
University Hospital, London, Ontario, Canada

In the past 10 years, over 700 intracerebral aneurysm patients have been operated upon with the aid of induced hypotension in the neurosurgical service of the University of Western Ontario Medical School.

The anaesthetic technique employed has been based on several assumptions. If these are valid, then I believe the method is logical and coherent. The first assumption is that hypotension is necessary in aneurysm surgery. I am assured by my neurosurgeon colleagues that a careful dissection of the aneurysm and its vicinity is essential in order that small feeding vessels and collateral branches are not incorporated in the repair. Moreover, the wall of an aneurysm can be very thin, and since it is composed largely of inelastic collagen a rise in blood pressure increases the stress upon it much more than in more elastic vessels. Hence, the aneurysm is prone to rupture even when gently handled, and when this occurs, a hurried and possibly unsatisfactory repair may be required.

In accordance with LaPlace's Principle, if the pressure within the aneurysm is lowered its radius is decreased and the tension of the aneurysm wall is reduced. The fact that this reduction is linear leads to a second assumption – that blood pressure should be taken to the lowest level consistent with the patient's well-being in order to offer the greatest protection against rupture of the aneurysm.

Occlusion of the arteries feeding the aneurysm produces the same effect of course. This requires the imposition of hypothermia if more than 3 min interruption of blood flow is required, and even then dissection must be periodically stopped to allow cerebral perfusion. Nor should the possibility of intimal damage by these manoeuvres be ignored, with its risk of subsequent emboli formation or thrombosis. I do not know of a study comparing the risk to the patient of hypotension versus hypothermia, though I suspect they are comparable. But hypotension has the merits of relative simplicity and decreased anaesthetic time, plus the fact that the surgeon can work without interruption for long periods.

Here, it is appropriate to briefly discuss blood pressure measurements. In the literature on hypotension, different authors have used different techniques and it is not easy to compare the blood pressure values they give. My own experience has led me to rely on direct measurement of mean arterial pressure in a peripheral artery. The radial is more easily cannulated, but the dorsalis pedis may be more accessible and is a useful alternative. It must be remembered that the blood pressure transducer, regardless of type, measures the pressure at its own level. If the brain is above the transducer, the cerebral blood pressure will be lower than the figures displayed. The variation is easily calculated by recalling that a column of water, or blood, 13 cm in height is equivalent to 10 mm Hg. In practice it seems simplest to put the transducer at the level of the cerebral cortex. Then, whatever the patient's position one is reading the pressure in the cortex and no extrapolation is needed. It has been possible on three occasions to measure the pressure within an aneurysm directly, and the values obtained agreed with those derived peripherally (Ferguson, 1972).

Having agreed upon a standard method of blood pressure measurement, the question may be raised, 'How far may blood pressure be safely lowered?' The answer must be that for a particular patient no one knows. Individuals vary greatly in their tolerance to hypotension depending on their age, physical status and the severity of brain damage following the subarachnoid haemorrhage. Clinical experience suggests that most healthy people, with no neurological deficit, will tolerate a mean arterial pressure of 40 Torr, with the cerebral cortex as reference point, for periods exceeding 3 hr, if certain conditions are met. These are, a normal or elevated arterial oxygen tension, a normal or slightly elevated arterial CO_2 tension, a light level of nitrous oxide, halothane anaesthesia, and hypotension produced with short-acting agents such as trimetaphan or sodium nitroprusside.

Using these criteria, Fitch et al. (1973) measured cerebral blood flow in baboons, and demonstrated that autoregulation of cerebral blood flow continued until mean pressures of 35–40 Torr were reached. In contrast, in a control series of animals anaesthetized with a narcotic-relaxant sequence, and hypotensed by exsanguination, autoregulation ceased at mean pressures of 60 Torr. This would seem to be laboratory confirmation of clinical experience.

But how is it to be recognized that a particular patient will tolerate hypotension at 40 Torr mean, and how can he be protected against errors in blood pressure measurement? The answer to this is a final assumption, that changes in signs of respiration will indicate when hypotension has exceeded a safe level.

It has long been known that respiration fails in the presence of severe cerebral hypoxia. Brierly and Excell (1966) reported experiments with monkeys where those animals whose blood pressure was reduced to the point of apnoea did not recover. If respiration did not fail, however, long periods of extreme hypotension were survived. If these observations are applicable to man, then a patient permitted to breathe spontaneously should show a change in his respiratory pattern if hypotension is too severe.

The most extreme change is respiratory arrest, which may be preceded by gasping respiration, or periodic breathing. These signs denote severe hypoxia and should not be allowed to develop. An earlier warning is given by the development of decreased tidal air and minute volume. I believe this represents a deepening of the level of anaesthesia as a result of hypoxia. Hypoxia per se is supposed to produce an increase in respiratory effort, but a lightly anaesthetized patient will respond to surgical stimuli by hyperventilation. Since the latter is the more common cause, I have not found hyperpnoea a useful sign. But any change in the respiratory pattern must be viewed as a possible sign of trouble. If there is any doubt, the blood pressure should be raised.

One wishes that there were better guides to the adequacy of cerebral perfusion. Changes in respiration indicate brain stem ischaemia, and are not obvious when small arteries are occluded or where retractor pressure deprives the underlying brain of blood. But at the present time, methods of monitoring the EEG, or measuring cerebral blood flow do not seem applicable to the clinical situation.

The concept of permitting spontaneous respiration for neurosurgical procedures is disturbing to most, if not all neurosurgical anaesthetists. They are well aware of the effects of hypercarbia on brain size, and are rightly concerned that underventilation can add to the tissue hypoxia which hypotension might produce. I am convinced that the value of the information obtained by letting the patient breathe on his own outweighs the danger of inadequate ventilation and as a rule, the patient's blood gases can be maintained within the normal range, and the surgeon can have satisfactory operating conditions without the use of controlled ventilation.

This must be qualified, of course. This type of anaesthesia should be employed only in those aneurysm patients who have recovered from the immediate effects of their haemorrhage and who again possess normal intracranial pressure. In most cases, at least a week must have passed. It is not applicable to those with a ventilatory defect or cardio-vascular disease, which in themselves contraindicate the use of maximal hypotension. However, since subarachnoid haemorrhage seems most common in early middle age and before, the majority of its victims are suitable candidates for the method.

A simple, standard form of anaesthesia is used. No premedication is given, since even in small amounts it increases respiratory depression. The preoperative visit should do as much, or more, to allay anxiety. Induction is accomplished with a 'sleep' dose of thiopentone. If subarachnoid haemorrhage was recent, or if there is a history of hypertension, it is prudent to deepen anaesthesia with several minutes of a 2–3% halothane concentration in order to reduce blood pressure, and to diminish the blood pressure rise which can occur during intubation. I have seen 5 patients re-bleed during induction and intubation with the thiopentone-succinylcholine sequence, and deeper anaesthesia seems the simplest way to avoid such disasters.

When a satisfactory fall in pressure is achieved, a small dose of succinylcholine facilitates intubation. I personally prefer to use a liberal amount of lidocaine spray to the larynx and trachea as well, to minimize the risk of straining as the relaxant wears off. Anaesthesia is then continued with nitrous oxide and halothane, but at a much lighter plane. Halothane concentrations below 1% are generally adequate. Any efficient circuit is satisfactory. At present, we are using a modified Mapleson 'D', with gas flows in excess of 70 ml/kg (Bain and Spoerel, 1972).

Blood pressure is monitored by cuff and auscultation, as well as the intra-arterial cannula. An ECG with chest leads permits observation of heart rate and rhythm, and may also display S-T segment changes if hypotension is too severe in the presence of coronary insufficiency. A healthy heart, however, will show little change in the ECG pattern, even if hypotension is low enough to produce apnoea. Body temperature is monitored, and a warming blanket is used to maintain normothermia.

Brain size is controlled by assuring adequate ventilation, by the use of 20% mannitol, and by lumbar spinal fluid drainage. The last has some interesting side effects which Dr. Barker has enlarged upon (*This Volume*, p. 763).

There are some general considerations in the use of hypotension in aneurysm surgery. Since one is using it to decrease tension in the aneurysm sac wall, rather than to produce a bloodless field, it is not induced until the surgeon is approaching the lesion. If the aneurysm is torn, the blood pressure may fall as a result of the haemorrhage, and the hypotensive drug must be discontinued. In addition, the patient should be normotensive before closure of the dura, so that no bleeding points are overlooked. The longer acting agents such as hexamethonium are thus contraindicated in favour of those of very short duration. The position of the patient required by the surgeon is not always the most advantageous for producing hypotension.

Because they must be in a light plane of anaesthesia to have satisfactory respiratory exchange, patients tend to be more resistant to the effects of the hypotensive agent. For the same reason, the possibility of using the hypotensive effects of deep halothane anaesthesia is denied.

My own experience has been confined to the use of trimetaphan (Arfonad) and sodium nitroprusside. Arfonad is primarily a ganglionic blocker, though in large doses it can produce histamine release. Unfortunately, it is rather unpredictable in action. Some patients require very little to achieve the desired response, while at the opposite extreme, others are almost totally resistant. Several factors appear to be involved. The degree of volaemia is important, and those patients who are hypovolaemic may be extremely responsive to the hypotensive drug. Treatment for hypertension preoperatively may include drugs which act at the same site, and compete with Arfonad. Larson (1964) reports that guanethidine will increase the histamine release effect. Propranolol will certainly hinder the development of the tachycardia ordinarily produced by Arfonad, and its accompanying rise in cardiac output. Finally, catecholamine release from surgical stimulation in a lightly anaesthetized patient may be sufficient to overwhelm the ganglionic blockade.

In spite of these shortcomings, I consider Arfonad a safe drug ('benign' might be a better term) and I prefer to try its effect initially. If this is not satisfactory one can then resort to sodium nitroprusside (Taylor et al., 1970). This agent, which contains the cyanide radical, is almost 10-times as potent as Arfonad on a weight basis. It works by direct action on the vascular smooth muscle to allow pooling of blood in the capacitance vessels, and as well, probably produces a fall in cardiac output, in spite of the tachycardia accompanying its use.

Because of its different mode of action, sodium nitroprusside can work very well where Arfonad has failed. But there is a group which resists even this drug: young, robust males primarily. And, in 'pushing' sodium nitroprusside on these people I have become concerned that the drug is not innocuous. On several occasions hyperpnoea has developed, and I have wondered if this could be due to hypoxia from the cyanide action on intracellular metabolism. I do not consider it as safe a drug as Arfonad.

In using either of these drugs one must establish the patient's response by introducing the agent slowly. It seems best to reduce blood pressure to the desired level over a period of 5–10 min to allow autoregulation of cerebral blood flow to take place. A precipitate fall may not permit this, and as well one may overshoot, overcorrect and have a very uneven blood pressure pattern. My own preference is for an infusion sufficiently concentrated that large amounts of fluid are not required, with an infusion control such as the Ivac 200 Controller.

What can be done to assist the induction of hypotension in the resistant group? Before sodium nitroprusside was available, it was helpful to deliberately permit a degree of hypovolaemia by withholding fluids and early blood loss replacement. The timing of mannitol infusion is important, so that hypotension is not competing with the stage of hypervolaemia which precedes diuresis. A few patients who I expected to be difficult had been given the β-blocker, propranolol, preoperatively. I was impressed with the absence of tachycardia and good response to the hypotensive agent. However, the possibility of bronchospasm induced by the combination of halothane, propranolol and perhaps Arfonad deters one from using it routinely. Positive airway pressure can certainly lower systemic blood pressure, but I am reluctant to use it for fear of inducing coughing in the lightly anaesthetized patient. As well, the increased central venous pressure may be transmitted to the cerebral veins.

I am more and more of the opinion however, that extreme resistance to efforts to produce hypotension is a signal from the patient that he cannot tolerate the degree you seek to impose on him. If his pressure is allowed to rise, he will often 'plateau' at a slightly higher level without difficulty.

The safety of induced hypotension has been long and inconclusively debated. There have been no deaths which were considered directly attributable to hypotension in our patients, but it is more difficult to assess morbidity. Gross neurologic deficits have had a surgical explanation in every instance. Personality and mental changes as an indication of minor degrees of impairment of cerebral function would appear to be the same as with other techniques used in aneurysm surgery. The incidence of cerebral vasospasm and oedema is likewise comparable.

We continue the use of induced hypotension in the belief that it makes the surgeon's task possible in a way that is relatively safe for the patient, and that the margin of safety is greatly enhanced by preserving the signs of respiration.

REFERENCES

Bain, J. A. and Spoerel, W. E. (1972): *Canad. Anaesth. Soc. J.*, *19/4*, 426.
Brierly, J. B. and Excell, B. J. (1966): *Brain*, *89*, 269.
Fitch, W., Ferguson, G. G., Sengupta, D. and Garibi, J. (1973): *Stroke*, *4*, 324.
Ferguson, G. G. (1972): *J. Neurosurg.*, *36/5*, 560.
Larson, A. G. (1964): *Anaesthesiology*, *25/5*, 682.
Taylor, T. H., Styles, M. and Lamming, A. J. (1970): *Brit. J. Anaesth.*, *42*, 859.

Management of acute head injuries by controlled ventilation

EMERIC GORDON

Department of Neuroanaesthesia, Karolinska Hospital, Stockholm, Sweden

Treatment of patients with head injuries hitherto was aimed at supervision sc that expanding intracranial processes could be detected in time and operative decompression or removal of these lesions performed. During the last decade, however, the nonoperative treatment of head-injury patients has become increasingly effective and a number of new methods for monitoring and combating increased intracranial pressure and tissue hypoxia have been developed.

The primary aim of treatment of head injuries is to prevent secondary brain-stem damage, caused by a vicious circle of increased intracranial pressure and ventilatory insufficiency which, if untreated, rapidly leads to irreversible coma or death. In this context, the care of the airway and adequate ventilation play a decisive role in the treatment and recovery of these patients.

RESPIRATION

One of the most common symptoms in patients with acute head injuries are respiratory disturbances. Early studies (Huang et al., 1963; Frowein et al., 1964) on this subject report respiratory acidosis, but this finding always indicates a very grave prognosis. Respiratory acidosis most often indicates direct damage to the respiratory centres in the brain stem, and forebodes impending respiratory standstill. However, it may, in some cases, result from severe pulmonary changes.

Later studies (Campan, 1968; Gordon and Rossanda, 1968, 1970; Katsurada et al., 1969; Brown, 1970; Frowein, 1970) pointed out the very striking but uneconomical hyperventilation with increasing respiratory frequency of more than 30/min. Hyperventilation was often accompanied by severe restlessness and decerebrate cramp attacks with resulting serious exhaustion of the patient. The reason for this severe spontaneous hyperventilation has been explained by several authors (Froman, 1968; Eichbaum, 1964; Simmons et al., 1969; Katsurada et al., 1973) on the basis of arterial hypoxaemia caused by pulmonary alterations (chest injuries, uneven ventilation-perfusion ratio, aspiration of blood or gastric contents, neurogenic pulmonary oedema caused by increased intracranial pressure). However, hypoxaemia of the above-mentioned aetiology responds favourably to treatment with oxygen, while most of the hyperventilating head-injury patients continue to hyperventilate despite the achievement of normal arterial oxygen content.

Many other workers (Stueck and Fischer, 1961; Froman and Crampton-Smith, 1966, 1967; Gordon and Rossanda, 1968, 1970; Kaasik and Zupping, 1969; Zupping et al., 1971) have presented experimental and clinical evidence showing that hyperventilation is initiated by severe intracerebral metabolic acidosis which is created by the brain lesion itself. Some of these workers (Zupping et al., 1971) have also shown that there are close correlations between the severity of intracerebral acidosis, brain injury and the degree of hyperventilation. The aim of vigorous spontaneous hyperventilation is thus a restitution of intracerebral pH towards normal levels by rapid elimination of carbon dioxide. The normal cerebral pH is an absolute requirement for restoration of normal vasomotor tone, decrease of brain oedema and intracranial pressure, and could lead to the restitution of blood supply to at least certain parts of the hypoxic brain, thus diminishing the area which might otherwise suffer irreversible damage.

Thus, although spontaneous hyperventilation seems to be a useful protective mechanism for the organism, it has several disadvantages. The extra work of breathing, severe restlessness and decerebrate cramps put a heavy burden on the heart which can lead to serious myocardial insufficiency and to cardiac standstill. Restlessness and cramps require adequate sedation which nearly always results in respiratory depression. Controlled ventilation is the only way in these circumstances both of relieving muscular overwork and of maintaining adequate respiratory gas exchange. In addition, the administration of a high concentration of oxygen, which is needed by the hypoxic brain, can be effectively and safely achieved.

The pressure-decreasing effect of controlled hyperventilation is now well-established. In cases with focal lesions this effect is perhaps even more pronounced than in the normal brain. The uneven flow situation is the basis for the paradoxical flow reaction or steal reaction. The general feature of the steal syndrome is that measures which normally enhance the flow, e.g. an increased P_{CO_2}, increase the perfusion only in the undamaged regions but further compromise the flow in the damaged areas. The counter-steal phenomenon, which occurs during hyperventilation, then decreases intracranial pressure by constricting normally reacting vessels in undamaged areas while arterioles in damaged areas are unable to change diameter due to the intense lactacidosis.

An important effect of hyperventilation is that it compensates, at least partially, for the low intracerebral pH caused by the brain lesion. As cerebrospinal fluid follows the changes in the blood, the chance that cerebral pH comes nearer to normal values is somewhat increased.

Many authors (Malette, 1959; Sugioka and Davis, 1960; Meyer and Gotoh, 1960; Plum and Posner, 1967; Granholm et al., 1969) were opposed to the use of this technique because of the risk of cerebral hypoxia from cerebral vasoconstriction caused by the low Pa_{CO_2}, and from the Bohr effect. However, most of these results emanated from experimental studies in animals or normal volunteers in whom Pa_{CO_2} was often lower than 20 mm Hg. The interpretation of these findings is not even accepted, and no clinical evidence is available of a deleterious effect of moderate controlled hyperventilation. On the contrary, a great number of clinical observations (Cohen et al., 1964; Wollman et al., 1965, 1967; Hunter, 1970) support the assumption that the reduction of CBF in normal regions of the brain does not jeopardize cerebral oxygenation.

CLINICAL MANAGEMENT

Initial treatment

When faced with an unconscious patient with acute brain lesion immediately after admission to the emergency unit, no time should be spent in prognostic and detailed diagnostic evaluations. The airway and ventilation must be controlled promptly and the safest way to do this is by endotracheal intubation and a ventilator. These measures must have the highest priority among those performed at the emergency station. After some hours of controlled ventilation the patient's condition may improve sufficiently so that the endotracheal tube and ventilator treatment may be withdrawn. Secondary deterioration can, however, always occur and therefore head-injury patients must be kept under close supervision until the possibility of further unconsciousness can be safely excluded.

In unconscious patients the treatment with controlled hyperventilation should be continued irrespective of operation. Patients with extradural or subdural haematomas without signs of serious brain tissue damage may emerge rapidly from anaesthesia after the evacuation of the haematoma, and can therefore be extubated. On the other hand, patients with unconsciousness preoperatively and/or more or less extensive brain laceration and oedema usually remain unconscious for several days or weeks. For this reason it is advisable to perform a tracheostomy immediately after the intracranial operation. The endotracheal tube is left in place only if the patient's condition has severely deteriorated during the operation – or, on the contrary, if there are signs of possible recovery within the next 48 hr. The endotracheal tube should not, however, be left in place beyond this period, as the care of the airway, in our experience, becomes increasingly troublesome.

Indications for cerebral angiography, particularly at the early stages of the illness, in the absence of operation, should be very generous. Controlled hyperventilation may temporarily improve the clinical condition even in the presence of an expanding haematoma, which should be evacuated as soon as possible. Sooner or later the potential for compensatory decrease in intracranial pressure is exhausted and a sudden, and sometimes irreversible, deterioration of the patient occurs.

Long-term respirator treatment

The patient is given equal amounts of air and oxygen and the respiratory volume is regulated to obtain a Pa_{CO_2} of about 25 mm Hg. When necessary small doses of phenoperidine are administered to control severe restlessness or decerebrate cramps. This drug is very effective and does not interfere with normal reflex movements or the levels of consciousness.

Weaning and final assessment

During treatment with automatic ventilation the patient's general condition, level of consciousness and pattern of spontaneous respiration are estimated during short periods when controlled ventilation is temporarily interrupted. The rapidity with which patients emerge from unconsciousness varies according to their age, the severity of lesion and many other unknown factors. In less severe lesions, however, recovery proceeds fast enough to be observed from day to day. In more severe lesions the clinical course is extremely slow and signs of amelioration, if any, can only be assessed by very close observation of the patient's neurological condition.

In patients where the clinical course shows a rapid or slow but continual improvement, ventilator treatment is continued until the patient's conscious level is such that there is reaction to simple commands; spontaneous respiration is normal, with normal blood gases after at least 30 min of breathing. Usually, ventilator treatment is used during the 1 or 2 nights following, unless the patient is in such a good condition that this is unnecessary. It is remarkable to see how rapidly blood gases adapt to the new situation and normal values are usually re-established within 24 hr. Generally, the process of weaning is surprisingly smooth even after several weeks of treatment, and relapse to a gravely abnormal respiratory pattern is very rare. This may be explained by the fact that ventilator treatment is not withdrawn until the patient's condition is near normal.

The tracheostomy tube remains in place for a further 3–4 days to ensure that recovery proceeds normally. When the pharyngeal and swallowing reflexes allow, normal per-oral nutrition can be resumed, decannulation is performed. If the swallowing reflex is defective, decannulation is usually postponed, until the risk of pulmonary complications has passed.

In some patients, a short period of unrest and unresponsiveness occurs after the respirator treatment is concluded. The exact cause of this is not clear, but it is considered to be a withdrawal syndrome after prolonged use of phenoperidine. This is not described in the literature, but it is possible that phenoperidine in common with other opiate derivatives, has such an effect. The problem is not serious and symptoms disappear after a couple of days. Diazepam or a phenothiazine can be used with a good effect.

The assessment of unconscious patients

In some cases, even if the patient shows an initial tendency towards improvement, this trend slows down and eventually stops after a period of 1–2 weeks, after which the clinical condition remains unchanged for a long time. In these patients, and in those where the clinical status has not changed during the entire period of treatment, controlled ventilation is gradually abandoned after approximately 1–2 weeks, even if the patient remains unconscious with or without normal spontaneous respiration. If these patients are followed after this period, most of them remain essentially in a 'persistent vegetative state'. In a limited number of cases, however, an astonishing degree of recovery towards normal consciousness occurs after periods of several months.

RESULTS AND DISCUSSION OF TREATMENT

The results of treatment of severe head injuries with controlled hyperventilation have been published previously (Gordon, 1971). The results obtained during 1970–73 are seen in Table 1 and the overall results during 1959–73 are summarized in Table 2.

Table 1. *Final outcome of treatment of 92 unconscious head-injury patients during 1970–1973 treated with controlled hyperventilation*

Patient category	No. of patients	%
1	26 ⎱ 60	28 ⎱ 65
2	34 ⎰	37 ⎰
3	12 ⎱ 32	13 ⎱ 35
4	20 ⎰	22 ⎰
Total	92	100

Category 1 = recovered totally; 2 = recovered consciousness with neurological sequelae; 3 = remained unconscious; 4 = died.

The number of patients with serious head injuries admitted to our clinic remained constant over this period of 14 years and was about 20–30 patients annually. It is, however, interesting to note that there seems to be a certain tendency towards selection of patients during the last 4–5 years, which results in an increasing percentage of more severely injured patients, while the less seriously injured, especially if there is no reason to suspect an expanding, intracranial lesion, remain in the smaller and more peripherally situated hospitals. This selection of patients may explain the somewhat increased mortality rate during the last 4-year period, as compared with the results noted during the years 1967–69. The results during 1970–73 are otherwise very similar to the previous period of 1967–69. The percentage of patients who totally recovered (Category 1) is somewhat diminished during 1970–73, but the difference between this group of patients and those not treated with ventilation is not significant, as is also the case when the whole series is considered (see Table 2). The percentage of patients who regained full consciousness but had persistent neurological deficits (Category 2) remained virtually unchanged (see Table 1). The percentage of useful recoveries (Categories 1 and 2) is thus essentially unchanged in the whole material of 143 patients (67%) and still shows a significantly better result compared with the group not treated with a ventilator (52%). It is also evident from the new data that the percentage of permanently unconscious patients has declined rather than increased during the last

Table 2. *Final outcome of treatment of 344 unconscious head-injury patients during 1959–1973*

Patient category	Group A		Group B	
	No. of patients	%	No. of patients	%
1	43	30 ⎱ 67	61	30 ⎱ 52
2	53	37 ⎰	45	22 ⎰
3	22	15.5 ⎱ 33	30	15 ⎱ 48
4	25	17.5 ⎰	65	33 ⎰
Total	143	100	201	100

Category 1 = recovered totally; 2 = recovered consciousness with neurological sequelae; 3 = remained unconscious; 4 = died.
Group A: Patients treated with controlled hyperventilation; Group B: Patients not treated with controlled hyperventilation.

4-year period. These data do not support the contention that ventilator treatment increases the number of 'vegetative survivals'. On the other hand, the mortality rate increased significantly during the last period of 4 years. A tentative explanation for these results was discussed earlier. Nevertheless, the overall mortality rate in the whole series is still only about half that of those not treated with controlled ventilation and thus the difference is statistically highly significant.

CONCLUSIONS

An analysis of an additional 92 patients with serious head injuries shows that our neuro-traumatological unit receives an unchanged number of such patients over the years. The clinical status, and probably also the anatomo-pathological lesion is, however, apparently more severe than in a previous series. Despite these facts the rate of recovery is still significantly higher and the mortality lower when compared with a similar group of patients not treated with controlled ventilation. It is believed therefore, that the treatment of unconscious patients with severe brain damage with prolonged controlled hyperventilation is useful and all effort should be made for the early institution of this treatment and its continuance according to the recommendations outlined above.

REFERENCES

Brown, A. S. (1971): In: *Head Injury Symposium*, p. 266. Churchill-Livingstone, Edinburgh – London.
Campan, L. (1968): *Ann. Anesth. franç.*, *9/4*, 677.
Cohen, P. J., Wollman, H., Alexander, S. C., Chase, P. E. and Behar, M. G. (1964): *Anesthesio ogy*, *25*, 185.
Eichbaum, F. W. (1964): *Virchows Arch. path. Anat.*, *338*, 78.
Froman, C. (1968): *Brit. J. Anaesth.*, *40*, 354.
Froman, M. B. and Crampton-Smith, A. C. (1966): *Lancet*, *1*, 780.
Froman, C. and Crampton-Smith, A. C. (1967): *Lancet*, *1*, 965.
Frowein, R. A. (1970): In: *Head Injury Symposium*, p. 156. Churchill-Livingstone, Edinburgh – London.
Frowein, R. A., Karimi-Nejad, A. and Euler, K. H. (1964): *Zbl. Neurochir.*, *25*, 39.
Gordon, E. (1971): *Acta anaesth. scand.*, *15*, 193.
Gordon, E. and Rossanda, M. (1968): *Acta anaesth. scand.*, *12*, 51.
Gordon, E. and Rossanda, M. (1970): *Acta anaesth. scand.*, *14*, 97.
Granholm, L., Lukjanova, L. and Siesjö, B. (1969): *Acta physiol. scand.*, *77*, 179.
Huang, C. T., Cook, A. W. and Lyons, H. A. (1963): *Arch. Neurol. (Chic.)*, *9*, 545.
Hunter, A. R. (1970): *Acta anaesth. scand. (Suppl.)*, *37*, 149.
Kaasik, A. E. and Zupping, H. (1969): In: *Cerebral Blood Flow*, p. 129. Editors: M. Brock, C. Fieschi, D. H. Ingvar, N. A. Lassen and K. Schürmann. Springer-Verlag, Berlin – Göttingen – Heidelberg – New York.
Katsurada, K., Sugimoto, T. and Onji, Y. (1969): *J. Trauma*, *9*, 799.
Katsurada, K., Yamada, R. and Sugimoto, T. (1973): *Surgery*, *73*, 191.
Malette, W. (1959): *Surg. Forum*, *9*, 208.
Meyer, J. S. and Gotoh, F. (1960): *Arch. Neurol. (Chic.)*, *3*, 539.
Plum, F. and Posner, J. B. (1967): *Amer. J. Physiol.*, *212*, 864.
Simmons, R. L., Martin, A. M., Heisterkamp III, C. A. and Ducker, T. B. (1969): *Ann. Surg.*, *170*, 39.
Stueck, G. H. and Fisher, R. G. (1961): *Bull. Johns Hopk. Hosp.*, *108*, 339.
Sugioka, K. and Davis, D. A. (1960): *Anesthesiology*, *21*, 135.
Wollman, H., Alexander, S. C., Cohen, P., Smith, T. C., Chase, P. E. and Van der Molen, R. A. (1965): *Anesthesiology*, *26*, 3.
Wollman, H., Alexander, S. C. and Cohen, P. J. (1967): In: *Clinical Anesthesia. Neurological Considerations*, p. 1. Editor: M. Harmel. Blackwell Scientific Publishers, Oxford.
Zupping, R., Kaasik, A. E. and Raudam, E. (1971): *Arch. Neurol. (Chic.)*, *25*, 35.

Neurosurgical intensive care

MARINA ROSSANDA

Department of Anaesthesia and Intensive Care, Ospedale Maggiore Ca' Granda, Milan, Italy

Intensive care of patients with severe cerebral and spinal lesions requires a special knowledge of the pharmacology and pathophysiology of the central nervous system. In some countries therefore, this is being developed as a special branch (Horton, 1965; Bozza-Marrubini, 1965; Tindal, 1971). However, there are only a few special units and actual experience of their management is still limited. This paper will outline the main problems affecting the choice of equipment, design and staffing, since they arise from prolonged practice in neurosurgical patients treated in a general Intensive Care Unit (ICU).

RESPIRATORY AND CIRCULATORY CARE

Airway toilet, humidification, artificial ventilation, control of body temperature, prevention and treatment of circulatory failure are fundamental tasks, requiring the classical equipment of any ICU.

The importance of artificial ventilation in unconscious patients is dealt with by Gordon elsewhere (*This Volume*, p. 784).

MONITORING

The monitoring equipment may be somewhat different in a neurosurgical ICU. A series of new systems for detection and recording of cardiac arrhythmia has been developed for coronary care units and postoperative care in cardiac surgery. It is questionable if they are of real use in neurosurgical patients. Although it is well-known that acute damage of the brain-stem and medulla can be associated with cardiac arrhmia, the author is not aware of any recommendation for arrhythmia monitors in neurosurgical intensive care. The occurrence of alterations of heart rhythm is not exceptional in patients with cerebral or spinal lesions, but no special need is felt for sophisticated instruments to check and treat them.

A frequent EEG recording may be of great use, to assist management of status epilepticus, the detection of deterioration in severe brain lesions, and finally, for the demonstration of cerebral death.

Computer-processing of the electroencephalogram (EEG) recorded at the bedside is being studied (Myers et al., 1973). Its wide application to intensive care is still hindered by two main difficulties; elimination of artefacts, and the large data capacity required. More generally, the use of computer-processing techniques in neurosurgical monitoring is still in an experimental stage, no adequate programme being available at present (Beduschi et al., 1972).

Monitoring of intracranial pressure by means of intraventricular, subdural or epidural sensors is now well-established as the most important contribution to both research and clinical management in neurosurgery. This subject is dealt with by Barker elsewhere (*This Volume*, p. 763).

Continuous monitoring of oxygen and carbon dioxide concentrations in the expired air might be exceedingly useful, given the importance of a careful respiratory control, but the instruments chosen should not be too sensitive to humidity. Anyhow, as changes of the ventilation/perfusion ratio are easily found in long-term unconsciousness and also in the acute stage of injuries, expired air monitoring will never abolish the basic need for frequent measurement of blood gas tensions in arterial samples.

METABOLIC CARE

Unconscious patients and patients with spinal lesions present complex metabolic problems.

High spinal lesions are frequently associated with paralytic ileus. In severe brain injuries a very acid gastric juice is produced and this should be drained away in order to prevent and cure gastric ulcers. As a consequence, tube feeding may be impossible for several days and parenteral nutrition cannot be avoided. It is easily performed by means of caval catheters, introduced via the basilic, the external jugular or the subclavian vein. Dextrose solutions of various concentrations, with addition of electrolytes and insulin, laevo-amino acid solutions, and human albumin are thus given by intravenous drip.

The daily intake is calculated and compared with the urinary loss of water, electrolytes (sodium, potassium and chloride), nitrogen. When a large amount of gastric juice is drained, its electrolyte content is also measured and taken into account. Perspiration is evaluated grossly.

The fluid and electrolyte balance thus calculated is obviously approximate, but in spite of this it is recommended because some important deviation may be detected which may be significant for therapy.

Lately, attention has been drawn to the frequent occurrence of hyponatraemia in neuro-surgical patients (Fox et al., 1971; Wise, 1972) and in other hospital patients (Flear and Singh, 1973). Ventilator treatment might enhance the development of plasma hypotonicity, which is most likely to be related to inappropriate ADH secretion, followed by body fluid expansion, lowered aldosterone secretion and high urinary sodium loss (salt wasting) (White and Bergland, 1972).

Serum hypotonicity may be very dangerous for patients with cerebral lesions, if their intracranial content is near the critical point of the pressure/volume curve, when a very little increase of volume is followed by a steep increase of pressure (Miller and Garibi, 1972).

In a review of 2 years' activity in one ICU, Boselli and Betto (1973) found that plasma hypotonicity with salt wasting was present in 25% of the injured patients (both cerebral and extra-cerebral injuries); dilution hypotonicity developed in another 20%, while only 7% of the brain injuries were associated with hyperosmolar syndromes and 50% showed no imbalance. A coincidence between the beginning of salt wasting and worsening of the neurological status was noticed in several cases.

Of 30 subjects studied with continuous monitoring of intracranial pressure, 12 developed increases of pressure a few days after the injury. In 4 of these cases the pressure rise was coincident with salt wasting and low serum sodium. The decrease in serum sodium concentration seems to be especially dangerous when associated with simultaneous increase of arterial carbon dioxide tension, due to reduced hyperventilation (Rossanda et al., 1974).

Fluid restriction is the only useful way of preventing and treating plasma hypotonicity. Therefore, a fluid restrictive policy is now being applied to brain lesions in our ICU, and the same careful attention is paid to arterial blood gas data and fluid balance.

It may be difficult to combine the policy of fluid restriction with high calorie intake if the solely parenteral route is available. In this case 30–50% glucose is given, with variable amounts of insulin. As the acute condition and the administration of corticoids are often associated with insulin resistance, determination of the dosage of insulin can be difficult, requiring frequent assessment of blood and urine sugar.

When the gastric route becomes available, nutrition is no longer a problem. However, in the present situation of several units, loss of weight and other nutritional complications cannot be frequently avoided, perhaps due to the high rate of infection and inefficient physiotherapy, that result from overcrowding and understaffing.

DESIGN OF THE UNIT

Neurosurgical patients often need a long stay in the ICU. This depends on the fact that recovery from a cerebral lesion is usually slow. The acute stage of respiratory dependence can be prolonged and also after this stage a long time is required for the patient to learn control feeding, excretion and movement. Mental and affective disorders are commonplace in the transition stages from coma to normality. During this phase there may be a long-lasting need for 'heavy nursing' and frequent laboratory control; all this can be provided more readily in an ICU than in general wards. During this phase the patients need continuous stimulation and intensive rehabilitation procedures, which conflicts with the isolation required for their protection from cross-infection.

Actually, the unconscious and patients with spinal injuries are easily infected even during a prolonged acute stage. A potential danger then exists for the other cases. The increasing use of ventricular indwelling catheters for intracranial pressure monitoring entails a serious risk of ventricular or meningeal sepsis, to be added to the well-known risk of lung and bladder infection.

On the basis of these considerations, a suggestion can be made concerning the design of a neurosurgical unit for intensive care. The ICU could be divided into 3 subunits. A short-stay subunit could admit postoperative or trauma patients requiring strict observation for 2–3 days. The design would be similar to that of a recovery room, with sufficient space to allow 'barrier nursing'.

The second subunit would represent the real ICU, including isolation facilities for long-term ventilator treatment, intracranial pressure monitoring and infected patients.

These 2 subunits ought to be carefully protected from external contamination, and traffic should be limited to people directly involved in therapy. The design of the subunits could allow visual and verbal communication between the isolated ward and an external system of rooms or corridors accessible to visitors.

The 3rd subunit could be used for the stage of treatment following the acute phase, when the patients are usually less sensitive to infection, but still require artificial feeding and control of artificial airways and there is a pronounced need for personal contacts with therapists and relatives in order to accelerate the process of rehabilitation.

In this part of the unit – more open to visitors – some ventilator places could be found for conscious patients bound to ventilators for very long periods (tetraparesis, muscular dystrophy).

The suggested scheme obviously does not solve all problems, but may represent an advancement in comparison with the usual arrangement, subjecting all patients to the same degree of isolation, which is generally too little for real protection from infection and entails serious psychological stress for conscious patients and relatives.

STAFFING

In a neurosurgical ICU neuroanaesthesiologists and neurosurgeons ought to work in strict collaboration for the best results to be obtained from intensive therapy.

A common language is not always easily found to describe neurological conditions and to determine a safe policy of diagnostic and therapeutic procedures. Sedation, for example, is an important feature in ventilator treatment, but the neurosurgeon should be aware of the kind of sedative drug used for a correct evaluation of the clinical course of his patient, while the neuroanaesthetist should know the side-effects of the drug on the cerebral circulation and the intracranial pressure.

A common language should also be found by the medical and the nursing staff. The nurses will need special training in order to recognise promptly the most significant changes of reactivity, to learn how to check the monitoring instruments and how to manage critically ill patients.

In a neurosurgical ICU a heavy psychological burden is imposed on the nurses even more than on the doctors. Mortality is often higher than in other ICUs, and even in the favourable cases recovery can be so slow that it cannot be appreciated by the nursing staff, who are not usually involved in after-care. This can give rise to frustration and render still more difficult the task of recruitment. The isolation with unconscious patients is a further negative factor, as is the role of the unit in preparation of donors for organ transplantation.

If a long-stay subunit with large space for rehabilitation procedures can be kept close to the acute ICU, as suggested above, the nursing staff can gain the opportunity of rotation, thus alleviating the strain without losing the advantage of maintaining special skills already acquired.

REFERENCES

Beduschi, A., Bozza-Marrubini, M. and Pinciroli, F. (1972): *Anest. Rianim., 13/1,* 83.

Boselli, L. and Betto, C. (1973): *J. neurosurg. Sci., 17/4,* 261.

Bozza-Marrubini, M. L., Gemelli, P. and Ghezzi, R. (1965): In: *Proceedings, Third International Congress of Neurological Surgery, Copenhagen 1965,* p. 250. Editor: A. C. de Vet. Excerpta Medica, Amsterdam.

Flear, C. T. G. and Singh, C. M. (1973): *Brit. J. Anaesth., 45/9,* 937.

Fox, J. L., Falik, J. L. and Shaloub, R. J. (1971): *J. Neurosurg., 34/4,* 506.

Horton, J. M. (1965): In: *Proceedings, Third International Congress of Neurological Surgery, Copenhagen 1965,* p. 313. Editor: A. C. de Vet. Excerpta Medica, Amsterdam.

Miller, J. D. and Garibi, J. (1972): In: *Intracranial Pressure,* Chapter 8, p. 270. Editors: M. Brock and H. Dietz. Springer Verlag, Berlin – Heidelberg – New York.

Myers, R. R., Stockard, F. F., Fleming, N. I., France, C. F. and Bickford, R. G. (1973): *Brit. J. Anaesth., 45/7,* 664.

Rossanda, M., Collice, M., Boselli, L. and Porta, M. (1974): In: *Proceedings, Second International Symposium on Intracranial Pressure, Lund.* In press.

Tindal, S. (1971): *Canad. Anaesth. Soc. J., 18/6,* 637.

White, W. A. and Bergland, R. M. (1972): *J. Neurosurg., 36/5,* 608.

Wise, B. L. (1972): *Preoperative and Postoperative Care in Neurological Surgery.* Charles C. Thomas, Springfield, Ill.

The effect of induction of anaesthesia on intracranial pressure*

R. GREENBAUM[1], R. COOPER[2], A. HULME[1] and I. P. MACKINTOSH[1]

[1]Frenchay Hospital, and [2]Burden Neurological Institute, Bristol, United Kingdom

There has been widespread concern with the increased intracranial pressure (ICP) found during general anaesthesia. Large rises in intracranial pressure with halothane, methoxyfluorane and trichloroethylene are particularly evident in patients who have a pre-existing pathologically high intracranial pressure (Jennett et al., 1969; Fitch et al., 1969). More recently, there have been several studies which have found that the induction of anaesthesia is associated with sudden and severe elevations in intracranial pressure, both due to noxious stimuli such as laryngoscopy (Shapiro et al., 1972), the administration of nitrous oxide (Henriksen and Jörgensen, 1973) and to a combination of these effects with minimal carbon dioxide retention (Hulme and Cooper, 1972). In these circumstances, cerebral perfusion pressure may fall to low levels and, therefore, lead to accentuation of intracranial pressure gradients leading to brain shifts, or mass displacement of the brain and brain stem ischaemia (Fitch and McDowall, 1971).

As neurosurgical patients with high intracranial pressures must have general anaesthetics, it is essential to choose an induction which minimises these risks. Unfortunately, the induction of anaesthesia involves several almost coincident events, each of which might be responsible for ICP changes: (1) the administration of an intravenous barbiturate; (2) the application of an anaesthetic circuit with its associated resistance to breathing and apparatus dead space; (3) the administration of nitrous oxide, with a change in inspired oxygen concentration; (4) the administration of a muscle relaxant and manual ventilation; (5) laryngoscopy and endotracheal intubation; (6) intermittent positive pressure ventilation and hypocapnia.

We, therefore, have used standardised induction sequences by means of which these factors can be separately assessed.

MATERIAL AND METHODS

In this report, measurements taken from 14 patients are presented. All had evidence of raised intracranial pressure due to tumours or other pathology (Table 1).

A burr hole was made under local anaesthesia for ventriculography or other diagnostic purposes, two or more days before general anaesthesia. Intracranial pressure was then measured either by the use of a miniature pressure transducer of the Konisberg P 22 type inserted into the subdural space (Hulme and Cooper, 1966), or, alternatively, by ventricular fluid pressure measurement using an external S.E. pressure transducer and catheter system. The reference for ICP was the midpoint of the cranium when using the external transducer, or transducer level with implanted transducers.

* This work has been supported by grants from the Research Funds of the South Western Regional Hospital Board and the Medical Research Council.

Table 1. *Details of patients studied*

Patient No.	Sex	Age	Diagnosis	Control ICP (mm Hg)
1	Female	58	Tentorial meningioma	10
2	Male	46	Tentorial meningioma	33
3	Male	49	Haemangioblastoma	30
4	Male	62	Post-subarachnoid hydrocephalus	40
5	Female	50	Post-meningitic hydrocephalus	35
6	Male	60	Posterior fossa tumour	25
7	Female	57	Posterior fossa metastasis	25
8	Male	60	Communicating hydrocephalus	20
9	Male	53	Posterior fossa dermoid	22
10	Male	61	Tumour third ventricle	40
11	Male	28	Cystic astrocytoma	25
12	Female	60	Posterior fossa tumour	45
13	Female	48	Post-subarachnoid hydrocephalus	20
14	Female	41	Posterior fossa metastases	12

Mean systemic arterial blood pressure was measured by radial artery cannulation and an S.E. pressure transducer, zero at heart level. This information was logged on magnetic tape and processed using a LINC-8 computer.

Cerebral perfusion pressure was derived from the difference between mean arterial blood pressure and mean ICP.

Arterial samples were taken for P_{CO_2} and P_{O_2} at each event during the anaesthetic induction. They were analysed using an I.L. 213 blood gas analyser.

Patients were premedicated with atropine 0.6 mg and, if nervous, diazepam 5–10 mg. All patients were studied in the supine position.

Induction of anaesthesia was performed in the following stages:

Stage 1. Mask – non-rebreathing system using Reuben valve and administration of 30% oxygen in nitrogen,

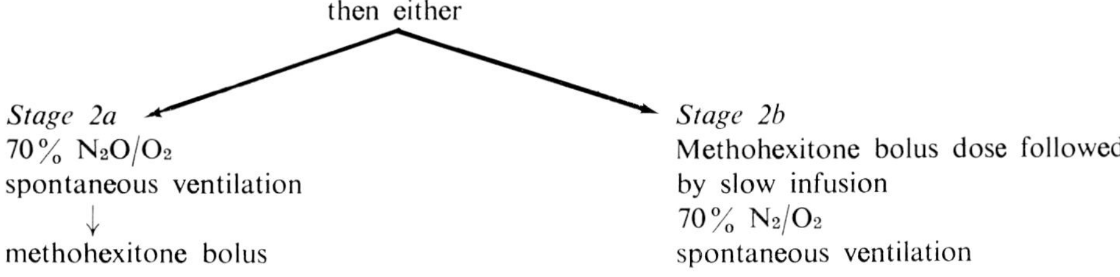

Stage 3. Muscle relaxant (alcuronium or pancuronium) and manual IPPV.
Stage 4. Laryngoscopy and endotracheal intubation.
Stage 5. Hyperventilation using a Manley ventilator.

In each of these stages, measurements have been taken from the records when a steady state of ICP and mean blood pressure has been achieved; in Stage 3, 4 min were allowed before laryngoscopy and intubation.

If there was an episode of hypoxia, or if it was thought necessary to drain off some CSF in the interests of the patient's safety, then the patient was excluded from the study from that stage in the induction sequence (Cases 1, 3 and 10). Patients 12, 13 and 14 had intubations using succinylcholine and, therefore, their Stages 3, 4 and 5 are not included in this report.

RESULTS AND DISCUSSION

Stage 1

It was important to establish a control value for intracranial pressure when the patient was breathing gas of the same inspired oxygen concentration as was to be used in the subsequent anaesthetic. Cerebral blood flow is influenced by the arterial oxygen tension (Smith and Wollman, 1972). It was also necessary to evaluate the effects of increased resistance to breathing and apparatus dead space of the anaesthetic circuit on intracranial pressure.

Table 2 shows that in 10 patients studied in this way, there was no significant change in arterial blood pressure or cerebral perfusion pressure; however, there was a small but statistically significant rise in ICP.

Table 2. *The influence of the anaesthetic circuit on ICP and mean blood pressure in 10 patients breathing 70% N_2/30% O_2 mixture*

Patient No.	Mean blood pressure (mm Hg) (a)	(b)	Change in blood pressure (a)–(b)	ICP (mm Hg) (a)	(b)	Change in ICP (a)–(b)	Change in perfusion pressure	Pa_{CO_2} (mm Hg) (a)	(b)
2	85	85	0	33	40	+ 7	− 7	36	36
3	140	140	0	30	30	0	0		
4	90	98	+ 8	40	43	+ 3	+ 5	35	35
5	105	105	0	35	33	− 2	+ 2		
6	82	83	+ 1	25	25	0	+ 1	28	30
7	110	100	−10	25	30	+ 5	−15	37	37
8	140	140	0	20	20	0	0	42	42
9	107	100	− 7	22	33	+11	−18		42
10	100	100	0	40	40	0	0	35	35
11	105	110	+ 5	25	30	+ 5 *	0		

(a)=control; (b)=breathing from anaesthetic circuit.
* mean+2.9; $p < 0.05$; mean increase in ICP.

Stage 2a

In all cases nitrous oxide anaesthesia led to a rise of ICP starting about 60 sec after commencing its administration (Fig. 1). ICP rose steeply to reach a plateau within 5 min and then gradually fell to a final value which, although less than the peak level, was significantly higher than the control (Table 3). The mean rise of ICP in the series was 27 mm Hg at peak and 18 mm Hg after levelling off. The mean arterial blood pressure was unchanged, so that these changes were associated with dangerously low cerebral perfusion pressure. There were no alterations in Pa_{CO_2}.

These findings confirm the study by Henriksen and Jörgensen (1973), who investigated 14 patients having 66% nitrous oxide in oxygen and found large rises in intracranial pressure which could be reversed by the administration of 100% oxygen. The effect of nitrous oxide could be due to its diffusion into any air in the ventricular system. However, this is unlikely as particular care was taken to avoid the possibility of residual air in the ventricles at the time of this study, and was not present in Henriksen's patients. It is likely that the initial rise in ICP is associated with a light plane of anaesthesia, and the persistent elevation in ICP is caused by cerebral vasodilatation.

The detection of such a change is only possible at normocapnia and in patients with

Table 3. *The influence of nitrous oxide (70%) on ICP and mean blood pressure*

Patient No.	Mean blood pressure (mm Hg)		Change in blood pressure (a)–(b)	ICP (mm Hg)			Change in ICP (a)–(b)	Change in perfusion pressure	Pa_{O_2} (mm Hg)	
	(a)	(b)		(a)	(b)	(c)			(a)	(b)
1	110	120	+10	10	50	60	+40	—30	40	40
5	105	105	0	25	33	40	+ 8	— 8		
12	95	95	0	45	60	70	+15	—15	40	40
13	140	140	0	20	30	50	+10	—10	39	39
14	100	110	+10	12	28	35	+16 *	— 6 **		

(a)=pre-nitrous oxide; (b)=after levelling of ICP during nitrous oxide; (c)=peak levels of ICP during nitrous oxide.

* Mean+18 mm Hg, p < 0.01; mean increase in ICP.

** Mean—14 mm Hg, p < 0.01; mean fall in perfusion pressure.

initially high ICP. Several studies have failed to show any effect of nitrous oxide on cerebral haemodynamics, but used controlled ventilation and produced hypocapnia (Saidman and Eger, 1965; Gordon and Greitz, 1970).

Stage 2b

The results (Table 4) show that in 9 patients studied there was no significant change in mean arterial blood pressure, ICP or cerebral perfusion pressure. The results show a wide variation in response; 4 patients have a useful fall in intracranial pressure (Cases 7, 9, 10 and 11); however, the hypotension in Case 9, led to a serious fall in cerebral perfusion pressure. Methohexitone was given as a bolus followed by a slow infusion and although great care was taken to avoid respiratory depression, in Cases 4, 6 and 8, the Pa_{CO_2} rose by from 2–10 mm Hg. This probably caused these patients to have elevations of ICP. Methohexitone was the barbiturate selected in this series, as it is reputed to cause less arterial hypotension than thiopentone (Dundee and Moore, 1961), and it is easier to avoid respiratory depression when using methohexitone as an infusion.

Table 4. *The influence of methohexitone on ICP and mean blood pressure*

Patient No.	Mean blood pressure (mm Hg)		Change in blood pressure (a)–(b)	ICP (mm Hg)		Change in ICP (a)–(b)	Change in perfusion pressure	Pa_{CO_2} (mm Hg)	
	(a)	(b)		(a)	(b)			(a)	(b)
2	85	85	0	40	50	+10	—10	36	36
3	150	150	0	20	30	+10	—10		
4	98	90	— 8	43	50	+ 7	—15	35	37
6	83	100	+17	25	40	+15	+ 2	30	40
7	100	60	—40	30	10	—20	—20	37	46
8	140	142	+ 2	20	30	+10	— 8	42	46
9	100	100	0	33	15	—18	+18	42	43
10	80	90	+10	40	30	—10	+20		
11	110	95	—15	32	20	—12	— 3	35	35

(a)=pre-methohexitone; (b)=during methohexitone infusion.

Shapiro and his colleagues used a bolus injection of thiopentone in patients with varying degrees of intracranial hypertension (2–50 mm Hg) (Shapiro et al., 1973). They found that thiopentone produced a large reduction in ICP and an improvement in cerebral perfusion pressure in those patients with the highest ICP. However, these patients were given fentanyl before thiopentone and, in our experience, this will produce a marked rise in ICP due to carbon dioxide retention when given to patients with high ICP. Thiopentone was, therefore, reducing an induced elevation of ICP. Shapiro et al. (1973) also had occasional cases of hypotension compromising cerebral perfusion. Barbiturates may have a place in reducing intracranial pressure, but this has not been shown to be without risk.

Stage 3

Relaxation was achieved using alcuronium or pancuronium and was usually accompanied by some carbon dioxide retention despite manual ventilation by experienced anaesthetists (Table 5), Pa_{CO_2} rises varying from 0–14 mm Hg. This rise in Pa_{CO_2} caused a significant rise in intracranial pressure and fall in cerebral perfusion pressure. It is unlikely that these muscle relaxant drugs have any direct pharmacological influence on cerebral haemodynamics.

Table 5. *The influence of muscle relaxant and manual ventilation on ICP and mean blood pressure*

Patient No.	Relaxant	Mean blood pressure (mm Hg) (a)	(b)	Change in blood pressure (a)–(b)	ICP (mm Hg) (a)	(b)	Change in ICP (a)–(b)	Change in perfusion pressure	Pa_{CO_2} (mm Hg) (a)	(b)
2	Alcuronium	85	75	—10	50	50	0	—10	36	36
4	Alcuronium	90	80	—10	40	45	+ 5	—15	37	40
6	Alcuronium	100	100	0	40	60	+20	—20	40	40
7	Pancuronium	80	100	+20	50	70	+20	0	40	54
8	Pancuronium	142	148	+ 6	30	50	+20	—14		
9	Alcuronium	100	100	0	15	30	+15	—15	43	46
10	Alcuronium	90	90	0	30	50	+20	—20	35	40
11	Alcuronium	95	90	— 5	20	20	0 *	— 5 **		

(a)=pre-relaxant; (b)=post-relaxant.
 * Mean increase in ICP 12.5 mm Hg, $p < 0.05$.
 ** Mean fall in perfusion pressure 12.4 mm Hg, $p < 0.05$.

Stage 4

Table 6 shows that intubation produces the well-known explosive increase in ICP and arterial blood pressure. There is no statistically significant change in cerebral perfusion pressure.

The intracranial pressure may go so high (Fig. 1*a*) during laryngoscopy and intubation that there is a great risk of intracranial focal or general ischaemia, or coning.

We, therefore, are currently investigating the possibility of preventing this change by the use of adrenergic β-receptor blockade using practolol (Fig. 1*b*).

It is presumed that the responses to laryngoscopy etc. are due to the loss of autoregulatory control and, therefore, a passive increase in cerebral blood flow and blood volume is caused by hypertension (Paulson, 1972). However, it is possible that the raised ICP occurs independently of the blood pressure elevation. If this is the case, our use of β-blockade will prove unsatisfactory.

Table 6. *The influence of laryngoscopy and endotracheal intubation in ICP and mean blood pressure*

Patient No.	Mean blood pressure (mm Hg)		Change in blood pressure (a)–(b)	ICP (mm Hg)		Change in ICP (a)–(b)	Change in perfusion pressure	Pa_{CO_2} (mm Hg)	
	(a)	(b)		(a)	(b)			(a)	(b)
2	75	100	+25	50	60	+10	+15	36	39
4	80	90	+10	45	50	+ 5	+ 5	40	45
5	105	110	+ 5	55	65	+10	— 5		
6	100	120	+20	60	100	+40	—20	41	38
7	100	130	+30	70	100	+30	0	34	
8	148	175	+27	50	60	+10	+17	46	47
9	100	130	+30	40	50	+10	+20	50	50
11	90	130	+40	20	100	+80	—40	40	40
			*			**	***		

(a)=pre-intubation; (b)=immediately after intubation.
   *   Mean increase in mean arterial pressure 23.4 mm Hg, $p < 0.01$.
 **   Mean rise in ICP 24.3 mm Hg, $p < 0.01$.
***   Not significant.

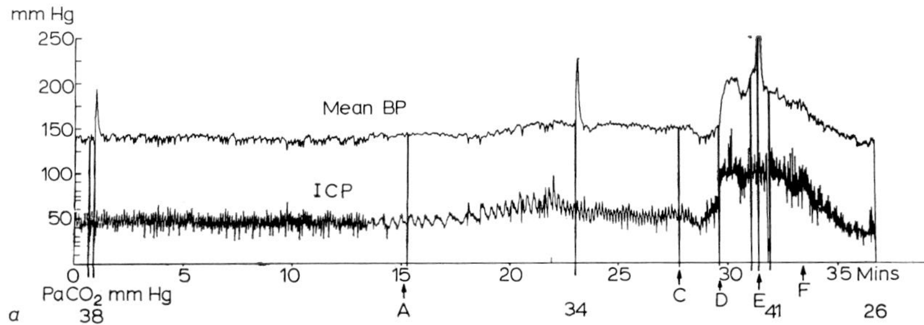

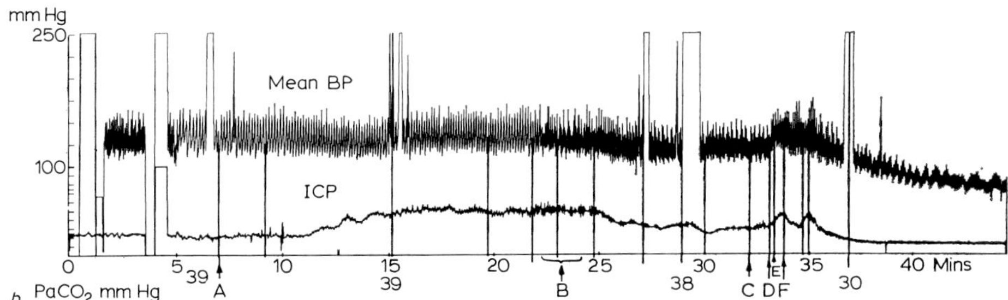

Fig. 1. *Records of ICP and mean blood pressure showing the characteristic increases in ICP during induction of anaesthesia with nitrous oxide and on endotracheal intubation. In (b), the patient was given atropine and practolol in an attempt to block the ICP and blood pressure changes on intubation. Event code as follows: (A) Nitrous oxide and oxygen by mask; (B) In (b), atropine 1 mg and practolol 25 mg; (C) Succinylcholine 100 mg; (D) Laryngoscopy and intubation; (E) Manual ventilation; (F) Hyperventilation using a Manley ventilator.*

Stage 5

Table 7 shows that hyperventilation and hypocapnia reduce ICP, although a moderate fall in blood pressure is produced in some cases. There is a large increase in cerebral perfusion pressure.

Table 7.   *The influence of hyperventilation and hypocapnia on ICP and mean blood pressure*

Patient No.	Mean blood pressure (mm Hg)		Change in blood pressure (a)–(b)	ICP (mm Hg)		Change in ICP (a)–(b)	Change in perfusion pressure	Pa_{CO_2} (mm Hg)	
	(a)	(b)		(a)	(b)			(a)	(b)
2	100	75	—25	60	35	—25	0	39	35
4	90	60	—30	50	33	—17	—13	45	30
5	110	100	—10	65	22	—43	+33		
6	120	110	—10	100	17	—83	+73	38	26
7	130	110	—20	100	15	—85	+65	54	31
9	130	150	+20	40	5	—35	+55	47	30
11	130	105	—25	100	40	—60	+35	40	25
			*			**	***		

(a)=pre-hyperventilation; (b)=during hyperventilation.
   *   Mean fall in mean blood pressure 14.3 mm Hg, p=0.07.
  **   Mean fall in ICP 49.8 mm Hg, p<0.01.
***   Mean increase in cerebral perfusion pressure 35.4 mm Hg, p<0.05.

Thus, hypocapnia completely corrects the abnormalities in cerebral perfusion which we had produced by nitrous oxide etc. This is in agreement with the findings of Henriksen and Jörgensen (1973). There is a restoration of autoregulation with hypocapnia which may protect the brain against oedema formation (Paulson et al., 1972).

CONCLUSION

When inducing anaesthesia in patients with raised intracranial pressure, there are several insults that must be avoided: (1) nitrous oxide induction; (2) carbon dioxide retention and, therefore, respiratory depressants and deep anaesthesia; and (3) slow or difficult intubation.

Therefore, the patient should have no respiratory depressant premedication and be encouraged to hyperventilate until he is given a sufficient dose of intravenous barbiturate to produce sleep without hypotension. He should be paralysed using succinylcholine, ventilated and then gently and expeditiously intubated and hyperventilated.

ACKNOWLEDGEMENTS

I would like to thank Drs D. F. Cochrane, D. P. G. Griffiths and J. S. M. Zorab for their help in anaesthetising these patients and Miss J. A. Foster for secretarial help.

REFERENCES

Dundee, J. W. and Moore, J. (1961): *Anaesthesia, 16,* 50.
Fitch, W., Barker, J., McDowall, D. G. and Jennett, W. B. (1969): *Brit. J. Anaesth., 41,* 564.

Fitch, W. and McDowall, D. G. (1971): *Brit. J. Anaesth.*, *43*, 904.
Gordon, E. and Greitz, T. (1970): *Brit. J. Anaesth.*, *42*, 2.
Henriksen, H. T. and Jörgensen, P. B. (1973): *Brit. J. Anaesth.*, *45*, 486.
Hulme, A. and Cooper, R. (1966): *J. Neurol. Neurosurg. Psychiat.*, *29*, 154.
Hulme, A. and Cooper, R. (1972): *Proc. roy. Soc. Med.*, *65*, 883.
Jennett, W. B., Barker, J., Fitch, W. and McDowall, D. G. (1969): *Lancet, 1*, 61.
Paulson, O. B. (1972): *Anaesthesiology*, *36*, 1.
Paulson, O. B., Olesen, J. and Christensen, M. S. (1972): *Neurology*, *22*, 286.
Saidman, L. J. and Eger II, E. I. (1965): *Anesthesiology*, *26*, 67.
Shapiro, H. M., Wyte, S. R., Harris, A. B. and Galindo, A. (1972): *Anesthesiology*, *37*, 399.
Shapiro, H. M., Galindo, S. R. and Harris, A. B. (1973): *Brit. J. Anaesth.*, *45*, 1057.
Smith, A. L. and Wollman, H. (1972): *Anesthesiology*, *36*, 378.

ECG effects of halothane hypotension for cerebral vascular surgery

B. KAY

Derbyshire Royal Infirmary, Derby, United Kingdom

This is a brief account of an extensive study of 202 patients undergoing surgery for cerebral aneurysm at Derbyshire Royal Infirmary. All the patients were operated on by the same surgeon, and the majority were anaesthetised by one of two anesthetists.

In more than half the patients the anaesthetist induced moderate hypotension during the surgical approach to the aneurysm, in order to reduce the possibility of rupture, or reduce the haemorrhage should a tear occur. Hypotension was induced by the use of halothane in the great majority of cases, otherwise by the use of pentolinium, reducing the systolic blood pressure to 90 mm Hg or less.

The purpose of this study was to assess the effects of halothane induced hypotension on the operative and postoperative course of the patient and in particular to note the effects on the ECG. From every patient an ECG record was obtained preoperatively, postoperatively, and during surgery.

Induction of anaesthesia was identical in all the patients. An intravenous barbiturate was followed by suxamethonium, then local anaesthetic to the vocal cords and trachea before endotracheal intubation. Anaesthesia was continued with nitrous oxide and oxygen with curare or pancuronium followed by moderate hyperventilation by IPPR. A majority of patients (74%) received intravenous mannitol during induction of anaesthesia, usually 500 ml of 20%.

All received a maintenance supplement, either halothane 0.5%, trichlorethylene 0.25%–0.5%, or intermittent fentanyl. There were thus 4 groups of patients (Table 1) of which Groups 1 and 4 (117 patients) received hypotension, 95 of these using halothane, and Groups 2 and 3 did not have hypotension induced.

Table 1. *Patients grouped according to maintenance supplement*

Group	Maintenance supplement	No. of patients
1	Halothane hypotension	95
2	Halothane without hypotension	45
3	Trilene and/or fentanyl	40
4	Trilene and/or fentanyl plus ganglion blocker	22

The groups are not statistically comparable. Not surprisingly, the anaesthetists involved tended to favour one technique or another, although both major anaesthetists used all techniques according to circumstance. Group 1 also has a significantly higher proportion of females than the other groups, and more patients with aneurysms of the internal carotid or anterior communicating arteries, the lesions producing the greatest incidence of morbidity and mortality. The average age was 46 years.

RESULTS

Table 2 shows the overall early mortality (up to 21 days). Two patients, both in Group 3, died during operation. No patients died between 10 and 21 days. A greater proportion of patients in Group 1 (halothane with hypotension) died than in Group 2 (halothane without hypotension) but there is little difference between halothane and non-halothane anaesthesia, or normotensive and hypotensive groups. The increased incidence of early death in Group 1 is entirely attributable to 12 patients who died from a further intracranial haemorrhage, compared with 1 dying from this cause in each of the other groups.

Table 2. *Overall early mortality*

Group	No.	%
1	17	18
2	4	9
3	7*	18
4	1	5

* Includes 2 deaths during operation.

Undoubtedly the major factor contributing to death was the presence of established preoperative disease (Table 3). 40 patients (20%) came into this category, equally distributed through the groups, and more than half died, twice the overall percentage mortality. Similarly, this 20% of patients with preoperative disease contributed 50% of the patients dying in the postoperative period (21 days). The commonest preoperative disease was established cardiovascular disease (not the hypertensive response to subarachnoid haemorrhage).

Table 3. *Effect of preoperative disease on mortality*

	No. of patients	Early death No.	(%)	Eventual death No.	(%)
Preoperative disease	40	14	(34)	21	(50)
No preoperative disease	162	15	(9)	25	(15)
Total	202	29	(14)	46	(23)

The most frequent operative complication was rupture of the aneurysm, shown in Table 4. Overall, there is surprisingly little difference between hypotensive and non-hypotensive groups, but hypotension was induced in 5 patients in Group 1 *after* rupture of the aneurysm during early dissection, in order to reduce haemorrhage and allow the operation to proceed.

Table 4.   *Rupture of aneurysm*

	Gross		Corrected	
Group	No.	(%)	No.	(%)
1	30	(31)	25	(25)
4	9	(41)	9	(41)
2 and 3	33	(39)	38	(43)

The only other point of interest during operation was the incidence of high intracranial pressure, which was similar in all groups. In the postoperative phase, also, all groups produced similar incidences of delayed recovery, neurological deficit, pulmonary and cardiovascular complications, except for the increased incidence of further intracranial haemorrhage found in the hypotensive groups, 15 (13.5%) against 3 (3.5%) in the normotensive groups.

The mean systolic blood pressures are shown in Table 5 and demonstrate a remarkable similarity of levels between techniques in the hypotensive and normotensive groups. Blood pressure was rarely intentionally reduced below 80 mm Hg, and in those patients where unintentional falls below this level occurred, there was a 50% mortality.

Table 5.   *Mean systolic blood pressure (mm Hg)*

	Group			
	1	2	3	4
Preoperative	153	159	156	144
Post-induction	116	127	129	117
Dissection of aneurysm	84	111	106	84
End-operation	117	125	126	114
Day after operation	145	146	148	141

ECG CHANGES

As in previously reported series we found a considerable proportion of ECG abnormalities associated with subarachnoid haemorrhage (Table 6), frequently simulating myocardial ischaemia.

All forms of anaesthesia produced certain modification of the ECG. As expected, there was a rise in pulse rate after induction of anaesthesia (Table 7), which remained noticeably raised in Group 4. Associated with the effects of atropine, all sinus bradycardia disappeared

Table 6.   *Major preoperative ECG abnormalities*
           (figures in %)

Sinus arrhythmias	35	Tall U-waves	22
Sinus bradycardia	26	T–U	35
Prolonged Q–T	13	Raised ST	15
L. ventricular hypertrophy	25	Lowered ST	21
L. axis deviation	11	T-wave inversion	23
Tall P-waves	7	T-wave flattening	10

Table 7. *Mean pulse rates*

	Group			
	1	2	3	4
Preoperative	67	65	69	72
Post-induction	93	94	87	98
Dissection of aneurysm	79	77	73	91
End-operation	74	75	72	80
Postoperative	77	79	81	82

after induction of anaesthesia, to reappear by the end of operation, and the incidence of sinus arrhythmias fell from 35%–6%. Also associated with this tachycardia, the incidence of tall P-waves increased from 7%–16% after induction of anaesthesia, gradually reducing thereafter. This effect is frequently seen after atropine and possibly due to a transient pulmonary hypertension.

The most striking effect of induction of anaesthesia was however the dramatic disappearance of tall U-waves, down to 2%, and T-U phenomena, down to 5%. This was not entirely associated with the tachycardia as the reduction persisted throughout anaesthesia and did not approach the preoperative incidence until the day after operation. Preoperatively these ECG changes seem to be associated with high circulating catecholamine levels, and possibly mediated a relative local hypokalaemia. Cell membrane stabilization, and potassium ion release by suxamethonium and transfused blood may be factors in changing this pattern during anaesthesia.

All the changes associated with anaesthesia were equally marked in all the four groups. The incidences of left ventricular hypertrophy and left axis deviation did not change with anaesthesia.

Table 8 shows the remaining major ECG changes. QTc changes were the most marked, with a very great increase in the presence of long QT intervals through the early phases of anaesthesia, persisting until after recovery. One speculates whether the effects of atropine and the tachycardia of the postinduction phase might not be concealing the full effects of anaesthesia displayed later.

Table 8. *Other ECG changes (figures in %)*

	Long QTc	ST ↑	ST ↓	T ↓
Preoperative	13	15	21	23
Post-induction	27	4	33	14
Dissection of aneurysm	66	8	26	18
End-operation	61	7	26	24
Postoperative	16	10	34	24

Induction of anaesthesia depresses the previously raised ST segment, with an initial disappearance of preoperatively inverted T-waves. T-wave inversion tends to recur however, and the signs of cardiac ischaemia, depressed ST segment and inverted T-wave persist postoperatively, gradually disappearing over weeks. Again, there is no difference between the groups.

Arrhythmias in association with the anaesthesia were rare and transient except in the case of Group 1.

Here, nodal rhythm, presumably halothane induced, doubled to 7% after induction of anaesthesia, and again to 16% during hypotension. However, by the end of operation the incidence was 9% and postoperatively down to 2%.

The results of this survey, although not statistically significant, raise the question of whether induced moderate hypotension really protects the life and postoperative state of the patient undergoing surgery on a cerebral aneurysm. There seems little difference between the anaesthetic techniques used so far as these results are concerned, and although the ECG changes are marked, again they were equally so in all 4 groups, hypotension producing no particular variation.

Intracranial ionic imbalance induced by halogenated anesthetics*

A. SCHETTINI

VA Wadsworth Hospital Center, Los Angeles, Calif., U.S.A.

INTRODUCTION

Halothane inhalation may cause a tight brain despite hyperventilation (Editorial, 1969). The increased subpial tension may be due to cerebral vascular expansion and possibly to increased brain water since halothane is a cerebral vasodilator (McDowall and Harper, 1965).

In clinical situations, it has been suggested that thiopental-hyperventilation induction minimizes the rise in cerebrospinal fluid (CSF) pressure with halothane inhalation (Adams et al., 1972). This normalization of CSF pressure, however, does not preclude vasodilatation because cerebral vascular expansion which primarily affects the subpial compartment is accompanied by compensatory CSF reduction. These changes can be detected directly by simultaneous monitoring of pressure and displacement during intracranial pressure measurements made epidurally (Schettini and Walsh, 1974). Once the two intracranial compartments have been identified for each animal, any pressure dissociation can be accurately recorded and the influence of anesthetics on brain mechanical properties quantitated.

This method of investigation coupled with measurement of both brain electrical impedance and CSF electrolytes was used to compare intracranial dynamic responses to halothane, enflurane (Ethrane),** and isoflurane (Forane).** Brain electrical impedance was monitored at 1 kHz to detect ionic shifts between brain extra- and intracellular space. Of the various brain viscoelastic functions, we elected to determine changes in brain relative stiffness (BRS) since earlier experiments suggested that this function reflects qualitative changes in cerebral blood volume (Schettini et al., 1972).

MATERIALS AND METHODS

Nine dogs (21 $\pm$ 1.5 kg) were chronically implanted for measurement of brain electrical impedance, intracranial pressures epidurally, and arterial blood pressure. Cisternal CSF samples were analyzed for Na and K by flame photometry and for Cl with a Cotlove chloridometer. Arterial blood samples were analyzed for gas tensions and pH with a microelectrode system; anesthetic concentrations were analyzed by gas chromatography. Subarachnoid CSF and surface brain pressure measurements were obtained at 15 min intervals from the pressure-depth-time response of the intracranial system (Schettini and Walsh, 1974). Brain

---

* Supported by Grant No. V.A. 7749–01, and by Ohio Medical Products, Airco Inc., Murray Hill, N.J., U.S.A.
** Ohio Medical Products, Inc.

Table 1. *Experimental findings (actual changes in means $\pm$ SD) in nine dogs during enflurane, isoflurane and halothane inhalation. All dogs were induced with a thiopental-hyperventilation sequence (at T_0)*

	Pa_{CO_2} (mm Hg)	Arterial anesthetic concentration (vol %)	P_{CSF} [1] (mm Hg)	P_B [2] (mm Hg)	Brain relative stiffness (dynes/m $\times 10^5$)	Brain electrical impedance [3] range of changes (%)	
						(Ohms)	Minimum/Maximum
Enflurane (9)							
Control	34.5 ± 3.0	–	6.0 ± 3.4	15.9 ± 2.9	1.10 ± 0.58	180.0 ± 70.0	
T_0	-6.5 ± 0.5	–	-1.5 ± 0.5	-2.0 ± 0.5	-0.0 ± 0.05	$+4.0 \pm 1.0$	
T_{15}	–	1.6 ± 0.2	$+3.4 \pm 2.0**$	$+5.3 \pm 4.5**$	-0.04 ± 0.68	$+11.7 \pm 11.3$	
T_{60}	-10.0 ± 0.8	1.2 ± 0.5	$+0.2 \pm 3.0$	$+2.6 \pm 3.2*$	$+0.34 \pm 0.67$	$+20.9 \pm 9.0$	$8.7 \rightarrow 28.3$
Isoflurane (9)							
Control	32.1 ± 2.6	–	5.8 ± 3.2	12.5 ± 1.4	0.87 ± 0.09	150.0 ± 40.0	
T_0	-6.0 ± 0.5	–	-3.0 ± 1.0	-1.5 ± 0.5	-0.01 ± 0.01	$+3.0 \pm 1.0$	
T_{15}	–	1.6 ± 0.6	$+2.2 \pm 5.4$	$+3.1 \pm 3.9*$	$+0.02 \pm 0.50$	$+6.6 \pm 3.0$	
T_{60}	-6.0 ± 0.5	1.2 ± 0.5	-0.8 ± 2.9	$+0.2 \pm 3.5$	$+0.3 \pm 0.60$	$+11.4 \pm 4.0$	$5.0 \rightarrow 13.9$
Halothane (9)							
Control	33.6 ± 2.6	–	6.0 ± 1.7	12.0 ± 1.7	0.96 ± 0.25	150.0 ± 60.0	
T_0	-6.0 ± 1.0	–	-2.0 ± 0.5	-3.0 ± 0.5	-0.0 ± 0.05	$+4.0 \pm 1.0$	
T_{15}	–	0.8 ± 0.1	-0.6 ± 3.0	$+2.7 \pm 1.5**$	$+0.16 \pm 0.50$	$+4.7 \pm 3.0$	
T_{60}	-6.0 ± 0.9	0.9 ± 0.3	-1.8 ± 2.5	$+1.3 \pm 1.3*$	$+0.38 \pm 0.40*$	$+16.3 \pm 4.0$	$6.9 \rightarrow 16.6$

[1] = Subarachnoid CSF (cranial vault). [2] = Surface brain pressure. [3] = Transfer factor for impedance probes: 4.5 ± 0.5.
* $p < 0.05$. ** $p < 0.01$.

relative stiffness (BRS) was estimated from pressure-displacement diagrams of ramp tests and expressed in dynes/cm $\times$ 10^5 after appropriate conversion into one unitary system (Schettini et al., 1972). Brain electrical impedance was measured at 1 kHz using the four electrode coated probe method (Ranck, 1966). Polarization impedance was eliminated by a circuitry of operational amplifiers. All measurements were recorded on an oscillograph-x-y graph-FM tape recording system (Schettini and Walsh, 1974).

The dogs were induced with thiopental (30 mg/kg), intubated, hyperventilated mechanically to a Pa_{CO_2} in the range of 26–28 mm Hg and then randomly exposed at 2-day intervals to one of the three inhalant anesthetics for 60 min. Enflurane in oxygen was vaporized via a copper kettle and administered in decreasing concentration (4.0–2.0%); halothane/oxygen (1.5–0.8%) and isoflurane/oxygen (2.5–1.5%) were administered through calibrated vaporizers (Fluotec-Cyprane, Ltd., Buffalo, N.Y.). Arterial pressure was maintained near control values (110 $\pm$ 15 mm Hg) with a 0.1% phenylephrine infusion. Statistical significance was determined by paired t-tests with significance at $p < 0.05$.

RESULTS

Intracranial pressures and brain relative stiffness (BRS)

The results are summarized in Table 1 and Figure 1. All control measurements are within normal limits. As expected, thiopental-hyperventilation induction produced nonsignificant changes. At 15 min of enflurane inhalation, CSF and surface brain pressures both increased ($p < 0.01$) while BRS decreased. At 60 min of anesthesia, CSF pressure was near normal whereas surface brain pressure remained elevated ($p < 0.05$) and BRS tended to increase. This was statistically nonsignificant. With halothane inhalation, CSF pressure decreased from the beginning while surface brain pressure increased significantly ($p < 0.01$) and BRS exhibited a more definitive trend toward an increase. At 60 min CSF pressure was below normal while brain pressure and BRS were above normal ($p < 0.05$). Isoflurane inhalation caused an initial (15 min) increase in CSF and surface brain pressures. Statistical significance was obtained only for the subpial pressure measurement ($p < 0.05$). At 60 min of anesthesia and hyperventilation ($Pa_{CO_2} = 26 \pm 2.5$ mm Hg) intracranial pressures were near normal while changes in BRS were not significant (Table 1).

Brain electrical impedance

Within 2–3 min of enflurane inhalation brain impedance changed, exhibiting a biphasic curve of increase and decrease. There was considerable variation among animals, as reflected in the large standard deviations (Table 1). With halothane and isoflurane the impedance rose gradually with less variability among animals as compared to enflurane. The percentage of impedance rise was greater with enflurane (9–28%) than with either halothane (7–17%) or isoflurane (5–14%).

CSF electrolytes

Na increased with halothane ($p < 0.05$) but not with enflurane or isoflurane. K decreased with all three agents. Statistical significance ($p < 0.05$) was obtained for all three drugs at 60 min and also at 45 min for both enflurane ($p < 0.01$) and halothane ($p < 0.05$). The tendency toward Cl decrease was not significant and probably reflected hyperventilation (increased lactate ion). Total osmolarity for CSF remained unchanged for all three agents (Fig. 1).

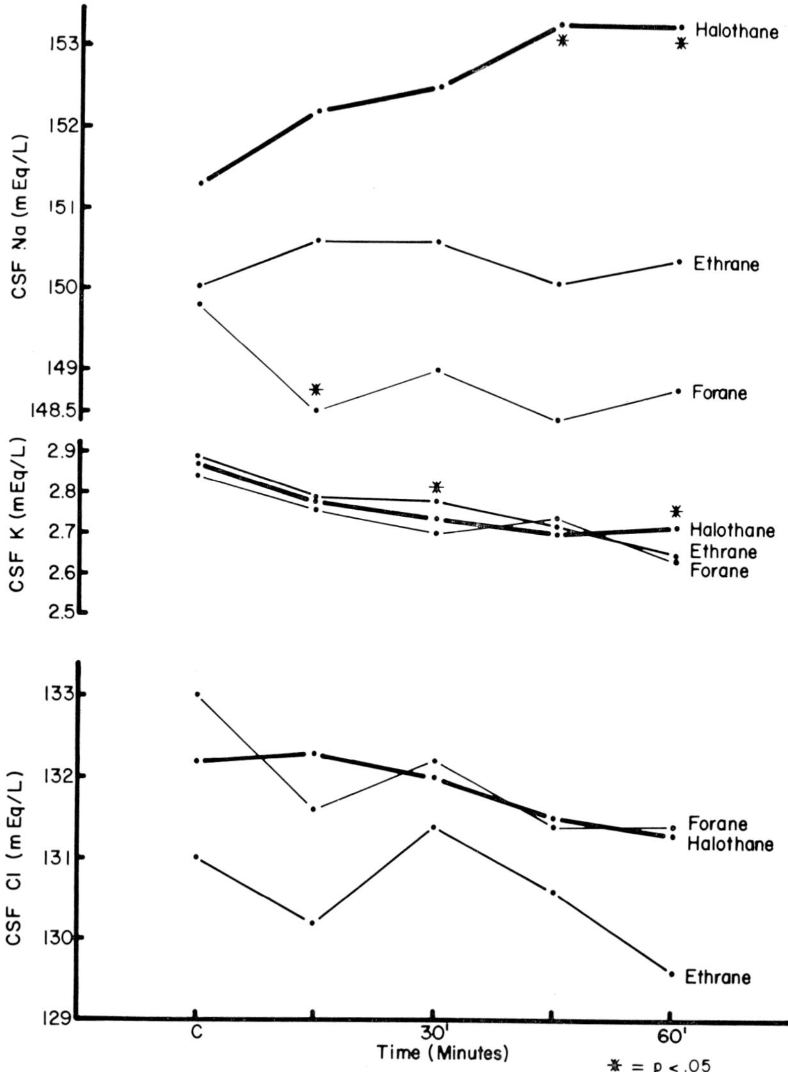

Fig. 1.   *Changes (means) in CSF electrolytes (Na, K, Cl) of 7 dogs during 60 min of enflurane, halothane, and isoflurane anesthesia (C=control).*

COMMENTS

The present study shows that even after thiopental-hyperventilation induction, volatile halogenated anesthetics may alter intracranial dynamics by causing a pressure dissociation between subarachnoid and subpial compartments. Although the observed changes are small, these dogs had normal intracranial tension. Such changes might be more significant in the presence of reduced spatial compensation.

The pressure dissociation could be due to the cerebral vasodilating properties of these volatile anesthetics. Under our experimental conditions (hypocarbia and normotensive arterial blood pressure) vasodilatation led to cerebral vascular expansion and was reflected in the increased surface brain pressure and brain relative stiffness. The effects of cerebral vascular expansion, however, were more pronounced with enflurane and halothane than with isoflurane. These findings support the view that intracranial dynamic responses cannot be properly assessed in the presence of cerebral circulatory changes unless the pressure-depth-time response of both the subarachnoid and subpial compartments is determined; the resultant pressure-displacement diagrams reflect the degree of spatial compensation of the intracranial system (Schettini and Walsh, 1974).

The mechanism underlying the anesthetic induced vasodilatation could be metabolic in origin. H^+ changes alone, in brain perivascular structure, cannot explain this vaso-dilatation. Repeated studies have failed to demonstrate unequivocally any significant role of brain interstitial pH by itself in normal autoregulation of cerebral blood flow (McDowall and Harper, 1970). An alternative explanation is that volatile halogenated anesthetics may cause both changes in H^+ and ionic imbalance (Ca, K) in brain ECS, leading to both, increased brain water and subpial pressure. The rise in brain electrical imbalance and concomitant decreased K CSF with all three inhalant agents tend to support this hypothesis. Considerable experimental evidence suggests that changes in brain electrical impedance at low frequency principally reflect ionic shifts between intra- and extracellular space (ECS) (Van Harreveld, 1966). Changes in CSF electrolytes in the present studies were consistent only for the decrease in K. This may reflect differences in ion kinetics and/or sampling site. Even so, the decrease in K may be significant by reason of the rigid mechanism controlling K CSF independent of blood K (Cserr, 1965).

The decrease in both conductivity (reciprocal of impedance) and K CSF may be inter-preted in terms of (1) ionic shifts between brain extra- and intracellular space, and (2) electrical inactivation of the ions in brain extracellular matrix. Both of these mechanisms could be due to the interaction between anesthetic molecule and cell membrane (Seeman, 1972). The impedance pattern of enflurane was biphasic and similar to that seen with chemical convulsants (Van Harreveld, 1966). When selected anticonvulsants preceded enflurane inhalation, the biphasic impedance pattern was converted into one of more gradual rise, as seen with halothane and isoflurane (Schettini and Wilder, 1974). The nature of these metabolic changes (H^+ and cationic shifts) however, needs further investigation since with isoflurane there was a dissociation between normalization of intracranial pressure and the decreased ionic conductivity and K CSF. This cannot be explained from our data. Possibly, there is a mediating mechanism (H^+, Ca^{++}) which is altered with enflurane and halothane but not with isoflurane.

Nevertheless, we conclude that volatile halogenated anesthetics induce variable degrees of transient CNS cationic permeability. This ionic imbalance may be responsible for the intracranial pressure gradient under conditions of normotensive arterial blood pressure. These factors may account for their unreliability in neurosurgical anesthesia when used in concentrations of one MAC or more.

REFERENCES

Adams, R. W., Gronert, G. A. and Sundt, T. M. et al. (1972): *Anesthesiology, 37*, 510.
Cserr, H. (1965): *Amer. J. Physiol., 209*, 1219.
Editorial (1969): *Brit. J. Anaesth., 41*, 277.
McDowall, D. G. and Harper, A. M. (1965): *Acta neurol. scand. (Suppl.), 14*, 146.
McDowall, D. G. and Harper, A. M. (1970): In: *Proceedings, Fourth World Congress of Anaesthesiologists, London 1968*, p. 542. Editors: T. B. Boulton, R. Bryce-Smith, M. K. Sykes, G. B. Gillett and A. L. Revell. Excerpta Medica, Amsterdam.
Ranck, J. B. (1966): *Exp. Neurol., 16*, 416.

Schettini, A., Mahig, J. and Moreshead, G. (1972): In: *Intracranial Pressure: Experimental and Clinical Aspects*, p. 27. Editors: M. Brock and H. Dietz. Springer Verlag, Berlin – Heidelberg – New York.
Schettini, A. and Walsh, E. K. (1974): *J. Neurosurg.*, *40*, 609.
Schettini, A. and Wilder, B. J. (1974): *Anesth. Analg. Curr. Res.*, *53*, 951.
Seeman, P. (1972): *Pharmacol. Rev.*, *24*, 584.
Van Harreveld, A. (1966): In: *Brain Tissue Electrolytes*, Chapter 2, p. 50. Editor: A. van Harreveld. Butterworths, Washington, D.C.

Sodium nitroprusside in cerebral aneurysm surgery

J. S. M. ZORAB *, B. H. CUMMINS *, R. GREENBAUM *, H. B. GRIFFITH *,
D. P. G. GRIFFITHS *, G. E. STADDON ** and D. G. WILKINS **

* Frenchay Hospital and ** United Bristol Hospitals, Bristol, United Kingdom

INTRODUCTION

The operation for the clipping of a cerebral aneurysm presents both the anaesthetist and the surgeon with a number of problems, not the least of which is the risk of rupture of the aneurysm during its dissection. It is now well established practice by many neurosurgical teams to use induced hypotension during this type of surgery because it is felt that, firstly, this will reduce the stress on the wall of the aneurysmal sac and thus make rupture less likely and, secondly, that, should rupture occur, the reduced arterial pressure will ease control of the subsequent bleeding.

In this Unit, the arterial pressure is allowed to remain at normal levels until the approach surgery is about to begin and the pressure is then lowered to a mean value of 60 mm Hg where it is maintained until the clip is in position. The pressure is then restored to normal and an immediate cerebral angiogram is performed.

In the course of a research project into changes in cerebral blood flow during this type of surgery, the opportunity was taken to study and assess the value of sodium nitroprusside as the means of inducing hypotension (Griffiths et al., 1974).

Sodium nitroprusside is a ferrous, hydrated, penta-cyano compound which was first described over 100 years ago. Although its hypotensive properties have been known for many years, its use to provide hypotension during surgery is a relatively recent development. It does not, so far, appear to be commercially available but its preparation is comparatively simple and well within the scope of many hospital pharmacies.

There are a number of features of sodium nitroprusside which make it particularly suitable for providing the kind of short-term hypotension that we find ideal for aneurysm surgery.

FEATURES OF SODIUM NITROPRUSSIDE

Rapid onset

Because the arterial pressure is maintained at normal levels until the surgeon is ready to approach the aneurysm, it is an advantage to have an agent with a quick onset of action. Sodium nitroprusside fulfils this need and the pressure begins to fall within one or two minutes of starting administration.

Continuous control

Sodium nitroprusside has a very brief duration of action. It has therefore, to be given

813

continuously and this allows the level of hypotension to be controlled by the rate of administration. In this respect, it is similar to trimetaphan but, in our experience, the level of hypotension is easier to control.

In the early stages of its use, a fairly concentrated solution was used and given with a variable speed electric syringe pump but this was not very satisfactory and it proved far too easy to give a bolus injection while setting up the apparatus.

A micro-drip apparatus is now preferred which gives very satisfactory results.

As with all methods of induced hypotension, accurate and, preferably, continuous measurement of the mean arterial pressure adds substantially to the safety margin of the technique. When the apparatus and technical help is available, electrical methods of measurement are ideal.

However, a simple aneroid manometer connected by an air and heparinised saline column to an arterial cannula is a simpler, cheaper and highly satisfactory device (Zorab, 1969).

No autonomic blockade

Sodium nitroprusside works by a direct effect on the vessel wall and its action is, therefore, independent of autonomic innervation. Indeed, it was this feature that first led to the investigation of its effect in cerebral blood flow. An additional benefit stemming from this feature is the absence of dilatation of the pupils which is seen with all the ganglion-blocking drugs and increases the problems during the postoperative assessment of these patients.

Little tachyphylaxis

Those who have used sodium nitroprusside for induced hypotension during surgery have been impressed by the consistency of patient response to this agent.

Low toxicity

Although sodium nitroprusside is broken down to form cyanide, it appears to be free from toxic effects in the doses used in clinical practice. Nevertheless, Vesey et al. (1974) have shown that a significant rise in plasma cyanide level does take place during nitroprusside therapy.

However, although a rise in cyanide level occurs, its significance still has to be interpreted. Since cyanide passes rapidly into the erythrocytes it is this red cell cyanide level that is most important and this may possibly affect oxygen transport because of the known effect of cyanide on cellular respiration. Vitamin B12, known as hydroxocobalamin, has been shown to be a potent antidote to cyanide. Vesey measured the erythrocyte cyanide levels in a patient on long-term nitroprusside therapy before and after hydroxocobalamin administration.

The steadily rising cyanide level was found to fall abruptly following 5 mg of hydroxocobalamin although the nitroprusside infusion was still in progress. From this and other published data, it appears that it may be wise to administer large doses of hydroxocobalamin before and during nitroprusside infusions, especially where long-term therapy is envisaged or where the patient might be expected to have low vitamin B12 levels.

Rapid recovery

The evanescent action of sodium nitroprusside to which reference has already been made, ensures that there is a rapid recovery of the arterial pressure following the cessation of administration. This is a valuable feature of the drug for, once the aneurysm clip is in position, the pressure is restored to normal as soon as possible for the peroperative angiogram that is done immediately after clipping.

MEASUREMENTS AND MONITORING

In the short research series of 20 cases, various measurements were made. Ventilation was controlled at 10 l/min with an inspired oxygen concentration of 30%. Carbon dioxide was added to the inspired mixture to produce an arterial P_{CO_2} of about 42 mm Hg and temperature loss was avoided by the use of water blankets.

The mean arterial pressures recorded before and during the administration of sodium nitroprusside revealed a fall from a mean of 115 to 67 – a drop of 48 mm Hg. This pressure drop was accompanied by an overall slight increase in heart rate from 62–70 – a scarcely significant difference. The central venous pressure fell slightly but, again, this was not significant.

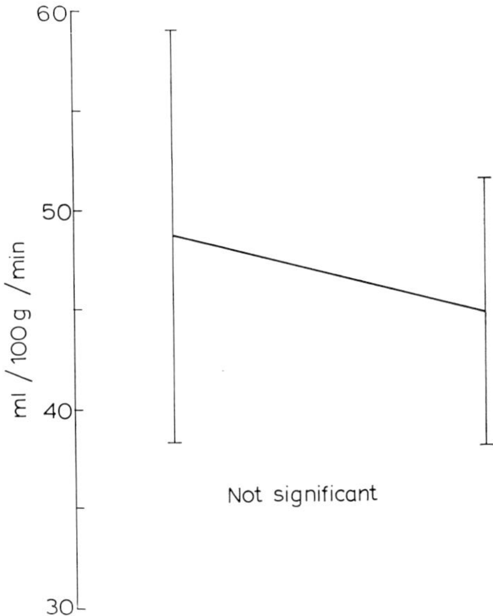

Fig. 1. *Cerebral blood flow before and during hypotension.*

The most important measurement in this context was the cerebral blood flow. This was expressed as grey flow measured as millilitres of blood per 100 grams of brain per minute and Figure 1 shows that, from the mean figures, no significant fall took place. Indeed, the percentage fall shown is of the order of 8.2%. However, if the percentage change of cerebral blood flow is studied (Fig. 2) in each of the 19 patients in whom successful measurements were made, it can be seen that there is a considerable scatter of change; some patients showing a marked increase in flow while others show a substantial decrease.

CONCLUSION

It is clear that there are other factors affecting the autoregulation of the cerebral blood flow besides the mean arterial pressure but, nevertheless, sodium nitroprusside has proved

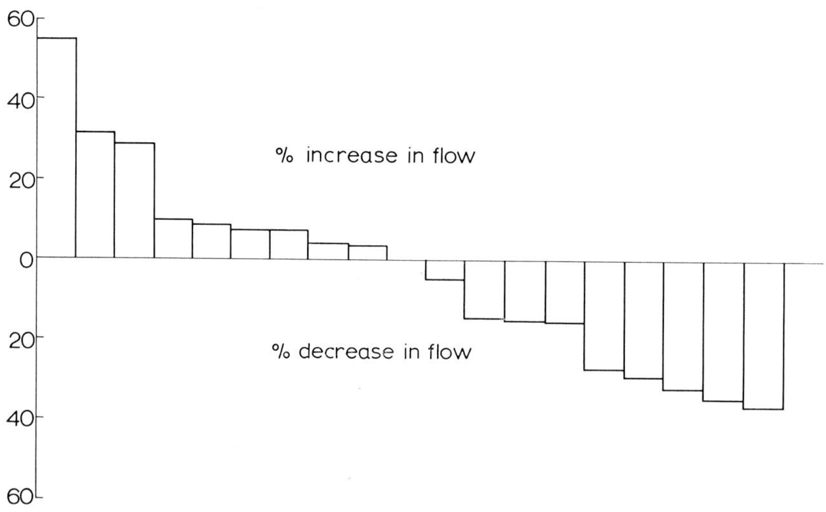

Fig. 2.   *Percentage change in cerebral blood flow.*

to be a useful agent and, at present, is being used as the drug of choice in this department for inducing hypotension in cerebral aneurysm surgery.

REFERENCES

Griffiths, D. P. G., Cummins, B. H., Greenbaum, R., Griffith, H. B., Staddon, G. E., Wilkins, D. G. and Zorab, J. S. M. (1974): *Brit. J. Anaesth.*, *46*, 641.
Vesey, C. J., Cole, P. V., Linnell, J. C. and Wilson, J. (1974): *Brit. med. J.*, *2*, 140.
Zorab, J. S. M. (1969): *Anaesthesia*, *24/3*, 431.

NOTE ADDED IN PROOF

Recently published case reports (*Brit. J. Anaesth.*, 1974, *46*, 324 and 952) suggest that some patients may be resistant to sodium nitroprusside and that the administration of a high dosage is required to obtain the desired degree of hypotension. It appears that such high dosages are harmful and that severe metabolic acidosis can occur, possibly as a result of high plasma cyanide levels. It would seem that alternative agents should be used in patients showing this type of response.

Anesthesia for microneurosurgery

FLOYD S. BRAUER

Department of Anesthesiology, Loma Linda University, Loma Linda, Calif., U.S.A.

The introduction of the operating microscope has opened new dimensions in neurosurgery. It is now possible to perform intracranial anastomoses of vessels of small caliber for treatment of vascular insufficiencies. Internal carotid artery blockage is treated surgically in our institution by an anastomosis of the superficial temporal artery (STA) to the middle cerebral artery (MCA) of the affected side. The anesthetic management of these operations is challenging because of unusual requirements of surgery and because of problems presented by these patients. The majority have a complete blockage of one internal carotid artery while a few have no flow in either internal carotid and the only blood supply to the brain flows via the vertebral arteries with possibly some collateral circulation through the external carotid. Preoperative cerebral blood flow studies on these patients show that frontal and parietal blood flows are 30–60% below normal values (Austin et al., 1972). Unless normal CO_2 levels are maintained at all times during surgery this blood flow will be reduced even further. Cerebral arterial vasoconstriction also increases the technical difficulties of this extremely delicate surgery.

Cerebral autoregulation cannot be depended upon to maintain flow in areas of ischemic brain or in the dissected and loose segments of superficial temporal artery. A steady adequate head of arterial pressure of about 100 Torr is necessary continually during surgery and in the postoperative period. A fall in blood pressure, even momentarily, can result in a stroke in these brittle patients. Hypertension may cause an increase in bleeding which without the microscope would probably not be detected but with 10–25 power magnification it can interfere with surgery. Any movement of the brain is also magnified and thus complicates and restricts surgical maneuvers. Even respiratory movements have to be minimized during the critical stages by manual ventilation at reduced volumes. Brain bounce from pulsatile blood flow is a constant annoyance to the surgeon. It is impossible to overcome this completely but it often can be minimized by reduced ventilation which reduces brain slack. Paradoxically an extremely slack brain has pronounced pulsatile movement.

ANESTHETIC MANAGEMENT

Candidates for superficial temporal to middle cerebral artery anastomosis are carefully evaluated. Cardiac, pulmonary, neurologic and psychiatric consultations are obtained and appropriate therapy instituted. Laboratory studies include radioisotope cerebral blood flow studies, brain scans, cerebral angiographies and electroencephalography. Surgery is not scheduled until the patient is in the best possible condition. A member of the anesthesia staff visits the patient several days before surgery and explains the anesthetic procedure in detail.

Premedication is light to avoid respiratory depression which may result in increased intracerebral pressure. Adequate sedation is achieved in stronger patients by intramuscular administration of one ml of Innovar and 0.4 mg of scopolamine one hr before operation.

Fragile patients may receive only 0.5–0.25 ml of Innovar and 0.2 mg of scopolamine. Innovar is used because droperidol, which it contains, reduces cerebral vascular resistance and may reverse the effects of cerebral insufficiency (Bloor, personal communication). In addition droperidol relieves apprehension and is an antiemetic. After arrival in the operating room an intravenous infusion of lactated Ringer's solution is started. Additional increments of Innovar may be given if necessary to relieve apprehension. These should be no more than 0.5 ml at one time as hypotension can ensue with 1 ml increments. Before anesthesia is induced an 18-gauge teflon catheter is placed percutaneously into the radial artery for continual blood pressure measurements using either a Statham strain gauge with a Grass polygraph or a 'Ram-tech' transducer and aneroid gauge. Tympanic and rectal temperature probes, EKG electrodes, esophageal stethoscope and urine catheter are introduced after induction of anesthesia.

Anesthesia is induced with small increments of sodium thiopental. Oxygen is administered by mask. The epiglottis, vocal cords and trachea are sprayed with 4% lidocaine. Intubation is performed with gallamine for relaxation, as it produces no rise in intracerebral pressure from muscular fasciculation and blood pressure levels are preserved during turning of the patient to the lateral position. A 'Lanz' low-pressure, large-volume cuff endotracheal tube is used to avoid the danger of tracheal pressure build-up from the diffusion expansion of nitrous oxide. Stanley and Kawamura (1973) and Wen-Hsein et al. (1973) have shown that cuff volumes in an endotracheal tube can more than double in over 4 hr of nitrous oxide anesthesia. After initial denitrogenation with high flows, anesthesia is maintained with nitrous oxide and oxygen 3:1 l/min and is supplemented during the 1st hr by small amounts of Innovar and during the remainder of the procedure by fentanyl given intravenously in fractional doses. Pancuronium 0.06–0.08 mg/kg is administered immediately prior to microdissection of the superficial temporal artery. The same dose of pancuronium is repeated just before the 2 vessels are anastomosed, usually about 4 hr after the 1st dose. Relaxants and narcotics are not used during the last 2 hr of surgery. The patient is allowed to move during closure.

Ventilation during the operation is by a volume-controlled respirator and is regulated by serial blood gas analysis at 30 min and later at 1 hr intervals to achieve a Pa_{CO_2} between 36 and 40 Torr and a Pa_{O_2} level in excess of 80 Torr. Large tidal volumes (about 850–950 ml) and slow respiratory rates (9–11/min) with addition of about 50 ml of dead space behind the endotracheal tube, result in normal Pa_{CO_2} levels and give better oxygenation than is obtained with more rapid rates with smaller tidal volumes.

Serial serum osmolalities are obtained and fluid replacement is based on these results and urine output. At the conclusion of surgery, atropine-neostigmine is given even if respiration appears adequate. In some of the early cases respiratory insufficiency developed in the recovery room when this was omitted.

RESULTS

In our first 50 cases no major anesthetic complications have been noted. There have been no intraoperative deaths or deaths in the first 5 postoperative days. Three late deaths have occurred, one with an intracranial serratius infection, one from preexisting cardiopulmonary complications, and one with a cerebral vascular accident. None of these were related to anesthesia. One patient developed a transient partial hemiparesis which persisted for 24 hr. This patient had a hypotensive episode for a short period early in the anesthetic course.

Almost all of these patients improved subjectively. Many returned to occupations they were unable to perform preoperatively because of cerebral insufficiency. Postoperative xenon cerebral blood flow studies show an average 25% improvement in the affected areas. Angiographic studies suggest that the anastomoses in 5 patients may not be patent.

There were two intraoperative anesthetic problems both involving endotracheal tubes. A leak developed around the cuff after approximately 4 hr of anesthesia. In one case an affixed cuff separated from the endotracheal tube and in the other the tube was pulled out somewhat during surgery so that the cuff was located between the vocal cords with resultant loss of seal. Both patients had to be reintubated while on their side, under the drapes, avoiding contamination of the surgical field.

DISCUSSION

Restriction of fluids before, during and immediately after intracerebral surgery is a common practice since dehydration is believed to result in a reduction of intracerebral volume. This may be permissible in cases of space-occupying lesions or where hypotensive anesthesia is used. But preoperative dehydration is not desirable in microneurosurgery because of the danger of hypotension. Fishman (1953) has pointed out that with surgical stress, dehydrated patients develop an antidiuresis from ADH output but that well-hydrated patients do not manifest this ADH outpouring. Without ADH interference, urine output becomes a more reliable guide to intravenous fluid administration. Our osmolality studies show that neurosurgical patients frequently arrive in the operating room slightly dehydrated, with osmolalities over 300 mOsm/l. If mannitol and steroids are then given while fluids are restricted, these patients may become severely dehydrated, with serum osmolality values as high as 335 mOsm/l. To prevent this, we administer up to one liter Ringer's lactate solution before surgery commences and then titrate intravenous fluids to urine output and serial osmolality studies. Ringer's lactate solution is preferable to dextrose in water in neurosurgery, because sugar is rapidly absorbed into cells, drawing water with it. This increases the brain mass (Gronert, 1973). With an intact blood/brain barrier, water in polyionic salt solutions does not pass into the brain cells as water is held in the extracellular fluid compartment by the Na ion.

Light anesthesia is maintained because immediate awakening after surgery is necessary. Neurological testing including motor function, vision and speech is performed immediately at the conclusion of surgery. Long-acting narcotics such as morphine and volatile anesthetic agents which are soluble in body tissues are therefore avoided. None of our patients have complained of awareness during surgery with flows of 3:1 N_2O/O_2.

Direct intraarterial blood pressure monitoring is usually not a routine practice in neurosurgery except for cerebral aneurysm. We consider it essential during STA-MCA anastomosis in order to diagnose and treat hypotension immediately. For this reason, arterial cannulation is performed prior to induction of anesthesia and before positioning of the patient. It is no more painful than venipuncture. Occasional transient hypotension responds to intravenous ephedrine 15 mg. Mean blood pressures over 110 mm Hg are lowered with an intravenous infusion of sodium nitroprusside (20 mg in 500 ml) via a minidrip device. Nitroprusside has the rapidity of action of trimetaphan camphorsulphonate but does not manifest the drawback of tachyphylaxis. Nitroprusside formerly was thought to have the disadvantage of rapid deterioration in solution; but when buffered to a pH of 4.2, it has an almost indefinite shelf life if stored at temperatures below 10° C and protected from light.

Blood loss is difficult to assess as copious amounts of irrigating solutions are used and the loss is directly into the surgical drapes. Our experience has been that total blood loss is usually considerably less than 20% of blood volume and that transfusion is not necessary with adequate volume replacement by fluids.

It is interesting to note the differences in temperatures as recorded at tympanic membrane, esophagus and the rectum. During intracranial surgery where irrigants are used the temperature recorded at the tympanic membrane may drop as much as 5° C below the esophageal temperature, whereas the rectal temperature reflects the room temperature and the amount of covers over the lower part of the body.

The use of halothane in neurosurgery has been a controversial subject since the article by Jennett et al. (1969) showing the rise in intracerebral pressure with halothane usage in patients with space-occupying lesions, and the subsequent editorial in the *British Journal of Anaesthesia* also in 1969. Inasmuch as intracranial volume is not increased in these patients, intracranial pressure elevations of a significant magnitude would not be expected and thus halothane would seem to have much to recommend it. Enflurane has also been suggested for neurosurgery. Halothane and enflurane were used in some of our early cases. We abandoned their use not because of intracranial pressure changes but because of hypotension during surgery and in the postoperative period. This hypotension often persisted many hours, required vasopressor infusions to keep the mean pressure at levels close to 100, and resulted in much anxiety the night after surgery. With adequate intraoperative fluid replacement and the discontinuance of the use of volatile anesthetic agents, no hypotension late in surgery or in the postoperative period has been noted. Our neurosurgeons feel that the abandonment of volatile anesthetic agents has been the most significant factor in reducing anesthetic and postanesthetic problems in these patients.

CONCLUSION

Microneurosurgery is an exciting and demanding new form of neurosurgery with its own anesthetic requirements which often differ from the anesthetic requirements of other intra-cranial surgery.

REFERENCES

Austin, G., Horn, N., Rouhe, S. and Hayward, W. (1972): *Europ. Neurol., 8*, 41.
Editorial (1960): *Brit. J. Anaesth., 41*, 277.
Fishman, R. A. (1953): *Arch. Neurol. (Chic.), 70*, 350.
Gronert, G. A. (1973): *American Society of Anesthesiologists Annual Refresher Course Lectures 107*.
Hayes, M. A., Brynes, W. P., Goldenberg, I. S., Greene, N. M. and Tuthill, E. (1959): *Surgery, 46*, 123.
Jennett, W. B., Barker, J., Fitch, W. and McDowall, G. D. (1969): *Lancet, 1*, 61.
Stanley, T. H. and Kawamura, R. (1973): In: *Abstracts of Scientific Papers, A.S.A. Annual Meeting, 1973*, p. 65.
Wen-Hsein, W. U., Il-Taik, Lim, Simpson, F. A. and Turndorf, H. (1973): *Crit. Care Med., 1–4*, 197.

Chapter XIX

Miscellaneous

Current paths of development in reanimatology

V. NEGOVSKY

Laboratory for Reanimation, U.S.S.R. Academy of Medical Science, Moscow, U.S.S.R.

When prehistoric man drew the outline of a mammoth on the walls of the Pindal cave in the Asturias (Spain), with a dark patch on the breast, the silhouette of a heart, he already had a vague idea that the life of man was connected with that organ. This is confirmed by the records of attempts to revive the hearts of people in ancient times. Many millenia had to pass, and a vast store of knowledge had to be accumulated, before a science of the law of dying and of resuscitation – reanimatology – developed in response to the direct demands of practice. In the Soviet Union it developed before anaesthesiology; in other countries within the framework of the latter, and in part, of other medical sciences. Today it is firmly established as the theoretical basis of reanimation and as an independent medical discipline with its own tasks and goals. Death and resuscitation have become the objects of study, such is one of the results of modern natural science. A view of clinical death as a reversible state distinguishable from both life and death has developed. There has also evolved, though not fully, an idea of the physiological mechanisms of the sequence of the decline and restoration of life; and an idea of postreanimation sickness, and of a new class of biological phenomena standing at the boundary between life and death, has developed.

In this paper only a fraction of the subject is considered; the most pressing problems and conclusions arising from study of cessation and restoration of the cardiovascular system, respiration, metabolism, and the central nervous system are discussed.

Detailed study of the pathophysiological patterns of the dying and resuscitation of the heart, and in particular of the dynamics of bioelectric activity, has enabled us to establish the basis for exact diagnosis and choice of optimum therapeutic action.

During clinical death alternate periods of sinus activity with periods of conduction block are observed for several minutes, with migration of the starting point of automaticity to different sectors of the conducting system of the heart. At the same time transmission of excitation from the conducting system to the myocardium ceases. During resuscitation the conducting system function is restored first, and then the transmission of excitation to the myocardium. This is seen in restoration of the activity of the sino-atrial node and of the specific shape of the ventricular complex.

During clinical death, and also during the first minutes after recommencement of myocardial contraction as a result of reanimatory procedures, the mechanisms of central regulation of the heart are depressed. Their restoration coincides, apparently, with the restoration of brain-stem function. This can be assessed, in particular, from the appearance of typical respiratory arrhythmia. There is plenty of experimental and clinical evidence which suggests that recommencement of central regulatory influences promotes stabilization of all haemodynamics.

One form of disturbance of cardiac contractile activity, fibrillation, is of special interest because the possibility of eliminating it determines, to a considerable extent, the outcome of reanimation. It has been established in principle that excitation may be synchronized by a strong electric stimulus; and on that basis the optimum duration of action has been determined as close to the 'useful' stimulation time for the heart. The electric impulse can be safe and extremely effective; electrical defibrillation can be performed without opening up the thorax. It has been demonstrated that the damaging effect of repeated defibrillation depends on the absolute strength of direct current, and the curative effect on the total amplitude of both half-waves of the oscillatory discharge. The results obtained have provided a basis for designing a defibrillator that generates a bipolar pulse, thus the threshold of defibrillation is lowered without loss of effectiveness. Some interest has been shown in recent years in the experimental observation that transconductance of the trailing edge of the pulse has a decisive influence on the process of defibrillation. It has been found that a pulse with a steep trailing edge of the first half-wave (40 A/msec) is more effective. Thus therapeutic effect must be assessed in relation to the pulse shape, duration and amplitude of the electric stimulus.

The restoration and maintenance of effective cardiac activity is one of the most important tasks of reanimation. After the recommencement of regular heart activity and an adequate level of arterial pressure, significant disturbances of circulation are observed which are important in the development of postreanimation sickness and govern the development of irreversible changes in the organs and tissues.

The state of the circulation in the early postreanimation period is conditioned by the interaction of pathological and compensatory processes. One compensatory reaction is the extremely strong beating of the heart. Another consists in the centralization of circulation and the increase of cerebral and coronary blood flow. Protracted compensation which sustains vital organs becomes a harmful factor aggravating the disturbances of regional blood flow and of microcirculation. Depression of compensatory mechanisms develops and the cardiac output is lowered by 40–50%, which may be due to reduction in myocardial contractility or as a result of disturbances in the peripheral circulation. The reduction of cardiac output is most marked when the outcome of resuscitation is unfavourable; but it is also noted when the restoration of vital functions is uncomplicated. The nature of the phenomenon needs detailed study, since clarification of the triggering mechanisms in the development of circulatory disturbances would enable the most rational treatment for the postreanimation period to be developed.

RESPIRATION

During the process of death the activity of the inspiratory and expiratory muscles increases, and the act of breathing involves accessory muscles. In the agonal period the expiratory muscles contract simultaneously with the inspiratory and accessory muscles during inhalation in consequence of disruption of the reciprocal relation between the inspiratory and expiratory centres. As a result the minute volume of respiration in this period, according to various authors, is between 40 and 15% of the initial volume. The cause of agonal breathing is hypoxia so that central control of the respiratory centre in the medulla oblongata is lost and hypoxaemic damage occurs in the brain stem.

Early restoration of spontaneous breathing is not only important for gas exchange, but is also vital because the focus of excitation in the region of the respiratory centre encourages arousal of other parts of the medulla. The inspiratory centre begins to function first. The expiratory centre recovers later since it is more sensitive to hypoxia. The respiratory centre reacts during the agonal phase and in the initial stage of the postreanimation period, to afferent impulses from receptors in the lungs and upper respiratory passages. The influence of the vagus nerve is restored several minutes after the activity of the inspiratory centre develops and affects the frequency of breathing, and accelerates the recovery of active expiration.

In the early restorative period independent breathing does not, as a rule, ensure adequate ventilation of the lungs. Increase in the electrical activity of the respiratory muscles, even with satisfactory blood-gas levels, is often a sign of respiratory insufficiency, since lung ventilation is being achieved because of strong stimulation from the respiratory centre. Artificial ventilation of the lungs should be continued until natural ventilation is fully restored, electrical activity in the accessory respiratory muscles disappears, haemodynamics are stabilized, and the most marked disturbances of the microcirculation and homeostasis are eliminated. Another indication for continued artificial ventilation is spontaneous hyperventilation (a minute volume greater than 170%), in spite of adequate arterial oxygen tensions and hypocapnia.

Difficulties often arise during adaptation of the patient to the respirator. The cause of out-of-phase breathing with the ventilator is inadequate minute volume ventilation.

It is not wise to abolish spontaneous ventilation if the cause of breathing out-of-phase has not been eliminated, that is hypoventilation, airway obstruction, pain, etc. Artificial ventilation during the acute period of respiratory insufficiency with moderate hyperventilation with an alveolar carbon dioxide partial pressure between 28 and 32 mm Hg should be continued. It seems that, when the circulation is disturbed, gaseous alkalosis in the arterial blood promotes the maintenance of normal acid-alkali balance in the tissues. Patients tolerate moderate hypocapnia better than normocapnia.

In patients with marked shunting in the lungs and significant increase in the alveolo-arterial oxygen difference, ventilation with 100% oxygen may not eliminate hypoxaemia. One way to overcome this dangerous situation is to ventilate the lungs artificially with constant positive pressure, which may cause a significant increase in oxygenation of the arterial blood and thus of the peripheral tissues. Hypoxia not amenable to ventilation with 100% oxygen with constant positive pressure is an indication for extracorporeal oxygenators.

METABOLISM

During the period of dying (from loss of blood, asphyxia, etc.) the brain tissues utilize carbohydrates by glycolysis: the levels of glucose, ATP, and creatine phosphate fall, and the levels of ADP, AMP, Pi, and lactic acid increase. Far-reaching changes in carbohydrate-phosphorus metabolism lead to disturbances in the metabolism of protein and nitrogen-containing compounds. The whole organism suffers acute oxygen lack, and unoxidized metabolites accumulate in the blood.

When the circulation is re-established the unoxidized metabolites, in particular the end product of glycolysis, lactic acid, begin to pass into the blood from the tissues. Uncompensated metabolic acidosis is observed in the blood. The maximum level of lactate, irrespective of the cause of the circulatory arrest, and of the duration of clinical death, rises to 70 or 80 mg/100 ml, and the lactate/pyruvate ratio increases sharply. During the period of clinical death the reserves of the substratum (glucose and glycogen) are apparently exhausted and glycolysis becomes attenuated. The maximum lactate value and L/P ratio therefore cannot serve as a criterion of the seriousness of the condition after clinical death, as it can in other states of shock of various aetiologies (Weil and Afif, 1970; and others).

When clinical death develops following prior hypotension (arterial pressure 40 mm Hg) the lactate value determined at the end of the second hour of hypotension may be used as an index of the severity of an animal's condition, and even as an index of non-reversibility.

All animals in which the lactate level is higher than 50 mg/100 ml die. Compensation of metabolic acidosis is observed within 90 min–2 hr of the postreanimation period. The compensated metabolic acidosis, combined with a significant loss of carbon dioxide, lasts for 6 hr; and disturbances of metabolism can still be observed for several days after resuscitation. At the end of the first hour of the postreanimation period the activity of alkaline phosphatase and lactate dehydrogenase begins to increase and remains at a raised level for 9 hr. The change in the activity of acid phosphatase is less obvious.

Oxidizing processes are not restored immediately in the brain; glycolysis continues for 20 or 30 min after the circulation is re-established, and in some areas of the brain possibly for even longer. The lactate level of the cerebrospinal fluid, which reaches 50 or 60 mg/100 ml in the fifth to eighth min after resuscitation, remains elevated for 6–9 hr.

The lysosome hydrolase of the grey matter becomes normal an hour after resuscitation. By the end of the first day secondary activation of acid phosphatase is noted in the mitochondrial fraction of the grey matter.

Thus the terminal state leads to marked disturbances of metabolic processes, which are unfavourable for the restoration of normal function.

In the overwhelming majority of clinical observations there is not complete cessation of the circulation. Therefore, despite the development of deep states of shock, the changes in acid-base balance are somewhat different from those of the experiments.

Patients with trauma, massive loss of blood, and with the phenomena of shock, develop progressive metabolic acidosis for the first 6–8 hr of treatment. Respiratory alkalosis, caused by hyperventilation, is also often present. By the end of the first day of active treatment and the beginning of the second, there is no base deficit, and the lactate and pyruvate levels are lowered. In the next 3–5 days the acid-base balance is within the normal limits, or tends to metabolic alkalosis, while the total organic acids are raised and the concentration of lactate and pyruvate is within or below the normal limits. The lactate/pyruvate ratio remains elevated for the whole period of observation.

In most patients breathing spontaneously arterial hypoxaemia is observed after 5 days, despite the absence of signs of respiratory insufficiency and stable arterial pressure. The reduction of oxygen reserves in the blood is apparently due to several mechanisms which include reduced haemoglobin concentration and disturbance of the oxygenation of the blood in the lungs as a result of the development of a 'lung-shock' syndrome.

Apart from the role of oxygen deficiency in the development of metabolic shifts in the postreanimation period, hypovolaemia and dehydration are involved, despite active transfusion therapy. Hypovolaemia, in particular when caused by disturbances of peripheral circulation, aggravates the inadequate tissue perfusion. In addition, it encourages increased liberation of potassium and retention of sodium by the kidneys. Accumulation of sodium leads to metabolic alkalosis, and hypopotassaemia results in the accumulation of hydrogen ions in the tissues; metabolic alkalosis in the blood is combined with intracellular metabolic acidosis.

In patients with massive blood loss and trauma, mixed hypoxia (anaemic, hypoxic, and circulatory) may persist for a long time. How serious it becomes depends on the seriousness of the patient's condition and the early therapy. Prophylaxis and treatment of hypoxia are two other problems facing present-day reanimatology. In patients with protracted arterial hypoxaemia ($Pa_{O_2} < 70$ mm Hg) the mortality is 4-times higher than in patients with analogous pathology but without arterial hypoxaemia.

Each derangement of metabolism should not be treated separately without removing the cause. Artificial ventilation of the lungs, rapid replacement of blood loss and oxygen lack, and the administration of drugs to improve the rheological properties of the blood, not only eliminate the existing shifts but also remove the preconditions for their subsequent development.

CENTRAL NERVOUS SYSTEM

Disturbances of the central nervous system have a special place in the clinical picture of postreanimation sickness ('the sickness of the resuscitated'), and it is this that determines whether or not the person will be a social asset, and consequently determines the expediency of reanimation. This is an important part of reanimatology, and can be called the neurology of the posthypoxic state, or the neurology of the terminal state. The need to develop this trend in reanimatology in order to treat postreanimation sickness can hardly be over-estimated.

It has been established that, with sudden cessation of the circulation, cerebral oedema greatly complicates posthypoxic restoration at first, but its development is not fatal. The literature indicates that the importance of cerebral oedema in cerebral pathology increases sharply after protracted hypercapnic hypoxia or with hypoxia complicated by venous stasis. Consequently, only direct indications justify dehydration therapy in the early post-reanimation period.

Clarification of the relative significance of intracerebral and extracerebral pathogenic factors in the development of irreversible changes in the brain after cessation of the circulation is an urgent problem. Comparison of the 2 models of stoppage (fibrillation of the heart and compressive ischaemia of the brain) has shown that the brain tolerates ischaemia twice as long in the second model. If the damage to the brain due to fibrillation is taken as 100%, there is a suggestion that the irreversible damage caused by direct damage to the brain is only 50%. Specially designed experiments have shown that around 25% of the irreversible changes in the brain following fibrillation depend on the blood retained in the brain and 25% result from hypoxic pathology of vital organs.

In spite of the extensive compensatory and adaptive mechanisms of the central nervous system secondary deterioration of the neurological state often develops 3–7 days after resuscitation. The reasons for this have not yet been established – it is possibly linked with the final death of some of the previously damaged neurons which occurs in this period.

Many authors, including the workers of our laboratory, report that an occasional prediction of a fatal outcome following resuscitation is possible in cases of temporary restoration of CNS function. The basis for such a prognosis is the duration, degree and character of the coma, the EEG, the presence or absence of convulsions, and other features of the neurological state.

The appearance on the EEG of continuous electrical activity and normal rhythm of the cortex in the first 20–40 min after resuscitation is usually observed in patients with a short period of clinical death; it correlates with full, stable restoration of CNS function.

Delay in the restoration of normal EEG rhythms, combined with separate clinical signs of disturbed higher nervous activity is an unfavourable sign. When delayed restoration of cortical function occurs persistent psychic defects may follow.

Unfortunately, it is not always possible to obtain early (in the first 15–30 min after resuscitation) any very valuable EEG information. Therefore study of the prognostic value of the various clinical neurological symptoms is necessary. A most unfavourable sign is generalized myoclonia on a background of a flat EEG, and in particular, myoclonia of the eyelids and eyes, which indicates serious brain damage. In addition to these signs in adult patients in a deep, usually atonic coma, horizontal movements of the eyeball (myoclonia of the eyes) have been observed, which outwardly resemble horizontal nystagmus. 42.1% of the total had fatal cases of myoclonia of the eyeball. This phenomenon has been observed in 3 patients who survived, but with profound psychic defects. Not a single patient with fully restored cortical function displayed even momentary myoclonia of the eyeballs.

Another bad prognostic sign is the development of spinal automatism in patients in a state of atonic coma: myoclonia of the orbital muscles and of the muscles of the upper shoulder girdle, and a myotonic reaction of separate groups of muscles arising in response to the stimulation of tendon reflexes and of the corneal reflex. This automatism, like the myoclonia of the eyeballs, has not been observed in patients with restoration of brain function.

CONCLUSIONS

At the beginning of the fourteenth century, one of the outstanding doctors of the Middle Ages, Arnoldo de Villanuova, who was born in the neighbourhood of Valencia, generalizing the work of the Salerno School in his famous Regimen sanitatis Salernitum or Medicina Salernitana, wrote: 'Contro forza di morte, non c'e medicina negli orti' (against the forces of death there is no medicine in the garden). He could not then foresee the whole progressive development of medical science, and could not know that 6 centuries would pass and as a result of the development of medicine there would be born a science of the resuscitation. Thousands of people who die prematurely can be given a second life. One of the holy of holies of nature, one of her most treasured secrets, has been discovered; and researchers into the problems of reanimatology experience great satisfaction from knowing that they are at the sources of this profoundly humane, infinitely complicated, and noble mystery of the struggle for the life of the dying man.

Response of myotonic patients to muscle relaxants and general anesthesia

BRANISLAV M. DRAGISIC

St. James Hospital, Chicago Heights, Ill., U.S.A.

Dystrophia myotonica is a hereditodegenerative disease characterized by muscle wasting, especially those of the face and neck, fatigue, cataracts, early baldness, testicular atrophy and inability to relax the muscle after a contraction (myotonia). The myotonia may precede the muscle wasting by many years or may occur independently. Occasionally the anesthesiologist may be privileged to diagnose dystrophia myotonica when the patient 'opens and closes' his hand before insertion of the needle.

SURGICAL AND ANESTHESIA RISK

Patients with dystrophia myotonica are sometimes presented for anesthesia particularly because of premature cataracts, or other surgical disease.

The principal precautions can be considered under 6 headings:

Pulmonary

Myotonia of the respiratory muscles commonly occurs in dystrophia myotonica. This may lead to a large reduction in the vital capacity and maximum breathing capacity. It has been stated that a patient with dystrophia myotonica is particularly susceptible to thiopentone, possibly due to a specific peripheral action of the drug, but further studies have not substantiated this. It is, however, true that a patient suffering from dystrophia myotonica is sensitive to thiopentone – 100 mg may cause apnea for 20 min or more. The effect is probably a central one and common to all respiratory depressant drugs. Weakness of the muscles of respiration may lead to respiratory inadequacy when depressant drugs are given, or when the work of breathing is increased. A period of artificial respiration may be necessary postoperatively, but myotonia of the respiratory muscles may make ventilation extremely difficult.

Cardiovascular

Diminished pulse-rate, increase of the auriculoventricular interval up to A-V block necessitates careful cardiac monitoring. It is interesting that adrenaline has a paradoxical effect on the heart (causes bradycardia).

Neuromuscular

The abnormality in dystrophia myotonica is believed to be an increase in sensitivity of the muscle fibre. The reaction to muscle relaxants is variable because the abnormality is in the muscle itself. Thiopentone does not influence neuromuscular transmission. Depolarizing drugs (succinylcholine) may increase the degree of myotonia whereas d-tubocurarine will block neuromuscular transmission without necessarily overcoming myotonia. Some authors described a case in which the myotonic episodes were directly attributable to the action of suxamethonium.

Pharmacology

Quinine hydrochloride prolongs refractory period of the muscle fibre after contraction. The quinine effect can be accentuated by calcium gluconate. Special precautions should be taken in the administration of neostigmine which may increase the degree of myotonia. Atropine sulfate has unpredictable results, usually little effect, but there are some reports that atropine causes an excessive reaction. Moreover non-depolarizing muscle relaxants are used, special precautions should be taken at the end of surgical procedure, to avoid the use of atropine and neostigmine. Procaine amide, quinine and Dilantin are very useful drugs in treating dystrophia myotonica.

Environment

It has been shown that cold increases the degree of myotonia and warm surroundings decrease the degree of myotonia; this clearly indicates the need for warmer operating room by several degrees.

Emotional

Preoperative rounds are of utmost importance to allay anxiety which reduces the degree of myotonia. The patient should be familiarized with forthcoming surgery and anesthesia, and everything should be explained. Tranquilizers may be used to reduce tension, but sedatives, narcotics, barbiturates or any central nervous system depressants should probably be avoided.

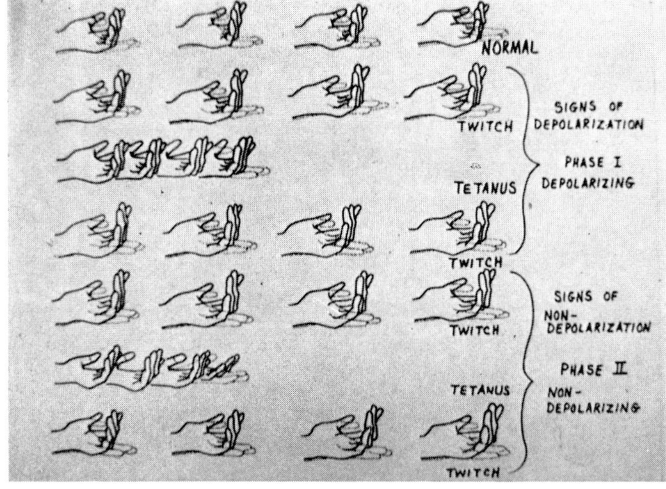

Fig. 1.   *Normal, 'depolarizing' and 'non-depolarizing' type of reaction to a nerve stimulus.*

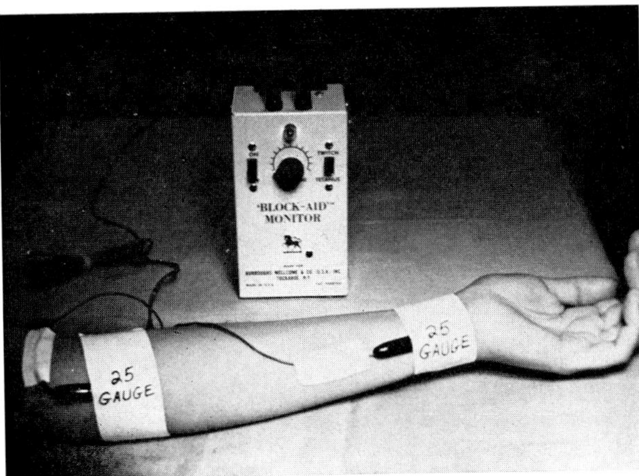

Fig. 2. *Nerve stimulator in place.*

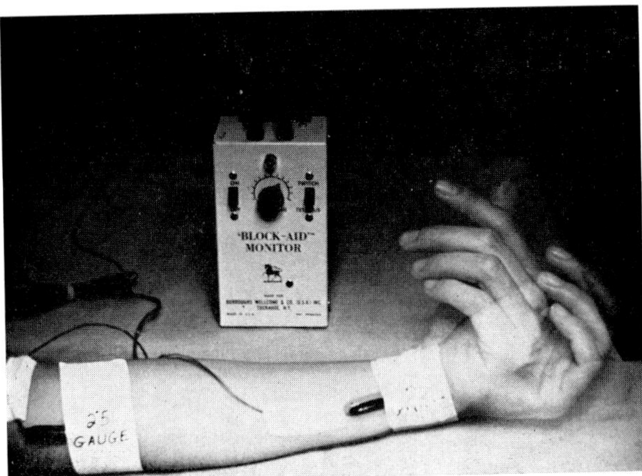

Fig. 3. *Twitch stimulus applied. Movement of the fingers is much more pronounced than in 'normal' reaction.*

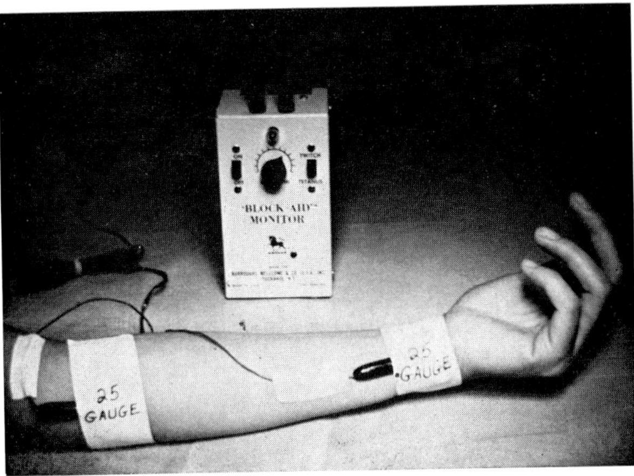

Fig. 4. *Position of the fingers after 5 sec; hand is not yet fully relaxed.*

CONDUCTION OF ANESTHESIA

Induction of anesthesia may be achieved very easily with a mask (halothane $+ N_2O + O_2$ technique) or with an intravenous technique using ketamine HCl as an induction agent, followed by halothane (tachycardia, commonly encountered by intravenous administration of ketamine HCl, has a desirable effect, because myotonic patients have a slow cardiac rate).

Careful monitoring of blood pressure, pulse, nerve stimulator, tidal volume and EKG are minimal requirements. The degree of myotonia is of special interest for anesthesiologists and can be monitored with a nerve stimulator.

MONITORING OF MUSCLE RELAXANT ACTION

The unmedicated response to a nerve stimulator and the response following 'depolarizing' and 'non-depolarizing' is shown in Figure 1. With myotonic patients relaxation time is strikingly slow. In the 'normal' patient the relaxation time following twitch stimuli is 0.1–0.5 sec. Relaxation time following tetanus stimuli in 'normal' patient is 0.4–1.5 sec. In the 'mytonic' patient the relaxation time following twitch stimuli is from 5–10 sec, and relaxation time following tetanus stimuli in 'myotonic' patient is up to 30 sec.

Figure 2 shows a patient's hand with the nerve stimulator in place. The stimulus is applied in Figure 3. Notice that movement of the fingers is much more pronounced than in 'normal' patients. After 5 sec the hand is not yet fully relaxed (Fig. 4). Notice wasting of the muscles of the hand (this is the hand of a 72 kg woman).

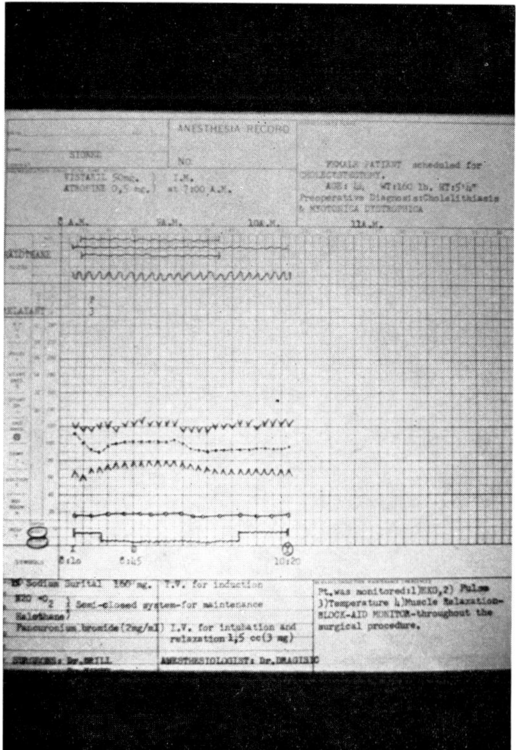

Fig. 5.   *An anesthesia record showing the uneventful course of anesthesia in a 'myotonic' patient.*

Other techniques of anesthesia are: regional, which is well-tolerated; local, with the precaution of non-use of any narcotic or CNS depressant, preoperatively or postoperatively. If general anesthesia is considered, halothane remains the anesthetic of choice.

The uncomplicated and uneventful course of anesthesia in severe dystrophia myotonica patient with halothane as major agent is shown in Figure 5. If muscle relaxants are being used, non-depolarizing agents are recommended like d-tubocurarine or pancuronium bromide. Depolarizing agents like succinylcholine or decamethonium should not be used under any circumstances.

General anaesthesia based on relaxants.
I. Personal technique

N. MIRCEA AND M. BALABAN

Department of Anaesthesia-Intensive Therapy, and
Department of Surgery, 'Victor Babeş' Hospital, Bucharest, Rumania

Although the anaesthetist has at his disposal a fairly small number of drugs, the technique of combined anaesthesia permits an impressive number of anaesthetic variants. Using only one of each class of the current drugs, the number of possible combinations reaches the striking figure of 3×10^4.

These combinations may be reduced to a single basic scheme of general anaesthesia (Fig. 1).

PREANAESTHESIA	INDUCTION		MAINTENANCE	REVERSAL BLOCK AND RECOVERY
	HYPNOTIC STARTER	INTUBATION		
ATROPINE PETHIDINE PROMETHAZINE DIAZEPAM THALAMONAL HYDROXYZINE	THIOPENTONE (PENTOTHAL) METHOHEXITONE DIAZEPAM DROPERIDOL FENTANYL	SUXAME-THONIUM	PIVOT OF INHALATION AGENTS HALOTHANE ETHER DIETHYL METHOXYFLURANE FLUROXENE NEUROMUSCULAR BLOCK GALLAMINE PIVOT OF INTRA-(FLAXEDIL) VENOUS AGENTS PANCURONIUM (BROMIDE) PETHIDINE d-TUBOCURARINE MORPHINE TOXIFERINE FENTANYL	ANTICHOLINESTERASE DRUGS ATROPINE NEOSTIGMINE NARCOTIC ANTAGONISTS TENSILON NIVALIN NALORPHINE
	O X Y G E N			
		NITROUS OXIDE		
	CONTROLLED RESPIRATION			

Fig. 1. *Basic scheme in the technique of combined general anaesthesia.*

The neuromuscular blocking drugs are the basic pharmacological elements in the technique called 'general anaesthesia on a pivot of relaxants'. The entire anaesthesia is based upon a competetive relaxant, used in a single very large dose, and the absence of premedication.

MATERIAL AND METHOD

1196 general anaesthetics based on relaxants were given. Preanaesthesia was completely excluded in our practice. Induction starts with rapid intravenous administration of a non-depolarising relaxant, followed by the rapid injection of a hypnotic.

The following basic relaxants were used: pancuronium (Pavulon) 0.15–0.35 mg/kg with a total maximum dose of 26 mg over 6 hr; gallamine (Flaxedil) 2.8–8.8 mg/kg with a maximum total dose of 700 mg; tubocurarine 1.3–2.8 mg/kg with a total maximum dose of 200 mg.

The endotracheal tube is passed after an interval of 1–4 min. During maintenance of the tube, the patient is hyperventilated with N_2O/O_2 manually or mechanically.

The following analgesics were used intravenously immediately after intubation in a single dose: pethidine 100 mg ± 100 mg (maximum 2.84 mg/kg); fentanyl 0.1–0.5 mg ± 25 mg (0.001–0.010 mg/kg).

Reversal of the neuromuscular block is essential – 1 mg atropine and 5 mg neostigmine is given. When this is not effective, a second antagonist is given (30 mg neostigmine).

Our technique is schematically represented in Figure 2.

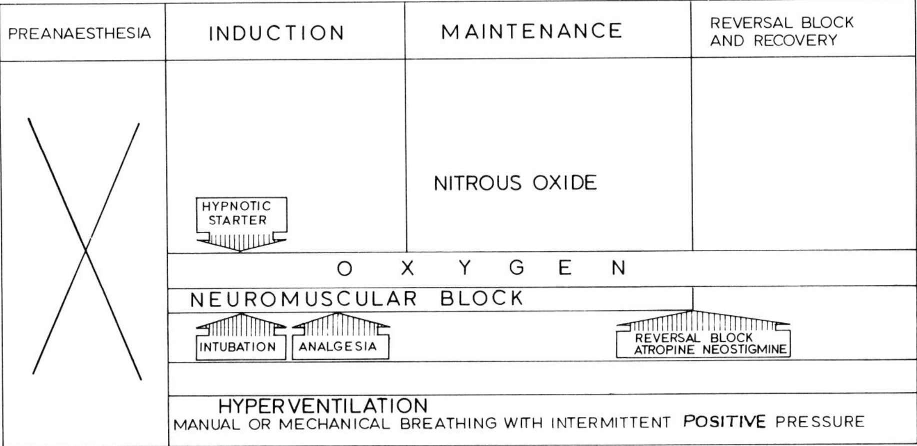

Fig. 2.   *Basic scheme in the technique of combined general anaesthesia on a pivot of muscle relaxants.*

	CLINICAL PARAMETER	PANCURONI-UM (PAVULOM)	GALLAMINE	d-TUBOCURARINE
1	CARDIOVASCULAR EFFECTS OF INITIAL DOSE	SYSTOLIC PRESSURE 0% — PULSE RATE 25% ↑	SYSTOLIC PRESSURE 20% ↑ — PULSE RATE 100% ↑	SYSTOLIC PRESSURE 36% ↓ — PULSE RATE 16% ↑
2	INTUBATION CONDITIONS	AVERAGE TIME TO INTUBATION 2′; EASY 95%; DIFFICULT 4%; IMPOSSIBLE 1%	AVERAGE TIME TO INTUBATION 4′; EASY 80%; DIFFICULT 20%; IMPOSSIBLE O	AVERAGE TIME TO INTUBATION 5′; EASY 65%; DIFFICULT 35%; IMPOSSIBLE O
3	HISTAMINE RELEASE (ERYTHEMA)	O	O	25%
4	CARDIOVASCULAR EFFECTS DURING ANAESTHESIA	SYSTOLIC PRESSURE O — PULSE RATE 15% ↑	SYSTOLIC PRESSURE 10-20 ↑ — PULSE RATE 100%	SYSTOLIC PRESSURE 20-30 ↓ — PULSE RATE 10% ↑
5	DOSAGE AND DURATION OF ACTION	CLASSICAL DOSE 0,1 mg/kg; TOTAL MAXIMAL DOSE 26 mg (0,35 mg/kg body weight)	CLASSICAL DOSE 2 mg/kg; TOTAL MAXIMAL DOSE 700 mg (10 mg/kg body weight)	CLASSICAL DOSE 0,5 mg/kg; TOTAL MAXIMAL DOSE 200 mg (2,8 mg/kg body weight)
6	REVERSAL BLOCK AND RECOVERY	GOOD	GOOD	GOOD

Fig. 3.   *Comparative clinical qualities of the relaxants used.*

Throughout the duration of anaesthesia a series of clinical parameters were followed either directly or by electronic monitoring (Fig. 3).

RESULTS

In this series there were no accidents, complications or deaths attributable to the anaesthetic technique.

Arousal, with recovery of muscle force, occurred at variable intervals ranging from immediate, sudden arousal after the administration of one antagonist (80% of the cases) to 30 min after the antagonist.

The immediate postoperative period was not associated with ventilatory insufficiency when a sufficient antagonist had been given.

The postoperative recovery was such that, a few hours after anaesthesia the patient could get up, pass urine spontaneously and in the same afternoon blood-gas was normal again (in more than 50% of the patients), provided that a blood volume was maintained with noncolloidal isotonic solutions.

CONCLUSIONS

General anaesthesia on pivot of relaxants is a simple technique and it provides marked haemodynamic stability throughout the duration of anaesthesia. Deep muscular relaxation during the anaesthesia allows easy ventilation with good oxygenation. Although used in a wide range of pathology, full satisfaction was only obtained in the aged patient, the patient with a high anaesthetic-surgical risk, in surgery of the chest, in endoscopies and arteriographies.

General anaesthesia based on relaxants. II. Justification

N. MIRCEA and M. BALABAN

Department of Anaesthesia-Intensive Therapy, and
Department of Surgery, 'Victor Babeş' Hospital, Bucharest, Rumania

The technique of anaesthesia based on relaxants, described in part I, is supported by current knowledge of physiology and pharmacology.

Premedication, including atropine is no longer justified, since it is not necessary to control the untoward effects of the drugs used in induction and maintenance.

Induction is the most important moment for the course of the entire anaesthesia. Relaxation and hypnosis must occur within as short a period as possible in order to avoid any momentary hypoxaemia. Rapid injection of the hypnotic immediately after tubocurarine prevents the painful sensation of relaxation and induces deep hypnosis which allows the operation to start immediately after intubation.

Muscular relaxation. Among modern anaesthetics, the neuromuscular blocking drugs produce, from the metabolic point of view, the mildest side-effects. Experimental use in doses several thousand times the apnea-inducing dose was not followed by major side-effects. The only harmful effects are those linked to ventilatory insufficiency and the resultant hypoxia, which are controlled by intubation and hyperventilation with O_2.

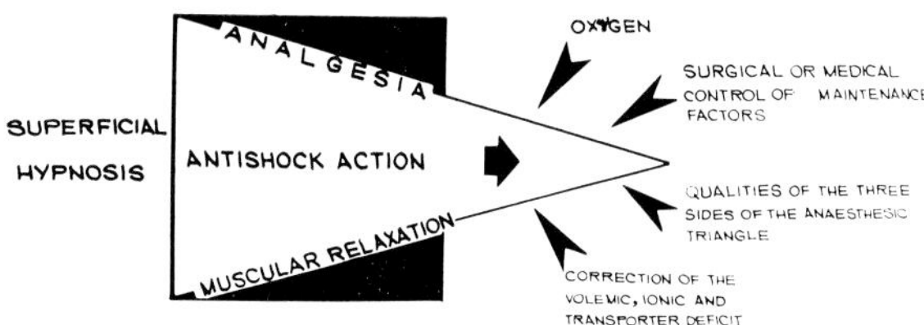

Fig. 1. *Convergence of antishock factors in general anaesthesia.*

The use of competitive neuromuscular blocking drugs has to be assessed statistically, since a progressive block is produced which is dose-dependent (that is, the ratio of acetylcholine to the blocking substance at the level of the receptors) and the mass ratio of the blocking drug to acetylcholine, which accounts for the different response to these drugs in the young and the old patient.

The dose of neuromuscular blocking drugs should be optimal from the beginning and administered in a single injection, since any reinjection is difficult, and the dose of antagonist is then uncertain.

Analgesia is obtained with our technique by combining the analgesic effects of N_2O with an intravenous analgesic, and the cerebral circulatory alterations induced by hyperventilation.

The amnesic effect of hyperventilation is due to its action at the level of the ascending reticular-activating system. Perception may probably be achieved at a lower neuronal level than that necessary for conserving the engram (permanent effect on new tissue) or subsequent ecphoria (active revival of an engram).

Hypnosis. With this technique sleep is superficial throughout maintenance and is stable, apart from the period of induction and immediately after loss of consciousness and amnesia. It is the result of the hypnotic side-effects of the analgesics used, of the residual effects of the induction and of hyperventilation.

Shock control. Although in modern combined anaesthesia 4 different aspects are differentiated (hypnosis, analgesia, muscular relaxation, shock control), it should be emphasized that there is no drug with a direct antishock action. The so-called specific antishock action, as considered in this technique, does not in fact exist. Shock control can be obtained by the complex number of measures taken over a long pre-, intra- and postoperative period.

In our opinion the antishock effect is the result of a sum of factors that combine to diminish and finally to cause failure of the autonomic-endocrine-metabolic-haemodynamic reaction, which occurs in response to trauma.

These factors are: (1) correct oxygenation of the patient under anaesthesia by efficient ventilation in the presence of muscular relaxation and endotracheal intubation; (2) surgical control of the factors maintaining shock (haemorrhage, perforation, septic focus); (3) correction of the blood volume and electrolytes; (4) the quality of the 3 aspects of anaesthesia.

The pharmacology of the substances used in anaesthesia plays a minor role for a brief period in minimizing shock during anaesthesia and surgery. This depends more on the efficiency and gentleness of ventilation, the amount and quality of the infusions and the hands of the surgeon who performs the operation quickly and gently.

Maintenance in this technique is simple, being characterized by haemodynamic stability and not requiring regular injection of drugs.

The colour of the blood in the wound is the most valuable sign for the correct management of anaesthesia, expressing synthetically O_2 partial pressure, the transporter capacity of the blood and haemodynamic parameters.

Reversal of the neuromuscular block, arousal and removal of the tube is the most difficult stage, at which the anaesthesia must be present. In this phase the patient is still under the residual action of relaxants whose specific antidote is anticholinesterase. Postoperative ventilatory insufficiency, a potential factor of morbidity and mortality in this technique, is avoided by the administration of equivalent amounts of an antagonist combined with hyperventilation up to recovery of efficient, spontaneous ventilation and muscular power.

CONCLUSIONS

Under present conditions, the use of large doses of neuromuscular blocking drugs appears less toxic and harmful than any other category of drugs. In recovery the patient is not under the cumulative influence of several drugs which have to be evaluated separately, but only under the residual action of neuromuscular blocking drugs which have a specific antagonist.

A. G. L. BURM, J. SPIERDIJK and V. REIJGER

Department of Anaesthesia, University Hospital Leiden, Leiden, The Netherlands

Several statistical studies into the health of anaesthetists and members of the nursing staff, as well as studies on the incidence of abortions in female anaesthetists and nurses who work in the operating room, have revealed a number of complaints which can be considered specific to anaesthesia (Askrog and Harvald, 1970; Bruce et al., 1968; Cohen et al., 1971; Corbett et al., 1973; Vaisman, 1967). Various authors have already pointed out that the observed complaints must be caused by some facet of the working conditions, specifically air pollution in the operating rooms due to narcotic gases and vapours. This pollution is a result of the fact that the gases which are exhaled by the patient are released into the room. In this way the members of the operating team are chronically exposed to these anaesthetics during their work in the operating room.

Although it is not justifiable to indicate pollution of the air as the only and direct cause, it is clear that an investigation of the influence of narcotic gases on the personnel is necessary. Studies in this field are being carried out in various countries at present. Key questions are: (1) How high are the concentrations of the narcotic gases in the operating rooms and how much of this is assimilated by personnel? (2) What is the effect of the narcotic gases on the personnel? (3) Should measures be taken to prevent or limit the pollution and if so, what methods are the most suitable?

The concentrations of narcotic gases in an operating room are in part dependent on the amount of gas released, the volume of the room and the ventilation of the room. If there is complete mixing of the narcotic gases with the air in the room and if the input of gases is constant, then the concentrations in the room can be calculated at any given time using the following formula:

$$c = \frac{60{,}000\ q}{a\ I}(1 - e^{-at}) \tag{1}$$

where,
c = concentration of the narcotic gas in ppm; q = input of the narcotic gas in l/min; a = ventilation rate in the room in hr^{-1}; I = volume of the room in m^3; e = base of natural logarithms ≈ 2.72; t = time in hr.

Mixing in the operating room is never complete so that the concentrations are dependent upon the location in the room. The differences in concentration are determined by the degree of mixing which in turn is dependent upon the air flow pattern. The concentrations cannot be calculated with sufficient accuracy and must be determined by measurement.

The concentrations of several anaesthetics, mainly halothane and nitrous oxide, have already been measured by different investigators. The concentrations reported in the literature vary for halothane from several ppm to more than 1000 ppm and for nitrous oxide from about 100 ppm to about 1% (Askrog and Petersen, 1970; Frey et al., 1973; Hallén et al.,

1970; Linde and Bruce, 1969; Schulze et al., 1969; Usubiaga et al., 1972; Whitcher et al., 1971). Halothane and nitrous oxide concentrations have been measured in two operating rooms at 3 different points, over several days using glass syringes every 0.5 hr during surgery. These samples were analyzed as quickly as possible by gas chromatography.

The results of the measurements are listed in Tables 1 and 2. In these tables the concentrations which would have been found if there had been complete mixing in the rooms are also shown. These concentrations are calculated from the known values of 'a' and 'I' and the estimated mean value of 'q' (see Formula 1).

Table 1.   *Concentrations of halothane and nitrous oxide in operating Room 1*

| Point of measurement* | Halothane | | | Nitrous oxide | | |
	Mean concentration (ppm)	Range (ppm)	Calculated concentration (ppm)**	Mean concentration (ppm)	Range (ppm)	Calculated concentration (ppm)**
A	1.76	0.79–2.36	$\pm$ 1.6	332	145–448	$\pm$ 210
B	5.31	1.31–22.2	$\pm$ 1.6	584	180–2040	$\pm$ 210
C	1.28	0.55–2.28	$\pm$ 1.6	245	124–409	$\pm$ 210

*A = breathing zone of the anaesthetist; distance from pop-off valve $\pm$ 1 m; B = distance from pop-off valve $\pm$ 0.5 m, height 1 m; C = distance from pop-off valve $\pm$ 5 m, height 1 m.
**$q_{hal} = \pm$ 0.05 l/min; $q_{N_2O} = \pm$ 6 l/min; a–I = 1800 m³/hr.

Table 2.   *Concentrations of halothane and nitrous oxide in operating Room 2*

| Point of measurement* | Halothane | | | Nitrous oxide | | |
	Mean concentration (ppm)	Range (ppm)	Calculated concentration (ppm)**	Mean concentration (ppm)	Range (ppm)	Calculated concentration (ppm)**
A	1.23	0.72–1.54	$\pm$ 1.2	188	81–502	$\pm$ 120
B	1.48	0.83–2.08	$\pm$ 1.2	185	94–403	$\pm$ 120
C	0.81	0.45–1.09	$\pm$ 1.2	109	40–157	$\pm$ 120

*A = breathing zone of the anaesthetist; distance from pop-off valve $\pm$ 1 m; B = distance from pop-off valve $\pm$ 1 m, height 1.5 m; C = distance from pop-off valve $\pm$ 5 m, height 1.5 m.
** $q_{hal} = \pm$ 0.04 l/min; $q_{N_2O} = \pm$ 4 l/min; a–I = 2000 m³/hr.

The tables show that the measured and calculated concentrations agree reasonably well. It also appears that the concentrations are dependent upon the location of the point of measurement. The concentrations distant from the pop-off valve are lower than those close to it. As previously mentioned this is related to the air flow in the operating room. An investigation of the distribution of narcotic gases in a model operating room showed that as the distance from the pop-off valve increases, the concentrations decrease (Spierdijk et al., 1974).

To obtain an accurate picture of the pollution, it is necessary that measurements be taken at several points; furthermore it is recommended that the air flow pattern be taken into consideration when these measurement points are chosen.

ACKNOWLEDGEMENT

The authors gratefully acknowledge the help of Mrs. J. H. Van Meeverden and Mr. A. W. M. Van Bijnen.

REFERENCES

Askrog, V. and Harvald, B. (1970): *Nord. Med.*, *83*, 498.
Askrog, V. and Petersen, R. (1970): *Nord. Med.*, *83*, 501.
Bruce, D. L., Eide, K. A., Linde, H. W. and Eckenhoff, J. E. (1968): *Anesthesiology*, *29/3*, 565.
Cohen, E. N., Bellville, J. W. and Brown, B. W. (1971): *Anesthesiology*, *35/4*, 343.
Corbett, T. H., Cornell, R. G., Lieding, K. and Endres, J. L. (1973): *Anesthesiology*, *38/3*, 260.
Frey, R., Gostomzyk, J. G., Gregori, M., Kapfhammer, H. and Spierdijk, J. (1973): *Verh. dtsch. Ges. inn. Med.*, *79*, 959.
Hallén, B., Ehrner-Samuel, H. and Thomason, M. (1970): *Acta anaesth. scand.*, *14*, 17.
Linde, H. W. and Bruce, D. L. (1969): *Anesthesiology*, *30/4*, 363.
Schulze, H. H., Kästner, D. and Lange, P. (1969): *Anaesthesist*, *18/11*, 378.
Spierdijk, J., Burm, A. G. L., Bossers, P. A., Van Beukering, F. C. and Van Gunst, E. (1974): *Paper presented at the* 'Workshop über Probleme der permanenten Konfrontation des Anästhesie-Personals mit Narkose-Gasen und -Dämpfen im Operationssaal', Städtischen Krankenhaus München-Neuperlach. In press.
Usubiaga, L., Aldrete, J. A. and Fiserova-Bergerova, V. (1972): *Anesth. Analg. Curr. Res.*, *51/6*, 968.
Vaisman, A. I. (1967): *Eksp. Khir. Anestheziol.*, *3*, 44.
Whitcher, C. E., Cohen, E. N. and Trudell, J. R. (1971): *Anesthesiology*, *35/4*, 348.

*Effects of halothane on lipid metabolism in human adipose tissue**

JARL BENNIS and ULF SMITH

Department of Anaesthesiology, Eastern Hospital, and Department of Medicine II,
Sahlgrens Hospital, University of Gothenburg, Gothenburg, Sweden

INTRODUCTION

Although halothane is a widely used anaesthetic and its clinical effects are well known, there is a great lack in our knowledge about the mechanisms involved. Clinical observations that vasodilatation, bronchial relaxation and uterine hypotonia accompany halothane anaesthesia emphasise the fact that halothane exerts effects similar to those produced by adrenergic β-receptor agonists. However, whether these effects are caused by a direct β-adrenergic receptor stimulation or not is presently unsettled. Klide et al. (1969) have found that halothane relaxes smooth muscles in different sites and species and that this effect can be abolished by β-receptor antagonists. Yang et al. (1973) on the other hand, showed that halothane stimulates the activity of adenylcyclase as well as that of phosphodiesterase in rat uterine muscle. These effects were not inhibited by β-receptor antagonists. In an attempt to study the possible effects on the β-adrenergic receptors the effect of halothane upon adipose tissue metabolism has been investigated.

It is now well-recognized that the lipolytic process in human adipose tissue is mediated by the level of cyclic adenosine 3′, 5′-monophosphate (cyclic AMP) (Carlson et al., 1970) induced by the β-receptor-adenylcyclase system (Östman and Efendic, 1970; Burns and Langley, 1970). The accessibility of adipose tissue makes it very convenient to study. Another advantage is that tissue specimens may repeatedly be obtained with only a slight trauma. Thus, it is possible to set up a model system for studying the effects of halothane upon the cyclic AMP system in human adipose tissue. Initially (Bennis and Smith, 1973) the metabolism of specimens of human adipose tissue obtained before and after halothane anaesthesia was studied. In an attempt to use a more well-defined system to study the effects of halothane an in vitro technique has been developed. The present communication summarizes the findings of these studies.

MATERIALS AND METHODS

Patients undergoing laparotomy for an isolated abdominal disorder were studied. All patients fasted overnight before operation. The patients were anaesthetized according to the normal procedure of the anaesthetic department. Anaesthesia was induced with a short-acting barbiturate, succinylcholine was given, the patient intubated and the anaesthesia

---

* Supported in part by grants from the Swedish Medical Research Council and Göteborgs Läkaresällskap.

was continued with nitrous oxide, oxygen and halothane plus a muscle relaxing agent. The incubation procedure used is a further development of that described by Smith (1970). Briefly, smaller fragments of the tissue specimens were incubated in Krebs Ringer bicarbonate buffer with 4% albumin added and in the presence of labelled glucose with or without the addition of recrystallized pork insulin or noradrenaline. In some experiments halothane (Fluothane®) was added to the medium at different concentrations from 10^{-6} M–10^{-2} M. As this anaesthetic cannot be dissolved in the incubation medium at concentrations higher than 4×10^{-2} M further uptake into the medium was reached by adding halothane at concentrations of 0.5%–3% to the gas above the medium. Incorporation of labelled glucose into the tissue triglycerides was determined.

The metabolic parameters are expressed in terms of the cellularity of the tissue specimens. Significance levels were calculated according to Student's t-test.

RESULTS

Halothane added in vivo

In some experiments specimens of the subcutaneous adipose tissue were excised before and 30 min after the addition of halothane. When the patients had been exposed to halothane the lipolysis of the tissue specimens was decreased. Furthermore, the antilipolytic effect of insulin was less pronounced while the effect of added catecholamines tended to be increased. Similar results were obtained when the release of free fatty acids (FFA) was determined. The incorporation of glucose into the lipids was similar in the specimens obtained before and after anaesthesia with halothane.

Halothane added to the incubation medium

In order to evaluate more directly the effect of halothane on adipose tissue metabolism the anaesthetic was added to the incubation medium or to the gas phase as described above. When halothane was added to the incubation medium a significant stimulating effect on the lipolysis was noted at concentrations below 10^{-3} M. This effect could be abolished by the addition of a β-receptor antagonist, propranolol (Table 1).

The presence of halothane in the incubation medium did not significantly change the antilipolytic effect of insulin or the lipolytic effect of noradrenaline.

The rate of incorporation of glucose into the lipids was not significantly changed by halothane and the effect of added insulin was similar whether halothane was present or not.

Table 1. *The effect of propranolol on the lipolysis in the presence of halothane in the medium*

Halothane concentration	Glycerol release (nmoles/10^5 cells)	
	Basal	+Propranolol
0	132.1 ± 32.9	158.6 ± 42.6
10^{-6}	177.4 ± 51.4	156.6 ± 47.2
10^{-5}	174.1 ± 29.7	143.2 ± 38.6
10^{-4}	161.9 ± 33.0	132.3 ± 30.8
10^{-3}	153.8 ± 54.4	150.8 ± 59.5
10^{-2}	170.1 ± 44.3	145.0 ± 44.1

Mean ± SEM; n = 4.

Halothane added to the gas phase

Halothane in the gas phase significantly inhibited the rate of lipolysis at all concentrations used (0.5%–3%). Only a slight further inhibitory effect was reached when the halothane concentration was raised beyond 0.5% (Fig. 1).

The inhibitory effect of insulin upon lipolysis was abolished in the presence of halothane. However, the stimulating effect of noradrenaline on lipolysis, expressed as percentage increase, was enhanced by the presence of halothane ($p < 0.05$) (Fig. 1). It should be noted, however, that even in the presence of the catecholamine the rate of lipid mobilization did not exceed the basal lipolytic rate found in the absence of halothane.

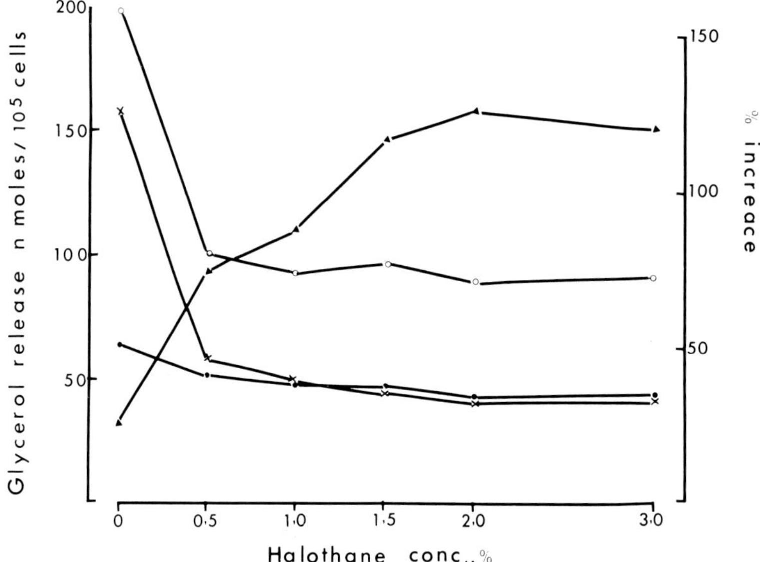

Fig. 1.   *Effects of different concentrations of halothane in the gas phase upon the lipolysis (n = 6)*
(× — × = basal values; ○ — ○ = insulin added; ● — ● = noradrenaline added; ▲ — ▲ = %
increase with noradrenaline).

A slight but significant reduction in the basal incorporation of glucose was found at all concentrations of halothane used ($p < 0.05$) exept at 1.0%. The effect of added insulin was similar whether halothane was present or not.

DISCUSSION

The lipolysis of adipose tissue specimens obtained from patients anaesthetized with halothane was decreased. Furthermore, the antilipolytic effect of insulin was less pronounced while the effect of added catecholamines tended to be increased. Using the in vitro technique described above we have been able to confirm these in vivo results. Mäkeläinen et al. (1973) recently reported that low concentrations of halothane stimulated the basal lipolysis of rat adipose tissue incubated in vitro and that this was due to a direct stimulating effect on the β-receptors. Similar results were obtained in our study when low concentrations of halothane were used. At higher concentrations halothane clearly inhibited the basal lipolytic process. It thus appears that halothane exerts different effects upon the lipolysis depending upon the concentrations used. The underlying mechanism for such dual effects of halothane is not known. However, Yang et al. (1972) have shown that halothane stimulates the adenylcyclase as well as the phosphodiesterase-activities in rat uterine muscle. If similar conditions apply to the adipose tissue it may then be that halothane at low concentrations stimulates the adenylcyclase activity to a greater extent than the phosphodiesterase, leading to an increased lipolysis. Support for this assumption is offered by our findings, and those of Mäkeläinen et al. (1973), that β-receptor antagonists may abolish the stimulatory effect of halothane. At higher concentrations of halothane a stimulating effect on the phosphodiesterase activity may predominate, leading to the inhibition of the lipolytic process.

The diminished lipolysis found in the present study would seem to be at variance with the fact that the plasma FFA levels only show minor alterations in connection with halothane anaesthesia alone (Oyama and Takazawa, 1971). However, these data are not conclusive since a decreased mobilization may be balanced by a decreased rate of utilization.

REFERENCES

Bennis, J. and Smith, U. (1973): *Acta anaesth. scand.*, *17*, 76.
Burns, T. W. and Langley, P. E. (1970): *J. Lab. clin. Med.*, *75*, 983.
Carlson, L. A., Butcher, R. W. and Micheli, H. (1970): *Acta med. scand.*, *187*, 525.
Klide, A. M., Penna, M. and Aviado, D. M. (1969): *Anesth. Analg. Curr. Res.*, *48*, 58.
Mäkeläinen, A., Vapaatalo, H. and Nikki, P. (1973): *Acta anaesth. scand.*, *17*, 179.
Östman, J. and Efendic, S. (1970): *Acta med. scand.*, *187*, 471.
Oyama, T. and Takazawa, T. (1971): *Brit. J. Anaesth.*, *43*, 573.
Smith, U. (1970): *Biochim. biophys. Acta (Amst.)*, *218*, 417.
Yang, J. C., Triner, L., Vulliemoz, Y., Verosky, M. and Ngai, S. H. (1973): *Anesthesiology*, *38*, 244.

Effects of controlled hyperventilation on cerebral blood flow in patients during anaesthesia

I. PICHLMAYR, R. SIPPEL, E. MASCHER AND R. PICHLMAYR

Institut für Anaesthesiologie, Medizinische Hochschule Hannover,
Hannover, Federal Republic of Germany

The aim of the study is to determine suitable volumes of ventilation during controlled ventilation in anaesthesia. The effects of controlled hyperventilation in comparison to normoventilation upon cerebral blood flow (CBF) acid-base status and peripheral circulation parameters have therefore been studied.

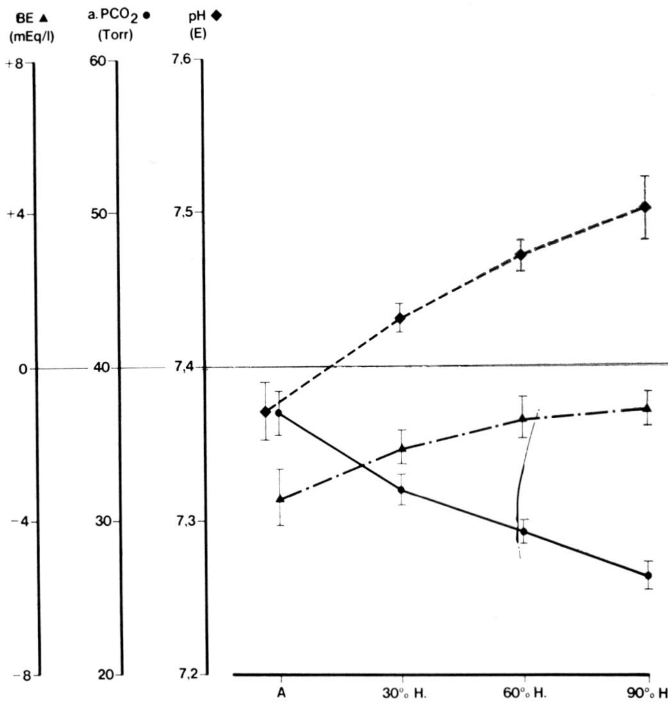

Fig. 1. *Changes of acid-base status in 18 patients during anaesthesia and hyperventilation (A = anaesthesia and normoventilation; H = hyperventilation).*

METHODS

Investigations have been made in 18 patients who underwent abdominal operations (mean age 63 ± 3 years). Neuroleptanalgesia (NLA) was used for deep anaesthesia together with muscle relaxation. Ventilation was carried out with a Pulmonat (Dräger) or with a Spiromat (Dräger). The volume of ventilation was determined according to the ventilation-nomogram of Engström, Herzog and Norlander. During anaesthesia the volume of ventilation was raised stepwise at intervals of 35–40 min from normoventilation up to 90% hyperventilation.

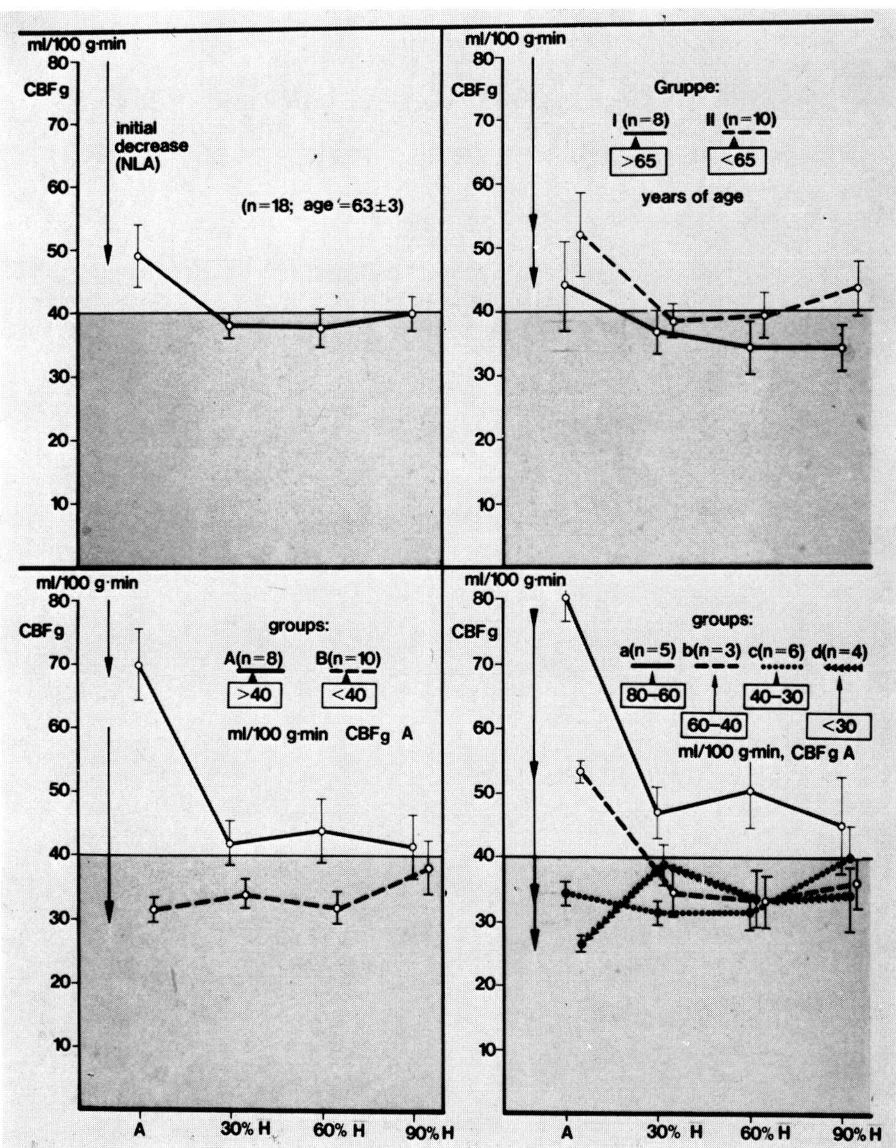

Fig. 2. *Effects of increasing degrees of hyperventilation upon CBFg (A = anaesthesia and normoventilation; H = hyperventilation).*

A series of measurements were made 20 min after each change of ventilation – measurement I: normoventilation; measurement II: 30% hyperventilation; measurement III: 60% hyperventilation; measurement IV: 90% hyperventilation.

The following parameters have been determined: (1) cerebral blood flow, total as well as fractions of grey and white matter (CBFm, CBFg, CBFw) by ^{133}Xe clearance; (2) cerebral vascular resistance in the different areas (CVRm, CVRg, CVRw); (3) arterial acid-base status (pH, Pa_{CO_2}, Pa_{O_2}, O_2-S, BE, BB, SBC, ABC); (4) Hb and HK; (5) blood pressure and pulse rate.

RESULTS

Figure 1 shows that the arterial P_{CO_2} decreased according to the increase of ventilation volume from normoventilation to 90% hyperventilation. Values of pH and base excess, show a slight metabolic acidosis, and an increase to respiratory alkalosis according to the increase of ventilation.

The initial values for CBFg are about 40% lower under the NLA as compared with normal values in unanaesthetized persons (Fig. 2). This is in accordance with the well-known effect of a 10–50% reduction of CBF by intravenous anaesthetics which is thought to be a consequence of an equivalent reduction of cerebral metabolism during anaesthesia.

Hyperventilation however influences autoregulatory mechanisms of CBF by changes of arterial P_{CO_2}. Cerebral hypoxia during continued extreme hyperventilation cannot be excluded. 30% hyperventilation produced a significant fall of 14% CBFg additionally to the reduction caused by anaesthesia which is a total reduction of about 50% of the normal

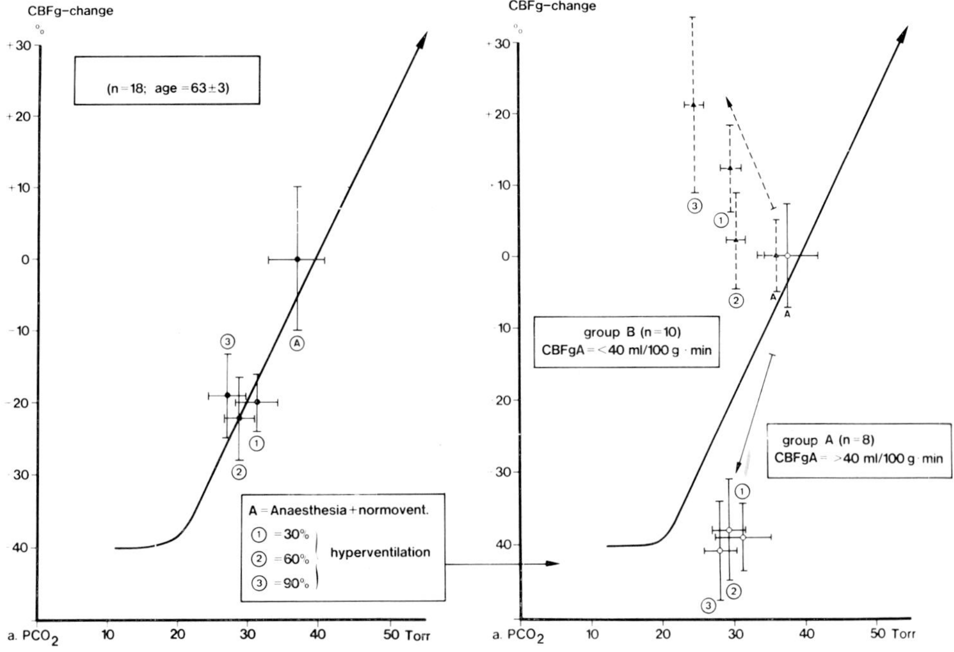

Fig. 3.   *Effects of hyperventilation on CBFg depending on initial values.*

CBFg. Higher degrees of hyperventilation (60% and 90%) did not increase this.

In evaluating 2 groups of patients according to their age below (I) and above (II) 65 years, it is evident that the decrease of CBFg is pronounced in the younger age-group only, whereas the decrease in the older group was statistically insignificant. In both groups higher ranges of hyperventilation did not influence CBFg values additionally.

Comparing the 2 groups of patients irrespective of age according to the initial CBFg values during anaesthesia (A = values above, B = values below 50% of the normal range) diminution of CBFg is present only in Group A. This is valid also if patients are subdivided additionally into Groups a–d according to the level of initial CBFg. Thus there is a strong correlation between the level of initial CBFg and its suppression by 30% hyperventilation.

Increased hyperventilation did not change CBFg any more. Peripheral circulation parameters as well as Hb and Hct remained unchanged during the entire anaesthesia. Cerebral vascular resistance changed in the opposite direction to CBF.

In Figure 3 the data is plotted against the nomogram of a P_{CO_2} dependent CBF variation. The mean values of all patients together are within this range, whereas the above mentioned groups A and B behave contrarily to each other. Changes in Group A are within the range of the nomogram but slightly more pronounced. But the changes in Group B do not follow the normal relationship between cerebral perfusion and arterial P_{CO_2}. Thus CBF in patients with initially reduced values (50%) is not dependent on changes of arterial P_{CO_2}.

DISCUSSION

In summary these results may account for finding the proper range of ventilation in the following way. If CBF already reduced during anaesthesia with normoventilation then hyperventilation does not produce an additional effect. Similarly CBFg is not reduced below the critical level of 40 ml/100 g min in any group. Nevertheless marked hyperventilation cannot be recommended as a routine. The depression in CBFg in patients with high initial CBFg values is significant. This diminution is independent of the cerebral metabolic rate and may be important in some patients with clinically undetected cerebrovascular disorders. Hypoxia is conceivable even without CBFg below 40 ml/100 g min.

Influence of anesthesia on regional cerebral blood flow (rCBF) measured by a 10-channel cerebrograph*

J. VAN AKEN and G. ROLLY

Department of Anesthesiology, University of Ghent Academic Hospital, Ghent, Belgium

Ingvar and Lassen published in 1961 (Ingvar and Lassen, 1972; Lassen and Ingvar, 1961) a method for measuring regional cerebral blood flow (rCBF) based on the clearance of an isotope from brain tissue after injection in the internal carotid artery. The equipment used to determine this clearance curve consists of measuring electronics, punch tape, a strip chart recorder with 4 channels and the collimator block with 10 scintillation counters.

The information from the 10 measuring probes is simultaneously passed to the punch tape and to the strip chart recorder. Four regions chosen in advance can be graphically reproduced in real time. The shape of these 4 curves gives direct information for routine, clinical diagnosis. The scintillation counters are fitted in a collimator block with guide channels. These guide channels are arranged so that the measuring fields of the 10 probes do not overlap.

In practice, measurement of the rCBF is carried out together with carotid angiography. As Herrschaft et al. (1974) and others have been able to show, angiography impairs the CBF for no longer than 5 min. Routinely after puncturing the common carotid artery, serial angiography in 2 planes is carried out. After 5 min a small teflon catheter is slipped in the needle and pushed into the internal carotid artery. To be sure that the catheter lies in the internal carotid artery, 1 ml of Evan's blue is injected which colours a small area of the face near the nose. The collimator block is then placed in the correct position and 2–3 mCi of ^{133}Xe dissolved in 2 ml saline solution is quickly injected into the internal carotid artery. The clearance of the isotope is measured over a period of 10 min with the 10 scintillation counters. The first measurement determines CBF at rest. A second measurement is made after the injection of thiopentone (Pentothal®). Calculation of rCBF is by the use of electronic data processing, using the computer program of Sveinsdottir (1974). This program yields among other values the rCBF ∞, or mean regional cerebral blood flow, extrapolated with respect to time for infinity.

In order to ensure constant conditions care must be taken to maintain a steady state during the measurements. Patients were premedicated with 1 mg/kg meperidine and 0.5 mg atropine. Induction is with 500 mg propanidid (Epontol®). According to Herrschaft and Schmidt (1973) the effect of propanidid on the cerebral blood flow disappears after 10 min and the metabolites have no cerebrovascular effect.

Anesthesia is maintained with 30% O_2, 70% N_2O and pancuronium (Pavulon®). Pancuronium has no cardiac effects and does not influence CBF and it is given in a dose sufficient to abolish all response to nerve stimulation. Patients were normoventilated with

* Supported by a grant from the Fonds voor Geneeskundig Wetenschappelijk Onderzoek, Brussels, Belgium.

an Engström respirator. This procedure provides a stable acid-base state with no statistically significant changes in P_{CO_2}, pH or standard bicarbonate (Table 1).

At T_0 the first CBF measurement is made under nitrous oxide, oxygen, curare anesthesia. Arterial blood samples are taken and systolic, diastolic and mean arterial pressure are recorded by means of a catheter inserted in the femoral artery. Central venous pressures are measured through a right atrium catheter inserted in a cubital vein. Cardiac output is measured by impedance cardiography. Two minutes after the injection of 4 mg/kg thiopentone at T_1, a second series of measurements is made. At the end of the second CBF measurement, blood gases, cardiac output and arterial and venous pressures are again recorded at T_2.

Table 1. *Blood gases* $(n=10)$

	T_0		T_1		T_2		T_0-T_1 (p)	T_0-T_2 (p)	T_1-T_2 (p)
	Mean	SEM	Mean	SEM	Mean	SEM			
Arterial blood									
P_{O_2} (mm Hg)	107.9	11.9	121.1	14.6	114.9	13.7	< 0.05	NS	NS
pH	7.415	0.022	7.416	0.024	7.416	0.028	NS	NS	NS
P_{CO_2} (mm Hg)	38.3	2.3	37.3	2.8	37.4	3.3	NS	NS	NS
Standard bicarbonate (mEq/l)	24.3	0.8	23.7	0.7	23.8	0.9	NS	NS	NS
Mixed venous blood									
P_{O_2} (mm Hg)	51.5	2.38	50.9	1.9	47.8	2.4	NS	NS	< 0.05
pH	7.399	0.020	7.399	0.022	7.395	0.028	NS	NS	NS
P_{CO_2} (mm Hg)	39.6	3.1	39.5	2.5	41.9	3.2	NS	NS	NS
Standard bicarbonate (mEq/l)	23.8	0.9	23.9	0.7	24.3	0.8	NS	NS	NS

T_0 = rest values; T_1 = 2 min after i.v. pentothal injection; T_2 = 10 min after i.v. pentothal injection; SEM = standard error of mean; T_0-T_1 = T_0 values compared to T_1 values; T_0-T_2 = T_0 values compared to T_2 values; T_1-T_2 = T_1 values compared to T_2 values; NS = no statistically significant change.

Table 2. *Blood pressures* $(n=10)$

	T_0		T_1		T_2		T_0-T_1 (p)	T_0-T_2 (p)	T_1-T_2 (p)
	Mean	SEM	Mean	SEM	Mean	SEM			
Arterial pressure									
Systolic (cm Hg)	17.3	0.7	14.0	0.9	14.3	0.5	< 0.0005	< 0.0025	NS
Diastolic (cm Hg)	9.1	0.4	8.2	0.6	8.2	0.5	< 0.05	< 0.05	NS
Mean (cm Hg)	12.0	0.5	10.1	0.6	10.4	0.4	< 0.005	< 0.0125	NS
Heart rate	85.3	6.4	86.9	5.5	74.8	5.0	NS	< 0.0125	< 0.0005
Cardiac output (l/min)	5.90	0.80	5.59	0.52	5.27	0.58	NS	NS	NS
Central venous pressure									
Systolic (cm H_2O)	20.1	2.1	20.6	1.3	20.5	1.2	NS	NS	NS
Diastolic (cm H_2O)	10.7	1.8	12.7	1.4	12.7	1.4	NS	NS	NS
Mean (cm H_2O)	15.5	1.9	16.8	1.3	16.8	1.3	NS	NS	NS

T_0 = rest values; T_1 = 2 min after i.v. Pentothal injection; T_2 = 10 min after i.v. Pentothal injection; SEM = standard error of mean; T_0-T_1 = T_0 values compared to T_1 values; T_0-T_2 = T_0 values compared to T_2 values; T_1-T_2 = T_1 values compared to T_2 values; NS = no statistically significant change.

Table 3. *Regional cerebral blood flow (ml/100 g/min) (n=10)*

Regions	T_0 Mean rCBF	SEM	T_1 Mean rCBF	SEM	T_0-T_1 (p)
Frontal	44.25	9.72	33.87	5.21	< 0.05
Precentral	45.31	10.84	31.87	7.03	< 0.025
Central	54.35	9.45	39.72	7.04	< 0.0005
Parietal	57.00	10.40	40.57	6.31	< 0.005
Parieto-temporal	53.94	13.87	39.46	8.47	< 0.05
Temporal	70.13	15.42	41.20	6.28	< 0.025
Fronto-basal	58.23	11.23	40.55	6.44	< 0.01
Precentral	46.37	9.30	35.15	5.51	< 0.025
Occipital	49.20	10.70	34.75	6.31	< 0.0225
Temporo-basal	44.32	9.22	31.52	6.43	< 0.01

T_0=rest values; T_1=2 min after i.v. Pentothal injection; SEM=standard error of mean; T_0-T_1= T_0 values compared to T_1 values; p: varies from almost significant to highly significant.

In Table 2 the effect of thiopentone on arterial pressures, heart rate, cardiac output and central venous pressures is shown. The central venous pressures did not change significantly, nor did cardiac output, but some changes in arterial pressure were significant.

Table 3 shows how rCBF decreased with varying significance according to the region.

The decrease in the CBF is probably due to a decrease of cerebral metabolism; these figures also show that autoregulation is not fully operative. The question is, which is the more important, the metabolic influence of thiopentone or the upset of autoregulation?

REFERENCES

Herrschaft, H. (1972): *Electromedica, 1,* 6.
Herrschaft, H., Gleim, F. and Schmidt, H. (1974): *Neuroradiology, 7,* 95.
Herrschaft, H. and Schmidt, H. (1973): *Anaesthesist, 22,* 486.
Ingvar, D. H. and Lassen, N. A. (1972): *Acta physiol. scand., 54,* 325.
Lassen, N. A. (1971): *Acta anaesth. scand., Suppl. 45,* 78.
Lassen, N. A. and Ingvar, D. H. (1961): *Experientia (Basel), 17,* 42.
Paulson, O. B. and Lassen, N. A. (1971): In: *Proceedings, III International Symposia Angiologica Santoriana, Fribourgh, 1970,* p. 202. S. Karger, Basel – New York – Berlin.
Sveinsdottir, E. (1974): *Acta neurol. scand., 14,* 69.

Influence of individual factors in the actions and duration of the hypnotic effect of Ro 5-4200

F. BENITO QUINTELA

Instituto Oftalmico Nacional, Madrid, Spain

Ro 5-4200 is a new benzodiazepine whose actions and hypnotic effects have already been studied by many authors. This study is on unselected cases for 50 eye surgeries (62% female and 38% male; age range 15–79 years; weight 47–80 kg).

The aim was to determine whether any individual factor (dose, speed of injection, age, weight, sex, general state and previous premedication administration) is unfavourable for the application of the substance. The efficiency of the drug as a hypnotic and its dangers are also studied.

Table 1 shows that blood pressure falls and that pulse rate and respiratory rate rise. These changes are minor and do not differ from the mean overall results of other authors. Figure 1 shows graphically the *effect on the palpebral, corneal and painful reflexes* of Ro 5-4200.

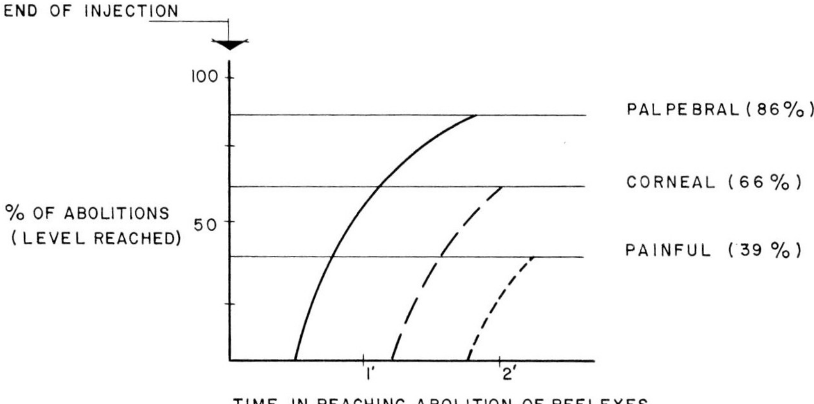

Fig. 1.   *Abolition of reflexes.*

It is clear that reflex abolition occurs firstly for the palpebral, secondly for the corneal and lastly for painful stimuli. At any given time the percentage of cases with abolished reflexes also decreases (86%, 66% and 39% respectively). This indicates that there is little analgesic effect.

The *hypnotic effect* is the most interesting aspect of this drug. To evaluate this the dose administered, the duration of injection, the instant at which sleep occurred, the age of the subject and the premedication must all be considered.

Table 1.   *Behavior of blood pressure, pulse and respiration after the administration of Ro 5-4200 in relation to various variables*

		Blood pressure systole/diastole (mm/Hg)			Pulse-rate/min			Respiration-rate/min		
		Before	After	Variation	Before	After	Variation	Before	After	Variation
Dose (mg)	2	137/80	119/73	—18/—7	89	95	+6	18.2	19.6	+1.4
	4	127/79	113/71	—14/—8	87	87	0	20.4	22.6	+2.2
Injection speed (secs)	5–25	136/81	121/74	—15/—7	82	92	+10	20.1	20.2	+0.1
	30–40	143/85.8	122/75.8	—10/—10	87.5	93	+ 5.5	19.6	22.2	+2.6
	60–90	129.6/76.9	115.7/71.9	—13.9/—5	102	100	— 2	17	16.8	—0.2
	120	130/75	118/72	—12/—3	86.9	88	+ 1.1	16.6	21.9	+5.3
Age (years)	10–29	118/71.5	111.5/66.9	—6.5/—4.6	84	91.6	+ 7.6	18.8	20.5	+1.8
	30–49	130.4/79.5	120/76.8	—10.4/—2.7	96.4	96.9	+ 0.5	19.4	18	—1.4
	50–69	147/85	122/75.4	—25/—9.6	87.5	93.3	+ 5.8	19.6	21.9	+2.3
	70–89	138/83.7	122/76.2	—16/—7.5	95	92.2	— 2.8	14.5	19.7	+5.2
Weight (kg)	45–54	132.7/72.7	112/66.8	—20.7/—5.9	93.3	92	— 1.3	19.2	20.3	+1.1
	55–64	136.9/76	122.5/74.4	—14.4/—1.6	89.3	96	+ 6.7	18.6	19.8	+1.2
	65–74	127.6/81.1	118/75.3	—9.6/—5.8	86.6	93	+ 6.4	18.5	19.8	+1.3
	75–84	146.8/86.2	123/78	—23.8/—8.2	87	91	+ 4	16.7	17.7	+1
Sex	M	129/77.9	117/71.6	—11.6/—6.3	90	95	+ 5	18.5	19.9	+1.4
	F	145/83.9	122/76.8	—23/—7.1	87.4	91	+ 3.6	19.4	21.3	+1.9
General state	(Good)	132.6/78.8	117/72.7	—15.6/—6.1	90.7	95.4	+ 4.7	18.3	20.5	+2.2
	(Medium)	146.5/85	121/76	—25.5/—9	84.8	87.3	+ 2.5	17.7	21.3	+3.6
	(Bad, 1 case)	150/85	165/85	—15/0	64	72	+ 8	22	26	+4
Previous premedication	(with)	131.8/79.3	115.6/72.9	—22.2/—6.4	96.7	104	+ 7.3	18.3	16.2	—2.1
	(without)	137.8/80.8	121.9/74.1	—15.9/—6.7	83.1	85.2	+ 2.1	19.2	23.1	+3.9

Table 2 shows that 28% went to sleep during injection and 68% after injection; 96% subjects went to sleep.

If injection is made slowly (over about one min) patients go to sleep during the same period; if the injection is made in less than one min sleep occurs after the injection. If the injection is made rapidly (5 sec), the patient goes to sleep after the injection, but more quickly if the injection rate is even faster. Young, healthy or heavy patients require increased doses. Sleep eventually occurs even if there is a delay – this is usually because the dose was inadequate.

Table 2.   *Sleep-effect of Ro 5-4200*

During the injection				After the injection			
Yes		No		Yes		No	
Frequency	%	Frequency	%	Frequency	%	Frequency	%
14	28	36	72	34	68	2	4

Total % of patients in whom sleep was induced = 96%.

If premedication is given a few minutes (from 5–15 min) before Ro 5-4200, the onset of sleep is rapid.

As far as the duration of sleep produced by Ro 5-4200 is concerned, only a small group of cases operated on with local anaesthesia who also received solely Ro 5-4200 can be considered since in the remaining cases several products were potentiated (premedication, general anaesthetics) and it was not possible to judge the hypnotic effect of a single substance. Sleep in this group lasted from 30–50 min, with an average duration of 40 min. Table 3 shows that sleep is briefest in the younger (even with a double dose) patients and in those in good general condition. In all these cases awakening was always prompt, complete and quiet.

Table 3.   *Response according to age and general state of health.*

	Case 1	Case 2	Case 3	Case 4	Case 5
Dose (mg)	4	2	2	2	2
Weight (kg)	60	52	57	54	59
Age (years)	22	40	43	60	66
Duration of sleep	30	48	35	50	40
Previous complications (general state)	–	C.V. Respirs. allergics.	–	Neurolg. Parkinson disease	–

From all the foregoing it may be concluded that Ro 5-4200 is efficient, very safe, almost innocuous; it produces hypnosis quietly but without analgesia, from which recovery is quiet and without problems. It is necessary to prescribe it on the basis of age and general physical state.

The effect of isoproterenol and dopamine on the fractional distribution of cardiac output and on the organ blood flow in the dog

HIROSHI IN-NAMI [1], TAHEI KAWAGUCHI [1], ISAO KOSUGI [2],
KAZUO OKADA [2], YOSHIHARU YAMAGUCHI [3] and HIDEO YAMAMURA [3]

[1] Department of Anesthesiology, Tokyo Teishin Hospital;
[2] Teikyo University School of Medicine; and [3] Tokyo University School of Medicine, Tokyo, Japan

The effects of isoproterenol and of dopamine on the systemic circulation and on the circulation of individual organs have been investigated extensively (Aviado, 1970; Goldberg, 1972). However, the effects of these agents on the distribution of cardiac output to individual organs have not been elucidated. This study was performed to investigate these effects in dogs using radioactive microspheres.

METHODS

Sixteen dogs were anesthetized with pentobarbital, and were allowed to breathe air spontaneously throughout the study. Arterial and venous catheterizations were performed for hemodynamic measurements, drug infusions and to obtain blood samples.

After a stabilization period, cardiac output and blood pressures were measured. Then the first dose of radioactive microspheres was injected into the left ventricle, and blood samples were taken for the analysis of blood gases and pH. Thereafter, the intravenous infusion of either isoproterenol (0.5 μg/kg/min) or dopamine (20 μg/kg/min) was started. Fifteen minutes after starting the drug infusion, the hemodynamic measurements and blood sampling were repeated, and the second injection of radioactive microspheres labeled with a different nucleide was performed.

Cardiac output was determined using the dye dilution method. Blood P_{O_2}, P_{CO_2} and pH were measured using suitably calibrated electrode systems. Radioactive microspheres used were 50 ± 10 (S.D.)μ in diameter, and were labeled either with ^{85}Sr or ^{141}Ce.

At the end of the experiment, each dog was sacrificed, organs and tissues were excised, and their radioactivities were determined. The fractional distribution of cardiac output and the organ or tissue blood flow were calculated by the method of Rudolph and Heymann (1967).

RESULTS

Pa_{O_2} and acid-base parameters were within normal limits in both the isoproterenol and dopamine groups during the control period. Pa_{CO_2} decreased significantly by 4 mm Hg in the isoproterenol group, while that in the dopamine group tended to increase (2 mm Hg).

With isoproterenol, mean arterial blood pressure fell from 149–101 mm Hg and pulse rate increased from 190–230 beats/min on an average, while mean arterial blood pressure and pulse rate remained unchanged during dopamine infusion. During the drug infusion, cardiac output increased in both the isoproterenol and dopamine groups, by 60% and 49%, respectively, and total peripheral vascular resistance decreased in both groups. Though approximately the same degree of increase in cardiac output was produced by

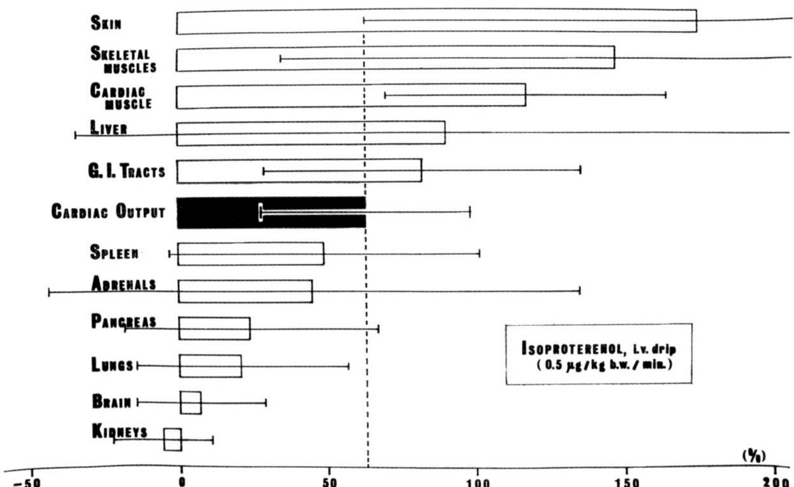

Fig. 1.   *Percent changes compared with respective control values in cardiac output and in the regional blood flow during the infusion of isoproterenol (0.5 μg/kg/min). Values are means and standard deviations obtained from 9 dogs under pentobarbital anesthesia (25 mg/kg, i.v.).*

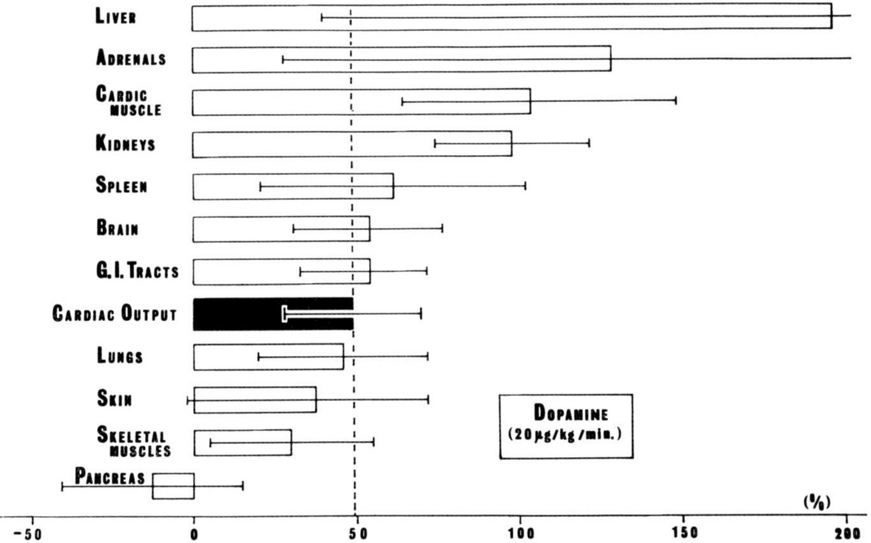

Fig. 2.   *The same percent changes as shown in Figure 1 during the infusion of dopamine (20 μg/kg/min). The data from 7 dogs under the same anesthesia as in Figure 1.*

each of the 2 agents, the patterns of redistribution of the increased cardiac output were different. With isoproterenol infusion (Fig. 1), the fraction of cardiac output to skin, skeletal and cardiac muscles, and gastrointestinal tracts increased significantly, while that to kidneys, brain, lungs (bronchial arteries) and pancreas decreased significantly. Moreover, the renal blood flow tended to decrease in spite of the increase in cardiac output.

With dopamine infusion (Fig. 2), the fraction of cardiac output to liver (hepatic arteries), adrenals, cardiac muscles and kidneys increased significantly, while that to pancreas and skeletal muscles decreased significantly. Furthermore, the pancreatic blood flow tended to decrease in spite of the increase in cardiac output.

DISCUSSION

The usefulness and validity of the microsphere method (Rudolph and Heymann, 1967) for determining the fractional distribution of cardiac output to various parts of the body have been confirmed by many investigators (Kaihara et al., 1968; Hoffbrand and Forsyth, 1969).

The systemic circulatory responses to both isoproterenol and dopamine found in the present study were similar to those described by previous investigators (Aviado, 1970; Goldberg, 1972). Cardiac output increased approximately 50% after the administration of each of the 2 agents, but the patterns of redistribution of the increased cardiac output were different. This difference might have resulted from the difference in the vasoactive property of each agent, especially from differences in direct and indirect vascular effects of each agent on individual organs and tissues.

A large number of β-adrenergic receptors have been found in blood vessels of cardiac and skeletal muscles, mesenteric viscera, while a few or none have been found in those of kidneys, brain and skin. Relatively abundant α-adrenergic receptors have been found in vessels of the skin, kidneys, mesenteric areas and skeletal muscles, while a few have been found in the brain (Green and Kepchar, 1959; Koelle, 1970). Specific dopamine receptors were demonstrated in renal and mesenteric arteries by Yeh et al. (1969), and Vatner et al. (1973) suggested that these also exist in coronary arteries.

Isoproterenol has been known to be a pure β-adrenergic stimulant. In the isoproterenol group, a significant increase in the fraction of cardiac output to skeletal and cardiac muscles and to gastrointestinal tracts occurred in spite of a fall in mean arterial pressure. These findings suggest that relatively dominant vasodilation might have occurred through stimulation of a large number of β-adrenergic receptors in these areas. A significant decrease in the fraction to kidneys, brain and pancreas might have been mainly due to less dominant vasodilation because of relative paucity in β-receptors in vessels of these organs. However, mechanisms other than β-receptor stimulation might have been involved in the increase in the fraction of cardiac output to the skin.

Dopamine is considered to be a 'mixed amine'. It produces vasoconstriction through stimulating α-adrenergic receptors and vasodilation through stimulating both β-adrenergic and dopamine receptors (Goldberg, 1972). Within a medium dose-range it also evokes a biphasic pressor-depressor effect on the artery in anesthetized dogs (McDonald and Goldberg, 1963). In the dopamine group, a selective increase in the fraction of cardiac output to the liver (hepatic arteries), adrenal, cardiac muscle and kidney suggests that dominant vasodilation might have occurred through stimulation of β-adrenergic or dopamine receptors in these organs, while a selective decrease in the fraction to the skeletal muscle and pancreas might be the results of its less dominant vasodilating or vasoconstricting effects in these areas.

A dose-related effect of isoproterenol on the fractional distribution of cardiac output was investigated by Hoffbrand et al. (1973), using a wide dose-range of the agent (0.06–0.9

kg/kg/min). Almost the same distributional pattern of cardiac output as found in the present study was observed in our previous study (In-nami et al., 1973), using a lower dose of dopamine (10 μg/kg/min). However, dose-dependent differences in the distribution of cardiac output would have been evoked, if studies with a wider dose-range of dopamine were carried out, because intravenous administration at a higher rate than 30 μg/kg/min of this agent was found to produce a norepinephrine-like effect upon blood vessels (Goldberg, 1972).

Changes in Pa_{CO_2} may affect the fractional distribution of cardiac output (In-nami et al., 1972). However, only a minimal change in Pa_{CO_2} was evoked by each agent, and the Pa_{CO_2} might not be a dominant contributing factor to the redistribution of cardiac output in this study. At the same time, Pa_{O_2} and body temperature remained unchanged, and the effects of these factors could be ruled out.

REFERENCES

Aviado, D. M. (1970): *Sympathomimetic Drugs*, p. 367, Charles C. Thomas, Springfield, Ill.
Goldberg, L. I. (1972): *Pharmacol. Rev., 24/1*, 1.
Green, H. D. and Kepchar, J. H. (1959): *Physiol. Rev., 39/4*, 617.
Hoffbrand, B. I. and Forsyth, R. P. (1969): *Cardiovasc. Res., 3*, 426.
Hoffbrand, B. I. et al. (1973): *Cardiovasc. Res., 7*, 664.
In-nami, H., Kawaguchi, T. and Kosugi, I. (1972): In: *Abstracts, V World Congress of Anaesthesiologists, Kyoto, 1972*, p. 45. Excerpta Medica, Amsterdam.
In-nami, H. et al. (1973): *Jap. J. Anesth., 22/10*, 1146.
Kaihara, S. et al. (1968): *J. appl. Physiol., 25/6*, 696.
Koelle, G. B. (1970): In: *The Pharmacological Basis of Therapeutics*, 4th ed., p. 402. Editors: L. S. Goodman and A. Gilman. The Macmillan Press Ltd., New York – Melbourne – London.
McDonald, R. H. and Goldberg, L. I. (1963): *J. Pharmacol. exp. Ther., 140/1*, 60.
Rudolph, A. M. and Heymann, M. A. (1967): *Circulat. Res., 21/2*, 163.
Vatner, S. F. et al. (1973): *J. Pharmacol. exp. Ther., 187/2*, 280.
Yeh, B. K. et al. (1969): *J. Pharmacol. exp. Ther., 168/2*, 303.

Myocardial depressant factor in shock

KAZUO OKADA [1], ISAO KOSUGI [1], YOSHIHARU YAMAGUCHI [1],
HIROSHI IN-NAMI [1], YASUO KAWASHIMA [2] and HIDEO YAMAMURA [3]

[1] Department of Anesthesiology, Teikyo University School of Medicine,
[2] Kanagawa Children's Hospital, and [3] Tokyo University School of Medicine, Tokyo, Japan

Whatever the cause of shock may be, there is always a marked decrease in splanchnic blood flow. A radioactive microsphere technique has been used to observe the distributional pattern of cardiac output in various forms of shock. Hypoperfusion of splanchnic viscera with concomitant hypoxia results in the disruption of cell structure and the release of some toxic substances into the peripheral plasma.

Lefer reported the impairment of myocardial performance and a causal relationship from the blood-borne toxic factor, called MDF (myocardial depressant factor). The aim of this present investigation is to confirm the existence of MDF in plasma and to study the origin of plasma MDF (Lefer and Martin, 1970; Lefer et al., 1973).

METHODS

Healthy mongrel dogs were anesthetized with pentobarbital. Arterial and venous catheterizations were performed to monitor hemodynamic parameters and to obtain blood samples. After taking a control blood sample, hemorrhagic shock was induced. Mean arterial blood pressure was kept at 50 mm Hg by Fine's method throughout the succeeding period. A second blood sample was taken 6 hr later, and then the pancreas, liver, small intestine and heart were excised.

Thirty ml of sampled blood was immediately centrifuged at $2250 \times G$ for 20 min at 4°C. The plasma was ultrafiltrated by a chamber with a DM-2 membrane to yield a molecular weight of less than 10,000. The ultrafiltrate was lyophilized to dryness, reconstituted to 2 ml with distilled water, and centrifuged again for 10 min. The supernatant fluid was applied to a column 500 mm $\times$ 18 mm containing Sephadex G-15 suspended with Krebs-Henseleit solution at flow rate of 60 ml/hr using a liquid chromatograph. The chromatography was conducted at 4°C, and the samples were collected by a fraction collector at 1-min intervals. Optical density of the elutes was measured by a spectrophotometer at 220 nm.

Sodium and potassium concentrations of each fraction were measured by flame-photometry. Four grams from every organ excised was homogenized in Krebs-Henseleit solution, and centrifuged at $2000 \times G$ for 20 min. The aliquots of their supernatant were treated by the same procedure as those from the blood samples.

Assays for MDF activity were performed on isolated cat papillary muscles. Immediately after removing the beating heart, papillary muscles were placed in a 30 ml chamber kept at $37 \pm 0.1°C$ in Krebs-Henseleit solution gassed with 95% O_2–5% CO_2. They were then stimulated at a frequency of 1/sec for a duration of 5 msec at 2 V above threshold voltage. Isometric contractions were continuously recorded by a force transducer. Each sample from both blood and organs was added to the chamber, and the effect on contractile force was determined.

RESULTS

Seven distinct fractions were obtained from the sample of blood and organs. They were termed peaks A through G in descending order of the molecular weights according to Lefer and Martin (1970).

A typical column elution pattern from the plasma ultrafiltrate of the control and of the shocked plasma from the same dog are shown in Figures 1*a* and *b*, respectively. Most of the peaks, especially C and D, increased in height in the shock stage. The molecular weight of peak D was confirmed between 700–1,000.

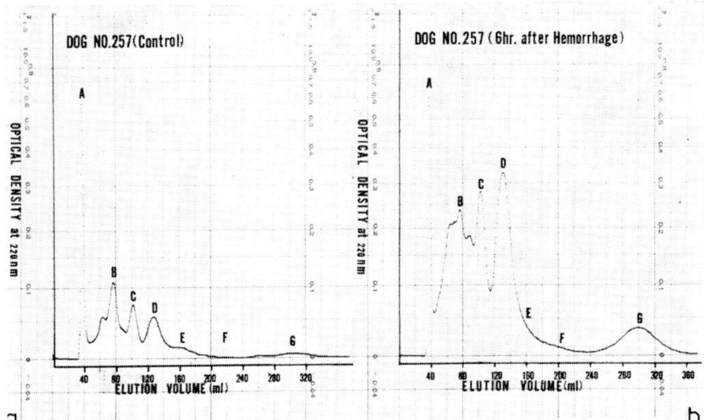

Fig. 1.   *(a) Typical column elution pattern from a sample of plasma from a dog in control stage; (b) typical column elution pattern from a sample of plasma from a dog in shock stage.*

Each peak of the ultrafiltrate taken from the pancreas was much higher than that from the plasma taken during the shock period. Peak C and D from the elution of liver also increased in size. The height of each peak from the cardiac muscle and the small intestine was almost the same as from the control plasma except for peak G. Most of the salt was found before peak D, and this peak had a normal Na ion concentration.

Figure 2 is a typical tracing of isometric contractions of the papillary muscle. At the arrow, the Krebs-Henseleit solution in the chamber was washed out and replaced with the fraction from a dog in shock containing peak D. A large decrease in developed tension was produced by the peak of the D fraction. A slight decrease in the tension was also produced by the peak C fraction from the same sample. However, the peaks of the control ultrafiltrate and the other peaks, other than C and D from the shock ultrafiltrate, did not exhibit any change in the developed tension.

DISCUSSION

There has been a continuing controversy about the production of a toxic substance which causes myocardial depression in the progress of shock. Lefer and Martin (1970) termed this substance as MDF and continued the work on the mechanism of its formation. Precise investigation was performed only by Lefer and his associates. Several investigators (Hinshaw , 1971; Wilson and Ebert, 1972), who denied the existence of MDF, did not follow method. This study confirms the presence of MDF in plasma and extracts of some in shocked dog by exactly following their method.

Seven distinct fractions were obtained from the plasma of a shocked dog and were termed A through G in descending order of their molecular weight.

The fraction containing peak D, which was prepared as the same concentration in plasma, depressed the contractile force of the cat's papillary muscle, and the proposal (Wangensteen et al., 1973) that MDF is salt is therefore denied. The elution pattern from the pancreas appeared to be identical to that from the plasma and each peak was much higher than that of the plasma. These findings probably support the concept that MDF is produced in the pancreas and is transported to the blood stream. However, the elution pattern from the liver in shock exhibited similar increase in peaks D through G. It is not clear, at this point, whether MDF is produced in the liver or trapped by its reticuloendothelial system. If MDF were produced in the liver, the total sum would be larger in the liver and might have a more important effect on its release to the blood stream, since the weight of the liver is 10-fold heavier than that of the pancreas. Further investigation on the elution from the spleen would clarify the activity of reticuloendothelial system in trapping MDF.

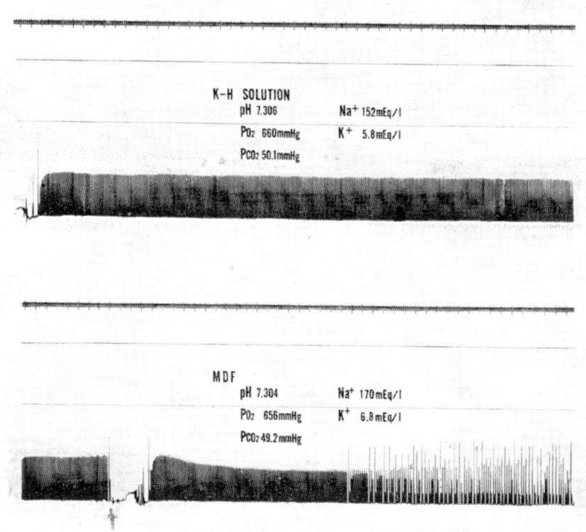

Fig. 2.   *Typical tracing of isometric contractions of papillary muscle pH, P_{O2}, P_{CO2}, Na^+, and K^+ concentration of each solution were indicated in this figure. At the arrow, the Krebs-Henseleit solution in chamber washed out and replaced with the peak D fraction from a dog in shock.*

The elution pattern in cardiac muscle did not show any increase in the peaks and this strongly suggests that MDF causing cardiac depression in this study is not produced by the heart itself but borne by the blood stream.

Corticosteroids were found to be effective in the treatment of various types of shock and several hypotheses have been formulated. Weissmann and Thomas (1962) and Lefer and Martin (1970), Lefer et al. (1973) proposed a stabilizing effect on lysosomal membranes in the splanchnic area. In another series of experiments, the pretreatment of dogs with 8 mg/kg of dexamethasone decreased the height of each peak both in plasma and in the pancreas, compared to the non-treated group (Okada et al., 1974). This adds to the suppo that corticosteroids are effective in maintaining the integrity of the lysosomal memb

Further studies are necessary to determine the role and significance of MDF in pr shock and in its reversibility.

REFERENCES

Hinshaw, L. B. et al. (1971): *Amer. J. Physiol.*, *221/2*, 504.
Lefer, A. M. and Martin, J. (1970): *Amer. J. Physiol.*, *218/5*, 1423.
Leffler, J. N. et al. (1973): *Amer. J. Physiol.*, *224/4*, 824.
Okada, K. et al. (1973): *Jap. J. Anesth.*, *22/6*, 511.
Okada, K. et al. (1974): *Jap. J. Anesth.*, *23/12*, 1170.
Wangensteen, S. L. et al. (1973): *J. Trauma*, *13/3*, 181.
Weissman, G. and Thomas, L. (1962): *J. exp. Med.*, *116/3*, 433.
Wilson, J. M. and Ebert, P. A. (1972): *Ann. Surg.*, *175/2*, 214.

A training scheme for resuscitation technique at Ullevål Hospital, Oslo, Norway

IVAR LUND and ANDREAS SKULBERG

Ullevål Hospital, Oslo, Norway

Teaching and training hospital personnel in resuscitation is an obvious obligation for every hospital. The teaching should be uniform and realistic to the extent that any employee of a hospital should be able to diagnose respiratory and cardiac arrest correctly, and, if need be, perform the necessary resuscitative measures immediately. To accomplish this the task of training and retraining is considerable, especially in a large hospital with a great turnover of personnel.

Some years ago, it was decided to try to improve our teaching in resuscitation by centralizing and standardizing our efforts, and an efficient, simple and inexpensive teaching system was sought. The Laerdal self-instruction system appeared to comply with the criteria, and it was decided to try this system with some slight modifications 2 years ago.

This system consists of the well-known training manikin for artificial ventilation and heart compression. A recording device is incorporated which displays a written tracing of the performance by the pupil. In addition there is a set of instructive illustrations and a tape recorder with an explanatory text. Our modification or addition to this system consists of a special teacher whose responsibility it is to organize the teaching sessions in the different wards and to keep the training equipment clean and in working order. The teacher is always present during the teaching sessions to give additional instruction and to answer questions from the class.

The routine is to have a group of 12 pupils for a teaching session which usually lasts for 1.5 hr. With this system it took us nearly 1.5 years to cover the hospital personnel of 3000 employees with a turnover of nearly 1500 persons per year.

In order to obtain an impression of the efficiency of this training scheme, 96 random pupils (nurses and nurses aids) who had had the regular instruction one year earlier were chosen for a test. Each of the pupils was tested individually. The teacher explained that the pupil was supposed to resuscitate the manikin *as if it was a person who suddenly had collapsed with no respiration and no detectable pulse.* When this was explained, the recorder of the manikin was started.

We found the following criteria to be of interest for the evaluation of the proficiency of the pupils: (1) adequacy of ventilation (> 8 l/min); (2) adequacy of external heart compression (4 cm depression); (3) correct ratio ventilation/compression (2/15); (4) delay in starting resuscitation (< 40 sec).

It appears from the figures that 89 and 88 respectively (92%) performed ventilation and cardiac compression satisfactorily. The correct ratio of ventilation and heart compression *for one rescuer* (2/15) was only carried out by 34 of the 96 pupils (35%), and only 45% started resuscitation within 40 sec. The teacher had the impression that most of the pupils were a little confused with the situation of having to resuscitate *alone.* They were apparently better prepared for a 2-rescuer technique (a ratio of one ventilation to 5 compression

This may also account for the low average score in starting within the 40-sec limit. Most of the pupils, however, started within one minute.

The test group was also given 39 written questions or statements about resuscitation to be answered as 'correct' or 'wrong'. These were not particularly difficult for a group who had received instruction in resuscitation before, and the average score was 33.4 correct answers of 39 possible (86%).

The same questions were also put to doctors in the Department of Anaesthesia who achieved a score of 35.5 (90.5%).

CONCLUSIONS

Our training scheme appears to be adequate as far as the technique of ventilation and cardiac compression is concerned. The results are not as good when it comes to carrying out a 'one-rescuer technique'. The fact that less than half of the pupils were able to start the resuscitation within the 40-sec limit, indicates that the time allotted for the training had been insufficient. It would probably be unfair to expect any better results from only 1.5 hr of instruction one year earlier. It is not known if any of the group might have received some training in resuscitation before the test, or if some of them had witnessed or taken part in a real resuscitation.

Although our pupils may have acquired good theoretical knowledge it is not known how these people would have behaved when faced with a situation where the life of a fellow man was at stake. It is justified to conclude however, that the teaching system is efficient and greatly facilitated the teaching of resuscitation to a group of several thousand people. This was essentially what our follow-up study was designed to test.

The use of Trasylol in fat embolism: Clinical experience and rationale

R. GREENBAUM

Frenchay Hospital, Bristol, United Kingdom

Some degree of pulmonary fat embolism is inevitable after fractures of long bones. In a small proportion of cases, severe cerebral and respiratory symptoms develop and, in such cases, the mortality rate has been estimated to be as high as 85%.

The symptoms usually develop on the third to fifth day after injury, but fulminating cases occur immediately after injury, indeed, variability is almost a characteristic of the syndrome. After the lucid interval, dyspnoea, tachypnoea and hyperventilation are usual, often accompanied by dull chest pain. Mental changes vary from mild euphoria, restlessness and drowsiness to profound coma. These symptoms may be masked by co-existent head injury or failure to recover consciousness after general anaesthesia.

Fever, tachycardia and skin petechiae are commonly seen. Often a severe and progressive anaemia develops which may be associated with haemolysis, fibrinolysis and thrombocytopenia.

Hypoxia is often severe and contributes to the deterioration of consciousness; it may prove fatal. This hypoxia is largely caused by increased pulmonary venous admixture, exacerbated by the increased oxygen consumption of pyrexia and increased respiratory work in those patients who are allowed to breathe spontaneously (Prys-Roberts et al., 1970).

The primary source of embolism appears to be from the traumatised area but possibly this is potentiated by fat globule formation in the blood, by platelet aggregates or by thrombi which may come from stored blood or from intravascular coagulation. These factors have provided an area of dispute, but are not incompatible and almost certainly act in unison to produce the syndrome. I believe that the prime source is marrow cells and marrow fat, and fat from adjacent adipose tissue which are liberated into the circulation after trauma, especially if there is a build up of local tissue pressure. The absorption of marrow fat is increased when treatment of blood loss is delayed or inadequate. In these circumstances, large amounts of marrow fat are probably transported via the lymphatic system and released into the circulation.

The alternative source of fat is that a change in plasma lipid colloid stability after injury leads to the presence in the blood of fat globules of over 8 μm in diameter (Gurd, 1970). It may be that the entry of marrow fat into the circulation triggers such chylomicron flocculation (Glas et al., 1955), or triggering may be due to the liberation of thromboplastic substances (Bergentz, 1961). Trauma and haemorrhage are associated with abnormal lipid metabolism, producing a lipaemia which is maximal at the same time as fat embolism usually occurs. This lipaemia is probably caused by catecholamine secretion and is inhibited by heparin. However, a casual relationship between posttraumatic lipaemia and fat embolism has not been established (Watson, 1970).

There is evidence that large numbers of platelet and leucocyte aggregates of over 50 μm in diameter accumulate during storage of blood for transfusion. This debris is inadequately filtered by normal blood administration sets with 170 μm filters and, when filtered by the

Table 1. *Summary of clinical features*

Patient	Age	Fractures	Other injuries	Estimated period trapped at accident	Interval before fat embolism	Level of consciousness	Time for recovery of consciousness	Units transfused	Platelet count
1	18	Bilateral femur, radius	None	None	48 hr	Coma	3 days	3	85,000
2	22	Right femur, skull	Swollen right frontal lobe (on carotid ateriography)	3 hr	24 hr	Deep coma decerebrate	7 days	7	134,000
3	24	Bilateral femur tibia, fibula, humerus, skull	Initially conscious and alert although fractured skull	3 hr	48 hr	Coma	5 days	12	Normal
4	20	Femur, radius and ulna, humerus, talus	Right pneumo-thorax, renal haematoma, given 30 mg morphine at roadside	1 hr	48 hr	Deep coma decerebrate	4 days	14	106,000
5	23	Bilateral tibia, radius and ulna	Initial aspiration blood and vomit	None	24 hr	Coma decerebrate	8 days	3	Normal
6	18	Right femur	Bilateral haemo-pneumothorax	0.5 hr upside down	Immediate	Coma	4 days then died 24 hr after recovery of consciousness	7	20,000

lungs produces vascular obstruction and has been associated with the development of 'shock lung' (Mosely and Doty, 1970).

Many patients also have several factors which are known to be associated with a high degree of risk of disseminated intravascular coagulation. Shock or oligaemic hypotension is known to be a cause of clotting defects and catecholamine release. Multiple transfusions, extensive trauma, haemolysis and infection are all likely in patients such as the group reported here. These patients, therefore, can be expected to develop a degree of disseminated intravascular coagulation (Hardaway, 1970).

ACTION OF EMBOLI

The emboli from any or all of the sources described produce a mechanical blockage of the pulmonary circulation which results in gross ventilation perfusion inequalities. This leads to increased venous admixture and an increased physiological dead space. However, the physiological dead space increase recovers more quickly than the venous admixture, the latter persisting due to alveolar damage. This may be caused by lipolysis of neutral fat into toxic free fatty acids which are known to produce haemorrhagic oedema and alveolar destruction.

Fat and platelet emboli may degenerate in the lungs, leading to a release of vasoactive polypeptides, histamine and serotonin, etc. These toxins would also cause breakdown of the alveolar capillary membrane and haemorrhagic oedema.

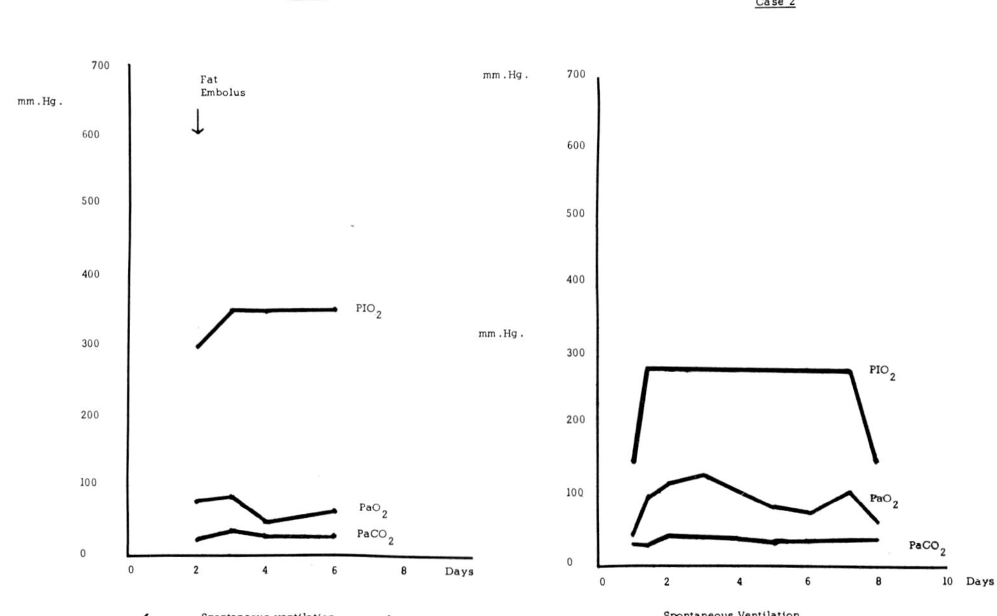

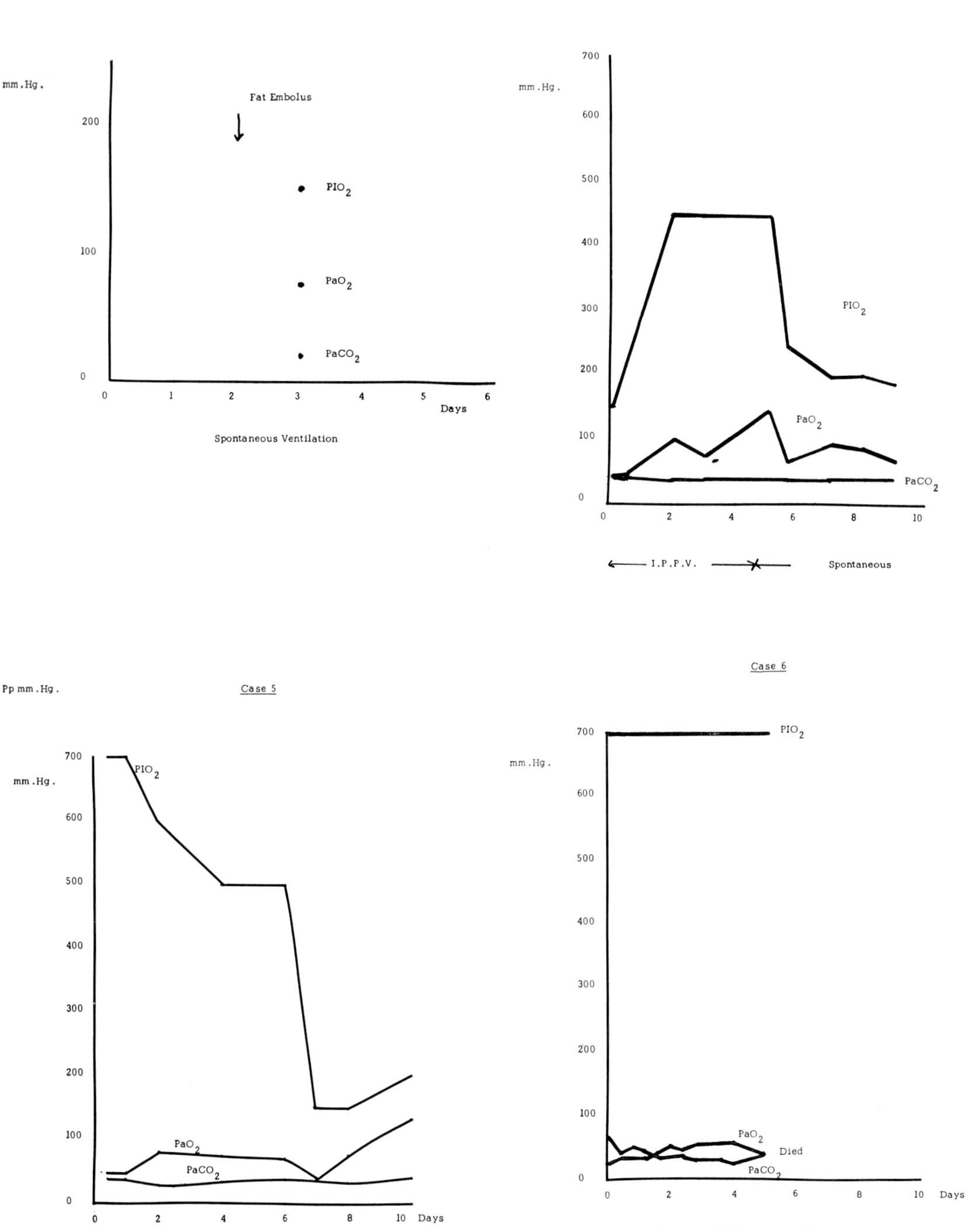

Fig. 1.   *The $P_{IO_2}/Pa_{O_2}/P_{CO_2}$ changes during the course of the therapy.*

TREATMENT

Therapy of fat embolism must include adequate and immediate replacement of blood loss in order to minimise lipid mobilisation, catecholamine release and the various other factors discussed.

Oxygen therapy is also mandatory. In mild cases this can be managed by simple masks, but severe anoxia and breathlessness necessitate the use of controlled ventilation with a high concentration of inspired oxygen to achieve safe levels of arterial oxygenation.

However necessary this therapy may be, it is only symptomatic and does not directly affect the actions or release of toxic chemicals in the lungs or fat, platelet and thrombus embolisation. It was, therefore, decided to use the proteinase inhibitor, Trasylol, in a series of cases of severe fat embolism.

Trasylol is a water soluble polypeptide, originally extracted from bovine parotid gland. It is a strong kallikrein inhibitor and also inhibits trypsin, chymotrypsin and plasmin; this effect prevents the release of vasoactive kinins into the plasma. Trasylol also has an inhibitory action on the Hageman factor and is, therefore, a minor anticoagulant affecting the thromboplastin mechanism. The prime action in clotting is as a plasmin inhibitor; therefore, Trasylol combines antifibrinolytic and antithromboplastic properties and is suitable for use in intravascular coagulation and clotting factor consumption states after trauma (Amris, 1966).

Trasylol also exerts an anti-oedematous effect which may be useful in fat embolism.

CLINICAL EXPERIENCE

We treated all patients, as soon as fat embolism was diagnosed, with Trasylol, 1,000,000 KIU in the first 24 hr, followed by 500,000 KIU daily, by intravenous infusion until recovery of consciousness and oxygenation was achieved.

The 6 patients are summarised in Table 1. All were young men who were involved in road traffic accidents. Four (Cases 2, 3, 4 and 6) were trapped in their vehicles, perhaps allowing a period of oligaemic shock before they could be freed and resuscitated.

Two patients had head injuries (Cases 2 and 3), 2 had pneumothoraces (Cases 4 and 6) and one patient had aspirated blood and vomitus before transfer to our hospital (Case 5). Every patient had characteristic skin petechiae and chest X-rays and all progressed into unconsciousness before eventual recovery. Recovery of consciousness took 3–8 days, although patients 2, 4 and 5 were deeply unconscious, decerebrate and had dilated pupils.

Pyrexia and tachycardia were present in every patient and usually improved with rising level of consciousness and arterial oxygenation. There was also the expected fall in haemoglobin concentration which averaged 2 g% in the 6 patients. Blood transfusions during the course of the illness ranged from 3-14 units.

Four patients demonstrated thrombocytopenia but only one patient (Case 6) developed evidence of increased fibrin degradation products and intravascular coagulation. This patient died 24 hr after recovering consciousness. Necropsy revealed an unexpected degree of myocardial contusion and intracardiac antemortem thrombus which was embolising peripherally.

Severe arterial hypoxia is demonstrated by the large P_{IO_2}-Pa_{O_2} difference in every patient (Fig. 1). Patient 6 arrived in hospital with Pa_{O_2} of 25 mm Hg. Patients 1, 2 and 3 were managed allowing spontaneous ventilation and 4, 5 and 6 were ventilated using a Cape ventilator. It was possible to maintain normal arterial P_{CO_2} levels in every patient.

Patients 1, 2, 3, 4 and 5 made complete recoveries and all were alert, orientated and breathing spontaneously on air within 8 days of the embolism.

DISCUSSION

It is clear that the treatment of anoxia alone will not cure every patient in coma due to fat embolism, although it is acknowledged to be an essential part of the symptomatic therapy (Sproule et al., 1964; Greenbaum et al., 1965; Prys-Roberts et al., 1970; O'Higgins, 1970).

Associated pulmonary or cerebral lesions which can exacerbate anoxia will increase the severity of the systemic embolism. The presence of a pneumothorax reduces the lethal dose of intravenous triolein in experimental animals (Szabo, 1970). Cases 2, 3, 4, 5 and 6 were, therefore, especially poor risks as they all had other anoxic factors at work.

These patients also received large volumes of blood transfusion, often had some delay in resuscitation and developed haemolysis and anaemia. It was, therefore, likely that catecholamine release, tissue anoxia and intravascular coagulation would take place.

The use of Trasylol in this series has been associated with a recovery of lung oxygenation function, less dramatic than that described by Gurd (1969) in experimental animals but this could have occurred by chance in this notoriously unpredictable disease.

The rapid recovery of consciousness in this series was more impressive and often preceded the attainment of raised arterial oxygen tension.

These results confirm the observations of Sevitt (1973) that the coma of fat embolism is not simply anoxic. Trasylol may be exerting a local effect on the cerebral vessels and their blood flow by blocking vasoactive kinins at this site, or by reducing postembolic cerebral oedema.

CONCLUSION

Rapid transfusion of adequately filtered blood for oligaemia, correction of anoxia and efficient splinting of fractures will minimise the risks of fat embolism. Trasylol appears to be a drug worthy of a larger trial in this condition, especially in those patients with cerebral symptoms.

REFERENCES

Amris, C. J. (1966): *Scand. J. Haemat.*, *3*, 19.

Bergentz, S. G. (1961): *Acta chir. scand.*, *Suppl. 282.*

Gias, W. W., Musselman, M. M. and Davis, H. L. (1955): *Arch. Surg.*, *71*, 600.

Greenbaum, R., Nunn, J. F., Prys-Roberts, C., Kelman, G. R. and Silk, F. F. (1965): *Brit. J. Anaesth.*, *37*, 554.

Gurd, A. R. (1969): *New Aspects of Trasylol Therapy.* F. K. Schattauer Verlag, Stuttgart–New York.

Gurd, A. R. (1970): *J. Bone Jt Surg.*, *52B/4*, 732.

Hardaway, R. M. (1970): *J. clin. Path.*, *23*, Suppl. 4, 110.

Mosely, R. V. and Doty, D. B. (1970): *Ann. Surg.*, *171*, 329.

O'Higgins, J. (1970): *Brit. J. Anaesth.*, *42*, 163.

Prys-Roberts, C., Greenbaum, R., Nunn, J. F. and Kelman, G. R. (1970): *J. clin. Path.*, *23*, *Suppl. 4*, 143.

Sevitt, S. (1973): *Brit. J. Hosp. Med.*, *9*, 784.

Sproule, B. J., Brady, J. S. and Gilbert, J. A. L. (1964): *Canad. med. Ass. J.*, *90*, 1243.

Szabo, G. (1970): *J. clin. Path.*, *23*, *Suppl. 4*, 123.

Watson, A. J. (1970): *J. clin. Path.*, *23*, *Suppl. 4*, 132.